Principles and Practice of Clinical Trials

Steven Piantadosi • Curtis L. Meinert
Editors

Principles and Practice of Clinical Trials

Volume 3

With 241 Figures and 191 Tables

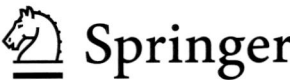

Editors
Steven Piantadosi
Department of Surgery
Division of Surgical Oncology
Brigham and Women's Hospital
Harvard Medical School
Boston, MA, USA

Curtis L. Meinert
Department of Epidemiology
School of Public Health
Johns Hopkins University
Baltimore, MD, USA

ISBN 978-3-319-52635-5   ISBN 978-3-319-52636-2 (eBook)
https://doi.org/10.1007/978-3-319-52636-2

© Springer Nature Switzerland AG 2022
This work is subject to copyright. All rights are reserved by the Publisher, whether the whole or part of the material is concerned, specifically the rights of translation, reprinting, reuse of illustrations, recitation, broadcasting, reproduction on microfilms or in any other physical way, and transmission or information storage and retrieval, electronic adaptation, computer software, or by similar or dissimilar methodology now known or hereafter developed.
The use of general descriptive names, registered names, trademarks, service marks, etc. in this publication does not imply, even in the absence of a specific statement, that such names are exempt from the relevant protective laws and regulations and therefore free for general use.
The publisher, the authors, and the editors are safe to assume that the advice and information in this book are believed to be true and accurate at the date of publication. Neither the publisher nor the authors or the editors give a warranty, expressed or implied, with respect to the material contained herein or for any errors or omissions that may have been made. The publisher remains neutral with regard to jurisdictional claims in published maps and institutional affiliations.

This Springer imprint is published by the registered company Springer Nature Switzerland AG.
The registered company address is: Gewerbestrasse 11, 6330 Cham, Switzerland

In memory of
Lulu, Champ, and Dudley

A Foreword to the Principles and Practice of Clinical Trials

Trying to identify the effects of treatments is not new. The *Book of Daniel* (verses 12–15) describes a test of the effects King Nebuchadnezzar's meat:

Prove thy servants, I beseech thee, ten days; and let them give us pulse to eat, and water to drink. Then let our countenances be looked upon before thee, and the countenance of the children that eat of the portion of the King's meat: and as thou seest, deal with thy servants. So he consented to them in this matter, and proved them ten days. And at the end of ten days their countenances appeared fairer and fatter in flesh than all the children which did eat the portion of the King's meat.

The requirement of comparison in identifying treatment effects was recognized in the tenth century by Abu Bakr Muhammad ibn Zakariya al-Razi (Persian physician):

When the dullness (thiqal) and the pain in the head and neck continue for three and four and five days or more, and the vision shuns light, and watering of the eyes is abundant, yawning and stretching are great, insomnia is severe, and extreme exhaustion occurs, then the patient after that will progress to meningitis (sirsâm)... If the dullness in the head is greater than the pain, and there is no insomnia, but rather sleep, then the fever will abate, but the throbbing will be immense but not frequent and he will progress into a stupor (lîthûrghas). So when you see these symptoms, then proceed with bloodletting. For I once saved one group [of patients] by it, while I intentionally neglected [to bleed] another group. By doing that, I wished to reach a conclusion (ra'y). And so all of these [latter] contracted meningitis. (Tibi 2006)

But it was not until the beginning of the eighteenth century before the importance of treatment comparisons was broadly acknowledged, for example, as in chances of contracting smallpox among people inoculated with smallpox lymph versus those who caught smallpox disease naturally (Bird 2018).

By the middle of the eighteenth century there were examples of tests with comparison groups, for example, as described by James Lind in relation to his scurvy experiment on board the HMS Salisbury at sea:

On the 20th of May 1747, I took twelve patients in the scurvy, on board the Salisbury at sea. Their cases were as similar as I could have them. They all in general had putrid gums, the spots and lassitude, with weakness of their knees. They lay together in one place, being a proper apartment for the sick in the fore-hold; and had one diet common to all, viz., watergruel sweetened with sugar in the morning; fresh mutton-broth often times for dinner;

> at other times puddings, boiled biscuit with sugar, etc; and for supper, barley and raisins, rice and currants, sago and wine, or the like. Two of these were ordered each a quart of cyder a-day. Two others took twenty-five gutts of elixir vitriol three times a day, upon an empty stomach; using a gargle strongly acidulated with it for their mouths. Two others took two spoonfuls of vinegar three times a day, upon an empty stomach; having their gruels and their other food well acidulated with it, as also the gargle for their mouth. Two of the worst patients, with the tendons in the ham rigid, (a symptom none of the rest had), were put under a course of seawater. Of this they drank half a pint every day, and sometimes more or less as it operated, by way of gentle physic. Two others had each two oranges and one lemon given them every day. These they eat with greediness, at different times, upon an empty stomach. They continued but six days under this course, having consumed the quantity that could be spared. The two remaining patients, took the bigness of a nutmeg three times a-day, of an electuary recommended by an hospital surgeon, made of garlic, mustard-seed, rad raphan, balsam of Peru, and gum myrrh; using for common drink, barley-water well acidulated with tamarinds; by a decoction of which, with the addition of cremor tartar, they were gently purged three or four times during the course.
>
> * * *
>
> The consequence was, that the most sudden and visible good effects were perceived from the use of the oranges and lemons; one of those who had taken them, being at the end of six days fit for duty. (Lind 1753)

Lind did not make clear how his 12 sailors were assigned to the treatments in his experiment. During the late nineteenth and early twentieth century, alternation (and sometimes randomization) became used to create study comparison groups that differed only by chance (Chalmers et al. 2011).

In 1937 assignment was discussed in Hill's book, *Principles of Medical Statistics*, in which he emphasized the importance of strictly observing the allocation schedule. Implementation of this principle was reflected in concealment of allocation schedules in two important clinical trials designed for the UK Medical Research Council in the 1940s (Medical Research Council 1944; 1948). Sir Austin Bradford Hill's 1937 book went into 12 editions, and his other writings, such as *Statistical Methods in Clinical and Preventive Medicine*, helped propel the upward methodological progression.

The United States Congress passed the Kefauver-Harris Amendments to the Food, Drug, and Cosmetic Act of 1938 in 1962. The amendments revolutionized drug development by requiring drug manufacturers to prove that a drug was safe and effective. A feature of the amendments was language spelling out the nature of scientific evidence required for a drug to be approved:

> The term "substantial evidence" means evidence consisting of adequate and well-controlled investigations, including clinical investigations, by experts qualified by scientific training and experience to evaluate the effectiveness of the drug involved, on the basis of which it could fairly and responsibly be concluded by such experts that the drug will have the effect it purports or is represented to have under the conditions of its use prescribed, recommended, or suggested in the labeling or proposed labeling thereof. (United States Congress 1962)

Post World War II prosperity brought sizeable increases in government funding for training and research. The National Institutes of Health played a major role in training biostatisticians in the 1960s and 1970s with its fellowship programs. By the

1980s clinical trial courses started showing up in syllabi of academic institutions. By the 1990s academic institutions started offering PhDs focused on design and conduct of trials with a few now offering PhD training in clinical trials.

The clinical trial enterprise is huge. There were over 25,000 trials registered on CT.gov starting in 2019. That number, assuming CT.gov registrations account for 70% of all registered trials, translates to 38,000 trials. That amounts to 2.3 million people studied when those trials are finished assuming a median sample size of 60 per trial.

Lind did his trial before IRBs and consents, before requirements for written protocols, before investigator certifications, before the Health Insurance Portability and Accountability Act (HIPAA), before data sharing, before data monitoring committees, before site visiting, and before requirements for posting results within 1 year of completion. Trials moved from the backroom of obscurity to front and center with trials seen as forms of public trust.

The act of trying progressed from efforts involving a single investigator to efforts involving cadres of investigators with training in medicine, biostatistics, epidemiology, programming, data processing, and in regulations and ethics underlying trials.

The size of the research team increases with the size and complexities of the trials. Multicenter trials may involve investigatorships numbering in the hundreds.

Enter trialists – persons with training and experience in the design, organization, conduct, and analysis of trials. Presently trialists are scattered, located in various departments in medical schools and schools of public health. They have no academic home.

The scattering works to the disadvantage of the art and science of trials in that it stymies communications and development of curricula relevant to trials. One of our motivations in undertaking this work is hope of speeding development of such homes.

The blessing of online publications is that works can be updated at will. The curse is that the work is never done. We hope to advance the science of trials by providing the trials world with a comprehensive work from leaders in the field covering the waterfront of clinical trials serving as a reference resource for novices and experts in trials for use in designing, conducting, and analyzing them.

13 May 2020   Steven Piantadosi and Curtis L. Meinert
Editors

Postscript

When we started this effort, there was no COVID-19. Now we are living through a pandemic caused by the virus leading us to proclaim in regard to trials, as Charles Dickens did in his *A Tale of Two Cities* in a different context, "the best of times, the worst of times."

"The best of times" because never before has there been more interest and attention directed to trials, even from the President. Everybody wants to know when there will be a vaccine to protect us from COVID-19.

"The worst of times" because of the chaos caused by the pandemic in mounting and doing trials and the impact of "social distancing" on the way trials are done now.

It is a given that the pandemic will change how we do trials, but whatever those changes will be, trials will remain humankind's best and most enduring answer to addressing the conditions and maladies that affect us.

Acknowledgment

We are indebted to Sir Iain Chalmers for his review and critical input in reviewing this piece. Dr. Chalmers is founder of the Cochrane Collaboration and first coordinator of the James Lind Library.

Events in the Development of Clinical Trials

Date	Author/source	Event
1747	Lind	Experiment with untreated control group (Lind 1953)
1799	Haygarth	Use of sham procedure (Haggard 1932)
1800	Waterhouse	Smallpox trial (Waterhouse 1802, 1800)
1863	Gull	Use of placebo treatment (Sutton 1865)
1918		First department of biostatistics; Johns Hopkins University, https://www.jhsph.edu/departments/biostatistics/about-us/history/
1923	Fisher	Application of randomization to experimentation (Fisher and MacKenzie 1923)
1931		Committee on clinical trials created by the Medical Research Council of Great Britain (Medical Research Council 1931)
1931	Amberson	Random assignment of treatment to groups of patients (Amberson et al. 1931)
1937	NIH	Start of NIH grant support with creation of the National Cancer Institute (National Institutes of Health 1981)
1944		Publication of multicenter trial on treatment for common cold (Patulin Clinical Trials Committee 1944)
1946		Nüremberg Code for Human Experimentation (Curran and Shapiro 1970) https://history.nih.gov/research/downloads/nuremberg.pdf
1948	MRC	Streptomycin TB multicenter trial published; BMJ: 30 Oct, 1948 (Medical Research Council 1948)
1962	Hill	Book: *Statistical Methods in Clinical and Preventive Medicine* (Hill 1962)
1962	Kefauver, Harris	Amendments to the Food, Drug, and Cosmetic Act of 1938 (United States Congress 1962)

Date	Author/source	Event
1964	NLM	MEDLARS® (MEDical Literature Analysis and Retrieval System) of the National Library of Medicine initiated
1966; 8 Feb	USPHS	Memo from Surgeon General of USPHS informing recipients of NIH funding of requirement for informed consent as condition for funding henceforth (Stewart 1966), https://history.nih.gov/research/downloads/surgeongeneraldirective1966.pdf
1966	Levine	Publication of U.S. Public Health Service regulations leading to creation of Institutional Review Boards for research involving humans (Levine 1988)
1966; 6 Sep	US govt	Freedom of Information Act (FOIA) signed into law by Lyndon Johnson 6 September 1966 (Public Law 89-554, 80 Statue 383); Act specifies US Governmental Agencies records subject to disclosure under the Act; amended and extended in 1996, 2002, and 2007, https://www.justice.gov/oip/foia_guide09/foia-final.pdf; 5 September 2009
1967	Tom Chalmers	Structure for separating the treatment monitoring and treatment administration process (Coronary Drug Project Research Group: 1973)
1974; 12 July	US govt	Creation of U.S. National Commission for the Protection of Human Subjects of Biomedical and Behavioral Research; part of the National Research Act (Public Law No. 93-348, § 202, 88 Stat. 342)
1974	US govt	US Code of Federal Regulations promulgated establishing Institutional Review Boards, https://www.hhs.gov/ohrp/humansubjects/guidance/45cfr46
1979	OPRR	Belmont Report (Ethical Principles and Guidelines for the Protection of Human Subjects of Research); product of the National Commission for the Protection of Human Subjects of Biomedical and Behavioral Research (Office for Protection from Research Risks Belmont Report 1979)
1979	Gorden	NIH Clinical Trials Committee (chaired by Robert Gorden) recommends that "every clinical trial should have provisions for data and safety monitoring" (National Institutes of Health 1979)
1979		Society for Clinical Trials established
1980		First issue of *Controlled Clinical Trials* (Meinert and Tonascia 1998)
1981	Friedman	Book: *Fundamentals of Clinical Trials* (Friedman et al. 1981)

Date	Author/source	Event
1983	Pocock	Book: *Clinical Trials: A Practical Approach* (Pocock 1983)
1986	Meinert	Book: *Clinical Trials: Design, Conduct, and Analysis* (Meinert and Tonascia 1986)
1990	ICH	International Conference on Harmonisation (ICH) formed (European Union, Japan, and the United States) (Vozeh 1995)
1990		Initiation of PhD training program in clinical trials at Johns Hopkins University
1992	FDA	Prescription Drug User Fee Act (PDUFA) enacted; allows FDA to collect fees for review of New Drug Applications (Public Law 102-571; 102 Congress; https://www.fda.gov/ForIndustry/UserFees/PrescriptionDrugUserFee/ucm200361.htm; 2002)
1993	US govt	Mandate regarding valid analysis for gender and ethnic origin treatment interactions (United States Congress 1993)
1993	UK	Cochrane Collaboration founded under leadership of Iain Chalmers; developed in response to Archie Cochrane's call for up-to-date, systematic reviews of all relevant trials in the healthcare field
1996	HIPAA	Health Insurance Portability and Accountability Act (HIPAA) enacted (Public Law 104-191; 104th US Congress; https://aspe.hhs.gov/admnsimp/pL10419.htm)
1996	NLM	PubMed (search engine for MEDLINE) made free to public
1996		Consolidated Standards of Reporting Trials (CONSORT) (Begg et al. 1996)
1997	US govt	US public law calling for registration of trials; Food and Drug Administration Modernization Act of 1997; Public Law 105-115; Nov 21, 1997 (https://www.govinfo.gov/content/pkg/PLAW-105publ115/pdf/PLAW-105publ115.pdf)
1997	Piantadosi	Book: *Clinical Trials: A Methodologic Perspective* (Piantadosi 1997)
2000	NIH	ClinicalTrials.gov registration website launched (Zarin et al. 2007)
2003	NIH	NIH statement on data sharing (National Institutes of Health 2003)
2003	UK	Launch of James Lind Library; marking 250th anniversary of the publication of James Lind's Treatise of the Scurvy (https://www.jameslindlibrary.org/search/)

Date	Author/source	Event
2004	ICMJE	Requirement of registration of trials in public registries as condition for publication for trials starting enrollment after 1 July 2005 by member journals of the International Committee of Medical Journal Editors (ICMJE) (DeAngelis et al. 2004)
2004; 3 Sep	NIH	NIH notice NOT-OD-04-064 (Enhanced Public Access to NIH Research Information) required "its grantees and supported Principal Investigators provide the NIH with electronic copies of all final version manuscripts upon acceptance for publication if the research was supported in whole or in part by NIH funding" for deposit in PubMed Central within six months after publication
2006	WHO	World Health Organization (WHO) launch of International Clinical Trials Registry Platform (ICTRP) (https://www.who.int/ictrp/en/)
2007	FDA	Requirement for investigators to post tabular results of trials covered under FDA regulations on ClinicalTrials.gov within one year of completion [Food and Drug Administration Amendments Act of 2007 (FDAAA)]
2007		Wiley Encyclopedia of Clinical Trials (4 vols) (D'Agostino et al. 2007)
2013		Standard Protocol Items: Recommendations for Interventional Trials (SPIRIT) (Chan et al. 2013)
2016	NIH	Final NIH policy on single institutional review board for multi-site research (NOT-OD-16-094)
2017	FDA	2007 requirement for posting results extended to all trials, whether or not subject to FDA regulations (81 FR64983)
2017	ICMJE	ICMJE requirement for data sharing in clinical trials (Ann Intern Med doi: 10.7326/M17-1028) (Taichman et al. 2017)

References

Amberson JB Jr, McMahon BT, Pinner M (1931) A clinical trial of sanocrysin in pulmonary tuberculosis. Am Rev Tuberc 24:401–435

Begg C, Cho M, Eastwood S, Horton R, Moher D, Olkin I, Pitkin R, Rennie D, Schulz KF, Simel D, Stroup DF (1996) Improving the quality of reporting of randomized controlled trials. The CONSORT statement. JAMA 276(8):637–639

Bird A (2018) James Jurin and the avoidance of bias in collecting and assessing evidence on the effects of variolation. JLL Bulletin: Commentaries on the history of treatment evaluation. https://www.jameslindlibrary.org/articles/james-jurin-

and-the-avoidance-of-bias-in-collecting-and-assessing-evidence-on-the-effects-of-variolation/

Chalmers I, Dukan E, Podolsky SH, Davey Smith G (2011) The advent of fair treatment allocation schedules in clinical trials during the 19th and early 20th centuries. JLL Bulletin: Commentaries on the history of treatment evaluation. https://www.jameslindlibrary.org/articles/the-advent-of-fair-treatment-allocation-schedules-in-clinical-trials-during-the-19th-and-early-20th-centuries/

Chan AW, Tetzlaff JM, Altman DG, Laupacis A, Gøtzsche PC, Krleža-Jeric K, Hróbjartsson A, Mann H, Dickersin K, Berlin JA, Doré CJ, Parulekar WR, Summerskill WSM, Groves T, Schulz KF, Sox HC, Rockhold FW, Drummond R, Moher D (2013) SPIRIT 2013 statement: defining standard protocol items for clinical trials. Ann Intern Med 158(3):200–207

Coronary Drug Project Research Group (1973) The Coronary Drug Project: design, methods, and baseline results. Circulation 47(Suppl I):I-1-I-50

Curran WJ, Shapiro ED (1970) Law, medicine, and forensic science, 2nd edn. Little, Brown, Boston

D'Agostino R, Sullivan LM, Massaro J (eds) (2007) Wiley encyclopedia of clinical trials, 4 vols. Wiley, New York

DeAngelis CD, Drazen JM, Frizelle FA, Haug C, Hoey J, Horton R, Kotzin S, Laine C, Marusic A, Overbeke AJPM, Schroeder TV, Sox HC, Van Der Weyden MB (2004) Clinical Trial Registration: A statement from the International Committee of Medical Journal Editors. JAMA 292:1363–1364

Fisher RA, MacKenzie WA (1923) Studies in crop variation: II. The manurial response of different potato varieties. J Agric Sci 13:311–320

Friedman LM, Furberg CD, DeMets DR (1981) Fundamentals of clinical trials, 5th edn, [2015]. Springer, New York

Haggard HW (1932) The Lame, the Halt, and the Blind: the vital role of medicine in the history of civilization. Harper and Brothers, New York

Hill AB (1937) Principles of medical statistics. Lancet

Hill AB (1962) Statistical methods in clinical and preventive medicine. Oxford University Press, New York

Levine RJ (1988) Ethics and regulation of clinical research, 2nd edn. Yale University Press, New Haven

Lind J (1753) A treatise of the scurvy (reprinted in Lind's treatise on scurvy, edited by CP Stewart, D Guthrie, Edinburgh University Press, Edinburgh, 1953). Sands, Murray, Cochran, Edinburgh

Medical Research Council (1931) Clinical trials of new remedies (annotations). Lancet 2:304

Medical Research Council (1944) Clinical trial of patulin in the common cold. Lancet 16:373–375

Medical Research Council (1948) Streptomycin treatment of pulmonary tuberculosis: a Medical Research Council investigation. Br Med J 2:769–782

Meinert CL, Tonascia S (1986) Clinical trials: design, conduct, and analysis. Oxford University Press, New York (2nd edn, 2012)

Meinert CL, Tonascia S (1998) Controlled Clinical Trials. Encyclopedia of biostatistics, vol 1. Wiley, New York, pp 929–931

National Institutes of Health (1979) Clinical trials activity (NIH Clinical Trials Committee; RS Gordon Jr, Chair). NIH Guide Grants Contracts 8 (# 8):29

National Institutes of Health (1981) NIH Almanac. Publ no 81-5. Division of Public Information, Bethesda

National Institutes of Health (2003) NIH data sharing policy and implementation guidance. http://grants.nih.gov/grants/policy/data_sharing/data_sharing_guidance.htm

Office for Protection from Research Risks (1979) The Belmont Report. Ethical principles and guidelines for the protection of human subjects of research, 18 April 1979

Patulin Clinical Trials Committee (of the Medical Research Council) (1944) Clinical trial of Patulin in the common cold. Lancet 2:373–375

Piantadosi S (1997) Clinical trials: a methodologic perspective. Wiley, Hoboken (3rd edn, 2017)

Pocock SJ (1983) Clinical trials: a practical approach. Wiley, New York

Stewart WH (1966) Surgeon general's directives on human experimentation. https://history.nih.gov/research/downloads/surgeongeneraldirective1966.pdf

Sutton HG (1865) Cases of rheumatic fever. Guy's Hosp Rep 11:392–428

Taichman DB, Sahni P, Pinborg A, Peiperl L, Laine C, James A, Hong ST, Haileamlak A, Gollogly L, Godlee F, Frizelle FA, Florenzano F, Drazen JM, Bauchner H, Baethge C, Backus J (2017) Data sharing statements for clinical trials: a requirement of the International Committee of Medical Journal Editors. Ann Intern Med 167(1):63–65

Tibi S (2006) Al-Razi and Islamic medicine in the 9th century; J R Soc Med 99(4): 206–207

United States Congress (103rd; 1st session): NIH Revitalization Act of 1993, 42 USC § 131 (1993); Clinical research equity regarding women and minorities; part I: women and minorities as subjects in clinical research, 1993

United States Congress (87th): Drug Amendments of 1962, Public Law 87-781, S 1522. Washington, Oct 10, 1962

Vozeh S (1995) The International Conference on Harmonisation. Eur J Clin Pharmacol 48:173–175

Waterhouse B (1800) A prospect of exterminating the small pox. Cambridge Press, Cambridge

Waterhouse B (1802) A prospect of exterminating the small pox (part II). University Press, Cambridge

Zarin DA, Ide NC, Tse T, Harlan WR, West JC, Lindberg DAB (2007) Issues in the registration of clinical trials. JAMA 297:2112–2120

Preface

The two of us have spent our professional lives doing trials; writing textbooks on how to do them, teaching about them, and sitting on advisory groups responsible for trials. We are pleased to say that over our lifetime trials have moved up the scale of importance to now where people feel cheated if denied enrollment.

Clinical trials are admixtures of disciplines: Medicine, behavioral sciences, biostatistics, epidemiology, ethics, quality control, and regulatory sciences to name the principal ones, making it difficult to cover the field in any textbook on the subject. This reality is the reason we campaigned (principally SP) for a collective work designed to cover the waterfront of trials. We are pleased to have been able to do this in conjunction with Springer Nature, both as print and e-books.

There has long been a need for a comprehensive clinical trials text written at a level accessible to both technical and nontechnical readers. The perspective is the same as that in many other fields where the scope of a "principles and practice" textbook has been defining and instructive to those learning the discipline. Accordingly, the intent of *Principles and Practice of Clinical Trials* has been to cover, define, and explicate the field in ways that are approachable to trialists of all types. The work is intended to be comprehensive, but not encyclopedic.

Boston, USA	Steven Piantadosi
Baltimore, USA	Curtis L. Meinert
April 2022	Editors

Acknowledgments

The work involved nine subject sections and appendices.

Section	Section editor	Affiliation
1 Perspectives on clinical trials	Steven N. Goodman Karen A. Robinson	Stanford University; Professor Johns Hopkins University; Professor
2 Conduct and management	Eleanor McFadden	Managing Director; Frontier Science (Scotland)
3 Regulation and oversight	Winifred Werther	Amgen; Epidemiologist
4 Bias control and precision	O. Dale Williams	Florida International University; Retired
5 Basics of trial design	Christopher S. Coffey	University of Iowa; Professor
6 Advanced topics in trial design	Babak Choodari-Oskooei Mahesh K. B. Parmar	University College London; Senior Research Associate University College London; Professor
7 Analysis	Stephen L. George	Duke University; Professor Emeritus
8 Publication and related issues	Tianjing Li	University of Colorado; Associate Professor
9 Special topics	Lawrence Friedman Nancy L. Geller	NIH:NHLBI; Retired NIH:NHLBI; Director, Office of Biostatistics Research
10 Appendices	Gillian Gresham	Cedars-Sinai Medical Center (Los Angeles); Assistant Professor

We are most grateful to the section editors in producing this work.

Thanks to Springer Nature in making this work possible.

Thanks for the guidance and council provided by Alexa Steele, editor, Springer Nature, and for the help and guidance provided by Rukmani Parameswaran and Swetha Varadharajan in shepherding this work to completion.

A special thanks to Gillian Gresham for her production of the appendices and her efforts as Senior Associate Editor.

Steven Piantadosi and Curtis L. Meinert
Editors

Contents

Volume 1

Part I   Perspectives on Clinical Trials 1

1   **Social and Scientific History of Randomized Controlled Trials** 3
    Laura E. Bothwell, Wen-Hua Kuo, David S. Jones, and Scott H. Podolsky

2   **Evolution of Clinical Trials Science** 21
    Steven Piantadosi

3   **Terminology: Conventions and Recommendations** 35
    Curtis L. Meinert

4   **Clinical Trials, Ethics, and Human Protections Policies** 55
    Jonathan Kimmelman

5   **History of the Society for Clinical Trials** 73
    O. Dale Williams and Barbara S. Hawkins

Part II   Conduct and Management 83

6   **Investigator Responsibilities** 85
    Bruce J. Giantonio

7   **Centers Participating in Multicenter Trials** 97
    Roberta W. Scherer and Barbara S. Hawkins

8   **Qualifications of the Research Staff** 123
    Catherine A. Meldrum

9   **Multicenter and Network Trials** 135
    Sheriza Baksh

| 10 | **Principles of Protocol Development** | 151 |

Bingshu E. Chen, Alison Urton, Anna Sadura, and
Wendy R. Parulekar

| 11 | **Procurement and Distribution of Study Medicines** | 169 |

Eric Hardter, Julia Collins, Dikla Shmueli-Blumberg, and
Gillian Armstrong

| 12 | **Selection of Study Centers and Investigators** | 191 |

Dikla Shmueli-Blumberg, Maria Figueroa, and Carolyn Burke

| 13 | **Design and Development of the Study Data System** | 209 |

Steve Canham

| 14 | **Implementing the Trial Protocol** | 239 |

Jamie B. Oughton and Amanda Lilley-Kelly

| 15 | **Participant Recruitment, Screening, and Enrollment** | 257 |

Pascale Wermuth

| 16 | **Administration of Study Treatments and Participant Follow-Up** | 279 |

Jennifer J. Gassman

| 17 | **Data Capture, Data Management, and Quality Control; Single Versus Multicenter Trials** | 303 |

Kristin Knust, Lauren Yesko, Ashley Case, and Kate Bickett

| 18 | **End of Trial and Close Out of Data Collection** | 321 |

Gillian Booth

| 19 | **International Trials** | 347 |

Lynette Blacher and Linda Marillo

| 20 | **Documentation: Essential Documents and Standard Operating Procedures** | 369 |

Eleanor McFadden, Julie Jackson, and Jane Forrest

| 21 | **Consent Forms and Procedures** | 389 |

Ann-Margret Ervin and Joan B. Cobb Pettit

| 22 | **Contracts and Budgets** | 411 |

Eric Riley and Eleanor McFadden

| 23 | **Long-Term Management of Data and Secondary Use** | 427 |

Steve Canham

Part III Regulation and Oversight 457

| 24 | **Regulatory Requirements in Clinical Trials** | 459 |

Michelle Pernice and Alan Colley

25	ClinicalTrials.gov Gillian Gresham	479
26	Funding Models and Proposals Matthew Westmore and Katie Meadmore	497
27	Financial Compliance in Clinical Trials Barbara K. Martin	521
28	Financial Conflicts of Interest in Clinical Trials Julie D. Gottlieb	541
29	Trial Organization and Governance O. Dale Williams and Katrina Epnere	559
30	Advocacy and Patient Involvement in Clinical Trials Ellen Sigal, Mark Stewart, and Diana Merino	569
31	Training the Investigatorship Claire Weber	583
32	Responsibilities and Management of the Clinical Coordinating Center Trinidad Ajazi	593
33	Efficient Management of a Publicly Funded Cancer Clinical Trials Portfolio Catherine Tangen and Michael LeBlanc	615
34	Archiving Records and Materials Winifred Werther and Curtis L. Meinert	637
35	Good Clinical Practice Claire Weber	649
36	Institutional Review Boards and Ethics Committees Keren R. Dunn	657
37	Data and Safety Monitoring and Reporting Sheriza Baksh and Lijuan Zeng	679
38	Post-Approval Regulatory Requirements Winifred Werther and Anita M. Loughlin	699

Volume 2

Part IV	**Bias Control and Precision**	**727**
39	Controlling for Multiplicity, Eligibility, and Exclusions Amber Salter and J. Philip Miller	729
40	Principles of Clinical Trials: Bias and Precision Control Fan-fan Yu	739

41	**Power and Sample Size** Elizabeth Garrett-Mayer	767
42	**Controlling Bias in Randomized Clinical Trials** Bruce A. Barton	787
43	**Masking of Trial Investigators** George Howard and Jenifer H. Voeks	805
44	**Masking Study Participants** Lea Drye	815
45	**Issues for Masked Data Monitoring** O. Dale Williams and Katrina Epnere	823
46	**Variance Control Procedures** Heidi L. Weiss, Jianrong Wu, Katrina Epnere, and O. Dale Williams	833
47	**Ascertainment and Classification of Outcomes** Wayne Rosamond and David Couper	843
48	**Bias Control in Randomized Controlled Clinical Trials** Diane Uschner and William F. Rosenberger	855
Part V	**Basics of Trial Design**	**875**
49	**Use of Historical Data in Design** Christopher Kim, Victoria Chia, and Michael Kelsh	877
50	**Outcomes in Clinical Trials** Justin M. Leach, Inmaculada Aban, and Gary R. Cutter	891
51	**Patient-Reported Outcomes** Gillian Gresham and Patricia A. Ganz	915
52	**Translational Clinical Trials** Steven Piantadosi	939
53	**Dose-Finding and Dose-Ranging Studies** Mark R. Conaway and Gina R. Petroni	951
54	**Inferential Frameworks for Clinical Trials** James P. Long and J. Jack Lee	973
55	**Dose Finding for Drug Combinations** Mourad Tighiouart	1003
56	**Middle Development Trials** Emine O. Bayman	1031

| 57 | **Randomized Selection Designs** | 1047 |

Shing M. Lee, Bruce Levin, and Cheng-Shiun Leu

| 58 | **Futility Designs** | 1067 |

Sharon D. Yeatts and Yuko Y. Palesch

| 59 | **Interim Analysis in Clinical Trials** | 1083 |

John A. Kairalla, Rachel Zahigian, and Samuel S. Wu

Part VI Advanced Topics in Trial Design 1103

| 60 | **Bayesian Adaptive Designs for Phase I Trials** | 1105 |

Michael J. Sweeting, Adrian P. Mander, and Graham M. Wheeler

| 61 | **Adaptive Phase II Trials** | 1133 |

Boris Freidlin and Edward L. Korn

| 62 | **Biomarker-Guided Trials** | 1145 |

L. C. Brown, A. L. Jorgensen, M. Antoniou, and J. Wason

| 63 | **Diagnostic Trials** | 1171 |

Madhu Mazumdar, Xiaobo Zhong, and Bart Ferket

| 64 | **Designs to Detect Disease Modification** | 1199 |

Michael P. McDermott

| 65 | **Screening Trials** | 1219 |

Philip C. Prorok

| 66 | **Biosimilar Drug Development** | 1237 |

Johanna Mielke and Byron Jones

| 67 | **Prevention Trials: Challenges in Design, Analysis, and Interpretation of Prevention Trials** | 1261 |

Shu Jiang and Graham A. Colditz

| 68 | **N-of-1 Randomized Trials** | 1279 |

Reza D. Mirza, Sunita Vohra, Richard Kravitz, and Gordon H. Guyatt

| 69 | **Noninferiority Trials** | 1297 |

Patrick P. J. Phillips and David V. Glidden

| 70 | **Cross-over Trials** | 1325 |

Byron Jones

| 71 | **Factorial Trials** | 1353 |

Steven Piantadosi and Susan Halabi

72	**Within Person Randomized Trials**	1377
	Gui-Shuang Ying	

73	**Device Trials**	1399
	Heng Li, Pamela E. Scott, and Lilly Q. Yue	

74	**Complex Intervention Trials**	1417
	Linda Sharples and Olympia Papachristofi	

75	**Randomized Discontinuation Trials**	1439
	Valerii V. Fedorov	

76	**Platform Trial Designs**	1455
	Oleksandr Sverdlov, Ekkehard Glimm, and Peter Mesenbrink	

77	**Cluster Randomized Trials**	1487
	Lawrence H. Moulton and Richard J. Hayes	

78	**Multi-arm Multi-stage (MAMS) Platform Randomized Clinical Trials**	1507
	Babak Choodari-Oskooei, Matthew R. Sydes, Patrick Royston, and Mahesh K. B. Parmar	

79	**Sequential, Multiple Assignment, Randomized Trials (SMART)**	1543
	Nicholas J. Seewald, Olivia Hackworth, and Daniel Almirall	

80	**Monte Carlo Simulation for Trial Design Tool**	1563
	Suresh Ankolekar, Cyrus Mehta, Rajat Mukherjee, Sam Hsiao, Jennifer Smith, and Tarek Haddad	

Volume 3

Part VII	**Analysis**	**1587**
81	**Preview of Counting and Analysis Principles**	1589
	Nancy L. Geller	
82	**Intention to Treat and Alternative Approaches**	1597
	Judith D. Goldberg	
83	**Estimation and Hypothesis Testing**	1615
	Pamela A. Shaw and Michael A. Proschan	
84	**Estimands and Sensitivity Analyses**	1631
	Estelle Russek-Cohen and David Petullo	

85	**Confident Statistical Inference with Multiple Outcomes, Subgroups, and Other Issues of Multiplicity** .... Siyoen Kil, Eloise Kaizar, Szu-Yu Tang, and Jason C. Hsu	1659
86	**Missing Data** .... Guangyu Tong, Fan Li, and Andrew S. Allen	1681
87	**Essential Statistical Tests** .... Gregory R. Pond and Samantha-Jo Caetano	1703
88	**Nonparametric Survival Analysis** .... Yuliya Lokhnygina	1717
89	**Survival Analysis II** .... James J. Dignam	1743
90	**Prognostic Factor Analyses** .... Liang Li	1771
91	**Logistic Regression and Related Methods** .... Márcio A. Diniz and Tiago M. Magalhães	1789
92	**Statistical Analysis of Patient-Reported Outcomes in Clinical Trials** .... Gina L. Mazza and Amylou C. Dueck	1813
93	**Adherence Adjusted Estimates in Randomized Clinical Trials** .... Sreelatha Meleth	1833
94	**Randomization and Permutation Tests** .... Vance W. Berger, Patrick Onghena, and J. Rosser Matthews	1851
95	**Generalized Pairwise Comparisons for Prioritized Outcomes** ... Marc Buyse and Julien Peron	1869
96	**Use of Resampling Procedures to Investigate Issues of Model Building and Its Stability** .... Willi Sauerbrei and Anne-Laure Boulesteix	1895
97	**Joint Analysis of Longitudinal and Time-to-Event Data** .... Zheng Lu, Emmanuel Chigutsa, and Xiao Tong	1919
98	**Pharmacokinetic and Pharmacodynamic Modeling** .... Shamir N. Kalaria, Hechuan Wang, and Jogarao V. Gobburu	1937
99	**Safety and Risk Benefit Analyses** .... Jeff Jianfei Guo	1961

100	Causal Inference: Efficacy and Mechanism Evaluation	1981
	Sabine Landau and Richard Emsley	
101	Development and Validation of Risk Prediction Models	2003
	Damien Drubay, Ben Van Calster, and Stefan Michiels	

Part VIII Publication and Related Issues 2025

102	Paper Writing	2027
	Curtis L. Meinert	
103	Reporting Biases	2045
	S. Swaroop Vedula, Asbjørn Hróbjartsson, and Matthew J. Page	
104	CONSORT and Its Extensions for Reporting Clinical Trials	2073
	Sally Hopewell, Isabelle Boutron, and David Moher	
105	Publications from Clinical Trials	2089
	Barbara S. Hawkins	
106	Study Name, Authorship, Titling, and Credits	2103
	Curtis L. Meinert	
107	De-identifying Clinical Trial Data	2115
	Jimmy Le	
108	Data Sharing and Reuse	2137
	Ida Sim	
109	Introduction to Systematic Reviews	2159
	Tianjing Li, Ian J. Saldanha, and Karen A. Robinson	
110	Introduction to Meta-Analysis	2179
	Theodoros Evrenoglou, Silvia Metelli, and Anna Chaimani	
111	Reading and Interpreting the Literature on Randomized Controlled Trials	2197
	Janet Wittes	
112	Trials Can Inform or Misinform: "The Story of Vitamin A Deficiency and Childhood Mortality"	2209
	Alfred Sommer	

Part IX Special Topics 2225

113	Issues in Generalizing Results from Clinical Trials	2227
	Steven Piantadosi	

114	Leveraging "Big Data" for the Design and Execution of Clinical Trials .... 2241 Stephen J. Greene, Marc D. Samsky, and Adrian F. Hernandez
115	Trials in Complementary and Integrative Health Interventions .... 2263 Catherine M. Meyers and Qilu Yu
116	Orphan Drugs and Rare Diseases .... 2289 James E. Valentine and Frank J. Sasinowski
117	Pragmatic Randomized Trials Using Claims or Electronic Health Record Data .... 2307 Frank W. Rockhold and Benjamin A. Goldstein
118	Fraud in Clinical Trials .... 2319 Stephen L. George, Marc Buyse, and Steven Piantadosi
119	Clinical Trials on Trial: Lawsuits Stemming from Clinical Research .... 2339 John J. DeBoy and Annie X. Wang
120	Biomarker-Driven Adaptive Phase III Clinical Trials .... 2367 Richard Simon
121	Clinical Trials in Children .... 2379 Gail D. Pearson, Kristin M. Burns, and Victoria L. Pemberton
122	Trials in Older Adults .... 2397 Sergei Romashkan and Laurie Ryan
123	Trials in Minority Populations .... 2417 Otis W. Brawley
124	Expanded Access to Drug and Device Products for Clinical Treatment .... 2431 Tracy Ziolek, Jessica L. Yoos, Inna Strakovsky, Praharsh Shah, and Emily Robison
125	A Perspective on the Process of Designing and Conducting Clinical Trials .... 2453 Curtis L. Meinert and Steven Piantadosi

Appendix 1	2475
Appendix 2	2477
Appendix 3	2481
Appendix 4	2489
Appendix 5	2493
Appendix 6	2499
Appendix 7	2503
Appendix 8	2509
Appendix 9	2513
Appendix 10	2515
Appendix 11	2523
Appendix 12	2525
Appendix 13	2529
Appendix 14	2535
Appendix 15	2557
Appendix 16	2563
Index	2565

About the Editors

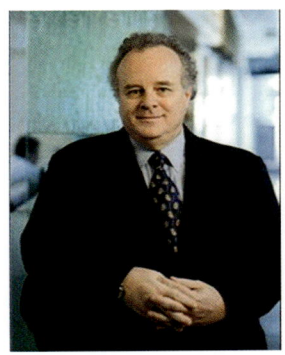

Steven Piantadosi, MD, PhD, is a clinical trialist with 40 years' experience in research, teaching, and healthcare leadership. He has worked on clinical trials of all types, including multicenter and international trials, academic portfolios, and regulatory trials. Most of his work has been in cancer; he also works in other disciplines such as neurodegenerative and cardiovascular diseases.

Dr. Piantadosi began his career in clinical trials early during an intramural Staff Fellowship at the National Cancer Institute's Clinical and Diagnostic Trials Section from 1982 to 1987. That group focused on theory, methodology, and applications with the NCI-sponsored *Lung Cancer Study Group*. Collaborative work included studies of bias induced by missing covariates, factorial clinical trials, and the ecological fallacy. In the latter years, the Branch was focused on Cancer Prevention, including design of the PLCO Trial, which would conclude 30 years later.

In 1987, Dr. Piantadosi joined the Johns Hopkins Oncology Center (now the Johns Hopkins Sidney Kimmel Comprehensive Cancer Center) as the first Director of Biostatistics and the CC Shared Resource. He also carried appointments in the Department of Biostatistics, and in the Johns Hopkins Center for Clinical Trials in the Department of Epidemiology in the School of Public Health (now the Johns Hopkins Bloomberg School). The division he founded became well diversified in cancer research and peer reviewed support, including the CCSG, 6 SPORE grants, PPGs, R01s, and many other grants. A program in Bioinformatics was begun jointly with the Biostatistics Department in Public Health, which would eventually develop into its own funded CCSG Shared Resource. The Biostatistics Division also had key responsibilities in Cancer Center teaching, the Protocol Review and Monitoring Committee, Clinical Research Office, Clinical Informatics, and Research Data Systems and Informatics.

From 1987 onward Dr. Piantadosi's work involved nearly every type of cancer, but especially bone marrow transplant, lung cancer, brain tumors, and drug development. In 1994, he helped to found the New Approaches to Brian Tumor Therapy Consortium (now the *Adult Brian Tumor Consortium*, ABTC), focused on early developmental trials of new agents. This group was funded by NCI for 25 years, was one of the first to accomplish multicenter phase I trials, and was an early implementer of the Continual Reassessment Method (CRM) for dose-finding.

Collaborations at Johns Hopkins extended well beyond the Oncology Department and included Epidemiology (Multi-Center AIDS Cohort Study), Biostatistics, Surgery, Medicine, Anesthesiology, Urology, and Neurosurgery. His work on design and analysis of brain tumor trials through the Department of Neurosurgery led to the FDA approval of BCNU-impregnated biodegradable polymers (Gliadel) for treatment of glioblastoma. He also maintained important external collaborations such as with the *Parkinson's Study Group*, based at the University of Rochester. He ran the Coordinating Center for the *National Emphysema Treatment Trial (NETT)* sponsored by NHLBI and CMS. Numerous important findings emerged from this trial, not the least of which was sharpened indications for risks, benefits, and efficacy of lung volume reduction surgery for emphysema. Dr. Piantadosi also participated actively in prevention trials such as the Alzheimer's Disease Anti-Inflammatory Prevention Trial (ADAPT) and the Chemoprevention for Barrett's Esophagus Trial, both employing NSAIDs and concluding that they were ineffective preventives. He worked with FDA, serving on the *Oncologic Drugs Advisory Committee*, and afterwards on various review panels, and as advisor to industry.

From 2007 to 2017, Dr. Piantadosi was the inaugural Director of the Samuel Oschin Cancer Institute at Cedars Sinai, a UCLA teaching hospital, Professor of Medicine, and Professor of Biomathematics and

Medicine at UCLA. Cedars is the largest hospital in the western USA and treats over 5000 new cancer cases each year, using full-time faculty, in-network oncologists, and private practitioners. Broadly applied work continued with activities in the *Long-Term Oxygen Treatment Trial* (LOTT), dose-finding designs for cancer drug combinations, neurodegenerative disease trial design, and support of the UCLA multi-campus CTSA. During this interval, numerous clinicians and researchers were recruited. Peer-reviewed funding increased from ~$1M to over $20M annually. A clinical trialist is an unusual choice for a Cancer Center director, but it represented an opportunity to improve cancer care in Los Angeles, strengthen the academics at the institution using the NCI P30 model, and serve as a role model for clinical trialists.

In 2018, Dr. Piantadosi joined the Division of Surgical Oncology at Brigham and Women's Hospital, as Professor in Residence, Harvard Medical School. Work at BWH, HMS, includes roles on the *Alliance* NCTN group Executive Committee as the Associate Group Chair for Strategic Initiatives and Innovation, as well as mentoring in the Alliance Statistics Office. He is currently course Co-director for Methods in Clinical Research at DFCI and Course Director for Advanced Clinical Trials (CI 726) in the Master of Medical Sciences in Clinical Investigation Program at Harvard Medical School.

Teaching and Education: In 1988, while at Hopkins Dr. Piantadosi began teaching Experimental Design followed by advanced Clinical Trials. This work formed the foundation for the textbook *Clinical Trials: A Methodologic Perspective*, first published in 1997 and now in its 3rd edition. His course was a staple for students in Biostatistics, Epidemiology, and the Graduate Training Program in Clinical Investigation, where he also taught a research seminar. Subsequently, he mentored numerous PhD graduate students and fellows and served on many doctoral committees. At UCLA, he continued to teach Clinical Trials in their Specialty Training and Research Program.

Dr. Piantadosi has also taught extensively in national workshops focused on training of clinical investigators in cancer, biostatistics, and neurologic disease. This began with the start of the well-known Vail Workshop, and similar venues in Europe and Australia. He was also the Director of several similarly structured courses solely for biostatisticians sponsored by AACR. Independent of those workshops, he taught extensively in Japan, Holland, and Italy.

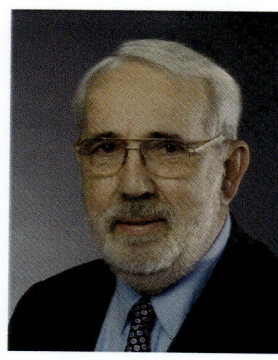

Curtis L. Meinert
Department of Epidemiology
School of Public Health
Johns Hopkins University
Baltimore, MD, USA

Professor Emeritus (Retired 30 June 2019)

I was born 30 June 1934 on a farm four miles west of Sleepy Eye, Minnesota.

My birthday was the first day of a three-day rampage orchestrated by Adolf Hitler known as the Night of the Long Knives. Ominous foreboding of events to come.

My first 6 years of schooling was in a country school located near the Chicago and Northwestern railroad line. There was no studying when freight trains got stuck making the grade past the school.

As was the custom of my parents, all four of us were sent to St John's Lutheran School in Sleepy Eye for our seventh and eighth years of schooling for modicums of religious training. After Lutheran School it was Sleepy Eye Public School, and after that it was the University of Minnesota.

Bachelor of Arts in psychology (1956)
Masters of Science in biostatistics (1959)
Doctor of Philosophy in biostatistics (1964) (Dissertation: Quantitation of the isotope displacement insulin immunoassay)

My sojourn in trials started when I was a graduate student at the University of Minnesota. It started when I signed on to work with Chris Klimt looking for someone to work with him developing what was to become the University Group Diabetes Program (UGDP).

Dr. Klimt decided to move to Baltimore in 1962 to take an appointment in the University of Maryland Medical School. He wanted me to move with him. I did, albeit reluctantly because I wanted to stay and finish my PhD dissertation.

Being Midwestern, Baltimore seemed foreign. People said we talked with an accent, but in our mind it was they who had the accents. A few days after we unpacked I told my wife we would stay a little while, but that I did not want to wake up dead in Baltimore. That surely now is my fate with all my daughters and grand children living here.

The UGDP begat the Coronary Drug Project (CDP; 1966) and it begat others.

I moved across town in 1979 to accept an appointment in the Department of Epidemiology, School of Public Health, Johns Hopkins University. The move led to classroom teaching, mentoring passels of doctoral students, several text books, and a blog site trialsmeinertsway.com.

It was Abe Lilienfeld, after I arrived at Hopkins, who rekindled my "textbook fire." I had taken a sabbatical a few years back while at Maryland to write a text on design and conduct of trials and produced nothing! The good news was that the "textbook bug" was gone – that is until Abe got a hold of me at Hopkins.

Trials became my life with the creation of the Center for Clinical Trials (now the Center for Clinical Trials and Evidence Synthesis) established in 1990 with the urging and help of Al Sommer, then dean of the school. The Center has done dozens and dozens of trials since its creation.

I lost my wife 20 February 2015. I met her at a Tupperware party on Washington's birthday in 1954. We married a year and half later. She was born and raised in Sioux Falls, South Dakota. Being 5'9" inches tall she was happy to be able to wear her 3" heels when we went out on the town and still be 6 in. shorter than her escort. Height has its advantages, but not when you are in the middle seat flying sardine!

I came to know Steve Piantadosi after he arrived at Hopkins in 1987. He started talking about a collective work as we are now involved in long before it had a name. For years I ignored his talk, but the "smooth talking North Carolinian" can be insidious and convincing.

So here I am, with Steve joined at the hip, trying to shepherd this work to the finish line.

About the Section Editors

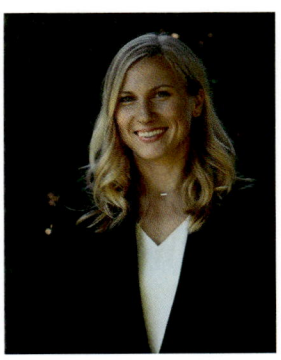

Gillian Gresham
Department of Medicine
Cedars-Sinai Medical Center
Los Angeles, CA, USA

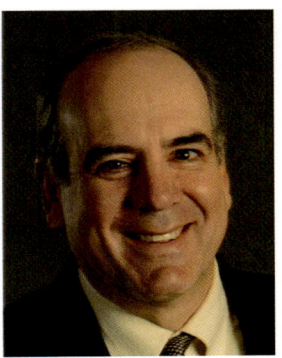

Steven N. Goodman
Stanford University School of Medicine
Stanford, CA, USA

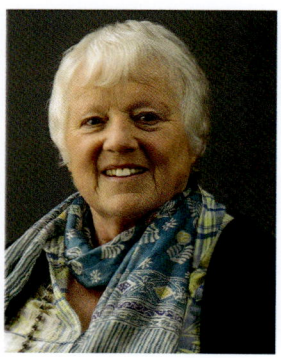

Eleanor McFadden
Frontier Science (Scotland) Ltd.
Kincraig, Scotland

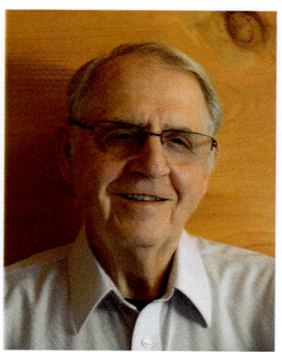

O. Dale Williams
University of North Carolina at Chapel Hill
Chapel Hill, NC, USA

University of Alabama at Birmingham
Birmingham, AL, USA

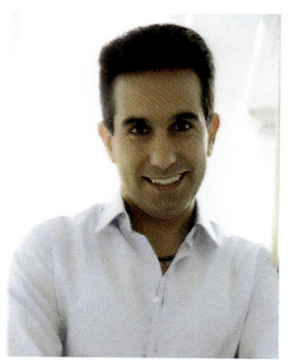

Babak Choodari-Oskooei
MRC Clinical Trials Unit at UCL
Institute of Clinical Trials and Methodology, UCL
London, UK

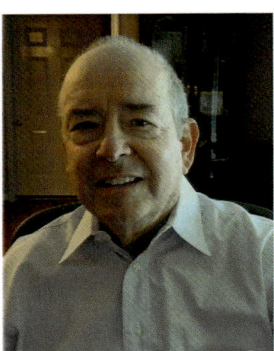

Stephen L. George
Department of Biostatistics and Bioinformatics
Duke University School of Medicine
Durham, NC, USA

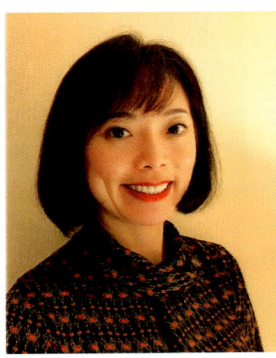

Tianjing Li
Department of Ophthalmology
School of Medicine
University of Colorado Anschutz Medical Campus
Colorado School of Public Health
Aurora, CO, USA

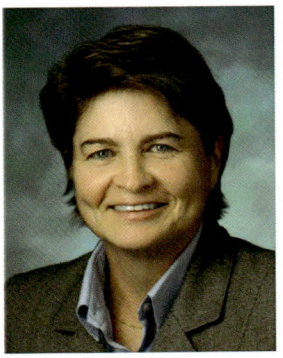

Karen A. Robinson
Johns Hopkins University
Baltimore, MD, USA

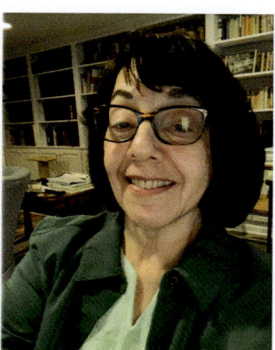

Nancy L. Geller
Office of Biostatistics Research
NHLBI
Bethesda, MD, USA

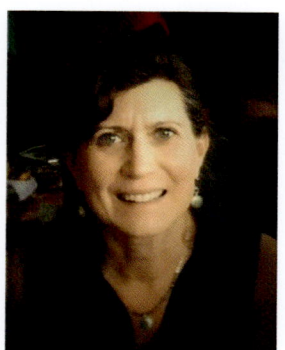

Winifred Werther
Amgen Inc.
South San Francisco, CA, USA

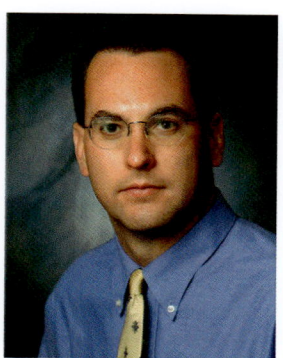

Christopher S. Coffey
University of Iowa
Iowa City, IA, USA

About the Section Editors

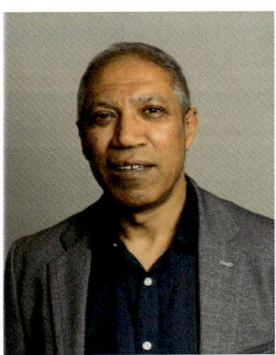

Mahesh K. B. Parmar
University College of London
London, England

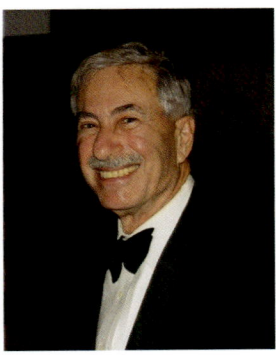

Lawrence Friedman
Rockville, MD, USA

Contributors

Inmaculada Aban Department of Biostatistics, University of Alabama at Birmingham, Birmingham, AL, USA

Trinidad Ajazi Alliance for Clinical Trials in Oncology, University of Chicago, Chicago, IL, USA

Andrew S. Allen Department of Biostatistics and Bioinformatics, Duke University, School of Medicine, Durham, NC, USA

Daniel Almirall University of Michigan, Ann Arbor, MI, USA

Suresh Ankolekar Cytel Inc, Cambridge, MA, USA
Maastricht School of Management, Maastricht, Netherlands

M. Antoniou F. Hoffmann-La Roche Ltd, Basel, Switzerland

Gillian Armstrong GSK, Slaoui Center for Vaccines Research, Rockville, MD, USA

Sheriza Baksh Johns Hopkins Bloomberg School of Public Health, Baltimore, MD, USA

Bruce A. Barton Department of Population and Quantitative Health Sciences, University of Massachusetts Medical School, Worcester, MA, USA

Emine O. Bayman University of Iowa, Iowa City, IA, USA

Vance W. Berger Biometry Research Group, National Cancer Institute, Rockville, MD, USA

Kate Bickett Emmes, Rockville, MD, USA

Lynette Blacher Frontier Science Amherst, Amherst, NY, USA

Gillian Booth Leeds Institute of Clinical Trials Research, University of Leeds, Leeds, UK

Laura E. Bothwell Worcester State University, Worcester, MA, USA

Anne-Laure Boulesteix Institute for Medical Information Processing, Biometry, and Epidemiology, LMU Munich, Munich, Germany

Isabelle Boutron Epidemiology and Biostatistics Research Center (CRESS), Inserm UMR1153, Université de Paris, Paris, France

Otis W. Brawley Johns Hopkins School of Medicine, and Johns Hopkins Bloomberg School of Public Health, Baltimore, MD, USA

L. C. Brown MRC Clinical Trials Unit, UCL Institute of Clinical Trials and Methodology, London, UK

Carolyn Burke The Emmes Company, LLC, Rockville, MD, USA

Kristin M. Burns National Heart, Lung, and Blood Institute, National Institutes of Health, Bethesda, MD, USA

Marc Buyse International Drug Development Institute (IDDI) Inc., San Francisco, CA, USA

CluePoints S.A., Louvain-la-Neuve, Belgium and I-BioStat, University of Hasselt, Louvain-la-Neuve, Belgium

Interuniversity Institute for Biostatistics and Statistical Bioinformatics (I-BioStat), Hasselt University, Hasselt, Belgium

Samantha-Jo Caetano Department of Mathematics and Statistics, McMaster University, Hamilton, ON, Canada

Steve Canham European Clinical Research Infrastructure Network (ECRIN), Paris, France

Ashley Case Emmes, Rockville, MD, USA

Anna Chaimani Université de Paris, Research Center of Epidemiology and Statistics (CRESS-U1153), INSERM, Paris, France

Cochrane France, Paris, France

Bingshu E. Chen Canadian Cancer Trials Group, Queen's University, Kingston, ON, Canada

Victoria Chia Amgen Inc., Thousand Oaks, CA, USA

Emmanuel Chigutsa Pharmacometrics, Eli Lilly and Company, Zionsville, IN, USA

Babak Choodari-Oskooei MRC Clinical Trials Unit at UCL, Institute of Clinical Trials and Methodology, London, UK

Joan B. Cobb Pettit Johns Hopkins Bloomberg School of Public Health, Baltimore, MD, USA

Graham A. Colditz Division of Public Health Sciences, Department of Surgery, Washington University School of Medicine, Saint Louis, MO, USA

Alan Colley Amgen, Ltd, Cambridge, UK

Julia Collins The Emmes Company, LLC, Rockville, MD, USA

Mark R. Conaway University of Virginia Health System, Charlottesville, VA, USA

David Couper Department of Biostatistics, Gillings School of Global Public Health, University of North Carolina, Chapel Hill, NC, USA

Gary R. Cutter Department of Biostatistics, University of Alabama at Birmingham, Birmingham, AL, USA

John J. DeBoy Covington & Burling LLP, Washington, DC, USA

James J. Dignam Department of Public Health Sciences, The University of Chicago, Chicago, IL, USA

Márcio A. Diniz Biostatistics and Bioinfomatics Research Center, Samuel Oschin Cancer Center, Cedars Sinai Medical Center, Los Angeles, CA, USA

Damien Drubay INSERM U1018, CESP, Paris-Saclay University, UVSQ, Villejuif, France

Gustave Roussy, Service de Biostatistique et d'Epidémiologie, Villejuif, France

Lea Drye Office of Clinical Affairs, Blue Cross Blue Shield Association, Chicago, IL, USA

Amylou C. Dueck Division of Biomedical Statistics and Informatics, Department of Health Sciences Research, Mayo Clinic, Scottsdale, AZ, USA

Keren R. Dunn Office of Research Compliance and Quality Improvement, Cedars-Sinai Medical Center, Los Angeles, CA, USA

Richard Emsley Department of Biostatistics and Health Informatics, King's College London, London, UK

Katrina Epnere WCG Statistics Collaborative, Washington, DC, USA

Ann-Margret Ervin Johns Hopkins Bloomberg School of Public Health, Baltimore, MD, USA

The Johns Hopkins Center for Clinical Trials and Evidence Synthesis, Johns Hopkins University, Baltimore, MD, USA

Theodoros Evrenoglou Université de Paris, Research Center of Epidemiology and Statistics (CRESS-U1153), INSERM, Paris, France

Valerii V. Fedorov ICON, North Wales, PA, USA

Bart Ferket Ichan School of Medicine at Mount Sinai, New York, NY, USA

Maria Figueroa The Emmes Company, LLC, Rockville, MD, USA

Jane Forrest Frontier Science (Scotland) Ltd, Grampian View, Kincraig, UK

Boris Freidlin Biometric Research Program, Division of Cancer Treatment and Diagnosis, National Cancer Institute, Bethesda, MD, USA

Patricia A. Ganz Jonsson Comprehensive Cancer Center, University of California at Los Angeles, Los Angeles, CA, USA

Elizabeth Garrett-Mayer American Society of Clinical Oncology, Alexandria, VA, USA

Jennifer J. Gassman Department of Quantitative Health Sciences, Cleveland Clinic, Cleveland, OH, USA

Nancy L. Geller National Heart, Lung and Blood Institute, National Institutes of Health, Bethesda, MD, USA

Stephen L. George Department of Biostatistics and Bioinformatics, Basic Science Division, Duke University School of Medicine, Durham, NC, USA

Bruce J. Giantonio The ECOG-ACRIN Cancer Research Group, Philadelphia, PA, USA

Massachusetts General Hospital, Boston, MA, USA

Department of Medical Oncology, University of Pretoria, Pretoria, South Africa

David V. Glidden Department of Epidemiology and Biostatistics, University of California San Francisco, San Francisco, CA, USA

Ekkehard Glimm Novartis Pharma AG, Basel, Switzerland

Jogarao V. Gobburu Center for Translational Medicine, University of Maryland School of Pharmacy, Baltimore, MD, USA

Judith D. Goldberg Department of Population Health and Environmental Medicine, New York University School of Medicine, New York, NY, USA

Benjamin A. Goldstein Department of Biostatistics and Bioinformatics, Duke Clinical Research Institute, Duke University Medical Center, Durham, NC, USA

Julie D. Gottlieb Johns Hopkins University School of Medicine, Baltimore, MD, USA

Stephen J. Greene Duke Clinical Research Institute, Durham, NC, USA

Division of Cardiology, Duke University School of Medicine, Durham, NC, USA

Gillian Gresham Samuel Oschin Comprehensive Cancer Institute, Cedars-Sinai Medical Center, Los Angeles, CA, USA

Jeff Jianfei Guo Division of Pharmacy Practice and Administrative Sciences, University of Cincinnati College of Pharmacy, Cincinnati, OH, USA

Gordon H. Guyatt McMaster University, Hamilton, ON, Canada

Olivia Hackworth University of Michigan, Ann Arbor, MI, USA

Tarek Haddad Medtronic Inc, Minneapolis, MN, USA

Susan Halabi Department of Biostatistics and Bioinformatics, Duke University Medical Center, Durham, NC, USA

Eric Hardter The Emmes Company, LLC, Rockville, MD, USA

Barbara S. Hawkins Johns Hopkins School of Medicine and Bloomberg School of Public Health, The Johns Hopkins University, Baltimore, MD, USA

Richard J. Hayes Faculty of Epidemiology and Population Health, London School of Hygiene and Tropical Medicine, London, UK

Adrian F. Hernandez Duke Clinical Research Institute, Durham, NC, USA
Division of Cardiology, Duke University School of Medicine, Durham, NC, USA

Sally Hopewell Centre for Statistics in Medicine, Nuffield Department of Orthopaedics, Rheumatology and Musculoskeletal Sciences, University of Oxford, Oxford, UK

George Howard Department of Biostatistics, University of Alabama at Birmingham, Birmingham, AL, USA

Asbjørn Hróbjartsson Cochrane Denmark and Centre for Evidence-Based Medicine Odense, University of Southern Denmark, Odense, Denmark

Sam Hsiao Cytel Inc, Cambridge, MA, USA

Jason C. Hsu Department of Statistics, The Ohio State University, Columbus, OH, USA

Julie Jackson Frontier Science (Scotland) Ltd, Grampian View, Kincraig, UK

Shu Jiang Division of Public Health Sciences, Department of Surgery, Washington University School of Medicine, Saint Louis, MO, USA

Byron Jones Novartis Pharma AG, Basel, Switzerland

David S. Jones Harvard University, Cambridge, MA, USA

A. L. Jorgensen Department of Health Data Science, University of Liverpool, Liverpool, UK

John A. Kairalla University of Florida, Gainesville, FL, USA

Eloise Kaizar The Ohio State University, Columbus, OH, USA

Shamir N. Kalaria Center for Translational Medicine, University of Maryland School of Pharmacy, Baltimore, MD, USA

Michael Kelsh Amgen Inc., Thousand Oaks, CA, USA

Siyoen Kil LSK Global Pharmaceutical Services, Seoul, Republic of Korea

Christopher Kim Amgen Inc., Thousand Oaks, CA, USA

Jonathan Kimmelman Biomedical Ethics Unit, McGill University, Montreal, QC, Canada

Kristin Knust Emmes, Rockville, MD, USA

Edward L. Korn Biometric Research Program, Division of Cancer Treatment and Diagnosis, National Cancer Institute, Bethesda, MD, USA

Richard Kravitz University of California Davis, Davis, CA, USA

Wen-Hua Kuo National Yang-Ming University, Taipei City, Taiwan

Sabine Landau Department of Biostatistics and Health Informatics, King's College London, London, UK

Jimmy Le National Eye Institute, Bethesda, MD, USA

Justin M. Leach Department of Biostatistics, University of Alabama at Birmingham, Birmingham, AL, USA

Michael LeBlanc SWOG Statistical Center, Fred Hutchinson Cancer Research Center, Seattle, WA, USA

J. Jack Lee Department of Biostatistics, University of Texas MD Anderson Cancer Center, Houston, TX, USA

Shing M. Lee Department of Biostatistics, Mailman School of Public Health, Columbia University, New York, NY, USA

Cheng-Shiun Leu Department of Biostatistics, Mailman School of Public Health, Columbia University, New York, NY, USA

Bruce Levin Department of Biostatistics, Mailman School of Public Health, Columbia University, New York, NY, USA

Fan Li Department of Biostatistics, Yale University, School of Public Health, New Haven, CT, USA

Heng Li Center for Devices and Radiological Health, U.S. Food and Drug Administration, Silver Spring, MD, USA

Liang Li Department of Biostatistics, The University of Texas MD Anderson Cancer Center, Houston, TX, USA

Tianjing Li Department of Ophthalmology, University of Colorado Anschutz Medical Campus, Aurora, CO, USA

Amanda Lilley-Kelly Clinical Trials Research Unit, Leeds Institute of Clinical Trials Research, University of Leeds, Leeds, UK

Yuliya Lokhnygina Department of Biostatistics and Bioinformatics, Duke University, Durham, NC, USA

James P. Long Department of Biostatistics, University of Texas MD Anderson Cancer Center, Houston, TX, USA

Anita M. Loughlin Corrona LLC, Waltham, MA, USA

Zheng Lu Clinical Pharmacology and Exploratory Development, Astellas Pharma, Northbrook, IL, USA

Tiago M. Magalhães Department of Statistics, Institute of Exact Sciences, Federal University of Juiz de Fora, Juiz de Fora, Minas Gerais, Brazil

Adrian P. Mander Centre for Trials Research, Cardiff University, Cardiff, UK

Linda Marillo Frontier Science Amherst, Amherst, NY, USA

Barbara K. Martin Administrative Director, Research Institute, Penn Medicine Lancaster General Health, Lancaster, PA, USA

J. Rosser Matthews General Dynamics Health Solutions, Defense and Veterans Brain Injury Center, Silver Spring, MD, USA

Madhu Mazumdar Director of Institute for Healthcare Delivery Science, Mount Sinai Health System, NY, USA

Gina L. Mazza Division of Biomedical Statistics and Informatics, Department of Health Sciences Research, Mayo Clinic, Scottsdale, AZ, USA

Michael P. McDermott Department of Biostatistics and Computational Biology, University of Rochester Medical Center, Rochester, NY, USA

Eleanor McFadden Frontier Science (Scotland) Ltd., Kincraig, Scotland, UK

Katie Meadmore University of Southampton, Southampton, UK

Cyrus Mehta Cytel Inc, Cambridge, MA, USA
Harvard T.H. Chan School of Public Health, Boston, MA, USA

Curtis L. Meinert Department of Epidemiology, School of Public Health, Johns Hopkins University, Baltimore, MD, USA

Catherine A. Meldrum University of Michigan, Ann Arbor, MI, USA

Sreelatha Meleth RTI International, Atlanta, GA, USA

Diana Merino Friends of Cancer Research, Washington, DC, USA

Peter Mesenbrink Novartis Pharmaceuticals Corporation, East Hannover, NJ, USA

Silvia Metelli Université de Paris, Research Center of Epidemiology and Statistics (CRESS-U1153), INSERM, Paris, France
Assistance Publique - Hôpitaux de Paris (APHP), Paris, France

Catherine M. Meyers Office of Clinical and Regulatory Affairs, National Institutes of Health, National Center for Complementary and Integrative Health, Bethesda, MD, USA

Stefan Michiels INSERM U1018, CESP, Paris-Saclay University, UVSQ, Villejuif, France

Gustave Roussy, Service de Biostatistique et d'Epidémiologie, Villejuif, France

Johanna Mielke Novartis Pharma AG, Basel, Switzerland

J. Philip Miller Division of Biostatistics, Washington University School of Medicine in St. Louis, St. Louis, MO, USA

Reza D. Mirza Department of Medicine, McMaster University, Hamilton, ON, Canada

David Moher Centre for Journaology, Clinical Epidemiology Program, Ottawa Hospital Research Institute, Canadian EQUATOR centre, Ottawa, ON, Canada

Lawrence H. Moulton Departments of International Health and Biostatistics, Johns Hopkins Bloomberg School of Public Health, Baltimore, MD, USA

Rajat Mukherjee Cytel Inc, Cambridge, MA, USA

Patrick Onghena Faculty of Psychology and Educational Sciences, KU Leuven, Leuven, Belgium

Jamie B. Oughton Clinical Trials Research Unit, Leeds Institute of Clinical Trials Research, University of Leeds, Leeds, UK

Matthew J. Page School of Public Health and Preventive Medicine, Monash University, Melbourne, VIC, Australia

Yuko Y. Palesch Data Coordination Unit, Department of Public Health Sciences, Medical University of South Carolina, Charleston, SC, USA

Olympia Papachristofi London School of Hygiene and Tropical Medicine, London, UK

Clinical Development and Analytics, Novartis Pharma AG, Basel, Switzerland

Mahesh K. B. Parmar MRC Clinical Trials Unit at UCL, Institute of Clinical Trials and Methodology, London, UK

Wendy R. Parulekar Canadian Cancer Trials Group, Queen's University, Kingston, ON, Canada

Gail D. Pearson National Heart, Lung, and Blood Institute, National Institutes of Health, Bethesda, MD, USA

Victoria L. Pemberton National Heart, Lung, and Blood Institute, National Institutes of Health, Bethesda, MD, USA

Michelle Pernice Dynavax Technologies Corporation, Emeryville, CA, USA

Julien Peron CNRS, UMR 5558, Laboratoire de Biométrie et Biologie Evolutive, Université Lyon 1, France

Departments of Biostatistics and Medical Oncology, Centre Hospitalier Lyon-Sud, Institut de Cancérologie des Hospices Civils de Lyon, Lyon, France

Gina R. Petroni Translational Research and Applied Statistics, Public Health Sciences, University of Virginia Health System, Charlottesville, VA, USA

David Petullo Division of Biometrics II, Office of Biostatistics Office of Translational Sciences, Center for Drug Evaluation and Research, U.S. Food and Drug Administration, Silver Spring, MD, USA

Patrick P. J. Phillips UCSF Center for Tuberculosis, University of California San Francisco, San Francisco, CA, USA

Department of Epidemiology and Biostatistics, University of California San Francisco, San Francisco, CA, USA

Steven Piantadosi Department of Surgery, Division of Surgical Oncology, Brigham and Women's Hospital, Harvard Medical School, Boston, MA, USA

Scott H. Podolsky Harvard Medical School, Boston, MA, USA

Gregory R. Pond Department of Oncology, McMaster University, Hamilton, ON, Canada

Ontario Institute for Cancer Research, Toronto, ON, Canada

Philip C. Prorok Division of Cancer Prevention, National Cancer Institute, Bethesda, MD, USA

Michael A. Proschan National Institute of Allergy and Infectious Diseases, Bethesda, MD, USA

Eric Riley Frontier Science (Scotland) Ltd., Kincraig, Scotland, UK

Karen A. Robinson Department of Medicine, Johns Hopkins University, Baltimore, MD, USA

Emily Robison Optum Labs, Las Vegas, NV, USA

Frank W. Rockhold Department of Biostatistics and Bioinformatics, Duke Clinical Research Institute, Duke University Medical Center, Durham, NC, USA

Sergei Romashkan National Institutes of Health, National Institute on Aging, Bethesda, MD, USA

Wayne Rosamond Department of Epidemiology, Gillings School of Global Public Health, University of North Carolina, Chapel Hill, NC, USA

William F. Rosenberger Biostatistics Center, The George Washington University, Rockville, MD, USA

Patrick Royston MRC Clinical Trials Unit at UCL, Institute of Clinical Trials and Methodology, London, UK

Estelle Russek-Cohen Office of Biostatistics, Center for Drug Evaluation and Research, U.S. Food and Drug Administration, Silver Spring, MD, USA

Laurie Ryan National Institutes of Health, National Institute on Aging, Bethesda, MD, USA

Anna Sadura Canadian Cancer Trials Group, Queen's University, Kingston, ON, Canada

Ian J. Saldanha Department of Health Services, Policy, and Practice and Department of Epidemiology, Brown University School of Public Health, Providence, RI, USA

Amber Salter Division of Biostatistics, Washington University School of Medicine in St. Louis, St. Louis, MO, USA

Marc D. Samsky Duke Clinical Research Institute, Durham, NC, USA
Division of Cardiology, Duke University School of Medicine, Durham, NC, USA

Frank J. Sasinowski University of Rochester School of Medicine, Department of Neurology, Rochester, NY, USA

Willi Sauerbrei Institute of Medical Biometry and Statistics, Faculty of Medicine and Medical Center - University of Freiburg, Freiburg, Germany

Roberta W. Scherer Department of Epidemiology, Johns Hopkins Bloomberg School of Public Health, Baltimore, MD, USA

Pamela E. Scott Office of the Commissioner, U.S. Food and Drug Administration, Silver Spring, MD, USA

Nicholas J. Seewald University of Michigan, Ann Arbor, MI, USA

Praharsh Shah University of Pennsylvania, Philadelphia, PA, USA

Linda Sharples London School of Hygiene and Tropical Medicine, London, UK

Pamela A. Shaw University of Pennsylvania Perelman School of Medicine, Philadelphia, PA, USA

Dikla Shmueli-Blumberg The Emmes Company, LLC, Rockville, MD, USA

Ellen Sigal Friends of Cancer Research, Washington, DC, USA

Ida Sim Division of General Internal Medicine, University of California San Francisco, San Francisco, CA, USA

Richard Simon R Simon Consulting, Potomac, MD, USA

Jennifer Smith Sunesis Pharmaceuticals Inc, San Francisco, CA, USA

Alfred Sommer Johns Hopkins Bloomberg School of Public Health, Baltimore, MD, USA

Mark Stewart Friends of Cancer Research, Washington, DC, USA

Inna Strakovsky University of Pennsylvania, Philadelphia, PA, USA

Oleksandr Sverdlov Novartis Pharmaceuticals Corporation, East Hannover, NJ, USA

Michael J. Sweeting Department of Health Sciences, University of Leicester, Leicester, UK

Department of Public Health and Primary Care, University of Cambridge, Cambridge, UK

Matthew R. Sydes MRC Clinical Trials Unit at UCL, Institute of Clinical Trials and Methodology, London, UK

Szu-Yu Tang Roche Tissue Diagnostics, Oro Valley, AZ, USA

Catherine Tangen SWOG Statistical Center, Fred Hutchinson Cancer Research Center, Seattle, WA, USA

Mourad Tighiouart Cedars-Sinai Medical Center, Los Angeles, CA, USA

Guangyu Tong Department of Sociology, Duke University, Durham, NC, USA

Xiao Tong Clinical Pharmacology, Biogen, Boston, MA, USA

Alison Urton Canadian Cancer Trials Group, Queen's University, Kingston, ON, Canada

Diane Uschner Department of Statistics, George Mason University, Fairfax, VA, USA

James E. Valentine University of Maryland Carey School of Law, Baltimore, MD, USA

Ben Van Calster Department of Development and Regeneration, KU Leuven, Leuven, Belgium

Department of Biomedical Data Sciences, Leiden University Medical Center, Leiden, The Netherlands

S. Swaroop Vedula Malone Center for Engineering in Healthcare, Whiting School of Engineering, The Johns Hopkins University, Baltimore, MD, USA

Jenifer H. Voeks Department of Neurology, Medical University of South Carolina, Charleston, SC, USA

Sunita Vohra University of Alberta, Edmonton, AB, Canada

Annie X. Wang Covington & Burling LLP, Washington, DC, USA

Hechuan Wang Center for Translational Medicine, University of Maryland School of Pharmacy, Baltimore, MD, USA

J. Wason Population Health Sciences Institute, Newcastle University, Newcastle upon Tyne, UK

MRC Biostatistics Unit, University of Cambridge, Cambridge, UK

Claire Weber Excellence Consulting, LLC, Moraga, CA, USA

Heidi L. Weiss Biostatistics and Bioinformatics Shared Resource Facility, Markey Cancer Center, University of Kentucky, Lexington, KY, USA

Pascale Wermuth Basel, Switzerland

Winifred Werther Center for Observational Research, Amgen Inc, South San Francisco, CA, USA

Matthew Westmore University of Southampton, Southampton, UK

Graham M. Wheeler Imperial Clinical Trials Unit, Imperial College London, London, UK

Cancer Research UK & UCL Cancer Trials Centre, University College London, London, UK

O. Dale Williams Department of Biostatistics, University of North Carolina, Chapel Hill, NC, USA

Department of Medicine, University of Alabama at Birmingham, Birmingham, AL, USA

Janet Wittes Statistics Collaborative, Inc, Washington, DC, USA

Jianrong Wu Biostatistics and Bioinformatics Shared Resource Facility, Markey Cancer Center, University of Kentucky, Lexington, KY, USA

Samuel S. Wu University of Florida, Gainesville, FL, USA

Sharon D. Yeatts Data Coordination Unit, Department of Public Health Sciences, Medical University of South Carolina, Charleston, SC, USA

Lauren Yesko Emmes, Rockville, MD, USA

Gui-Shuang Ying Center for Preventive Ophthalmology and Biostatistics, Department of Ophthalmology, Perelman School of Medicine, University of Pennsylvania, Philadelphia, PA, USA

Jessica L. Yoos University of Pennsylvania, Philadelphia, PA, USA

Qilu Yu Office of Clinical and Regulatory Affairs, National Institutes of Health, National Center for Complementary and Integrative Health, Bethesda, MD, USA

Fan-fan Yu Statistics Collaborative, Inc., Washington, DC, USA

Lilly Q. Yue Center for Devices and Radiological Health, U.S. Food and Drug Administration, Silver Spring, MD, USA

Rachel Zahigian Vertex Pharmaceuticals, Boston, MA, USA

Lijuan Zeng Statistics Collaborative, Inc., Washington, DC, USA

Xiaobo Zhong Ichan School of Medicine at Mount Sinai, New York, NY, USA

Tracy Ziolek University of Pennsylvania, Philadelphia, PA, USA

Part VII

Analysis

Preview of Counting and Analysis Principles 81

Nancy L. Geller

Contents

Introduction	1590
Who Counts? Everyone Randomized	1590
What Happens when Things Are Not Perfect?	1591
Missing Outcome Data	1591
Analyses Other than Intention to Treat	1592
Analysis Principles in Complex Trials	1593
Other Analyses	1594
Summary and Conclusion	1595
Key Facts	1595
Cross-References	1595
References	1596

Abstract

This chapter provides an introduction to the Section on Analysis. The chapters in this section range from elementary design and analysis considerations to many more advanced topics. In this preview, each chapter is briefly mentioned in turn and the reader is invited to delve more deeply into the individual chapter for details.

Keywords

Analysis of clinical trials · Intention to treat · Missing outcome data · Non-compliance · Statistical analysis plan · Analyses other than intent-to-treat

---

N. L. Geller (✉)
National Heart, Lung and Blood Institute, National Institutes of Health, Bethesda, MD, USA
e-mail: gellern@nhlbi.nih.gov

© Springer Nature Switzerland AG 2022
S. Piantadosi, C. L. Meinert (eds.), *Principles and Practice of Clinical Trials*,
https://doi.org/10.1007/978-3-319-52636-2_112

Introduction

This chapter covers a broad range of topics some elementary, and with some advanced. The first section gives a broad overview of the chapter brief reference to the contents of each of the sections

Who Counts? Everyone Randomized

A fundamental tenet of clinical trial methodology is that the analysis of a clinical trial should account for everyone randomized. The basic principle of including all randomized subjects in the primary analysis according to their randomized treatment assignment (and not according to treatment received) is known as the intention-to-treat (ITT) principle. Good discussions on this topic are found in Lachin (2000) and Friedman et al. (2015). A summary of ITT and alternatives is given in ▶ Chap. 82, "Intention to Treat and Alternative Approaches," by Goldberg. There are also three other chapters in this book that briefly discuss ITT: ▶ Chaps. 100, "Causal Inference: Efficacy and Mechanism Evaluation," ▶ 93, "Adherence Adjusted Estimates in Randomized Clinical Trials," and ▶ 84, "Estimands and Sensitivity Analyses."

Because randomization assures balance on average in baseline factors, both known and unknown, an ITT analysis is an unbiased comparison between the treatments among all randomized subjects, presumably defined by the eligibility criteria of the trial. An ITT analysis evaluates a treatment policy. It ignores non-adherence, withdrawal from the trial, and treatment stoppages (even if the protocol allows them). Even dropping randomized subjects who receive no treatment can lead to biased results; for example, in a trial of treatment compared to placebo, those assigned to active treatment who do not take the treatment makes treatment look more like placebo. Further, It is likely that adherers differ from non-adherers in ways that are difficult to assess.

A proper ITT analysis requires outcomes on all randomized subjects and one should do as best as is possible to get these outcomes, no matter whether the subject remains on trial or takes assigned treatment as planned.

In some trials, subjects have been excluded from the trial after they are randomized (whether or not they received their assigned treatments). This may well lead to spurious results. A classic example of excluding randomized subjects from analysis is the Anturane reinfarction trial (The Anturane Reinfarction Trial Research Group 1978, 1980) which was a double-blind placebo-controlled trial of sulfinpyrazone in recent post-myocardial infarction (post-MI patients. The primary endpoint was sudden cardiac death within six months. Only those who received therapy for at least seven days were considered "analyzable." Of the 1620 patients randomized, this eliminated 145 patients, more-or-less equally distributed in the two treatment groups. Results reported were overwhelmingly positive for sulfinpyrazone. Since sulfinpyrazone was an approved drug only for gout, the sponsor went before the FDA to have the drug approved for a new indication, sudden cardiac death in patients who were within 6 months post-MI. The FDA review of the data revealed that the results depended on after-the-fact exclusions of events. Although the exclusions were equally distributed in the two treatment groups, the exclusions eliminated many more events in the sulfinpyrazone group. Including all randomized patients in the analysis completely changed the results and the new indication was not granted (Temple and Pledger 1980).

What Happens when Things Are Not Perfect?

Much can go wrong, making the ITT principle not so easy to implement, even in the two-armed randomized comparison with a well-defined single endpoint. Two simple examples are missing outcome data and non-compliance. Often when there are only a few subjects with missing outcome data, they are censored at their last follow up. This inherently assumes that the reason for the missing is unrelated to treatment assignment, which usually has no basis. Non-compliance can make the outcomes of the treatments look more alike. Of course a pharmaceutical company in interested in the effect of their product in those who take it.

These two issues have led to a great deal of statistical methodology to evaluate clinical trial results accounting for missing outcome data and non-compliance.

Missing Outcome Data

Many trials ignore missing outcome data, often citing that only a small percent of those randomized have been lost to follow up and have missing outcomes. Such an analysis assumes that data are missing completely at random (MCAR), that is, that the trial results would not change if we did have those missing data. That is a strong assumption, as subjects are "lost" for reasons often related to treatment assignment. Examples vary from experiencing toxicity (whether or not related to the trial) to just being "sick and tired" of all of the necessary visits, to development of other conditions that require the subject's attention. One way in which the MCAR assumption is justified is to compare baseline data of those missing outcome data to those with outcome data. Of course, not finding a difference does not guarantee there is no difference.

In a case where a few subjects provide baseline data and no follow up (i.e., subjects drop out after baseline) and, further, there is balance in drop outs between treatment arms, the Guidance for Clinical Trials (1998) suggested justifying the dropping of such patients from the trial analysis. This is acceptable in some cases (c.f. Choi et al. 2020), but usually there is some data beyond baseline even when subjects are lost to follow up. There is a vast literature dealing with the problem of missing outcome data, starting with the classical book by Little and Rubin (2002, second edition). An introduction to methods for missing data is given in ▶ Chap. 86, "Missing Data," by Tong, Li, and Allen.

A common way to deal with missing outcome data is to use the data in the trial to substitute or *impute* values for the missing data. A simple way to do this is to consider the best and worst case scenarios. That is, the best case scenario would give the most favorable values (among trial outcomes) for one treatment group and the least favorable values for the other treatment group. The worst case scenario would do the reverse. If there are few missing outcomes, these two methods could lead to the same trial result, which would be highly satisfying. However, these simple methods can give vastly different estimates of treatment effect, more so with more missing data. They also underestimate the standard errors because the uncertainty in the missing values is not considered. Methods that substitute one value for missing data are called *single imputation* methods.

Rather than replacing missing data with one substituted value, the distribution of observed values may be used by devising models to predict the outcome variable based on the complete data and then using these models to estimate the missing outcome data. Doing this multiple times yields an estimate of each outcome as well as a better estimate of its standard error than single imputation methods. There are several different multiple imputation methods that may be used (Sterne et al. 2009). Others advocate supervised learning as far superior for imputation (Chakrabortty and Cai 2018). Thus, there is no definitive way to deal with missing outcome data. Six different methods are described by Badr (2019). All methods require some statistical assumptions and thus will often be controversial. The best that investigators can do is to set forth the primary method that will be used for the primary analysis, as well as a number of sensitivity analyses to give confidence to the primary results. How to interpret results if some sensitivity analyses lead to a different trial outcome also should be considered. Most important is to plan for how missing data will be dealt with in the statistical analysis plan, because missing data are almost inevitable.

Some still call an analysis which ignores missing data (e.g., patient was lost to follow up and dropped from the primary analysis) an ITT analysis, which is both misleading and a misuse of the term.

Analyses Other than Intention to Treat

Many who undertake clinical trials, notably in the pharmaceutical industry, are interested in other analyses than ITT analyses because the ITT estimates of treatment effect "may not provide an intuitive or clinically meaningful estimate of treatment effects" (Ruberg and Akacha 2017).

A treatment effect of primary interest, which may not be the ITT estimate, is called an *estimand*. A description of estimands, including the need for careful definition and for planning sensitivity analysis is provided in ► Chap. 84, "Estimands and Sensitivity Analyses," by Russek-Cohen and Petullo. Adherence-adjusted analyses are also discussed in ► Chap. 92, "Statistical Analysis of Patient-Reported Outcomes in Clinical Trials," by Mazza and Dueck, and causal estimands are discussed in ► Chap. 100, "Causal Inference: Efficacy and Mechanism Evaluation," by Landau and Emsley.

Ruberg and Akacha suggest that ITT analyses do not adjust for confounding factors post-randomization (such as drug discontinuation or addition of rescue medication). They require an explicit definition of what treatment effect is of primary interest ("relevant and meaningful"), which they call the *estimand*. They define four estimands other than the ITT estimand. One is based on a composite variable which combines a change in a symptom score with discontinuation of study drug due to an adverse event. "Success" is improvement in symptom score and completion of taking the study drug. A second estimand is the treatment effect if all subjects adhered to study medication for the period of the trial. A third is what is the effect on those who can take the study drug(s) without adverse events. The fourth is the treatment effect for each subject before an adverse event or discontinuation.

Ruberg and Akacha claim that the probability of discontinuation of a study drug due to either adverse events or lack of efficacy (or both) may be quantified and treatment comparisons made using usual statistical methods if reasons for discontinuation are carefully defined. They do not consider "physician choice" or "loss to follow up" to be sufficiently detailed. They consider administrative discontinuation (e.g., the patient moves away from the center) to be missing completely at random, so that they don't include such patients. To estimate efficacy and safety for those able to adhere to study treatment, adherence must be first defined and would be trial specific, perhaps taking 70% or 80% of the drug. The authors claim that this combination of probability of discontinuing study drug due to AE, probability of discontinuation for lack of efficacy and efficacy in adherers provides a more complete and meaningful description of drug effect that the ITT estimate.

While the FDA demands an ITT analysis, perhaps allowing other analyses, the European Medicines Agency (EMA), has produced ICH E9 (R1), Addendum on estimands and sensitivity analysis in clinical trials to the guideline on statistical principles for clinical trials (ema.europa.eu/documents/scientific-guideline/ich-e9-r1-addendum-estimands-sensitivity-analysis-clinical-trials-guideline-statistical_en.pdf). EMA allows treatment effect to be specified through an estimand (rather than through the ITT estimate):

> The definition of a treatment effect, specified through an estimand, should consider whether values of the variable after an intercurrent event are relevant, as well as how to account for the (possibly treatment-related) occurrence or non-occurrence of the event itself. More formally, an estimand defines in detail what needs to be estimated to address a specific scientific question of interest.

Analysis Principles in Complex Trials

Several chapters deal with elementary statistical methods to perform hypothesis tests and parameter estimation. (See the ▶ Chaps. 83, "Estimation and Hypothesis Testing," ▶ 87, "Essential Statistical Tests," ▶ 88, "Nonparametric Survival Analysis." So why is there need for so much more statistical methodology?

Over time, clinical trials have become more complex and often attempt to answer more complicated questions than two-armed trials with one primary endpoint. In many cases, incorporating covariates into the primary analysis increases the power to detect differences. An introduction to regression methods for dichotomous or polychotomous data is given in ▶ Chap. 91, "Logistic Regression and Related Methods," by Diniz and Magalhães and for censored data is given in ▶ Chap. 88, "Nonparametric Survival Analysis," by Lokhnygina. Extensions beyond the Cox Proportional Hazards Model are summarized in ▶ Chap. 89, "Survival Analysis II," by Dignam.

Multiple endpoints and/or multiple treatments (multi-armed trials) are also frequently of interest. Combined with these may be multiple subgroup analyses. Such complex trials have several null hypotheses, and so give rise to the *multiplicity problem*: what type of error control is needed for each null hypothesis and for all or several of them simultaneously? ▶ Chapter 85, "Confident Statistical Inference with Multiple Outcomes, Subgroups, and Other Issues of Multiplicity," by Kil, Kazar, Tang, and Hsu address several types of error control for multiplicity problems in the context of personalized medicine and carefully outline how to obtain *Strong* control of Type I error. This means that the probability of *rejecting at least one true null* hypothesis is controlled, even if some null hypotheses are false.

A simplifying approach to multiple outcomes in the two sample case is possible when the outcomes can be prioritized (e.g., death is worse than recurrence without death) so that patients in each treatment arm may be compared to one another. In the two sample case, a Mann-Whitney Wilcoxon test may be performed to decide if two treatments differ. This methodology is described in ▶ Chap. 95, "Generalized Pairwise Comparisons for Prioritized Outcomes," by Buyse and Peron.

Recent work has considered multiplicity problems in the context of longitudinal outcomes when covariates are also considered and linearity of the outcome over time is not assumed (e.g., Jeffries et al. 2018). The joint analysis of survival and longitudinal data is summarized in ▶ Chap. 90, "Prognostic Factor Analyses," by Li.

Patient reported outcomes often include many of these multiplicity problems. These are described in ▶ Chap. 92, "Statistical Analysis of Patient-Reported Outcomes in Clinical Trials," by Mazza and Dueck.

The main analysis principle is that the primary analysis should allow investigators to properly answer the primary question of the trial, no matter how complex, and maintain a prefixed type 1 error, preferably with strong control.

Other Analyses

Potential prognostic factors are among the data collected in clinical trials for use in the primary analysis or for modeling response. In Sect. 7.10, Li presents insight into the process of finding prognostic factors as well as suggesting use of prognostic factors to increase the power of the primary statistical analysis. The stability of statistical models may be assessed by resampling procedures and this is described by Sauerbrei and Boulesteix (▶ Chap. 96, "Use of Resampling Procedures to Investigate Issues of Model Building and Its Stability"). ▶ Chapter 101, "Development and Validation of Risk Prediction Models," describe risk prediction models and how to develop and validate them.

Several other statistical problems require specialized analyses. The nonlinear nature of pharmacokinetic and pharmacodynamic processes require special analyses to relate drug exposure to response and several methods are described in ▶ Chap. 98, "Pharmacokinetic and Pharmacodynamic Modeling," by Kalaria, Wang, and Gobburu. The potential for adverse events after a drug or device receives marketing approval has led to pharmacovigilance, the study of adverse effects of drugs post-marketing. ▶ Chapter 99, "Safety and Risk Benefit Analyses," by Guo describes many methods of benefit-risk analysis.

The main analysis principle here is that the analysis should reflect the specific goals of the question being answered. There are often multiple methods that might be used and the onus is on the investigators, in particular the statistical investigators, to choose the one she or he considers most suitable, or even to derive new methods. Although controversial, ▶ Chap. 94, "Randomization and Permutation Tests," advocate randomization tests for many situations, in particular, for when the assumptions of the usual approaches are unlikely to be met.

Summary and Conclusion

Clinical trials should be well designed to test a carefully posed primary hypothesis and/or estimate a well-defined primary parameter. A statistical analysis plan (SAP) should describe the methodology that will be used to answer the questions posed, both primary and secondary. The plan should account for all randomized patients, even if some are missing outcome data. The SAP should be completed before the data are unblinded. There are many choices for statistical analysis for a given situation and they are mentioned here and further described in the following chapters.

Key Facts

From the simple two-armed randomized trial with a single primary endpoint, clinical trials have become more complex, with investigators working in broad research areas, such as longitudinal data, multiple endpoints, multiple treatment arms, and data with special characteristics, such as safety data and quality of life data. This chapter covers many aspects of basic clinical trial analysis as well as many recent developments.

Cross-References

- ▶ Adherence Adjusted Estimates in Randomized Clinical Trials
- ▶ Causal Inference: Efficacy and Mechanism Evaluation
- ▶ Confident Statistical Inference with Multiple Outcomes, Subgroups, and Other Issues of Multiplicity
- ▶ Development and Validation of Risk Prediction Models
- ▶ Essential Statistical Tests
- ▶ Estimands and Sensitivity Analyses
- ▶ Estimation and Hypothesis Testing

- Generalized Pairwise Comparisons for Prioritized Outcomes
- Intention to Treat and Alternative Approaches
- Joint Analysis of Longitudinal and Time-to-Event Data
- Logistic Regression and Related Methods
- Missing Data
- Pharmacokinetic and Pharmacodynamic Modeling
- Prognostic Factor Analyses
- Randomization and Permutation Tests
- Safety and Risk Benefit Analyses
- Statistical Analysis of Patient-Reported Outcomes in Clinical Trials
- Survival Analysis II
- Use of Resampling Procedures to Investigate Issues of Model Building and its Stability

References

Badr W (2019) 6 different ways to compensate for missing values in a dataset (Data Imputation with examples). https://towardsdatascience.com/6-different-ways-to-compensate-for-missing-values-data-imputation-with-examples-6022d9ca0779

Chakrabortty A, Cai T (2018) Efficient and adaptive linear regression in semi-supervised settings. Ann Stat 46:1541–1572. https://doi.org/10.1214/17-AOS1594

Choi IJ, Kim CG, Lee JY, Young-Il Kim Y-I, Myeong-Cherl Kook MC, Park B, Joo J (2020) Family history of gastric cancer and *Helicobacter pylori* treatment. N Engl J Med 382:427–436. https://doi.org/10.1056/NEJMoa1909666

Friedman LM, Furberg CD, DeMets D, Reboussin DM, Granger CB (2015) Fundamentals of clinical trials, 5th edn. Springer. Chapter 18. ISBN 978-3-319-18539-2

ICH E9 (R1), Addendum on estimands and sensitivity analysis in clinical trials to the guideline on statistical principles for clinical trials. http://ema.europa.eu/documents/scientific-guideline/ich-e9-r1-addendum-estimands-sensitivity-analysis-clinical-trials-guideline-statistical_en.pdf

ICH Harmonized Tripartite Guideline Statistical Principles for Clinical Trials E9 (1998). https://database.ich.org/sites/default/files/E9_Guideline.pdf

Jeffries NO, Troendle JF, Geller NL (2018) Detecting treatment differences in group sequential longitudinal studies with covariate adjustment. Biometrics 74:1072–1081. https://doi.org/10.1111/biom.12837

Lachin JM (2000) Statistical considerations in the intent-to-treat principle. Control Clin Trials 21:167–189

Little RJA, Rubin DB (2002) Statistical analysis with missing data, 2nd edn. Wiley, Hoboken

Ruberg SJ, Akacha M (2017) Considerations for evaluating treatment effects from RCTs. Clin Pharmacol Ther. https://doi.org/10.1002/cpt.869

Sterne JAC, White IR, Carlin JB, Spratt M, Royston P, Kenward MG, Wood AM, Carpenter JR (2009) Multiple imputation for missing data in epidemiological and clinical research: potential and pitfalls. Br Med J 338:b2393. https://doi.org/10.1136/bmj.b2393

Temple R, Pledger G (1980) The FDA's critique of the Anturane Reinfarction trial. N Engl J Med 303:1488–1492

The Anturane Reinfarction Trial Research Group (1978) Sulfinpyrazone in the prevention of cardiac death after myocardial infarction – the Anturane Reinfarction trial. N Engl J Med 298:289–295

The Anturane Reinfarction Trial Research Group (1980) Sulfinpyrazone in the prevention of sudden death after myocardial infarction. N Engl J Med 302:250–256.

Intention to Treat and Alternative Approaches

82

Judith D. Goldberg

Contents

Introduction	1598
Randomized Controlled Clinical Trials (RCTs)	1600
Examples of RCTs	1600
Example: Salk Vaccine Trial – Vaccine Efficacy	1600
Example: The HIP Breast Cancer Screening Study – Screening for Early Detection of Disease	1601
Example: The Polycythemia Vera Study Group PVSG-01 – A Randomized Multicenter Trial (Open Label) for Chronic Disease	1602
Example: Randomized Phase III Trial in Chronic Disease – MPD-RC 112 Phase III Trial of Frontline Pegylated Interferon Alpha-2a (PEG) Versus Hydroxyurea (HU) in High-Risk Polycythemia Vera (PV) and Essential Thrombocythemia (ET): NCT01258856	1604
ITT Principle	1604
Alternatives to ITT Population for Analysis	1606
Missing Data	1607
Alternative Approaches to Analysis	1608
Noninferiority and Equivalence Trials	1609
Cluster Randomized Trials	1610
Example: Cluster Randomized Trials and IIT – Online Wound Electronic Medical Record to Reduce Lower Extremity Amputations in Diabetics – A Cluster Randomized Trial [AHRQ: R01 HS019218-01]	1610
Some Additional Design Considerations for ITT Analyses	1610
Summary and Conclusions	1611
Key Facts	1612
Cross-References	1612
References	1612

J. D. Goldberg (✉)
Department of Population Health and Environmental Medicine, New York University School of Medicine, New York, NY, USA
e-mail: Jd.goldberg@nyulangone.org

© Springer Nature Switzerland AG 2022
S. Piantadosi, C. L. Meinert (eds.), *Principles and Practice of Clinical Trials*,
https://doi.org/10.1007/978-3-319-52636-2_113

Abstract

"Intention to treat" or "intent to treat" (ITT) is the principal approach for the evaluation of the treatment or intervention effect in a randomized clinical trial (RCT). In an RCT, patients or subjects are randomized to one or more study interventions according to a formal protocol that describes the entry criteria, study treatments, follow-up plans, and statistical analysis approaches. In an ideal trial, all randomized patients or subjects have the correct diagnosis, are randomized correctly, comply with the treatment, and are evaluated according to the study plan. These patients would have complete data and follow-up. In this case, the ITT analysis that respects the randomization principle provides unbiased tests of the null hypothesis that there is no treatment or intervention effect. The goal in many cases is to establish the efficacy of a treatment or intervention: does the planned treatment work? In practice, however, because of the many ways in which the ideal is not the reality, an ITT analysis provides a comparative evaluation of the effectiveness of the randomized intervention strategy (does the strategy work), rather than of the efficacy of the planned intervention itself. Examples of blinded, unblinded, screening, and drug clinical trials are provided. Approaches to handling deviations from ideal are described.

Keywords

Intent to treat (intention to treat) · Randomized controlled trial (RCT) · Compliance · Protocol · Efficacy · Effectiveness · Causality · Missing data

Introduction

The randomized clinical trial (RCT) is the gold standard that is used to establish the efficacy or effectiveness of a new treatment or intervention. In an RCT, participants (subjects or patients) are assigned to one or more treatment or intervention groups using a random assignment mechanism, that is, patients or subjects are allocated to the one or more treatment or intervention groups using a prespecified random allocation scheme where allocation, ideally, is double blind; both participants and treating (and evaluating) staff are blinded (masked) to treatment assignment. Further, under these ideal circumstances, only subjects who have met all of the eligibility criteria for entry into the trial would be randomized as close to the initiation of the treatment or intervention as possible. This set of all randomized patients or subjects comprises what is generally defined as the "intent-to-treat" or "intention-to-treat" (ITT) population. The ITT population is included in the analysis in the group to which they were assigned (see, e.g., Ellenberg 1996; Piantadosi 1997; DeMets 2004; Goldberg and Belitskaya-Levy 2008a; Friedman et al. 1998). Adherence to intention to treat in the analysis requires that all randomized patients or subjects be included in the analyses regardless of whether or not they received the assigned treatment, complied with the trial requirements, completed the trial, or even met the entry criteria for the trial. This approach is preferred for the analysis of RCTs since it respects the principle of randomization and provides unbiased tests of the null hypothesis that there is no treatment or intervention effect, although the estimate of the treatment effect may still be biased (Harrington 2000). There are, however, multiple ways in which the actual deviates from the ideal. RCTs come in many flavors, have different objectives, and are conducted with varying levels of quality. Different trial objectives, issues in trial implementation and conduct that include missing data, patient/subject noncompliance, and differing degrees of follow-up lead to deviations from the ideal that have to be recognized and handled in the analysis of such trials.

Under the ITT principle, in a randomized trial, patients remain in the trial under the following circumstances which have implications for analysis and interpretation (Goldberg and Belitskaya-Levy 2008a, b):

- If the patient is found to not have the disease under study. This can occur when final verification of disease status is based on special tests that are completed after randomization or on a central review of patient eligibility.
- If the patient never receives a single dose of the study drug.
- If the patient does not comply with the assigned treatment regimen or does not compete the course of treatment.
- If the patient withdraws from the study for any reason.

This chapter reviews concepts for randomized trials, the issues regarding implementation of the operational definition of ITT in specific trials, and the implications of the operational definition on the statistical analysis as the trial proceeds. These issues range from evaluation of the impact of the deviation from the ITT model to the consideration of other potential paradigms based on differing definitions of the population included in the analysis. These alternatives range from various modifications of ITT (mITT), such as all treated patients, to all treated patients with the correct diagnosis and to all treated patients who complied with assigned treatment, among others. Further, errors in treatment allocation and diagnosis at the time of randomization as well as missing outcomes and errors or misclassification of outcomes and errors of measurement or misclassification of covariates including stratification factors, multicenter deviations and heterogeneity, and missing data of all kinds need to be considered.

Traditional approaches to handle these issues as well as recent alternative approaches to analysis are described. Note that the deviations from the planned randomization and the ITT paradigm move the randomized clinical trial to an observational trial setting that leads to additional considerations in analysis.

Examples that illustrate the evolution of the concept of "intention to treat" and its implications are provided to frame these issues. In addition, the interpretation of ITT in non-inferiority and equivalence RCTs are discussed as are analogues to ITT analyses in non-randomized trials and observational studies.

The discussion in this chapter also includes considerations for the statistical analysis under the ITT paradigm for different types of clinical trials with different types of objectives.

Randomized Controlled Clinical Trials (RCTs)

In the context of medical research and the search to improve treatments or other interventions to improve outcomes for patients or participants, the RCT provides the controlled experimental setting to evaluate the efficacy or effectiveness of the "new" treatment or intervention compared to control (either placebo or another active treatment) in an unbiased, ideally blinded manner. An RCT is conducted under a clinical protocol that explicitly defines the trial objectives; the primary outcome(s); how, when, and on whom the outcome(s) will be measured; and the measures of the effects of the intervention (National Research Council 2010) with a focus on prevention of missing data of all types. The benefits of this controlled experimental approach are that any observed differences between the two (or more) groups with respect to the outcome are attributable to the intervention. Both confounding and selection bias are removed since neither the subject nor the investigator chooses the treatment assignment (see, e.g., Harrington 2000). In what follows, several examples of RCTS are provided. These trials illustrate many of the issues that arise in the analysis and interpretation in the ITT framework and its alternatives.

Examples of RCTs

Example: Salk Vaccine Trial – Vaccine Efficacy

The Salk polio vaccine trial, a classic example of a prevention trial, established the efficacy of the new killed virus vaccine to provide protection against paralysis or death from poliomyelitis (Brownlee 1955; Francis et al. 1955; Meier 1957, 1989). While there were safety issues associated with the use of a killed virus vaccine (Meier 1957, 1989), the National Foundation for Infantile Paralysis (NFIP) advisory committee agreed that the Salk vaccine was safe and could produce desired antibody levels in children who had been tested. Thus, "it remained to prove that the vaccine actually would prevent polio in exposed individuals. It would be unjustified to release such a vaccine for general use without convincing proof of its effectiveness, so it was determined that a large-scale 'field-trial' should be undertaken" (Meier 1989).

Various approaches to the design of such a trial were considered that included the vital statistics approach, an observed control approach, and lastly, an RCT with randomization to a placebo control group. While the ideal design was the RCT, the general reluctance to randomize children to placebo injections led to the choice of an observed control study in which children in grade 2 would receive the vaccine and children in grades 1 and 3 would be observed for the occurrence of polio. The final study, however, also included a double blind RCT in which 750,000 children were randomized to injections with placebo or with the vaccine. The trial was conducted in a relatively short timeframe with endpoints observed within the time period. While the results of the observed control portion of the trial favored the vaccine, the results of the RCT portion were unequivocal and provided compelling evidence of the effectiveness of the vaccine. The primary results of the RCT were based on the ITT analysis of all randomized children who were included in their assigned treatment group regardless of whether or not they received the injections as planned; that is, the primary comparison included those subjects who were randomized to be vaccinated (including those who were not vaccinated) with the polio vaccine or the placebo in each of the randomized groups. In the observed control study, it was known who received and who did not receive the vaccination among the intervention subjects, but not among the control subjects. The control group then inherently could consist of subjects who would have received the vaccine and those who would not have received it, so any fair comparison must consider all subjects in each group.

Example: The HIP Breast Cancer Screening Study – Screening for Early Detection of Disease

A classic example of a randomized trial of screening for the early detection of breast cancer is the HIP Breast Cancer Screening Study. This RCT was designed to evaluate the effectiveness of mammography, at the time an untested tool for early detection, in combination with a clinical examination, to be compared with "usual care." The primary question was whether a screening program that incorporated mammography could reduce mortality from breast cancer. The study was conducted in the Health Insurance Plan of Greater New York, one of the first health maintenance organizations (HMO) in the USA. Sixty-two thousand women were randomly chosen across all of clinical sites in New York City. Of these women, approximately 30,000 were randomized to be invited for an initial screening examination and 3 subsequent annual examinations. The remaining 30,000 women were followed for diagnosis of and mortality from breast cancer. This trial, initiated in 1963, predates the requirements for Institutional Review Board approvals and informed consent requirements that have since become the norm. The trial design and results are described by Shapiro et al. (1974, 1988).

Of the 30,000 women who were randomized to be invited for screening, 20,000 accepted the initial invitation; 59% of these women completed all 4 examinations. In the 5 years of the screening study, 299 cases of breast cancer were diagnosed among the women randomized to the screening group: 225 of these cases were detected among women who had a screening examination; 74 cases were detected among those who refused the invitations. There were 285 cases detected in the control group (Shapiro et al. 1974). Table 1 shows the cumulative numbers of deaths in the first 5 years: those women who refused screening have a higher observed death rate from breast cancer than those women who were screened; death rates for all causes reflect the same phenomenon. The primary results of the trial rest on the comparison of the

Table 1 HIP Breast Cancer Screening Study: cumulative deaths in the first 5 years from entry

Group	Number of women	# BC deaths	BC deaths/ 1000	# All other deaths	All deaths/ 1000
Total randomized to screening	31,000	39	**1.3**	837	27
Screened	20,200	23	1.1	428	21
Refused	10,800	16	1.5	409	38
Total randomized to control	31,000	63	**2.0**	879	28

5-year death rates in the total screened group (1.3/1000) compared with total control group rate (2.0/1000).

The control group consists of a group of women who would have accepted the invitation to be screened and those who would have refused. Within the control group, who falls into each of these groups is unknown, and, therefore, the only fair comparison is of the rates in the total randomized groups, the ITT comparison. Fink et al. (1968) studied the "reluctant" participants who refused screening in the randomized to screening group and identified differences between those who did and not participate that were related to socioeconomic status and education as well as presence of other health issues that took priority for them. While this trial was randomized, it was not blinded in the sense that it is known which women were in each group; the control group received usual care. Outcomes could more readily be evaluated because of the nature of the HMO that did have medical records for all participants. There was central review of biopsy and surgery records. Follow-up was carried out for all women in the trial from these records and from death records.

Screening trials have additional considerations that will not be discussed here. Note, however, that self-selection of participants, handled primarily through the ITT primary analysis, can still be an issue in interpretation. Other issues that impact the analysis and interpretation of the results of these trials include the distinctions between diagnosis at an initial screen, reflecting disease prevalence, and diagnosis at subsequent screens, identifying incident cases; the definition of a positive screen in a multi-modality setting; the lack of true follow-up of negatives on screening (false negatives); lead time bias; length-biased sampling; and misclassification of disease status.

Example: The Polycythemia Vera Study Group PVSG-01 – A Randomized Multicenter Trial (Open Label) for Chronic Disease

In 1967, the National Cancer Institute supported an international multicenter randomized clinical trial to compare treatment with a radiotherapeutic agent, ^{32}P, administered as a monthly injection, a chemotherapeutic agent (chlorambucil, an alkylating agent), and phlebotomy (at the time, standard of care) for patients with polycythemia vera (PV). PV is a relatively rare chronic disease characterized by an elevated hematocrit. This phase III clinical trial (Goldberg 2006; Goldberg and Shao

2008) was designed to evaluate the available treatments to develop definitive recommendations for care. Stroke, hemorrhage, leukemia, and death were the expected negative outcomes. Patients were randomized between 1967 and 1974 from more than 40 institutions in 4 countries. While treatment was randomly assigned, there was no blinding, and the timing and route of delivery differed for each treatment. Diagnostic criteria were ill-defined, and capabilities for diagnosis varied across centers and regions. The trial was planned to evaluate multiple endpoints over a lengthy period of follow-up. Over this follow-up period, treatment changed, compliance (or lack of compliance) was not well captured, and supportive care changed. Frequent interim analyses (every 6 months) were conducted for the semi-annual investigator meetings with reviews of patient accrual, patient eligibility, and outcomes. The concept of ITT had not been developed; patients who were randomized without any follow-up or who were found to be ineligible were excluded from the analyses of "evaluable" patients. Randomized treatment assignments were provided in sealed envelopes to each center; web-based study management was not yet available.

Four hundred seventy eight patients were randomized; 431 patients comprised the randomized, eligible patient population. The results, reviewed regularly, were fraught with issues of timeliness in reporting, multiple analyses of "dirty data," and center and regional variability in all aspects of implementation and follow-up of patients.

The primary study endpoint was time to first occurrence of a major endpoint (major thrombotic event, development of acute leukemia or lymphoma, development of nonhematologic cancer, or death). Follow-up was intensive through 1981, was updated in 1987 with all events reported as of January 1, 1987, and again in 1993 (Berk et al. 1981, 1995). At the time of the 1987 update, 16.3% of the initial 431 randomized, eligible patients were still alive and actively in follow-up, 50.8% had died while on study, 29.0% of the initial population had been removed from the study for a variety of reasons including major protocol violations, and 3.9% were irretrievably lost to follow-up.

Ineligibility rates after central review varied by treatment group (14% on phlebotomy, 9% on chlorambucil, and 6% on ^{32}P) and by region (4% in the US region and 18% in the major non-US region). In particular, the early loss to follow-up rates differed by region with the largest losses in the phlebotomy arm in the same non-US region (23%) with the highest ineligibility rate (Goldberg and Koury 1989).

In summary, this trial illustrates all of the complexities associated with a long enrollment period, ongoing treatment over time, lack of blinding at randomization, difficulties with respect to long-term follow-up during which changes in treatment and supportive care occur, relatively high ineligibility rates, differential follow-up across treatment groups, and nonblinded data monitoring. The major results of the trial included the identification of excess risks of leukemia and nonhematologic malignancies associated with treatment with chlorambucil. To the extent possible, sensitivity analyses to evaluate the effects of these many issues did not change the interpretation of the results. Nevertheless, the lessons learned serve to inform the design and conduct of trials and the use of the ITT paradigm for the analysis of the primary objectives in randomized controlled trials.

Example: Randomized Phase III Trial in Chronic Disease – MPD-RC 112 Phase III Trial of Frontline Pegylated Interferon Alpha-2a (PEG) Versus Hydroxyurea (HU) in High-Risk Polycythemia Vera (PV) and Essential Thrombocythemia (ET): NCT01258856

In this randomized open label (unblinded) phase III trial, the primary objective was to compare complete hematologic response rates determined by blinded central review in patients randomized to treatment by PEG (new treatment) and HU (standard of care, readily available by prescription) by the end of 12 months of therapy with planned analyses in each of the two disease strata (PV and ET). Patients were to be within 1 year of initial diagnosis and to be treatment naïve with less than 3 months of HU therapy. The trial was originally designed to randomize 612 patients with 2 planned interim analyses, the first when 25% of accrual with adequate time on study to be evaluable for response. Randomization began in September 2011 and continued through June 2016 at 24 centers in 6 countries. The study was amended multiple times because of slow enrollment to a final sample size of 170 patients across the 2 disease strata with 1 interim analysis planned to be conducted when 75 patients were evaluable for response. Entry criteria were relaxed so that allowable prior duration of disease was lengthened from less than 1 year in the original protocol to less than 5 years in a situation where the diagnosis of the disease could be made only at the time of an identified complication. Thus, this amendment would enroll more patients with indolent disease who did not have an early complication that would have rendered them ineligible for the study. This trial illustrates many additional difficulties in the conduct of an RCT when one of treatments is the current standard of care available outside of the trial. In fact, the sponsor of the experimental arm stopped drug supply for administrative reasons. While treatment assignments were implemented using a blinded randomization scheme, the actual assigned treatment was known to both the investigators and patients because of the different methods of delivery. In this trial, 7% of the 86 HU patients never received any treatment, while all of the 82 PEG patients received treatment. When the study was closed with the reduced sample size, the final ITT CR rates were 37.2% in the HU group and 35.4% in the PEG group (Mascarenhas et al. 2018).

ITT Principle

The International Conference on Harmonization ICH E9 (1998) guideline for statistical principles in randomized trials defines ITT as "the principle that the effect of a treatment policy can be best assessed by evaluating on the basis of the intention to treat a subject (i.e., the planned treatment regimen) rather than the actual treatment given. It has the consequence that participants allocated to a treatment group should be followed up, assessed, and analyzed as members of that group irrespective of their compliance to the planned course of treatment" (See Little and Kang 2015; ICH E9 1998). ITT is the gold standard for the analysis of randomized trials. Many authors have reviewed the issues that surround the use of ITT over recent years (see, for some discussions, Goldberg and Belitskaya-Levy 2008a, b, c; Ellenberg 1996, 2005; DeMets 2004).

The analysis of a randomized trial based on the ITT principle can be considered a comparison of the planned treatments, or of the treatment strategies as planned. The general assumption is that the ITT analysis in a superiority or difference trial is conservative. All patients who do not satisfy the conditions of the study at randomization or during the trial are effectively treatment "failures" when they are included as randomized. When subjects or patients are distributed equally among the different treatment groups, then any differences between the groups are, in general, reduced, and the effective sample size is reduced. If the results of the trial still favor superiority, while the estimate of the treatment effect (or effectiveness) may be attenuated, the conclusion would remain unchanged. On the other hand, if there are differential effects associated with treatment group, the ITT analysis can inflate the estimated effectiveness (Goldberg 1975).

The ITT paradigm yields an estimate of the difference or the relative difference in the effectiveness of the planned treatment strategies in the simple two-arm randomized trial rather than of the actual efficacy in patients who met the entry criteria, complied with the treatment, and had complete outcome data. For example, if 90% of those randomized to a new treatment refused to comply with the treatment, even if the success rate in the remaining 10% of patients was 100%, the estimated effectiveness for the ITT analysis would be 10% which may be lower than under the rate for the standard treatment strategy with a higher compliance rate.

Historically, trials were often planned with an increased sample size to allow some flexibility for missing data of various kinds. However, even with an inflation in planned sample size, the issues of the impact of missing data of all types still remain to be addressed. The National Research Council report on "The Prevention and Treatment of Missing Data in Clinical Trials" (2010) outlines the key issues and provides some recommendations to deal with these issues. Recent reviews of publications of randomized controlled clinical trial results in various therapeutic areas suggest that the ITT principle is used less often than would be expected and that attention to the implications of missing data in the analyses is limited. For example, Royes et al. (2015) reported that of 91 trials published in 5 major musculoskeletal journals over 2 years, only 38% used a complete ITT analysis for the primary outcome. Bell et al. (2014) in a recent review of handling of missing data in 77 RCTs in top medical journals published within a 6-month period following the NRC report indicated that 95% of these trials reported some missing outcome data with a median of 9% and maximum of 70%. Further, complete case analysis was the most common approach to handing missing data in the primary analysis (45%) followed by simple imputation and then model-based methods and multiple imputation. Most of the trials used an ITT or modified ITT analysis with only 35% of trials reporting sensitivity analysis.

The NRC report recommends a primary analysis under the assumption that data are missing at random, followed by sensitivity analyses that weaken assumptions to include data not missing at random.

Alternatives to ITT Population for Analysis

The alternatives frequently used in place of the ITT principle to define the study population for comparison in an RCT include modifications to the ITT (mITT), per protocol (PP), as treated (AT), and variations among these and other options to define the groups that are being compared in a trial. Each of these alternatives requires careful definition within a trial protocol to ensure that there is clarity with respect to the details.

mITT is often only vaguely defined and requires specificity to even evaluate how it would operationally impact the analysis of an RCT. For example, patients randomized as eligible, but subsequently found to be ineligible, could be excluded. Or, the modification could be just to include all patients randomized to a trial who actually received at least one dose of study treatment as randomized. The closest to the ITT paradigm would be to include these patients as randomized. In randomized trials of infectious diseases, a modified ITT approach is often used. In this case, outcomes in the two treatment groups are compared for patients who actually have diseases caused by organisms sensitive to the treatments. But, in practice, treatment is given presumptively since the results of sensitivity testing are often not available at the initiation of treatment. In this case, the ITT approach provides an approximation to the treatment strategy that would be implemented in practice.

Per protocol (PP) populations are defined to include patients who met the protocol criteria for entry, complied with the treatment regimen based on the trial definition of compliance and completed follow-up for the outcome. PP approach includes analysis of patients evaluable for response in oncology trials, for example, in which only those patients who received sufficient treatment to be evaluated at the primary response outcome assessment are included in the analysis, eliminating those patients who might have deteriorated on treatment and went on to other treatments or died prior to the evaluation time. Clearly, this can provide misleading results depending on the distributions of these patients in the treatment groups being compared.

As treated (AT) populations would include patients with assignment to the treatment actually received rather than assignment to treatment as randomized. An as-treated (AT) analysis assigns subjects or patients to the treatment-taken group regardless of the randomized assignment. As Ellenberg (1996) points out, these AT analyses assign subjects to groups based on their compliance in the randomized trial. And the definition of compliance to the assigned treatment can be subjective. In an AT analysis, for example, a subject assigned to the new treatment may actually take the standard treatment. In a blinded RCT, subjects can take only the standard if available outside the trial, a common issue in trials that use available treatments as the standard. In the absence of blinding, when one or both treatments are available outside the trial setting (such as MPD-RC 112 with both hydroxyurea and PEG interferon available outside the trial), the problem is exacerbated. In fact, patients and/or their physicians will comply with the assigned treatment only if it is not available to them in other ways. In these settings, compliance rates on the randomized regimen often differ for the two (or more) treatment arms. The ITT analysis in this setting provides an unrealistic assessment of the treatment effects, but any other analyses are biased by the selection process associated with compliance.

Note that safety analyses, however, are conducted appropriately on an AT basis with subjects assigned to the regimen actually taken, as distinct from the ITT approach for effectiveness.

While there are multiple variants of these broad approaches to identifying the populations for analysis in an RCT, each of which has limitations, if these multiple analyses do not differ in any substantive way, the risk of incorrectly attributing efficacy (or lack of efficacy) to a new treatment are reduced.

In the setting of a noninferiority or equivalence trial, the use of the ITT population for analysis reduces any differences between the two groups favoring the conclusion of noninferiority or equivalence (see, e.g., Kim and Goldberg 2001; Sanchez and Chen 2006).

Missing Data

The consensus among clinical trialists is that the gold standard remains the ITT analysis for the randomized trial. The primary source of deviation from the ITT paradigm arises from missing data of some type. That said, the NRC report (2010) and many other authors focus on the need to develop a careful protocol that considers primary outcomes and includes plans to minimize missing data of all kinds. Missing data can occur at every stage of a trial with differing implications for analysis.

That missing data are unrelated to treatment or outcome and are missing completely at random (MCAR) is generally not the case in RCTs. Rather, missingness can be related to treatment but not outcome, missing at random (MAR), a possible scenario. Such an assumption can lead to overly optimistic estimates of treatment effects (see ▶ Chap. 84, "Estimands and Sensitivity Analyses") but can be useful. Lastly, missingness can be related to both treatment and outcome, that is, not missing at random (NMAR), a scenario as noted in ▶ Chap. 84, "Estimands and Sensitivity Analyses," that is a more likely occurrence than one would like. The ▶ chapter 86, "Missing Data" provides details of approaches to incorporate missing data into the analysis of an RCT.

Patients can be randomized to the incorrect treatment, in incorrect strata, or with incorrect diagnoses at the outset. In some trials, randomization and treatment occur based on a presumptive diagnosis while additional testing and review of the entry criteria continue. At the study design stage, the goal is to randomize as close to the initiation of treatment as possible with as much confirmed information as possible. The handling of these types of errors impacts the analysis. In the ITT paradigm, subjects or patients remain in the trial as randomized. Similarly, if the subject or patient never receives the randomized treatment, the subject remains in the analysis as randomized. If the patient does not comply with the assigned treatment, the patient remains as randomized. And, if the patient withdraws from the study for any reason at any point, the patient remains in the trial as randomized.

The emphasis in the NRC report (2010) is on minimizing missing data of any kind. Some baseline data can be missing in any trial. Trials with a single treatment or intervention encounter and an immediate assessment of the outcome have the smallest potential for missing data. As the duration of the intervention increases, the potential for missing data increases and includes subject withdrawal for many potential reasons that may be related to the intervention (e.g., side effects). As the length of the follow-up period after the completion of treatment increases, the potential for loss to follow-up as well as for the use of alternative treatments increases. Short-term treatment and follow-up minimize missing data; long-term treatment with end of treatment follow-up or long-term post treatment follow-up. Post-randomization missing data can become a major problem of analysis and interpretation (NRC 2010; Little and Kang 2015) after long-term post treatment follow-up provide more opportunities for increased missing data.

In short-term trials with, for example, a one-time intervention (e.g., vaccine, screening test) and a short-term single outcome assessment, missing outcome data should not pose a major problem. Most clinical trials, however, involve multiple dosing or treatments over time with follow-up at planned intervals during the active intervention phase and then long-term follow-up after the intervention is complete. Because the likelihood that complete data are obtained as planned is reduced, there is recent interest in extending the concept of the ITT approach through a focus on how to evaluate the multiple objectives, including the primary objective, of the trial and choice of the appropriate outcomes (measurements) to be used for these evaluations.

▶ Chapter 84, "Estimands and Sensitivity Analyses," provides an overview and summarizes the strategies for the choice of "estimands" for different scenarios beyond the ITT analysis. In this context, the ITT estimand estimates the effect of the randomization to treatment on outcome. Among strategies to address intercurrent events (post randomization) including compliance/noncompliance (Little et al. 2009) are treatment policy estimands similar to the ITT approach, composite endpoints that include intercurrent events on treatment, hypothetical estimands, principal stratification causal estimates (Fragakis and Rubin 2002; Little and Rubin 2000), and on-treatment estimates. Compliance can be incorporated into analyses in various ways including as a covariate. However, the definition of compliance has to be clear and consistent and defined in the protocol. These concepts are elucidated from a regulatory standpoint in ICH E9 R1 (2017) and elsewhere.

Alternative Approaches to Analysis

The primary ITT analysis in an RCT provides as we note above an estimate of the treatment strategy defined by a protocol that includes all randomized patients as randomized. The reality in a trial is often quite different. In addition, different kinds of trials have different requirements. The AT and PP populations can be analyzed, but each has different interpretations with respect to trial results. Composite endpoints can provide a single summary in an ongoing trial that includes events on treatment. For example, such an endpoint in a survival-type trial could be based on progression-free survival, the time to disease progression or death, whichever occurs first. The analysis of long-term outcomes can also be confounded with use of rescue medications, side effects, and response or lack of efficacy itself if there any of these events contribute to missing data, particularly with differential rates in the groups being compared. Of course, it is still possible to have incomplete information with respect to the earlier endpoint so that there is bias introduced when the first event is death that may or may not have been preceded by disease progression. Analyses of multiple endpoints and competing risk analyses can shed some light on these potential biases.

In longitudinal trials with repeated measurements of outcomes such as blood pressure over time, mixed effects regression models and general estimating equation models can be used. However, again, the assumptions of such methods (e.g., missing at random) can easily be violated by differences in the distributions and types of intercurrent events between the treatment groups (Little and Kang (2015). Hogan et al. (2004) summarize approaches to handling dropouts in the longitudinal setting.

Various approaches to analysis of the different populations (AT, PP, compliers) have been traditionally employed with known limitations. For example, single imputation in an analysis based on PP patients can be viewed as a variant of what is known as a "completers" or "complete case" analysis. The other extreme of this approach is to use the first observation carried forward, best observation carried forward, or "last observation carried forward" (LOCF) to replace missing outcome data. In an LOCF analysis, the last available observation is used for each subject in the analysis; this observation could even be the baseline pre-treatment observation. These kinds of analyses are flawed and yield results that are biased in different ways. While these methods have mostly been replaced by mixed effects regression models and various other approaches, the differences in the results from all of these methods can provide useful sensitivity analyses (see Thabane et al. 2013).

Other approaches that have been proposed for the analysis of RCTs that address many of these issues are beyond the scope of this chapter. Bayesian methods can be used to incorporate additional treatment information such as rescue medication for treatment failure using data augmentation algorithms (Shaffer and Chinchilli 2004). Selection models allow formal incorporation of potential outcomes and pattern mixture models to model associations between observed exposures and outcomes (Goetghebuer and Loeys 2002). Causal effect models can be used for realistic treatment assignment rules when the expected treatment assignment (ETA) is violated (Van der Laan and Petersen 2007).

Noninferiority and Equivalence Trials

In the case of noninferiority or equivalence trials, an ITT analysis can bias the results in favor of noninferiority or equivalence. This occurs because the effective sample size is reduced by the inclusion of ineligible and noncompliant patients and the difference between the groups is decreased favoring "no difference." Hybrid ITT/PP analyses that exclude noncompliant patients and incorporate the impact of missing data in this setting have been proposed by Sanchez and Chen (2006).

Cluster Randomized Trials

Example: Cluster Randomized Trials and IIT – Online Wound Electronic Medical Record to Reduce Lower Extremity Amputations in Diabetics – A Cluster Randomized Trial [AHRQ: R01 HS019218-01]

The Online Wound Electronic Medical Record (OWEMR) was an informatics tool that synthesizes diabetic foot ulcer (DFU) data to inform treatment decisions. The primary objective of this two-arm cluster RCT was to assess the impact by 6 months of the OWEMR and standard of care (OWEMR+SOC) compared to SOC alone on lower limb amputation or death. In a cluster randomized trial, intervention or treatment assignment is randomized to a group of individuals defined, for example, by a classroom, a school, or a center in a multicenter trial. In such a trial, the cluster or group is randomized, and all members of the group or unit receive the same treatment assignment. Thus, the unit of randomization is the cluster. Sample size is based on the number of clusters and, only in part, on the number of observations within a cluster. Analyses are based on the cluster summary and can also be based on the individual observations nested within cluster. In a cluster randomized trial, the ITT analysis can be thought of as the analysis of all randomized clusters. However, there can be instances in which within a cluster, individuals do not uniformly adhere to the assigned treatment. Within a cluster, individual outcomes are often correlated.

This RCT was originally designed to include 3504 patients in 12 centers (clusters; 292 patients/cluster) each of which would be randomized to the tool+SOC or SOC alone. Enrollment began in August 2011 and was expected to complete in September 2013. Six of the original 12 study sites were closed for poor accrual. Additional sites were identified; 16 study sites (ranging in size from 0 to 295 patients) were included in this study. Of the 1608 subjects who signed informed consent in these sites, 47 were screen failures and 1561 were enrolled in the trial. OWEMR+SOC centers enrolled 1 to 295 subjects (total, 977; outcome rate, 14.7%), and SOC alone centers enrolled 0 to 169 subjects (total, 584; primary outcome rate, 11.8%). When early terminations were included as failures, the composite failure rates were, respectively, 36.9% and 42.1%. For the primary endpoint, the results favored SOC, but the dropout and early termination rates were, in fact, higher in the SOC arm. This illustrates the difficulty in attracting centers (and patients) to remain on a trial when they are not randomized to the new intervention.

Some Additional Design Considerations for ITT Analyses

Careful consideration to all of the design details in the RCT protocol can facilitate analysis and interpretation of the results. Some possible design modifications could retain the features of the planned ITT analyses.

Often in RCTs, substudies using new and potentially expensive technologies are incorporated into the trial. Frequently, these substudies are carried out in convenience samples or "wherever data are available." While a relatively large sample size is often required for the primary and secondary endpoints, the inability to measure all variables on all subjects/patients introduces missing data that may or may not be missing at random. Nested random subsamples of the overall study population can be used to measure these more expensive classes of variable with smaller subsamples as the cost of collection increases. These SMAR-type designs (Belitskaya-Levy et al. 2008; Goldberg 2006) enable integrated analyses in a setting of planned monotone missingness with data missing at random.

In RCTs with response-dependent changes in treatment, patients can be randomized to complete regimens at the initial randomization with a treatment strategy randomization that incorporates treatment arms that randomize patients to continue treatment or to receive additional treatment if required. For example, in combination therapy trials for hypertension, patients could be randomized to the new treatment, standard treatment, or placebo at the initial stage. Subsequent randomizations would allow various combinations within each of the original treatment groups. Such a design would allow an unbiased comparison within each original randomization group of patients with and without additional therapy after the first stage.

Sequential Multiple Assignment Randomized Trials (SMARTs) allow the comparison of dynamic treatment strategies (DTS) or sets of decision rules for patient management (see Almirall et al. 2014). In the SMART framework, patients are randomized to different treatment branches that separate DTSs. In the classic ITT framework, randomization occurs at the start of the trial with subsequent treatment changes after the initial randomization that are not governed by randomization. The DTS ITT converts to SMART by using randomization when treatment decisions would change. Patient information would contribute to one or more DTSs until the patient leaves the DTS. These designs are gaining traction particularly in areas such as behavioral intervention trials for smoking cessation.

Summary and Conclusions

Intention to treat (ITT) is the preferred approach for the statistical analysis of randomized clinical trials. A careful, unambiguous protocol should be developed prior to the trial initiation, and a plan for statistical analysis should be in place prior to the conclusion of the trial and its unblinding. Investigators must provide a careful accounting of all patients randomized, all patients treated, and all post-randomization exclusions (if any) for lack of efficacy, lack of compliance, or lack of safety (see, e.g., DeMets 2004; Begg 2000; Lachin 2000). The ITT principle provides a paradigm for the conduct of RCTs that focuses on reducing any biases in patient/subject assignment or evaluation of outcomes. That said, the realities of clinical trial conduct often make it necessary to carefully consider deviations from the ideal model in the analysis. The NRC report (2010) and the IHC E9 guidance (2017) review the alternatives for analysis based on the goals of the specific trial and advantages and limitations of these alternatives. Regardless of the primary method of analysis, sensitivity analyses should be conducted to evaluate the effects of missing and/or erroneous data at all stages of the trial process from randomization errors to missing outcome data as well as the impact of lack of compliance.

Key Facts

- **Randomized clinical trial (RCT)**. An **RCT** is the gold standard experimental paradigm to test a null hypothesis that a treatment or intervention effect is 0 versus the alternative that this effect is not equal to 0 in the 2 group trial.
- **Blinding**. An RCT ideally should be blinded for treatment assignment and outcome assessments and to patients or subjects. In practice, variations of this occur.
- **Intention to treat (ITT)**. ITT is the principle for the statistical evaluation of an RCT that includes all subjects or patients in the analysis with assignment to their randomized treatment or intervention group regardless of whether or not they received the planned regimen.
- **Efficacy**. An RCT that includes all subjects randomized and all data from these subjects should ideally compare the actual treatment effect if delivered as planned.
- **Effectiveness**. An ITT analysis of an RCT evaluates the effectiveness of the planned treatment as assigned regardless of the deviations from the plan as the trial progresses.
- **Missing data in RCTs**. Data can be missing in any RCT for multiple reasons. The extent and nature of missing data in an RCT can impact results and interpretation under the ITT paradigm and alternative analyses.

Cross-References

- ▶ Adherence Adjusted Estimates in Randomized Clinical Trials
- ▶ Causal Inference: Efficacy and Mechanism Evaluation
- ▶ Estimands and Sensitivity Analyses
- ▶ Missing Data
- ▶ Prevention Trials: Challenges in Design, Analysis, and Interpretation of Prevention Trials
- ▶ Screening Trials
- ▶ Sequential, Multiple Assignment, Randomized Trials (SMART)

References

Almirall D, Nahum-Shani I, Sherwood NE, Murphy SA (2014) Introduction to SMART designs for the development of adaptive interventions: with application to weight loss research. Transl Behav Med 4:26–274. PMCID: PMC4167891

Begg CB (2000) Commentary: ruminations on the intent-to-treat principle. Control Clin Trials 21:241–243

Belitskaya-Levy I, Shao Y, Goldberg JD (2008) Systematic missing-at-random (SMAR) design and analysis for translational research studies. Int J Biostat 4(1):Article 15. https://doi.org/10.2202/1557-4679.1046. PubMed PMID: 20231908; PubMed Central PMCID: PMC2835456

Bell ML, Fiero M, Horton NJ, Hsu C-H (2014) Handling missing data in RCTs; a review of the top medical journals. BMC Med Res Methodol 14:118

Berk PD, Goldberg JD, Silverstein MN et al (1981) Increased incidence of acute leukemia in polycythemia vera associated with chlorambucil therapy. NEJM 304:441–447

Berk PD, Wasserman LR, Fruchtman SM, Goldberg JD (1995) Treatment of polycythemia vera; a summary of clinical trials conducted by the polycythemia vera study group. In: Wasserman LR, Berk PD (eds) Polycythemia vera and the myeloproliferative disorders. Chapter 15. N. Saunders, Berlin, pp 166–194

Brownlee KA (1955) Statistics of the 1954 polio vaccine trials. J Am Stat Assoc 50(272): 1005–1013

DeMets DL (2004) Statistical issues in interpreting clinical trials. J Intern Med 255:529–537

Ellenberg J (1996) Intent-to-treat analysis vs as-treated analysis. Drug Inf J 30:535–544

Ellenberg J (2005) Intention to treat analysis: basic. Encyclopedia of biostatistics. John Wiley and Sons, Ltd

Fink R, Shapiro S, Lewison J (1968) The reluctant participant in a breast cancer screening program. Public Health Rep 83(6):479–490

Fragakis CE, Rubin DB (2002) Principal stratification in causal inference. Biometrics 58:21–29

Francis T Jr et al (1955) An evaluation of the 1954 poliomyelitis vaccine trials – summary report. Am J Public Health 45(5):1–63

Friedman LM, Furberg CD, DeMets DL (1998) Fundamentals of clinical trials, 3rd edn. Springer, New Year

Goetghebuer E, Loeys T (2002) Beyond intention to treat. Epidemiol Rev 24:85–90

Goldberg JD (1975) The effects of misclassification on the bias in the difference between two proportions and the relative odds in the fourfold table. J Am Stat Assoc 70:561–567

Goldberg JD (2006) The changing role of statistics in medical research: experiences from the past and directions for the future. Invited paper, Proc Amer Stat Assoc. 1963–1969

Goldberg JD, Belitskaya-Levy I (2008a) In: Melnick E, Everitt BS (eds) Intent-to-treat principle. Encyclopedia of quantitative risk assessment. Wiley, Chichester

Goldberg JD, Belitskaya-Levy I (2008b) In: Melnick E, Everitt BS (eds) Randomized controlled trials. Encyclopedia of quantitative risk assessment. Wiley, Chichester

Goldberg JD, Belitskaya-Levy I (2008c) In: Melnick E, Everitt BS (eds) Efficacy. Encyclopedia of quantitative risk assessment. Wiley, Chichester

Goldberg JD, Koury KJ (1989) In: Berry DA (ed) Design and analysis of multicenter trials. Chapter 7 in statistical methodology in the pharmaceutical sciences. Marcel Dekker, New York, pp 201–237

Goldberg JD, Shao YS (2008) In: Melnick E, Everitt BS (eds) Comparative efficacy trials (phase III studies). Encyclopedia of quantitative risk assessment. Wiley, Chichester

Harrington DB (2000) The randomized clinical trial. J Am Stat Assoc 95:312–315

Hogan JW, Roy J, Korkontzelou C (2004) Tutorial in biostatistics: handling drop-out in longitudinal studies. Stat Med 23:1455–1497

ICH (1998) E9: guideline on statistical principles for clinical trials. www.ich.org

ICH (2017) E9 R1: Addendum on estimands and sensitivity analyses in clinical trials. Step 2. www.ich.org

Kim MY, Goldberg JD (2001) The effects of outcome misclassification and measurement error on the design and analysis of therapeutic equivalence trials. Stat Med 20(14):2065–2078. PubMed PMID: 1143942

Lachin JM (2000) Statistical considerations in the intent-to-treat principle. Control Clin Trials 21:167–189

Little R, Kang S (2015) Intention-to-treat analysis with treatment discontinuation and missing data in clinical trials. Stat Med 34:2381–2390

Little RJA, Rubin DB (2000) Casual effects in clinical and epidemiological studies via potential outcomes: concepts and analytical approaches. Annu Rev Public Health 21:121–145

Little RJA, Long Q, Lin X (2009) A comparison of methods for estimating the causal effects of a treatment in randomized clinical trials subject to noncompliance. Biometrics 65:640–649

Mascarenhas J et al (2018) Results of the myeloproliferative neoplasms – research consortium (MPN-RC) 112 randomized trial of pegylated interferon alfa-2a (PEG) versus hydroxyurea

(HU) therapy for the treatment of high risk polycythemia vera (PV) and high risk essential thrombocythemia (ET). Blood 132:577. https://doi.org/10.1182/blood-2018-99-111946

Meier P (1957) Safety testing of poliomyelitis vaccine. Science 125:1067–1071. https://doi.org/10.1126/science.125.3257

Meier P (1989) The biggest public health experiment ever: the 1954 field trial of the Salk poliomyelitis vaccine. In: Tanur JM, Mosteller F, Kruskal WH, Lehmann EL, Link RF, Pieters RS, Rising GR (eds) Statistics: a guide to the unknown, 3rd edn. Duxbury

National Research Council (2010) The prevention and treatment of missing data in clinical trials. The National Academies Press, Washington, DC

Piantadosi S (1997) Clinical trials: a methodologic perspective. Wiley-Interscience, New York

Royes J, Sims J, Ogollah R, Lewis M (2015) A systematic review finds variable use of the intention-to-treat principle in musculoskeletal randomized controlled trials with missing data. J Clin Epidemiol 68:15–24

Sanchez MM, Chen X (2006) Choosing the analysis population in non-inferiority studies. Stat Med 25:1169–1181

Shaffer M, Chinchilli V (2004) Bayesian inferences for randomized clinical trials with treatment failures. Stat Med 23:1215–1228

Shapiro S, Goldberg JD, Hutchison GB (1974) Lead time in breast cancer detection and implications for periodicity of screening. Am J Epidemiol 100(5):357–366. PubMed PMID: 4417355

Shapiro S, Venet W, Strax P, Venet L (1988) Periodic screening for breast cancer: the health insurance plan project and its sequelae, 1963–1986. Johns Hopkins, Baltimore

Stuart EA, Perry DF, Le H-N, Ialongo NS (2008) Estimating intervention effects of prevention programs: accounting for noncompliance. Prev Sci 9:288–298

Thabane L, Mbuagbaw L, Zhang S, Samaan Z, Marcucci M, Ye C, Thabane M, Giangregorio L, Dennis B, Kosa D, Debana VB, Dillenburg R, Fruci V, Bawor M, Lee J, Wells G, Goldsmith CH (2013) A tutorial on sensitivity analyses in clinical trials: the what, why, when and how. BMC Med Res Methodol 13:92. http://www.biomedcentral.com/1471-2288/13/92. Accessed 28 Apr 2018

US FDA (2016) Non-inferiority clinical trials to establish effectiveness: guidance for industry. https://www.fda.gov/downloads/Drugs/Guidances/UCM202140

Van der Laan MJ, Petersen ML (2007) Causal effect models for realistic individualized treatment and intention to treat rules. Int J Biostat 3(1):Article 3. http://www.bepress.com/ijb/vol3/iss1/3

Estimation and Hypothesis Testing

83

Pamela A. Shaw and Michael A. Proschan

Contents

Introduction	1616
Estimation and Uncertainty for Continuous Endpoints	1617
Estimation and Uncertainty for Noncontinuous Outcomes	1618
Estimation of the Difference Between Groups	1619
Hypothesis Testing	1620
Special Topics in Hypothesis Testing	1623
Exact Tests and Other Considerations for Choosing a Hypothesis Test	1623
Multiple Comparisons	1625
Noninferiority Versus Superiority	1626
Controversies in Hypothesis Testing	1627
Two-Sided Versus One-Sided Controversy	1627
The P-Value Controversy	1628
Summary and Conclusion	1629
Key Facts	1629
Cross-References	1630
References	1630

Abstract

This chapter presents basic elements of parameter estimation and hypothesis testing. The reader will learn how to form confidence intervals for the mean, and more generally, how to calculate confidence intervals for the one parameter setting and for the difference between two groups. Principles of hypothesis testing are detailed, including the choice of the null and alternative hypotheses, the significance level, and implications for choosing a one-sided versus two-sided

---

P. A. Shaw (✉)
University of Pennsylvania Perelman School of Medicine, Philadelphia, PA, USA
e-mail: shawp@upenn.edu

M. A. Proschan
National Institute of Allergy and Infectious Diseases, Bethesda, MD, USA
e-mail: proscham@niaid.nih.gov

© Springer Nature Switzerland AG 2022
S. Piantadosi, C. L. Meinert (eds.), *Principles and Practice of Clinical Trials*,
https://doi.org/10.1007/978-3-319-52636-2_114

test. The p-value is defined and a discussion of controversies that have arisen over its use are included. After reading this chapter, the reader will have a better understanding of the necessary steps to set up a hypothesis test and make valid inference about the quantity of interest. Other topics in this chapter include exact hypothesis tests, which may be preferable for small sample settings, and the choice of a parametric versus nonparametric test. The chapter also includes a brief discussion of the implications of multiple comparisons on hypothesis testing and considerations of hypothesis testing in the setting of noninferiority trials.

Keywords

Confidence interval · Hypothesis testing · Noninferiority trial · Parameter · p-value · Power · Significance · Standard error · Test statistic · Type I error · Type II error

Introduction

Suppose a trial of two interventions aimed at helping individuals lose weight is conducted. Individuals on Intervention A lose more weight on average than those on intervention B. Can one conclude that Intervention A is better? What information is needed to be fairly certain that if an independent clinical trial of these interventions were conducted, its data would lead to the same conclusion? Suppose the data in the original trial showed that individuals on arm A lost 6 pounds and individuals on arm B lost 2 pounds, on average. Could one now conclude Arm A was definitively better? The answer is, it depends. It depends on whether 4 lb. is an important clinical difference in weight change. It also depends on whether the found 4 lb. difference between groups is larger than the natural variability in average weight loss on each arm.

This chapter considers two principal goals of statistical analysis: (1) estimating a parameter that summarizes the outcome of interest, e.g., effect of treatment on weight change and (2) testing whether the value of the parameter of interest is different in different groups, for example, is the effect of treatment on weight change different for treatment A versus B. Both of these activities rely on quantifying the amount of uncertainty in the estimate of the parameter of interest. This allows calculation of the likelihood of a difference between two groups at least as large as what was observed if treatment truly has no effect. We describe a number of common summary statistics (mean, proportion, etc.) and their measures of uncertainty, i.e., the statistic's variance. We define and present methods to calculate confidence intervals that summarize the range of plausible parameter values. Finally, we describe a formal framework for hypothesis testing that helps determine whether signals observed in data can be distinguished from chance. Statistical inference is the process of making statements from data about a parameter of interest. Confidence intervals and hypothesis tests are the primary tools of statistical inference.

Estimation and Uncertainty for Continuous Endpoints

The principal goal in a randomized clinical trial is to summarize the effect of an intervention using data gathered from trial participants. The primary outcome chosen to summarize the drug's effect focuses on safety in early phase trials and efficacy in later phase trials. To reliably quantify the degree of certainty about statements of safety or efficacy of an intervention, one must specify in advance in the protocol and statistical analysis plan the specific parameter of interest, and methods to estimate its value. The parameter can be thought of as the true underlying value for a population under study, such as the true average change in weight after 3 months of intervention A. In this section, we focus on what is probably the most common parameter estimate used in clinical trials for a continuous outcome, the mean, to illustrate the general approach to summarizing an intervention effect.

Return to the example of the weight loss trial. The primary outcome is weight change from baseline to end of trial. The distribution of weight change may look like the bell curve of a normal distribution, or it may be skewed. The Central Limit Theorem says that as the sample size increases, the distribution of the arithmetic mean tends towards the normal distribution. This holds regardless of how weight change is distributed, provided only that its variance is finite. This means we can use attributes of the normal distribution to make statements about the mean. In particular, with 95% probability, a normally distributed statistic will take on a value that is within approximately two standard deviations of its mean. A normal distribution is completely characterized by its mean and standard deviation. This underlying principle is used to construct what is known as the confidence interval for the unknown parameter of interest, say μ_A, the underlying mean weight change for intervention A. Specifically, if the trial were repeated thousands of times, approximately 95% of such intervals would contain the true parameter value μ_A. The 95% confidence interval can be approximated by $\bar{x} \pm 1.960 \times SE$, where SE is the estimated standard error and 1.960 (−1.960) is the upper (lower) 2.5% quantile of a standard normal distribution. As shown in Fig. 1, for the standard normal distribution (mean 0, standard deviation 1), 2.5% of the values are above the value 1.960. Thus, $z_{.025} = 1.960$ for this distribution and, by symmetry, 95% of the values are between

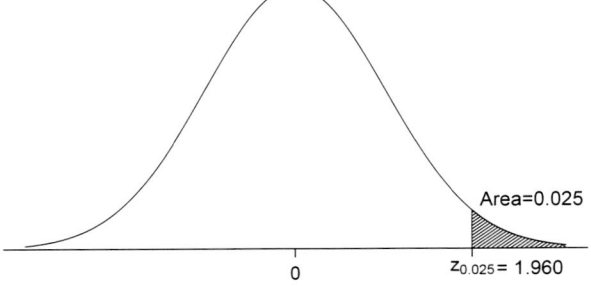

Fig. 1 The standard normal distribution, which has mean 0 and standard deviation 1, is shown along with its upper 2.5% quantile, denoted by $z_{0.025}$ where $z_{0.025} = 1.960$. The probability that values from this distribution exceed 1.960 is 2.5%

−1.960 and 1.960. For a sample mean of n independent observations with the same underlying variance, the SE is estimated by $s/\sqrt{n}$, where s is the sample standard deviation. Suppose in the weight loss trial there are 100 individuals on intervention A, the sample mean is 6 and $s = 20$. Then the SE for the sample mean is SE = 2.0, and the 95% confidence interval for μ_A is approximately (2.08, 9.92). One can construct a confidence interval of arbitrary confidence level L (e.g., 0.95) by adding and subtracting $z_{\alpha/2} \times$ SE to $\bar{x}$ when the sample size is large, where $z_{\alpha/2}$ is the upper $\alpha/2$ quantile of the normal distribution and SE is the standard error for the mean.

In the weight loss trial, as is typical, the sample standard deviation had to be estimated. This extra imprecision needs to be taken into account for the 95% confidence interval to preserve its property of covering the true value 95% of the time (particularly with modest sample sizes).

Quantiles from the t-distribution with n-1 degrees of freedom ($t_{n-1,\alpha}$), instead of the normal distribution, will account for this extra uncertainty for a sample of size n. Thus, confidence intervals are generally formed with $\bar{x} \pm t_{n-1,0.025} \times$SE. For large n, $t_{n-1,0.025}$ quickly becomes indistinguishable from $z_{.025}$. For example, for $n = 100$, $t_{99,0.025} = 1.984$, and for $n = 500$, $t_{499,0.025} = 1.965$. The t-statistic applies here specifically because the standardized quantity $(\bar{x} - \mu)/SE$ follows a t-distribution with $n-1$ degrees of freedom. This t-distribution is symmetric about 0, like the normal, but with wider tail probabilities. The t-distribution is sometimes referred to as Student's t distribution, named after the pseudonym under which William Sealy Gosset first published the distribution for the standardized sample mean (Wendl 2016).

Estimation and Uncertainty for Noncontinuous Outcomes

Two other common parameters of interest for clinical trials are proportions from binary outcomes and hazard ratios from time-to-event outcomes. For these parameters, the principles of the CI are the same. We can again rely on the Central Limit Theorem and form the confidence interval by adding and subtracting the desired quantile multiple of the appropriate SE. For proportions, the sample mean of the binary outcome is the estimated proportion $\hat{p}$ and the estimated SE is $[\hat{p}(1-\hat{p})/n]^{1/2}$. The 95% confidence interval for a population proportion is thus $\hat{p} \pm 1.960[\hat{p}(1-\hat{p})/n]^{1/2}$. The log hazard ratio $(\hat{\beta})$ and its SE can be directly estimated from the Cox model, and it is on the log-scale that the hazard ratio estimator is approximately normal (Cox 1972; Hosmer et al. 2011). One can form the 95% confidence interval by $\hat{\beta} \pm 1.960$ SE. This is also referred to as the Wald confidence interval for the log-hazard ratio. For this and other statistics estimated with likelihood techniques, there are other methods besides the Wald approach to estimate confidence intervals, such as those that rely on the score or the likelihood ratio statistics (Casella and Berger 2002). While for large sample sizes, these three methods will produce similar results, at smaller sample sizes there will be noticeable differences. The score statistic can be a more efficient method than the more commonly used Wald technique; that is, with the same data set, the score interval can be narrower, which is a desirable feature for a confidence interval. See Lin et al. (2016) for a comparison of the different methods of hazard ratio confidence interval estimation.

For discrete data that take on many values that have a natural order, such as count data or an outcome taken from an ordinal scale, such as the Likert scale, it is common to treat these outcomes like a continuous outcome to summarize a treatment effect. That is, the mean value $\bar{x}$ and sample standard deviation s are calculated for each arm and a 95% confidence interval is formed using methods for a continuous outcome, seen in the previous section. For an ordinal scale, one must first assign numeric values; most commonly the positive integers are used. For example, for the 5-level Likert scale, one can assign 1 = strongly disagree, 2 = disagree, 3 = neither agree nor disagree, 4 = agree, and 5 = strongly agree. For data such as these, that start off far from normally distributed, it may take larger sample sizes for the estimate of interest, say $\bar{x}$, to be well-approximated with a normal distribution. An alternative approach, called nonparametric statistics, is discussed in a later section of this chapter.

Estimation of the Difference Between Groups

A formal comparison of the difference between two arms of a clinical trial is often desired. For quantities like the sample mean or proportion, which are approximately normally distributed, this will be relatively straightforward. The difference is approximately normally distributed, as any linear combination of two (jointly) normal statistics will also be normally distributed. Thus, we can apply our general confidence interval technique to form the CI for the difference. We can then examine this confidence interval and see whether it contains the value 0, which would indicate the data are consistent with no difference in the parameter of interest between groups.

For example, suppose in the weight loss trial the mean weight change from baseline is $\bar{x} = 6$ for arm A and $\bar{y} = 2$ for arm B. Suppose further arm A has a sample standard deviation $s_x = 20$ and $m = 100$ people and arm B has standard deviation $s_y = 15$ and $n = 90$ people. The estimated mean weight change difference between arms is $\bar{x} - \bar{y} = 4$. If we assume the true SD in each arm may be different, then the SE for this difference is calculated by the square root of the sum of the variances for each mean, $s_{\bar{x}-\bar{y}} = \sqrt{20^2/100 + 15^2/90} = 2.550$. An approximate 95% CI could be formed again using quantiles from a t distribution, but in this case, the degrees of freedom (df) for the difference of means must be estimated. The common approach is to use Satterthwaite's formula (Rosner 2015), which yields

$$df = \left(\frac{s_x^2}{m} + \frac{s_y^2}{n}\right)^2 \left(\frac{\left(\frac{s_x^2}{m}\right)^2}{m-1} + \frac{\left(\frac{s_y^2}{n}\right)^2}{n-1}\right)^{-1}.$$

The 95% confidence interval is then $4 \pm t_{182.2371, 0.0.025}$ (2.550), or $(-1.03, 9.03)$. The confidence interval includes 0, which does not support the conclusion that there is a difference in weight loss between the two arms. If one assumed that the two arms had a common true variance, one could use a more efficient estimate of the common variance by pooling data from the two arms and estimating a single SD. Since we generally do not know whether arms have a common SD, the Satterthwaite method is preferable. A common, yet faulty, approach is to use the same data to first conduct a hypothesis test for equal variances between the two arms and then, based on results of that test, decide which estimate of the SE to use. This procedure can yield slightly anti-conservative confidence intervals.

In the case of paired differences for a continuous outcome, one can first form the within person difference d = x-y for each individual and then follow the usual procedure for confidence intervals for a single continuous outcome.

For a clinical trial with binary outcomes, we can take a similar approach to forming the confidence interval for the difference in proportions between two independent groups. Denote the difference in sample proportions by $\hat{p}_x - \hat{p}_y$. Since each $\hat{p}$ is approximately normally distributed, so is the difference in proportions. The SE for $\hat{p}_x - \hat{p}_y$ can be estimated as $SE_{\hat{p}_x - \hat{p}_y} = \sqrt{\frac{\hat{p}_x(1-\hat{p}_x)}{m} + \frac{\hat{p}_y(1-\hat{p}_y)}{n}}$, and the 95% CI becomes $\hat{p}_x - \hat{p}_y \pm 1.960\ SE_{\hat{p}_x - \hat{p}_y}$. To determine whether the data are consistent with no between-arm difference, one can again consider whether the CI contains the value zero.

When estimating the difference between intervention groups for other outcomes, one simply needs to formulate a parameter in a statistical model which represents this difference and estimate it. The 1-α confidence interval could be formed with the upper and lower α/2 quantile of the probability distribution appropriate for that statistical model. A common approach parameterizes this difference in a regression model. Estimates for both the parameter and its SE are straightforward. For censored survival data, the hazard ratio is inherently a parameter for the difference between arms, in this case a ratio. For a ratio, the value representing no difference between arms is 1. Consequently, a confidence interval for the HR containing 1, or equivalently a confidence interval of the log-hazard containing 0, is consistent with no difference between arms.

Hypothesis Testing

In the previous section, the confidence interval was used to answer questions about the parameter such as whether data were consistent with no difference between two intervention arms. We can also directly answer questions about the value of a parameter with a process called hypothesis testing. Confidence intervals and hypothesis testing are intimately linked. In fact, as will be explained below, in many situations, there is a 1–1 correspondence between the conclusion made from a confidence interval for the value of a parameter (such as whether a value of zero is consistent with the data) and the results of a hypothesis test. The hypothesis testing framework provides a way to formalize the language and process for drawing conclusions about parameter values from the data.

The hypothesis test can be described as consisting of five steps:

1) Formulate the null hypothesis
2) Formulate the alternative hypothesis
3) Set a level of significance
4) Evaluate a test statistic for the hypothesis
5) Estimate the p-value for the test statistic.

The null hypothesis is a statement about a value for the parameter, for which data will be collected to assess. For the parameter of interest μ, the null value is represented μ_0. For example, if $\mu = \mu_A - \mu_B$ is the parameter for the difference in the average weight change between arms A and B, one may set the null to be one of no difference, i.e., $H_0: \mu_0 = 0$. For this one-dimensional parameter, the alternative hypothesis (H_A) can take on three possible forms: (i) $\mu < 0$ (individuals on Arm A have smaller weight change), (ii) $\mu > 0$ (individuals on Arm A have bigger weight change), and (iii) $\mu \neq 0$ (the average weight change for arm A and B is different).

The first two are examples of "one-sided" (also called "one-tailed") alternative hypotheses and the third is a "two-sided" alternative hypothesis. This distinction will matter in terms of evaluating the strength of evidence against the null hypothesis. In a randomized clinical trial, even though showing a difference in one direction is more of interest (such as that the novel intervention A is superior to intervention B), it is most typical to have a two-sided hypothesis. The issue of one-sided versus two-sided has been the source of continued debate and some controversy, as will be explained later in this chapter.

The basic idea of conducting a hypothesis test is to calculate a test statistic that estimates how far the sample estimate of the parameter of interest is from its target value under the null hypothesis (μ_0). The assumed probability distribution for the data is used to calculate the likelihood of a test statistic value at least as extreme as the observed value, assuming the null hypothesis is true. This probability is called the *p-value*. R.A. Fisher is attributed to having given the p-value its dominance in the scientific literature with his seminal book in 1925 (Fisher 1925; Kyriacou 2016). For approximately normal data, we can measure the departure from the null hypothesis in terms of numbers of standard errors. That is, we form the statistic $t = (\hat{\mu} - \mu_0)/\text{SE}$, where $\hat{\mu}$ is the sample value for the parameter of interest and SE is the standard error for $\hat{\mu}$. When $\hat{\mu}$ is a mean or difference of means, the test statistic t has an approximate t distribution, with degrees of freedom that can again be approximated by the Satterthwaite formula. In other settings, it is common to rely on the approximate normality of t to calculate the p-value. Test statistics can also take on different functional forms, for which their likelihood must be derived in order to calculate the p-value.

For the weight loss trial, one can set up the null and alternative hypotheses for the between-arm difference in average change in weight (μ). The null and alternative hypotheses are $H_0: \mu = 0$ and $H_A: \mu \neq 0$, respectively. Recall $\hat{\mu} = \bar{x} - \bar{y} = 4$ and

SE = 2.550. Relying on approximate normality of the sample means in the two groups, we form the test statistic t = (4–0)/2.550 = 1.569. The reference distribution is the student t distribution, using the Satterthwaite formula again, with 182.2371 degrees of freedom. The percentile for 1.569 for the $t_{182.2371}$ distribution is 0.9408. The p-value is 2(1–0.9408) = 0.1184, which is the probability that t is at least as extreme as 1.569 (t < −1.569 or t > 1.569). Note that here, p < 0.05 would have happened only if the magnitude of test statistic were larger than $t_{182.2371, 0.025}$, or equivalently, if the difference in sample means were more than $t_{182.2371, 0.025}$ standard errors away from the null value of 0. Thus, two-sided hypothesis testing of the null hypothesis is the same as checking whether the confidence interval includes the null value μ_0.

A significance level is chosen prior to conducting a hypothesis test, and if the p-value is smaller than this extreme value, the null hypothesis is rejected in favor of the alternative. If the p-value is larger than the significance level, one fails to reject. This does not mean that the null hypothesis is proven to be true. Though this language is common, it is not correct to accept the null hypothesis as true. If the p-value is greater than the significance level, as in the weight loss trial example, one can conclude only that there was not enough evidence in the data to reject the null. The null hypothesis might be true or the true difference might be too small to be reliably detected. Alternatively, the null hypothesis may be true, but a rare event was observed, and the null hypothesis was falsely rejected.

In a hypothesis test, two possible errors are: type I error (with probability denoted by α), namely rejecting the null hypothesis when it is really true and type II error (with probability β), namely failing to reject the null hypothesis when it is really false. The significance level, known as the alpha level, is the maximum type I error probability. The typical value set for alpha is 0.05. R.A. Fisher stated in the theoretical development of experimental design "...If one in twenty does not seem high enough odds, we may, if we prefer it, draw the line at one in fifty or one in a hundred. Personally, the writer prefers to set a low standard of significance at the 5 per cent point, and ignore entirely all results which fail to reach this level. A scientific fact should be regarded as experimentally established only if a properly designed experiment rarely fails to give this level of significance..." (Fisher 1925; Hackshaw and Kirkwood 2011). Though popular, the significance level of 0.05 may not be appropriate for every setting. For example, in a definitive phase III study, one may choose to set alpha = 0.01. In an early phase drug development, where the goal is only to gather preliminary evidence and avoid type II error, alpha = 0.10 is one common value.

An important concept in hypothesis testing is power, which is the probability of rejecting the null hypothesis given the alternative is true. Power is the same as 1 minus the type II error rate, i.e., $1-\beta$, and in order to calculate power, one must specify a specific alternative hypothesis. For example, in the weight loss trial, suppose during the design of the trial investigators expected to enroll 190 subjects, in a 1:1 ratio, onto two arms and expected the SD for weight loss to be 10 lb. in both arms. Assuming weight change is normally distributed, there would be 92.9% chance of having a significant difference between the arms at the 0.05 level if the true between-arm difference in average weight change was 5 lb. Having good power helps interpret a null result. For an adequately powered study, one with a high chance of rejecting the null in favor of the alternative of interest, a null result indicates the data are not consistent with that alternative. If power was 92.9% in the weight loss trial, and the null was not rejected, this is reasonably strong evidence that the between-arm difference in weight change is smaller than 5 lb. In this example, the observed sample standard deviations were 15 and 20 lb. on the two arms. If the true underlying SD on each arm were 18 lb. and the true treatment difference 5 lb., power with 95 per arm would be only 48%. Thus, with such low power, it is equally likely to reject or not reject the null. Therefore, failure to reject the null in this trial would not provide reliable evidence that the alternative was false. In many settings, the sample size is chosen so that power for an alternative of interest is at least 80% (20% type II error rate). In definitive settings, such as a large phase III trial, 90% power is often desirable.

Special Topics in Hypothesis Testing

Exact Tests and Other Considerations for Choosing a Hypothesis Test

The validity of a hypothesis test relies on choosing the correct method or probability distribution for the test statistic. This will depend on the distribution of the variables being measured and the study design. For instance, if data are highly skewed and the sample size is small, then using the t-test will likely result in an incorrect p-value. Even if data are not severely skewed, small samples may mean that one cannot rely on approximate normality of the test statistic to calculate the p-value. In this case, it would be better to consider an exact method – one that does not rely on approximate normality but rather uses the correct probability distribution of the test statistic.

One exact test is based on permuting the labels of treatment and control observations. Consider the strong null hypothesis that treatment has no effect on anyone. The idea is to fix the data at their observed values, permute the treatment labels, and compute the value of the test statistic assuming the permuted treatment labels were the actual ones. After all, under the null hypothesis of no effect of treatment, the same data would have been observed regardless of treatment received. Repeat this process for all possible, or at least a large number of, permutations to generate a reference distribution for the test statistic under the null hypothesis. The p-value is the proportion of test statistic values in the reference distribution at least as extreme as the observed test statistic value. For a one-sided test to determine whether treatment produces larger outcome values than control, reference values "at least as extreme" are those that are at least as large. For example, if the observed value of the test statistic is 2.5, and only 1% of the reference distribution is 2.5 or larger, the p-value is 0.01.

The permutation test can be used in many settings. When the outcome is binary and the test statistic is the difference in sample proportions, the permutation reference distribution can be computed theoretically using probability, and the permutation test is equivalent to Fisher's exact test. If the sample size is large, the permutation test is nearly identical to the z-test of proportions, which is equivalent to the chi-squared test. When the outcome is continuous and the test statistic is the difference in sample means, the permutation test is nearly identical to the t-test if the sample size is large. The advantage of the permutation test is that, without any further assumptions, it provides a valid test of the strong null hypothesis that treatment has no effect on anyone.

A disadvantage of permutation tests is that, although they give nearly the same answer as t-tests or z-tests of proportions when sample sizes are large, they can be quite conservative for smaller sample sizes. For instance, with only 3 patients per arm, the smallest possible two-sided p-value is 0.10 (i.e., a statistically significant result at the conventional alpha level of 0.05 is impossible). Many would say that such conservatism is appropriate if the sample sizes are that small.

A common error when determining the distribution of a test statistic is failure to account for correlation between observations. For example, suppose one were interested in comparing the efficacy of two weight loss interventions and married couples were recruited and assigned to the same intervention. Since married individuals tend to share meals, their weight loss may be positively correlated. Failure to account for the correlation leads to a higher than intended probability of falsely declaring benefit of a diet. Interestingly, a permutation test that adheres to the original randomization (i.e., both members of the couple receive the same treatment) automatically accounts for such correlation and provides a valid p-value. Further discussion of permutation tests is provided in the section on ▶ Chap. 94, "Randomization and Permutation Tests" in the Analysis chapter.

Nonparametric Versus Parametric Analysis

Two classes of statistical analysis are *parametric* and *nonparametric* methods. Parametric methods make more assumptions, e.g., that the data are normally distributed. Nonparametric analyses make fewer assumptions. For example, the Wilcoxon rank sum test comparing two arms is valid regardless of the shape of the distribution of data; the only assumption is that the distribution is shifted in one arm relative to the other. Other popular nonparametric methods include the Kruskal–Wallis test, instead of the parametric one-way ANOVA, and rank regression instead of linear regression. The reward for using parametric analysis is that, **if the underlying assumptions are true**, power is better and conclusions may be stronger. On the other hand, if those assumptions are false, the parametric analysis may lead to incorrect conclusions.

Many people feel that clinical trials should provide valid results with as few assumptions as possible. This would argue for nonparametric analysis of data. Nonparametric analyses are often nearly as powerful as parametric analyses if sample sizes are large. For example, the sample size required for a desired level of power is only about 5% smaller for the t-test relative to the Wilcoxon rank sum test when data actually are normally distributed. If data are not normally distributed, the t-test may give invalid results. Even if data have a symmetric distribution, power for a t-test can be substantially lower than that of a Wilcoxon test. The advantage of the t-test seems outweighed by its disadvantages.

Transformations of data are common. A log transformation can greatly reduce skew. Sometimes square roots or other monotone transformations (meaning that if x < y, the transformed x is also less than the transformed y) are used. It is reasonable to assume that **some** transformation of the data will result in approximate normality. The ranks of the monotone transformed data are identical to those of the original data, so a nonparametric test reaches the same conclusion for any monotone transformation. Therefore, a nonparametric test may be viewed as first finding a transformation that "normalizes" the data, then applying a test to compare means of transformed data. This is equivalent to comparing medians of untransformed data.

A disadvantage of nonparametric methods is that they do not naturally facilitate analyses that adjust for baseline imbalances in covariates. Parametric methods do facilitate such an analysis. For instance, a linear regression model can incorporate covariates, and it simplifies to a t-test when there are no covariates other than treatment. A nonparametric analog, known as rank regression, is not as appealing because ranks are inherently discrete. Regression parameters for rank regression, which summarize covariate effects on the rank of the outcome, are generally more difficult to interpret than those for parametric regression methods where the parameter of interest relates to the outcome on a more natural scale (such as the mean value).

Multiple Comparisons

The problem that multiple comparisons create for hypothesis testing is best illustrated with the following analogy. In the popular game of darts, a circular target board is placed at a certain distance from a player, which makes throwing a dart and hitting a target difficult. The bullseye, a small ring in the center of the board, is worth the most points. Compare two players. One hits the bullseye on the first attempt and one takes 100 attempts to hit the bullseye. Though the first player could have been lucky, it seems clear that the second player is not particularly good at hitting the target. If the second player reported that he hit the target without specifying how many attempts it had taken him, it would be difficult to conclude how good a player he was. One might even incorrectly assume he had only thrown the dart once. Similarly, suppose a large study examining whether a certain compound was efficacious at preventing cancer reported that treatment had a significantly lower incidence of stomach cancer than control. It would be important for investigators of this study to disclose for how many different cancers was a hypothesis test done to compare that treatment with control. Looking at 10 cancers increases the probability that one hypothesis test would be significant by chance alone, even if the risk for none of the cancers was influenced by the treatment. The alpha level, below which a p-value is declared significant, must be adjusted for multiple comparisons in order to preserve the type I error rate. Many methods exist for adjusting the testing procedure to accommodate multiple comparisons so that it maintains the desired type I error rate (Hochberg and Tamhane 1987). Issues of multiple comparisons are considered further in the section on ▶ Chap. 85, "Confident Statistical Inference with Multiple Outcomes, Subgroups, and Other Issues of Multiplicity" in the Analysis chapter.

Noninferiority Versus Superiority

Sometimes the goal of a clinical trial is to show not that the new treatment is superior to, but rather that it is almost as good as, the standard treatment. Such a design is called a *noninferiority trial*. Noninferiority trials are appealing if the standard treatment is onerous or has serious side effects. Even if the new treatment is almost as good as the standard, it may be preferred by patients. The ACTG 076 trial in the United States and France had already demonstrated the preventive benefit of a longer course of AZT, but the longer course was prohibitively expensive for developing countries. A superiority trial randomizing HIV-infected mothers to a shorter course of AZT or placebo drew criticism on ethical grounds (Lurie and Wolfe 1997). Some critics argued that a trial demonstrating noninferiority of the short course to the longer course was more ethical and could have indirectly shown that the short course was superior to placebo.

In a noninferiority trial, a new treatment N is compared to a standard treatment S. In a noninferiority setting, S has already been shown superior to placebo in a previous trial by some amount M_1. That is, if p_S and p_0 denote the proportions with events, say a heart attack, in the standard and placebo arms in the previous trial, $p_0 - p_S = M_1 > 0$. Suppose one can show that N is not worse than S by more than a prespecified noninferiority margin M, i.e., $p_N - p_S \leq M$. Then $p_N - p_0 = p_N - p_S + p_S - p_0 \leq M - M_1$. As long as M is smaller than M_1, one can conclude that N would have beaten the placebo (that is, $p_N - p_0 < 0$), had the current trial used a placebo. The noninferiority design begins by prespecifying a noninferiority margin M. A common choice for the noninferiority margin is half of the known effect of S relative to placebo, $M = M_1/2$. That way, demonstration of noninferiority shows that the new treatment preserves at least half of the benefit of the standard treatment seen in the previous trial.

The null and alternative hypotheses are essentially reversed in a noninferiority trial. The null hypothesis is that the new treatment is worse than the standard by more than M: H_0: $p_N - p_S > M$, and the alternative is that treatment is worse than the standard by no more than M: H_1: $p_N - p_S \leq M$. Rejection of the null in favor of the alternative hypothesis at the given alpha level demonstrates noninferiority. The procedure is equivalent to constructing a $1-2\alpha$ confidence interval for $p_N - p_S$ and declaring noninferiority if the upper limit of the interval is M or less. For example, if the alpha level of the test of noninferiority is 0.05, the procedure is equivalent to constructing a 90% confidence interval and declaring noninferiority if the upper limit of the interval is M or less.

One of the biggest drawbacks of noninferiority designs is that things that ought to be bad in a clinical trial actually help demonstrate noninferiority. For instance, suppose that the new drug is so ineffective that 100% of patients in arm N abandon the new treatment and start taking the standard treatment. Then the observed difference between N and S will be close to 0, making it easier to establish noninferiority. That can't be good! For this reason, even though intent-to-treat is the primary analysis method for superiority trials, an as-treated analysis is often the primary analysis in noninferiority trials. Another downside of noninferiority trials is that it assumes that the effect of the standard treatment relative to placebo is unchanged from the previous to the current trial, the so-called *constancy assumption*. That is why the noninferiority margin is often taken to be half of the "known" effect of S relative to placebo.

Because noninferiority trials are inherently problematic, they should be avoided whenever the question can be answered in another way. For example, when a placebo is considered unethical, one could provide everyone the standard treatment and test whether the new treatment has additional benefit. Another alternative to a noninferiority design is a superiority design in patients who do not benefit from, or cannot tolerate, the standard treatment. Noninferiority designs are also discussed further in the "Equivalence and Noninferiority Designs" section in the Advanced Topics in Trial Design chapter.

Controversies in Hypothesis Testing

Two-Sided Versus One-Sided Controversy

In 1988, many cardiologists believed that patients with a prior heart attack and cardiac arrhythmias could reduce their risk of cardiac arrest and sudden death by suppressing those arrhythmias. After all, studies showed clearly that heart attack patients with arrhythmias were at increased risk of sudden death. Therefore, when the Cardiac Arrhythmia Suppression Trial (CAST) tested the "suppression hypothesis," their original alternative hypothesis was that the antiarrhythmic arm would have a lower risk of cardiac arrest/sudden death than the placebo arm. More specifically, with λ denoting the log-hazard ratio for sudden death/cardiac arrest in the antiarrhythmic arm relative to placebo, the null and alternative hypotheses were $H_0: \lambda = 0$ (no effect) and $H_1: \lambda < 0$ (the antiarrhythmic arm is superior). As described in Friedman et al. (1993), at its first review meeting, the Data and Safety Monitoring Board (DSMB) recommended switching to the two-sided alternative hypothesis $H_1: \lambda \neq 0$, which allows a decrease or increase in the risk of cardiac arrest/sudden death in the antiarrhythmic arm. This was a prescient move; the trial stopped early because the event rate was much higher in the antiarrhythmic arm (CAST Investigators 1989). CAST reminds us that interventions can cause harm. The prevailing view is that one should always use a two-sided alternative hypothesis. Some medical journals have gone so far as not allowing one-sided testing.

A counter-argument to two-sided testing is that there is no interest in proving harm. If results in the treatment harm were going the wrong way, the trial would be stopped before the evidence was sufficient to show actual harm. But this was not true in CAST. The widespread misconception about the benefits of suppression of cardiac arrhythmias needed to be dispelled before medical practice could change.

A better argument against two-sided tests is that the two errors, (1) falsely declaring treatment beneficial and (2) falsely declaring treatment harmful, are very different with vastly different consequences. Declaring a drug harmful when it actually has no effect may not have serious consequences because that drug should not be used anyway. On the other hand, declaring a drug beneficial when it is ineffective is problematic because patients may eschew truly effective treatments for the ineffective treatment. Therefore, it is important to consider each of the one-sided error rates.

The P-Value Controversy

P-values have been viewed in the medical literature as the definitive measure of evidence for many years. A counter-movement is underway to eliminate them. Both viewpoints can be viewed as overreactions.

One must first understand what a p-value is and what role it plays. Imagine 10 people exposed to a level of radiation that is known to be 95% fatal. They are given a new treatment, and half survive. How compelling is the evidence that the new treatment saves lives? Are observed results consistent with chance? It can be shown that the probability of 5 or more people out of 10 surviving a condition that is 95% fatal is only 0.00006. The two possible conclusions are (1) the new treatment saves lives or (2) the new treatment does not save lives, but an incredibly rare event occurred. Chance is not a plausible explanation for the observed results. A small p-value does not necessarily imply that the treatment effect was large. For instance, suppose that 1,000 people had been exposed to a radiation level that is known to be 95% fatal, and 80 people survived. The p-value in that case would be 0.00003, yet 92% still died. The observed treatment effect was small, but it was large enough to effectively rule out chance. The sole purpose of a p-value is to see whether results are consistent with chance; it is imperative to supplement p-values with estimates and confidence intervals for the size of the treatment effect to appreciate whether the effect is both statistically significant and clinically important.

A criticism commonly levied against the p-value is that it is not reproducible. If we repeat the same trial, the p-value may be completely different. This is especially true if the true treatment effect is small. For example, if treatment has no true effect, the p-value for many tests is uniformly distributed between 0 and 1, meaning that it is equally likely to be large, medium, or small. Therefore, if treatment has no true effect, we might see a relatively small p-value in the first trial and a much larger one in the next trial. The p-value is less variable if treatment is truly effective. Reproducibility worries are somewhat ameliorated by the common practice of lumping p-values above 0.05, declaring them "not statistically significant." One must bear in mind that the purpose of a p-value is to determine whether chance provides a plausible explanation for observed results.

Another criticism of the p-value is that it depends not only on the observed results but also on what action we would have taken if other results had been observed. In other words, to compute a p-value, one must define what results are at least as extreme as the observed results. Critics question the logic of computing the probability of the actual result **or a more extreme result**, when no more extreme result occurred.

The p-value has limitations. Nonetheless, the p-value is useful for its intended purpose. Its primary competitor is Bayesian methodology, which has its own criticisms. Although not covered in this chapter, Bayesian methodology has received considerable attention in clinical trials (Berry et al. 2010).

Summary and Conclusion

Two principal aims of statistics are to use data to (1) provide an estimate of a population parameter and (2) to test whether two populations may be different with respect to this parameter. Sample estimates have uncertainty that can be expressed with their associated confidence interval. Hypothesis testing is used to make statements about the value of a parameter, such as whether treatment A is superior to treatment B. To conduct a reliable hypothesis test, one must specify in advance the null and alternative hypothesis for the parameter of interest and choose a study design that has good power to reject the null in favor of the specified alternative. The p-value summarizes the evidence against the null hypothesis. The validity of the hypothesis test relies on calculating the p-value with a correctly specified probability distribution. The study design and distribution of the study outcome will determine which distribution is appropriate. In some cases, an exact or nonparametric test may be desired to avoid unnecessary assumptions. When interpreting results, one must remember that no reasonable hypothesis test has zero type I or type II error. In many settings, other evidence, such as results from other clinical trials or mechanistic laboratory studies, are useful to evaluate the totality of evidence for the question under study.

Key Facts

- The confidence interval contains values of the parameter that are consistent with study data. For a study repeated many times, the 95% confidence interval is expected to contain the true value 95% of the time.
- A hypothesis test requires specifying a null and alternative hypothesis for the parameter.
- The p-value is the proportion of test statistic values in the reference distribution at least as extreme as the observed test statistic value. The chosen alternative hypothesis determines whether this is a one-sided or two-sided p-value.
- Type I error rate, denoted by α, is the probability of rejecting the null hypothesis when it is true. Type II error rate, denoted by β, is the probability of failing to reject the null hypothesis when it is false.
- Power helps us interpret a null result; if power was high and the null was not rejected, we can be reasonably confident that the effect was not as strong as originally hypothesized. If the trial was not well-powered, a null result is difficult to interpret.

Cross-References

▶ Confident Statistical Inference with Multiple Outcomes, Subgroups, and Other Issues of Multiplicity
▶ Randomization and Permutation Tests

References

Berry SM, Carlin BP, Lee JJ, Muller P (2010) Bayesian adaptive methods for clinical trials. CRC Press, Boca Raton

Cardiac Arrhythmia Suppression Trial (CAST) Investigators (1989) Preliminary report: effect of encainide and flecainide on mortality in a randomized trial of arrhythmia suppression after myocardial infarction. NEJM 321(6):406–412

Casella G, Berger RL (2002) Statistical inference. Duxbury, Pacific Grove

Cox DR (1972) Regression models and life-tables. Journal of the Royal Statistical Society: Series B (Methodological) 34(2):187–202

Fisher RA (1925) Statistical methods for research workers. Oliver and Boyd, Edinburgh

Friedman LM, Bristow JD, Hallstrom A et al (1993) Data monitoring in the cardiac arrhythmia suppression trial. Online J Curr Clin Trials, Doc. No. 79 [5870 words; 53 paragraphs]

Hackshaw A, Kirkwood A (2011) Interpreting and reporting clinical trials with results of borderline significance. BMJ 343:d3340

Hochberg Y, Tamhane AC (1987) Multiple comparison procedures. Wiley, Hoboken

Hosmer DW Jr, Lemeshow S, May S (2011) Applied survival analysis: regression modeling of time-to-event data. Wiley, Hoboken

Kyriacou DN (2016) The enduring evolution of the p value. JAMA 315(11):1113–1115

Lin DY, Dai L, Cheng G et al (2016) On confidence intervals for the hazard ratio in randomized clinical trials. Biometrics 72(4):1098–1102

Lurie P, Wolfe SM (1997) Unethical trials of interventions to reduce perinatal transmission of the human immunodeficiency virus in developing countries. NEJM 337(12):853–856

Rosner B (2015) Fundamentals of biostatistics. Brooks/Cole, Boston

Wendl MC (2016) Pseudonymous fame. Science 351(6280):1406–1406

Estimands and Sensitivity Analyses

84

Estelle Russek-Cohen and David Petullo

Contents

Introduction	1632
Randomization and Randomized Clinical Trials	1634
Causal Inference	1635
Estimand Framework	1635
Intent to Treat	1636
Types of Trials and Measurements in Trials	1636
Strategies for Addressing Intercurrent Events when Formulating Estimands	1637
Treatment Policy Strategy	1638
Hypothetical Strategy	1639
Principal Stratification Strategy: Estimands and Causal Inference	1639
Some Cautions	1641
Other Considerations	1643
Importance of Selecting an Estimand at the Planning Stage	1643
Role of Covariates	1644
Types of Missingness	1644
Estimands and Safety	1645
Estimands in Studies with Time-to-Event Endpoints	1645
Estimands in Complex Designs	1646

This chapter reflects the views of the authors and should not be construed to FDA's views or policies.

E. Russek-Cohen (✉)
Office of Biostatistics, Center for Drug Evaluation and Research,
U.S. Food and Drug Administration, Silver Spring, MD, USA
e-mail: russekcohen.estelle@gmail.com

D. Petullo
Division of Biometrics II, Office of Biostatistics Office of Translational Sciences,
Center for Drug Evaluation and Research, U.S. Food and Drug Administration,
Silver Spring, MD, USA
e-mail: David.Petullo@fda.hhs.gov

© This is a U.S. Government work and not under copyright protection in the U.S.;
foreign copyright protection may apply 2022
S. Piantadosi, C. L. Meinert (eds.), *Principles and Practice of Clinical Trials*,
https://doi.org/10.1007/978-3-319-52636-2_115

Estimands and Meta-Analysis	1646
Network Meta-Analysis	1646
Estimands in Non-inferiority (NI) Studies	1647
Going from Estimand to Estimator	1647
Benefit Risk	1648
Sensitivity Analyses	1648
An Example	1649
Challenges for Clinical Trials to Evaluate Pain Medications	1650
Estimands, Estimation, and Sensitivity Analysis Illustrated Using an FDA Example	1651
An Estimand, Estimate, and a Tipping Point Analysis	1653
Conclusion	1654
Key Facts	1655
Cross-References	1655
References	1655

Abstract

An estimand is a quantity used to define a treatment effect in a clinical trial. In many cases, clinical trial planners skipped the step of defining the estimand in their rush to pick a test statistic and calculate planned sample size(s). This would sometimes lead to ambiguity on how results of a trial were to be interpreted. In this chapter we describe estimands in detail and explain the importance of defining estimands when planning randomized trials and doing this before picking a test statistic to use in evaluating trial outcomes. The estimand is key to defining the scientific question the trial needs to address. When patients drop out or fail to follow a planned regime within a randomized clinical trial and stakeholders disagree on how this impacts the analysis of the trial, interpretability of this trial can be called into question. A clear definition of treatment effect ought to capture how dropouts and protocol violators will be handled.

In this chapter sensitivity analyses are tied to the definition of the estimand in a trial. In practice, sensitivity analyses are often ad hoc and only addressed after a study is completed. Considering both estimands and sensitivity analyses in planning will improve the interpretation of results from completed randomized trials. While regulators (e.g., the US Food and Drug Administration) have been particularly interested in advancing these ideas, utilization of these ideas ought to improve the interpretability of randomized trials more generally.

Keywords

Intent to treat · Intercurrent events · Protocol violations · Tipping point analyses · Treatment effect

Introduction

In other parts of this text, considerable attention is made to planning of clinical trials, estimation of key summary measures, and finally reporting of clinical trial results. The topic of an estimand may never enter into those discussions, and in clinical trial textbooks written over a decade ago, it seems unlikely that the topic of an estimand would be covered. Yet estimands are defined as quantities used to capture treatment effects within a clinical trial, and they are not always carefully considered during the planning stage. Sensitivity analyses may be something you have seen before but, as with estimands, are not often covered in a systematic way in textbooks. Discussions on estimands force a clinical trial planning team to define the scientific question to be answered in the trial. Sensitivity analyses are often used at the end of a trial to confirm the results and the assumptions of any statistical methods used, but ought to follow from first defining the estimand of interest. A systematic approach to sensitivity analyses set up prior to starting the study is preferable to generating a laundry list of data analyses after the study is over. This chapter stresses the importance of selecting an appropriate estimand(s) and sensitivity analyses at the planning stage to allow for a cleaner interpretation of results once the study is completed.

If all studies went exactly "as planned" and everyone completed the trial without exception to protocol guidelines, defining an estimand could be a trivial task and possibly left till the end. However, as noted in a survey by Fletcher et al. (2017), the overwhelming majority of clinical trials have missing data or protocol deviations. Waiting till the study is over to decide how these issues will be addressed when determining treatment effects is not good science and frankly, pretty naive. Furthermore, to the extent that clinical trials mimic real-world use of a product, dropouts and failure to take doses as prescribed are a common occurrence and one should not be surprised by this at the end of the study. Regulators such as the US Food and Drug Administration (FDA) and companies wanting to market a medical product often negotiate success criteria for a clinical trial. The choice of an estimand and showing how an estimate of treatment effect follows from it will be important. However, if both groups are not on the same page, it would be painful to discover this after a rather expensive clinical trial has been completed. So the desire to prespecify estimands is of importance to regulators. It should be noted in some cases, there could be more than one acceptable estimand, so regulators and companies need to communicate early in the development process.

The FDA commissioned a report by the National Academy of Sciences (NAS) and its research arm, the National Research Council (NRC 2010), dealing with the prevention and treatment of missing data in clinical trials. One motivation for the NAS report was the arbitrary use of "last observation carried forward" (LOCF) as a way of filling in missing values when subjects drop out of a clinical trial submitted to the FDA. It was easy to calculate and there may be settings in which LOCF made sense but the option was often used without justification. One general recommendation that came out of the NAS document was that one should design trials that minimize the amount of missing data and estimands ought to be defined when planning the trial. However, in spite of the NAS report, regulators realized that current practice had not moved forward (LaVange and Permutt 2016). In 2014 multiple regulatory agencies and their industry counterparts under the umbrella of the International Council for Harmonisation (ICH) agreed to develop an addendum to an important international guideline on statistical principles in clinical trials (ICH 1998, 2014). The focus of the addendum is estimands and sensitivity analyses.

While regulators and their industry counterparts are now considering estimands earlier in their deliberations, it would be unfortunate to think these discussions are solely related to medical product approval. There are many clinical trials sponsored by others (e.g., National Institutes of Health) that have public health impacts and thinking about how results will be interpreted as one plans a study should improve the science. Practices such as increasing the sample size to account for an expected dropout rate without thinking about why dropouts occur are a missed opportunity to plan a better study.

Randomization and Randomized Clinical Trials

The majority of clinical trials reported in a drug or medical device label are randomized, and such trials are considered the gold standard in establishing treatment differences. In this chapter, for simplicity, we focus on clinical trials with two treatment groups, most commonly a treatment group and a control group. However, the principles here ought to have relevance to other kinds of trials, e.g., traditional trials with more than two arms, pragmatic clinical trials (Ford and Norrie 2016) that may harness electronic health records, and/or relax eligibility requirements to assess something closer to real-world effectiveness of an intervention and to trials that rely more heavily on data from other sources (e.g., using external control data).

Randomization in most trials should result in comparability of subjects in the two treatment groups with respect to baseline characteristics, but comparability can be lost depending on events that occur post-randomization. What is often missing from the characterization of a treatment effect is how post-randomization events were handled. The new ICH E9 R1 document defines events such as leaving a study early, use of rescue medications, and so on as "intercurrent" events. When these events are not balanced across treatment arms or the reasons for why these occur are not the same, the interpretability of the study may be problematic. Therefore, when choosing an estimand, one should consider all relevant intercurrent events. In many therapeutic areas, these can impact a substantial portion of the study subjects. The NAS report (NRC 2010) encourages FDA to explore which post-randomization events (i.e., intercurrent events) are common and in what settings so future clinical trials can be better planned. This kind of activity is still going on at FDA.

Randomized clinical trials have appeal because one can attribute causation, namely, if the randomization was done appropriately and the study went according to plan, observed significant treatment differences can be attributed to the difference in treatments under investigation. However, in long-term studies or any trial where there are more than a few dropouts and/or protocol violators, treatment effects are harder to interpret. The issue is worse if the number of dropouts or the reasons for dropouts and protocol violations differs among treatment arms. For example, a dropout on a placebo arm could be due to ineffectiveness of the intervention, but dropouts on the arm with a new drug could be due to serious side effects.

Causal Inference

The term estimand appears in the literature associated with causal inference (Little and Rubin 2000) where one recognized the role of confounding and interpreting treatment effects in something other than a randomized clinical trial had to be done with caution. At the heart of many causal inference discussions, the reader is asked to imagine how the same subject would respond if they were assigned to one treatment group and then if they were assigned to the other treatment and think of the treatment effect for that subject as the difference in the two values (Y(trt)-Y(control)). The value for that subject in the unobserved arm is the unobserved potential outcome. In most instances one only gets to observe the outcome on one treatment, but under randomization, one could imagine the two groups being comparable at baseline and treatment effect could logically be interpreted to be the mean of the subject level treatment effects.

Estimand Framework

An estimand should be thoroughly vetted among the interdisciplinary team and could be stated in words so that both clinicians and statisticians can comprehend what is needed. After deciding on a clinically relevant estimand, one can decide on how to estimate it, referred to as an estimator. This estimator can be defined using words or using formulas as appropriate. In statistical terms, this would be the parameter of interest. An estimate is derived from the clinical trial data, and if possible, an unbiased estimate of treatment effect is desired.

There can be more than one estimand in a trial. For example, trials may have multiple key endpoints, or multiple stakeholders may view the results of a trial differently. However, the process of picking the estimand, the estimator, and estimate would need to be repeated for each estimand. Some estimands can be regarded primary, while others may be considered as supportive (e.g., involving a different handling of dropouts or protocol violators).

In Table 1, we see the components of an estimand defined. Previous clinical trial textbooks focused on the need to define the population and the variable of interest along with a summary statistic without specifically indicating how intercurrent events are reflected in the estimand and estimator. This is new. In this definition, a different consideration of intercurrent events would result in a different estimand even for the same trial.

When different parties have different objectives, there may be different estimands. For example, regulators primarily want to establish efficacy and safety in a specific context, namely, the drug or device working. Insurers may interpret the results of a study differently since cost of a therapeutic intervention or the cost of follow-up in the event of treatment failure may not be considered by regulators like the FDA.

Table 1 Elements of an estimand (ICH 2017)

Population for which we want to address as a scientific question;
Variable, which consists of the measurements taken in a time period or at a certain time point (e.g., blood pressure 24 weeks after randomization) or functions thereof (e.g., change from baseline to 24 weeks in blood pressure) and could be a composite measure that incorporates several individual components;
Intervention effect describing how intercurrent events are reflected in the scientific question;
Summary measure for the variable on which the treatment effect will be based (e.g., variable mean)

It is common to see a statistical analysis plan (SAP) state that because the trial sponsor anticipated a 20% drop out rate, they would increase the sample size by some corresponding value (e.g., using 125% of the calculated sample size), ignoring why missing data occurs or that it may be imbalanced among the treatment arms. This is incorrect even if one does need an increase in sample size, since a failure to account for intercurrent events may still result in an uninterpretable trial. Others involved in planning trials may ignore missing data issues altogether. Sponsors of clinical trials would regularly use terms like intent to treat (ITT) that were interpreted differently by other stakeholders. Some interpreted ITT as only recording data while on treatment, yet others would follow subjects till the end irrespective of whether they complied with the assigned treatment regime. In reality, many analysis plans did not consider the basis of missing data and instead picked a method that used simpler and possibly unrealistic assumptions such as missing completely at random (see section "Types of Missingness"; Little and Rubin 2014).

Intent to Treat

The term "intent to treat" or ITT became much more commonly used in the clinical trial literature after the publication of the ICH E9 document Statistical Principles in Clinical Trials in 1998. This ICH guideline is used globally to assist companies in designing clinical trials to generate evidence in support of drug approval. However, people used the term ITT inconsistently after the 1998 document was published and confused two concepts, namely, the need to account for all subjects enrolled in a trial and the need to randomize subjects to avoid confounding due to imbalances in baseline covariates. The new ICH document (ICH 2017) distinguishes these concepts to add clarity to what treatment effect is being measured. See chapter on "Intent to Treat."

Types of Trials and Measurements in Trials

While there are many kinds of clinical trials, the topic of estimands has gained more attention in the context of longitudinal studies where patients are randomized to one of two (or more) treatments at baseline and patients are repeatedly assessed using the same measurement at fixed time points prespecified in the protocol (e.g., every month for 6 months). In O'Neill and Temple (2012), these have been called symptom trials though the outcomes could be laboratory measurements. For example, glycosylated hemoglobin or hemoglobin A1C (HgA1C) is measured at scheduled visits after subjects are randomized to treatment arms in trials that evaluate drugs to treat diabetes. Subjects may drop out at various times, but most are likely to stay until the end. These types of longitudinal studies are common in the assessment of treatments for diabetes, depression, pain, allergies, and other possibly chronic disorders. For such studies, the estimand is often defined in terms of a treatment effect at the end of the observed time period (e.g., the difference in average HgA1C after 6 months on assigned treatment). Information collected at earlier times may improve the precision of the estimate of treatment effect, particularly when a subject discontinues before 6 months on treatment. For other settings, perhaps the interest may be the average treatment difference over the observed time period (e.g., evaluating a treatment for symptom relief for seasonal allergies).

One alternative class of trials would be outcome trials (O'Neill and Temple 2012), and these focus on a single event for each subject but may fall into two categories based on the endpoint utilized. For example, in infectious disease trials, the primary focus may be on whether the treatment cures a subject of a disease and outcomes correspond to subject status at a given time point (disease present or not at 6 months after start of therapy). Dropouts are often regarded as treatment failures, and dropouts are an important consideration when evaluating a trial. For several therapeutic areas, including oncology, time to a prespecified major clinical event is the most common form of endpoint used, but, for example, it could be time until disease progression (with an agreed to basis of how this is defined) or time until death due to any cause (overall survival) (FDA-NIH 2018). In some instances (e.g., in drug trials in cardiology), time to event is a composite outcome (e.g., time until stroke, heart attack, or death, whichever comes first). In these settings, when subjects have not had the event of interest, an observation is considered censored. How protocol violators are handled or whether some of these events can be treated as censored should be considered when planning a trial much as intercurrent events are addressed in a longitudinal symptom trial.

Strategies for Addressing Intercurrent Events when Formulating Estimands

The ICH E9 R1 addendum (2017) defines a set of five strategies for selecting estimands. These are referred to as treatment policy, composite, hypothetical, principal stratum, and while on treatment. Statisticians, clinicians, and others with an understanding of the disease including epidemiologists may need to weigh in on the choice of an estimand. This would include selection of meaningful endpoints, identifying clinically relevant intercurrent events likely to occur and then defining the estimands in the presence of these intercurrent events. These strategies are discussed below.

The strategies presented are not exhaustive nor are they mutually exclusive. For example, Mallinckrodt et al. (2012) define de Jure and de Facto estimands with de Jure focusing on what might have been if subjects completed the planned course of treatment and de Facto estimands focusing on what is actually observed. However, these do not directly correspond to the five categories we provide below. The paper by Phillips et al. (2017) states that even though Mallinckrodt implies de Jure estimands are equated to efficacy and de Facto estimands are equated to effectiveness, given the restricted nature of who enrolls in trials relative to who may use a particular intervention once in practice, effectiveness may not be characterized in the most common clinical trials. Others have provided approaches that may not be defined exactly as we have below (Permutt 2016).

Treatment Policy Strategy

The occurrence of intercurrent events is irrelevant, and so in the context of Table 1, one would not need to state how each intercurrent event would be handled. The value for the variable of interest will be the endpoint of interest (e.g., HgBA1c at 6 months) regardless of whether an intercurrent event occurs. So all subjects are accounted for whether or not there is an intercurrent event. A key consideration for choosing this estimand is subjects need to be followed even if they start using rescue medication or fail to follow the treatment regime as described in the protocol. In studies where subjects are exposed to treatments that are relatively short in duration and assessments come with few missing data values, this may be the most sensible. In areas where use of rescue medication is quite common, an estimand that is the result of the treatment policy strategy may be hard to interpret if your goal is assessing the impact of a new drug. This is because you are comparing treatment+ rescue medications versus control+ rescue medications, and the effect will be influenced not only by the treatment under investigation but will be impacted by rescue medications taken by study participants.

A treatment policy strategy could be acceptable if the only intercurrent events were subjects crossing over to another treatment in the same trial. If rescue medications are designed to keep side effects down or are considered as appropriate with the treatments under study, perhaps these are not intercurrent events that require special attention in the definition of an estimand. But when subjects use various rescue medications decided on by the subjects or their providers rather than the trial sponsor, the estimand may no longer reflect the impact of the investigational drug. This is particularly true if the "rescue medication" is another treatment for the same indication.

When trial sponsors agree to a treatment policy strategy, all efforts should be made to keep subjects in the study (NRC 2010). This could mean providing incentives for subjects to stay in the trial and not miss visits. For those that are genuinely lost to follow-up, one may need to consider a hybrid of a treatment policy strategy and one of the strategies below.

In trials where overall survival is the endpoint of interest, a treatment policy estimand would have some advantages. There is little subjectivity involved in whether a person is alive or not though sponsors of a trial would need to determine the status of subjects that may be lost to follow-up. Sometimes to reduce missing data information external to the trial is used to determine the date of death for these study participants.

Hypothetical Strategy

A scenario is envisaged in which the intercurrent event would not occur. One would choose a value to reflect the scientific question of interest assuming a particular hypothetical scenario, i.e., what a subject's pain score would have been at the end of the study had they completed 12 weeks of treatment. Assuming a subject is comparable to a placebo subject once treatment is discontinued (Mehrotra et al. 2017) or was never on a treatment (as might be implied when using baseline observation carried forward (BOCF)) (Phillips et al. 2017) may be sensible. However, each of these approaches to dealing with an intercurrent event is distinct, and treatment estimates that follow from each of these estimands may result in different estimates of treatment effect.

Principal Stratification Strategy: Estimands and Causal Inference

Principal stratification is a means of adjusting for variables that are observed after randomization. An overview of these methods is provided by Fragakis and Rubin (2002), but several basic tutorials are available (e.g., Baker et al. 2016; Stuart et al. 2008; Dunn et al. 2005). Methods vary depending on the context of the study, the kind of post-randomization event, and the properties of the variable that describes the post-randomization event (e.g., dichotomous or continuous) and the primary outcome variable for the trial. However, the theory behind principal stratification relies heavily on the concept of causal estimands which we described briefly earlier. Namely, one needs to imagine there is a potential outcome for every subject on each treatment, but one only gets to observe one of them. Additional assumptions specific to principal stratification imply the potential outcomes for each person do not depend on the treatment status of others in the study. If subjects were not blinded to their treatment assignment, their behavior could be influenced by the outcomes of others. This section briefly describes some simpler examples.

Compliance as a Post-randomization/Intercurrent Event

In the estimand definition presented, failure to comply with the assigned treatment would be an intercurrent event. Baker et al. (2016) and Stuart et al. (2008) focus on randomized trials with two treatments (an active treatment and a control), and compliance is modeled as an all or none event, namely, subjects will either follow one treatment or the other. Dunn et al. (2005) start off with this same setting but then adds discussions on missing data. The context for these is where patients can either agree to be part of the treatment group they are assigned to via randomization ("compliers") or some may show some distinct preferences, namely, some subjects would always stay with an active treatment ("always takers") even if assigned to the control and those that would always stay with a control treatment (the latter are called "never takers" in the literature implying they would never take the active treatment). Their models also imply that there are no subjects that are "defiers." Defiers would always go to the other treatment irrespective of which treatment they are assigned to. The model assumes the distribution of always takers, never takers, and compliers is the same in the two treatment arms, a logical result of randomization. An additional assumption is that "always takers" and "never takers" will not contribute to an overall treatment effect. Namely, the subject specific causal estimand is zero for an "always taker" and zero for a "never taker." The estimate of treatment effect in compliers is then an estimate of the treatment policy estimand (namely, an estimate of treatment effect in everyone) divided by the estimate of the fraction that would comply with their randomization assignment. Generally, the treatment effect in compliers is expected to be larger than one derived using a treatment policy estimand. This very basic model does not account for dropouts, loss to follow-up, and so on. However, it does not require that we label a subject as a complier prior to randomization.

A hypothetical example in Dunn et al. (2005) illustrates the concepts. Patients are randomized to be cared for as a day patient or an inpatient, whereas the treatment received is either to be cared for as a day patient or an inpatient. Patients could in theory elect to choose a treatment option other than that assigned via randomization, and this could be the result of previous experience, costs, severity of the condition being treated, ability to get to and from day care, etc. This in turn could impact their outcome (e.g., going back to work within a week or not, a dichotomous outcome). Compliance is all or none (they do comply with one of the two treatments and they do not switch between day care and inpatient once they start a particular treatment). This may not always be realistic so one should think through the assumptions before selecting a model. Dunn et al. (2005) only consider compliance (and not the factors that may drive compliance) and a binary response variable. The latent classes for this problem are as in the paragraph above but translated to this particular problem. Compliers will stay with the randomized treatment. "Always takers" will be those that are day patients irrespective of how they were assigned, and "never takers" are those that are inpatient no matter how they were assigned via randomization. As with Stuart et al. (2008) and Baker et al. (2016), closed form equations for an estimate of the causal effect are presented with the same assumption that only compliers have a subject-specific treatment effect that is non-zero.

Stuart et al. (2008) point to a two-stage regression model that can be used to generalize beyond this simple example including incorporation of covariates that can predict participation with assigned treatments and covariates that impact the outcome or variable of interest. These have been implemented in statistics packages but are beyond the scope of this chapter.

Noncompliance and Attrition as Post-randomization (Intercurrent) Events

In reality, as noted earlier in this chapter, many studies have dropouts. Dunn et al. (2005) provide two approaches to handling missing data. One builds on the simple day care example with six categories of subjects. The six categories are determined by the latent compliance variable (always takers, compliers, and never takers) by treatment assigned via randomization. They assume that the mean outcome in each of six categories is the same as that determined by those that are observed. This may be an improvement over ignoring missing data but may not take advantage of what else is known about each subject in the study. This is called latent ignorability since one does not know the true designation of compliance status for each subject. Dunn et al. (2005) present closed form equations in this setting for a causal estimate of treatment effect in the simple case of a dichotomous outcome.

A more general approach when developing causal estimands in this setting is to develop a set of regression models:

1. One needs regression equation(s) to predict probability of being a complier for each subject even though this is a latent variable. This could be a logistic regression if one assumes compliance is described as compliers and never takers. Note: When the trial involves a novel treatment, subjects that are "always takers" will not have access to the novel treatment when assigned to the control. So they may not participate, and compliance may be regarded as a dichotomous variable.
2. A second regression equation is used to predict who is likely to drop out or not in studies in which dropouts are a concern and includes terms associated with treatment assignment and the latent compliance variable in addition to baseline variables.
3. A third equation predicts the response or outcome variable and includes both baseline covariates and variables that relate to compliance class and treatment assignment.

The covariates in each model need not be the same since there may be covariates that drive one to stay in the trial and other covariates that help predict the outcome variable. The model is fit iteratively, and Dunn et al. have proposed an approach based on a variant of maximum likelihood called "ML EM." The nice part is that one can fit such models in a number of statistical packages though the fitting options are apt to vary.

Some Cautions

Since latent variables are not "observed," these approaches could be challenged in that different assumptions regarding latent variables could yield different causal estimates of treatment effect. However, ignoring imbalances in dropouts or arbitrarily using a treatment policy estimand without thinking about compliance is not sensible. So, these models provide estimates of treatment effect allowing one to challenge the robustness of treatment effect in the presence of certain intercurrent events. When compliance is partial or dropouts are not adequately described by the models used, the models are more approximate (Stuart et al. 2008; Baker et al. 2016).

Death Before a Fixed Time as a Post-randomization (Intercurrent) Event

If the treatment is designed to improve the quality of life (QOL) in a serious chronic disease, mortality during the trial can make assessing the QOL endpoint a challenge. If the QOL measure is taken at 12 months on the treatment, and the person dies before then, one can treat survival as a dichotomous variable depending on whether the person is alive and can be evaluated at 12 months. If the assumption that mortality is not influenced by the treatment is plausible, one could elect to use a "while on treatment" strategy which is described later on. However, if this is unknown, one option is to use a principal stratification method that includes a sensitivity analysis that looks at the impact of survival on estimates of treatment effect (Chiba and Vanderweele 2011), i.e., by comparing those that are likely to survive under either treatment. In practical terms, if mortality were higher in the active treatment arm, survivors in the active group may be healthier to begin with, and better QOL values may not be attributable to the treatment under study. Note that this form of sensitivity analysis is quite different from the sensitivity analyses we present later. However, it is an analysis designed to help the evaluator gain a better understanding of what is attributable to the intervention of interest. Thus, it is in the same spirit as the sensitivity analyses we discuss later. Large differences in survival can make interpreting a QOL endpoint challenging in any case.

With death as an intercurrent event, a treatment policy estimand could be an issue. However, a treatment policy estimand could be fine if overall survival is the endpoint of interest. Context matters.

Per Protocol Analyses

In the original ICH E9 (1998), there is a discussion of a per protocol analysis. Although not following the protocol is a post-randomization event, the simple exclusion of protocol violators from an analysis would not be an example of a principal stratification since there is no effort to break the data down by principal strata in the analysis and try and develop a causal estimate of treatment effect. In real terms, the nature of dropouts could vary by treatment arm, and the proportion dropping out could be considerably different. Causal estimates are designed to compare outcomes among similar individuals. See chapter on "Intent to Treat."

Composite strategy

The occurrence of intercurrent event is taken to be a component of the variable, i.e., the intercurrent event is integrated with one or more other clinical measures of interest. For example, in a rare disease setting, the focus is on a treatment to treat multiple symptoms of the disease (e.g., headaches, diarrhea, etc.). The estimand may be defined in terms of the average number of days per week without a symptom. The use of rescue medications to alleviate any one symptom could be considered a day with a symptom. Assuming the rare disease is chronic (so subjects may be on the medication for a very long time in practice), one may wish to focus on the change from baseline versus the last week on a treatment for a weekly average number of days without symptoms.

Another approach that falls within a composite strategy would be a "responder" analysis that bins subjects into two classes, namely, success and failure. Multiple features can be considered in defining success or failure but dropouts are considered failures. While this results in a loss of information and reduced power, how treatment effect will be captured is quite clear. This should not be the sole consideration in picking an estimand. Several estimands including composite estimands are illustrated in an example later in this chapter.

While on Treatment Strategy

This would be a case where one is only interested in information prior to an intercurrent event. For example, if the treatment is a palliative treatment (e.g., for pain) in late-stage cancer, one would not want to consider data after a patient dies. Analyses that treat values after death as missing rather than nonexistent can be somewhat nonsensical. As in the section on a "Principal Stratification Strategy: Estimands and Causal Inference," if the treatment impacted survival in addition to pain, an estimand based on this strategy could be hard to interpret.

A discussion of estimands when longitudinal data and survival are in the same study can be found in Kurland et al. (2009).

Other strategies. One can combine strategies. For example, in a chronic pain trial where pain is assessed daily, use of rescue medication can be part of a composite strategy by assuming the "worst pain over the past 24-hours" is not impacted by short-term use of rescue medications. But treatment dropouts could be handled by (1) either collecting data on all subjects whether or not they take the assigned regime or more likely (2) treating subjects that leave the study as treatment failures. However, these need to be carefully considered early on as they may have ramifications for what data needs to be collected in a protocol and which statistical analyses make sense. Simulations may be necessary to see what impact decisions on intercurrent events have on operating characteristics and sample size requirements.

Other Considerations

Importance of Selecting an Estimand at the Planning Stage

By acknowledging which estimands are to be assessed, one can properly state what data needs to be collected in the protocol. Choice of an estimand may mean one needs to document why subjects leave, and trial sponsors may need to consider incentives to keep subjects in the trial. Some advice on protocol writing is on an NIH website, but it is geared for investigators needing to come to FDA to have their study plan approved (NIH-FDA 2017). It is common practice to have a protocol complete prior to finalizing an SAP. But it is logical to say an initial draft of an SAP ought to be evaluated with the protocol to be sure the right information will be collected. In the early stages of most clinical trials, both the protocol and SAP are refined, but they should be in sync with respect to the primary analyses.

Role of Covariates

The elements of an estimand (see Table 1) do not explicitly call for covariates. One can consider covariates when the estimator or the estimate of treatment effect is defined. Use of appropriate covariates can greatly improve the precision of an estimate of treatment effect and the power of a test of hypotheses. However, consider covariates that are reliably collected at screening or baseline so that use of covariates does not generate a bigger missing data issue. Covariates can also be very useful when deciding among approaches for imputing missing data (Little and Rubin 2014).

Types of Missingness

When selecting an estimand, one needs to think through the analysis options and various anticipated patterns of missing data that may occur. This could be influenced by the type of intercurrent events that are anticipated and the factors that influence whether or not these occur. Of course, estimands that do not rely on data after a patient stops taking their assigned medication means data at that stage is not considered missing and may not always be collected (nor should it be imputed). Similarly, there is no need to impute values for life after death in a sensible estimand. See "▶ Chap. 86, Missing Data," and Little and Rubin (2014).

Missing completely at random (MCAR) usually results in an analysis that ignores the reason for the missing data. As we have discussed in the section on "Principal Stratification Strategy: Estimands and Causal Inference," if missing data is thought to be unrelated to treatment assignment, intercurrent events may still impact the precision of treatment effects, but the resulting estimator and estimate may still be sensible. However, in most settings, this may be the least realistic. Missing at random (MAR) usually means the chance of being missing is a function of terms measured during the trial and incorporated into the analysis. Mehrotra et al. (2017) suggest that MAR in a longitudinal study with repeated measures involves the assumption that subjects that drop out are like the subjects that had the same values until the time drop out occurs. In drug trials subjects often drop out because they are not doing especially well on their assigned treatment group, so this assumption can be misleading and can result in an overly optimistic estimate of treatment effect. One of the most common approaches in analyzing the longitudinal studies we describe here uses a mixed model with repeated measures (noted as MMRM), which does not explicitly impute the gaps in the dataset. However, because the analysis is consistent with assuming the data is MAR, it typically generates an overly optimistic estimate of treatment effect.

Missing not at random (MNAR) is missing data that is not MAR or MCAR and is probably more common than one would like to admit. In studies with large amounts of missing data, an analysis that is consistent with an MAR assumption would be especially problematic even though one sees this in the literature on a regular basis. The reality is values that would have occurred after a subject leaves a study are at best a guess since these values do not really exist, so analysis methods that minimize the assumptions made for unobserved values are the most appropriate.

For longitudinal studies, sometimes the term "monotone missingness" is used. In the section on "Sensitivity Analysis," an approach that assumes monotone missingness (as the primary source of missing data in a trial) is discussed. Once a subject drops out, they will no longer contribute data, and they do not return. If clinicians are likely to use certain laboratory measurements to take a subject off a treatment, how that information is reflected in the data analysis should be thought out, but it would be inappropriate to consider that data as MCAR (Holzhauer et al. 2015).

Although estimands ought to be spelled out prior to selecting an estimator, there likely will be an iterative process involved. Missing data and/or protocol violations will have to be part of the conversation. This is normal when planning a clinical trial.

Estimands and Safety

There can be one estimand (or more) for efficacy and other estimands for safety. For example, in vaccine trials submitted to FDA in support of vaccines for healthy subjects, only subjects completing a prescribed regimen are typically included in the efficacy calculations. Those included in the safety assessments are those who receive at least one dose of the treatment assigned. So, efficacy and safety estimands differ and the resulting estimates may not involve using data from the same subjects.

For trials where safety is a primary outcome, such as a safety study to rule out an elevated cardiovascular risk for a drug to treat diabetes (FDA 2008), the estimand may be defined in terms of an intent to treat policy strategy where all subjects are included, whether or not they adhere to the assigned treatment regimen. This could differ from a study in which a more traditional efficacy endpoint is being used, and there are no prespecified hypotheses associated with safety.

Estimands in Studies with Time-to-Event Endpoints

In oncology and many cardiovascular trials, time to event data, such as time until death from any cause (overall survival), are common endpoints of interest. The most common measure of treatment efficacy in that setting is a hazard ratio (e.g., using a Cox proportional hazards regression). It would be hard to represent the hazard ratio as a causal estimand (see section on "Causal Inference"). But it would be inappropriate to think that some of the principles we have identified here do not apply. In many time-to-event studies, not all the patients will die (or have the event of interest) by the time the study is ended and that must be considered in the analysis. Administrative censoring refers to subjects not having the event of interest at the time the study is over and that would likely be considered non-informative (namely, the time to event and the time at which censoring occurs are regarded as independent). However, one would need to specify how other types of censoring are considered, e.g., how would one treat patients that move onto another treatment because of disease progression in a trial with overall survival as an endpoint. One may want to treat results differently if (1) patients moved onto another active treatment for the indication in question may be considered differently than (2) patients moving from the active treatment to the control arm.

Clarity in endpoints and reasons for censoring can be relevant in other time to event settings (FDA-NIH 2018). Planning in advance for how these are handled is also better science.

Estimands in Complex Designs

Adaptive designs are more common today, and some designs can alter the estimand after the start of the trial. One obvious case of this would be adaptive enrichment (Rosenblum et al. 2016) where an interim analysis is planned. Based on the interim analysis, restrict future recruitment to a prespecified subgroup of patients, e.g., those with more severe disease. This may change the estimand in that this changes the intended population; it may also alter the frequency of certain outcomes (e.g., deaths may occur at a higher frequency in a study of severely ill patients). The decision to study a subgroup should not jeopardize the overall integrity of the study (FDA 2019).

Estimands and Meta-Analysis

Meta-analyses are common when there are multiple trials designed to answer similar questions. One common objective in a meta-analysis is to provide a global estimate of treatment effect, combining information from several trials. It would be challenging to include trials with different estimands (and perhaps a different consideration of intercurrent events) into a meta-analysis. Trials of different duration are a challenge particularly if effect size is apt to change with duration. In addition, intercurrent events could be more likely if patients are observed over a longer time period. It may be necessary to obtain line data and reanalyze the data with a common estimand and a consistent approach to handling missing data in mind. This could be a challenge since many meta-analyses use summary measures from journal articles. Note this concern is distinct from the issue of relying solely on published studies.

Network Meta-Analysis

Network meta-analysis (Efthimiou et al. 2016) is often used in comparative effectiveness studies because it allows comparisons of therapies not in the same trial, but when a different population or different handling of intercurrent events occurs, the resulting analysis may make no sense. These share the same concerns as traditional meta-analyses.

Estimands in Non-inferiority (NI) Studies

NI studies are common in a regulatory environment where one wants to allow drugs and other medical products to compete with other products on the market by showing comparability rather than superiority (see chapter on "Non-inferiority").

NI studies use an already established therapy (e.g., a medical product already approved at FDA) to serve as an "active control." Previous studies are used to formulate a margin, namely, (1) considering how the active control compares to a placebo and (2) defining how to compare a new treatment to an active control. "The margin needs to be small enough to demonstrate that the novel treatment is still effective relative to placebo and part of planning can involve trying to capture what proportion of that effect needs to be conserved with the new product." The US guidance on NI studies for drugs and biologics (FDA 2016) provides advice on determining an NI margin though in other settings, the margin can be determined in other ways. In the guidance, the margin is often determined using a meta-analysis that compares a proposed active control arm to a placebo. It would be useful to have all the trials used in the meta-analysis and the planned trial to use the same estimand or at least factor the use of different estimands into which trials are or are not included when the margin is determined.

Because having a treatment effect that is close to zero is usually declared a success in this setting, non-inferiority studies with large numbers of intercurrent events could be suspected, and minimizing intercurrent events is critical (Rothmann et al. 2011).

Going from Estimand to Estimator

Different estimands may result in different estimators. However, a choice of a single estimand could result in more than one estimator that is in alignment with the estimand. As part of the estimand decision, someone may decide that data after a patient goes off treatment is not missing and therefore does not need to be collected or imputed. A choice of estimand may also limit the choice of strategies for estimating missing values via an imputation method (Phillips et al. 2017; see "▶ Chap. 86, Missing Data"). Different choices of estimands and estimators are possible and may vary even within the same broad therapeutic area. An extensive discussion of picking estimators and subsequent choices of estimation in the context of type 2 diabetes is in Holzhauer et al. (2015). They note that some estimators that are the result of a particular choice of estimand may impact the distribution of test statistics and ought to be evaluated using simulations in advance of a study. Mehrotra et al. (2017) show more than one analysis approach to addressing a specific estimand and illustrate using multiple datasets.

Estimands need to be selected such that once a trial is completed and one uses estimators consistent with an estimand, the results are interpretable. Regulators are obligated to approve products that are both safe and effective, and estimates of treatment effect will drive decision-making. However, in medical practice, there may be an interest in comparing different treatments for a given patient. Different estimands and different ways of estimating treatment effects could hamper using summary data from various trials to decide which treatments are best.

Benefit Risk

While most trials may handle effectiveness and safety separately, there is use in considering benefit and risk together. So, if one were treating patients for certain types of heart disease, drugs that reduce the risk of clots can come with an elevated risk of serious bleeding, and one may wish to define an endpoint and an estimand that formally weighs both kinds of events. Literature in this space is limited.

Sensitivity Analyses

As noted earlier, sensitivity analyses are often performed at the completion of a clinical trials. Prior to the ICH addendum (ICH 2017), sensitivity analyses were often used but not always with an explicit tie to an estimand. Common sensitivity analyses could include different treatment of outliers or challenging the distributional assumptions of an analysis (e.g., using a nonparametric method in place of a t-test). Sensitivity analyses were focused on the data analysis aspects but not always with a formal consideration of intercurrent events. There is a wealth of literature on methods for imputing missing data and many robust methods to minimize the impact of outliers. However, sponsors of a trial should be proactive in minimizing missing data when designing the trial and anticipating what data needs to be collected to provide an estimate consistent with a proposed estimand. Anticipated protocol violations and how they will be addressed need to be described in the SAP and considered when developing a sensitivity analysis.

Sensitivity analyses can challenge various aspects of the primary analysis. Our common use of covariates in randomized trials should improve the analysis while not impacting the estimand. However, in those cases where qualitative treatment by covariate interactions arise, the new treatment may be better for some while harmful for others; some common sense needs to be there. Subgroup analyses are inevitable in clinical trials (Alosh et al. 2015), but these are normally not considered part of a sensitivity analysis associated with a specific estimand.

By tying sensitivity analyses to the prespecified estimand, the sensitivity analysis is tied to the underlying research question to be answered. Scharfstein et al. (2014) have divided sensitivity analyses into ad hoc, local, and global forms of sensitivity analyses. Ad hoc sensitivity analyses correspond to the more basic assessments of assumptions of the statistical analyses just described (though such analyses do not have to be considered ad hoc), while global assessments look at the impact of dropouts on the conclusions regarding the treatment effect. This method relies on monotone missingness, namely, once a patient skips a visit, they do not come back later. This a major source of missing data in many longitudinal studies.

Leuchs et al. (2015) discuss sensitivity analyses but refer to use of alternative estimands as a type of sensitivity analyses. In the ICH E9 R1 guidance addendum (ICH 2017), these analyses are regarded as supportive analyses. So, terminology in this space is evolving.

If sensitivity analyses are prespecified, there are likely to be fewer analyses. A clearer interpretation of the trial is more likely. Studies with a large degree of noncompliance with a protocol are likely to fail certain sensitivity analyses, and all sides involved in the planning ought to discuss what that might mean before the study is over.

When one analyzes data assuming dropouts equate to a failure (e.g., assigning dropouts as the worst rank using a rank-based test), it may be reasonable to assume the analysis is regarded as primary and a sensitivity analysis using the same estimand may not be warranted. A primary analysis that still addresses intercurrent events but is accompanied with a tipping point analysis is another approach. Ouyang et al. (2017) describe "tipping point analyses used to explore how extreme and detrimental outcomes among subjects with missing data need to be to overturn the positive treatment effect attained in subjects with complete data." There have been multiple approaches to tipping point analyses, but they often involve challenging a primary analysis by deciding what changes in values associated with intercurrent events lead to a different conclusion regarding study success (e.g., Mehrotra et al. 2017; Scharfstein et al. 2014; Campbell et al. 2011). Approaches differ by how missing data and protocol violators are handled. Tipping point analyses minimize reliance on methods that ignore the reasons for the missing data, or possibly make conservative assumptions regarding likely values that substitute for a missing value. Most tipping point results are captured in a table or graph and would require subject matter experts to interpret.

There are sensitivity analyses specific to time to event analyses, but these are beyond the scope of this chapter. Distinguishing a primary analysis from a sensitivity analysis when reporting results would be important.

An Example

An example from the US FDA is presented (authors are not permitted to share the line data). It illustrates the discussions presented on estimands and sensitivity analyses (namely, tipping point analyses) in the context of formal decision-making. First some issues that arise when designing clinical trials to evaluate pain medications are discussed first.

Challenges for Clinical Trials to Evaluate Pain Medications

Pain can be categorized according to duration, acute or chronic, as well as other characteristics such as breakthrough pain (i.e., acute episodes of pain that occur on a background of well-controlled chronic pain). Acute pain is defined as pain that is self-limiting and generally requires treatment for no more than a few weeks (e.g., postoperative pain after various types of surgeries). In contrast, chronic pain is defined as pain persisting longer than 3 months (e.g., chronic lower back pain and pain associated with spinal cord injuries (SCI)). See the Initiative on Methods, Measurements, and Pain Assessments in Clinical Trials (IMMPACT 2011) and Analgesic, Anesthetic, and Addiction Clinical Trial Translation, Innovations, Opportunities, and Network (ACTTION 2002) websites for more information regarding different trial designs.

Pain, the primary efficacy endpoint of interest, is subjective in nature and is measured by a subject self-reporting their pain. It is often measured daily on an 11-point numerical rating scale (NRS) where a score of 0 indicates no pain and 10 is the worst pain possible. Other scales may be acceptable. In chronic pain, these conditions could last a lifetime, but a randomized double-blind, adequate, and well-controlled trial where each subject is on study medication for about 12 weeks has been accepted as a reasonable assessment of long-term use. To ensure subjects have adequate pain and to demonstrate an effect, subjects are generally required to have a minimum pain score of at least 4 over a given timeframe to be eligible for randomization into the trial. To determine if a drug is working, mean change from baseline pain at the end of an agreed to time is used as a primary summary statistic, though a difference in trimmed means (Permutt and Li 2017) could also be considered. Measurements recorded between baseline and the agreed to time can improve the efficiency of the analysis or possibly provide a basis for imputing missing values. Often an MMRM analysis is conducted where a difference in adjusted means at week 12 is the comparison of interest.

Chronic pain trials often have 30–50% of subjects discontinuing due to lack of efficacy (placebo group) and/or intolerability (active drug). Two methods are commonly utilized to minimize these discontinuations:

- Allow subjects to use rescue medication to minimize study discontinuations due to lack of efficacy. The protocol should specify the type and amount of rescue medication that will be allowed during the study. Rescue medication use needs to be done in a manner that does not interfere with scheduled pain assessments. In chronic pain trials, short-term use of rescue medication is often not considered when evaluating pain since the worst pain experienced in the previous 24 h includes pain assessed prior to taking rescue medication. All use of rescue medications is recorded. It would be a concern if treatment arm subjects used more rescue medications than those on the placebo arm (Dworkin et al. 2005).
- To minimize discontinuations due to intolerability to study drug, during the first 2–3 weeks of the trial, often in an open-label fashion, subjects are titrated to an effective dose of study drug. Only subjects who achieve an effective dose of

the experimental drug are randomized into the double-blind treatment phase. Randomized subjects either stay on active treatment or switch to the control group. If the control group is a placebo, subjects are tapered off the active drug to minimize discontinuations due to withdrawal symptoms and to assist in maintaining the blinding of the study. This is referred to as an enriched enrollment withdrawal design. Even with this design, subjects still discontinue active treatment for lack of efficacy and adverse events (Katz 2009).

In chronic pain trials, subjects that discontinue treatment will most likely switch to other therapies. This makes an estimand based on a treatment policy strategy difficult to interpret since it measures the impact of "treatment plus other therapies" versus "placebo plus other therapies." An estimand using a composite strategy that considers treatment discontinuations as failures is more commonly used. The focus is on the difference in the two treatments at week 12 as this is a chronic condition although subjects may stay on a drug considerably longer if approved.

Sometimes one sees a responder analysis in this setting. A responder is a subject that shows a prespecified improvement in baseline pain, such as a 30% or 50% improvement which has been deemed to be clinically relevant. This responder definition may also include use of rescue medication such as no use or less than a specific amount. For example, if a subject uses rescue medication for 7 consecutive days or longer, they are considered a non-responder in the primary analysis (Dworkin et al. 2005). So, subjects are either a responder or a non-responder. This approach has often been criticized as having less power, but it is easy to implement.

A method that retains more information than a dichotomy of response utilizes a continuous responder curve with an appropriate corresponding analysis. We illustrate this in our FDA example below.

Estimands, Estimation, and Sensitivity Analysis Illustrated Using an FDA Example

This example was submitted to FDA in a New Drug Application (NDA). Statistical and clinical reviews are provided by FDA at the Drugs@FDA weblink (FDA 2020). The study will be briefly described along with a discussion of possible estimands and estimators along with corresponding estimates of treatment effect. These were previously presented (Petullo 2016).

This was an 18-week (4-week dose-adjustment phase, 12-week fixed-dose maintenance phase, 1-week taper phase, 1-week follow-up phase) randomized, double-blind, placebo-controlled, multicenter trial. Subjects were started on 150 mg per day or placebo and titrated to a target dose range of 150–600 mg per day. Subjects were required to have a diagnosis of traumatic SCI of at least 1-year duration with central neuropathic pain that had persisted continuously for at least 3 months or with remissions and relapses for at least 6 months. Concomitant analgesics were allowed if subjects were on a stable dose regimen prior to randomization. Subjects must have had an average daily pain score of at least 4 (0–10 NRS) during the 7 days prior to randomization.

The study randomized 219 subjects, 108 subjects in the placebo arm and 111 in the active arm. There were approximately 15% of subjects with missing data at Week 16 (15% in the placebo arm and 17% in the active arm). There were similar numbers dropping out for adverse events and lack of efficacy in both treatment arms.

When this study was planned, conducted, and reviewed by FDA, a primary estimand of interest was not explicitly stated, but the estimand that corresponds to the analysis to support approval is presented along with how it was estimated.

A **composite strategy was used to define an estimand**, i.e., to define the effect of the active drug for treating neuropathic pain associated with SCI. Use of this estimand did not require follow-up of subjects after treatment discontinuation as they are considered treatment failures or non-responders. The four components of this estimand are described below:

(A) Population: Subjects with traumatic SCI of at least 1-year duration with central neuropathic pain that had persisted continuously for at least 3 months or with remissions and relapses for at least 6 months.
(B) Variable: Change from baseline pain score Week 16. (Baseline pain was defined as the pain prior to the OL titration phase.)
(C) Intercurrent Event: Subject did not complete 16 weeks of treatment. Subjects that experienced the intercurrent event were considered as having no improvement in baseline pain.
(D) Population-Level Summary: Difference in mean change in baseline pain at Week 16 comparing subjects with neuropathic pain associated with spinal cord injuries assigned to active drug versus those assigned to placebo.

The analysis used to estimate the population-level summary was an analysis of covariance (ANCOVA) with treatment as a fixed effect and baseline pain as a covariate. Subjects that discontinued were assigned the baseline value as the Week 16 value (i.e., a BOCF strategy). Results from the ANCOVA analysis gave an estimated mean change from baseline at Week 16 of 1.1 and 1.7 for placebo and active drug, respectively. The estimated difference of 0.6 (95% CI: 0.1, 1.1) was significant with a p-value<0.01 (FDA 2020). This was considered the primary analysis at the time of review.

An alternative estimand based on a composite strategy is also feasible. Parts A. and B. of the estimand above are the same as above, but parts C. and D. are changed:

(C) Intercurrent Event: Patient failed to complete 16 weeks of treatment. Subjects that fail to complete are assigned a poor outcome.
(D) Population-Level Summary: Difference in mean change from baseline pain at Week 16 in the best 80% of subjects from each treatment arm comparing subjects with neuropathic pain associated with spinal cord injuries (a logical

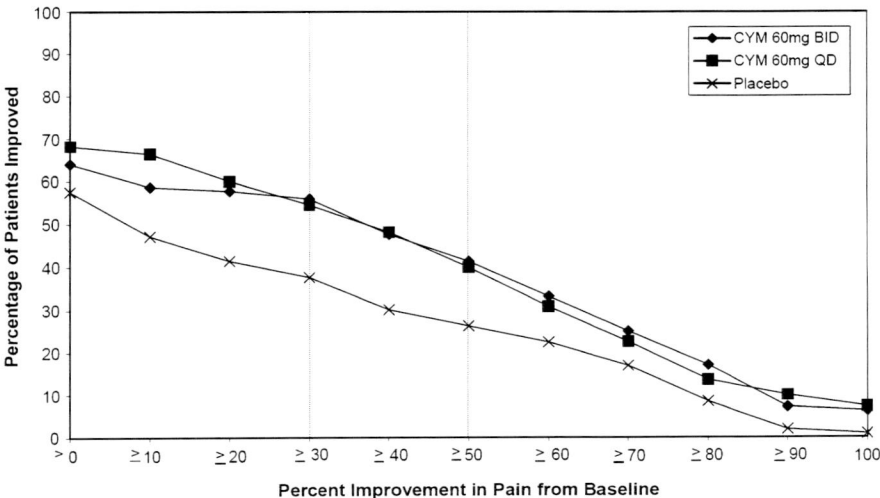

Fig. 1 Continuous responder curves – composite estimand

graphical display of the data in support of a trimmed mean analysis could be continuous responder curves; see Fig. 1).

As noted above, 15% of placebo subjects discontinued versus 17% of active subjects. Therefore, trim at least 17% of the data from both treatment arms. To simplify, a 20% trimmed mean was selected. It is important to note that this should be prespecified and should at a minimum trim all dropouts. Compare the differences in trimmed means using a permutation test though if one only wanted a p-value rather than an estimate of treatment effect, one could use a rank test with failures being assigned the worst rank.

The 20% trimmed mean for placebo was −0.9 and −1.9 for the active arm. The difference in trimmed means in this example was −1.0 (95% CI: −1.4, −0.5). Using a permutation test, the difference was considered significant, with a p-value less than 0.001. The continuous responder curve in Fig. 1 is a useful way of graphically displaying results when a trimmed mean is used (see Farrar et al. 2006).

An Estimand, Estimate, and a Tipping Point Analysis

For the estimands in the example above, subjects that discontinued treatment were considered as treatment failures, and imputation was simple. If the primary analysis uses a more optimistic assumption, namely, that those that dropped out were like those that stayed in up until they left an analysis consistent with an MAR assumption can be the primary analysis. A tipping point analysis evaluating how sensitive the results was to this assumption is worth considering. Starting from a MAR

Table 2 Tipping point analysis (Petullo et al. 2016)

Shift in mean change from baseline at Week 16: difference from placebo: mean (95% CI)							
		Placebo					
		0	0.5	1.0	1.5	2.0	2.5
Lyrica	0	0.8 (0.3, 1.4)	0.9 (−0.4, 1.5)	1.0 (0.4, 1.5)	1.1 (0.5, 1.6)	1.1 (0.6, 1.7)	1.2 (0.7, 1.8)
	−0.5	0.8 (0.2, 1.3)	0.8 (−1.4, −0.3)	0.9 (0.4, 1.5)	1.0 (0.4, 1.5)	1.1 (0.5, 1.6)	1.1 (0.6, 1.7)
	−1.0	0.7 (0.1, 1.2)	0.8 (−1.3, −0.2)	0.8 (0.3, 1.4)	0.9 (0.3, 1.5)	1.0 (0.4, 1.5)	1.1 (0.5, 1.6)
	−1.5	0.6 (0.0, 1.2)	0.7 (0.1, 1.2)	0.7 (0.2, 1.3)	0.8 (0.3, 1.4)	0.9 (0.3, 1.5)	1.0 (0.4, 1.5)
	−2.0	0.5 (0.1, 1.1)	0.6 (0.0, 1.1)	0.7 (0.1, 1.2)	0.7 (0.2, 1.3)	0.8 (0.2, 1.4)	0.9 (0.3, 1.5)
	−2.5	0.4 (−0.1, 1.0)	0.5 (−0.1, 1.0)	0.6 (0, 1.21.2)	0.7 (0.1, 1.2)	0.7 (0.1, 1.3)	0.8 (0.2, 1.4)

assumption, the tipping point analysis varies the pains scores for subjects with missing outcomes. The missing outcomes on each treatment arm are allowed to vary independently and includes scenarios where dropouts on the active arm have worse outcomes than dropouts on control. The goal is to explore the plausibility of missing data assumptions under which there is no longer evidence of a treatment effect. As seen in Table 2, the analysis only tips, i.e., p-value >0.05, if missing data for active subjects are assumed to have a much worse outcome than missing data for placebo subjects. In this example, the various analyses did not appear to impact the final conclusions. When it does, those involved in the analysis and interpretation of the trial need to determine what this means. The choice of a particular primary analysis and sensitivity analysis could depend on the degree of missing data anticipated, and MAR as a starting assumption for data analysis could be quite plausible in settings where dropouts are not all that frequent. It may not be ideal in pain studies where dropouts are common.

Conclusion

The importance of considering both estimands and sensitivity analyses and their role in planning of clinical trials was described here. It is possible to have more than one plausible estimand and more than one analysis. But it is anticipated that all those involved in the trial planning and assessment will understand what is going to be presented when a trial is completed.

It is hoped that greater considerations at the planning stage of things that can go awry will lead to better writing of protocols and analysis plans. Thinking through the options before a study starts could impact what data needs to be collected, what is regarded as missing, and will limit the number and kinds of analyses that are reasonable given the question of interest. It is recognized that one cannot anticipate all things that can happen in a clinical trial, but that does not mean planning to prevent or minimize problems that have occurred in related trials is unimportant. Some of the attention to this topic has been motivated by regulators, but the principles described are not solely applicable to trials for medical product approvals.

Finally, we recognize that more complex analytical approaches to handling missing data exist. See "▶ Chap. 86, Missing Data."

Key Facts

- When the patterns of intercurrent events occurring after treatment assignment differ by treatment arm, interpretation of treatment effects can be challenging or even misleading.
- If one formulates an estimand without considering how intercurrent events will factor into the estimand, the study may not answer the question the trial is intended to answer.
- The **statistical analysis plan** ought to address how intercurrent events will impact the estimated treatment effects to be calculated and the estimate ought to follow logically from the proposed estimand.
- Sensitivity analyses designed to challenge the assumptions associated with a primary set of analyses are best understood if planned in conjunction with the formulation of an estimand.
- Methods to minimize intercurrent events are important in clinical trials.

Cross-References

► Missing Data

References

ACTTION (2002) Analgesic, Anesthetic, and Addiction Clinical Trial Translations, Innovations, Opportunities, and Networks (ACTTION). www.acttion.org. Accessed Jan 2019

Alosh M, Fritsch K, Huque M, Mahjoob K, Pennello G, Rothmann M, Russek-Cohen E, Smith F, Wilson S, Yue L (2015) Statistical considerations on subgroup analysis in clinical trials. Stat Biopharm Res 7:286–303

Baker SG, Kramer BS, Lindemen KS (2016) Latent class instrumental variables: a clinical and biostatistical perspective. Stat Med 35:147–160

Campbell G, Pennello G, Yue L (2011) Missing data in the regulation of medical devices. J Biopharm Stat 21:180–195

Chiba, Vanderweele (2011) A simple method for principal strata effects when the outcome is truncated due to death. Am J Epidemiol 173:745–751

Dunn G, Maracy M, Tomenton B (2005) Estimating treatment effects from randomized clinical trials with noncompliance and loss to follow-up: the role of instrumental variable methods. Stat Methods Med Res 14:369–395

Dworkin RH, Turk DC, Farrar JT, Haythornthwaite JA, Jensen MP, Katz NP, Kerns RD, Stucki G, Allen RR, Bellamy N, Carr DB, Chandler J, Cowan P, Dionne R, Galer BS, Hertz S, Jadad AR, Kramer LD, Manning DC, Martin S, McCormick CG, McDermott MP, McGrath P, Quessy S, Rappaport BA, Robbins W, Robinson JP, Rothman M, Royal MA, Simon L, Stauffer JW, Stein W, Tollett J, Wernicke J, Witter J (2005) Core outcome measures for chronic pain trials: IMMPACT recommendations. Pain 113(1–2):9–19

Efthimiou O, Debray TPA, van Valkenhoef G, Trelle S, Panaidou K, Moons KGM, Reitsma JB, Shang A, Salanti G et al (2016) GetReal in network meta-analysis: a review of the methodology. Res Synth Methods 7:236–263

Farrar JT, Dworkin RH, Max MB (2006) Use of the cumulative proportion analysis graph to present data over a range of cut-off points: making clinical trial data more understandable. J Pain Symptom Manag 31(4):369–377

FDA (2020) Drugs@FDA https:// HYPERLINK. http://www.accessdata.Fda.gov/scripts/cder/daf

FDA-NIH Biomarker Working Group BEST (Biomarkers, Endpoints, and other tools) Resource (Internet). Silver Spring, Glossary Created 2016 Jan 28 (Updated 2018 May 2) Co-published by National Institutes of Health (US), Bethesda

Fletcher C, Tsuchiya S, Mehrotra D (2017) Current practices in choosing Estimands and sensitivity analyses in clinical trials: results of the ICH E9 survey. Therapeutic Innovation and Regulatory. Science 51:69–76

Ford I, Norrie J (2016) Pragmatic trials. NEJM 375:454–463

Fragakis CE, Rubin DB (2002) Principal stratification in causal inference. Biometrics 58:21–29

Holzhauer B, Akacha M, Bermann G (2015) Choice of estimand and analysis methods in diabetes trials with rescue medication. Pharm Stat 14:433–447

ICH (1998) E9: Guideline on statistical principles for clinical trials. http://www.ich.org

ICH (2014) E9 concept paper on estimands and sensitivity analyses. http://www.ich.org

ICH (2017) E9 R1: Addendum on estimands and sensitivity analyses in clinical trials. Step 2. www.ich.org

IMMPACT (2011) Initiative on methods, measurement, and pain assessment in clinical trials (IMMPACT). www.immpact.com. Accessed Jan 2019

Katz N (2009) Enriched enrollment randomized withdrawal trial designs of analgesics: focus on methodology. Clin J Pain 25(9):797–807

Kurland BF, Johnson LL, Egleston BL, Diehr PH (2009) Longitudinal data with follow-up truncated by death: match the analysis method to research aims. Stat Sci 24:211–222

Lavange LM, Permutt T (2016) A regulatory perspective on missing data in the aftermath of the NRC report. Stat Med 35:2853–2864

Leuchs A, Zinserling J, Brandt A, Wirtz D, Benda N (2015) Choosing appropriate estimands in clinical trials. Therapeutic innovation and Regulatory. Science 49:584–592

Little RJA, Rubin DB (2000) Casual effects in clinical and epidemiological studies via potential outcomes: concepts and analytical approaches. Annu Rev Public Health 21:121–145

Little RJA, Rubin DB (2014) Statistical analysis with missing data, 2nd edn. Wiley, New York. 408pp

Mallinckrodt CH, Lin Q, Lipkovich I, Molenberghs (2012) A structured approach to choosing estimands in longitudinal clinical trials. Pharm Stat 11:456–461

Mehrotra D, Liu F, Permutt T (2017) Missing data in clinical trials: control based mean imputation and sensitivity analysis. Pharm Stat 16:378–392

National Research Council (2010) The prevention and treatment of missing data in clinical trials. National Academies of Science Press, Washington, DC

O'Neill RT, Temple R (2012) The prevention and treatment of missing data in clinical trials: an FDA perspective on the importance of dealing with it. Clin Pharmacol Ther 91:550–554

Ouyang J, Carroll KJ, Koch G, Li J (2017) Coping with missing data in phase III pivotal registration trials: Tolvaptan in subjects with kidney disease, a case study. Pharm Stat 16:250–266

Permutt T (2016) A taxonomy of Estimands for regulatory clinical trials with discontinuations. Stat Med 35:2865–2864

Permutt T, Li F (2017) Trimmed means for symptom trials with dropouts. Pharm Stat 16:20–283

Petullo D (2016) Statistical review and evaluation. https://www.accessdata.fda.gov/drugsatfda_docs/nda/2012/021446Orig1s028StatR.pdf

Petullo D, Permutt T, Li F (2016) An alternative to data imputation in analgesic clinical trials. American Pain Society Conference on Analgesic Trials, Austin Texas

Phillips A, Abellan-Andres J, Soren A, Bretz F, Fletcher C, FranceI GA, Harris R, Kjaer M, Keene O, Morgan D, O'Kelley M, Roger J (2017) Estimands: discussion points from the PSI estimands and sensitivity expert group. Pharm Stat 16:6–11

Rosenblum M, Qian T, Du Y, Qiu H, Fisher A (2016) Multiple testing procedures for adaptive enrichment designs: combining group sequential and reallocation approaches. Biostatistics 17(4):650–662

Rothmann MD, Wiens BL, Chan ISF (2011) Design and analysis of non-inferiority trials. Chapman & Hall/CRC, CRC Press lists Boca Raton, FL, 454p

Scharfstein D, McDermott A, Olson W, Wiegand F (2014) Global sensitivity analyses with informative dropouts: a fully parametric approach. Stat Biopharm Res 6:338–348

Stuart EA, Perry DF, Le H-N, Ialongo NS (2008) Estimating intervention effects of prevention programs: accounting for noncompliance. Prev Sci 9:288–298

US FDA (2008) Guideline for industry: diabetes mellitus-evaluating cardiovascular risk in new antidiabetic therapies to treat Type 2 diabetes. Dec 2008. https://www.fda.gov/downloads/Drugs/Guidances/UCM071627

US FDA (2016) Non-inferiority clinical trials to establish effectiveness: guidance for industry. Nov 2016. https://www.fda.gov/downloads/Drugs/Guidances/UCM202140

US FDA (2018) Product label for Cymbalta. https://www.accessdata.fda.gov/drugsatfda_docs/label/2008/022148lbl.pdf. Accessed Jan 2019

US FDA (2019) Adaptive designs for clinical trials for drugs and biologics: guidance for industry. https://www.fda.gov/media/78495/download. Accessed 24 April 2020

US National Institutes of Health-Food and Drug Administration (2017) NIH-FDA Protocol template. https://osp.od.nih.gov/clinical-research/clinical-trials. Accessed 9 Nov 2018

Confident Statistical Inference with Multiple Outcomes, Subgroups, and Other Issues of Multiplicity

85

Siyoen Kil, Eloise Kaizar, Szu-Yu Tang, and Jason C. Hsu

Contents

Introduction	1660
Patient Targeting for a Targeted Therapy	1660
Strength of Error Rate Controls in Patient Targeting	1661
Respecting Logical Relationships	1664
Three Kinds of Outcome Measures	1664
A Common Misconception	1665
Binary Outcome	1666
Time-to-Event Outcome	1669
The Subgroup Mixable Estimation (SME) Principle	1671
Effect of the Prognostic Factor on Permutation Tests	1672
Data Model	1672
Predictive Null Hypothesis	1673
Test Statistic and Reference Distributions	1674
Numerical Study	1675
Summary and Conclusions	1678
Key Facts	1678
Cross-References	1678
References	1679

S. Kil
LSK Global Pharmaceutical Services, Seoul, Republic of Korea

E. Kaizar
The Ohio State University, Columbus, OH, USA
e-mail: kaizar.1@osu.edu

S.-Y. Tang
Roche Tissue Diagnostics, Oro Valley, AZ, USA
e-mail: tang.142@buckeyemail.osu.edu

J. C. Hsu (✉)
Department of Statistics, The Ohio State University, Columbus, OH, USA
e-mail: jch@stat.osu.edu

© Springer Nature Switzerland AG 2022
S. Piantadosi, C. L. Meinert (eds.), *Principles and Practice of Clinical Trials*,
https://doi.org/10.1007/978-3-319-52636-2_116

Abstract

This chapter starts with a thorough discussion of different multiple comparison error rates, including weak and strong control for multiple tests and noncoverage probability for confidence sets. With multiple endpoints as an example, it describes which error rate controls would translate to incorrect decision rate controls. Then, using targeted therapy as the context, this chapter discusses a potential issue with some efficacy measures in terms of respecting logical relationships among the subgroups. A statistical principle that helps avoid this issue is described. As another example of multiplicity-induced issues to be aware of, it is shown that permutation test for patient targeting may not control Type I error rate in some situations. Finally, a list of the key points and a summary of the conclusions are given.

Keywords

Subgroups · Multiple comparisons · Prognostic effect · Permutation tests

Introduction

Multiplicity issues arise in clinical trials due to having multiple treatments, endpoints, and subgroups. Using precision medicine as the context, this chapter describes multiple comparison principles that help ensure proper error rate control. To start, the extent of each multiple comparison Type I error rate control ensures control of the incorrect decision rate is discussed. Then, which efficacy measures that respect natural logical relationships among patient subgroups are enumerated. The Subgroup Mixable Estimation (SME) principle for achieving statistical inference that respects such logic is described. It is also shown that permutation testing is a technique that should be avoided, as it does not produce a valid null distribution with a discrete outcome even with only one subgroup classifier. Finally, a list of key points is given, and a summary of the conclusions is provided.

Patient Targeting for a Targeted Therapy

Targeted therapies, which as Woodcock (2015) states are sometimes called "personalized medicine" or "precision medicine," target specific pathways.

Suppose a companion diagnostic test (CDx) divides patients into a marker-positive (g^+) subgroup and its complementary marker-negative (g^-) subgroup. Call the entire patient population $\{g^+, g^-\}$ "all-comers." If all-comers or a patient subgroup can confidently be inferred to receive clinically meaningful efficacy, then a decision is made to target all-comers or that subgroup. If no patient group can be identified as receiving clinically meaningful efficacy, then development of that therapy has failed.

With a biomarker that may be predictive of treatment response, for every potential cut-point value c of the biomarker, efficacy is assessed in the marker-positive patients (g_c^+ patients, those with values $>c$), marker-negative patients (g_c^- patients, those with values $<c$), and in the all-comer $\{g^+, g^-\}$ population.

Statistical methods for patient targeting should control the probability of incorrect targeting, the probability that a targeted patient group does not derive clinically meaningful efficacy from the treatment it is given.

Strength of Error Rate Controls in Patient Targeting

A statistical error rate control has meaning only if it translates to an incorrect decision rate control.

Consider a two-arm randomized clinical trial (RCT). Denote "treatment" and "control" by Rx and C, and assume there is no differential propensity in treatment assignment, so that under the Rx and the C arms, the prevalence of the g^+ subgroup is the same in the *population* by γ^+.

In this setting with multiple subgroups and potentially multiple endpoints, multiple comparisons are made. Tukey (1953), which has been reprinted as Tukey (1994), defined three kinds of multiple comparison error rates: *per comparison*, *per family*, and *familywise*. For confirmatory studies, the familywise error rate (FWER) is most relevant. Inference in Tukey (1953) is in the form of confidence intervals, and FWER is defined as the (maximum) probability that at least one of the simultaneous confidence intervals fails to cover its true value. When FWER is applied to tests of null hypotheses, there has been some confusion as to what it is. We explain, in a test of hypotheses setting, what FWER control needs to be, in order to control the rate of incorrect decision-making.

Null Control

Some methods for patient targeting offer error rate control under what can be called the *null* null hypothesis. The *null* null hypothesis is that Rx has exactly the same effect as C for all biomarker subgroups. In other words, there is no treatment effect or biomarker effect whatsoever.

If the outcome is survival time, say, then under the *null* null, all patients come from a single group with the same survival curve, regardless of whether they are given Rx and C, or what biomarker value they have.

In a lucid paper written before the adoption of modern concepts of multiple comparison error rate control, Miller and Siegmund (1982) suggest forming 2×2 tables of Rx vs. C and responder vs. nonresponder at every cut-point and then selecting the cut-point with the maximum chi-square statistic value. Their critical value calculation for testing that the *observed* differential efficacy between the g^+

patients and g^- patients at the *sample* maximum chi-square statistic is not just due to random sample fluctuation is under the *null* null hypothesis.

As John W. Tukey would say, "controlling the Type I error rate testing a *null* null is a null guarantee," because there will surely be some difference between Rx and C effects, if measured to enough decimal places. A *null* null is even more restrictive than a *complete* null used in weak control.

Weak Control

The *complete* null is where *all* the null hypotheses are true. Controlling the Type I error rate under the *complete* null is termed *weak* control.

When there are subgroups, the null hypothesis for each subgroup is Rx and C have the same effect in that subgroup. So, under the *complete* null, the biomarker can have an effect (a *prognostic* effect), but effects of Rx and C do not differ in each of the subgroups.

Thus, weak control controls the probability of inferring Rx and C have different effects in at least one subgroup, when in fact Rx and C have the same effect in all the subgroups.

Suppose there is originally a single primary endpoint E1. If only weak Type I error rate control is required, then one can game the system by artificially introducing a second primary endpoint E2, a co-primary endpoint so that Rx is approved only if its efficacy relative to C is shown in both endpoints E1 and E2. It would seem that adding E2 would not make getting Rx approved easier.

Suppose the Statistical Analysis Plan (SAP) is a two-step process, as follows:

Step 1 Test, at the 5% level, the complete null hypothesis that there is no difference between Rx and C for either endpoint; if the complete null hypothesis is rejected, then go to Step 2; otherwise Stop.
Step 2 Infer Rx is better than C.

This procedure controls the Type I error rate weakly at 5%, but what is its incorrect decision rate?

Suppose E2, a clinically meaningless endpoint, is chosen on the basis that it is a sure bet that efficacy in this endpoint can be proven. Then, at the end of the study, the complete null will surely be rejected, and Rx is guaranteed to be approved by this procedure (regardless of what the data indicates). If Rx is in fact slightly worse than C on endpoint E1, then the probability of an incorrect decision can in fact be close to one-half. Clearly, weak control of the Type I error rate may not translate to control of the incorrect decision rate. Requiring strong control ameliorates this concern.

Similarly, weak control is insufficient to control the incorrect targeting rate, because it does not control the probability of inferring Rx is better than C for g^- patients when they have the same effect in g^-, if it is true that Rx is better than C for g^+ patients, for example.

Even with these known limitations, some methods for subgroup identification rely on weak control. The machine learning approach of Lipkovich et al. (2011) and the likelihood ratio testing approach of Jiang et al. (2007) compute the *null* distributions by *permutation* which, as explained in Xu and Hsu (2007) and Kaizar et al. (2011), requires the subtle MDJ (marginals-determine-the-joint) assumption to control Type I error rate weakly (The crux of the matter is that permutation generates a null distribution assuming the *joint* distribution of observations are identical under *Rx* and *C* across all biomarker values, while the complete null only specifies that the *marginal* distributions are the same.).

MDJ If a subset of the null hypotheses that state under *Rx* and *C* the *marginal* distributions of the observations are identical are true, then the *joint* distributions of the observations are identical under *Rx* and *C* for that subset as well.

In applying any permutation-based technique, whether MDJ holds should be checked.

Strong Control

Strong control of Type I error rate means that even if some of the null hypotheses are false, the probability of *rejecting at least one true null* hypothesis is controlled.

Strong control would control the probability of incorrect decision if the null hypotheses are appropriately formulated.

Confident Directional Control

Actionable inferences are *directional* in nature: *Rx* is better than *C*, or *Rx* is worse than *C*. As explained in Section 5 of Lin et al. (2019), basing directional decisions on confidence intervals automatically controls the directional error rate: if one infers $\mu > 0$ when its 95% confidence interval is entirely larger than zero, then the probability of inferring $\mu > 0$ when in fact $\mu \leq 0$ is at most 5%. Such methods are what Tukey (1953) calls *confident direction* methods.

It is an incorrect perception that stepwise testing methods do not have confidence sets. Actually, so long as the union of the null hypotheses being tested by a multiple test covers the entire parameter space, the Partitioning Principle (as described, e.g., in Huang and Hsu 2007) can be used to pivot the test to a corresponding confidence set (The name *The Partitioning Principle* was officially coined by Finner and Strassburger (2002). Historically, this principle was independently developed by Helmut Finner and associates as well as Takeuchi (1973, 2010) and Stefansson et al. (1988).). See Stefansson et al. (1988), Hayter and Hsu (1994), Hsu (1996), and Hsu and Berger (1999) for examples of using the pivoting technique, and Finner and Strassburger (2007) and Strassburger and Bretz (2008) for additional examples. We thus urge more attention be paid to checking whether proposed multiple tests have associated confidence sets.

Respecting Logical Relationships

Subgroups can be defined by biomarkers or by other characteristics such as regions. In the former case, decision-making involves assessing efficacy in the subgroups and their mixtures. In the latter case, typical practice is to adjust for baseline differences in the subgroups in assessing a presumed common efficacy across the subgroups, though therapies are approved separately for each region. This chapter focuses on the former situation.

Let $\mu^{Rx}(x)$ and $\mu^C(x)$ denote the true effect of Rx and C at each biomarker value x. Recall $p(x)$ is the density of patient biomarker values in the population which, in our RCT setting, is the same for Rx and C. Suppose a biomarker cut-point value c divides the entire population into two subgroups, $g_c^+\{x \geq c\}$ and $g_c^-\{x < c\}$.

Denote the true (unknown) efficacy in g_c^+, g_c^-, and all-comers $\{all\}$ by $\eta_{g_c^+}, \eta_{g_c^-}, \eta_{\{all\}}$, respectively. Since all-comers are a mixture of g_c^+ and g_c^-, it seems desirable for efficacy measures to meet the criterion that efficacy for all-comers lies between the efficacies of the complementary subgroups:

Definition : An efficacy measure is logic−respecting if

$$\eta_{\{all\}} \in [\eta_{g_c^-}, \eta_{g_c^+}] \forall c \in (a, b) \tag{1}$$

Note that *logic-respecting* is a property of an efficacy measure, not a property of the type of data that quantifies outcome, or a statistical model for such data.

Three Kinds of Outcome Measures

Outcome measures in some therapeutic areas are continuous in nature (To be precise, by "continuous" outcome, we mean the observed response is modeled linearly with iid Normally distributed errors.). For Type 2 diabetes, *change* in hemoglobin A1c from baseline A1c is the usual clinical measure of a treatment's effect. For schizophrenia, *change* in Positive and Negative Syndrome Scale from baseline is a typical clinical measure of a treatment's effect. For Alzheimer's disease, *change* in Alzheimer's Disease Assessment Scale-Cognitive Subscale from baseline is a common measure of a treatment's effect.

In oncology, a typical primary endpoint for phase 3 studies is overall survival (OS), while for phase 2 oncology studies, the primary endpoint may be progression-free survival (PFS) or objective response rate (ORR). OS and PFS are time-to-event endpoints, while ORR is a binary endpoint.

There seems to be a belief that, based on asymptotic normality, knowledge about continuous outcome automatically carries over to binary or survival outcomes. Indeed, examples of applications of multiple comparison methods in Hsu (1996) are almost all for continuous outcomes. However, analyzing precision medicine data made us realize that reality is more complex.

Denote by $\mu_{g^+}^{Rx}, \mu_{g^-}^{Rx}, \mu_{g^+}^{C}, \mu_{g^-}^{C}$ the true *expected* outcomes in the g^+ and g^- subgroups for each treatment arm and denote by μ^{Rx} and μ^{C} the true *expected* outcome over the entire patient population if the entire population had received Rx or C, respectively. In therapeutic areas such as Type 2 diabetes and Alzheimer's disease with continuous outcome measures, traditionally efficacy of Rx vs. C is measured by the *difference* of *mean* treatment and control effects, so

$$\eta_{g^+} = \mu_{g^+}^{Rx} - \mu_{g^+}^{C} \text{ and } \eta_{g^-} = \mu_{g^-}^{Rx} - \mu_{g^-}^{C}$$

represent efficacy of Rx vs. C in the g^+ and g^- subgroups. In our RCT setting, with population prevalence of the g^+ subgroup being γ^+,

$$\mu^{Rx} = \gamma^+ \times \mu_{g^+}^{Rx} + (1 - \gamma^+) \times \mu_{g^-}^{Rx}, \qquad (2)$$

$$\mu^{C} = \gamma^+ \times \mu_{g^+}^{C} + (1 - \gamma^+) \times \mu_{g^-}^{C}. \qquad (3)$$

Therefore, in the case of efficacy being a difference of means, efficacy in the combined population is

$$\eta_{\{g^+,g^-\}} = \mu^{Rx} - \mu^{C} = \gamma^+ \times \eta_{g^+} + (1 - \gamma^+) \times \eta_{g^-}, \qquad (4)$$

and is therefore logic-respecting.

A Common Misconception

So, for efficacy measured as a *difference* of *means*, efficacy in all-comers $\eta_{\{g^+,g^-\}}$ can be determined by efficacies η_{g^+} and η_{g^-} in the subgroups (an average of differences equals a difference of averages). This fact seems to have led to the common misconception that, for any efficacy measure, efficacy in all-comers $\eta_{\{g^+,g^-\}}$ can be determined by efficacies η_{g^+} and η_{g^-} in the subgroups. But this is not true, because in general efficacy in all-comers depends not only on comparing Rx on g^+ vs. C on g^+ and Rx on g^- vs. C on g^- but also on comparing Rx on g^+ vs. C on g^- and Rx on g^- vs. C on g^+.

Consider the case that efficacy is measured by a *ratio* of *means*. Then within each treatment arm, treatment effect in all-comers is still its average effect on g^+ and g^- patients weighted by prevalence, as in (2) and (3). However, efficacy in all-comers is

$$\eta_{\{g^+,g^-\}} = \frac{\gamma^+ \times \mu_{g^+}^{Rx} + (1 - \gamma^+) \times \mu_{g^-}^{Rx}}{\gamma^+ \times \mu_{g^+}^{C} + (1 - \gamma^+) \times \mu_{g^-}^{C}}$$

which cannot be determined by efficacies $\mu_{g^+}^{Rx}/\mu_{g^+}^{C}$ and $\mu_{g^-}^{Rx}/\mu_{g^-}^{C}$ in the subgroups alone (an average of mean outcome ratios in subgroups does not equal a ratio of mean outcomes in the two arms).

Currently, stratified analyses in computer packages assess all-comer efficacy as a weighted average of efficacies in the subgroups. Least Squares means analysis weights by $\gamma^+ = \frac{1}{2}$ by default, while the observed marginals (OM) option in SAS estimates γ^+ from the data. While this practice is correct for continuous outcomes with efficacy measured as a difference of means, it does not typically represent efficacy in the combined $\{g^+, g^-\}$ population for binary and time-to-event outcomes, because of *confounding* by the *prognostic effect*.

We first define what prognostic and predictive biomarkers are.

Prognostic and Predictive Biomarkers

The Merriam-Webster dictionary definition of "prognostic" is "something that foretells." So a biomarker is **prognostic** of a therapy if its value has some ability to foretell the outcome for a patient given that therapy. A biomarker is thus *not* prognostic of a therapy if its value has no such ability, that is, patients form a single population under that therapy.

Our definition of a "prognostic" biomarker is perhaps more refined than some traditional definitions in the sense that ours is treatment arm specific. This is to distinguish between the situation where the marker is not prognostic in one arm but is prognostic in the other (as in Fig. 1a) and the situation where the marker is equally prognostic in both arms (as in Fig. 1b).

A biomarker is **predictive** if its value has some ability to differentiate between the effect of Rx from the effect of C (i.e., it has some ability to foretell the *efficacy* of Rx vs. C). We might say the biomarker is *purely predictive* in the case of Fig. 1a, while we say the biomarker is *purely prognostic* in the case of Fig. 1b.

The reason we make such fine distinctions is that it is simpler to relate efficacy in subgroups and their mixtures in the *purely predictive* case, while the *purely prognostic* situation implies some efficacy measures cannot be logic-respecting.

Binary Outcome

Denote by RR_{g^+}, RR_{g^-}, and $\overline{RR}$ the relative response for the g^+, g^- subpopulations, and the mixture $\{g^+, g^-\}$ all-comers population, respectively, so, in terms of the marginal responder probabilities in Table 1,

$$RR_{g^+} = \frac{p_{g^+}^{Rx}}{p_{g^+}^{C}}, RR_{g^-} = \frac{p_{g^-}^{Rx}}{p_{g^-}^{C}}, \overline{RR} = \frac{p^{Rx}}{p^{C}}. \tag{5}$$

Note intuitively and crucially that natural mixing is in terms of responder probabilities **within each arm**. With population prevalence of the g^+ subgroup being γ^+, the responder rates in the mixture $\{g^+, g^-\}$ population are:

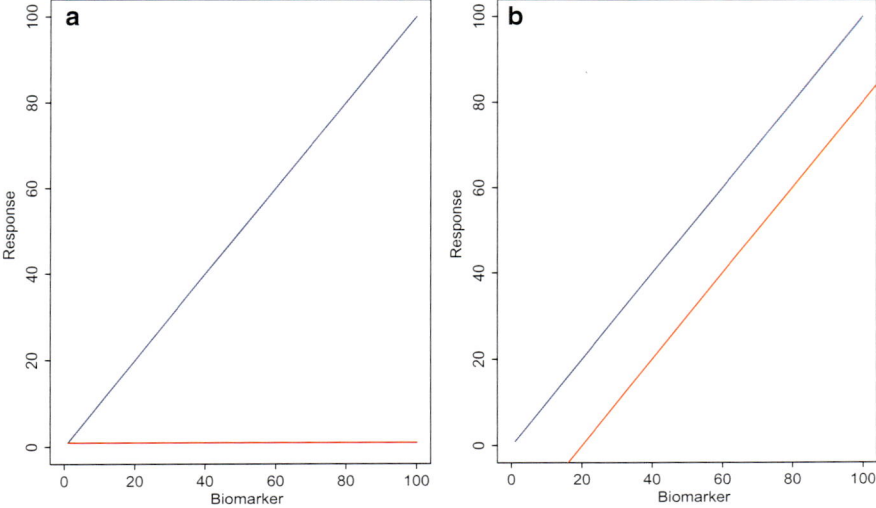

Fig. 1 Predictive marker (left panel) vs. non-predictive marker (right panel)

Table 1 Conditional response probability given treatment Rx or C for patients in the g^+ and g^- biomarker subgroups and marginal probability in the all-comers population

	g^+ subpopulation			g^- subpopulation			Population		
	R	NR		R	NR		R	NR	
Rx	$p^{Rx}_{g^+}$	$1 - p^{Rx}_{g^+}$	1	$p^{Rx}_{g^-}$	$1 - p^{Rx}_{g^-}$	1	p^{Rx}	$1 - p^{Rx}$	1
C	$p^{C}_{g^+}$	$1 - p^{C}_{g^+}$	1	$p^{C}_{g^-}$	$1 - p^{C}_{g^-}$	1	p^{C}	$1 - p^{C}$	1
	p_{g^+}	$1 - p_{g^+}$	1	p_{g^-}	$1 - p_{g^-}$	1	p	$1 - p$	1

$$p^{Rx} = \gamma^+ \times p^{Rx}_{g^+} + (1 - \gamma^+) \times \left(p^{Rx}_{g^-}\right) \qquad (6)$$

$$p^{C} = \gamma^+ \times p^{C}_{g^+} + (1 - \gamma^+) \times \left(p^{C}_{g^-}\right) \qquad (7)$$

But (5), (6), and (7) from the marginal probabilities in Table 1 are insufficient to reveal the relationships among RR_{g^+}, RR_{g^-}, and $\overline{RR}$. For that, one needs Table 2, which gives *in the total population* the logical relationship between responder probabilities in the g^+ and g^- subpopulations under Rx and C and their combined probabilities in the mixture $\{g^+, g^-\}$ population. In terms of Table 2,

Table 2 Joint probabilities of response (R) or nonresponse (NR) in the total population, with prevalence γ^+ and $\gamma^- (= 1 - \gamma^+)$ for the g^+ and g^- subgroups. The table on the right displays the correct marginal probabilities when the g^+ and g^- subgroups are combined, so that the sum of the probabilities in corresponding cells of the two tables at the left equals the probability in the corresponding cell of the right-hand table

	g^+ subpopulation				g^- subpopulation				Population		
	R	NR			R	NR			R	NR	
Rx	$p_{g^+}^{Rx}(R)$	$p_{g^+}^{Rx}(NR)$	$\gamma^+\tau^{Rx}$	$+$	$p_{g^-}^{Rx}(R)$	$p_{g^-}^{Rx}(NR)$	$\gamma^-\tau^{Rx}$	$=$	$p^{Rx}(R)$	$p^{Rx}(NR)$	τ^{Rx}
C	$p_{g^+}^{C}(R)$	$p_{g^+}^{C}(NR)$	$\gamma^+\tau^{C}$	$+$	$p_{g^-}^{C}(R)$	$p_{g^-}^{C}(NR)$	$\gamma^-\tau^{C}$	$=$	$p^{C}(R)$	$p^{C}(NR)$	τ^{C}
	$p_{g^+}(R)$	$p_{g^+}(NR)$	γ^+	$+$	$p_{g^-}(R)$	$p_{g^-}(NR)$	γ^-	$=$	$p(R)$	$p(NR)$	1

$$RR_{g^+} = \frac{p_{g^+}^{Rx}(R)/(\gamma^+\tau^{Rx})}{p_{g^+}^{C}(R)/(\gamma^+\tau^{C}_{g^+})}, \quad RR_{g^-} = \frac{p_{g^-}^{Rx}(R)/(\gamma^-\tau^{Rx}_{g^-})}{p_{g^-}^{C}(R)/(\gamma^-\tau^{C}_{g^-})},$$

$$\overline{RR} = \frac{p^{Rx}(R)/\tau^{Rx}}{p^{C}(R)/\tau^{C}}. \tag{8}$$

Since

$$\frac{p_{g^+}^{C}(R)}{p_{g^+}^{C}(R) + p_{g^-}^{C}(R)} \frac{p_{g^+}^{Rx}(R)/\tau^{Rx}}{p_{g^+}^{C}(R)/\tau^{C}} + \frac{p_{g^-}^{C}(R)}{p_{g^+}^{C}(R) + p_{g^-}^{C}(R)} \frac{p_{g^-}^{Rx}(R)/\tau^{Rx}}{p_{g^-}^{C}(R)/\tau^{C}} = \frac{p^{Rx}(R)}{p^{C}(R)} \frac{\tau^{C}}{\tau^{Rx}}, \tag{9}$$

the true mixture relative response $\overline{RR}$ can be represented as

$$\overline{RR} = \frac{p_{g^+}^{C}(R)}{p^{C}(R)} \times RR_{g^+} + \frac{p_{g^-}^{C}(R)}{p^{C}(R)} \times RR_{g^-}. \tag{10}$$

So $\overline{RR}$ is in fact a mixture of RR_{g^+} and RR_{g^-} weighted by $\frac{p_{g^+}^{C}(R)}{p^{C}(R)}$ and $\frac{p_{g^-}^{C}(R)}{p^{C}(R)}$, the population proportion of responders **under** C who are g^+ and g^-, respectively. Therefore, the efficacy measure relative response RR is logic-respecting.

If the biomarker is not prognostic, then the (joint) responder rates under C and in g^+ or g^- (i.e., $p_{g^+}^{C}(R)$ and $p_{g^-}^{C}(R)$) would be proportional to the overall responder rate under C, therefore $p_{g^+}^{C}(R) = \gamma^+ \times p^{C}(R)$ and $p_{g^-}^{C}(R) = (1 - \gamma^+) \times p^{C}(R)$, in which case

$$\overline{RR} = \gamma^+ \times RR_{g^+} + (1 - \gamma^+) \times RR_{g^-}. \tag{11}$$

Note, however, as pointed out in Lin et al. (2019), deviation of the mixing coefficient $M^+ = \frac{p_{g^+}^{C}(R)}{p^{C}(R)}$ from the prevalence γ^+ is actually the biomarker's *prognostic* effect. If the biomarker has a prognostic effect, then (11) would not equal (10), and

Table 3 Hypothetical probabilities of treatment assignment (Rx or C), biomarker subgroup (g^+ or g^-), and response (responders (R) or nonresponders (NR)), with $\Sigma = 4$, demonstrating OR is not logic-respecting

	g^+ subpopulation				g^- subpopulation				Population		
	R	NR			R	NR			R	NR	
Rx	$0.25/\Sigma$	$0.75/\Sigma$	$1/\Sigma$	+	$0.75/\Sigma$	$0.25/\Sigma$	$1/\Sigma$	=	$1/\Sigma$	$1/\Sigma$	$2/\Sigma$
C	$0.1/\Sigma$	$0.9/\Sigma$	$1/\Sigma$		$0.5/\Sigma$	$0.5/\Sigma$	$1/\Sigma$		$0.6/\Sigma$	$1.4/\Sigma$	$2/\Sigma$
	$0.35/\Sigma$	$1.65/\Sigma$	$2/\Sigma$		$1.25/\Sigma$	$0.75/\Sigma$	$2/\Sigma$		$1.6/\Sigma$	$2.4/\Sigma$	1

$\overline{RR}$ in the all-comers population cannot be determined by RR in the g^+ and g^- subpopulations and the prevalence γ^+, knowledge of M^+ is needed.

OR, the ratio of the odds of response between the treatment and control groups, is also a commonly used efficacy measure for binary outcomes. Similar to what we did with RR, one can work out a relationship between the ORs in the g^+ and g^- subgroups and the overall population (which involves the prognostic effect). However, in contrast to the linear relationship (10) for RR, the relationship for OR is nonlinear, and OR turns out to be *not* logic-respecting, as the scenario depicted in Table 3 illustrates. In this example, OR equals exactly 3 for both the g^+ and the g^- subgroups, but the true $\overline{OR}$ for the overall population equals $2\frac{1}{3}$.

So it is not the involvement of the prognostic effect in the efficacy for all-comers per se that causes an efficacy to not be logic-respecting. It is *how* the prognostic effect is involved that matters.

Time-to-Event Outcome

A survival function is defined by its probability of survival at each time point. Comparison of a family of survival curves would be simplified tremendously if the curves can be indexed by a single parameter. One way of indexing a family of survival curves by a single parameter is to assume, *on the time scale*, each curve is a multiple of a reference curve, which leads to the accelerated failure time model.

Alternatively, to index a family of survival curves by a single parameter *on the survival probability scale*, since every survival curve must start with probability one at time zero and ends with probability zero at time infinity, one might assume each curve is a reference curve raised to some power. Such families of distributions or survival functions are said to form a Lehmann Family, and this was indeed the original definition of a family of survival functions with proportional hazard (PH), on page 23 of Cox and Oakes (1984). The power that the reference survival function is raised to is in fact the hazard ratio (HR). Suppose we denote the survival function of a new treatment Rx by $S_{Rx}(t)$ and the survival function of a control treatment C by $S_C(t)$. Then $S_{Rx}(t)$ and $S_C(t)$ have PH if

$$S_{Rx}(t) = [S_C(t)]^p \forall t$$

for some ρ, and the power ρ is in fact the hazard ratio (HR) of the survival function S_{Rx} relative to S_C, HR $= \rho$. From this definition, it is easy to prove that, if the biomarker does anything, that is, if it is either *prognostic* or *predictive*, then all-comers will not have PH.

So we consider efficacy measures that are well defined, such as ratio of median survival times. We discuss this efficacy measure in the framework of a Weibull model, because it provides a link between the HR and the ratio of the mean (or median) survival time. (Weibull is the only model with both a proportional hazard interpretation and an accelerated failure time interpretation.)

Thus assume the time-to-event data fit the following Cox PH model:

$$h(t|Trt, M) = h_0(t) \exp\{\beta_1 Trt + \beta_2 M + \beta_3 Trt \times M\}, \tag{12}$$

where $Trt = 0$ (C) or $Trt = 1$ (Rx), $M = 0$ (g^-) or $M = 1$ (g^+), and $h_0(t) = h(t|C, g^-)$ is the hazard function for the g^- subgroup receiving C, and we assume that the survival function $S_0(t)$ for C, g^- is from a Weibull distribution with scale λ and shape k, i.e.,

$$S_0(t)\left(= S_{g^-}^C(t)\right) = e^{-(t/\lambda)^k}, t \geq 0.$$

Denote by v^{Rx} and v^C the true median survival times over the entire patient population (randomized to Rx and C, respectively). Denote by $v_{g^+}^{Rx}, v_{g^-}^{Rx}, v_{g^+}^C, v_{g^-}^C$ the corresponding median survival times in the g^+ and g^- subgroups. Denote $\theta_1 = e^{\beta_1}$, $\theta_2 = e^{\beta_2}$, and $\theta_3 = e^{\beta_3}$. Note that θ_1, θ_2, and θ_3 all >0.

By the PH property, the survival function for each of the subgroups has the following form:

$$S_{g^-}^C(t) = e^{-(t/\lambda)^k}, \quad S_{g^-}^{Rx}(t) = e^{-\theta_1(t/\lambda)^k},$$
$$S_{g^+}^C(t) = e^{-\theta_2(t/\lambda)^k}, \quad S_{g^+}^{Rx}(t) = e^{-\theta_1\theta_2\theta_3(t/\lambda)^k}.$$

Note that θ_2 is the *prognostic* effect. Under C, if $\theta_2 = 1$ ($\beta_2 = 0$), then the hazard is unaffected by marker status M and $S_{g^-}^C = S_{g^+}^C$, i.e., there are no subgroups under C.

Ding et al. (2016) showed that the ratio of median for the mixture group $\bar{r} \equiv v^{Rx}/v^C$ is a function of (λ, k, θ_1, θ_2, θ_3) which implicitly involves θ_2 the *prognostic* effect. Nevertheless, they proved

Theorem 4.1 *If efficacy is defined as the ratio of median survival times (between Rx and C), then under a Weibull model, efficacy of the mixture is always guaranteed to stay within the interval of the subgroups' efficacies.*

So ratio of median is logic-respecting (The logic-respecting property in RCT is related to the collapsibility property discussed in causal inference, in Greenland et al.

(1999), for example. An association/efficacy measure being *not* collapsible implies it is not logic-respecting. There is awareness that HR is not collapsible (Martinussen et al. 2018).). See also Buyse and Péron ▶ Chap. 95, "Generalized Pairwise Comparisons for Prioritized Outcomes" for examples of other measures of efficacy.

The Subgroup Mixable Estimation (SME) Principle

Despite the fact that, except for efficacy measured as a difference of means, efficacy in all-comers involves the prognostic effect, to estimate efficacy in $\{g^+, g^-\}$, computer packages by and large start by comparing Rx with C within g^+ and g^- and then take a linear combination of the efficacy estimates weighted by prevalences, ignoring the prognostic effect.

What (6) and (7) highlight is outcome measures naturally mix *within each of the Rx and C arms*, weighted by prevalence of the subgroups. Subgroup Mixable Estimation (SME) in Ding et al. (2016) and Lin et al. (2019) is a principled approach that produces correct inferences for efficacy in the mixture by reversing the process: mix g^+ and g^- within each arm first and then compare Rx with C. A three-step process, SME takes the LSmeans estimates for the (canonical) parameters in models appropriate for the CRT data (e.g., logistic, log-linear, Weibull) to whatever space appropriate for mixing (e.g., responder probability or survival probability) within each arm and then calculate efficacy in g^+, g^-, and $\{g^+, g^-\}$:

1. Fit a model for the clinical outcome and obtain LSmeans estimates for the model parameters and their estimated variance-covariance matrix.
2. *Within each of the Rx and C arms*, estimate the effects in the g^+ and g^- subgroups as appropriate functions of the model parameters. Additionally, estimate the effects (be it response probability or median survival time) in $\{g^+, g^-\}$ *within each of the Rx and C arms*, mixing in accordance to prevalence in the intended patient population (Some stratified studies are "enriched," so that the proportion of g^+ patients in the study is γ_E^+ instead of the prevalence γ^+ in the intended patient population. For such studies, estimation of the effects in Step 2 of SME should be based on γ^+ in the intended patient population, not γ_E^+ .). Obtain estimated variance-covariance matrices for the estimates by the delta method.
3. Estimate efficacy in g^+, g^- subgroups and in all-comers $\{g^+, g^-\}$ by comparing Rx with C, deriving the estimated variance-covariance matrix of these estimates by the delta method.

While SME naturally takes the prognostic effect into account, it will not magically transform a non-collapsible efficacy measure into a logic-respecting one. One should usually start with a logic-respecting efficacy measure and then apply the SME principle to it.

Effect of the Prognostic Factor on Permutation Tests

Prognostic biomarkers also unexpectedly affect the results of hypothesis tests based on permutation. Suppose the data come from a RCT and that we have a single biomarker (or other explanatory variable) that divides the population into two subgroups. While some multiple testing procedures might test for efficacy in both subgroups and in the overall population, we focus on the test of homogeneity of effect size across the two subgroups.

Data Model

We assume that a prospectively designed RCT involving N patients is conducted so that by design a known number of subjects (usually half) are assigned to Rx, and the remaining subjects are assigned to C. At the end of the trial, a binary response (Y) is measured for each subject without any error. After the trial, a single binary biomarker X (such as the genotype at a single location, or a gene classified as "wild" or "mutated") is measured without error for each subject in the trial. Within each treatment group, we classify the subjects into one of four subgroups according to their biomarker/response combination. Given a known sample size for each treatment group, each treatment-specific vector of cross-classified counts ($\mathbf{n}_{Rx}$ and $\mathbf{n}_C$) can be independently modeled with an extension of the binomial distribution called the multinomial distribution:

$$\mathbf{n}_i \mid N_i \stackrel{\text{ind}}{\sim} \text{Multinomial}(N_i, \mathbf{p}_i),$$

for $i = Rx, C$. The vector of probabilities $\mathbf{p}_i$ can be somewhat defined by exploiting the independent random assignment so that the probability of a positive biomarker, $Pr(X = +) = \pi$, is the same for both treatment groups. The remaining definition relies on the conditional probability of response given the treatment and biomarker, $\gamma_{ik} = Pr(Y = 1 | T = i, X = k)$, for $i = Rx, C$ and $k = +, -$ (We use new notations to facilitate the presentation in this section, but note γ_{ik} corresponds to p_k^i in Table 1.). In summary, the vector of probabilities of each outcome-biomarker cross-classification for treatment group i is

$$\mathbf{p}_i = (p_{i0-}, p_{i1-}, p_{i0+}, p_{i1+})$$
$$= ((1-\pi)(1-\gamma_{i-}), (1-\pi)\gamma_{i-}, \pi(1-\gamma_{i+}), \pi\gamma_{i+}),$$

where p_{ijk} is the probability that a participant had response j and biomarker k, given that they received treatment i. These conditional probabilities are also displayed in Table 4. Note that if $\gamma_{i+} = \gamma_{i-}$ for all i, then the biomarker is not prognostic.

Again exploiting the independence of the responses in the two treatment groups, we note that the joint distribution of the number of subjects who fall within each treatment-response-biomarker cross-classification, conditional on the total number

Table 4 Conditional probabilities of each biomarker-response pair given a known treatment assignment. Note that probabilities sum to one across the two rows

Treatment	$X = -$		$X = +$	
	$Y = 0$	$Y = 1$	$Y = 0$	$Y = 1$
$T = C$	$(1-\pi)(1-\gamma_{0-})$	$(1-\pi)\gamma_{0-}$	$\pi(1-\gamma_{0+})$	$\pi \gamma_{0+}$
$T = Rx$	$(1-\pi)(1-\gamma_{1-})$	$(1-\pi)\gamma_{1-}$	$\pi(1-\gamma_{1+})$	$\pi \gamma_{1+}$

of subjects assigned to control and treatment, is a product multinomial distribution, i.e., the product of two multinomial distributions, each with probability vector $\mathbf{p}_i$.

We also note that if we further condition on the number of subjects in the treatment by biomarker group ($n_{i \cdot k}$), where the count n_{ijk} is the number of subjects in treatment group i with response j and biomarker k and a '·' in the subscript denotes summation over the possible values of that subscript, the conditional distribution of response Y can be represented by a logistic regression:

$$n_{i1k} \mid n_{i \cdot k} \stackrel{\text{ind}}{\sim} \text{Binomial}\left(n_{i \cdot k}, \frac{p_{i1k}}{p_{i \cdot k}}\right) \tag{13}$$

$$\text{logit}\left(\frac{p_{i1k}}{p_{i \cdot k}}\right) = \beta_0 + \beta_i^{(T)} + \beta_k^{(X)} + \beta_{ik}^{(TX)} \tag{14}$$

In this formulation, $\beta_{ik}^{(TX)}$ is the parameter that quantifies the predictive value of the biomarker and thus is the parameter of interest.

We are interested in constructing tests for the hypothesis of homogeneous drug effect sizes across biomarker groups. How we formulate this hypothesis depends on which measure of effect size we choose to use. We focus on the odds ratio.

Predictive Null Hypothesis

Based on measuring effect size with the odds ratio, the null hypothesis of interest is that the effect of treatment is the same in the marker-positive and marker-negative subgroups:

$$H_0 : \{\text{Odds ratio for } X = -\} = \{\text{Odds ratio for } X = +\}$$
$$: \frac{\gamma_{0-}/(1-\gamma_{0-})}{\gamma_{1-}/(1-\gamma_{1-})} = \frac{\gamma_{0+}/(1-\gamma_{0+})}{\gamma_{1+}/(1-\gamma_{1+})} \tag{15}$$

It is important to note that there are four γ parameters that define the effect size in the two groups, and the hypothesis only imposes a single restriction on this four-dimensional space. That is, even when the null hypothesis is true, the parameter space is a restricted space in three dimensions. Thus, the "marginal" null hypothesis does not determine the joint distribution of all the cross-classified counts.

Test Statistic and Reference Distributions

A commonly used test statistic is the maximum likelihood estimator from the logistic regression described in Eqs. (13) and (14), denoted $T_{ML} = \widehat{\beta}_{ik}^{(TX)}$. Values far from zero (where "far" is defined by a reference distribution for the test statistic when the null hypothesis is true) are strong evidence against the null hypothesis.

The correct or true reference distribution can be calculated if the true parameter values γ are known. Of course, the true parameters are not known in practice, and it is tempting to construct a reference distribution using permutation. However, we will see that this permutation reference distribution is not guaranteed to be a good approximation of the true reference distribution with known parameters.

To build a reference distribution for T_{ML}, we first calculate the probability of observing any particular table of cross-classified counts according to permutation. Here we consider permuting the biomarker label (X). Permuting the treatment label (T) would yield similar results. When the biomarker labels are permuted, we can again summarize the sample in a $2 \times 2 \times 2$ table. For each permutation, we simply shuffle the X labels, so we do not change the marginal count of patients in each of the four treatments by response combinations, or the total count of patients in each biomarker subgroup. Thus, the calculated reference probabilities of each possible table of cross-classified counts based on permutation is conditioned on those fixed margins. The permutation probability of a single observed table (denoted **n**) can be defined in terms of only the counts among those with a negative biomarker ($X = -$) conditioned on the fixed margin constraints:

$$P^{\text{prem}}(\mathbf{n} | \text{fixed } T \text{ by } Y \text{ marginal and } X \text{ total counts})$$
$$= \frac{\# \text{ permutations that result in } \mathbf{n}}{\# \text{ permutations}}$$
$$= \frac{\binom{n_{C0\cdot}}{n_{C0-}} \binom{n_{C1\cdot}}{n_{C1-}} \binom{n_{Rx0\cdot}}{n_{Rx0-}} \binom{n_{Rx1\cdot}}{n_{Rx1-}}}{\binom{N}{n_{\cdot\cdot-}}} = \frac{Q(\mathbf{n})}{S(\mathbf{n})}, \quad (16)$$

where $Q(\mathbf{n}) = [n_{\cdot\cdot-}! \, n_{\cdot\cdot+}! \prod_{i=C,Rx} \prod_{j=0,1} n_{ij\cdot}!]/N!$ depends only on the T by Y marginal and X total counts and $S(\mathbf{n}) = \prod_{i=C,Rx} \prod_{j=0,1} n_{ij-}! \, (n_{ij\cdot} - n_{ij-})!$ depends on all of the three-way cross-classified counts.

We also consider the corresponding true probability distribution of the observed table of counts when the null hypothesis (Eq. (15)) is true. To obtain a comparable probability distribution, we condition on the same marginal and total counts as for the permutation probability using the definition of conditional probability and the probability mass function f defined by the product multinomial distribution.

$$P^{\text{true}}(\mathbf{n}|\text{fixed } T \text{ by } Y \text{ marginal and } X \text{ total counts})$$

$$= \frac{f(\mathbf{n}|\text{Count in each treatment group})}{\sum_{\mathbf{n}* \in \Xi} f(\mathbf{n}*|\text{Counts in each treatment group})} = \left[\frac{R(\mathbf{n})}{\sum_{\mathbf{n}* \in \Xi} \frac{R(\mathbf{n}*)}{S(\mathbf{n}*)}} \right] / S(\mathbf{n}), \tag{17}$$

where $R(\mathbf{n}) = \left(\frac{1-\gamma_{0-}}{1-\gamma_{0+}}\right)^{n_{C0-}} \left(\frac{\gamma_{0-}}{\gamma_{0+}}\right)^{n_{C1-}} \left(\frac{1-\gamma_{1-}}{1-\gamma_{1+}}\right)^{n_{Rx0-}} \left(\frac{\gamma_{1-}}{\gamma_{1+}}\right)^{n_{Rx1-}}$ and Ξ is the set of all possible table cross-classifications $\mathbf{n}^*$ whose marginal counts match the fixed marginal counts in the original table $\mathbf{n}$.

By comparing Eqs. (16) and (17), we can readily determine a sufficient condition on the true parameters that results in permutation reference distributions that match true reference distributions and thus results in tests that properly control Type I error. When this condition holds, the numerator in Eq. (17) reduces to the normalizing constant $Q(\mathbf{n})$, and the two functions are equal. This sufficient condition is $\gamma_{0-} = \gamma_{0+}$ and $\gamma_{1-} = \gamma_{1+}$. We note that although this sufficient condition appears to involve two equalities, it is actually a single constraint when the null hypothesis in Eq. (15) is true:

$$\gamma_{1+} \overset{H_0}{=} \left(1 + \frac{\frac{\gamma_{0-}}{1-\gamma_{0-}}}{\frac{\gamma_{0+}}{1-\gamma_{0+}} \frac{\gamma_{1-}}{1-\gamma_{1-}}}\right)^{-1} \overset{\gamma_{0-}=\gamma_{0+}}{=} \gamma_{1-}. \tag{18}$$

The meaning of this sufficient condition is also readily apparent. Permutation-based tests of treatment effect homogeneity are guaranteed to appropriately control Type I error if the probability of a positive response ($Y = 1$) for each treatment group is homogeneous across biomarker groups. That is, a permutation-based test for a *predictive* biomarker is guaranteed to control Type I error at the nominal level when that marker is *not prognostic*. If the marker is indeed prognostic, the permutation probability (16) will not always equal the probability (17), and thus permutation-based tests are not guaranteed to control Type I error rate.

Of course, this comparison is for the distribution of the entire $2 \times 2 \times 2$ table of counts. Proposed tests for subgroup discovery are based on the sampling distribution of a test statistic, such as T_{ML} or another one of those presented in section "Test Statistic and Reference Distributions" above. These sampling distributions are of complex form, and so we turn to a numerical study to demonstrate the same result holds: if a biomarker is prognostic, permutation-based tests are not guaranteed to control Type I error rate.

Numerical Study

We focus our numerical study on one particular "toy" example, with 20 subjects in the marker-negative group and 20 in the marker-positive group. These 40 subjects

Table 5 Observed marginal counts for a study where 20 participants are marker negative and 20 are marker positive

	$Y = 0$	$Y = 1$	Total
$T = C$	10	10	20
$T = Rx$	10	10	20
Total	20	20	40

are observed to be equally divided among the four treatment-by-response cross-classifications, so that we observe the marginal table displayed in Table 5. These counts are relatively small but allow for quick exact calculation of the sampling distributions of the test statistics, rather than forcing us to rely on a numerical approximation.

We consider the true study parameters to reflect the case of a relatively common biomarker, $P(X = +) = \pi = 0.75$, measured in a randomized experiment, $P(T = C) = 0.5$ and X independent of T. We further suppose a highly prognostic marker, where the prognosis in the two treatment subgroups is identical at a risk difference of $0.9 - 0.1 = 0.8$ or odds ratio of $\{0.9 \times (1 - 0.1)\}/\{0.1 \times (1 - 0.9)\} = 81$:

$$\gamma_{0-} = \gamma_{1-} = P(Y = 1 | T = Rx, X = -) = 0.9$$
$$\gamma_{0+} = \gamma_{1+} = P(Y = 1 | T = Rx, X = +) = 0.1 \quad (19)$$

We also note that this choice of conditional distribution for the response satisfies our null hypothesis of no interaction between marker and treatment (Eq. (15)). That is, for these parameter values, the odds ratio between response and treatment is constant across the biomarker levels (X). We chose such an extreme example so that the difference in estimation would be apparent even in the small sample size for our numerical study.

For these particular values, we can calculate the cumulative distribution function of the test statistic defined in section "Test Statistic and Reference Distributions" by calculating its exact pmf both under the assumption that the pmf for **n** follows from permutation as defined in Eq. (16) and under the true pmf that follows from the product multinomial distribution. We accomplish this via the following algorithm:

1. Enumerate all $2 \times 2 \times 2$ tables of counts consistent with 20 participants in each biomarker level and the marginal totals in Table 5.
2. For each table, calculate the permutation probability using Eq. (16) and the true probability using Eq. (17).
3. For each table, calculate the value of T_{ML}, adjusted as described below.
4. For each probability measure (P^{perm} and P^{true}), sum the probabilities from Step 2 for each unique value of T_{ML} to find its exact probability mass function.

In Step 3 of the algorithm, we make an adjustment for T_{ML} where there are no observations in some combination of X and T in the $2 \times 2 \times 2$ table. In this case, the

85 Confident Statistical Inference with Multiple Outcomes, Subgroups...

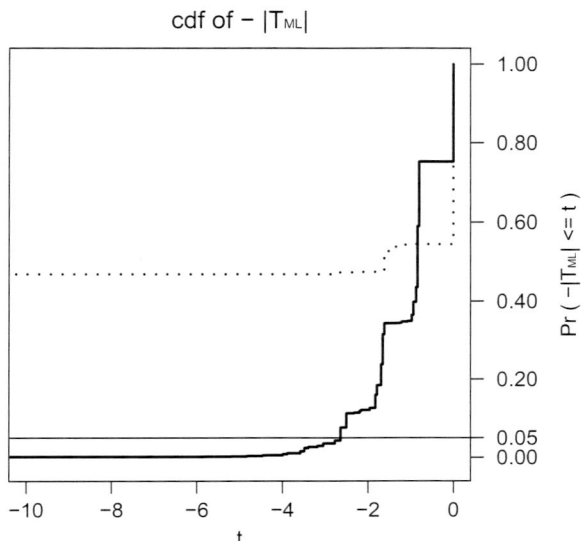

Fig. 2 Reference CDF of $-|T_{ML}|$, with P^{perm} as a solid line and P^{true} as a dotted line, assuming the parameters in Eq. (19) are true with margin constraint in Table 5

probability that $Y = 1$ cannot be estimated, or even bounded. Thus, in this case we assigned the least extreme value (0) as the value of the test statistic. In addition, T_{ML} is not guaranteed to be finite for certain patterns of "zero" counts in the $2 \times 2 \times 2$ table. To adjust for this phenomenon, we first determined the shape of the appropriate likelihood function and then assigned the test statistic to be $\pm\infty$ for monotone likelihoods and 0 for flat likelihoods. Finally, we are interested in a two-sided test, and so we also take the negative of the absolute value of the test statistic T_{ML}, so that the CDFs correspond to p-values.

Figure 2 demonstrates that there is a big gap between the reference distribution from permutation and the true reference distribution. In the CDF of $-|T_{ML}|$, the permutation reference distribution (solid line) suggests an enhanced drug effect for one targeted subgroup for any statistic value smaller than -2.7, but the true reference distribution (dotted line) does not imply any significant drug effect using $\alpha = 0.05$. That is, the critical region for the permutation distribution is $\{t: t \leq -2.7\}$, while the critical region for the true distribution is empty. Figure 2 is an example that shows permutation does not always control the Type I error rate.

Even though Fig. 2 is only for the extreme parameter values we posited in Eq. (19), we have explored the control of Type I error for additional combinations of parameters, and the message remains the same: permuting subgroup membership labels does not reliably produce a valid null distribution for the test statistics in a randomized clinical trial with discrete response, even with only one subgroup classifier.

Summary and Conclusions

Strong control of the familywise Type I error rate of appropriately formulated null hypotheses is required to control the incorrect decision rate in clinical trials. The closed testing principle is the most commonly applied technique to construct multiple tests with strong control. However, even strong control of testing null hypotheses of *equalities* may not necessarily control the rate of directional errors.

The Partitioning principle can be applied to construct multiple tests that not only control the familywise Type I error rate strongly but also have confidence sets. Making decisions based on confidence sets automatically control the directional error rate.

When there are subgroups defined by biomarkers, respecting logical relationships among the parameters is desirable. The Subgroup Mixable Estimation (SME) is a principled approach that ensures estimates of efficacy are logic-respecting for logic-respecting efficacy measures such as relative response (RR) and ratio of median survival times. One should however be aware that even in a randomized clinical trial (RCT), odds ratio and hazard ratio are not logic-respecting and are affected by the prognostic effect. One should also be aware that permutation tests for equality of treatment effect across subgroups may not control the Type I error rate, if the biomarker has a *prognostic* effect.

Key Facts

- In making a decision by testing multiple hypotheses, only controlling the maximum probability of *rejecting at least one true null* hypothesis (even if some of the null hypotheses are false), called *strong* Type I error rate control, controls the probability of an *incorrect decision*.
- With strong control, one can be confident that the *directional* error rate is controlled if the null hypotheses are not just equalities but in fact partition the entire parameter space.
- The efficacy measures odds ratio and hazard ratio are not logic-respecting/collapsible, but relative response and ratio of median survival times are logic-respecting/collapsible in randomized clinical trials.
- Permutation tests for equality of treatment effect across subgroups may fail to control the Type I error rate even if the (marginal) null hypothesis is true, if the biomarker has a *prognostic* effect.
- Subgroup Mixable Estimation is a principled approach that works with least squares means to facilitate logical assessment of efficacy in subgroups and their mixtures.

Cross-References

▶ Generalized Pairwise Comparisons for Prioritized Outcomes

References

Cox DR, Oakes D (1984) Analysis of Survival Data. Chapman and Hall

Ding Y, Lin H-M, Hsu JC (2016) Subgroup mixable inference on treatment efficacy in mixture populations, with an application to time-to-event outcomes. Stat Med 35:1580–1594

Finner H, Strassburger K (2002) The partitioning principle: a powerful tool in multiple decision theory. Ann Stat 30:1194–1213

Finner H, Strassburger K (2007) Step-up related simultaneous confidence intervals for MCC and MCB. Biom J 49(1):40–51

Greenland S, Robins JM, Pearl J (1999) Confounding and collapsibility in causal inference. Stat Sci 14(1):29–46

Hayter AJ, Hsu JC (1994) On the relationship between stepwise decision procedures and confidence sets. J Am Stat Assoc 89:128–136

Hsu JC (1996) Multiple comparisons: theory and methods. Chapman & Hall, London

Hsu JC, Berger RL (1999) Stepwise confidence intervals without multiplicity adjustment for dose response and toxicity studies. J Am Stat Assoc 94:468–482

Huang Y, Hsu JC (2007) Hochberg's step-up method: cutting corners off Holm's step-down method. Biometrika 22:2244–2248

Jiang W, Freidlin B, Simon R (2007) Biomarker-adaptive threshold design: a procedure for evaluating treatment with possible biomarker-defined subset effect. J Natl Cancer Inst 99:1036–1043

Kaizar EE, Li Y, Hsu JC (2011) Permutation multiple tests of binary features do not uniformly control error rates. J Am Stat Assoc 106:1067–1074

Lin H-M, Xu H, Ding Y, Hsu JC (2019) Correct and logical inference on efficacy in subgroups and their mixture for binary outcomes. Biom J 61:8–26

Lipkovich I, Dmitrienko A, Denne J, Enas G (2011) Subgroup identification based on differential effect search – a recursive partitioning method for establishing response to treatment in patient subpopulations. Stat Med 30:2601–2621

Martinussen T, Vansteelandt S, Andersen PK (2018) Subtleties in the interpretation of hazard ratios. arXiv:1810.09192v1

Miller R, Siegmund D (1982) Maximally selected Chi-square statistics. Biometrics 38:1011–1016

Stefansson G, Kim W, Hsu JC (1988) On confidence sets in multiple comparisons. In: Gupta SS, Berger JO (eds) Statistical decision theory and related topics IV, vol 2. Springer, New York, pp 89–104

Strassburger K, Bretz F (2008) Compatible simultaneous lower confidence bounds for the holm procedure and other Bonferroni-based closed tests. Stat Med 27(24):4914–4927

Takeuchi K (1973) Studies in some aspects of theoretical foundations of statistical data analysis (in Japanese). Toyo Keizai Shinposha, Tokyo

Takeuchi K (2010) Basic ideas and concepts for multiple comparison procedures. Biom J 52:722–734

Tukey JW (1953) The problem of multiple comparisons. Dittoed manuscript of 396 pages, Department of Statistics, Princeton University

Tukey JW (1994) The problem of multiple comparisons, Chapter 1. In: Braun HI (ed) The collected works of John W. Tukey, vol VIII. Chapman & Hall, New York/London, pp 1–300

Woodcock J (2015) FDA Voice. Posted 23 Mar 2015

Xu H, Hsu JC (2007) Using the partitioning principle to control the generalized family error rate. Biom J 49:52–67

Missing Data

86

Guangyu Tong, Fan Li, and Andrew S. Allen

Contents

Introduction	1682
Missing Data Mechanism	1683
Likelihood-Based Approach	1684
Weighting Methods	1686
Inverse Probability Weighting	1686
Doubly Robust Inference	1689
Imputation-Based Method	1690
Regression Imputation	1690
Multiple Imputation	1692
Joint Modeling Approach (MCMC)	1694
Fully Conditional Specification (MICE)	1696
Sensitivity Analysis	1697
Summary and Conclusion	1698
Key Facts	1699
Cross-References	1700
References	1700

G. Tong
Department of Sociology, Duke University, Durham, NC, USA
e-mail: guangyu.tong@duke.edu

F. Li
Department of Biostatistics, Yale University, School of Public Health, New Haven, CT, USA
e-mail: fan.f.li@yale.edu

A. S. Allen (✉)
Department of Biostatistics and Bioinformatics, Duke University, School of Medicine, Durham, NC, USA
e-mail: asallen@duke.edu

© Springer Nature Switzerland AG 2022
S. Piantadosi, C. L. Meinert (eds.), *Principles and Practice of Clinical Trials*,
https://doi.org/10.1007/978-3-319-52636-2_117

Abstract

Missing data are commonly seen in randomized clinical trials. When missingness is not completely random, a complete-case analysis that ignores the missing data process often leads to biased estimates of the average treatment effect. This chapter defines different missing data mechanisms, discusses their impact on inference, and presents statistical methods that address missing data, including likelihood-based analysis, inverse probability weighting, and imputation. Each of these methods either models the missingness process or the observed outcome distribution. A more robust approach that combines the virtue of each of these modeling approaches is also introduced. This approach is doubly robust such that it yields a consistent estimate of the average treatment effect if either one of the missingness model or the outcome model is correctly specified, but not necessarily both. The chapter concludes with a brief discussion of sensitivity analyses used to assess the impact of unmeasured factors that affect both the missingness and outcomes. Throughout, statistical and practical considerations are discussed in the context of randomized clinical trials where the primary analysis is to compare two treatments and to estimate the average comparative effect among the enrolled population.

Keywords

Average treatment effect · Randomized clinical trials · Doubly robust · Inverse probability weighting · Likelihood · Missing at random · Markov Chain Monte Carlo · Multiple imputation · Sensitivity analysis

Introduction

Randomized clinical trials (RCTs) are routinely conducted to evaluate the effectiveness of new drugs or medical interventions based on human participants. Random allocation of treatment tends to balance both observed and unobserved factors across comparison groups, which allows causal inference on the intervention effect on the outcome. However, missing data frequently occur in RCTs because of patient dropout. If patients who dropped out from the study differ systematically in the outcome of interest from the patients who completed the study, biased group comparison may result, and the subsequent causal statement for the intervention effect becomes invalid (Mallinckrodt 2013).

The National Research Council (NRC) Report recommended approaches tailored to various missing data scenarios (Little et al. 2010). Simple methods such as complete-case analysis (i.e., only using cases with complete outcome and covariates in analysis) and last observation carried forward (i.e., the future observations of a dropout case are all assumed to be equal to the last observed value in a longitudinal clinical trial (Kenward and Molenberghs 2009)) are not recommended. The central aim of this chapter is to introduce the use of mainstream statistical methods to handle missing data, in accordance with the suggestions in the NRC Report and ICH E9 guidelines for medical research (International Conference on Harmonization 1998).

Missing Data Mechanism

It is important to understand the nature of missing data to make valid statistical inference. Researchers often consider plausible missing data mechanisms based on substantive knowledge from the trial. A missing data mechanism is characterized by the conditional distribution of missingness given both observed and unobserved (i.e., missing) data. In practice, the missing data mechanism is unknown, and assumptions are required to characterize the missingness process. The validity of these assumptions in any given data analysis affects which statistical approaches will lead to correct inference and which will not.

The missingness mechanism is often classified into three types (Rubin 1976): (i) missing completely at random (MCAR), (ii) missing at random (MAR), and (iii) missing not at random (MNAR). MCAR assumes that the probability of missingness does not depend on any observed or unobserved variables. MAR relaxes the MCAR assumption and states that the missingness is related to observed but unrelated to any unobserved variables. If the missingness mechanism is neither MCAR nor MAR, the missingness is MNAR. The validity of subsequent statistical analysis depends on whether the assumptions on the missingness mechanism hold for the study of interest. The following example is used to illustrate the definitions of missing data mechanisms.

Consider a trial evaluating the effect of a new drug in reducing the blood pressure of patients. Let us assume a total of n patients are recruited in the trial; half of them are randomly assigned to receive the new drug and the rest to receive placebo. Write the binary variable $G_i = 1$ if the ith patient receives the new drug and $G_i = 0$ otherwise. Let Y_i denote the blood pressure measurement of the ith patient at the end of the study and X_i be a collection of covariates that are not of primary interest (e.g., demographic information of patients, blood pressure measurement taken at the start of the trial, etc.). In this chapter, the focus will be data with missing outcomes, and therefore let us assume the covariates are fully observed. Let R_i denote the missingness indicator with $R_i = 1$ representing that Y_i is observed and $R_i = 0$ if Y_i is missing. The full data can be written by $(Y_i, X_i, G_i, i = 1, \ldots, n)$, which are the collection of data that would have been observed in the absence of missing data. In contrast, the observed data is represented by $(R_i, R_i Y_i, X_i, G_i, i = 1, \ldots, n)$ with the outcome of interest, Y_i, only fully observed when the missingness indicator is equal to one. In the present trial, the goal of inference is the average treatment effect that compares the average difference in the blood pressure between the treatment and the placebo groups (see Chap. 4 for alternative definitions of estimands). A complete-case estimator that only compares the average observed outcomes between the two groups is

$$\hat{\mu}^{CC} = \hat{\mu}_1^{CC} - \hat{\mu}_0^{CC} = \frac{\sum_{i=1}^{n} R_i G_i Y_i}{\sum_{i=1}^{n} R_i G_i} - \frac{\sum_{i=1}^{n} R_i (1 - G_i) Y_i}{\sum_{i=1}^{n} R_i (1 - G_i)}.$$

If the missingness probability,

$$P(R_i = 0|Y_i, X_i, G_i) = \pi, \quad \text{for all } i = 1, \ldots, n,$$

where π is a constant value unrelated to Y_i and X_i, or treatment G_i, then the missingness is MCAR. For both the treatment and placebo groups, MCAR suggests that the expectation of observed outcomes is equal to that of the full outcomes. In this case, $\hat{\mu}^{CC}$ provides an unbiased estimate of the average treatment effect of the new drug. In other words, MCAR ensures the inference based on the observed data can inform that of the full data without any bias.

If the missingness probability,

$$P(R_i = 0|Y_i, X_i, G_i) = P(R_i = 0|X_i, G_i), \quad \text{for all } i = 1, \ldots, n,$$

depends on the observed covariates X_i and treatment G_i but is free of the potentially unobserved value of Y_i, then the missingness is MAR. MAR implies that the distribution of missing Y_is is the same as that of the corresponding observed Y_is within each stratum of X_i, given the same treatment G_i. In this case, the complete-case estimator $\hat{\mu}^{CC}$ will lead to a biased estimator of the average treatment effect. Finally, if the missingness probability is a function of the unobserved values of the outcome variable, then the missingness is MNAR, and the complete-case estimator $\hat{\mu}^{CC}$ is also biased.

It is evident that these different assumptions on the missing data process have different implications for the analysis of trial data. Unfortunately, these assumptions are not testable based on the observed data, and an argument supporting a specific missingness mechanism is often a substantive one and should be informed by discussions with trialists. In some cases, the plausibility of the missingness assumption can be indirectly assessed, such as comparing the baseline characteristics for participants with missing outcomes to those without. However, the MNAR assumption cannot be formally ruled out with such indirect examinations. If MCAR is considered plausible, complete-case analysis provides an unbiased estimate of the average treatment effect. However, randomized trials often collect a range of baseline covariates, and it may be more plausible to assume the missing data are MAR. As will be seen in due course, under MAR, adjusting for observed patient characteristics is sufficient to obtain an unbiased estimate of the average treatment effect. Finally, since MNAR involves unobserved missing outcomes, more complicated statistical methods are required in this case. As this chapter mainly focuses on methods that address missing data under the MAR assumption, we will refer the discussions of MNAR elsewhere (Carpenter and Kenward 2012).

Likelihood-Based Approach

Likelihood-based methods are widely used in statistical problems as the resulting maximum likelihood estimator (MLE) is asymptotically efficient when the likelihood is correctly specified (see Chap. 15 for additional details of likelihood). This optimality carries over to the randomized clinical trial setting with missing data. An important result regarding the likelihood approach is that, under MAR, the observed data likelihood can factor and therefore allow the missingness model to be ignored. In other words, the MLE obtained from the observed data likelihood is approximately unbiased to the target parameter in large samples.

To make such ideas more concrete, let us consider the previous RCT example which evaluates the effect of a new drug in reducing patient's blood pressure (Y_i). Recall that the interest is in estimating the average treatment effect $\mu = \mu_1 - \mu_0 = E[Y|\ G = 1] - E[Y|\ G = 0]$, where G_i is the treatment status (active drug or placebo). In what follows, let us consider the estimation of μ_1 when the outcome is missing at random, since the logic for estimating μ_0 is exactly the same. Suppose there is no missing outcome, one could parametrically specify the joint probability for each observation in the treatment group as

$$f(Y, X|G = 1, \theta) = f(Y|X, G = 1, \theta_1) f(X|G = 1, \theta_2),$$

and $\theta = (\theta_1^T, \theta_2^T)^T$ is the unknown vector of parameters with θ_1 for the outcome model and θ_2 for the covariate model. From the Law of Iterated Expectation, suppose $\hat{\theta}$ is an unbiased estimator for θ, then $\hat{\mu}_1$ can be identified through

$$\hat{\mu}_1(\hat{\theta}) = \int \int Y f(Y|X, G = 1, \hat{\theta}_1) f(X|G = 1, \hat{\theta}_2) dY dX.$$

For the case of missing outcomes under MAR, it can be shown that the joint probability of the observed data can be represented as follows:

$$[f(Y, X, R = 1|\ G = 1)]^{I(R=1)} [f(X, R = 0|\ G = 1)]^{I(R=0)}$$
$$= [f(Y|X, G = 1, \theta_1)]^{I(R=1)} f(X|G = 1, \theta_2) [f(R = 1|X, G = 1, \eta)]^{I(R=1)} [f(R = 0|X, G = 1, \eta)]^{I(R=0)},$$

where η is now the parameter indexing the missingness model (R-model), namely, a model for the missingness indicator R as a function of baseline covariate X and treatment status G. In the above factorization, the first two components $[f(Y|X, G = 1, \theta_1)]^{I(R=1)} f(X|G = 1, \theta_2)$ are parameterized by θ and are therefore of interest, while the latter two components concern the missingness process. As long as the parameter η is distinct from θ, the above factorization suggests that one could safely ignore the missingness model when the primary interest is in θ. In other words, the observed likelihood for the collection of observations in the treatment group could be maximized to obtain the MLE $\hat{\theta}$, and then $\hat{\mu}_1(\hat{\theta})$ can be estimated based on the aforementioned integral without additional assumptions on the missingness process. This likelihood estimator $\hat{\mu}_1(\hat{\theta})$ is consistent to μ_1 when the parametric model $f(Y, X|G = 1, \theta)$ is correctly specified. In this case, $\hat{\mu}_1$ is also asymptotically efficient in a sense that it achieves the lower bound of the large-sample variance among all consistent estimators of μ_1. With μ_0 estimated in the same manner, the average treatment effect of a new drug in reducing patient's blood pressure can be obtained. Notice that in simple cases where the likelihood model is multivariate normal, $\hat{\mu}_1(\hat{\theta})$ may have a closed form representation and the computation is straightforward. However, a limitation of this approach is that when the likelihood model is complicated, the resulting estimator $\hat{\mu}_1(\hat{\theta})$ involves a multidimensional integral and may demand intensive computation.

The above example is a simple illustration of the likelihood-based approach. In fact, the likelihood-based approach provides a general solution for a broader class of missing data problems and is not necessarily restricted to the MAR assumption. As in the above example, the key idea is to specify a joint likelihood for the full data and then make the inference based on the induced likelihood for the observed data. Let Y denote the generic full data (without distinguishing between outcome and covariates); then one could define the joint density of the full data as $L(\theta|\ Y) = f(Y|\ \theta)$ for some unknown parameter θ, which often includes a known function of the target parameter. Write $Y = (Y_{obs}, Y_{mis})$ where Y_{obs} denotes the observed part of Y and Y_{mis} denotes the unobserved or missing part. The induced likelihood for the observed data could be defined by integrating or marginalizing over the missing part

$$L(\theta|Y_{obs}) = \int f(Y_{obs}, Y_{mis}|\theta) dY_{mis}.$$

It is easy to see that once a joint model for Y is specified ($f(Y_{obs}, Y_{mis}|\ \theta)$), the maximum likelihood inference could then proceed by maximizing $L(\theta|\ Y_{obs})$.

In simple cases where $\int f(Y_{obs}, Y_{mis}|\ \theta) dY_{mis}$ has a closed form, such as when the joint model is multivariate normal, the MLE $\hat{\theta}$ could be found via Newton-Raphson or Fisher scoring algorithms, both of which require the second-order derivatives of the log-likelihood, $l(\theta|\ Y_{obs})$. For more general cases where the integral of the above equation does not come in closed forms, a more computationally tractable approach that does not require the calculation of the second-order derivatives – the expectation-maximization (EM) algorithm – has been developed to maximize $l(\theta|\ Y_{obs})$ based on the complete data log-likelihood $l(\theta|\ Y)$. A more detailed introduction to the EM algorithm and related approaches can be found in Dempster et al. (1977) and Little and Rubin (2014).

Weighting Methods

Inverse Probability Weighting

Inverse probability weighting (IPW) has long been established as a standard approach to estimate population quantities in survey sampling, which dates to the seminal work of Horvitz and Thompson (1952). From a missing data perspective, estimating population quantities from an observed survey sample involves addressing missing data by design, as the nonresponses in a survey can affect the population-level inference. By weighting each unit using the inverse of the known selection probability, the weighted pseudo-population coincides with the target population from which the sample is taken, and one can recover the population quantity of interest by analyzing the weighted sample. In RCTs, if the missing outcome is MAR, the IPW approach could be used in a similar fashion to recover the full data from the observed part.

To illustrate the idea of IPW, consider our RCT example with two treatments (a new drug versus placebo) and a cross-sectional continuous outcome, the blood pressure. In the absence of missing data, the difference-in-means estimator $\hat{\mu} = \hat{\mu}_1 - \hat{\mu}_0 = \frac{\sum_{i=1}^n G_i Y_i}{\sum_{i=1}^n G_i} - \frac{\sum_{i=1}^n (1-G_i) Y_i}{\sum_{i=1}^n (1-G_i)}$ provides an unbiased quantification of the average treatment effect. Here, we illustrate how IPW provides an unbiased estimator for $\mu_1 = E[Y| G = 1]$. Similar logic follows for μ_0. Under MAR, one could first estimate the probability of observing the complete data $P(R_i = 1| Y_i, X_i, G_i) = P(R_i = 1| X_i, G_i) = \pi(X_i, G_i)$. We refer to $\pi(X_i, G_i)$ as an R-model. Estimating parameters in the R-model can, for example, proceed by fitting a logistic regression model to the entire data consisting of $(R_i, X_i, G_i)_{i=1,\ldots,n}$,

$$\pi_i(X_i; \psi) = \frac{\exp\left(\psi_0 + X_i^T \psi_1 + G_i \psi_2 + G_i X_i^T \psi_3\right)}{1 + \exp\left(\psi_0 + X_i^T \psi_1 + G_i \psi_2 + G_i X_i^T \psi_3\right)}, \quad i = 1\ldots n,$$

where $\psi = (\psi_0, \psi_1^T, \psi_2, \psi_3^T)^T$ are the model parameters. We refer the readers to Chap. 11 for additional expositions on the logistic regression model. Notice that the treatment-by-covariate interactions are often included to allow for differential missingness across treatment groups. If the above R-model is correctly specified, then the MLE, $\hat{\psi}$, is a consistent estimator for ψ, and $\hat{\pi}_i = \pi(X_i; \hat{\psi})$ is a consistent estimator for $\Pr(R_i = 1| X_i, G_i)$. Hence, an IPW estimator for μ_1 takes the form

$$\hat{\mu}_1^{IPW} = \frac{\sum_{i=1}^n R_i G_i Y_i / \hat{\pi}_i}{\sum_{i=1}^n R_i G_i / \hat{\pi}_i}.$$

Note that $\hat{\mu}_1^{IPW}$ is a weighted average of the observed outcomes among the treated group, where the weights are proportional to $1/\hat{\pi}_i$, the inverse of the predicted probability of observing the case based on the above logistic regression model.

Under MAR, when the missingness probability is accurately predicted from a correct logistic model, the IPW estimator $\hat{\mu}_1^{IPW}$ is a consistent estimator of μ_1. Similarly, we can also show that $\hat{\mu}_0^{IPW} = \frac{\sum_{i=1}^n R_i (1-G_i) Y_i / \hat{\pi}_i}{\sum_{i=1}^n R_i (1-G_i) / \hat{\pi}_i}$ is a consistent estimator of μ_0. Thus, the IPW estimator, $\hat{\mu}^{IPW} = \hat{\mu}_1^{IPW} - \hat{\mu}_0^{IPW}$, is a consistent estimator for the true average treatment effect. Intuitively, IPW weights the observed cases with $1/\hat{\pi}_i$ to adjust for their representation in the population and creates a pseudo-population that has the same covariate distribution as the full data.

The variance estimator of $\hat{\mu}^{IPW}$ can be obtained by using both semi-parametric and nonparametric approaches. For the semi-parametric approach, one could use the M-estimation theory to derive a sandwich estimator. For interested readers, a simple sketch of derivation of the variance is provided here; others can skip this paragraph without loss of continuity. Additional details on M-estimation can be found in Lunceford and Davidian (2004) and Tsiatis (2007). Denote the collection of parameters $\theta = (\mu_1, \mu_0, \psi)^T$, $\hat{\mu}_1^{IPW}$ can be viewed as the solution to the estimating equation $\sum_{i=1}^n \widetilde{U}_{1i}(\mu_1, \psi) = \sum_{i=1}^n \frac{G_i R_i (Y_i - \mu_1)}{\pi_i} = 0$ and that $\hat{\mu}_0^{IPW}$ can be viewed as the solution to the estimating equation $\sum_{i=1}^n \widetilde{U}_{0i}(\mu_0, \psi) = \sum_{i=1}^n \frac{(1-G)_i R_i (Y_i - \mu_0)}{\pi_i} = 0$. Further denote $S_i(\psi)$ as the individual score function of the logistic R-model, and the estimator $\hat{\theta}$ can be viewed as a solution to the joint estimating equations $\sum_{i=1}^n U_i(\hat{\theta}) = 0$, where

$$U_i(\theta) = \begin{pmatrix} \widetilde{U}_{1i}(\mu_1, \psi) \\ \widetilde{U}_{0i}(\mu_0, \psi) \\ S_i(\psi) \end{pmatrix}$$

is the stacked estimating function. Denote the true value of θ as θ^*. The sandwich estimator is obtained by a Taylor series expansion. One obtains $\sqrt{n}(\hat{\theta} - \theta^*) \approx A_n(\theta^*)^{-1} B_n(\theta^*) \left[A_n(\theta^*)^{-1} \right]^T$, where $A_n(\theta^*) = -\frac{1}{n} \sum_{i=1}^n \frac{\partial U_i(\theta^*)}{\partial \theta'}$ and $B_n(\theta^*) = \frac{1}{n} \sum_{i=1}^n U_i(\theta^*) U_i^T(\theta^*)$. Since $\hat{\theta}$ consistently estimates θ^*, a plug-in variance estimator is obtained as

$$\widehat{Var}(\hat{\theta}) = n^{-1} A_n(\hat{\theta})^{-1} B_n(\hat{\theta}) \left[A_n(\hat{\theta})^{-1} \right]^T.$$

Because $\hat{\mu}^{IPW}$ is a function of $\hat{\theta}$, the variance of $\hat{\mu}^{IPW}$ can then be easily estimated by the Delta method (Oehlert 1992). Such a sandwich variance estimator takes into account the uncertainty in estimating the R-model and therefore provides an adequate characterization of the variability of the treatment effect.

A more flexible approach to estimate the variance of $\hat{\mu}^{IPW}$ is the nonparametric bootstrap (Efron and Tibshirani 1994). To proceed, one could write the data vector as $\widetilde{Z} = \{R, RY, X\}$, where X includes the treatment variable G. Define $F_n(\widetilde{Z})$ as the empirical distribution function of the data vector $\widetilde{Z}$. Then one could sample with replacement from the empirical distribution $F_n(\widetilde{Z})$ to obtain the bth ($b = 1, \ldots, B$) bootstrap replicate, $\{\widetilde{Z}_j^b, j = 1, \ldots, n\}$, from which the IPW estimator $\hat{\mu}^{IPW,b}$ is computed. A consistent variance estimator is then obtained as the variance of the bootstrap sample $\{\hat{\mu}^{IPW,1}, \ldots, \hat{\mu}^{IPW,B}\}$. Compared to the sandwich variance estimator, the bootstrap estimator is easier to implement and generally more flexible without relying on model assumptions, although it may become computationally intensive for large datasets.

In finite samples, one crucial condition for the IPW estimator to perform well is positivity, which means that π_i should always be bounded away from zero. In other words, within each strata of covariate X, the probability of observing a case (or non-missingness) should be strictly positive. In practice, extreme probabilities $\hat{\pi}_i$ close to zero usually leads to a biased IPW estimator with excessive variance, and one could consider excluding the units with extreme probabilities to improve the efficiency of the IPW estimator. Similar concerns are also discussed in length in the causal inference literature (see, e.g., Li et al. 2018).

Doubly Robust Inference

A critical condition for the IPW estimator to be unbiased is that the R-model $\pi(X_i; \psi)$ should be correctly specified. If this model is misspecified, $\hat{\mu}^{IPW}$ may be an inconsistent estimator of the average treatment effect μ. To address this concern, the doubly robust estimator has been developed to combine the virtue of weighting (R-model) and regression. The regression model, which is also referred to as the Y-model, regresses the observed values of outcome on covariates so that the missing outcome data can be directly imputed or predicted. More details of regression imputation are explained in the next section. Here, for the doubly robust estimator, one could augment the IPW estimator using a regression imputation estimator as

$$\hat{\mu}_1^{DR} = \hat{\mu}_1^{IPW} - \frac{\sum_{i=1}^n \{R_i - \hat{\pi}_i\} G_i m_1(X_i; \hat{\beta})/\hat{\pi}_i}{\sum_{i=1}^n \frac{R_i G_i}{\hat{\pi}_i}},$$

where $m_1(X_i; \hat{\beta})$ is a regression imputation estimator for the treatment group. The name "doubly robust" is coined since $\hat{\mu}_1^{DR}$ is consistent to μ_1 as long as one of the two models – $\pi(X_i; \psi)$ or $m_1(X_i; \beta)$ – is correctly specified, but not necessarily both. In addition, $\hat{\mu}_1^{DR}$ is locally efficient for μ_1 when both $\pi(X_i; \psi)$ and $m_1(X_i; \beta)$ are correctly specified. Intuitively, the efficiency gain comes from the fact that the regression imputation estimator $m_1(X_i; \hat{\beta})$ leverages additional information from the incomplete cases. Similarly, one could construct an augmented IPW estimator for μ_0 as

$$\hat{\mu}_0^{DR} = \hat{\mu}_0^{IPW} - \frac{\sum_{i=1}^n \{R_i - \hat{\pi}_i\}(1 - G_i) m_0(X_i; \hat{\gamma})/\hat{\pi}_i}{\sum_{i=1}^n R_i(1 - G_i)/\hat{\pi}_i}$$

and estimate the average treatment effect by $\hat{\mu}^{DR} = \hat{\mu}_1^{DR} - \hat{\mu}_0^{DR}$, for which the doubly robust and efficiency properties similarly apply. Variance estimation for $\hat{\mu}^{DR}$ could proceed as outlined above for $\hat{\mu}^{IPW}$ with a slight modification for the sandwich variance estimator as one needs to incorporate the score functions for the regression models m_1 and m_0 into the joint estimating function $U_i(\theta)$.

Outside of the missing data applications, the doubly robust estimator is also popular in the causal inference literature (Chap. 21 provides an introduction of causal inference methods). The doubly robust estimator improves the weighting estimator since it offers two chances to consistently estimate the average treatment effect. On the other hand, it also provides two chances to incorrectly specify the model, and, therefore, a limitation of this estimator is that when both models are incorrectly specified, the bias could be substantial and oftentimes exceeds the bias of the simple IPW estimator (Kang and Schafer 2007; Ridgeway and McCaffrey 2007; Tsiatis and Davidian 2007). A lively stream of research is devoted to developing bias-corrected doubly robust estimators that improve the bias and variance properties of $\hat{\mu}^{DR}$. A technical exposition on these new estimators is omitted due to limited space, and details on recent developments could be found in a recent review by Seaman and Vansteelandt (2018).

Imputation-Based Method

Regression Imputation

For an RCT with missing outcomes, one sensible approach is to fill in these missing outcome data by exploiting the relationship between the observed values of the outcome and baseline covariates. This is often done using an outcome regression model or a Y-model. The regression imputation is a special type of simple imputation method that provides a convenient solution to the missing data problem. The core idea of this approach is to fill in the missing data and then allows analysts to use any valid statistical methods to analyze the RCT as if the full data have been observed (Little and Rubin 2002).

The unbiasedness of regression imputation relies on the MAR assumption. Consider an outcome regression model that specifies the parametric relationship between outcome Y and covariate X within each treatment group as $f(Y|X, G, \theta)$, where θ is a collection of unknown parameters. Had one known the value of θ, one could characterize the dependency of Y on X and could then fill in the missing values of the outcome by a best "guess" from the distribution $f(Y|X, G, \theta)$ – for example, by the conditional expectation $E(Y|X, G, \theta)$. In practice, the value of θ is unknown and must be estimated. Under the assumption of MAR, it is easy to show that

$$f(Y|X, G, \theta) = f(Y|X, G, R = 1, \theta),$$

where R is the missingness indicator. The above relationship suggests that θ can be consistently estimated by using only the complete cases. Once an estimator $\hat{\theta}$ is obtained, the missing outcomes could be predicted by $E(Y|X, G, \hat{\theta})$ to construct a full dataset for subsequent analysis.

To illustrate the idea of regression imputation, consider our previous RCT, which is conducted to evaluate the effect of a new drug in reducing patients' blood pressure. Consider the n_1 patients in the treatment group ($G_i = 1$). In this group, let us assume that the first s_1 patients have complete observations for this outcome, and the remaining $n_1 - s_1$ patients have missing values in the outcome. One could then use a normal model with a multiple linear regression form to represent the conditional density function of the observed blood pressure:

$$Y_i \mid X_i, G_i = 1 \sim N(\alpha + X_i^T \beta, \sigma^2), i = 1 \ldots s_1.$$

Here, $\theta = (\alpha, \beta^T, \sigma^2)^T$, where α is the intercept, β is the slope parameter, and σ^2 is the residual variance. In other words, the above normality representation implies a multiple linear regression for the mean of blood pressure on the covariate vector as $E(Y_i|X_i, G_i = 1) = \alpha + X_i^T \beta$, and the parameters can be estimated by ordinary least squares (OLS). With the OLS estimates $\hat{\alpha}$ and $\hat{\beta}$, each missing outcome Y_j can be imputed with a random draw from a normal distribution with estimated mean, $\hat{\alpha} + X_j^T \hat{\beta}$, and estimated variance $\hat{\sigma}^2$, for $j = s_1 + 1 \ldots n_1$. The same steps could be carried out to impute the missing outcomes in the control group and hence to obtain a full dataset for the RCT. Assume that the Y-model is correctly specified and the imputed value $\hat{Y}_j$ is a consistent estimator for the true and unobserved value under MAR. Therefore, the imputed full dataset is an approximately unbiased representation of the true but unobserved full dataset, and subsequent analysis of the imputed dataset can give an approximately unbiased point estimate of the average treatment effect.

The same logic carries over to the analysis of binary outcomes. Suppose that the secondary endpoint is the event indicator of hypertension such that $Y_i = 1$ or 0 dpending the occurrence of hypertension at the end of the study. In the treatment group, let us still assume that the first s_1 patients have fully observed outcomes and the remaining $n_1 - s_1$ patients have missing outcomes. One can specify a logistic regression model for this group:

$$\log\left(\frac{\Pr(Y_i = 1|X_i, G_i = 1)}{1 - \Pr(Y_i = 1|X_i, G_i = 1)}\right) = \alpha + X_i^T \beta, i = 1 \ldots s_1.$$

Once the regression coefficients are estimated by maximum likelihood, the missing outcomes can then be filled by drawing from the Bernoulli distribution with event probability:

$$\Pr(Y_j = 1 | X_j, G_j = 1) = \frac{\exp\left(\hat{\alpha} + X_j^T \hat{\beta}\right)}{1 + \exp\left(\hat{\alpha} + X_j^T \hat{\beta}\right)} \quad \text{for } j = s_1 + 1 \ldots n_1.$$

There are two known limitations of regression imputation. First, regression imputation is an example of single imputation, which fills in the missing data once. Because single imputation fails to acknowledge all sources of uncertainty, the variance of subsequent analysis will overstate the certainty of the treatment effect, leading to an inflated type I error rate. Specifically, in the linear regression imputation model, the uncertainty in estimating the parameters $\hat{\alpha}$, $\hat{\beta}$, and $\hat{\sigma}^2$ has not been properly accounted for, and hence analysis based on the imputed dataset tends to underestimate the true variability (Rubin 1996, 2004). Second, the validity of regression imputation critically depends on the correct specification of the imputation model. To guard against model misspecification, researchers have the liberty to choose more advanced nonparametric regression without restrictive parametric assumptions. For example, one can impute the missing entries with observed entries from similar units (e.g., hot deck approach (Hanson 1978)) or more generally define the similarity between units based on their covariate distance and impute missing Ys using the mean outcomes of their k nearest neighbors (Cochran and Rubin 1973). These approaches are similar to the matching approach in the causal inference literature (Imbens and Rubin 2015). The regression imputation methods can also be extended to the cases with missing covariates (Little 1992), although they are not often used in practice to deal with them. Finally, another ad hoc approach called "unconditional imputation" or "mean imputation" is also a special case of regression imputation in which the imputation model only includes an intercept. Such a method can be difficult to justify in RCT applications as it implicitly assumes the more restrictive MCAR assumption.

Multiple Imputation

While single imputation usually fails to properly acknowledge all sources of variation in the imputation process, multiple imputation can properly account for uncertainty by providing multiply imputed datasets (Rubin 1976, 1996, 2004). Multiple imputation fills in the missing data with an imputation model that resembles the data generating process. The imputation model describes the relationships across all observed variables in the data by specifying a joint model on them. By contrast, the outcome regression model or Y-model described earlier for the regression imputation represents a simple model of imputation, which has limited use in handling complex missing data scenarios where both covariates and outcomes are missing.

In brief, multiple imputation includes three steps. First, missing data entries are imputed multiple (m) times based on a joint model of variables, and m complete datasets $D_1 \ldots D_k \ldots D_m$ are generated. Second, one analyzes each imputed dataset using any pre-specified statistical method as if there is no missing data to obtain m point estimates $\hat{\theta}^{(1)}\ldots\hat{\theta}^{(k)}\ldots\hat{\theta}^{(m)}$ and their corresponding variance estimates $V^{(1)}\ldots V^{(k)}\ldots V^{(m)}$. Third, the final point estimate and variance are obtained using Rubin's rule (Rubin 2004):

$$\hat{\theta}^{MI} = \frac{1}{m}\sum_{k=1}^{m}\hat{\theta}^{(k)}$$

$$V^{MI} = W + B = \frac{\sum_{k=1}^{m} V^{(k)}}{m} + \left(1 + \frac{1}{m}\right)\sum_{k=1}^{m}\frac{\left(\hat{\theta}^{(k)} - \hat{\theta}^{MI}\right)^2}{m-1}.$$

For the variance term, W is the within-imputation variance and B is the between-imputation variance. Statistical test for $H_0: \theta = \theta^*$ could then be carried out based on

$$\frac{\hat{\theta}^{MI} - \theta^*}{\sqrt{V^{MI}}} \sim t_v,$$

where the degrees of freedom are

$$v = (m-1)\left(1 + \frac{m}{m+1}\frac{W}{B}\right)^2.$$

However, this test is derived under the assumption that the degrees of freedom for the full data $v_{full} = \infty$, which is not always attenable (Barnard and Rubin 1999). If the sample size is relatively small, the degree of freedom for the full data v_{full} can also be small (such as pilot studies evaluating the safety and efficacy of new medications). A more appropriate degree of freedom or the adjusted degree of freedom is provided as

$$v^* = \frac{1}{v} + \frac{1}{\hat{v}_{obs}} \leq v_{full},$$

where

$$\hat{v}_{obs} = \left(\frac{v_{full}+1}{v_{full}+3}\right)v_{full}\left(1 + \frac{m+1}{m}\frac{B}{W}\right)^{-1}.$$

The building block of multiple imputation is the specification of a reasonable imputation model that mimics the data generating procedure. To obtain a complete dataset, both frequentist and Bayesian methods can be used. Specifically, one could partition the full data into (Y_{mis}, Y_{obs}) and factorize the joint distribution of $(Y_{mis},$

$Y_{obs} \mid \theta)$ as $f(Y_{mis} \mid Y_{obs}, \theta) f(Y_{obs} \mid \theta)$. Note that here the role of outcome and covariates is not distinguished for notational simplicity. In other words, Y is used to represent a generic data vector including both outcomes and covariates. From the frequentist point of view, θ is the data feature shared by both the observed and missing data. Therefore, Y_{mis} can be drawn from the imputation model $f(Y_{mis} \mid Y_{obs}, \hat{\theta})$ with $\hat{\theta}$ estimated from a model characterizing $f(Y_{obs} \mid \theta)$. However, such imputation model is considered "improper" because the uncertainty in $\hat{\theta}$ is not accounted for during the imputation process. A proper imputation procedure that accounts for all sources of uncertainty is desired and often necessary to allow the use of Rubin's rules to obtain valid results (Rubin 2004).

By contrast, it is relatively more straightforward to proceed within the Bayesian framework because the imputed data can be randomly drawn from the posterior predictive distribution. More specifically, the Bayesian approach iteratively samples θ and Y_{mis} from their conditional posterior distributions as follows:

$$Y_{mis}^{(t+1)} \sim f\left(Y_{mis} \mid Y_{obs}, \hat{\theta}^{(t)}\right)$$

$$\hat{\theta}^{(t+1)} \sim f(\theta \mid Y_{mis}^{(t+1)}, Y_{obs}),$$

where the superscript t represents the iteration count. In what follows, we provide a more focused discussion on how multiple imputation is carried out and mention a few practical issues.

Joint Modeling Approach (MCMC)

The joint modeling approach is based on a full data model, in which the missing data are treated as an unknown parameter. In other words, one could formulate a joint model for (Y_{mis}, Y_{obs}), parameterized by θ. All unknown parameters in the joint model are then estimated by Markov Chain Monte Carlo (MCMC), a computational algorithm to iteratively update parameters until convergence. Since Y_{mis} is treated as the unknown and updated in each iteration, such an approach is also referred to as data augmentation (Schafer 1997).

Suppose missing data exist for both the outcomes and covariates except for the treatment assignment. Write $\left(Y_{mis}^1, Y_{obs}^1\right)$ and $\left(Y_{mis}^0, Y_{obs}^0\right)$ as the missing and observed data in the treatment and control groups. Since the outcome model is likely to be different for the treated and control groups, the imputation model may differ between groups. One could either specify a joint model allowing for treatment-by-covariate interactions or simply carry out imputation separately for each group. Below we will focus on the latter strategy. Let us mainly look at the imputation for the treatment group and omit the superscript for $\left(Y_{mis}^1, Y_{obs}^1\right)$ to reduce notation. For the treatment group, one could assume $(Y_{i,\,mis}, Y_{i,\,obs})$ is jointly multivariate normal with mean μ and variance Σ and express the joint density by $f(Y_{i,\,mis}, Y_{i,\,obs} \mid \mu, \Sigma)$. If there is no missing data (i.e., Y_{mis} is fully observed), the posterior distribution for (μ, Σ) can be obtained as the product of data likelihood and prior distributions for (μ, Σ). Frequently, the use of multivariate normal models could greatly simplify the calculation in the posterior distribution due to the conjugacy property, which refers to the fact that the prior distribution and the posterior distribution are within the same parametric family (Press 2005). Specifically, by assuming the following prior distributions,

$$\mu \sim N(\mu_0, \Lambda_0), \quad \Sigma \sim \text{inverse} - \text{Wishart}\left(\nu_0, S_0^{-1}\right),$$

the posterior distribution for μ is also multivariate normal, and the posterior distribution for Σ is also inverse-Wishart. One can thereby construct a Gibbs sampler to iteratively update μ and Σ. However, because $Y_{i,\,mis}$ is also unknown, the iteratively process should include an additional step to augment $Y_{i,\,mis}$ from $f(Y_{i,mis}|Y_{i,obs}, \mu, \Sigma) = N\left(\widetilde{\mu}, \widetilde{\Sigma}\right)$, where

$$\widetilde{\mu} = \mu_{mis} + \Sigma_{[mis,obs]} \left(\Sigma_{[obs,obs]}\right)^{-1} (Y_{obs} - \mu_{obs})$$

$$\widetilde{\Sigma} = \Sigma_{[mis,mis]} - \Sigma_{[mis,obs]} \left(\Sigma_{[obs,obs]}\right)^{-1} \Sigma_{[obs,mis]}.$$

The full Gibbs sampler scheme is summarized as follows. One first supplies a set of starting values for $\left(\left\{Y_{i,mis}^{(0)}\right\}_{i:G_i=1}, \mu^{(0)}, \Sigma^{(0)}\right)$, and then the following updates are iterated until convergence:

1. Sample $\mu^{(t+1)}$ from $f(\mu | \{Y_{i,mis}^{(t)}, Y_{i,obs}\}_{i:G_i=1}, \Sigma^{(t)})$
2. Sample $\Sigma^{(t+1)}$ from $f\left(\Sigma | \{Y_{i,mis}^{(t)}, Y_{i,obs}\}_{i:G_i=1}, \mu^{(t+1)}\right)$
3. Sample $Y_{i,mis}^{(t+1)}$ from $f(Y_{i,mis} | Y_{i,obs}, \mu^{(t+1)}, \Sigma^{(t+1)})$ for each i with $G_i = 1$

With a large enough number of iterations, the chain will converge, and one can obtain a stable posterior sample for (Y_{mis}, μ, Σ). Once the chain has converged, the posterior sample could be used to impute missing entries. Since the consecutive draws for the MCMC tend to have non-negligible serial correlations, thinning is often recommended as a strategy to obtain relatively independent posterior draws. For example, to obtain $m = 20$ multiply imputed datasets, one could take the posterior predictive draws every ten iterations after the chain has converged. The thinning parameter could also be decided by examining autocorrelation plots (Hoff 2009). The stability of the multivariate normal model for imputing missing data has been demonstrated in a range of scenarios (Schafer 1997).

The multivariate normal model can also be extended to impute binary variables under a latent variable representation, $U_i \sim N(\eta, 1)$, such that $Y_i = 1$ if $U_i > 0$ (Albert and Chib 1993). With the introduction of the additional latent parameter η, the multivariate normal theory could still be useful. However, for ordinal outcomes or time-to-event outcomes, a more sophisticated MCMC algorithm – the Metropolis-Hastings algorithm – may be used to update parameters since the full conditional posterior distributions often do not have closed-form solutions (Browne 2006). Despite the usefulness of the Metropolis-Hastings algorithm in more general settings, it requires a careful selection of the proposal distributions.

One apparent limitation for the joint modeling approach is that the imputation model becomes difficult to specify in the presence of a mix of continuous, categorical, ordinal, and count variables. The multivariate normal model naturally accommodates continuous variables but may find limited use for categorical, ordinal, and time-to-event variables. Although prior simulations have shown that the multivariate normal model may not necessarily produce biased results when it was used to impute binary variables (i.e., postulating a normal distribution for the binary outcome) (Schafer 1997), the imputed values are not guaranteed to satisfy the natural bounds for probabilities (i.e., between 0 and 1).

Fully Conditional Specification (MICE)

Instead of specifying a joint distribution of data, an alternative approach is to specify the full conditional distribution for each variable with missing entries. In other words, each variable is modeled as a function of all other variables in the imputation process so that traditional forms of regression models (e.g., linear, logistic, multinomial logistic, etc.) can be applied to assist the specification of the full conditional distributions. This framework of imputation is called the "multiple imputation using chained equations" (MICE) and was firstly developed by van Buuren and Groothuis-Oudshoorn (2011) and Raghunathan et al. (2001). MICE can not only incorporate data-type information but also allow for flexible model choices that include higher-order terms and interactions. Because of its flexibility in imputation, MICE has been widely used in practice.

In fact, the implementation of MICE resembles the steps involved in the joint modeling approach, since the joint modeling approach also requires iterative updates from the posterior full conditionals. MICE requires that each variable with missing entries is imputed based on a regression model that specifies its relationship to other variables. The parameters in each conditional model are estimated and updated in each iteration. To initiate MICE, starting values for missing entries are required, but starting values for model parameters are no longer necessary. The implementation of MICE is available in existing statistical software, such as the "mice" package in R (van Buuren and Groothuis-Oudshoorn 2011) and PROC MI in SAS.

Despite its popularity, a known limitation of MICE is the lack of theoretical underpinnings. The performance of MICE is largely justified based on its ad hoc statistical performance in providing adequate imputed values. Simulation studies have demonstrated that the performance of MICE and the joint modeling approach are largely similar, while MICE tends to be more flexible (Akande et al. 2017). However, the computational cost of MICE can increase if many binary or categorical variables need to be imputed. Often, the imputation of these variables relies on multinomial or ordered logistic regression models, which may be rather difficult to compute when the dimension of covariates is large.

Model choice in multiple imputation, especially in MICE, can be challenging. In clinical trials, one may have many covariates to be included in the imputation model, and model specification, such as the inclusion of higher-order terms and interactions, can be hard to determine. While no panacea is available to tackle these challenges, it is generally agreed that substantive knowledge of a specific study is necessary to determine an adequate imputation model. It is also worth noting that the imputation of missing data belongs to the "design" phase of a study, as its aim is to provide multiply imputed datasets for subsequent analysis. The choice of imputation model should ideally be consistent with the analytical considerations. The compatibility or congeniality between imputation model and analysis model has been extensively discussed by Meng (1994).

Another practical issue is to determine the number of imputed datasets (m) for the actual analysis. While m should ideally be large, the early work by Rubin (1978) suggests 3–5 imputations can provide efficient results, and the additional efficiency gain by increasing m is limited. Even if 50% of the data is missing, 91% relative efficiency can be achieved with $m = 5$, and 95% relative efficiency can be achieved with $m = 10$. However, recent literature suggests the validity of imputation should not only be assessed based on the point estimate. The variation incurred by the Monte Carlo procedure can create quite different imputed datasets that lead to point estimates with large confidence intervals (White et al. 2011). Based on prior simulation studies, it is recommended that m should be proportional to the fraction of missing information (F) in a dataset. A rule of thumb is to obtain no less than $100 \times F$ imputed datasets to achieve a sufficient reduction in the Monte Carlo error.

Sensitivity Analysis

As the MAR assumption is often untestable from data, sensitivity analysis may be necessary to assess how different the estimates would be from the observed estimate under less restrictive missingness assumptions. While there are many ways to assess sensitivity in various contexts, here we only sketch a general idea for clinical trials with a cross-sectional outcome. Recall that the MAR assumption serves as the basis for most of the approaches we have discussed so far. When the missing data mechanism is MNAR, analysis based on any of those approaches may be biased, and sensitivity analysis could provide a sense of how large such bias could be. The most typical sensitivity analysis assumes the existence of an unmeasured covariate that is associated with both the missingness indicator and the outcome (we will call such a covariate an unmeasured confounder following the nomenclature in causal inference). Analyses are then conducted ignoring such a covariate, and these results

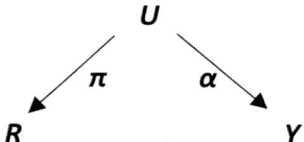

Fig. 1 A schematic illustration of the sensitivity analysis that assesses the influence of an unmeasured confounder. R missingness indicator, Y outcome, U unmeasured confounder, π relationship between U and R, α relationship between U and Y

are then compared with the primary analysis. For example, one could create a hypothetical covariate U and postulate its relationship – characterized by sensitivity parameter π, α – on the missingness mechanism (R) and outcome (Y). The direction and magnitude of π and α should ideally be informed by the substantive knowledge of the study. More than one set of π, α is often necessary to simulate the covariate U. The schematic illustration of the sensitivity analysis is provided in the Fig. 1. One needs to simulate U based on each set of (π, α) and repeat the primary analysis assuming U is unobserved. Comparing the set of results under various assumptions of (π, α) could provide a sense of validity in the primary analysis.

Another type of sensitivity analysis focuses on the diversified reasons underlying the missingness. In RCTs, missing outcomes can also arise from treatment noncompliance and death, among others, and the corresponding missingness processes may be distinguished. To handle missing data in such cases, a good starting point is to define the sensible causal estimand. To do so, the following questions would be instructive. Is the intention-to-treat analysis that reflects the effect of the assigned treatment of primary interest? Are the missing responses due to death of research interest, or equivalently, should these participants be included in the target population? If the answers are both yes, pattern mixture models or the framework of principle stratification may provide more defensible statistical solutions than the complete-case analysis (Angrist et al. 1996; Hollis and Campbell 1999; Frangakis and Rubin 2002).

Summary and Conclusion

This chapter explains different missing data mechanisms (MCAR, MAR, and MNAR) and introduces likelihood-based, weighting, and imputation methods to handle missing data in RCTs. For the past decades, the field has moved from the simplest, ad hoc approaches (e.g., complete-case analysis, single imputation) to more statistically rigorous, flexible approaches (e.g., doubly robust inference and multiple imputation). Due to the limited space, this chapter only discusses the basic scenario with a single type of missing data, while in clinical studies, multiple types of missing data may arise from patient dropout, censoring by death and treatment noncompliance, among others. For example, Little (2014) and Little and Kang (2015) studied missing data methods to differentiate multiple types of missingness and offered practical recommendations for trialists. In practice, we strongly encourage a careful design of trials to prevent the occurrence of missing data in order to minimize the risk of selection bias; this task requires a joint effort between stakeholders, trialists, implementation scientists, and statisticians and should precede any treatment of missing data. In studies where missing data are challenging to prevent, the tools presented in the current chapter may be useful to reduce the selection bias. Since these statistical approaches rely on assumptions on the missingness mechanisms, additional sensitivity analysis is often necessary and has been increasingly emphasized in applications (Little et al. 2016).

Key Facts

- Three types of missing data mechanisms are distinguished, missing completely at random (MCAR), missing at random (MAR), and missing not at random (MNAR). The true missing data mechanism is unknown and could not be tested based on data. Substantive considerations often support the assumption of missing data mechanism.
- Likelihood-based methods provide statistically efficient estimators in the presence of missing data when the likelihood model is correctly specified. Oftentimes, a joint likelihood for the entire data is difficult to specify in the presence of different data types, such as continuous, categorical, count, and ordinal variables.
- Single imputation, such as regression imputation, may generate unbiased imputed values if the model is correctly specified. However, single imputation often underestimates the variability in the imputed process and may lead to inflated type I error rate in testing for the treatment effect.
- Inverse probability weight (IPW) models the missingness process and is easy to implement. The unbiasedness of IPW relies on the correct specification of the missingness model. Combining weighting and regression imputation leads to a doubly robust estimator with improved statistical properties.
- Multiple imputation appropriately acknowledges all sources of uncertainty and leads to unbiased results when the imputation model is correctly specified. Joint modeling approach (MCMC) and the fully conditional specification (MICE) represent two widely used approaches to handle missing data.
- A typical sensitivity analysis assesses how unmeasured factors (confounders) could alter the observed estimate of the average treatment effect. To do so, one would motivate the sensitivity parameters in the RCT context, repeat the pre-specified analysis under each assumed sensitivity parameter, and assess the difference relative to the primary analysis.
- A careful design of trials is strongly encouraged to prevent the occurrence of missing data; such a task requires a joint effort between stakeholders, trialists, implementation scientists, and statisticians and should precede any treatment of missing data. In studies where missing data are challenging to prevent, the tools presented in the current chapter may be useful to reduce the selection bias due to missing data.

Cross-References

▶ Causal Inference: Efficacy and Mechanism Evaluation
▶ Estimands and Sensitivity Analyses
▶ Logistic Regression and Related Methods

References

Akande O, Li F, Reiter J (2017) An empirical comparison of multiple imputation methods for categorical data. Am Stat 71:162–170

Albert JH, Chib S (1993) Bayesian analysis of binary and polychotomous response data. J Am Sat Assoc 88:669–679

Angrist JD, Imbens GW, Rubin DB (1996) Identification of causal effects using instrumental variables. J Am Stat Assoc 91:444–455

Barnard J, Rubin DB (1999) Miscellanea. Small-sample degrees of freedom with multiple imputation. Biometrika 86:948–955

Browne WJ (2006) MCMC algorithms for constrained variance matrices. Comput Stat Data Anal 50:1655–1677

Carpenter J, Kenward M (2012) Multiple imputation and its application. Wiley, London

Cochran WG, Rubin DB (1973) Controlling bias in observational studies: a review. Sankhyā Indian J Stat Ser A 35:417–446

Dempster AP, Laird NM, Rubin DB (1977) Maximum likelihood from incomplete data via the EM algorithm. J R Stat Soc Ser B Methodol 39:1–38

Efron B, Tibshirani RJ (1994) An Introduction to the Bootstrap. Chapman and Hall/CRC, New York

Frangakis CE, Rubin DB (2002) Principal stratification in causal inference. Biometrics 58:21–29

Hanson RH (1978) The current population survey: design and methodology. Department of Commerce, Bureau of the Census

Hoff PD (2009) A first course in Bayesian statistical methods. Springer Science & Business Media, New York

Hollis S, Campbell F (1999) What is meant by intention to treat analysis? Survey of published randomised controlled trials. BMJ 319:670–674

Horvitz DG, Thompson DJ (1952) A generalization of sampling without replacement from a finite universe. J Am Stat Assoc 47:663–685

Imbens GW, Rubin DB (2015) Causal inference in statistics, social, and biomedical sciences. Cambridge University Press, New York

International Conference on Harmonization (1998) Statistical principles for clinical trials E9. https://www.ich.org/fileadmin/Public_Web_Site/ICH_Products/Guidelines/Efficacy/E9/Step4/E9_Guideline.pdf

Kang JD, Schafer JL (2007) Demystifying double robustness: a comparison of alternative strategies for estimating a population mean from incomplete data. Stat Sci 22:523–539

Kenward MG, Molenberghs G (2009) Last observation carried forward: a crystal ball? J Biopharm Stat 19:872–888

Li F, Thomas LE, Li F (2018) Addressing extreme propensity scores via the overlap weights. Am J Epidemiol. https://doi.org/10.1093/aje/kwy201

Little RJ (1992) Regression with missing X's: a review. J Am Stat Assoc 87:1227–1237

Little RJA, Rubin DB (2002) Statistical Analysis with Missing Data, Second Edition. John Wiley & Sons, Inc., Hoboken, New Jersey

Little RJ (2014) Dropouts in longitudinal studies: methods of analysis. Wiley StatsRef: Statistics Reference Online

Little R, Kang S (2015) Intention-to-treat analysis with treatment discontinuation and missing data in clinical trials. Stat Med 34:2381–2390

Little RJ, Rubin DB (2014) Statistical analysis with missing data. Wiley, Hoboken

Little RJ, D'Agostino R, Dickersin K et al (2010) The prevention and treatment of missing data in clinical trials. Panel on handling missing data in clinical trials. In: Committee on national statistics, division of behavioral and social sciences and education. The National Academies Press, Washington DC

Little RJ, Wang J, Sun X, Tian H, Suh EY, Lee M et al (2016) The treatment of missing data in a large cardiovascular clinical outcomes study. Clin Trials 13:344–351

Lunceford JK, Davidian M (2004) Stratification and weighting via the propensity score in estimation of causal treatment effects: a comparative study. Stat Med 23:2937–2960

Mallinckrodt CH (2013) Preventing and treating missing data in longitudinal clinical trials: a practical guide. Cambridge University Press, New York

Meng X-L (1994) Multiple-imputation inferences with uncongenial sources of input. Stat Sci 9:538–558

Oehlert GW (1992) A note on the delta method. Am Stat 46(1):27–29

Press SJ (2005) Applied multivariate analysis: using Bayesian and frequentist methods of inference. Dover Publications, INC. Mineola, New York

Raghunathan TE, Lepkowski JM, Van Hoewyk J, Solenberger P (2001) A multivariate technique for multiply imputing missing values using a sequence of regression models. Surv Methodol 27:85–96

Ridgeway G, McCaffrey DF (2007) Comment: demystifying double robustness: a comparison of alternative strategies for estimating a population mean from incomplete data. Stat Sci 22:540–543

Rubin DB (1976) Inference and missing data. Biometrika 63:581–592

Rubin DB (1978) Multiple imputations in sample surveys-a phenomenological Bayesian approach to nonresponse. In: Proceedings of the survey research methods section of the American Statistical Association. American Statistical Association, pp 20–34

Rubin DB (1996) Multiple imputation after 18+ years. J Am Stat Assoc 91:473–489

Rubin DB (2004) Multiple imputation for nonresponse in surveys. Wiley, New York

Schafer JL (1997) Analysis of incomplete multivariate data. Chapman and Hall/CRC, New York

Seaman SR, Vansteelandt S (2018) Introduction to double robust methods for incomplete data. Stat Sci Rev J Inst Math Stat 33:184–197

Tsiatis A (2007) Semiparametric theory and missing data. Springer Science & Business Media, New York

Tsiatis AA, Davidian M (2007) Comment: demystifying double robustness: a comparison of alternative strategies for estimating a population mean from incomplete data. Stat Sci 22:569–573

van Buuren S, Groothuis-Oudshoorn K (2011) MICE: multivariate imputation by chained equations in R. J Stat Softw 45:1–67

White IR, Royston P, Wood AM (2011) Multiple imputation using chained equations: issues and guidance for practice. Stat Med 30:377–399

Essential Statistical Tests

87

Gregory R. Pond and Samantha-Jo Caetano

Contents

Introduction	1704
Common Statistical Tests	1706
Tests for Continuous Outcomes	1706
T-Test	1706
Non-parametric Tests in Lieu of T-Tests	1708
Multiple Groups	1710
Non-parametric Tests for Multiple Groups	1711
Tests for Contingency Tables	1711
χ^2 Test	1711
Non-parametric Tests for Categorical Variables	1713
Summary	1715
Key Facts	1715
Cross-References	1716
References	1716

Abstract

This chapter summarizes the basic steps involved in performing commonly used statistical hypothesis tests for continuous and categorical outcomes in randomized clinical trials and further describes the statistical test procedures. Statistical hypothesis tests generally fall into two broad categories, parametric and non-parametric statistical tests. Parametric tests are statistical tests that require the assumption that the data follows some known distribution. These include t-tests, analysis of

G. R. Pond (✉)
Department of Oncology, McMaster University, Hamilton, ON, Canada

Ontario Institute for Cancer Research, Toronto, ON, Canada
e-mail: gpond@mcmaster.ca

S.-J. Caetano
Department of Mathematics and Statistics, McMaster University, Hamilton, ON, Canada
e-mail: caetans@math.mcmaster.ca

© Springer Nature Switzerland AG 2022
S. Piantadosi, C. L. Meinert (eds.), *Principles and Practice of Clinical Trials*,
https://doi.org/10.1007/978-3-319-52636-2_118

variance (ANOVA), and χ^2 tests. Non-parametric tests do not require this assumption, and are robust to misspecification, but are generally more conservative. Commonly used non-parametric tests include the signed-rank test, Wilcoxon rank sum test, Kruskal-Wallis test, and Fisher's exact test. While not an exhaustive list, this chapter will describe each of these tests in detail and give an overview of their use.

Keywords

Hypothesis test · Parametric · Non-parametric · T-test · Chi-square · ANOVA

Introduction

The essential principle behind randomized clinical trials is that patients are randomly allocated to receive one of two or more interventions so that the interventions can be compared. In a simplistic scenario, the health of all individuals who receive one intervention would improve, while all those who receive a competing intervention would worsen, clearly showing that the first intervention is superior. Unfortunately, real-life clinical trials rarely, if ever, have extreme results such as this. It is not always straightforward to determine which intervention is superior or if all interventions are more or less equally efficacious. Statistical hypothesis tests are therefore needed to make inferences about the observed data in a randomized clinical trial.

Simplistically, one must perform a series of design, conduct, and analysis steps to perform a statistical hypothesis test. In the design of the hypothesis test, one must (1) define the outcome of interest, (2) specify the hypotheses to be tested, (3) define the test statistic to be used, and (4) define a decision rule based on the test statistic. Then, to conduct the analysis, one must (5) collect the data and (6) interpret results based on the observed data and the pre-defined decision rule. These steps have to occur in order to be statistically sound. Although the majority of this chapter will focus on defining the test statistic, a brief summary of each of these steps is needed. For a more thorough review, the reader is referred to one of the many published articles on the subject, for example, Guyatt et al. (1995).

The process of performing a statistical hypothesis test starts by defining the outcome. A good outcome measure is one which is objectively measured and quantifiable and has clinical relevance. Examples such as the objective tumor response rate, 90-day surgical mortality rate, or survival time (time from randomization to death) are commonly used outcomes. The type of outcome is generally defined as either continuous, categorical, or time-to-event, and common statistics, such as the mean, median, or proportion, are used to quantify the data.

In a clinical trial, investigators are usually interested in whether an "average" patient does better when given one intervention or the other. Intuitively, they just compare the "average" observed value between interventions (i.e., do patients receiving intervention A have a higher response rate, or a shorter median time in hospital, than patients who received intervention B?). However, to formalize the decision-making process, investigators must pre-define their initial hypotheses, typically referred to as the null hypothesis (H_0) and the alternative hypothesis (H_1 or H_A). The null hypothesis is generally the default position, and evidence is collected which allows investigators to test the validity of H_0. The alternative hypothesis is the result that investigators wish to prove. Generally, the alternative hypothesis must be true if H_0 is false. Initially, one assumes that H_0 is true by default, and the conclusion of the hypothesis test will be based on whether the data provides compelling evidence to reject H_0 or not. If a test results in a rejection of the null hypothesis, then there is compelling evidence in favor of the alternative hypothesis.

A test statistic is defined based on the type of data being measured, which allows one to quantify how consistent the observed data is with the different hypotheses. The test statistic is principally a measure of the effect of the intervention (or difference in outcomes between interventions) relative to its variability (i.e., ratio of signal-to-noise). A decision rule is used to define a "critical region" (or sometimes referred to as a "rejection region"). The critical region contains all values of the test statistic that are considered to be "extreme" given the initial assumption of H_0 being true. Thus, the critical region is the set of possible values of the test statistic that are unlikely, under the null hypothesis, which can be calculated because one knows the distribution of the test statistic. Therefore, one can calculate the probability that the value of the test statistic will be in the critical region given H_0 is true. Further, after acquiring data and calculating the test statistic using the observed data, one can calculate the probability of results being as extreme, or more extreme, than the observed data under the assumption of H_0 being true. This is called the p-value. If the p-value is small, then the probability is small that one could get results as extreme as the observed if the null hypothesis were correct; this would therefore give evidence against H_0. Statisticians define a threshold p-value (e.g., 0.05) prior to collecting the data, so that if the p-value is less than this threshold, they would reject H_0. Equivalently, this threshold is the probability of the test statistic falling in the critical region of possible values considered extreme, given the initial assumption of H_0 being true.

Since research studies use a sample of patients in an attempt to make inferences regarding the larger population, there is the potential for drawing an incorrect conclusion. For instance, it is possible that observed results provide little evidence to reject H_0. Investigators might then conclude that H_0 is plausible, when the truth is that H_0 is false. In this case, the investigators would have made an erroneous conclusion, specifically a type II error. The rate of committing a type II error is denoted as β. Alternatively, investigators may conclude the observed data is not consistent with H_0; therefore they reject H_0 in favor of H_1. However, it could be in truth that the interventions are actually similar and H_0 should not be rejected. The investigators mistakenly rejected H_0 in this scenario and made a type I error. The rate of committing a type I error is denoted as α. One should keep both error rates as low as possible, but there is a trade-off between the two. Increased sample sizes will decrease the possibility of making a type I or type II error, but there is always a chance the study conclusion could be incorrect, no matter how large is the study sample size.

The rest of this chapter will focus on the basic types of statistical tests that are used in clinical trials and the creation of the test statistic. It will be assumed that one has already defined the type of outcome measure to be used for analysis; details on how to identify and define outcomes are described in detail in a separate chapter. Further, this chapter will only focus on continuous and categorical outcomes. Tests for time-to-event outcomes, including time-to-death (overall survival), are sufficiently important that they warrant two chapters on its own (see ▶ Chaps. 88, "Nonparametric Survival Analysis," by Y. Lokhnygina and ▶ 89, "Survival Analysis II," by J. Dignam).

Common Statistical Tests

Despite the increasing sophistication of statistical methods used in the medical literature (Sato et al. 2017), basic statistical tests remain commonly employed. In fact, contingency tables (which includes χ^2, Fisher's exact, and McNemar tests) for categorical data were used in over half of all original and special articles published in the *New England Journal of Medicine* in 2015 (Gosho et al. 2017). Only power analyses and survival methods, whose use has rapidly increased over the past 30 years, were used more frequently. T-tests for continuous data were used in almost 1/3 of studies, while analysis of variance (ANOVA) was used in another 1/4 of studies. The use of t-tests has declined slightly over time, while the use of non-parametric tests has increased (Fagerland 2012). Non-parametric tests are those tests based on statistics that do not have a known or easily specified distribution, such as analyses where the primary outcome is the median, or the sample size is small, and the central limit theorem (CLT) cannot be used. The CLT is one of the most important theorems in statistics and states that the sampling distribution of the sample mean will converge to a normal distribution as the sample size gets larger (e.g., >30), regardless of the underlying shape of the population distribution. Use of the t-test requires the assumption of normality for the sampling distribution, demonstrating the importance of the CLT. Because of the CLT and the simplicity of the t-test, it is clear why the use of the t-test remains common in the scientific literature.

This chapter will focus on essential statistical tests for contingency tables, t-tests for continuous data, and non-parametric tests. Other statistical techniques which were reported as frequently as these tests (i.e., power analysis, survival methods, sensitivity analyses, epidemiology statistics – i.e., logistic regression and regression) are discussed in other chapters (see for example ▶ Chaps. 41, "Power and Sample Size", ▶ 89, "Survival Analysis II", ▶ 91, "Logistic Regression and Related Methods").

Tests for Continuous Outcomes

T-Test

The Student's t-test is named after the pseudonym "Student," used by William Sealy Gosset, a chemist working for the Guinness brewery in Dublin, Ireland, who published the seminal paper introducing the t-statistic in 1908 (Zabell 2008). The t-test encompasses a set of statistical tests, where the test statistic is assumed to follow a t-distribution under the null hypothesis. There are two key versions of the t-test. The first is a two-group, unpaired t-test and the second is a one-group, or paired, t-test. In both cases, the outcome is a continuous variable. Since randomized clinical trials inherently involve comparing patients from two separate groups, the two-group, unpaired t-test will be discussed first.

The two-group, unpaired t-test is used to compare whether the mean value of one group is different from the mean of the second group. For instance, one might be interested to see if the mean change in blood pressure from baseline to month 3 is different between patients randomized to two different treatments. The null hypothesis for the two-sample t-test is $H_0: \mu_A = \mu_B$, where μ_i is the population mean for group i. Note that if H_0 is true, then $\mu_A = \mu_B = \mu_{(A+B)}$, where $\mu_{(A+B)}$ is the mean of both groups combined. Under the null hypothesis, the t-statistic can be calculated as $t = \frac{\bar{x}_A - \bar{x}_B}{SE_{Diff}}$, where $\bar{x}_i$ is the sample mean for group i and SE_{Diff} is the standard error of the difference (of the group means). Note that the actual calculation of SE_{Diff} differs slightly depending on the scenario (i.e., whether groups A and B have equal sample size or equal variance), and the specifics of this calculation will not be discussed here. If $|t|$ is large, then the probability of the data occurring when H_0 is actually true would be small (i.e., the p-value would be small), and one could reject H_0.

In the usual clinical trial scenario, it can be assumed that the sampled groups come from independent populations, one group of patients receiving one intervention and one group receiving a different intervention. In this instance, there is no relationship between the patients who received intervention one and those patients who received intervention two; thus, they are statistically independent. A different scenario occurs if one sample was obtained for a group of patients prior to an intervention, and the second sample was obtained from the same patients but only after the intervention. In this situation, the two groups are not independent because the value for a given individual after the intervention is likely related to the value before the intervention; for example, a patient with high blood pressure prior to the start of an intervention will tend to have high blood pressure after the intervention. In this case, one can pair the outcome of the two groups (before intervention and after intervention) by patient and use the paired t-test – which is fundamentally the same as the one-group t-test.

Although the one-group or paired t-test is not a primary test used to compare interventions in a randomized clinical trial, it is sometimes used in non-randomized clinical studies, so details are provided for completeness. The one-group or paired t-test is used to compare whether the mean value of one group is different from some value. Often, interest lies in testing whether the mean differs from 0 (i.e., no change in effect when looking at paired data). For instance, one might be interested to see if there is a change in the mean blood pressure from baseline to month 3 in a single cohort of individuals who are given an intervention. If the change in blood pressure is not different from 0, then it can be assumed that no change occurred over time and the intervention has no effect on blood pressure. The null hypothesis for the one-sample t-test is $H_0: \mu = 0$, and the t-statistic can be calculated as $t = \frac{\bar{x}}{SE}$, where $\bar{x}$ is the sample mean and SE is the standard error of the sample mean. Note the similarities in the equation to the two-group t-test, as both are a measure of signal-to-noise ratio.

It is assumed for t-tests that the outcome data comes from a normal distribution. This means that in the two-group situation, the outcome data is normally distributed within both groups, and in a one-group situation, the outcome data (or the difference – in the paired t-test) is normally distributed overall. This assumption can be assessed formally (methods to do this are not discussed in this chapter), but it can also be assumed to be true if the sample size is sufficiently large, due to the CLT described earlier. The t-test is also fairly robust to the assumption of normality, so results from t-tests are generally believed to be relatively reliable even if there are minor deviations from normality. However, there are situations when the assumption of normality is violated, such as when there are outliers in the data or when the data comes from a distribution that is known to be not symmetric (such as the distribution of the median). Similarly, if the sample size is small, it might not be reasonable to assume the data comes from a normal distribution (e.g., a rule of thumb is if there are <30 data points).

Non-parametric Tests in Lieu of T-Tests

As mentioned, there are situations where the normality assumption of the t-test is violated and the t-test cannot be used, or researchers may simply desire not to make assumptions about the shape of the sampling distribution. In these cases one may use a non-parametric test which does not assume any known distribution for the parameter. Since they require fewer assumptions, non-parametric tests are typically more conservative than parametric tests and are preferred in general by some statisticians. Some of the more common non-parametric tests include the sign test, Mann-Whitney-Wilcoxon rank sum test, and Wilcoxon signed-rank test.

The sign test can be used to evaluate data from a single group, when there is paired data, such as comparing patient scores before and after an intervention (similar to the one-group or paired t-test). Here, one would assume that if the intervention had no effect on patient scores, that roughly half the pre-intervention scores would be more than the post-intervention scores, and roughly half would be less. Thus, this test looks at the signs of the difference of each pair of data points. The magnitude of the difference is not important in this scenario. To illustrate, assume there are eight patients and the first patient has a risk score of 52% before the intervention and a risk score of 47% after the intervention, then this patient's difference is -5% (47–52), which is a negative difference score. One repeats this process for all eight patients, and investigators simply count the number of cases where there is a positive (or negative) difference score. The sign test has the following null hypothesis: $H_0: p = 0.5$, where $S = p*n$ and p is the probability of half the differences being greater than 0. The test statistic is simply s, the number of positive scores. The p-value, by definition, is the probability of observing s differences (or a more extreme amount than s) in n patients, under the assumption that $p = 0.5$. This can be calculated using a binomial distribution. For instance, if eight patients were in a study, and only one of them had a higher post-intervention score (i.e., only one positive difference), then the p-value = Prob(0 or 1 of 8 | $p = 0.5$) = 0.004 + 0.031 = 0.035.

One weakness of the sign test is that it does not include the magnitude of the differences. Intuitively, one might give greater credence to an intervention in reducing scores if the difference between pre- and post-intervention scores was small for the patient with a positive score and large for the other patients, than if there was a large positive difference for one patient and only very small negative differences for the rest. In this case, the Wilcoxon signed-rank test can be used, based on the absolute difference, or rank, in scores.

If H_0 is assumed to be true, the proportion and rank of negative scores should be approximately equal to the proportion and rank of positive scores. The test statistic for the Wilcoxon signed-rank test is then based on the number and rank of positive and negative scores. This is illustrated using an example (see Table 1). In this example, of the eight patients in this cohort, only one (patient 5) had a positive difference in pre- and post-intervention scores; the rest all had post-intervention scores that decreased. The only information used for the sign test is the fact that seven of eight patients had a decreased score, indicated by the "sign" row. The signed-rank test now includes information on the rank in addition to the sign. The absolute value of the sum of signed ranks is $W = |\text{-}3\text{-}4\text{-}1\text{-}8 + 2\text{-}5\text{-}6\text{-}7| = |\text{-}32| = 32$. Under the assumption of no difference, i.e., the sum of the negative rank scores equals the sum of positive rank scores, then H_0: $W = 0$. One can use a reference table or computer program to calculate the p-value, which for the test presented in Table 1 is 0.023. Note the importance of rank in the Wilcoxon signed-rank test; if patient 5 post-score was 73 instead of 53, indicating an increase of +20 (instead of +2), the sign test p-value of 0.035 does not change; however the Wilcoxon signed-rank test p-value would change dramatically to 0.195.

The Mann-Whitney test, or Wilcoxon rank sum test, extends the signed-rank test to two groups. Similar to the signed-rank test, the rank sum test is based on ranked observations, and the underlying assumption is that if there is no difference between groups, i.e., the sum of ranks for one group would be the same as the sum of ranks in the other group. The test statistic is not straightforward to define, but in essence, one ranks all individuals from both groups and then sums the ranks within each group. If the sum of ranked values for either group is either sufficiently high or low compared to the expected value, then one can conclude that the ranks are not equally distributed between the two groups. This would then allow the investigator to reject the hypothesis that the two groups are equal. Alternatively, if the sum of ranked values

Table 1 Example of Wilcoxon signed-rank test

Patient	1	2	3	4	5	6	7	8
Pre-score	52	46	41	72	51	46	51	55
Post-score	47	39	40	53	53	38	41	40
Difference	−5	−7	−1	−19	+2	−8	−10	−15
Absolute value	5	7	1	19	2	8	10	15
Sign	−	−	−	−	+	−	−	−
Rank	3	4	1	8	2	5	6	7
Signed rank	−3	−4	−1	−8	+2	−5	−6	−7

for either group is relatively close to the expected value, then investigators may conclude that the distributions of the two groups are similar (i.e., one would not reject the null hypothesis).

Multiple Groups

Occasionally, randomized clinical trials will be performed which involve a comparison among three or more different interventions with a continuous outcome. In this setting, one would perform an analysis of variance, commonly called ANOVA. Conceptually, an ANOVA is based on quantifying the different variance components. Variance exists between subjects within each group (or intervention), and variance exists between the different groups. The total amount of variance is just comprised of the sum of the variance of these two components. If the amount of variance between groups is high (relative to the amount of variance between subjects within groups), then one can conclude that the means of the groups are different and did not come from the same distribution, which is the null hypothesis.

Specifically, an ANOVA is performed to test $H_0: \mu_1 = \mu_2 = \ldots = \mu_k$, where μ_i is the mean of each group i (for groups 1, 2, ..., k) versus $H_1: \mu_i \neq \mu_j$ for any two different groups i and j. It is important to note that H_0 assumes that the mean of every group is the same; if just one group has a different mean (regardless of which group, or the number of different groups that are tested), then one would reject H_0 in favor of H_1. In other words, if one is testing, say, the differences in the mean between five different groups, and four of them are the same but one is different, this test should result in a rejection of H_0. The rejection of H_0 does not specify which group is different or by how much, only that at least one of the groups has a different mean compared to at least one other group.

Lay readers may wish to skip the remainder of this paragraph and peruse the article by Altman and Bland (Altman and Bland 1996) which provides a non-technical overview of the ANOVA methods. Results from an ANOVA are presented in tabular format, such as illustrated in Table 2, and start by calculating the sum of squares, which is a measure of variability. The sum of squares for treatment is a measure of the variability between treatment groups (specifically the sum over all treatment groups, of the squared difference between the treatment group mean and the overall mean). The sum of squares error is a measure of the variability within each treatment group (specifically the sum over all observations of the squared difference between the observation and the treatment group mean), and the sum of squares total is a measure of the variability not accounting for the different treatment

Table 2 ANOVA results

	SS	df	MS	F-test	p-value
Treatment	SS_T	df_T	MS_T	$F = MS_T/MS_E$	$Pr(F_{df_T, df_E} > F)$
Error	SS_E	df_E	MS_E		
Total	SS_{Tot}	df_{Tot}			

SS sum of squares, *df* degrees of freedom, *MS* mean squares, *T* treatment, *E* error groups (specifically the sum over all observations of the squared difference between the observation mean and the overall mean). The sum of squares total also happens to be the sum of the other two sums of square values; hence it is called sum of squares "total." The degrees of freedom for the treatment (df_T) is one less than the number of groups, and the degrees of freedom total (df_{Tot}) is one less than the total sample size. Thus, the error degrees of freedom (df_E) can be calculated as $df_E = df_{Tot} - df_T$. The mean square is simply the SS/df, for each respective type of variation. The ratio of mean square errors follows an F-distribution with df_E and df_T degrees of freedom. The test statistic of an ANOVA is then the ratio of mean square errors: $F = MS_T/MS_E$, which is essentially a measure of the amount of variability across the treatment means relative to the amount of variability across all observations not accounting for treatment group. Furthermore, the F-distribution is related to the Student-t in that $F \sim T^2$ where $T \sim t(\nu)$ is the t-distribution with ν degrees of freedom. So an ANOVA is often thought of as an extension of the t-test.

Non-parametric Tests for Multiple Groups

Generally, when performing an ANOVA, one needs to assume that the data of each group is normally distributed and the variance of the different groups are similar. These assumptions may not be reasonable, and in this case, performing a non-parametric test is appropriate. The Kruskal-Wallis test (Kruskal and Wallis 1952) is a commonly used non-parametric test for assessing differences in the data patterns of two or more groups. This test is an extension of the Mann-Whitney but can be applied to more than two groups.

The Kruskal-Wallis test procedure starts by ranking all the observations of all groups and accounts for ties by using an average between the potential ranks of the tied observations. The null hypothesis is the same as the ANOVA test. The non-parametric test statistic is formulaically complex but is essentially intended to look at the variation in the rank scores within the different groups. Similar to a parametric ANOVA, if the rank variances within the different groups are similar to the rank variances between the different groups, then one can assume that the distributions of the different groups are similar. In this case the investigators would fail to reject the null hypothesis. Alternatively, if the rank variances between the groups are much greater than within the groups, then there is evidence to suggest that the group distributions are different, thus H_0 would be rejected.

Tests for Contingency Tables

χ^2 Test

The Pearson χ^2 (chi-square) test is named after Karl Pearson who first investigated it over 100 years ago (Pearson 1900). The χ^2 test can be used when the outcome of interest is categorical, and it is of interest to see if the populations come from one overall population or whether they arise from two or more different populations.

This is the same as testing whether the categorical outcome variable of interested is independent of some other categorical variable.

The simplest form of this test is when there are two groups (e.g., intervention versus control) and a dichotomous outcome (e.g., response versus no response). Here one may be interested in investigating whether response is independent of treatment; in other words, the response rate is different for patients receiving one intervention compared with the other. This is illustrated in Table 3, which is a 2×2 contingency table.

The null hypothesis for this scenario would be H_0: $p_i = p_c$, where p is the population proportion of patients (i.e., B/N_i or D/N_c) with a response for group *intervention* or *control*, and the alternative hypothesis is H_1: $p_i \neq p_c$. Note that if H_0 is true, then $p_i = p_c$. Looking at Table 3, if H_0 is correct, then it would be expected that B/(A+B) is approximately equal to D/(C+D) (and ultimately = (B+D)/N) as the sample sizes get large. If the observed proportion of "responses" is different from the expected proportion, then this would give evidence against H_0.

Formally, this can be tested using the test statistic $\chi^2 = \sum_{i=1}^{r} \sum_{j=1}^{c} \frac{(O_{ij} - E_{ij})^2}{E_{ij}}$, where O_{ij} is the observed number of events with outcome *j* for group *i* and E_{ij} is the expected number of events. Since the proportion of patients with a response would be expected to be similar in both groups, assuming H_0 is true, then this would lead to situations where O_{ij} is close to E_{ij} for every cell, and the test statistic, χ^2, would be close to 0. If the test statistic is large, this indicates that O_{ij} is not close to E_{ij} and a potential violation of the assumption that H_0 is true. Formally, the test statistic follows the χ^2 distribution. Similar to the t-distribution, the χ^2 distribution is actually a series of distributions, based on the number of degrees of freedom. The df for a χ^2 test is calculated as $(r-1)*(c-1)$ with r = number of rows (i.e., groups) and c = number of columns (outcome variables). Therefore, for the 2×2 contingency table in Table 3, there are two rows and two columns, giving $(2-1)*(2-1) = 1$ degree of freedom.

It is assumed that the categories of the group and outcome variables are mutually exclusive for the χ^2 test. In other words, patients can be in one, and only one, group, and their outcomes must similarly be categorized into one, and only one, of the outcome categories. Similarly, under the null hypothesis, the group and outcome variables are initially assumed to be independent of one another. While the example above was for a 2×2 contingency table, the χ^2 test can be generalized to larger contingency tables, provided the above assumptions hold. Finally, the χ^2 test is a parametric distribution that only holds for large sample sizes. As a rule of thumb, one can use the χ^2 test if the expected number of events within every cell is at least 5.

Table 3 Example of a 2×2 contingency table

	No response	Response	Total
Intervention group	A	B	A+B
Control group	C	D	C+D
Total number	A+C	B+D	A+B+C+D

One common modification to the basic χ^2 test is called Yates' correction (Yates 1984). This correction is intended to account for the fact that the test is based on categorical outcomes, while the underlying χ^2 distribution is continuous. It should be noted that there is considerable debate as to whether this correction is required. Yates' correction is simply to add 0.5 to the observed number of events within each cell and then perform the χ^2 test on the resulting values.

Non-parametric Tests for Categorical Variables

Exact, non-parametric statistical tests can be used in lieu of the χ^2 test, which are particularly relevant when sample sizes are small (Agresti 2011), for example, when the cell sizes are less than 5. The most common non-parametric test used on 2×2 contingency tables is Fisher's exact test. Fisher's exact test has been criticized as being overly conservative; however, corrections similar to Yates' correction for the χ^2 test, called the "mid-p" correction, have also been proposed for Fisher's exact test (Routledge 1994). Although an extension of Fisher's exact test can be used for larger contingency tables, it is rarely used in practice. This is partly due the complexity of results and interpretability.

For Fisher's exact test (Fisher 1922), one observes results and enters them in a 2×2 contingency table similar to what was observed in Table 3. The exact probability of observing such a matrix can be calculated based on the hypergeometric distribution, if one knows the number of individuals in each group (i.e., N_I and N_C) and the total number of responders and non-responders ($N_{Response}$ and $N_{No\ Response}$). That is, the probability of this exact contingency table of observations is $P(contingency\ table) = \frac{\binom{A+B}{B}\binom{C+D}{D}}{\binom{A+B+C+D}{B+D}} = \frac{(A+B)!(C+D)!(A+C)!(B+D)!}{A!B!C!D!N!}$. To calculate the p-value, one simply adds up the probabilities of all possible contingency tables that are equal to or more extreme than the observed results.

For instance, assume one has the 2×2 contingency table observed in Table 4. Assume that the row and cell totals are fixed, that is, that $N_I = 11$, $N_C = 8$, $N_{Response} = 14$, and $N_{No\ Response} = 5$. Then, if A = 0, one can uniquely calculate the values in each of the other cells (i.e., B = 11, C = 5, and D = 3). The probability of this contingency table can be calculated using $P(contingency\ table) = 0.0048$. Since this contingency table is "more extreme" than the observed contingency table, this probability is summed with all other contingency tables that are "as extreme or more extreme" than the observed one to calculate the p-value. The observed

Table 4 Example of results for a 2×2 contingency table

	No response	Response	Total
Intervention group	1	10	11
Control group	4	4	8
Total N	5	14	19

contingency table has *P(contingency table)* = 0.0662, and if A = 5 (which is the maximum possible value since $N_{No\ Response}$ = 5), then *P(contingency table)* = 0.0397. The sum of the probabilities of these three contingency tables is 0.0048 + 0.0662 + 0.0397=0.1107, and this is the p-value using Fisher's exact test (or 0.0758 if the mid-p correction was used).

Note that the χ^2 test (uncorrected) p-value is 0.0456 and corrected (using Yates' correction) is 0.14. As the sample sizes get larger, the p-values will become more and more similar to each other, but this example illustrates the problems that occur if the incorrect statistical test is used. Specifically, one test, the uncorrected χ^2 test, yielded a statistically significant result at the conventional α = 0.05 level of significance, while the other three tests were not statistically significant. To avoid reliability issues, the specific test used must be defined clearly in advance of any analysis and relevant to the available data. Finally, this example also illustrates that the use of "statistical significance" should not be overinterpreted. By itself, statistical significance does not imply clinical importance, and one always needs to interpret any statistical results in the context of all available data. If nothing else, one should be wary about claiming a statistically significant and clinically meaningful result in a trial with only 19 patients included!

It is always also important to interpret results with an understanding of the magnitude of effect as well. The simplest method is to convert the numbers into proportions/percentages and calculate the difference; in Table 4, 10/11 or 90.9% of patients had a response, compared with 4/8 or 50.0% in the control group, leaving an absolute risk difference of 40.9%. Because there is an upper and lower bound on percentages (i.e., one could never have an absolute increase in response rate of >100%), the absolute difference in percentage may not be sufficient to understand the magnitude of effect. The relative risk (or risk ratio) is the response percentage in one group divided by the percentage in the second group. In the stated example, the risk ratio is (10/11)/(4/4)= 90.9%/50.0% = 1.82. Hence, the probability of response is 1.82 times greater among patients given the intervention. Finally, one might also be interested in determining the odds ratio (described in more detail in the ▶ Chap. 91, "Logistic Regression and Related Methods," by M. Diniz), where odds is the relative likelihood of having a response to not having a response. Among patients given the intervention, there were ten responses observed for every non-responder (10 to 1), while in the control group, the odds were 1 to 1 (an equal number of individuals had a response as did not have a response). The odds of having a response in the intervention group is then ten times greater than in the control group, and the odds ratio is 10 (calculated as (B∗C)/(A∗D) from Table 3). Note, however, that the relative magnitude of effect changes drastically depending on the base percentage; if the probability of response in the control group was only 5% and there was an equivalent absolute increase of 40.9% in the intervention group (to 45.9%), the relative risk would be 45.9%/5.9% = 7.8, and the odds ratio would be (95 ∗ 45.9)/(54.1 ∗ 5) = 16.1. Certainly while the absolute risk difference was the same, the importance of going from a response rate of 5% to 45.9% is much greater, which is demonstrated in the relative risk and odds ratio.

Another notable and common non-parametric test, used in lieu of the χ^2 test, is the Cochran-Mantel-Haenszel test (Mantel 1963). It can be used when the data is set up as a 2×2 contingency table; however, there are strata within each intervention group (e.g., if randomization of patients to treatment arm was stratified by age or by treatment center). Derivation of this test will not be described here. The only additional step is that one should perform a test of homogeneity, which tests whether contingency tables are similar between different strata. If there are differences, then one would need to perform separate analyses for each different stratum. Otherwise, the hypotheses H_0 and H_1 and ultimate inferences for the Cochran-Mantel-Haenszel test are similar to the χ^2 test except they incorporate an adjustment for stratification factors.

Summary

This overview provides a summary of the most common types of statistical tests used in clinical trials. This includes parametric tests such as the t-test, χ^2 test, and ANOVA and basic non-parametric tests such as the Wilcoxon rank sum test, signed-rank test, Fisher's exact test, and Cochran-Mantel-Haenszel test. This is not an exhaustive list. Other common tests, such as the log-rank test, or regression methods, such as linear, logistic, or proportional hazards, are also commonly employed and are described elsewhere. Given the plethora of possible statistical tests, choosing the correct test for the particular clinical trial requires knowledge of the clinical scenario, statistical aspects, assumptions, and potential deficiencies. Despite this complexity, the fundamental steps behind performing any statistical test remain the same. It is imperative, before the trial protocol is finalized, that the primary outcome, hypotheses, and statistical test to be used are clearly defined. The decision rule must be clear, based on the defined tolerable error rates. Having clearly defined hypotheses, tests and decision rules ensures unambiguous interpretation of the final results, and ensure that valid inferences are made from the trial based on the statistics.

Key Facts

- Most common statistical tests fall into two broad categories: parametric tests, which assume the data follow some known distribution, and non-parametric tests.
- The most frequently used parametric tests are t-tests, analysis of variance (ANOVA), and χ^2 tests.
- The most frequent non-parametric tests are the signed-rank test, Wilcoxon rank sum test, Kruskal-Wallis test, and Fisher's exact test.
- Although non-parametric tests do not require an assumption about the distribution of the data, they are generally more conservative.

Cross-References

► Estimands and Sensitivity Analyses
► Logistic Regression and Related Methods
► Power and Sample Size
► Survival Analysis II

References

Agresti A (2011) Exact inference for categorical data: recent advances and continuing controversies. Stat Med 20:17–18

Altman DG, Bland JM (1996) Statistics notes: comparing several groups using analysis of variance. BMJ 312:1472. https://doi.org/10.1136/bmj.312.7044.1472

Fagerland MW (2012) T-tests, non-parametric tests, and large studies – a paradox of statistical practice? BMC Med Res Meth 12:78. https://doi.org/10.1186/1471-2288-12-78

Fisher RA (1922) On the interpretation of χ^2 from contingency tables, and the calculation of P. J Royal Stat Soc 85(1):87–94. https://doi.org/10.2307/2340521

Gosho M, Sato Y, Nagashima K, Takahashi S (2017) Trends in study design and statistical methods employed in a leading general medicine journal. J Clin Pharm Therapeutics. https://doi.org/10.1111/jcpt.12605

Guyatt G, Jaeschke R, Heddle N, Cook D, Shannon H, Walter S (1995) Basic statistics for clinicians: 1. Hypothesis testing. Can Med Assoc J 152(1):27–32

Kruskal WH, Wallis WA (1952) Use of ranks in one-criterion variance analysis. J Am Stat Assoc 47(260):583–621. https://doi.org/10.1080/01621459.1952.10483441

Mantel N (1963) Chi-square tests with one degree of freedom; extensions of the mantel-Haenszel procedure. J Am Stat Assoc 58:690–700. https://doi.org/10.1080/01621459.1963.10500879

Pearson K (1900) On the criterion that a given system of deviations from the probable in the case of a correlated system of variables is such that it can be reasonably supposed to have arisen from random sampling. Philos Mag 50(302):157–175. https://doi.org/10.1080/14786440009463897

Routledge RD (1994) Practicing safe statistics with the mid-p. Can J Stat 22(1):103

Sato Y, Gosho M, Sato Y, Nagashima K, Takahashi S, Ware JH, Laird NM (2017) Statistical methods in the *journal* – an update. N England J Med 376(11):1086–1087. https://doi.org/10.1056/NEJMc1616211

Yates F (1984) Contingency tables involving small numbers and the chi-square test. J Royal Stat Soc 1:217–235

Zabell SL (2008) On Student's 1908 article "the probable error of a mean". J Am Stat Assoc 103(481):1–7

Nonparametric Survival Analysis

Yuliya Lokhnygina

Contents

Introduction	1718
Examples of Survival Data in Clinical Trials	1718
Example 1	1718
Example 2	1719
Basic Terminology and Concepts	1719
Examples of Some Popular Parametric Models for Survival Data	1721
Nonparametric Estimation	1722
Kaplan-Meier Estimator of the Survival Function	1722
Life-Table Estimator of the Survival Function	1726
Nelson-Aalen Estimator of the Cumulative Hazard Function	1727
Estimators of the Hazard Function	1728
Analyses of Truncated Data	1729
Hypothesis Testing	1734
Logrank Tests	1734
Logrank Test for Comparison of Multiple Groups	1737
Stratified Logrank Test	1738
Logrank Test for Trend	1739
Further Reading	1740
Summary and Conclusion	1740
Key Facts	1741
Cross-References	1741
References	1741

Abstract

Survival or time-to-event data are ubiquitous in clinical trials research. The presence of censoring requires specialized methods for the analysis of this type of data. This chapter describes the methods for nonparametric analyses of

---

Y. Lokhnygina (✉)
Department of Biostatistics and Bioinformatics, Duke University, Durham, NC, USA
e-mail: Yuliya.Lokhnygina@duke.edu

© Springer Nature Switzerland AG 2022
S. Piantadosi, C. L. Meinert (eds.), *Principles and Practice of Clinical Trials*,
https://doi.org/10.1007/978-3-319-52636-2_119

survival data, including estimation of the key survival quantities of interest and hypothesis testing.

Keywords

Survival · Time to event · Censoring · Kaplan-Meier · Logrank

Introduction

Survival or time-to-event data are encountered frequently in clinical trials research. These data are recorded as a pair of variables, 1) the time to a certain event, such as death or disease relapse, measured from some common time origin, and 2) the event status, describing whether an event occurred or not. Because survival times are often *censored*, specialized methods are required for the analysis of time-to-event data. The most common type of censoring in clinical trials is *right censoring*, where an event is not observed for a subject within the duration of a study. This could happen because the study ended (administrative censoring), or because the subject withdrew consent to be followed further, or was lost to follow-up (moved, or did not respond to the contact attempts by the study investigators, etc.) Other types of censoring include *left censoring*, when it is known that the subject had an event prior to a certain point in time, and *interval censoring*, when it is only known that the subject's event occurred within some time interval, such as the interval between consecutive clinic visits.

Most statistical software packages have capabilities for the analysis of survival data. Some of the most popular packages include SAS (SAS Institute, Cary, NC, USA), R (R Core Team, 2017), Stata (StataCorp), and S-Plus (TIBCO Software Inc.). Data examples in this chapter were analyzed using packages survival and muhaz in R version 3.6.2, and proc lifetest in SAS software version 9.4.

Examples of Survival Data in Clinical Trials

Example 1

The Platelet Glycoprotein IIb/IIIa in Unstable Angina: Receptor Suppression Using Integrilin Therapy (PURSUIT) Trial was conducted to test the hypothesis that the addition of an antiplatelet drug eptifibatide (Integrilin) to a standard therapy of aspirin and heparin reduced the incidence of adverse outcomes such as death and myocardial infarction (MI) in patients with acute coronary syndromes including unstable angina or non-ST-segment elevation MI (PURSUIT Trial Investigators 1998). The study was double-blind, randomized, and placebo controlled. A total of 10,948 patients were enrolled at 726 hospitals in 27 countries between November 1995 and January 1997; 1487 patients were randomly assigned to the low-dose eptifibatide arm, 4722 to the high-dose eptifibatide arm, and 4739 to the placebo arm. The primary efficacy outcome was a composite of death or nonfatal MI at 30 days; secondary outcomes included all-cause mortality within 30 days, a first or recurrent MI within 30 days, a composite of death or nonfatal MI at 96 h and at 7 days, as well as bleeding complications according to two commonly used scales of severity.

The primary outcome data from PURSUIT were reanalyzed to illustrate the application of the methods described in this chapter. The de-identified dataset was provided by the Duke Clinical Research Institute (Durham, NC, USA).

Example 2

Angiotensin-converting enzyme (ACE) inhibitors have been shown to reduce mortality and cardiovascular morbidity after MI. The Valsartan in Acute Myocardial Infarction trial (VALIANT) was designed to evaluate the clinical hypothesis that treatment with valsartan, an angiotensin-receptor blocker, alone or combined with captopril, an ACE inhibitor, would reduce mortality compared to treatment with captopril alone. This randomized, double-blind study was conducted at 931 centers in 24 countries. Between December 1998 and June 2001, a total of 14,808 patients with MI complicated by left ventricular systolic dysfunction, heart failure, or both were randomized in 1:1:1 ratio to valsartan monotherapy, captopril monotherapy, or valsartan in combination with captopril. The primary endpoint was mortality from any cause; secondary outcomes included cause-specific mortality, recurrent MI, and hospitalization for heart failure and stroke, among others. Two primary treatment comparisons were: 1) valsartan versus captopril and 2) valsartan plus captopril versus captopril alone. The study was designed to continue patient follow-up until at least 2700 deaths had occurred; the resulting median patient follow-up was 24.7 months. Because of the protocol violations, 105 patients from one site were not included in the analyses, leaving 4909 patients in the valsartan group, 4909 in the captopril group, and 4885 in the valsartan plus captopril group (Pfeffer et al. 2003).

The data for the secondary outcome of stroke, first reported in McMurray et al. (2006), were reanalyzed to demonstrate the application of the various nonparametric survival analysis methods described in this chapter. The de-identified dataset was provided by the Duke Clinical Research Institute (Durham, NC, USA).

Basic Terminology and Concepts

To describe the fundamental quantities used in survival analysis, some notation is necessary. Let T denote time to the event of interest and C time to censoring. Note that for a subject in a study either T or C can be observed, but not both. Further, let U denote the observed subject time in a study, which mathematically can be expressed as $U = \min(T, C)$, and let Δ be a censoring indicator, taking a value of 1 if a subject experienced an event in a study (i.e., $U = T$), or a value of 0 if a subject was censored (i.e., $U = C$). Mathematically, Δ can be expressed using an indicator function: $\Delta = I(T \leq C)$.

For all methods described in this chapter, it is assumed that time to event T and censoring time C are independent. Methods for the situations when this assumption does not hold are discussed in Emura and Chen (2018).

Basic quantities used to describe the distribution of time-to-event data include the distribution (or cumulative distribution) function, the survival (or survivor) function, and the hazard function.

The *distribution function* of T, denoted by $F(t)$, is the probability that the event occurs no later than time t:

$$F(t) = \Pr(T \leq t).$$

If T is a continuous random variable, then its distribution has an associated *density function* $f(t)$, which is related to $F(t)$ through the following equations:

$$f(t) = \frac{dF(t)}{dt},$$

$$F(T) = \int_0^t f(u)du.$$

The complement of the distribution function is the *survival function*, the probability of an event occurring beyond time t:

$$S(t) = 1 - F(t) = \Pr(T > t).$$

It is easy to see that when T is a continuous random variable, $S(t)$ and $f(t)$ are related as

$$f(t) = -\frac{dS(t)}{dt}.$$

An important property of $S(t)$ is that it is a nonincreasing function taking a value of 1 at the time origin and having a limit of 0 as time goes to infinity.

Another quantity used to describe the distribution of T is the *hazard function*, or hazard rate $h(t)$, defined as

$$h(t) = \lim_{\delta t \to 0} \frac{\Pr[t \leq T < t + \delta t | T \geq t]}{\delta t}$$

The hazard rate can be viewed as the instantaneous rate of an event at time t, conditional on the event not having occurred prior to t. It is important to note that the hazard rate is not a probability and does not have to be less than 1. It is, however, a nonnegative function. The quantity $h(t)\delta t$ can be interpreted as the approximate probability of having an event in the time interval $(t, t + \delta t)$.

The *cumulative* or *integrated hazard function* is defined as

$$H(t) = \int_0^t h(u)du.$$

Quantities $h(t)$, $f(t)$, $H(t)$, and $S(t)$ are connected via the relationships

$$h(t) = \frac{f(t)}{S(t)},$$

$$S(t) = \exp\{-H(t)\}.$$

Examples of Some Popular Parametric Models for Survival Data

Parametric distributions commonly used for modeling survival data are typically characterized by the shape of their hazard function. The simplest model is the one where the hazard rate is constant over time, corresponding to an *exponential* distribution:

$$h(t) = \lambda \quad (\lambda > 0),$$
$$S(t) = \exp(-\lambda t),$$
$$f(t) = \lambda \exp(-\lambda t).$$

The mean and the median of the exponential distribution are $\frac{1}{\lambda}$ and $\frac{\ln 2}{\lambda}$, respectively. This model may be appropriate for describing the mechanism of failure in a chronic disease. Another distribution widely used in modeling survival data is the *Weibull* distribution:

$$h(t) = \alpha \lambda t^{\alpha-1} \quad (\alpha, \lambda > 0),$$
$$S(t) = \exp(-\lambda t^\alpha),$$
$$f(t) = \alpha \lambda t^{\alpha-1} \exp(-\lambda t^\alpha).$$

The mean and the median of the Weibull distribution are $\lambda^{-1/\alpha}\Gamma(1 + 1/\alpha)$ and $\lambda^{-1/\alpha}(\ln 2)^{1/\alpha}$, respectively, where $\Gamma(b)$ is the gamma function, defined as

$$\Gamma(b) = \int_0^\infty x^{b-1} e^{-x} dx.$$

Depending on the values for α and λ, the Weibull hazard rate can be monotonically increasing or monotonically decreasing with time. Models where the hazard

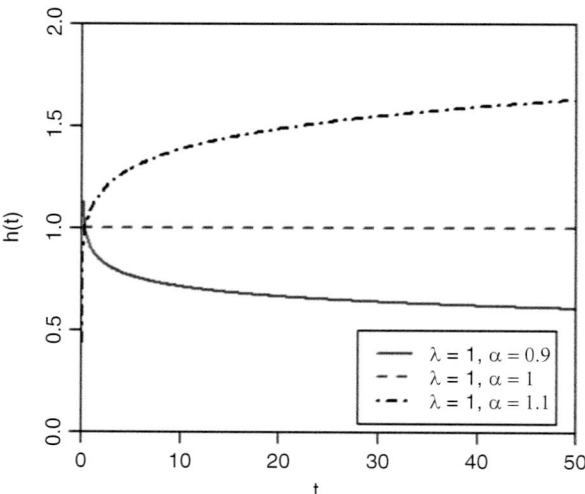

Fig. 1 Examples of the Weibull hazard function

rate increases over time may be suitable for describing processes associated with aging. Decreasing hazard functions may arise when there is an early high risk of failure which then decreases over time, such as, for example, the hazard of death after a complex life-saving surgical procedure. Some examples of the Weibull hazard function for various values of α and λ are given in Fig. 1.

Nonparametric Estimation

Kaplan-Meier Estimator of the Survival Function

Oftentimes, analysis of censored survival data from one or more groups starts with estimation of the survival distribution. The most common method used for that is the Kaplan-Meier method, also known as the Product-Limit method (Kaplan and Meier 1958).

Suppose time is divided into intervals $[t_{(j-1)}, t_{(j)})$, $j = 1, \ldots r$, where $t_{(1)}, \ldots, t_{(r)}$ are event times, $t_{(0)}$ is time origin, and $t_{(r+1)} = \infty$. Let n_j denote the number of subjects at risk just before $t_{(j)}$ and d_j denote the number of events at $t_{(j)}$. If a censored observation occurs at $t_{(j)}$, by convention, this censored observation is included in n_j, i.e., censoring in that case is assumed to occur just after $t_{(j)}$. Applying the probability chain rule consecutively, for $t_{(k)} \leq t < t_{(k+1)}$ it follows that

$$S(t) = \Pr(T > t) = \Pr(T > t, T > t_{(k)}) = \Pr(T > t | T > t_{(k)}) \Pr(T > t_{(k)}) =$$
$$\Pr(T > t | T > t_{(k)}) \Pr(T > t_{(k)} | T > t_{(k-1)}) \Pr(T > t_{(k-1)}) = \ldots = \quad (1)$$

$$\Pr(T > t | T > t_{(k)}) \Pr(T > t_{(k)} | T > t_{(k-1)}) \ldots \Pr(T > t_{(1)} | T > t_{(0)}) \Pr(T > t_{(0)}),$$

where $\Pr(T > t_{(0)}) = 1$. The conditional probability $\Pr(t_{(j)} \geq T > t_{(j-1)} | T > t_{(j-1)})$ of having an event in the time interval $(t_{(j-1)}, t_{(j)}]$, conditional on not having an event prior to or at $t_{(j-1)}$, can be estimated as $\frac{d_j}{n_j}$; consequently, probability $\Pr(T > t_{(j)} | T > t_{(j-1)})$ can be estimated as $1 - \frac{d_j}{n_j}$. Since no events occurred in the interval $(t_{(k)}, t]$, $\Pr(T > t | T > t_{(k)}) = 1$ and from (1), the survival function can be estimated as

$$\widehat{S}_{KM}(t) = \prod_{j=1}^{k} \frac{n_j - d_j}{n_j},$$

for $t_{(k)} \leq t < t_{(k+1)}$, $k = 1, \ldots, r$. When $t < t_{(1)}$, $\widehat{S}_{KM}(t) = 1$. In the case of no censoring, $n_{j+1} = n_j - d_j$ ($j = 1, \ldots, r$) and the Kaplan-Meier estimator is identical to the empirical survival function estimator:

$$\widehat{S}_{KM}(t) = \frac{n_2}{n_1} \frac{n_3}{n_2} \ldots \frac{n_{k+1}}{n_k} = \frac{n_{k+1}}{n_1}.$$

The standard error of $\widehat{S}_{KM}(t)$ can be estimated using Greenwood's formula (Greenwood 1926):

$$s.e.\left[\widehat{S}_{KM}(t)\right] = \widehat{S}_{KM}(t) \sqrt{\sum_{j=1}^{k} \frac{d_j}{n_j(n_j - d_j)}} \qquad (2)$$

Pointwise $(1-\alpha)100\%$ Wald confidence intervals for any estimate $\widehat{S}(t)$ of the survival function can be constructed as

$$\widehat{S}(t) \pm Z_{\alpha/2} * s.e.\left[\widehat{S}(t)\right],$$

where $Z_{\alpha/2}$ is the upper 1-sided $\alpha/2$-percentile of the standard normal distribution. This approach, however, can lead to confidence intervals that lie outside the (0,1) interval. An alternative procedure that avoids this issue is to first transform $\widehat{S}(t)$ to a function with values in $(-\infty, \infty)$, find confidence limits for the transformation, and then apply the back-transformation to the calculated confidence limits to obtain a confidence interval for $\widehat{S}(t)$. The logit transformation $\log\{S(t)/[1 - S(t)]\}$ and the complementary log-log transformation $\log\{-\log S(t)\}$ are most often used with this approach.

Example 3

To illustrate the application of the Kaplan-Meier method to estimation of the survival function, consider the primary outcome data from the PURSUIT study, described in Example 1. In this clinical trial, patients were enrolled in the hospital if they had ischemic chest pain within the previous 24 h. Occurrence of the myocardial infarction, which was one of the components of the primary outcome, was actively monitored using electrocardiograms and cardiac enzymes tests, and some of the deaths occurred while in the hospital. This meant that the timing of the events could have been ascertained down to the hour and the minute, and some patients had the primary outcome within minutes of being enrolled in the study. The primary comparison was between the high-dose eptifibatide group (that will be further called "eptifibatide" group, for brevity) and the placebo group. For this analysis, the subject follow-up was restricted to 30 days and all the data after 30 days were censored. Of the 4721 patients in the eptifibatide group (1 observation was deleted due to missing time value), there were 671 composite death or nonfatal MI events within 30 days from randomization, compared to 743 events among the 4739 patients in the placebo group. The data were analyzed using the function survfit() in the R package survival. The estimated event incidence rate at 30 days was 14.2% in the eptifibatide group and 15.7% in the placebo group. Estimated Kaplan-Meier survival curves for the two groups are shown in Fig. 2 and the partial output for the Kaplan-Meier estimates (KM) of the survival functions with 95% confidence limits (CL) is shown in the table below. The survival probability plot shows that the survival curves for the two groups start diverging at approximately 2 days and continue to separate until 30 days, indicating a possible difference in the distributions of time to event of interest between eptifibatide and placebo. Later on, this difference will be tested using the logrank test.

Placebo						
Time (days)	# At risk	# Events	KM	Standard error	Lower 95% CL	Upper 95% CL
0.01	4739	2	1.000	0.000298	0.999	1.000
0.02	4737	1	0.999	0.000365	0.999	1.000

(continued)

Fig. 2 Kaplan-Meier estimates of freedom from death and nonfatal MI up to 30 days for eptifibatide and placebo groups (PURSUIT study)

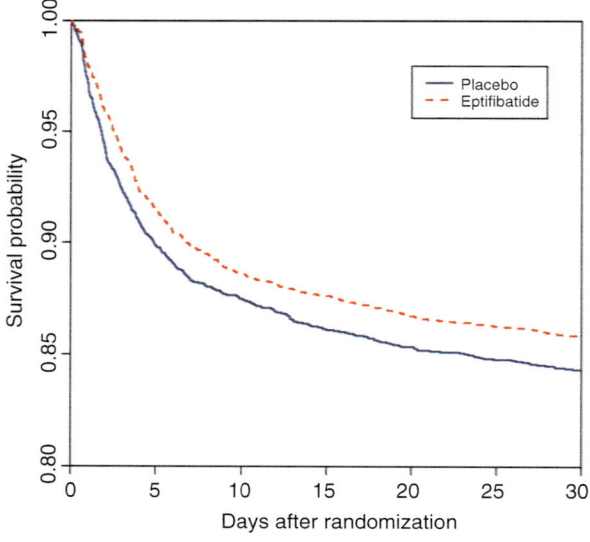

Placebo						
Time (days)	# At risk	# Events	KM	Standard error	Lower 95% CL	Upper 95% CL
...						
29.52	3988	1	0.843	0.005281	0.833	0.854
29.71	3987	1	0.843	0.005284	0.833	0.854
Eptifibatide						
Time (days)	# At risk	# Events	KM	Standard error	Lower 95% CL	Upper 95% CL
0.05	4721	1	1.000	0.000212	0.999	1.000
0.06	4720	1	1.000	0.000299	0.999	1.000
...						
29.70	4045	1	0.858	0.005082	0.848	0.868
29.85	4044	1	0.858	0.005085	0.848	0.868

Example 4

Consider the secondary outcome of stroke in the VALIANT study, described in Example 2. Among the patients included in the analyses, 157 of 4909 patients in the valsartan group, 166 of 4909 in the captopril group, and 140 of 4885 in the valsartan plus captopril group experienced a stroke event. Estimated Kaplan-Meier survival curves for the treatment groups are shown in Fig. 3 and the partial output for the Kaplan-Meier estimates (KM) of the survival functions with 95% confidence limits (CL) is shown in the table below. The data were analyzed using the function survfit() in the R package survival.

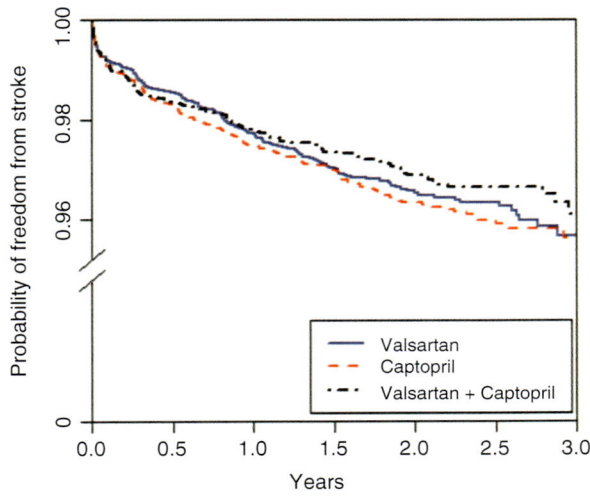

Fig. 3 Kaplan-Meier estimates of freedom from stroke for valsartan, captopril, and valsartan+captopril groups (VALIANT study)

Valsartan							
Time (years)	# At risk	# Events	KM	Standard error	Lower 95% CL	Upper 95% CL
0.0027	4909	2	1.000	0.000288	0.999	1.000
0.0055	4891	6	0.998	0.000577	0.997	0.999
...						
2.77	726	1	0.959	0.003703	0.951	0.966
2.89	509	1	0.957	0.004147	0.949	0.965
Captopril						
Time (years)	# At risk	# Events	KM	Standard error	Lower 95% CL	Upper 95% CL
0.0027	4909	5	0.999	0.000455	0.998	1.000
0.0055	4892	2	0.999	0.000539	0.998	1.000
...						
2.54	1242	1	0.958	0.003374	0.952	0.965
2.92	458	1	0.956	0.003963	0.948	0.964
Valsartan + captopril						
Time (years)	# At risk	# Events	KM	Standard error	Lower 95% CL	Upper 95% CL
0.0027	4885	1	1.000	0.000205	0.999	1.000
0.0055	4876	5	0.999	0.000502	0.998	1.000
...						
2.87	556	1	0.963	0.003644	0.956	0.971
2.95	407	1	0.961	0.004336	0.953	0.970

Life-Table Estimator of the Survival Function

When the survival data are interval censored, the Kaplan-Meier estimate of the survival function may be biased. The *life-table estimator*, also known as the *actuarial estimator* of the survival function, is more suitable in such cases. It is obtained by first dividing the time into a series of m time intervals $[t_{j-1}, t_j)$, $j = 1, \ldots, m$, where $t_0 = 0$ and $t_{m+1} = \infty$. Let n_j be the number of subjects at risk at the beginning of the jth interval, and let d_j and c_j be the number of events and the number of censored survival times, respectively, in the jth interval. The life-table method uses an *actuarial assumption* for the censoring process: It assumes that censoring times are distributed uniformly throughout each time interval, so that the average number of subjects at risk in the jth interval, sometimes called the effective sample size, is $n'_j = n_j - c_j/2$. The conditional probability of having an event in the jth interval among those at risk in the interval can be estimated as $q_j = d_j/n'_j$, and so the conditional probability of being event free throughout the interval among those at risk can be estimated as

$p_j = 1 - q_j = 1 - d_j/n'_j$. Using (1), the life-table estimator of the survival function can then be constructed as

$$\widehat{S}_{LT}(t) = \prod_{j=1}^{k} \frac{n'_j - d_j}{n'_j}, \quad t_k \leq t < t_{k+1}, \ m \geq k \geq 1,$$

$$\widehat{S}_{LT}(t) = 1, \ 0 \leq t < t_1.$$

The standard error of $\widehat{S}_{LT}(t)$ can be estimated using Greenwood's formula (2) with n_j substituted by n'_j.

Nelson-Aalen Estimator of the Cumulative Hazard Function

Cumulative hazard function $H(t)$ has multiple applications in the survival analysis. Survival function can be estimated as exponential of the negative estimate of $H(t)$. Cumulative hazard function can help to evaluate the proportional hazards assumption, common in many survival analysis applications, and it is also a basis for calculating various types of residuals that can be used to examine the fit of the Cox proportional hazards regression model, discussed in ▶ Chap. 89, "Survival Analysis II."

An estimator of the cumulative hazard function was separately proposed by Nelson (1972) and Aalen (1978). Using the notation from section "Kaplan-Meier Estimator of the Survival Function," the Nelson-Aalen estimate of the cumulative hazard function at time t $(t_{(k)} \leq t < t_{(k+1)}; k = 1, \ldots, r)$ is

$$\widehat{H}_{NA}(t) = \sum_{j=1}^{k} \frac{d_j}{n_j}.$$

When $t < t_{(1)}$, $\widehat{H}_{NA}(t) = 0$. Because of the relationship between the survival and cumulative hazard functions, a corresponding estimator for the survival function can be constructed:

$$\widehat{S}_{NA} = \exp\left\{-\widehat{H}_{NA}(t)\right\} = \prod_{j=1}^{k} \exp\left(-\frac{d_j}{n_j}\right).$$

Likewise, a cumulative hazard function estimator corresponding to the Kaplan-Meier estimator of the survival function is

$$\widehat{H}_{KM}(t) = -\log\left\{\widehat{S}_{KM}(t)\right\} = -\sum_{j=1}^{k} \log\left(\frac{n_j - d_j}{n_j}\right).$$

Example 5

Figure 4 shows Nelson-Aalen estimates of the cumulative hazard functions for death and nonfatal MI up to 30 days for the two treatment groups in the PURSUIT study. The data were analyzed using SAS proc lifetest with option method = breslow. SAS first calculates the estimates of the survival function, and the cumulative hazard function estimates are then obtained by taking the negative log of the survival

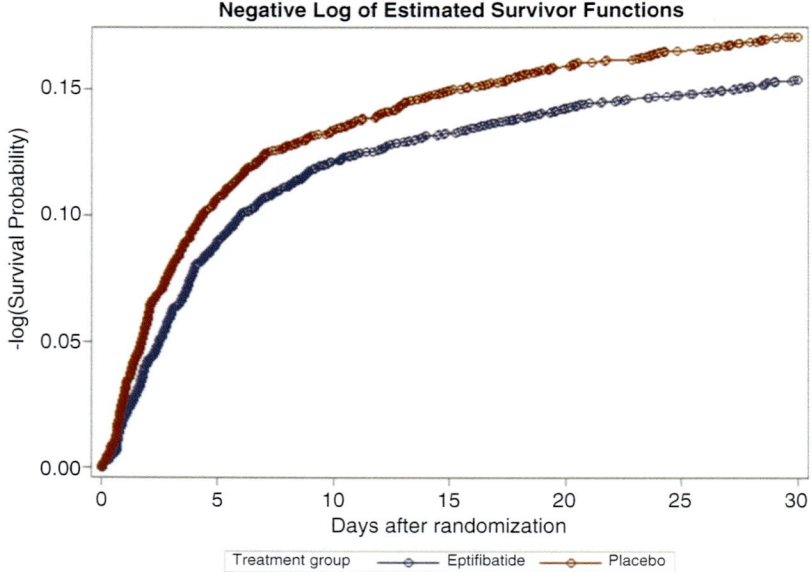

Fig. 4 Nelson-Aalen estimates of the cumulative hazard of death and nonfatal MI up to 30 days for eptifibatide and placebo groups (PURSUIT study)

function estimates (hence the title of the plot). Circles in the plot indicate censored observations.

Estimators of the Hazard Function

Occasionally, the investigators may be interested in estimating the hazard function, especially when trying to decide on the parametric model for the survival data. Both the Kaplan-Meier and the Nelson-Aalen estimators of the hazard function have the form

$$\widehat{h}_{KM}(t) = \frac{d_j}{n_j \tau_{(j)}},$$

for $t_{(j-1)} \leq t < t_{(j)}, j = 1, \ldots, r$. Here $\tau_{(j)} = t_{(j)} - t_{(j-1)}$ is the length of the jth time interval; notation is defined in section "Kaplan-Meier Estimator of the Survival Function."

Using the notation from section "Life-Table Estimator of the Survival Function," a life-table estimator of the hazard function is

$$\widehat{h}_{LT}(t) = \frac{d_j}{\left(n'_j - d_j/2\right)\tau_j},$$

for $t_{j-1} \leq t < t_j$, $(j = 1, \ldots, m)$, where $\tau_j = t_j - t_{j-1}$.

In practice, plots of the estimates of the hazard function calculated using the formulas described above tend to be rather erratic and hard to read. For this reason, most applications use smoothed versions of the hazard function estimators, typically obtained using so-called kernel smoothing functions which are defined on the interval $[-1,1]$. Briefly, a kernel-smoothed estimator of the hazard function at time t is a weighted average of the jumps of the Nelson-Aalen estimator of the cumulative hazard function $\left\{\widehat{H}_{NA}\left(t_{(j)}\right) - \widehat{H}_{NA}\left(t_{(j-1)}\right)\right\}$, over the event times that are within some bandwidth distance b of t. The weights are determined by the choice of the kernel function. For example, one of the most popular kernel functions is the Epanechnikov kernel (Epanechnikov 1969), defined as

$$K_E(x) = 0.75(1 - x^2), \quad -1 \leq x \leq 1,$$

and the corresponding Epanechnikov kernel-smoothed estimator of the hazard function with bandwidth b as the expression

$$\widehat{h}(t) = \frac{1}{b}\sum_{j=1}^{r} K_E\left(\frac{t - t_{(j)}}{b}\right)\frac{d_j}{n_j},$$

where $b \leq t \leq t_{(r)} - b$. Since the kernel function $K_E(x)$ is defined on an interval $[-1,1]$, only events in the interval $[t - b, t + b]$ contribute to the weighted average. For $t < b$ and $t_{(r)} - b < t \leq t_{(r)}$, corresponding asymmetric kernels are used in place of $K_E(x)$ (Gasser and Müller 1979); see Klein and Moeschberger (2006) for details.

Example 6

Figure 5 shows smoothed estimates of the hazard functions for death and nonfatal MI up to 30 days for the two treatment groups in the PURSUIT study. The estimates were obtained using the function muhaz() in the R package muhaz and then plotted using a custom plotter function written in R. The smoothing was performed with the Epanechnikov kernel with a bandwidth of 5 for the placebo group and 5.1 for the eptifibatide group (those were the values automatically chosen by the muhaz() function). The estimates show that for both treatment groups, the hazard was highest in the first day after randomization, declined sharply until approximately day 10 and then declined at much slower rate.

Analyses of Truncated Data

Truncation arises when only subjects whose observation times lie within a certain interval are included in the study. Unlike censoring, which occurs when there is no precise information on the timing of the event of interest for some study subjects, truncation can be viewed as a type of a sampling bias, leaving some subjects out of the study altogether. *Left* truncation can occur when a certain event happens that

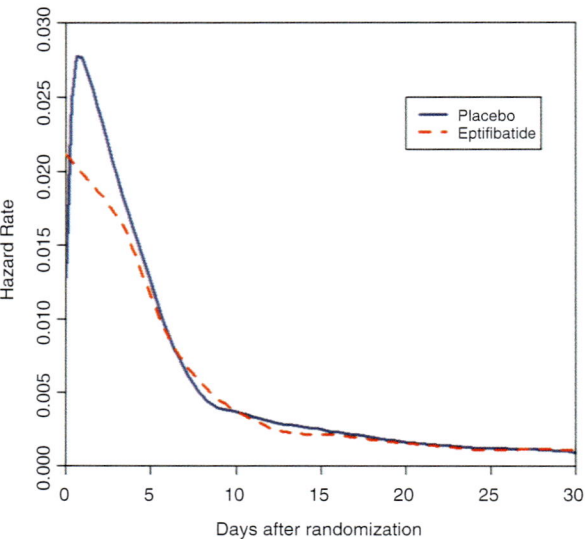

Fig. 5 Epanechnikov kernel-smoothed estimates of the hazard of death and nonfatal MI up to 30 days for eptifibatide and placebo groups (PURSUIT study)

precludes inclusion of a subject in the study. For example, consider a study of the risk of spontaneous abortion where pregnant women are included in the study only after a certain gestational age, known to be associated with high risk of spontaneous abortion. In such a study, the risk of spontaneous abortion would be underestimated because women who had spontaneous abortion prior to the gestational age used as an entry criterion for the study would be excluded. *Right* truncation occurs when only subjects who experience a certain event are included in the study. For instance, suppose the investigators are interested in estimating the distribution of time from blood transfusion to HIV diagnosis using a sample of HIV-positive patients whose infection was traced to the time when they received a blood transfusion. Because this study does not include subjects who received an HIV-contaminated blood transfusion but have not yet received a diagnosis of HIV, the estimated distribution of time from blood transfusion to HIV diagnosis will be biased. Other examples of truncated survival data are presented, for example, in Cole and Hudgens (2010) and in Lamarca et al. (1998).

Estimation for Left-Truncated Data

All estimators discussed in sections "Kaplan-Meier Estimator of the Survival Function," "Life-Table Estimator of the Survival Function," "Nelson-Aalen Estimator of the Cumulative Hazard Function," and "Estimators of the Hazard Function" are applicable in case of left-truncated data, under the assumption that truncation times are independent of survival times, with the following modification. Suppose the ith subject enters the study at time E_i. Just as before, $t_{(1)}, \ldots, t_{(r)}$ denote the event times and d_j is the number of events at $t_{(j)}$. In the previous sections, all subjects entered the study at time $t_{(0)}$ and n_j was the number of subjects still at risk just before $t_{(j)}$. For left-truncated data, we need to define the number of subjects at risk just before $t_{(j)}$ as the number of subjects who have entered the study prior to $t_{(j)}$ and were still at risk just before $t_{(j)}$, that is, the number of subjects with $E_i \leq t_{(j)} \leq U_i$, where U_i is the observed subject time, defined in section "Basic Terminology and Concepts." The interpretation of the estimators will have to change as well. For example, the Kaplan-Meier estimator will now estimate the *conditional* survival probability

$$\Pr(T > t | T > E) = \frac{\Pr(T > t)}{\Pr(T > E)},$$

where $E = \min_i E_i$ is the earliest of the entry times. It should also be noted that because subjects enter the study at different times, the number of subjects at risk in a study with left-truncated data does not have to monotonically decrease over time. In fact, the number at risk can be very low for small values of $t_{(j)}$, and if for some event time $t_{(j)}$ the number at risk n_j is equal to the number of events d_j, the Kaplan-Meier estimator will be zero for all $t \geq t_{(j)}$ even if subjects continue to enter the study after $t_{(j)}$.

Survival function estimates for left-truncated data can be obtained using function survfit() in the R package survival, or using SAS macro %lt_lifetest (Hu 2019).

Example 7

Consider again the VALIANT study, described in Example 2. Suppose now that we are interested in estimating $\Pr(T > t | T > 45)$, the probability of being stroke free as a function of age in patients aged 45 years or older by treatment group.

There were 4657 patients in the valsartan group, 4644 in the captopril group, and 4599 in the valsartan plus captopril group who were aged 45 years or older when they entered the study. Of those patients, 154, 164, and 135 experienced a stroke event, respectively. Estimated Kaplan-Meier survival curves by treatment group are shown in Fig. 6 and the partial output for the Kaplan-Meier estimates (KM) of the conditional survival functions with 95% confidence limits (CL) is shown in the table below. The data were analyzed using the function survfit() in the R package survival.

Valsartan						
Age (years)	# At risk	# Events	KM	Standard error	Lower 95% CL	Upper 95% CL
47.9	116	1	0.991	0.00858	0.975	1.000
48.0	181	1	0.986	0.01016	0.966	1.000
48.1	175	1	0.980	0.01158	0.958	1.000
...						
88.0	39	1	0.460	0.03477	0.397	0.533
88.1	37	1	0.448	0.03602	0.382	0.524

(continued)

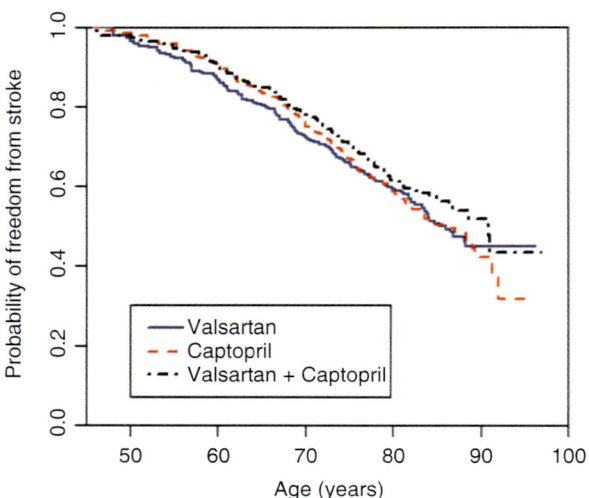

Fig. 6 Kaplan-Meier estimates of freedom from stroke as a function of age for patients aged 45 years or older randomized to valsartan, captopril, and valsartan +captopril groups (VALIANT study)

Valsartan						
Age (years)	# At risk	# Events	KM	Standard error	Lower 95% CL	Upper 95% CL
Captopril						
Age (years)	# At risk	# Events	KM	Standard error	Lower 95% CL	Upper 95% CL
46.5	112	1	0.991	0.00889	0.974	1.000
48.5	157	1	0.985	0.01085	0.964	1.000
51.0	197	1	0.980	0.01189	0.957	1.000
...						
91.3	8	1	0.368	0.06131	0.266	0.510
92.0	7	1	0.316	0.07397	0.199	0.500
Valsartan + captopril						
Age (years)	# At risk	# Events	KM	Standard error	Lower 95% CL	Upper 95% CL
46.1	103	1	0.990	0.00966	0.972	1.000
46.5	99	1	0.980	0.01380	0.954	1.000
50.2	181	1	0.975	0.01475	0.946	1.000
...						
90.9	13	1	0.476	0.05247	0.383	0.590
91.0	11	1	0.432	0.06259	0.326	0.574

Estimation for Right-Truncated Data

Estimation of the survival function in case of right-truncated data can be converted to an estimation problem involving left-truncated data by reversing the time scale. In a situation with right truncation, only subjects who experience an event are included in the study. Suppose the ith subject enters the study at the chronologic time E_i and has an event at the chronologic time $E_i + T_i$, where E_i and T_i are assumed to be independent. Suppose that the data (E_i, T_i) are obtained from a random sample of n subjects, where all values of E_i and $E_i + T_i$ lie in some chronologic time interval $[0, \tau]$. Denote $R_i = \tau - T_i$. Values of R_i are left truncated because for all subjects included in the sample $R_i \geq E_i$. Therefore, the Kaplan-Meier estimator with modified risk sets discussed in the previous section can be used to estimate the probability $\Pr(R > t|\, R > 0)$, which corresponds to the probability $G(t) = \Pr(T < \tau - t|\, T < \tau)$ on the original time scale. In "reverse" time R, the number "at risk" corresponding to a value $\tau - t_{(j)}$, where $t_{(1)} < \ldots < t_{(n)}$ denote the ordered event times $T_1, \ldots, T_n$, is the number of subjects i with $R_i \geq \tau - t_{(j)} \geq E_i$. On the original time scale, the number at risk is the number of subjects who entered the study no later than the chronologic time $\tau - t_{(j)}$ and who had event times no greater than $t_{(j)}$.

Example 8

Lagakos et al. (1988) reported the data from a study of 258 adults and 37 children who received contaminated blood transfusion and developed AIDS by June 30, 1986. The dates of infection and AIDS induction were grouped into 3-month intervals starting with April 1, 1978, so that $E = 0$ corresponds to an infection that occurred between April 1, 1978 and June 30, 1978. Time from infection to AIDS induction is measured in years. All infections and inductions occurred within 8 years from April 1, 1978, thus $\tau = 8$. The distribution of the induction times, conditional on being less than 8 years, is presented in Fig. 7 and in the table below, separately for children and for adults. The data were analyzed using the function survfit() in the R package survival.

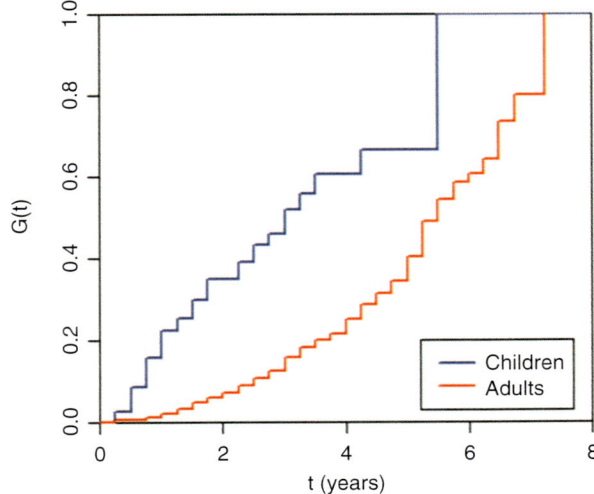

Fig. 7 Conditional distribution of the induction times for 258 adults and 37 children with transfusion-related AIDS

Children							
t (years)	$\tau - t$	# At risk	# Events	$G(t)$	Standard error	Lower 95% CL	Upper 95% CL
0.25	7.75	2	2	0	–	–	–
0.50	7.50	7	5	0.024	0.020	0.0048	0.123
0.75	7.25	13	6	0.085	0.049	0.028	0.260
...							
4.25	3.75	11	1	0.606	0.254	0.266	1.000
5.50	2.50	3	1	0.667	0.272	0.300	1.000
Adults							
t (years)	$\tau - t$	# At risk	# Events	$G(t)$	Standard error	Lower 95% CL	Upper 95% CL
0.25	7.75	6	6	0	–	–	–
0.50	7.50	8	2	0.0034	0.0018	0.0012	0.0094
0.75	7.25	21	13	0.0046	0.0022	0.0018	0.0116
...							
6.75	1.25	12	1	0.733	0.176	0.458	1.000
7.25	0.75	5	1	0.800	0.179	0.516	1.000

Hypothesis Testing

Logrank Tests

The logrank test is arguably the most popular of many nonparametric tests that are available for the comparison of two groups of survival data. It arose as a natural extension of the methods of analyzing 2×2 contingency tables. The logrank test is directly related to the Cox proportional hazards regression model discussed in chapter 9; when there are no tied observations, the logrank test is equivalent to the score test derived from this model. This relationship makes the logrank test a natural choice when the alternative hypothesis assumes "proportional hazards," that is, that at any point in time, the hazard of an event for a subject in one group is proportional to the hazard at that time for a subject in another group.

Consider two treatment groups, with group 0 denoted by $Z = 0$ and group 1 denoted by $Z = 1$. The null hypothesis is usually the one of no difference between the groups:

$$H_0 : S_0(t) = S_1(t), \quad t \geq 0,$$

or, equivalently

$$H_0 : h_0(t) = h_1(t), \quad t \geq 0.$$

The alternative hypothesis may be one sided:

$$H_1 : S_1(t) \geq S_0(t),$$

for $t \geq 0$, with strict inequality for some t, or it may be two sided:

H_1: either $S_1(t) \geq S_0(t)$, or $S_1(t) \leq S_0(t)$, for $t \geq 0$, with strict inequality for some t.

Suppose $t_{(1)} < t_{(2)} < \ldots < t_{(r)}$ are distinct event times across the two groups. Denote d_{ij} and n_{ij} ($i = 0, 1$) as the number of events at time $t_{(j)}$ and the number at risk just before $t_{(j)}$, respectively, in groups 0 and 1. Also denote the total number of events at time $t_{(j)}$ as $d_j = d_{0j} + d_{1j}$ and the total number at risk as $n_j = n_{0j} + n_{1j}$. At each event time $t_{(j)}$, the disposition of the study subjects can be summarized by the following table:

Group	Number of events at $t_{(j)}$	Number remaining event-free past $t_{(j)}$	Number at risk just before $t_{(j)}$
0	d_{0j}	$n_{0j} - d_{0j}$	n_{0j}
1	d_{1j}	$n_{1j} - d_{1j}$	n_{1j}
Total	d_j	$n_j - d_j$	n_j

Considering d_j, n_{0j}, n_{1j} as fixed, under the null hypothesis H_0, the number of events in Group 1 follows a hypergeometric distribution:

$$\Pr(\text{number of events in Group 1 at time } t_{(j)} \text{ is } d_{1j}) = \frac{\binom{d_j}{d_{1j}} \binom{n_j - d_j}{n_j - n_{1j}}}{\binom{n_j}{n_{1j}}},$$

where

$$\binom{d_j}{d_{1j}} = \frac{d_j!}{d_{1j}!(d_j - d_{1j})!}.$$

The hypergeometric distribution implies that the mean of d_{1j} can be calculated as $E(d_{1j}) = e_j = \frac{n_{1j}}{n_j} d_j$. Using the Cochran-Mantel-Haenszel method of combining information over a series of 2×2 tables, the logrank test is constructed as the ratio $L = \frac{U^2}{V}$, where

$$U = \sum_{j=1}^{r} (d_{1j} - e_{1j}), \tag{3}$$

$$V = \text{Var}(U) = \sum_{j=1}^{r} v_{1j}, \tag{4}$$

$$v_{1j} = \frac{n_{0j} n_{1j} d_j (n_j - d_j)}{n_j^2 (n_j - 1)}.$$

Under the null hypothesis, the logrank test follows the chi-square distribution with 1 degree of freedom.

The logrank test belongs to a class of weighted logrank tests of the form

$$\frac{U_W^2}{V_W},$$

where

$$U_w = \sum_{j=1}^r w_j(d_{1j} - e_{1j}),$$

$$V_W = \text{Var}(U_w) = \sum_{j=1}^r w_j^2 v_{1j}.$$

For the logrank test, all weights w_j take a value of 1. Another popular test from this class is the Wilcoxon (also known as Gehan-Wilcoxon, or Breslow) test, constructed using weights $w_j = n_j$. It can be shown that the logrank test is the most powerful of the class of weighted logrank tests when the alternative hypothesis is one of proportional hazards:

$$H_1 : h_1(t) = \varphi h_0(t), \quad t \geq 0,$$

where φ is some constant. The Wilcoxon test may be more suitable when the differences between the groups occur early in the follow-up, since earlier differences receive larger weights $w_j = n_j$ in the calculation of U_w.

Example 9

Let us return to the example of the PURSUIT study. The null hypothesis of no difference in the distribution of time to death or nonfatal MI up to 30 days between eptifibatide and placebo groups was analyzed with the logrank test using the function survdiff() in the R package survival. The absolute difference between the observed and expected numbers of events was 40 and the logrank test statistic was calculated as 4.48, with the corresponding p-value of 0.034. Therefore, at the significance level of 0.05 there is sufficient evidence that eptifibatide treatment is associated with reduced risk of death or nonfatal MI up to 30 days, as compared to placebo.

Example 10

In VALIANT, there were two primary comparisons of interest: valsartan versus captopril and valsartan plus captopril versus captopril alone. For the outcome of stroke, these two comparisons were analyzed with the logrank test using the function survdiff() in the R package survival. For the comparison of valsartan versus captopril, the absolute difference between the observed and expected numbers of events was 5 and the logrank test statistic was calculated as 0.3, with the corresponding p-value of 0.61. When valsartan plus captopril and captopril groups were compared, the absolute difference between the observed and expected numbers of events was 13, with the logrank test statistic equal to 2.1 and the corresponding p-value of 0.15. Thus, neither of the new treatments was shown to reduce the risk of stroke, as compared to captopril alone. These results support the visual analysis of the survival curves shown in Fig. 3 (Example 4).

Logrank Test for Comparison of Multiple Groups

The logrank test is easily extended to a situation where the comparison of interest involves $K \geq 3$ groups. Denote the survival function for group i as $S_i(t)$ ($i = 1, \ldots, K$). The null hypothesis of no difference between the groups is:

$$H_0 : S_1(t) = S_2(t) = \ldots = S_K(t), \quad t \geq 0,$$

and the two-sided alternative hypothesis can be stated as:

$$H_1 : S_i(t) \neq S_l(t),$$

for some $i \neq l$ and for some $t > 0$. As before, consider the distinct event times $t_{(1)} < t_{(2)} < \ldots < t_{(r)}$ across the K groups. Extending the notation from the previous section, at each event time $t_{(j)}$, the number of events and the number at risk in each group can be summarized by the table:

Group	Number of events at $t_{(j)}$	Number "surviving" past $t_{(j)}$	Number at risk just before $t_{(j)}$
1	d_{1j}	$n_{1j} - d_{1j}$	n_{1j}
2	d_{2j}	$n_{2j} - d_{2j}$	n_{2j}
...	...	,,,	...
K	d_{Kj}	$n_{Kj} - d_{Kj}$	n_{Kj}
Total	d_j	$n_j - d_j$	n_j

Assuming that d_j and n_{ij} ($i = 1, \ldots, K$) are fixed, under the null hypothesis H_0, the $K \times 1$ vector $\mathbf{d}_j = (d_{1j}, d_{2j}, \ldots, d_{Kj})^T$ follows a multivariate hypergeometric distribution, so that the mean and variance of the number of events in group i at time $t_{(j)}$ can be estimated as

$$E(d_{ij}) = e_{ij} = \frac{n_{ij}}{n_j} d_j,$$

$$Var(d_{ij}) = \frac{n_{ij}(n_j - n_{ij})d_j(n_j - d_j)}{n_j^2(n_j - 1)},$$

and the covariance between the numbers of events in groups i and l at time $t_{(j)}$ as

$$Cov(d_{ij}, d_{lj}) = -\frac{n_{ij}n_{lj}d_j(n_j - d_j)}{n_j^2(n_j - 1)}.$$

Consider a $(K - 1) \times 1$ vector $\mathbf{U} = (U_1, U_2, \ldots, U_{(K-1)})^T$, where

$$U_i = \sum\nolimits_{j=1}^{r} (d_{ij} - e_{ij}).$$

Note that the term U_K is not included in **U** because of redundancy, since U_K is completely determined from $U_1, U_2, \ldots, U_{K-1}$. It is easy to verify that

$$U_1 + U_2 + \ldots + U_{K-1} + U_K = 0.$$

The K-sample logrank test statistic is then given by the expression.

$$L^K = \mathbf{U}^T \mathbf{V}^{-1} \mathbf{U},$$

where **V** is the covariance matrix of **U**, with diagonal elements $V_{ii} = \sum_{j=1}^{r} Var(d_{ij})$ and off-diagonal elements $V_{il} = \sum_{j=1}^{r} Cov(d_{ij}, d_{lj})$. Under the null hypothesis, the K-sample logrank test statistic has an asymptotic chi-square distribution with $(K-1)$ degrees of freedom.

Example 11

To illustrate the use of the logrank test in the case of multiple groups, let us test the null hypothesis of no difference in the risk of stroke between the three treatment groups in the VALIANT study. Output from the function survdiff() in the R package survival showed that the logrank test statistic was equal to 2.1, and when compared to the chi-square distribution with 2 degrees of freedom, a p-value of 0.35 was obtained. Based on this result, we can conclude that the risk of stroke was similar in all three groups: valsartan, captopril, and valsartan plus captopril.

Stratified Logrank Test

When two or more groups of survival data are compared, especially in non-randomized studies, the apparent relationship (or lack of it) between the survival and the groups may be confounded by presence of other factors, in situations when unequal distribution of these factors between the groups makes them prognostically different. In such cases, one approach is to adjust for possible imbalances between the groups using a stratified version of the logrank or weighted logrank (e.g., Wilcoxon) test. In randomized studies that use stratified randomization in order to reduce the possibility of chance imbalance between the treatment groups, stratified tests are typically used as well.

As the first step in calculating stratified logrank test, the investigators need to define the strata, possibly using combinations of factors, within which subjects are expected to be more prognostically similar. In randomized studies with stratified randomization, this step may be unnecessary since such strata have been already defined. Then, U- and V-statistics discussed earlier in this chapter have to be calculated separately for each stratum and then combined across the strata. For the comparison of two groups, suppose U_k is the statistic calculated for the kth stratum using Eq. (3), with variance V_k calculated using (4) ($k = 1, \ldots, S$). Then the stratified logrank test statistic is

$$L_S = \frac{\left(\sum_{k=1}^{S} U_k\right)^2}{\sum_{k=1}^{S} V_k}.$$

To test the null hypothesis of no difference between the groups, this test statistic can be compared to the percentiles of the chi-squared distribution with one degree of freedom.

The stratified logrank test statistic can be extended to the comparison of more than two groups; however, the calculations in this case become much more cumbersome and are not presented here. Interested readers are referred to Klein and Moeschberger (2006) for further details.

Logrank Test for Trend

In some studies of more than two groups of survival data, the groups have a natural ordering, such as low, medium, or high treatment doses, or stages of disease of increasing severity. In such circumstances, the investigators may be interested in testing of the ordered alternatives, that is, alternatives of the form

$$H_1 : S_1(t) \leq S_2(t) \leq \ldots \leq S_K(t), \quad t \geq 0,$$

with at least one strict inequality for some t versus the null hypothesis

$$H_0 : S_1(t) = S_2(t) = \ldots = S_K(t), \quad t \geq 0.$$

These hypotheses can be evaluated using the logrank test for trend. Let $t_{(1)} < t_{(2)} < \ldots < t_{(r)}$ be the distinct event times across the K groups. Using the notation introduced in the discussion of the logrank test for comparison of multiple groups, consider the statistic

$$U_{Ti} = \sum_{j=1}^{r} W_i(t_{(j)}) \left(\frac{d_{ij}}{n_{ij}} - \frac{d_j}{n_j}\right), \quad i = 1, \ldots, K.$$

Here, $W_i(t)$ is a positive-valued weight function such that $W_i(t_{(j)}) = 0$ when $n_{ij} = 0$. In practice, this weight function is usually defined using some function $W(t)$ common to all groups as $W_i(t_{(j)}) = n_{ij} W(t_{(j)})$. Then, the expression for U_{Ti} can be written as

$$U_{Ti} = \sum_{j=1}^{r} W(t_{(j)}) \left(d_{ij} - \frac{n_{ij}}{n_j} d_j\right) = \sum_{j=1}^{r} W(t_{(j)}) (d_{ij} - e_{ij}), \quad i = 1, \ldots, K.$$

The test statistic for trend is constructed using a selected sequence of scores $a_1 < a_2 < \ldots < a_K$. Any increasing sequence can be used, but in most applications, the scores are defined as $a_i = i$. The logrank test for trend is then defined as

$$L_T = \frac{U_T^2}{V_T},$$

where

$$U_T = \sum_{i=1}^{K} a_i U_{Ti},$$

$$V_T = Var(U_T) = \sum_{i=1}^{K} \sum_{l=1}^{K} a_i a_l v_{il},$$

and the variance-covariance terms v_{il} are defined as

$$v_{ii} = \sum_{j=1}^{r} [W(t_{(j)})]^2 e_{ij}\left(1 - \frac{n_{ij}}{n_j}\right)\left(\frac{n_j - d_j}{n_j - 1}\right), \quad i = 1, \ldots, K$$

$$v_{il} = -\sum_{j=1}^{r} [W(t_{(j)})]^2 \frac{e_{ij} e_{lj}}{d_j}\left(\frac{n_j - d_j}{n_j - 1}\right), \quad i \neq l.$$

Under the null hypothesis, the test statistic L_T has an asymptotic chi-square distribution with 1 degree of freedom.

Further Reading

Many textbooks and journal review articles provide an introduction to the survival analysis methods, including those discussed in this chapter, illustrated with real data examples. Machin et al. (2006) present many common survival analysis techniques in a nontechnical way, with applications in clinical trials. Collett (2015) offers a comprehensive guide to the survival analysis at an intermediate level, which could be useful to a variety of audiences. Singh and Mukhopadhyay (2011) introduce the reader to the terminology and most often used methods in the survival analysis. Muenz (1983a, b) provide a review of common survival analysis methods, aimed at nonstatisticians. Freedman (2008) discusses various aspects of application of life tables and Kaplan-Meier estimators, as well as Cox proportional hazards model, using several observational studies as examples. Finally, a comprehensive guide to the SAS software used for survival analysis can be found in Allison (2010).

Summary and Conclusion

Nonparametric inference is usually the first step in the analysis of survival data from clinical trials. In this chapter, the main nonparametric methods for the analysis of survival data were presented, including the Kaplan-Meier estimator for the survival function, the Nelson-Aalen estimator for the cumulative hazard function, and the logrank test.

Key Facts

- Survival or time-to-event data often arise in clinical trials, especially in the fields like cardiology and cancer research.
- Specialized methods are needed for the analysis of survival data because of the presence of censoring.
- The key quantities used in survival analysis include the survival function, the hazard rate, and the cumulative hazard function.
- The common nonparametric methods for the analysis of survival data include the Kaplan-Meier estimator for the survival function, the Nelson-Aalen estimator for the cumulative hazard function, and the logrank test for the comparison of two or more groups of survival data.

Cross-References

▶ Essential Statistical Tests
▶ Estimation and Hypothesis Testing
▶ Logistic Regression and Related Methods
▶ Survival Analysis II

References

Aalen O (1978) Nonparametric inference for a family of counting processes. Ann Stat 6(4):701–726
Allison PD (2010) Survival analysis using SAS: a practical guide, 2nd Edition. Cary, NC: SAS Institute, Inc.
Cole SR, Hudgens MG (2010) Survival analysis in infectious disease research: describing events in time. AIDS (London, England) 24(16):2423
Collett D (2015) Modelling survival data in medical research, 3rd Edition. CRC press, Boca Raton, FL
Emura T, Chen YH (2018) Analysis of survival data with dependent censoring: Copula-based approaches. Springer, Singapore
Epanechnikov VA (1969) Non-parametric estimation of a multivariate probability density. Theory Probab Appl 14(1):153–158
Freedman DA (2008) Survival analysis: a primer. Am Stat 62(2):110–119
Gasser T, Müller HG (1979) Kernel estimation of regression functions. In: Smoothing techniques for curve estimation. Springer, Berlin/Heidelberg, pp 23–68
Greenwood M (1926) The "errors of sampling" of the survivorship tables. In: Reports on public health and medical subjects, number 33, Appendix 1. HMSO, London
Hu Z-H (2019) Using SAS® macros to analyze lifetime data with left truncation. In: SAS global forum 2019, Dallas
Kaplan EL, Meier P (1958) Nonparametric estimation from incomplete observations. J Am Stat Assoc 53(282):457–481
Klein JP, Moeschberger ML (2006) Survival analysis: techniques for censored and truncated data, 2nd Edition. Springer Science & Business Media, New York, NY
Lamarca R, Alonso J, Gomez G, Muñoz Á (1998) Left-truncated data with age as time scale: an alternative for survival analysis in the elderly population. J Gerontol Ser A Biol Med Sci 53(5): M337–M343

Machin D, Cheung YB, Parmar M (2006) Survival analysis: a practical approach, 2nd Edition. John Wiley & Sons, Chichester, West Sussex, England

McMurray J, Solomon S, Pieper K, Reed S, Rouleau J, Velazquez E, ... Køber L (2006) The effect of valsartan, captopril, or both on atherosclerotic events after acute myocardial infarction: an analysis of the Valsartan in Acute Myocardial Infarction Trial (VALIANT). J Am Coll Cardiol 47(4):726–733

Muenz LR (1983a) Comparing survival distributions: a review for nonstatisticians. I. Cancer Investig 1:455–466

Muenz LR (1983b) Comparing survival distributions: a review for nonstatisticians. II. Cancer Investig 1:537–545

Nelson W (1972) Theory and applications of hazard plotting for censored failure data. Technometrics 14(4):945–966

Pfeffer MA, McMurray JJ, Velazquez EJ, Rouleau JL, Køber L, Maggioni AP, ... Leimberger JD (2003) Valsartan, captopril, or both in myocardial infarction complicated by heart failure, left ventricular dysfunction, or both. N Engl J Med 349(20):1893–1906

PURSUIT Trial Investigators (1998) Inhibition of platelet glycoprotein IIb/IIIa with eptifibatide in patients with acute coronary syndromes. N Engl J Med 339(7):436–443

R Core Team (2017) R: a language and environment for statistical computing. R Foundation for Statistical Computing, Vienna. https://www.R-project.org/

Singh R, Mukhopadhyay K (2011) Survival analysis in clinical trials: basics and must know areas. Perspect Clin Res 2(4):145

Lagakos SW, Barraj LM, Gruttola VD (1988) Nonparametric analysis of truncated survival data, with application to AIDS. Biometrika 75(3):515–523

Survival Analysis II

89

James J. Dignam

Contents

Introduction	1744
Statistical Models for Time to Event Data	1745
Semi-Parametric Model	1746
Evaluating the Proportional Hazards Assumption	1750
Extensions of the Cox Model	1752
Alternate Approaches and Models	1754
Additional Modeling Considerations	1755
Competing Risks	1756
Competing Risks Observations	1757
The Nonidentifiability Problem	1757
Estimable Quantities	1758
Estimators	1759
Nonparametric Tests in Competing Risks Data	1761
Regression Models for Competing Risks	1765
Summary	1767
Key Facts	1767
Cross-References	1768
References	1768

Abstract

Survival analysis modeling is integral to clinical trial analysis, as even in well-designed randomized trials where the primary inference is to be based on fundamental quantities such as estimated survival distributions and nonparametric tests, survival models offer additional insights and succinct treatment effect summaries. The ubiquitous Cox proportional hazards model has numerous variations and extensions to fit specific analytic needs and has become a mainstay of

J. J. Dignam (✉)
Department of Public Health Sciences, The University of Chicago, Chicago, IL, USA
e-mail: jdignam@uchicago.edu

© Springer Nature Switzerland AG 2022
S. Piantadosi, C. L. Meinert (eds.), *Principles and Practice of Clinical Trials*,
https://doi.org/10.1007/978-3-319-52636-2_120

biomedical and clinical trial data analysis. However, other models and treatment effect metrics are increasingly available and should be adopted in cases where model assumptions are not met.

A natural extension of survival analysis pertains to the case where multiple potential causes of failure may be in effect. When these causes of failure are mutually exclusive, then competing risks observations are encountered, while in other cases, there may be multiple failures per individual. Methods that address these extensions of time to event data are needed to (a) assess of value of treatment in the presence of events that may preclude observation of the disease process of interest, (b) evaluate risks and benefits of treatment in a way that reflects patient experience, and (c) provide tools for study of factors related to different failure types and model more complex multi-event failure processes.

Keywords

Survival modeling · Hazard regression · Proportional hazards · Competing risks · Cause-specific hazard · Subdistribution hazard · Cumulative incidence

Introduction

Beyond the empirical survival and hazard function estimators and associated statistical tests presented in the last chapter ("Survival Analysis I"), there is a large body of more advanced survival analysis methods relevant to clinical trials. Two of these, survival modeling and competing risks analysis, are presented here. While clinical trial designs, and in particular randomized trials, seek to diminish the need for statistical modeling methods, survival models nonetheless play a key role in analysis of trials. Modeling methods can enhance the presentation of results and aid in addressing complexities that inevitably arise during trial conduct and subsequent analysis. A second important body of analysis methodology pertains to situations where, while observing patients for failure events of a specific type (e.g., disease recurrence), there are multiple other potential types of failure that may occur (e.g., onset of or death from another disease). These *competing risks* observations are frequently encountered in analysis of time to event outcomes in clinical trials. Extensions of survival analysis methods provide tools to correctly analyze and interpret competing risks data.

Methods described in this chapter are illustrated using data from four randomized clinical trials in cancer. NSABP B-14 evaluated the efficacy the anti-estrogen agent tamoxifen in early-stage breast cancer, with over 2800 women randomized to either tamoxifen or placebo after surgery for lymph node-negative, estrogen receptor-positive breast tumors; the trial later examined further the duration of tamoxifen therapy (Fisher et al. 1996). RTOG 9802 was a randomized trial of a multidrug chemotherapy regimen after surgery and radiotherapy for low-grade glioma (Buckner et al. 2016) among 251 patients. In RTOG 0825, over 600 patients with glioblastoma undergoing standard radiotherapy and chemotherapy were randomized to either bevacizumab or placebo (Gilbert et al. 2014). The randomized trial RTOG 9202 investigated whether longer duration of androgen deprivation therapy after radiotherapy for localized prostate cancer was more efficacious that short-duration treatment (Lawton et al. 2017).

Statistical Models for Time to Event Data

Statistical models for time to event data are a useful tool to (a) improve treatment effect estimation and obtain succinct summaries with reduced bias, which can arise even in carefully designed studies; (b) identify factors individually and collectively related to risk of failure and survival time, including synergistic and antagonistic effect of such factors on treatment response; and (c) make predictions of outcome based on treatment and other factors.

To relate covariates (treatment or other factors) to survival outcomes, a metric must be specified upon which to build the model. Relating covariates to the survival probability via the survivor function $S(t)$ directly is intuitively appealing but less straightforward than it would appear, as valid estimation would require multiple constraints ($S(t)$ is a strictly non-increasing function over t and takes on only valid probability values). Instead, using the fact that the cumulative hazard function $\Lambda(t)$ uniquely identifies the survival function via the relation

$$\Lambda(t) = -\log(S(t))$$

one can formulate a relationship between covariates and survival outcomes via the hazard of failure $\lambda(u) = d\Lambda(t)/dt$, which is defined on numerical range $(0, \infty)$ and can be non-monotonic over time. Moreover, formulating the model in terms of factors that influence the hazard, which heuristically represents the probability of failure at any given small interval of time among those failure-free thus far, is a naturally comprehensible way to characterize covariates in relation to survival histories. Additional details of the form of the model, in terms of how the effects manifest in the survival history, will determine how the estimates are interpreted.

To motivate the modeling approach most commonly used, a simple construct that relates the effect of a covariate on survival via the hazard is as follows. The exponential survival model is characterized by a single parameter λ that determines the failure rate and thus the survival probability over time.

$$S(t) = e^{-\lambda(t)}$$

Here, the hazard function is the failure rate parameter λ, which itself does not vary over time and is estimated by total events/total person time observed. The failure rate may differ between two groups, say treatment arms A and B, in which case the difference in hazard can be expressed as

$$\lambda_B(t) = \lambda_A(t) e^{\beta z}$$

where $z = 0$ for treatment A and 1 for treatment B. Note that the relative increment in risk from treatment A to treatment B is $\exp(\beta) = \theta$, a time-invariant constant that represents the multiplicative change in risk of failure between the two groups. (exp( ) is used for convenience since it is always nonnegative and thus a valid hazard rate quantity.) Equivalently, this effect can be expressed as the *hazard ratio*

$$\theta = \lambda_B(t)/\lambda_A(t)$$

and can be estimated from the failure rate ratio in the observed data. This model construct is known as having a *proportional hazards* property, owing to the constant proportional difference in risk of failure between groups over time. Figure 1a illustrates an approximate proportional hazards effect between two survival curves. Note that $S(t)$ curves for the two groups diverge over time, but at any given time point, the ratio of hazards between groups is approximately constant. This is difficult to directly assess, and thus proportionality can be checked via a diagnostic plot of $\log_e(-\log_e(S(t)))$ versus $\log_e(\text{time})$, which will result in approximately equidistant curves under proportional hazards (Fig. 1b).

The model can be extended to include additional covariates and conveniently forms a linear model on a (natural) log scale. In fact, early survival modeling approaches in the biomedical setting arose from applications in engineering reliability using the exponential model (Feigl and Zelen 1965; Byar et al. 1974). With both a time-invariant hazard and constant relative effect of covariates over time, this model is overly simplistic in many instances, but has nonetheless proven useful. More expansive parametric model forms that, for example, permit time-varying hazards are available in the survival and engineering reliability literature (Lawless 2002). In the biomedical context, a rich class of flexible parametric models have been developed and implemented in commonly used statistical software (Royston and Parmar 2002). However, in the great majority of survival modeling applications in the biomedical literature, parametric models have been forgone in favor of a more general model that preserves one key aspect, namely, the constant hazard ratio, of the simple exponential approach.

Semi-Parametric Model

Generalizing from the exponential survival regression model, one can specify the hazard function for a given subject with covariates $(Z_1, Z_2, \ldots Z_p)$ as

$$\lambda_1(t) = \lambda_0(t)e^{\beta Z}$$

where $\lambda_0(t)$ is left unspecified as to its form. For a single covariate Z as specified earlier (coded 0 or 1 for two treatment groups), the model again yields the time-invariant hazard ratio for the treatment effect e^β without a need to specify the hazard function form for either group. This semi-parametric model offers more flexibility than parametric models while preserving the proportional hazards property for

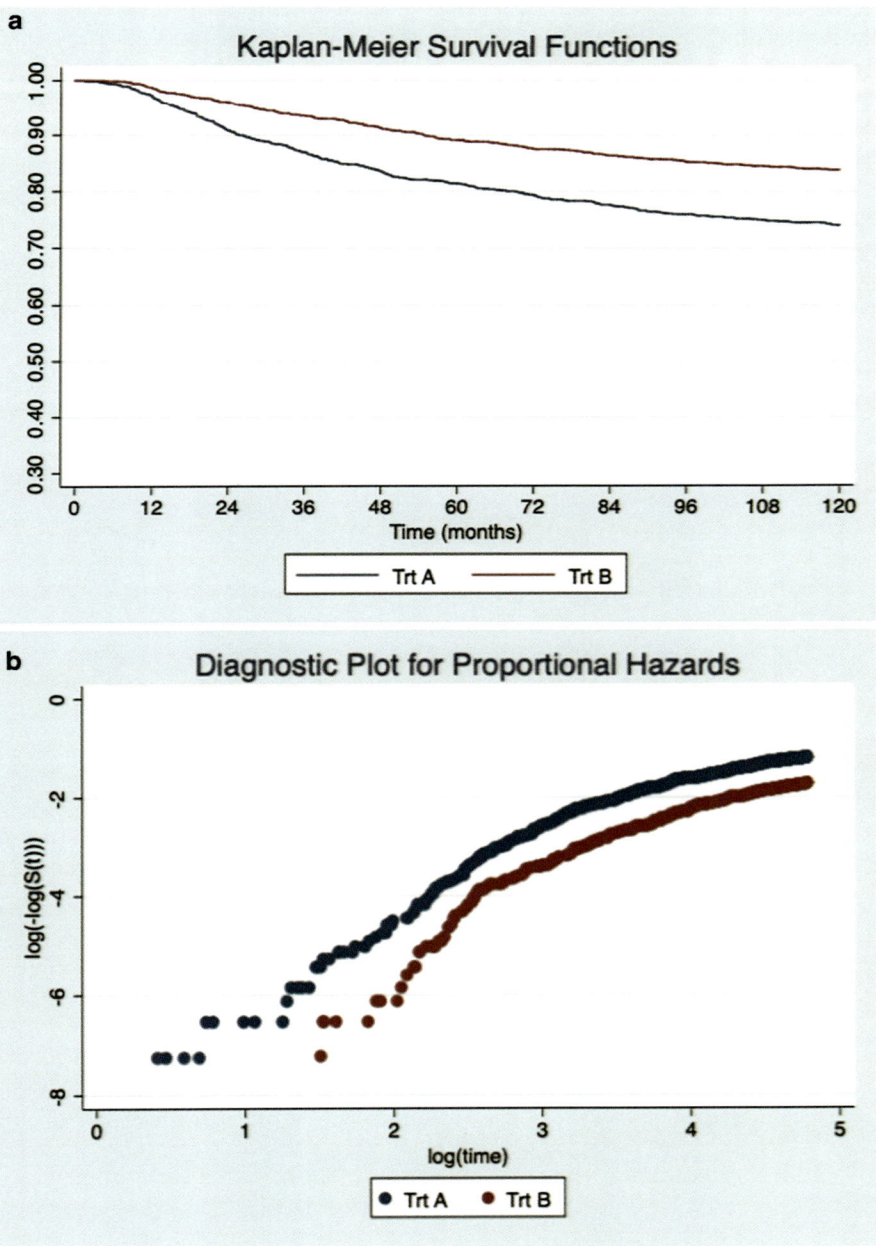

Fig. 1 (a) Survival curves exhibiting the proportional hazards property. (b) A diagnostic plot of curves transformed to hazard estimates, which when plotted against $\log_e(\text{time})$, will show approximately equidistant curves for the two groups

covariates (note that hazards need not be constant, but rather just the ratios of hazards for two contrasting covariate values, to satisfy proportional hazards). This model was among other related general forms proposed for survival data (Cox 1972), and perhaps owing to its straightforward form (although the theoretical justification is technically involved (Cox 1975; Tsiatis 1981)), and because the relative hazard measure produced is analogous to relative risk metric from epidemiology, the Cox proportional hazards model has become ubiquitous in biomedical applications and clinical trial analysis. The model also has natural links to common nonparametric analysis methods such as the logrank test. Following early theoretical work establishing properties, later developments led to many extensions and associated diagnostic tools for the model (Aalen 1978a; Fleming and Harrington 1991; Andersen et al. 1993).

In Table 1 (first panel), analysis of a clinical trial in breast cancer using the model is shown. The hazard ratio for patients assigned to receive tamoxifen versus placebo treatment is 0.66, indicating a 34% reduction in failure hazard (for the endpoint of time-free of disease recurrence, a second cancer of another type, or death from any cause). A 95% confidence interval provides an estimate of precision on the effect and an implicit test of whether the HR differs from unity (at 5% significance). Effects for other relevant covariates are interpreted in the same manner as described.

While primary interest in survival modeling is in the relative hazard estimates, one can also generate representative survival curves from the fitted model. These can be useful to visually depict outcomes for patient groups defined by one or more covariates, although it should be noted that generated curves conform to the assumptions of the model, and thus, for example, (perfect) proportionality will be imposed between curves generated from models having the proportional hazards property. For parametric survival models, estimates for the survival curves, and related quantities such as quantiles, are fully specified and easy to generate (Lawless 2002). For the Cox model, because of the minimal additional assumptions in the model, model curves are heuristically extensions of nonparametric estimators with proportional shifts (on the Y axis) in the curves depending on covariate values. The survivor function for a given covariate set values $Z = (z_1, z_2, \ldots z_p)$ takes the form

$$S(t; Z) = S_0(t)^{\exp(\beta Z)}$$

where $S_0(t)$ is a "baseline" survival function analogous to a nonparametric (i.e., Kaplan-Meier or based on a nonparametric estimate of $H(t)$) estimator at covariate value zero. There are various estimators for $S_0(t)$ available in statistical packages for the Cox model, all of which yield similar estimates under reasonable sample size.

Alternatively, one can use a method that in effect provides survival curve estimates by treatment group from the model if the two groups had identical distributions of other covariates, equivalent to the direct adjusted survival method from life-table analysis (Chang et al. 1982; Makuch 1982). This approach can provide a better visual summary of how the groups differ after multiple covariate adjustment without having to show several covariate combination-based curves. It also correctly depicts summary curves estimating population expected survival for a

Table 1 Examples of effect estimates from the Cox proportional hazards model

Ex. 1 Cox model with fixed effects – effect of tamoxifen and baseline patient/disease features in breast cancer

Covariate	Beta	Hazard ratio	95% CI	Interpretation
Treatment	−0.415	0.66	0.59–0.74	34% relative failure reduction for tamoxifen
Menopausal status	0.092	1.10	0.96–1.25	~10% relative failure increase among postmenopausal women
Tumor size	0.018	1.02	1.01–1.02	Approximate 2% failure increase per mm in tumor size

Ex. 2 Cox model with time-varying *covariate* – effects of androgen deprivation (AD) duration therapy, baseline patient/disease features, and PSA failure status in prostate cancer

Covariate	Beta	Hazard ratio	95% CI	Interpretation
Treatment	−0.032	0.97	0.86–1.09	3% relative reduction in risk of death for long-term AD
High Gleason score	0.295	1.34	1.05–1.72	34% increased relative risk for tumor Gleason 8–10 versus 7 or below
Age at diagnosis	0.048	1.05	1.04–1.06	5% increase in risk of death per year of age older (at diagnosis)
PSA failure status	0.547	1.73	1.53–1.95	For patients with PSA failure at any time in first 2 years, death risk increases by 73% relative to those without PSA failure

Ex. 3 Cox model with time-varying *coefficient* – effect of chemotherapy and other patient/disease features in low-grade glioma

Covariate	HR	95% CI	Interpretation
Chemotherapy			Large reduction in mortality hazard after 1 year for chemotherapy vs. not
< 1 year	1.15	0.30–4.33	
> 1 year	0.35	0.19–1.66	
Age (< 40 vs. 40+)	0.50	0.29–0.87	50% lower mortality risk for younger patients
IDH1-R132H mutation (absent vs. present)	0.66	0.39–1.12	Absence of mutation suggestive of better prognosis

group of patients with various covariate values, unlike an estimator obtained by specifying the mean value for each covariates (and in particular can accommodate adjustment for a discrete factor such as sex). To produce adjusted estimates by treatment group, specify a covariate Z_1 and vector of other covariates $\mathbf{Z_2}$. The model is first fit among all patients using Z_1 and $\mathbf{Z_2}$ as predictors. The quantity estimated for treatment $Z_1 = 1$ is then

$$S_1(t; Z_1 = 1, \mathbf{Z_2}) = \frac{1}{n} \sum_{l=1}^{n} S_l(t; Z_1 = 1, \mathbf{Z}_{2i})$$

This quantity is an average of all estimated survival curves for the group, weighted by the relative frequency of all covariate value combinations observed for $\mathbf{Z}_2$. A survival curve is then calculated for treatment group $Z_1 = 2$. In the resulting plot, the curves will reflect the treatment effect "adjusted" for other covariate effects, which are now perfectly balanced between groups. It should be noted that the curves still represent a model-dependent construct for treatment and other covariates (e.g., proportionality of the curves compared is assured regardless of any deviation in the actual data). Nonetheless, this underused graphical approach may be preferable to empirical survival curves in the presence of covariate imbalances. To illustrate, Fig. 2a shows a subset of patients from the glioblastoma trial, where the important prognostic factor MGMT gene methylation is imbalanced. Overall, 28% of patients have MGMT-methylated tumors, which confers a more favorable prognosis. In the placebo group of this subset, about 50% of patients in the bevacizumab treatment arm have MGMT-methylated tumors, which magnifies the apparent effect (unadjusted hazard ratio = 0.68). The adjusted hazard ratio is 0.79, and Fig. 2b shows a plot of model-based outcomes where the methylation status is identical between the two groups, showing a more modest treatment effect (MGMT was balanced in the study as a whole, and the hazard ratio was 0.79, 95% confidence interval 0.66–0.94 (Gilbert et al. 2014)).

Evaluating the Proportional Hazards Assumption

While the proportional hazards model provides considerable flexibility, the time-invariant effect for covariates is a restrictive assumption that must be evaluated to determine if it reasonably holds. One might indeed inquire as to why treatment should exert a constant hazard reduction effect over time, as it is well established that effects for some covariates may appear to change over time. For example, strong prognostic factors in cancer such as tumor size are diminished in importance among patients who have survived a certain duration of follow-up, and it is indeed logical that once a patient reaches long-term follow-up, the size of the original tumor becomes immaterial. Nonetheless, an assumed constant proportional effect can provide a valid summary of important factors, including treatment benefits, over clinically relevant timespans. Evaluation for any degree of deviation from proportionality remains important when presenting results in the form of time-invariant hazard ratios, particularly for the treatment effect in a comparative clinical trial. Numerous diagnostics are available, ranging from simple graphical evaluations as described earlier (Fig. 1b) to tests such as that of Grambsch et al. (1995), which may furthermore provide information on the functional form by which the effect is time-varying. Figure 3 illustrates some cases of nonproportionality of varying degrees that arise in clinical trials. In the case of modest deviations, such as where the treatment effect attenuates slightly in late follow-up (Fig. 3a), or when curves converge very late in follow-up where there are few patients remaining at risk, the hazard ratio nonetheless provides an interpretable summary metric. When curves converge more profoundly (Fig. 3b) or cross, a single hazard ratio might be reported but may not

89 Survival Analysis II

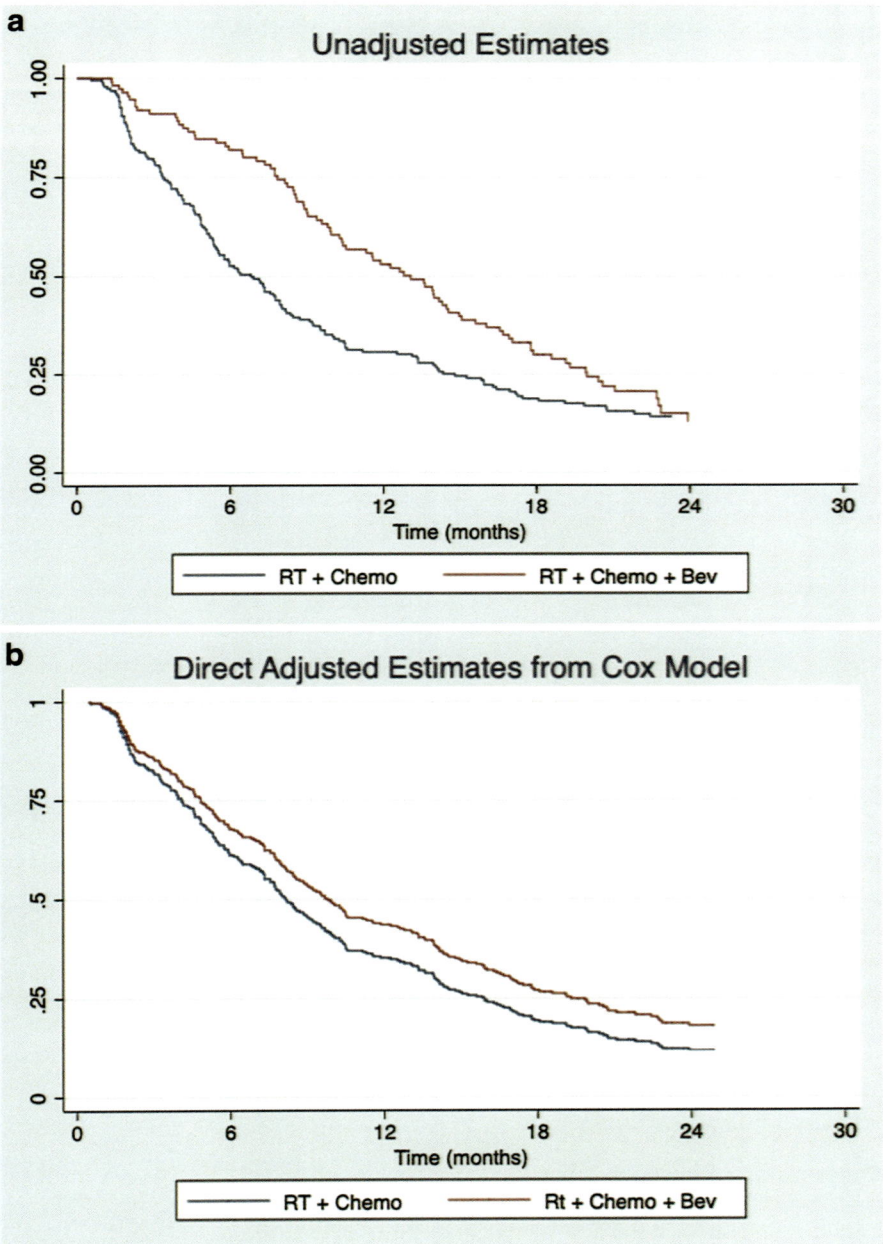

Fig. 2 (**a**) Unadjusted (Kaplan-Meier) survival curves comparing treatment groups in the glioblastoma trial. There is an imbalance in an important prognostic factor (MGMT gene methylation), which influences the apparent treatment difference. (**b**) Direct adjusted survival curves generated after fitting the Cox model with treatment and MGMT status, showing a more modest treatment effect

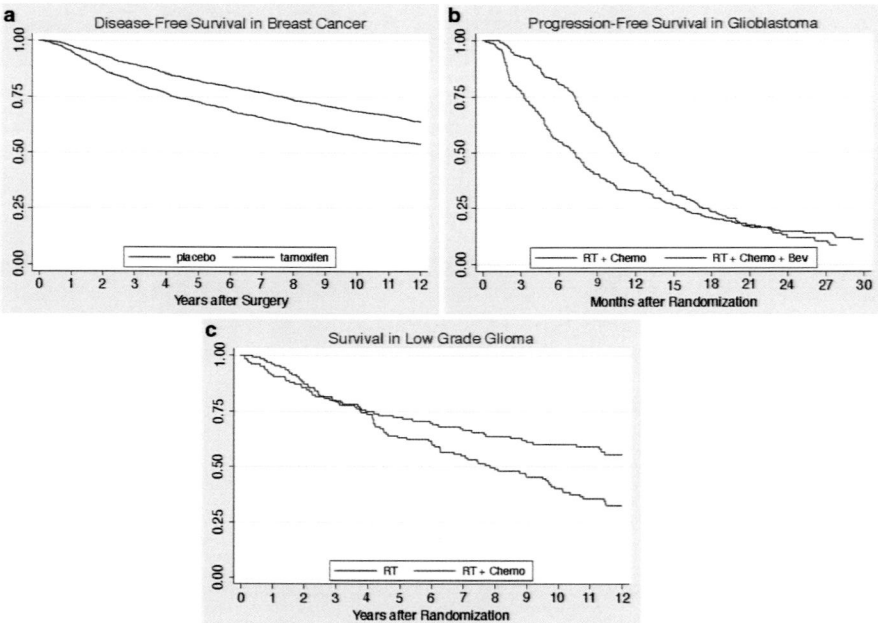

Fig. 3 Examples of patterns in survival curves: (**a**) disease-free survival in early breast cancer, showing approximately proportional hazards; (**b**) progression-free survival in glioblastoma, showing converging curves as underlying hazards converge; and (**c**) survival in low-grade glioma, with a late difference emerging between treatment groups

adequately summarize the effect. Late emerging differences represent another case where a single time-invariant hazard ratio does not suffice to summarize the effect (Fig. 3c).

The ubiquity of the Cox model and the (time-invariant) hazard ratio metric in the medical literature is being increasingly challenged. In addition to extensions of the model (described below), for problems that require it, alternate methods that explicitly provide estimates and inference for time-dependent hazard ratio function are available (e.g., Gilbert et al. 2002). Also, alternate metrics to hazard ratios such as the restricted mean survival time, which have been studied and advocated for many years, are increasingly gaining consideration (Karrison 1997; Zhao et al. 2016).

Extensions of the Cox Model

There are numerous variations on the basic Cox model form that extend capabilities to better suit specific data and research questions.

Stratified model – It may be the case that for some factors/covariates, there is no reasonable expectation of proportionality, or there may be interest in permitting a different background failure risk (still unspecified) in different subgroups, for example, by enrolling center, demographic factor, or disease feature. One can fit the model stratified by the factor(s) of interest. Note that this model dispenses with the proportional hazards assumption for the stratifying factor(s) and the model still produces a single common hazard ratio effect across strata for each model covariate. To further evaluate whether this is an appropriate model, interaction effects between strata and covariates need to be evaluated in the unstratified model. Analyses seeking to determine variation in outcomes by very large numbers of strata, say, examining variation in outcome by individual enrolling center in a large multi-center study, are best addressed using more advanced methods (such as frailty models, described in Therneau and Grambsch 2000).

Time-varying covariates – Covariates are in most instances time-fixed characteristics that are assigned values at the inception of follow-up. Covariates for which the value evolves over time (such as a disease response state, change in body weight, serial blood marker measures, etc.) can be accommodated (Cox 1972), provided these covariates $Z(t)$ are correctly specified in the model, which has the form

$$\lambda_1(t) = \lambda_0(t)e^{\beta Z + \beta Z(t)}$$

To fit the model correctly, the time-varying covariate values $Z(t)$ must be updated at each failure time t for all patients, so that the risk set in the estimation equation can be correctly specified (it is incorrect to assign values $Z(t)$ at follow-up initiation ($t = 0$) that are realized only after some amount of follow-up time has elapsed). The effect in the model represents the increment in risk for a unit change in the covariate value, contrasting those having had the covariate change to those whose value has not changed. As an example, Table 1 shows a model estimating the effect of treatment and a biochemical failure indicator (meaning that prostate-specific antigen level has risen to meet certain failure criteria) on survival among men randomized to different durations of androgen deprivation therapy for localized prostate cancer. There is a 54% relative increment in mortality risk among men who experienced biochemical failure compared to those who did not. Note that while the covariate is dynamic, the effect is still time-independent, in that a single β and thus hazard ratio is estimated and thus the risk increment is the same regardless of when the intermediate event occurs. A related but distinctly different approach that offers greater flexibility conversely has a time-fixed covariate (e.g., value assigned at beginning of follow-up) but incorporates a time-varying coefficient β *effect*.

$$\lambda_1(t) = \lambda_0(t)e^{\beta Z + \beta(t)X}$$

Some degree of time dependence in effects might be expected for patient/disease covariates as mentioned earlier, but may not warrant this more complex model. More often, consideration of a dynamic time-varying effect is required to adequately characterize treatment benefit or other covariate effects in clear cases of non-proportionality. Choices for how $\beta(t)$ is specified include simple step functions, whereby the time axis is partitioned into segments in which different β estimates are in effect to more complex functional forms suggested by model diagnostics

(Grambsch et al. 1995; Gray 1994). Results of one such analysis, estimating the treatment effect shown in Fig. 3c, are shown in Table 1. Here, a simple approach was taken, whereby hazard ratios were estimated in separate time intervals determined by a criterion used to select a partition of the time axis. This is tantamount to a treatment by (discrete) time interaction effect. Identification of the appropriate function is a complex statistical problem, and consequently, expanding the Cox model in this way for treatment effect estimation should be undertaken carefully.

Alternate Approaches and Models

An alternate approach to survival modeling, with a less familiar but in some ways intuitively more appealing treatment effect metric, is the accelerated failure time model. In this type of model, the treatment (or other covariate) effect is expressed in terms of a lengthening or shortening of time to specific survival time landmarks, such as the median (50th) or 75th percentile of the survival time distribution. This is contrasted with the proportional hazards model as follows, where θ represents a covariate effect and $S_0(t)$ is the reference survival curve:

$$\text{Proportional hazards}: S(t;\theta) = S_0(t)^\theta$$

$$\text{Accelerated failure time}: S(t;\theta) = S_0(\theta t)$$

For example, suppose that at time $t = 5$ years, $S_0(t)$ (patients in group 0) equals 50% (median survival time), and the estimated θ is 0.75. Under the proportional hazards model, patients in group 1 would have $S(t) = 0.59$ at this same time t (a better outcome). As the parameterization of the accelerated failure time model is different, so is the meaning of the covariate, in both direction of effect and how it reflects the outcome. If one obtained an estimated θ of 0.75 when fitting the accelerated failure time model, this would imply that patients in group 1 reach median survival at θt years or have a 25% decrease in median survival time (a worse outcome). Thus, both models will reflect how covariates manifest on the failure process, whether by the familiar hazard ratio metric (where $\theta < 1$ would imply decreased failure rate for group 1 relative to group 0), or the acceleration factor metric (where $\theta < 1$ indicates decreased time to a given survival landmark, and $\theta > 1$ indicates lengthening of time to failure), but in somewhat different ways. Use of the latter metric is less common but intuitively appealing and may be more appropriate for survival curves that maintain separation but do not adhere to proportional hazards.

While semi-parametric model forms for the accelerated failure time model have been proposed, these are not as reliable or easy to work with, and it is preferable to assume a suitable parametric model. However, the available options provide flexibility, and further developments in available software have provided ready access to highly flexible models for both accelerated failure time and proportional hazards

Table 2 Example of analysis using accelerated failure time (AFT) model and time ratio metric – tamoxifen and patient/disease features in breast cancer

Covariate	Beta	Time ratio	95% CI	Interpretation
Treatment	0.438	1.551	1.368–1.757	Patients receiving tamoxifen have time to survival curve quantiles (such as median) extended by about 56%
Menopausal status	−0.100	0.985	0.798–1.036	Postmenopausal patients reach survival quantiles about 1.5% earlier (nonsignificant)
Tumor size	−0.019	0.988	0.975–0.985	Time to survival quantile shortened by about 1% per mm tumor size

modeling in a parametric framework (Royston and Parmar 2002). The accelerated failure time model can be a good option when a constant shift in survival quantiles appears to be in effect (an assumption that can be checked graphically). When proportional hazards do not hold, either the Cox model extension for time-varying effects described earlier or the models discussed here can provide an appropriate alternative.

Table 2 shows an analysis of the data from Fig. 3a (and Table 1, first panel) using the accelerated failure time model. The model parameter for treatment suggests that tamoxifen treatment extends the time to a given survival landmark by about 55% relative to placebo. Increasing tumor size shortens time to failure landmarks by about 1% per millimeter. In this example, material conclusions are similar to that of the proportional hazards model.

Additional Modeling Considerations

Sample Size for Clinical Trials and Related Prognostic/Predictive Factor Studies

Survival models play an integral role in trial design, in that the exponential model described earlier often serves as the basis for sample size calculations in clinical trials with time to event endpoints. Specifically, either a difference in $S(t)$ between groups at some time t or a shift in median survival time (t where $S(t) = 0.5$) is posited, which implies a given hazard ratio (again time-invariant and thus implying proportional hazards is in effect), from which the sample size in terms of precision for detecting that effect is derived. In fact, the sample size formula for the typically used for the Cox model shares similarities with that of the standard logrank test (Schoenfeld 1983). The exponential model approach can provide at least the approximate sample size and study duration when further aspects of the clinical trial design such as staggered accrual rate and patient loss rate are incorporated (Rubinstein et al. 1981). This approach, which assumes proportional constant hazards, may require extension for time-varying hazard rates, which can be accomplished via software that permits these variations, often in a straightforward way by specifying time interval-specific hazard rates and ratios. The determination of sample size, discussed elsewhere in this work (▶ Chaps. 41, "Power and Sample Size" and ▶ 62, "Biomarker-Guided Trials"), additionally may need to incorporate noncompliance, treatment crossover, and other aspects of practical trial conduct.

Prognostic Modeling

Statistical models are often used to provide concise summary estimates of treatment effects in subclasses of patients, by estimating hazard ratios in independent strata of specific patient and disease features. These are typically presented in graphical form (estimates with confidence bounds) in a so-called forest plot. The primary goal of this analysis and display is to demonstrate consistency (or lack thereof) of treatment effect among patients with different features deemed important in clinical care. While this goal is laudable, it should be noted that natural variations in apparent benefit will invariably appear, and detection of true differential benefit is typically challenged by lack of adequate statistical power (Peterson and George 1993). Nonetheless, these analyses have become a staple of clinical trial presentations, particularly those of trials with potentially practice-changing results. Furthermore, with the advent of personalized or precision medicine, interest has heightened in the identification of factors imparting selective benefit, and thus such subgroup analyses are increasingly need to be a component of trial design (Polley et al. 2013). A more detailed discussion of other aspects of modeling and biomarker incorporation into clinical trials is discussed elsewhere (▶ Chaps. 62, "Biomarker-Guided Trials" and ▶ 90, "Prognostic Factor Analyses").

Competing Risks

For analysis of time to event data, a specific event type of interest is specified. However, before that event is observed, some precluding event may occur. Competing risks methods, which have a long history in demography, engineering, and medical studies, address this problem. Perhaps the most familiar example in the human health context is cause of death, where one may aim to estimate and make inference on time to death from disease-related cause, while deaths due to other causes will inevitably occur.

When competing events for a given primary failure cause endpoint are infrequent, treating those observations simply as censored may be reasonable and yield correct inferences, although even in this case, competing risks methods are useful. For example, one may wish to correctly estimate the cumulative probability over time for primary failure events and competing cause failures, which cannot be achieved without alternate estimators to the familiar Kaplan-Meier curve. In many settings, such as early-stage cancer, other-cause deaths are not at all infrequent, and thus methods addressing competing risks must be applied. Fortunately, there are straightforward and accessible methods that will enhance the interpretability of treatment effect evaluation in clinical trials.

Competing Risks Observations

Typical competing risks data is as follows: For $i = 1,2,\ldots,m$ individuals, there are K *mutually exclusive* event types with associated potential event times (Y_{i1}, Y_{i2}, … Y_{iK}), as well as an independent censoring time C_i, so that no failure is observed when all $Y_i > C_i$. We observe the minimum of these potential failure times $T_i = \min(Y_i, Y_{i2},\ldots,Y_{iK},C_i)$ and $\delta_i = k$ (with $\delta_i = 0$ for censored observations) indicating the type of failure that occurred.

Note that time to event endpoints may frequently have a competing risks representation, as oftentimes composites of multiple event types comprise a single endpoint in clinical trials. Examples include all-cause mortality and so-called disease-free survival in cancer (time to any of recurrence, second cancer, or death from other causes). Disease recurrence may be further broken down into anatomic site-specific types (local, regional, distant metastatic), for which there may be critical interest in evaluating the effect of treatment on each. These are not inherently mutually exclusive, but take on this property when defined as time to first failure site, as is frequently the case in clinical trials, because any first failure may prompt additional interventions.

The Nonidentifiability Problem

In competing risks observations, partial information on each failure time is available; for example, if the failure time for cause 1 (and thus time T) is 40 months, it is known that the failure time for others causes is at least 40 months, even though at most one complete failure time is observed. The crux of the competing risks problem is the determination of what can be learned about the failure process for all failure types from (T, δ). Quantities of interest include the multivariate survivor function,

$$S(y_1, y_2, \ldots, y_K) = \Pr(Y_1 > y_1, Y_2 > y_2, \ldots, Y_K > y_K),$$

historically referred to as the multiple-decrement survivor function, which refers to joint process by which individuals fail, including any dependence (e.g., correlation) among times for different failure types. The associated marginal survivor functions $S^j(y_j) = \Pr(Y_j > y_j)$ conceptually isolate the failure process to the failure type of interest. These distributions may be thought of as pertaining to hypothetical situations where other failure types are eliminated and can no longer preclude observation of the failure type of interest.

While demographers and others with long-standing interest in this problem have found workable solutions, developments in competing risks theory beginning in the 1950s have established what quantities can be uniquely estimated from competing risks observations. The overarching result is that the information contained in (T, δ) is more limited with respect to the multivariate failure process than may intuitively appear. Cox (1959) described problems in interpreting estimates from bivariate survival data specifically that the dependence structure between failure times Y_1

and Y_2 (and thus the joint and marginal distributions) cannot be uniquely determined from observation of the minimum failure time (e.g., competing risks data). The *nonidentifiability* theorem of Tsiatis (1975) and similar work by Gail (1975) established more formally that for competing risks observations, while one can formulate a bivariate competing risks model (i.e., with joint distribution fully specified) that would produce observations (T, δ), there always exists another model where failure times are independent that would produce the identical (T, δ) observations. Thus, uniquely estimable quantities are limited (Peterson 1976; Moeschberger and Klein 1995; Crowder 1991). In summary, competing risks data (T, δ) cannot uniquely identify quantities such as the marginal survival distributions, as the data will always be consistent with the independent risks model, which cannot be verified and is generally unrealistic in the biomedical context.

Estimable Quantities

Despite the above limitations, a significant portion of competing risks development has concerned itself with models for "latent" failure times (unobservable quantities representing time to failure that may have been realized had not a precluding failure event occurred) and means to undertake analysis under plausible albeit unverifiable assumptions. Alternatively, methods that deal strictly with estimable quantities offer a practical solution in many cases (Prentice et al. 1978). For purposes of clinical trial design and analysis, this chapter will concentrate on estimable quantities from competing risk data, which offer much in terms of providing an informative analysis of clinical trial results.

The survivor function (and associated hazard function) of the minimum failure time T (i.e., $S(t) = \Pr(T > t)$) can be estimated, as this is simply the survivor function for the composite endpoint of "time to any failure type," for example, all-cause mortality in the case where one is interested in death by cause. Furthermore, with K causes of failure, the overall hazard function (for any of the mutually exclusive failure types) can be decomposed into the cause-specific hazard functions, defined as

$$\lambda_k(t) = \lim_{\Delta t \to 0} \frac{\Pr(t < T_i < t + \Delta t, \delta = k | T_i > t)}{\Delta t}$$

These quantities heuristically represent the probability of failure from cause k in a small interval of time, given that one remains at risk (has not failed from any cause). For the K cause-specific hazards at time t, $\lambda(t) = \lambda_1(t) + \lambda_2(t) + \ldots + \lambda_K(t)$, equaling the hazard function for T. Cumulative cause-specific hazards $\Lambda_k(t)$ are similarly additive and relate to $S(t)$ via the identity

$$\exp\left(-(\Lambda_1(t) + \Lambda_2(t) + \ldots \Lambda_K(t))\right) = \exp\left(-\Lambda(t)\right) = S(t)$$

$S(t)$ is thus a product of the K components $S_k(t) = \exp(-\Lambda_k(t))$, which individually resemble but cannot in general be interpreted as survivor functions without the additional unverifiable assumption that the risks are independent.

Estimators

Nonparametric cause-specific hazards provide a useful visual summary of the relative intensity of different event types over time. For unique ordered failure times (due to any cause) $t_{(1)}, t_{(2)}, \ldots, t_{(J)}$, define $N_k(s)$ as the number of failures of type k at time s and $Y(s)$ as the number of patients remaining at risk as of that time. The nonparametric cumulative cause-specific cumulative hazard estimator is (Nelson 1972; Aalen 1978a)

$$\widehat{H}_k(t) = \sum_{j:t_{(j)}<t} \frac{N_k(t)}{Y(t)}$$

The increments in the estimator $H_k(t) - H_k(t-)$ can be taken as the hazard function estimate, although this quantity is highly variable, and a hazard estimate "binned" into time intervals or smoothed is more informative and interpretable.

A related simple tabular summary uses the incidence rate or average failure rate partitioned by cause, computed simply as events of type k/total person years,

$$\widehat{I}_k(t) = \frac{\sum N_k(t_{\max})}{\sum_i T_i}$$

These quantities, which are the maximum likelihood hazard rate estimates for the simple exponential hazards model described earlier, are also additive to the total failure hazard for the composite endpoint (i.e., time to first of any of a set of mutually exclusive first failure types). An example (Table 3) shows the endpoint disease-free survival (DFS) in early-stage breast cancer partitioned into event types comprising it, many of which are of interest with respect to the benefits and risk of tamoxifen. The summary conveniently shows how event type frequencies and relative failure rates differ between treatment groups, contributing to the overall DFS benefit for

Table 3 Summary of competing risks outcomes via average annual failure rates and rate ratios

	Placebo		Tamoxifen		
First event type	N events	Hazard[a]	N events	Hazard	Rate ratio
Tumor recurrence:					
Local	147	10.82	69	4.53	0.42
Regional	36	2.65	21	1.38	0.52
Distant	254	18.70	186	12.20	0.65
Contralateral breast tumor	105	7.73	81	5.31	0.69
Second primary cancers	92	6.77	140	8.91	1.31
Endometrial cancer					
Deaths prior to any of above	89	6.55	102	6.69	1.02
All first events	723	53.22	599	39.02	**0.73**

[a]Average annual rates per 1000

tamoxifen. This type of estimator can also be computed within disjoint time intervals (e.g., by year) as a means to better characterize changes in the failure rate over time.

In addition to the cause-specific hazards and average failure rate, a key quantity of interest is the cumulative probability over time of a given event type k occurring in the presence of competing events that may preclude it. Note that this quantity does not equal the marginal survival distribution for event type k as described above (except under unverifiable assumption). The quantity has been estimated as $1 - S_k(t)$, where $S_k(t)$ is estimated via, for example, the Kaplan-Meier estimator treating cause k failures as events and failure from other causes as censored observations. This quantity overestimates the quantity of interest, as it does not take into account competing events, for which one must remain free of in order to be at risk for failure due to cause k. Even if one can consider events other than k to act as independent censoring, one still obtains an overestimate and also a logical inconsistency in that

$$\sum_k (1 - S_k(t)) > 1 - S(t),$$

that is, the sum of probabilities of failing from each of the event types exceeds that of failing from any one of the event types, and the sum can even exceed 1.0 (an invalid value for $S(t)$ or its complement).

The correct estimator, known by numerous names and long appearing in survival analysis literature, is most commonly now referred to as the cumulative crude incidence or cumulative incidence function (Korn and Dorey 1992; Gaynor et al. 1993) and has the form

$$F_k(t) = \int_0^t S(u-)\lambda_k(u)du$$

The cumulative incidence function correctly equals the cumulative probably of event k in the presence of competing events, as heuristically it can be seen that in order to fail from cause k at time t, one must first remain event-free until that time point (represented by $S(u-)$) and then experience the relevant failure (via hazard for cause k). The set of $F_k(t)$ for the mutually exclusive and exhaustive failure types 1 ... K correctly sum at each time to the cumulative probability of failure from any cause (complement of all-cause failure function), or

$$\sum_k (1 - F_k(t)) = 1 - S(t)$$

Practically, the cumulative incidence function has a simple estimator that is a function of the constituent quantities: a Kaplan-Meier estimator of the "at-risk" probability $S(t-)$ and a hazard estimator for cause k at time t, such as the increment increase of the Nelson-Aalen estimator. The nonparametric estimator of the cumulative incidence function is thus

$$\widehat{F}_k(t) = \sum_{j:t_{(j)} \leq t} \widehat{S}(t_{(j-1)}) \frac{\Delta N(t_{(j)})}{Y(t_{(j)})}$$

Properties of this estimator, including variance expressions, are described in numerous sources (Aalen 1978b; Korn and Dorey 1992; Pepe and Mori 1993; Gaynor et al. 1993; Lin 1997).

Cumulative incidence functions provide a highly effective visual summary for contrasting groups with respect to cause-specific events comprising total failure risk, as the example in Fig. 3 illustrates. These plots identify which event types differ by group and also depict any shift in proportionate representation of different failure types in total failure risk over time, which could be due directly to treatment (say, if treatment were associated with specific adverse outcomes or strong efficacy against a specific failure type) or indirectly, as one event type may be necessarily increased in a given treatment group as other event types are decreased and all patient eventually fail. For example, if disease-specific mortality is decreased, other-cause mortality will eventually replace the events after long follow-up. In the example shown (Fig. 4), for early-stage breast cancer receiving tamoxifen, cumulative incidence of disease recurrence and opposite breast tumors were decreased (Fig. 4b), while incidence of other-cause deaths and second primary cancers other than endometrial cancer were not impacted (as seen in hazard rates in Table 3). With sufficiently lengthy follow-up, there may eventually be more of these events in the tamoxifen group (as those patients remain at risk for these events, having avoided breast cancer events). Endometrial cancer is an adverse effect of tamoxifen use, and as can be seen, cumulative incidence of this event is increased over time, reaching about 1.5% (Fig. 4b) versus 0.5% in the placebo group (Fig. 4a).

Nonparametric Tests in Competing Risks Data

From estimable quantities, inference via tests analogous to the usual single failure type case is available.

Logrank Test

The logrank statistic is the most commonly used method for comparing survival histories between two groups in the case where there is a single cause of failure ($K = 1$), with independent censoring. The test evaluates the hypothesis that the hazard of failure $\lambda(t)$ over t is identical in groups A and B, and expressed in the general form (Fleming and Harrington), sums

$$\int_0^t w(u)(\lambda_A(u) - \lambda_B(u))du$$

In the case where there are K types of failure and the groups are to be compared with respect to the hazard of failure due to a specific cause k, the same logrank test

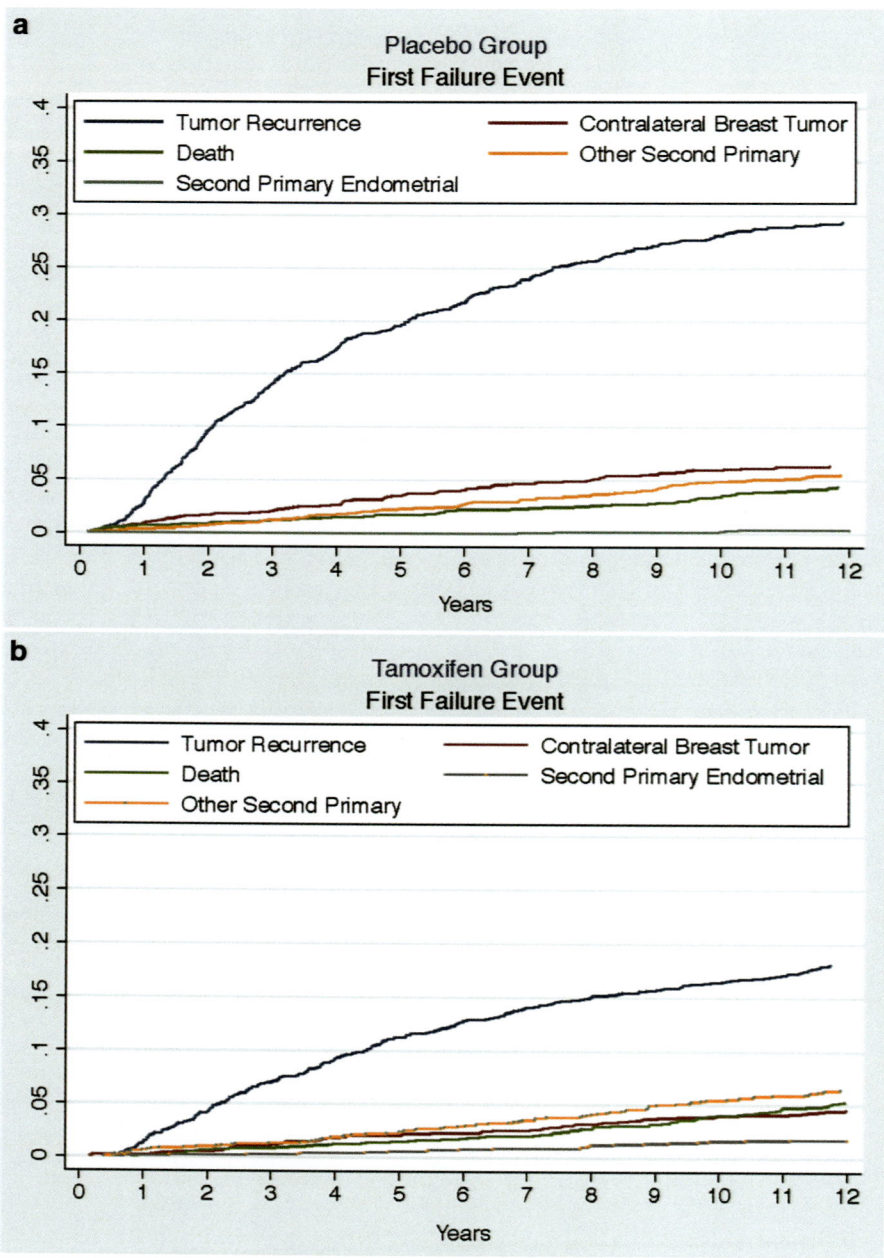

Fig. 4 Cumulative incidence of events comprising event-free survival in early-stage breast cancer undergoing surgery and randomized to (a) placebo or (b) tamoxifen

can be computed treating type-k failures as events and all other failures as censored (i.e., these subjects exit the at-risk group at the time of the competing event). When competing risks are present, the independent censoring assumption may not hold and is in any case cannot be tested (as indicated earlier, dependence between event types is non-identifiable). However, this procedure is a valid test for the equality of the cause-k-specific hazards between groups. It is recommended, however, that as in the case of the cause-specific incidence rates, testing for a difference in cause-specific hazard be carried out for competing cause failures in exhaustive fashion to fully characterize differences in failure history between groups.

Gray's Test

To compare cumulative incidence functions between groups, a number of tests have been developed, including weighted area between curves (Pepe and Mori 1993) and analogues to nonparametric tests for contrasting cumulative distribution functions (Lin 1997). However, the most common test is an analogue of the logrank test, adapted to the time to event distribution for a specific cause of failure in the presence of precluding failure causes (Gray 1988). The test has the same form as the logrank test, but contrasts the *subdistribution hazards* between groups. The subdistribution hazard is the "hazard function" uniquely defining a given cumulative incidence function, analogous to the relationship between the hazard and survivor functions more generally in survival analysis. Defined as

$$\lambda_k^*(t) = \frac{dF_k(t)}{1 - F_k(t)} \text{ for cumulative incidence function } Fk(t),$$

the subdistribution hazard can also be conceptualized as the hazard function for a random variable T^*, defined as follows:

$$T^* = \begin{cases} T \text{ (failure time)} & \text{if cause of failure} = k \\ \infty & \text{if cause of failure} \neq k \end{cases}$$

The test statistic is of the same form as the logrank test for contrasting hazard functions, with the relevant quantity being the sum over time. Gray's test is thus a logrank test for the subdistribution hazard.

The computational framework for the cause-specific logrank and Gray's tests resembles that of the single-cause logrank test, in that for unique failure times ordered from $t_1 \ldots t_M$, 2×2 tables cross-classifying treatment groups (A/B) with failed/did not fail are formed (Mantel 1966):

Outcome	Group A	Group B	
Failed	D_{1m}	D_{2m}	D_m
Did not fail	$Y_{1m} - D_{1m}$	$Y_{2m} - D_{2m}$	$Y_m - D_m$
At risk	Y_1	Y_2	Y_m

As individuals fail or are censored, they exit the risk set (Y_m). The quantity $D_{1m} - D_m Y_1/Y_m$ equals the "observed minus expected" failures in Group A under the null hypothesis of no difference between groups (for the unweighted form, $w(\ ) = 1$) and is summed over all tables indexed by unique failure times and divided by the relevant variance expression to form the test.

To understand how the logrank and Gray's tests differ, consider the case where there is no administrative censoring or loss to follow-up (i.e., all patients are observed to failure). For the logrank test, patients who fail from causes other than k simply exit the at-risk group when the failure occurs (and are absent from tables at t_{m+1} and beyond). The Gray's test computation is identical to that of the logrank test, but rather computed on T'. In that case, individuals who fail from a cause other than k "live forever" with respect to cause k and do not leave the risk in tables subsequent to t_m. Thus, the key distinction between the two tests for a given failure type is in how other-cause failures are handled, which influences the computational result. In simulated and actual data where there is *no difference* in failure hazard for a primary event k of interest while other-cause failure hazard differs between groups, different inferential results for the logrank and Gray's tests are readily demonstrated (Dignam and Kocherginsky 2008; Freidlin and Korn 2005). In general (except under cases of extreme correlation between event times in the true underlying bivariate distribution), the cause-specific logrank test reflects whether or not there is a difference in hazard between groups for a given failure cause k, whether or not the competing cause failure hazard differs between groups. The cumulative incidence test will reflect a difference in cumulative occurrence of event k failures, whether or not this is due to a difference in event k cause-specific hazards or competing causes of failure.

An example of the two tests is shown for competing causes of death in prostate cancer (Fig. 5). For men undergoing long-term androgen deprivation after radiotherapy, both the cause-specific hazard and cumulative incidence of prostate cancer death are reduced, and the result of the logrank and Gray's test is similar (left column plots). For the competing event of other-cause death, the logrank test indicates no difference, as the plot of the cumulative cause-specific hazard indicates. However, the cumulative incidence of other-cause deaths exceeds that of prostate cancer death, and Gray's test indicates a modest (statistically nonsignificant) difference between groups. In light of the lack of difference in cause-specific hazards for this event, one might interpret the excess of other-cause deaths as incidental to the reduction in prostate cancer deaths, rather than an excess in risk caused by long-term androgen deprivation (although this remains a topic of research for specific conditions such as heart disease and fractures).

While tests on subdistribution hazards and cause-specific hazards can result in different results, which are attributable to different aspects of the multiple event type failure process, both are informative, and one or the other may be preferred depending on the research question. For putative treatment or biomarker effects, it is desirable to isolate the effect to the cause of interest, and the logrank test is preferred and performs well except under the condition of strong dependence between event times (a condition that is not evaluable in competing risks data, but it may be reasonable to assume is not the case in many problems). On the other hand,

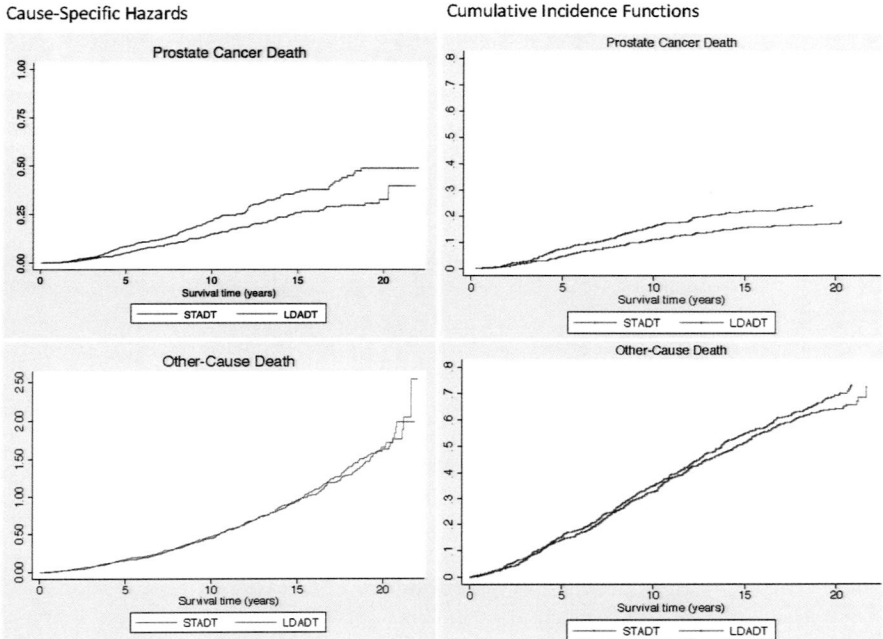

Fig. 5 Cumulative cause-specific hazard (left column) and cumulative incidence (right column) for prostate cancer deaths and other-cause deaths

a treatment may exert the same cause-specific hazard relative reduction, but if competing event hazards are large (e.g., in elderly vs. younger patients, other-cause mortality may be much greater), then the net benefit will be diminished. The subdistribution hazards test will better reflect the actual benefit realized in a given patient group.

Regression Models for Competing Risks

Competing risks methods naturally extend to modeling and, in fact, provide a means for extending time to event data to a more general representation as a multistate process, where individuals begin in an initial state upon study entry and treatment, and then may transition through one or more follow-up disease status states. These models can even incorporate reversible conditions, such as a transient affected and disease-free states (Andersen et al. 1993). The competing risks observations as described earlier are a special case of these general models, variations on which also pertain to clinical trials, providing a more informative analysis (Le-Rademacher et al. 2018).

Analogous to the case of summary estimators and tests between groups, modeling in competing risks can be approached from a focus on the cause-specific hazard or the cumulative incidence function. Prentice et al. (1978) provided a comprehensive overview of competing risks data and presented the Cox model for cause-specific failure, with estimation straightforwardly carried out by considering each of k causes separately

$$\lambda_{1k}(t) = \lambda_{0k}(t)e^{\beta_k Z}, k = 1, 2, \ldots K$$

Here, baseline hazard and covariate effects are specific for a given failure type being examined, reflecting treatment or other covariate effects on the cause-specific hazard in question. These can differ from the effect on other events or overall (composite of all competing event types). For example, in the analysis of disease-free survival in breast cancer shown in Table 1, increased age at diagnosis is associated with greater risk of failure (mostly due to increasing all-cause mortality with age), whereas in an analysis specifically for breast cancer recurrence, younger age is associated with significantly greater failure risk, a well-known phenomenon in that early-onset disease tends to be more aggressive.

Modeling in competing risks can also be undertaken via incorporation of covariates into the cumulative incidence function estimator. As it can be expressed as a function of all-cause-specific hazards in effect, one approach is to parameterize these (specifying parametric or semi-parametric cause-specific hazards models for the different failure types) and then construct an estimator (Benichou and Gail 1990; Cheng et al. 1998; Bryant and Dignam 2004). Alternatively and perhaps more straightforwardly, a model can be constructed directly on the cumulative incidence function or its transforms. Two main approaches have been suggested, one adapting the data to fit a generalized regression modeling framework (Klein and Andersen 2005) and the other proposing a proportional hazards form of model for the subdistribution hazard function (Fine and Gray 1999). The latter model has become the dominant approach in competing risks regression model applications. The model is of the form

$$\lambda_{1k}^*(t) = \lambda_{0k}^*(t)e^{\beta_k Z}, \quad k = 1, 2, \ldots K$$

As in the case of tests described earlier, different inferential results and estimates of the effects of treatment and covariates may be realized when alternatively using one of the two modeling metrics (Dignam et al. 2012). As an illustration, cause-specific endpoints in prostate cancer are modeled on the cause-specific hazard and cumulative incidence (subdistribution hazard) scale (Table 4). For prostate cancer deaths, treatment and other covariate effect estimates are similar in the two models. For other-cause deaths, there is a small nonsignificant excess risk for treatment for the subdistribution hazards model, likely as a consequence of decreased risk of prostate cancer deaths. It is also noted that variables associated with *increased* risk of prostate cancer death (high Gleason score, high PSA at diagnosis) are "protective" for other-cause death on the subdistribution hazards scale. Again, this is a consequence of these patients being more like to succumb to prostate cancer death, removing them from risk for other-cause death.

Considering how these models differ can help to guide choice of which to use depending on the questions of interest (Dignam et al. 2012). Cause-specific hazards

Table 4 Modeling cause-specific hazard and subdistribution hazard

	Prostate cancer deaths		Other-cause deaths	
	Cox hazard ratio	Fine-gray subdistribution hazard ratio	Cox hazard ratio	Fine-gray subdistribution hazard ratio
Long versus short ADT	0.70(0.55–0.88)	0.71(0.56–0.90)	0.96 (0.84–1.09)	1.06(0.94–1.21)
Age at diagnosis	0.97(0.96–0.99)	0.95(0.94–0.97)	1.07(1.06–1.09)	1.07(1.06–1.08)
High Gleason score	2.44(1.92–3.09)	2.26 (1.77–2.87)	1.06 (0.90–1.24)	0.76(0.64–0.90)
High baseline PSA	1.41(1.12–1.79)	1.43 (1.13–1.81)	0.95 (0.83–1.10)	0.89 (0.77–1.03)

models may better isolate the effects of treatment and other covariates on failure types of interest. On the other hand, modeling via cumulative incidence functions may be more appropriate when constructing nomogram to predict outcomes based on treatment and other covariates, as the model correctly downweights the realized benefit of treatment based on factors such as advanced age, which increases the probability of dying from causes other than that to which the treatment is directed.

Summary

The traditional Cox model approach and hazard ratio metric, a mainstay of clinical trial reporting, remains highly relevant, but extensions and alternatives should be considered when more informative or required due to failure to meet key assumptions on which the method is based. These methods have much to offer and are well facilitated by modern and readily available statistical software.

When competing risks are present, it is necessary to accurately characterize benefits and risks of treatment according to different failure types. Competing risks methods arise as a natural extension of survival analysis and have become a standard component of analysis software.

Key Facts

- Survival models are integral to the analysis of time to event data in clinical trials, as models provide succinct summaries of treatment effects and other information about patient histories. The proportional hazards construct remains a dominant and broadly useful approach in modeling.

- Extensions of the proportional hazards model offer opportunities to address problems such as heterogenous baseline failure risk, time-varying prognostic covariates, and time-varying effects of covariates. Alternative model constructs and summaries are increasingly available and should be considered.
- Competing risks observations, where one of multiple potential failure types occurs, are frequently encountered in clinical trials, and appropriate specialized survival analysis methods must be applied to correctly summarize and interpret outcomes.

Cross-References

▶ Biomarker-Guided Trials
▶ Essential Statistical Tests
▶ Power and Sample Size
▶ Prognostic Factor Analyses

References

Aalen O (1978a) Nonparametric estimation of partial transition probabilities in multiple decrement models. Ann Stat 6:534–545

Aalen O (1978b) Nonparametric inference for a family of counting processes. Ann Stat 6:701–726

Andersen PK, Borgan O, Gill R, Keiding N (1993) Statistical methods based on counting processes. Springer, Berlin

Benichou J, Gail MH (1990) Estimates of absolute cause-specific risk in cohort studies. Biometrics 46:813–826

Bryant J, Dignam JJ (2004) Semiparametric models for cumulative incidence functions. Biometrics 60:182–190

Buckner J, Shaw EG, Pugh S et al (2016) Radiation plus procarbazine, CCNU, and vincristine in low-grade glioma. N Engl J Med 374:1344–1355

Byar D, Huse R, Bailar JC et al (1974) An exponential model relating censored survival data and concomitant information for prostatic cancer patients. J Natl Cancer Inst 52:321–326

Chang IM, Gelman R, Pagano M (1982) Corrected group prognostic curves and summary statistics. J Chronic Dis 35:669–674

Cheng SC, Fine JP, Wei LJ (1998) Prediction of cumulative incidence function under the proportional hazards model. Biometrics 54:219–228

Cox DR (1959) The analysis of exponentially distributed life-times with two types of failure. J Roy Stat Soc B 21:411–421

Cox DR (1972) Regression models and life tables. J Roy Stat Soc B 34:187–220

Cox DR (1975) Partial likelihood. Biometrika 62:269–276

Crowder M (1991) On the identifiability crisis in competing risks analysis. Scand J Stat 18:223–233

Dignam JJ, Kocherginsky MN (2008) Choice and interpretation of statistical tests used when competing risks are present. J Clin Oncol 26:4027–4034

Dignam JJ, Zhang Q, Kocherginsky MN (2012) The use and interpretation of competing risks regression models. Clin Cancer Res 18:2301–2308

Feigl P, Zelen M (1965) Estimation of exponential survival probabilities with concomitant information. Biometrics 21:826–838

Fine JP, Gray RJ (1999) A proportional hazards model for the subdistribution of a competing risk. J Am Stat Assoc 94:496–509

Fisher B, Dignam J, Bryant J et al (1996) Five versus more than five years of tamoxifen therapy for breast cancer patients with negative lymph nodes and estrogen-receptor positive tumors. J Natl Cancer Inst 88:1529–1542

Fleming TR, Harrington DP (1991) Counting processes and survival analysis. Wiley, New York

Freidlin B, Korn EL (2005) Testing treatment effects in the presence of competing risks. Stat Med 24:1703–1712

Gail M (1975) A review and critique of some models used in competing risk analysis. Biometrics 31:209–222

Gaynor JJ, Feuer EJ, Tan CC, Wu DH, Little CR, Straus DJ, Clarkson BD, Brennan MF (1993) On the use of cause-specific failure and conditional failure probabilities: examples from clinical oncology data. J Am Stat Assoc 88:400–409

Gilbert PB, Wei LJ, Kosorok MR, Clemens JD (2002) Simultaneous inferences on the contrast of two hazard functions with censored observations. Biometrics 58:773–780

Gilbert M, Dignam JJ, Armstrong TS et al (2014) A randomized trial of bevacizumab for newly diagnosed glioblastoma. N Engl J Med 370:699–708

Grambsch P, Therneau T, Fleming TR (1995) Diagnostic plots to reveal functional form for covariates in multiplicative intensity models. Biometrics 51:1469–1482

Gray RJ (1988) A class of K-sample tests for comparing the cumulative incidence of a competing risk. Ann Stat 16:1141–1154

Gray RJ (1994) Spline-based tests in survival analysis. Biometrics 50:640–652

Karrison TG (1997) Use of Irwin's restricted mean as an index for comparing survival in different treatment groups – interpretation and power considerations. Contemp Clin Trials 18:151–167

Klein JP, Andersen PK (2005) Regression modeling of competing risks data based on pseudovalues of the cumulative incidence function. Biometrics 61:223–229

Korn EL, Dorey FJ (1992) Applications of crude incidence curves. Stat Med 11:813–829

Lawless JF (2002) Statistical models and methods for lifetime data, 2nd edn. Wiley, New York

Rubinstein LV, Gail MH, Santner TJ (1981) Planning the duration of a comparative clinical trial with loss to follow-up and a period of continued observation. J Chron Dis 34(9–10):469–479

Lawton C, Lin X, Hanks GE et al (2017) Duration of androgen deprivation in locally advanced prostate cancer: long-term update of NRG oncology RTOG 9202. Int J Radiat Oncol Biol Phys 98:296–303

Le-Rademacher JG, Peterson RA, Therneau TM, Sanford BL, Stone RM, Mandrekar SJ (2018) Application of multi-state models in cancer clinical trials. Clin Trials 15:489–498

Lin DY (1997) Nonparametric inference for cumulative incidence functions in competing risks studies. Stat Med 85:901–910

Makuch RW (1982) Adjusted survival curve estimation using covariates. J Chronic Dis 35:437–443

Mantel N (1966) Evaluation of survival data and two rank order statistics in its consideration. Cancer Chemother Rep 50:163–170

Moeschberger ML, Klein JP (1995) Statistical methods for dependent competing risks. Lifetime Data Anal 1:195–204

Nelson W (1972) Theory and application of hazard plotting for censored failure data. Technometrics 19:945–966

Pepe MS, Mori M (1993) Kaplan-Meier, marginal, or conditional probability curves in summarizing competing risks failure time data? Stat Med 12:737–751

Peterson AV (1976) Bounds for a joint distribution function with fixed subdistribution functions: applications to competing risks. Proc Natl Acad Sci 73:11–13

Peterson B, George SL (1993) Sample size requirements and length of study for testing interaction in a 2 x k factorial design when time-to-failure is the outcome [corrected]. Control Clin Trials 14:511–522. Erratum in: Control Clin Trials 1994 15:326

Polley MY, Freidlin B, Korn EL et al (2013) Statistical and practical considerations for clinical evaluation of predictive markers. J Natl Cancer Inst 105:1677–1683

Prentice RL, Kalbfleisch JD, Peterson AV, Flournoy N, Farewell VT, Breslow NE (1978) The analysis of failure times in the presence of competing risks. Biometrics 34:541–554

Royston P, Parmar MK (2002) Flexible parametric proportional-hazards and proportional-odds models for censored survival data, with application to prognostic modeling and estimation of treatment effects. Stat Med 21:2175–2197

Schoenfeld D (1983) Sample-size formula for the proportional hazards regression model. Biometrics 39:499–503

Therneau TM, Grambsch PM (2000) Modeling survival data: extending the Cox model. Springer, New York

Tsiatis AA (1975) A non-identifiability aspect of the problem of competing risks. Proc Natl Acad Sci 72:20–22

Tsiatis AA (1981) A large sample study of Cox's regression model. Ann Stat 9:93–108

Zhao L, Claggett B, Tian L et al (2016) On the restricted mean survival time curve in survival analysis. Biometrics 72:215–221

Prognostic Factor Analyses

90

Liang Li

Contents

Introduction	1772
Improvement in Statistical Efficiency	1773
Exploration of Treatment Effect Heterogeneity	1775
Statistical Models for Prognostic Factor Analysis	1777
Collapsibility	1777
Stratified Analysis	1779
Post-randomization Variables	1779
Selection of Prognostic Factors	1781
Pre-specification	1781
Variable Selection	1781
Imbalance in Baseline Prognostic Factors	1782
Stratified Randomization	1784
Adjustment for Covariate Imbalance	1784
Summary and Conclusion	1785
Key Facts	1785
References	1786

Abstract

Prognostic factor analysis refers to the adjustment of covariates when comparing treatments in a randomized clinical trial. This chapter covers various methodological issues related to prognostic factor analysis, including its importance to the randomization and primary analysis of the trial, statistical model building, selection of prognostic factors, and the study of interactions and subgroups, among

---

L. Li (✉)
Department of Biostatistics, The University of Texas MD Anderson Cancer Center, Houston, TX, USA
e-mail: LLi15@mdanderson.org

© Springer Nature Switzerland AG 2022
S. Piantadosi, C. L. Meinert (eds.), *Principles and Practice of Clinical Trials*,
https://doi.org/10.1007/978-3-319-52636-2_121

others. Methodological discussion is illustrated with data examples, and some commonly made mistakes in statistical practice are identified and discussed. This chapter is intended to provide readers with practical advice on how to use prognostic factors in the design, analysis, and reporting of randomized clinical trials.

Keywords

Analysis of covariance · ANCOVA · Baseline covariate · Covariate adjustment · Regression model · Stratified analysis · Stratified randomization · Subgroup analysis

Introduction

In the analysis of clinical trials with randomized treatments, *prognostic factors* refer to subject-level variables that are strongly associated with the outcome, and *prognostic factor analysis* refers to the adjustment of prognostic factors when studying the treatment effect on the outcome variable. Prognostic factors are usually baseline variables that are measured before randomization, such as age at randomization, tumor type, or disease stage in a study on cancer therapy after diagnosis. They also can include subject-specific characteristics that do not change throughout the study, such as gender, race, and the clinical center where the study participant receives the randomized treatment. When the outcome variable changes over time, its value at baseline also can be included as a prognostic factor when its value at a post-randomization time is the primary outcome of the study. For example, the primary outcome may be the quality of life score 6 months after the surgery, and the prognostic factor the quality of life score before the surgery.

When the outcome variable is continuous and modeled by a general linear model, and the prognostic factor is a continuous variable, this analysis also is called analysis of covariance or ANCOVA (Friedman et al. 2010; Walker 2002). When the outcome variable is continuous and the prognostic factor is a categorical variable, this analysis is called an *analysis of variance* or ANOVA (Walker 2002). When the prognostic factor is a categorical variable, this analysis can also be called a stratified analysis of an RCT, where each category of the prognostic factor is a stratum (Friedman et al. 2010; Kahan and Morris 2012b). Since all of the aforementioned analyses are regression models of treatment group indicator, with prognostic factors as additional covariates, such analyses also are called *covariate-adjusted analysis* or *adjusted analysis* in this chapter.

The discussion in this chapter focuses on randomized controlled trials (RCT) with two treatments, although the general principles apply to more than two treatments. Each of the following sections focuses on one specific methodological issue related to prognostic factor analysis, often illustrated with data examples. This chapter is intended both to stress the importance of prognostic factor analysis to clinical trials and to provide practical advice on its conduct. The most important take-home messages from this chapter are highlighted at the end in the "Summary and Conclusion" and "Key Facts" sections.

Improvement in Statistical Efficiency

In an RCT, the statistical power and sample size calculation are often performed in the context of a two-sample comparison on the outcome variable, such as t-test for continuous variables, chi-square test for dichotomous variables, or log-rank test for time-to-event variables. Accordingly, at the completion of the trial, the primary analysis often is based on a similar two-sample comparison, without adjusting for other covariates. This is called the *unadjusted analysis* throughout this chapter. However, numerous studies have shown that adjusting for prognostic factors as covariates can notably increase the efficiency and hence the statistical power of the analyses (Hernandez et al. 2004, 2006a, b; Kahan et al. 2014; Lingsma et al. 2010; Thompson et al. 2015). Increased statistical power can translate into reduced sample size and hence reduced costs of the trial. For example, Hernandez et al. reported that adjusting for strong prognostic factors of the outcome could lead to a 25% reduction in sample size requirements in traumatic brain injury trials (Hernandez et al. 2006). This is one of the reasons for recommending that prognostic factor analysis be given full consideration in the design and primary analysis of an RCT (European Medicines Agency 2013; Pocock et al. 2002; Robinson and Jewell 1991; Yu et al. 2010).

We illustrate this point using data from a small, simulated RCT, as shown in Fig. 1. In this trial, 15 participants are randomized to receive an experimental treatment, while another 15 are randomized to receive the placebo control. We assume that there is a continuous covariate that is strongly correlated with the outcome. Data for the outcome (Y), covariate (X), and the treatment indicator (Z) are generated from the following linear regression model:

$$Y = \beta_0 + \beta_1 Z + \beta_2 X + \epsilon, \tag{1}$$

where $\beta_0 = -1$, $\beta_1 = 2$, $\beta_2 = 0.5$, and $Z = 1$ or 0 indicate whether a subject receives the treatment or a placebo. The covariate X has a uniform distribution between -5 and 5, and ϵ is a random residual with a mean of 0 and a standard deviation of 0.5. Figure 1a plots the covariate against the outcome, where the "+" symbols represent subjects receiving the experimental treatment and the open circles represent subjects receiving the placebo. The solid and dashed straight lines represent the linear model that characterizes the relationship between the covariate and the outcome within the treatment and control groups, respectively. Since there is no interaction between the treatment and covariate, the two lines are parallel.

A covariate-adjusted comparison can be viewed conceptually as a two-sample comparison on the adjusted outcome, defined as $\tilde{Y} = Y - \beta_2 X$. In Fig. 1b, we plot the adjusted outcome against the covariate for the treatment and control groups. Since the systematic influence of the covariate on the outcome is removed, within

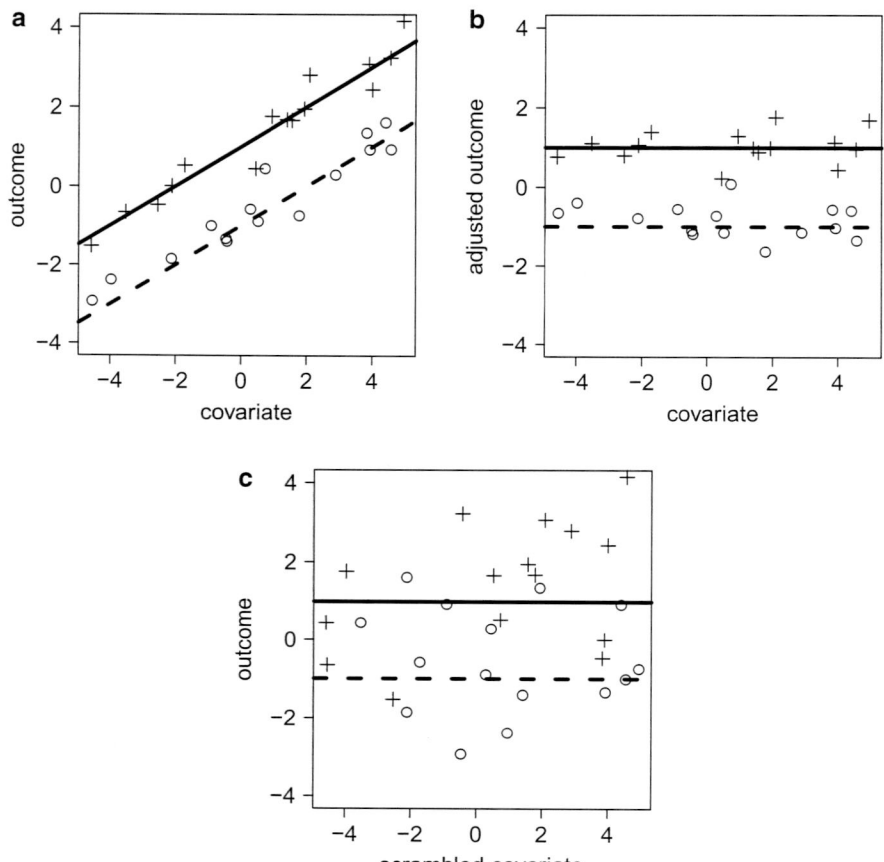

Fig. 1 Illustration of prognostic factor adjustment and statistical efficiency

each group the data points randomly scatter around a horizontal line that represents the group mean of the adjusted outcome.

In an unadjusted analysis, the covariate data are ignored. We illustrate this comparison in Fig. 1c, where the outcome variable is plotted against scrambled covariates for each of the two comparison groups. Since the covariate data are scrambled randomly, there is no systematic horizontal trend.

The group means of adjusted and unadjusted outcomes are the same in Fig. 1b, c, but the variability of the data around the group means is notably higher in the latter of the two. This suggests that an adjusted two-sample comparison is expected to have more statistical efficiency, which implies a more precise treatment effect estimator, higher power in statistical inference, and possibly a reduced sample size in similarly designed studies.

A more elaborate explanation of the above phenomenon is that the adjusted outcome $\tilde{Y} = Y - \beta_2 X = (\beta_0 + \beta_1 Z) + \epsilon$, according to the linear model (1), while the unadjusted outcome $Y = (\beta_0 + \beta_1 Z) + \beta_2 X + \epsilon$. The variability of the latter comes from both $\beta_2 X$ and ϵ, and hence is larger than the variability of the adjusted outcome, which includes only the variation in the residuals ϵ, because the effect of the covariate has been removed from the outcome. Note that in the actual data analysis, the adjusted treatment effect β_1 is estimated not via a two-sample comparison of the adjusted outcomes, but through a maximum likelihood or least squares algorithm, together with the rest of the model parameters in one step, but the conceptual explanation of the stated efficiency difference still applies.

The illustration above is made in the context of linear regression for continuous outcomes. The gain in statistical power mainly comes from a reduction in residual variation and hence an improvement in the precision of the estimated treatment effect. The point estimator itself, however, exhibits little change with the adjustment. Similar statistical power gain has been shown to hold more broadly in other regression models for RCT data, such as logistic regression for binary outcomes and time-to-event regression (Akazawa et al. 1997; Hauck et al. 1998; Hernandez et al. 2004; Lingsma et al. 2010; Robinson and Jewell 1991; Steyerberg et al. 2000). In the case of logistic regression, however, adjusting for prognostic covariates actually decreases the precision of the estimated log odds ratio of the treatment group, contrary to the linear model case above. But such an adjustment also increases the magnitude of the treatment effect. The overall consequence is that the statistical power still increases with the covariate adjustment (Robinson and Jewell 1991).A similar result holds for the Cox model for time-to-event data (Hauck et al. 1998; Kahan et al. 2014).

There are situations in which adjusting for prognostic factors might lead to a reduction in statistical power, though such situations are less common in practice (Kahan et al. 2014). For a fixed sample size, adding covariates to the model increases the "degrees of freedom" consumed by the model building, and hence increases the standard errors of the estimated model parameters, including parameters that quantify the treatment effect. This can lead to a loss in statistical power. In large trials with a small number of prognostic factors in the adjustment, the model degrees of freedom is relatively small compared with the sample size, and the benefit of adjusting for prognostic factors outweighs the consequence of increasing the degrees of freedom of the model. However, in small trials with a large number of prognostic factors, incorporating additional of these may not be desirable, from a statistical power perspective. See section "Pre-specification" for more discussion on this issue from a model specification perspective.

Exploration of Treatment Effect Heterogeneity

Another benefit of prognostic factor analysis is that it can be used to explore treatment effect heterogeneity (i.e., how the treatment effect varies with covariates or subgroups). This issue is of both scientific and clinical interest, but cannot be studied by averaging within each treatment group, as done in an unadjusted analysis. It can only be studied by prognostic factor analysis, where the outcome is regressed on treatment indicators and covariates, with or without their interactions.

Model (1) can be used to study the effect of a covariate, which is quantified by β_2, and this effect is assumed to be the same, regardless of which treatment the subject receives. Likewise, Model (1) also assumes that the treatment effect is the same for all subjects in the study, regardless of their covariate values. Alternatively, we can incorporate a cross-product interaction term $Z \times X$ into the model:

$$\begin{aligned} Y &= \beta_0 + \beta_1 Z + \beta_2 X + \beta_3 Z \times X + \epsilon \\ &= (\beta_0 + \beta_2 X) + (\beta_1 + \beta_3 X) \times Z + \epsilon \\ &= (\beta_0 + \beta_1 X) + (\beta_2 + \beta_3 Z) \times X + \epsilon. \end{aligned} \qquad (2)$$

In Model (2), the effect of Z is $\beta_1 + \beta_3 X$, which is allowed to vary with X in a subject-specific manner. Since the covariate may change the effect of the treatment when $\beta_3 \neq 0$, such a covariate is called a *treatment effect modifier*. Likewise, the effect of X on the outcome is $\beta_2 + \beta_3 Z$, which also is allowed to vary with Z when $\beta_3 \neq 0$, enabling us to study whether the treatment changes the magnitude of association between the covariate and outcome.

Model (2) is a regression model with both treatment group indicator and prognostic factors. It also can be used as a prediction tool. Given a new patient with prognostic factor X and receiving treatment Z, the model calculates an expected outcome. Prediction is very important to clinical practice. An extensive discussion of statistical prediction models can be found in Steyerberg (2009). However, one should be cautious that RCT data may not be the ideal data source for prediction model development and validation, because the study population may be different from the target population to which the prediction model will be applied. This is due to the restriction of the inclusion-exclusion criteria of the trial. As a result, model calibration (Steyerberg 2009) and generalizability assessment (Stuart et al. 2015) may need to be performed before the model can be used in practice.

Although the discussion above focuses on prognostic factor models with interactions, it should be emphasized that, from a study design perspective, the primary analysis of a confirmatory RCT ideally should use a model without covariate-by-treatment interaction. An RCT is designed to estimate the average treatment effect in a population. The averaging is better justified when the treatment effect is relatively homogeneous across various subgroups. If a strong treatment by covariate interaction is anticipated during the planning of a trial, then the design may need adjustment to accommodate separate estimation of the treatment effects within each covariate-defined subgroup or to focus on certain subgroups that benefit most from the treatment. If a strong treatment by covariate interaction is discovered in post hoc analysis, then the result should be viewed as exploratory analysis that suggests new directions for future research, and the overall treatment effect should be interpreted with caution (European Medicines Agency 2013).

Statistical Models for Prognostic Factor Analysis

A prognostic factor analysis is essentially a regression analysis of the outcome variable on the treatment group indicator and prognostic factors. Depending on the type of outcome, various regression models can be used, such as a linear model, generalized linear model, time-to-event model, and longitudinal data model, among others. A detailed description of these models is beyond the scope of this chapter. Interested readers may refer to standard reference books on regression analysis (Harrell 2015; Walker 2002) or other chapters of this book (e.g., chapters on logistic regression and survival regression). The following subsections are devoted to selected methodological issues that are particularly relevant to prognostic factor analysis.

Collapsibility

Models (1)and (2) are linear models for prognostic factor analysis with continuous outcomes. For binary outcomes, logistic regression is commonly used:

$$\text{logit}\{P(Y=1|Z,X)\} = \beta_0 + \beta_1 Z + \beta_2 X. \tag{3}$$

Here, the logit function is $\text{logit}(x) = \log(x/(1-x))$ for $x \in (0, 1)$. This model expresses the log odds ratio of having a positive outcome ($Y = 1$) as a linear combination of Z and X. The effect of the randomized treatment is quantified by β_1, the *conditional* log odds ratio of Z, which is interpreted as the difference in the log odds of having a positive outcome ($Y = 1$) between a treated subject ($Z = 1$) and a control subject ($Z = 0$), randomly selected from the subpopulation with covariate X.

In an unadjusted analysis, one fits the following logistic regression model without adjusting for the covariate X:

$$\text{logit}\{P(Y=1|Z)\} = \alpha_0 + \alpha_1 Z. \tag{4}$$

The effect of the randomized treatment is quantified by α_1, the marginal log odds ratio, which is interpreted as the difference in the log odds of having a positive outcome between a treated subject and a control subject, randomly selected from the population under study.

The modeling assumption of Model (4) is automatically satisfied. To see this, let pi denote the probability of having a positive outcome, if all the subjects receive the treatment, and p_0 the corresponding probability of the controls. Then it can be shown that Model (4) holds with $\alpha_0 = \text{logit}(p_0)$ and $\alpha_1 = \text{logit}(p_1) - \text{logit}(p_0)$. Suppose we further assume that the modeling assumption of Model (3) also holds. If one performs an unadjusted analysis to estimate α_1 and then performs an adjusted analysis to estimate β_1, then the two estimators are not expected to be similar, though they both measure the association between the treatment and the binary outcome. This is shown in the derivation below:

$$P(Y=1|Z) = E(Y|Z) = E\{E(Y|Z,X)|Z\} = \int \frac{\exp(\beta_0 + \beta_1 Z + \beta_2 X)}{1 + \exp(\beta_0 + \beta_1 Z + \beta_2 X)} f(X) dX.$$

The equality on the second line uses the fact that in a randomized trial, the conditional density of X given Z, $f(X|Z)$, is the same as the marginal density of X, $f(X)$, due to randomization. The above equation does not, in general, equal to:

$$\frac{\exp(\gamma + \beta_1 Z)}{1 + \exp(\gamma + \beta_1 Z)},$$

regardless of what constant is used for γ. This result implies that the regression coefficient in an adjusted analysis is not the same as the regression coefficient from an unadjusted analysis. In such a situation, the regression coefficient of the adjusted analysis is called *non-collapsible* (Guo and Geng 1995). In contrast to the logistic regression, the regression coefficients of a linear regression model are collapsible. To see this, we write the means of the adjusted and unadjusted linear model as:

$$E(Y|Z,X) = \beta_0 + \beta_1 Z + \beta_2 X$$
$$E(Y|Z) = \alpha_0 + \alpha_1 Z.$$

Since $E(Y|Z) = E\{E(Y|Z,X)|Z\} = \{\beta_0 + \beta_2 E(X|Z)\} + \beta_1 Z$, we have $\alpha_0 = \beta_0 + \beta_2 E(X|Z) = \beta_0 + \beta_2 E(X)$ and $\alpha_1 = \beta_1$. Therefore, the adjusted (β_1) and unadjusted (α_1) treatment effects are equal.

A key aspect that leads to the difference in collapsibility in these two models is that logistic regression is a generalized linear model with a nonlinear link function (i.e., the logit function), while the linear regression has an identity link function. Among the commonly used generalized linear models, the linear regression, with identity link function, and the Poisson regression, with log link function, are the only two that have collapsible regression coefficients (Gail et al. 1984). The implication of this result for a prognostic factor analysis is that the adjusted and unadjusted analyses are often expected to produce different point estimators of the treatment effect.

The unadjusted analysis and adjusted analysis have different interpretation. The choice should be made during the study design, as part of the pre-specified statistical analysis plan. The choice depends on the scientific rationale, as well as statistical consideration, as discussed in sections "Improvement in Statistical Efficiency" and "Exploration of Treatment Effect Heterogeneity." Although these two analyses do not always produce similar numerical results, the findings are expected to agree with each other qualitatively. If the adjusted and unadjusted analyses produce conflicting results, then the related data should be investigated, and proper interpretation of the trial results should be provided.

Stratified Analysis

When the outcome is time-to-event, it is common to use the log-rank test or a Cox model with hazard function $\lambda_0(t)$ exp.$(\alpha_1 Z)$ for the unadjusted analysis, where $\lambda_0(t)$ denotes the baseline hazard and α_1 is the log hazard ratio of the treatment. The Cox model can incorporate additional covariates for the adjusted analysis: $\lambda_0(t)$ exp.$(\beta_1 Z + \beta_2 X)$. Similar to the logistic regression, the regression coefficients of a Cox model are not collapsible (Austin et al. 2007). Therefore, it is possible to obtain notably different estimators of α_1 and β_1, even when both models fit the data properly.

Many RCTs are multicenter studies. It is common practice to treat the centers as a prognostic factor in the adjusted analysis. This can be accomplished by creating a number of dummy variables that represent each center, including them in the model either as fixed or random effects. In the context of a Cox model, one can fit a stratified Cox model with the hazard function: $\lambda_{0k}(t)$ exp.$(\beta_1 Z + \beta_2 X)$. This model allows each of the K centers to have its own baseline hazard function $\lambda_{0k}(t)$ ($k = 1$, 2,..., K). A distinct baseline hazard function per center is sometimes justified, because the patient populations are different across centers, as are their respective average survival probabilities. This stratified Cox model takes a more flexible form than the Cox model with centers entered as covariates, but it requires a larger sample size per center to reliably estimate all of the model parameters.

With binary outcomes, the stratified analysis can be performed with the Cochran-Mantel-Hanzel (CMH) test (Agresti 2002; Walker 2002), instead of logistic regression. The CMH test produces an average odds ratio as a measure of the association between the binary outcome and the dichotomous treatment groups.

Regardless of which approach is used, it is recommended that an overall treatment effect across all centers be reported in the primary analysis of the RCT data. An effective treatment should work well in all centers. The center-specific treatment effects should be explored by an interaction analysis or subgroup analysis, but they are of less scientific relevance, less likely to be generalizable, and estimated with less precision. In the situation that the treatment demonstrates strong between-center heterogeneity, then the result should be discussed, and a possible explanation should be provided.

Post-randomization Variables

The prognostic factors are usually baseline variables, measured before the assignment of the randomized treatments. For the purpose of studying the causal effect of the randomized treatments, any data collected after randomization (i.e., post-randomization variables) are considered outcome variables, because they may be affected by the treatments. In general, it is not appropriate to adjust for a post-randomization variable in the prognostic factor analysis. Since the effect of the treatment may have already been captured in the post-randomization variable, such adjustment produces biased result.

This phenomenon is illustrated below through a simple numerical experiment. We simulated 100 subjects, half receiving the treatment ($Z = 1$) and half receiving the control ($Z = 0$). For each control subject, we simulated the outcome (Y) and post-randomization variable (S) from a bivariate normal distribution with zero mean, unit variance, and a correlation of ρ. For each treated subject, a similar joint distribution of Y and S was used, but the means of Y and S were set at 0.5, implying that the treatment causes an increase in both the outcome and post-randomization variable, and the causal effect of the treatment on the outcome is 0.5. We compared two approaches: an unadjusted analysis, in which Y is regressed on Z in a linear regression, and an adjusted analysis, in which Y is regressed on both Z and S. In all scenarios, we found that the unadjusted analysis produced unbiased estimators for the treatment effect, but the estimated effects in the adjusted analysis are 0.50, 0.30, and 0.10, respectively, when ρ equals to 0, 0.4, and 0.8. This result shows that when the treatment has a causal effect on both the outcome and post-randomization variable, adjusting for the post-randomization variable introduces bias, due to the correlation between the two variables; the magnitude of the bias increases with the level of correlation. The intuition behind this result is that in the adjusted regression analysis $Y \sim S + Z$, the total treatment effect of Z on Y is captured in both the effect of Z on S and the incremental effect of Z conditional on S. Hence, the latter is biased for the total treatment effect of Z.

Many RCTs collect both longitudinal data (repeated measures) and time-to-event data as end points or for other purposes. One should be cautious to not include post-randomization variables in the analysis that studies the causal effect of the randomized treatments. For example, in the AASK trial (Agodoa et al. 2001), the investigators compared three medications (i.e., ramipril, amlodipine, and metoprolol) on hypertensive renal disease progression. The primary outcome was the rate of change in a renal function biomarker, called the glomerular filtration rate (GFR). This biomarker was measured repeatedly after randomization, specifically at clinical visits scheduled every 6 months. The subject-specific rate of change in GFR is modeled by a linear mixed model. The primary analysis of the AASK trial incorporated pre-specified covariates, including proteinuria, history of heart disease, mean arterial pressure, sex, age, and clinical center, all of which were baseline variables. The trial also has a secondary analysis with time-to-new onset of proteinuria as the outcome. A Cox model with treatment indicator and baseline covariates was used. No time-dependent covariates were involved in this analysis, though the Cox model can incorporate time-dependent covariates, and abundant longitudinal data were collected in this trial. Cox models with time-dependent covariates may be used in secondary analyses for studying the association between the time-dependent longitudinal variable and time-to-event (Elashoff et al. 2016).

Selection of Prognostic Factors

This section discusses which prognostic factors should be used in a prognostic factor modeling, with an emphasis on two methodological issues. The first is whether it is appropriate to propose a large number of candidate prognostic factors and use a data-adaptive model selection algorithm to determine the set of variables in the final model. The second is related to how to use prognostic factor models to reduce the effect of imbalance in baseline covariates. The latter issue is an important benefit of using prognostic factor analysis.

Pre-specification

In a confirmatory RCT, the primary analysis needs to be pre-specified prior to the study. That includes the pre-specification of prognostic factors in the adjusted analysis and the type of model used (Raab et al. 2000). The prognostic factors should be variables that are known to be strongly associated with the outcome, based on existing literature and preliminary data. The stronger the association, the more likely that adjusting for this prognostic factor will lead to efficiency gains (Hernandez et al. 2004, a, b) and the more important that exploring treatment effect heterogeneity could be.

It is desirable to adjust for a small number of strong prognostic factors (European Medicines Agency 2013). Including too many covariates in the model increases the possibility of model misspecification, which is undesirable for the primary analysis of an RCT. To aid the interpretation of results, the model should be kept in the simplest possible form, adding interactions or nonlinear terms of covariates only when justified by substantial statistical and clinical evidence. As discussed in section "Exploration of Treatment Effect Heterogeneity," ideally the treatment effect should be relatively homogeneous across subgroups. Results indicating strong subgroup heterogeneity should be investigated and interpreted with caution. For small trials in particular, incorporating an excessive number of prognostic factors in the model may cause the model to be unstable (Heinze and Schemper 2002) or reduce statistical power, due to large degrees of freedom consumed by the model estimation (section "Improvement in Statistical Efficiency").

Variable Selection

Data-driven algorithms are available to select important covariates into the final model among a large pool of candidate covariates. Examples include backward, forward, and stepwise model selection procedures (Harrell 2015). However, these algorithms are not needed, even if some pre-specified prognostic factors are not statistically significant, for the following reasons. First, a statistically nonsignificant result does not necessarily indicate that the prognostic factor has no effect on the outcome. It may suggest that the study does not have adequate statistical power to reach a statistically significant result for this particular covariate-outcome relationship. Note that the sample size of the trial is chosen to study the association between the treatment and the outcome, not the prognostic factor and the outcome. Second, the research focus is to estimate the treatment effect conditional on pre-specified prognostic factors. In models with non-collapsible regression coefficients, the conditional treatment effect is expected to vary with the set of covariates in the adjustment. The interpretation of the trial result would be difficult if that set was adaptive. Third, and most importantly, the usual statistical test of the treatment effect is designed to properly account for the sampling variability of data with a fixed set of covariates. It does not account for the extra variability introduced by the variable selection process. Therefore, if the model specification depends on the statistical significance of the prognostic factors, as many data-driven model selection algorithms do, the statistical test of the treatment effect is not expected to preserve its usual statistical properties, and the p-value may be incorrect (Kahan et al. 2014).

Pre-specification of prognostic factors requires some knowledge of the association between prognostic factors and the outcome, which comes either from the previous literature or preliminary data. In situations where such association is not well understood, a prognostic factor analysis can be specified as the secondary or exploratory analysis of the RCT. A large number of prognostic factors can be incorporated into the model for exploration purposes, and methods for variable selection (Harrell 2015) can be used in that context.

Imbalance in Baseline Prognostic Factors

Randomization is expected to ensure balance in all covariates, measured or unmeasured, between the two randomized groups. Here the "balance" specifically means that the sample distributions of the covariates are very close. In practice, we often examine balance in distribution through certain sample statistics, such as the sample mean for continuous variables and sample proportions for categorical variables. Due to sampling variability, these sample statistics are not expected to be the same, unless a special randomization procedure is used to ensure exact balance (Friedman et al. 2010). If the randomization has been done properly, as can be adjudicated by reviewing the randomization records, then any difference in the sample statistics reflects only a chance imbalance.

While simple descriptive statistics (e.g., sample mean and sample proportions) have intuitive meanings, the relative magnitude of the imbalance can be better assessed by rescaling. For example, suppose that two RCTs, one conducted among elementary school children and the other conducted among the general population, both have a difference of 1.5 years in the mean baseline ages of the randomized groups. This imbalance is perhaps more prominent and noteworthy in the trial on school children, because the age range is smaller. For this reason, standardized differences have been recommended in some literature as a measure of imbalance (Austin 2009). Let $\bar{x}_1$ and $\bar{x}_0$ denote the sample mean of a covariate in the treated and control groups, respectively. Let s_1^2 and s_0^2 denote the corresponding sample standard deviations. The standardized difference, expressed as a percentage, is defined as:

$$\frac{100 \times |\bar{x}_1 - \bar{x}_0|}{\sqrt{\frac{s_1^2 + s_0^2}{2}}}.$$

This is the absolute mean difference, expressed as a percentage of the average standard deviation. It places the difference in sample means against the backdrop of the data variation. Note that the standardized difference is fundamentally different from the Z-test statistic, because the latter has the standard error of the mean, instead of the standard deviation of the data, in the denominator (Walker 2002).

Since covariate imbalance arises by chance, it can go in either direction. If the covariate is correlated with the outcome, the difference in outcome between the treatment groups also fluctuates around its expectation in either direction. Therefore, chance imbalance does not cause bias in the RCT, in the sense that if we repeat the similar trial many times, the average estimated treatment effect will be unbiased. Since the statistical test or confidence interval already accounted for the sampling variability in the data, the statistical inference and p-values are correct. Hence, it is unbiased in the probability sense. However, if we examine the result of a single trial and find a sizable imbalance in an important prognostic factor, this may suggest that the point estimator of the treatment effect from that particular trial has large deviation from the true treatment effect. Therefore, it is desirable to reduce covariate imbalance. While this is best done through an appropriate randomization procedure, as described later, a prognostic factor analysis also can help with removing the effect of that imbalance through modeling.

What standardized difference would suggest considerable imbalance? There is no consensus criteria for this question. This is partially because the observed magnitude of imbalance is only part of the concern. Another important aspect is the strength of the association between the covariate and the outcome. For a very strong prognostic factor, a small imbalance may have a notable influence on the estimated treatment effect; for a weak prognostic factor, a larger imbalance may not matter. Therefore, to reduce the influence of covariate imbalance, it is important to identify strong prognostic factors at the study design stage, and use proper randomization procedures to ensure their balance by design. This issue will be discussed in more detail in section "Stratified Randomization." In situations where notable covariate imbalance is observed after the completion of the trial data collection, prognostic factor modeling can help mitigate the effect of the imbalance, but one should be careful about some pitfalls, as discussed in section "Adjustment for Covariate Imbalance."

Two-sample tests cannot be used to check for balance in baseline covariates between the two treatment groups (Senn 1994; de Boer et al. 2015). Such a test is illogical, because the null hypothesis is known to be true due to randomization (Begg 1990). Hence, any statistically significant result is known to be false positive. Following this argument, the usual "Table 1" of a publication of the randomized trial data, which presents descriptive statistics of covariates for each treatment group, should not include p-values from a two-sample test of each covariate (Austin, et al. 2010).

Stratified Randomization

Suppose one prognostic factor is known to have a strong influence on the outcome, based on previous research; we turn it into a categorical variable with K levels, if it is a continuous variable. Randomization can be done separately within each of the K strata, ensuring that approximately half of the subjects receive either treatment. This simple stratified randomization procedure can effectively eliminate chance imbalance of the prognostic factor, compared with simple randomization without stratification (Friedman et al. 2010). In multicenter trials, clinical centers are commonly used as strata. Other more sophisticated randomization methods are available for various contexts (Scott et al. 2002), though a detailed survey of these methods is beyond the scope of this chapter.

It is important to point out that, if a prognostic factor has been used in stratified randomization, the primary analysis of the trial must be a prognostic factor analysis with that variable in the adjustment (Kahan and Morris 2012a, b). Simple unadjusted analysis should not be used.

Adjustment for Covariate Imbalance

If the trial has already completed and some covariate imbalance is identified, is it necessary to adjust for these covariates in a prognostic factor analysis? Note that such observations are not pre-specified prognostic factors; rather, they are identified as post hoc.

First, if the imbalance is determined as chance occurrence (i.e., not by any systematic errors in the randomization, upon the examination of randomization records), then it remains valid to proceed with the pre-specified analysis, including unadjusted two-group comparison or adjusted analysis with pre-specified prognostic factors. The typical statistical procedures can all properly account for a random variation leading to such an observed imbalance. Hence, any chance variation in the covariate or outcome data is already properly incorporated in the estimation and inference procedures.

Second, adjusting for prognostic factors identified post hoc will actually inject an additional source of variation into the primary analysis of the trial, which standard statistical inference procedures are not designed to handle. That is the uncertainty in the model form, depending on which prognostic factors are identified post hoc. As a result, the statistical inference, such as the p-value, may not have the desired performance that it is designed to have. In the case of statistical models with non-collapsible coefficients, it also causes the estimated treatment effect to vary as a result of the list of covariates in the adjustment.

Third, the covariates that turn out to exhibit a larger chance imbalance are random, and they may not be the covariates that have strong associations with the outcome. Consequently, this approach may lead to unnecessary adjustment for covariates that are not important, which decreases the statistical power.

For these reasons, it is generally recommended that the prognostic factors be pre-specified in the primary analysis, based on their strength of association with the outcome, but not on a post hoc imbalance (European Medicines Agency 2013). The analysis that adjusts for post hoc imbalance should be used, at best, as a sensitivity analysis to explore whether or to what extent the imbalance might have affected the result.

Summary and Conclusion

In the design and analysis of randomized clinical trials, prognostic factors (i.e., subject-level variables that are strongly associated with the outcome variable) must be routinely considered in the development of randomization scheme and statistical analysis plan. The prognostic factor analysis is important, because it improves the statistical power in comparison with models that do not adjust for prognostic factors, offers insight into treatment effect heterogeneity and subgroup analysis, and corrects for chance imbalance among the treatment groups at baseline. The prognostic factors and their analysis plan must be pre-specified for the primary analysis at the study design stage. This chapter offers practical advice on how to conduct a prognostic factor analysis.

Key Facts

- In a randomized clinical trial, a prognostic factor usually refers to a subject-level variable that is strongly associated with the outcome. The prognostic factor analysis refers to the adjustment of prognostic factors in the primary analysis of the trial.
- Prognostic factors should be routinely considered in the protocol development and analysis of the randomized clinical trials. They can be used to increase the statistical power of studying the treatment effect and explore treatment effect heterogeneity.
- Prognostic factors and the related statistical analysis plan must be pre-specified prior to the launch of the study. Randomization with stratification on important prognostic factors can effectively reduce or eliminate chance imbalance. Prognostic factors involved in stratified randomization must be adjusted in the primary analysis.
- Covariates with chance imbalance at baseline should be investigated in a sensitivity analysis.
- Adjusting for post-randomization variables is discouraged.

References

Agodoa LY, Appel L, Bakris GL, Beck G, Bourgoignie J, Briggs JP, Charleston J, Cheek D, Cleveland W, Douglas JG, Douglas M, Dowie D, Faulkner M, Gabriel A, Gassman J, Greene T, Hall Y, Hebert L, Hiremath L, Jamerson K, Johnson CJ, Kopple J, Kusek J, Lash J, Lea J, Lewis JB, Lipkowitz M, Massry S, Middleton J, Miller ER 3rd, Norris K, O'Connor D, Ojo A, Phillips RA, Pogue V, Rahman M, Randall OS, Rostand S, Schulman G, Smith W, Thornley-Brown D, Tisher CC, Toto RD, Wright JT Jr, Xu S, African American Study of Kidney Disease and Hypertension (AASK) Study Group (2001) Effect of ramipril vs amlodipine on renal outcomes in hypertensive nephrosclerosis: a randomized controlled trial. J Am Med Assoc 285(21):2719–2728

Agresti A (2002) Categorical data analysis. Wiley, Hoboken

Akazawa K, Nakamura T, Palesch Y (1997) Power of log-rank test and Cox regression model in clinical trials with heterogeneous samples. Stat Med 16:583–597

Austin PC (2009) Balance diagnostics for comparing the distribution of baseline covariates between treatment groups in propensity-score matched samples. Stat Med 28(25):3083–3107

Austin PC, Grootendorst P, Normand SL, Anderson GM (2007) Conditioning on the propensity score can result in biased estimation of common measures of treatment effect: a Monte Carlo study. Stat Med 26(4):754–768

Austin PC, Manca A, Zwarenstein M, Juurlink DN, Stanbrook MB (2010) A substantial and confusing variation exists in handling of baseline covariates in randomized controlled trials: a review of trials published in leading medical journals. J Clin Epidemiol 63(2):142–153

Begg CB (1990) Significance tests of covariate imbalance in clinical trials. Control Clin Trials 11 (4):223–225

de Boer MR, Waterlander WE, Kuijper LD, Steenhuis IH, Twisk JW (2015) Testing for baseline differences in randomized controlled trials: an unhealthy research behavior that is hard to eradicate. Int J Behav Nutr Phys Act 12(4)

Elashoff R, Li G, Li N (2016) Joint modeling of longitudinal and time-to-event data. Chapman & Hall/CRC

European Medicines Agency Committee for Medicinal Products for Human Use (2013) Guideline on adjustment for baseline covariates in clinical trials. European Medicines Agency, EMA/CHMP/295050/2013

Friedman LM, Furberg CD, DeMets DL (2010) Fundamentals of clinical trials, 4th edn. Springer Science + Business Media, LLC, New York

Gail MH, Wieand S, Piantadosi S (1984) Biased estimates of treatment effect in randomized experiments with nonlinear regressions and omitted covariates. Biometrika 71:431–444

Guo J, Geng Z (1995) Collapsibility of logistic regression coefficients. J Royal Statistical Soc Ser B 57(1):263–267

Harrell FE Jr (2015) Regression modeling strategies: with applications to linear models, logistic and ordinal regression, and survival analysis, 2nd edn. Springer, New York

Hauck WW, Anderson S, Marcus SM (1998) Should we adjust for covariates in nonlinear regression analyses of randomized trials? Control Clin Trials 19:249–256

Heinze G, Schemper MA (2002) A solution to the problem of separation in logistic regression. Stat Med 21(16):2409–2419

Hernandez AV, Steyerberg EW, Habbema JD (2004) Covariate adjustment in randomized controlled trials with dichotomous outcomes increases statistical power and reduces sample size requirements. J Clin Epidemiol 57:454–460

Hernandez AV, Eijkemans MJ, Steyerberg EW (2006a) Randomized controlled trials with time-to-event outcomes: how much does prespecified covariate adjustment increase power? Ann Epidemiol 16(1):41–48

Hernandez AV, Steyerberg EW, Butcher I, Mushkudiani N, Taylor GS, Murray GD, Marmarou A, Choi SC, Lu J, Habbema JD, Maas AI (2006b) Adjustment for strong predictors of outcome in traumatic brain injury trials: 25% reduction in sample size requirements in the IMPACT study. J Neurotrauma 23(9):1295–1303

Kahan BC, Morris TP (2012a) Improper analysis of trials randomised using stratified blocks or minimisation. Stat Med 31(4):328–340

Kahan BC, Morris TP (2012b) Reporting and analysis of trials using stratified randomisation in leading medical journals: review and reanalysis. BMJ 345:e5840. https://doi.org/10.1136/bmj.e5840

Kahan BC, Jairath V, Dore CJ, Morris TP (2014) The risks and rewards of covariate adjustment in randomized trials: an assessment of 12 outcomes from 8 studies. Trials 15:139

Lingsma H, Roozenbeek B, Steyerberg E (2010) Covariate adjustment increases statistical power in randomized controlled trials. J Clin Epidemiol 63:1391–1393

Pocock SJ, Assmann SE, Enos LE, Kasten LE (2002) Subgroup analysis, covariate adjustment and baseline comparisons in clinical trial reporting: current practice and problems. Stat Med 21(19):2917–2930

Raab GM, Day S, Sales J (2000) How to select covariates to include in the analysis of a clinical trial? Control Clin Trials 21(4):330–342

Robinson LD, Jewell NP (1991) Some surprising results about covariate adjustment in logistic regression models. Int Stat Rev 59:227–240

Scott NW, McPherson GC, Ramsay CR, Campbell MK (2002) The method of minimization for allocation to clinical trials. A review. Control Clin Trials 23(6):662–674

Senn S (1994) Testing for baseline balance in clinical trials. Stat Med 13(17):1715–1726

Steyerberg EW (2009) Clinical prediction models: a practical approach to development, validation, and updating. Springer, New York

Steyerberg EW, Bossuyt PM, Lee KL (2000) Clinical trials in acute myocardial infarction: should we adjust for baseline characteristics? Am Heart J 139:745–751

Stuart EA, Bradshaw CP, Leaf PJ (2015) Assessing the generalizability of randomized trial results to target populations. Prev Sci 16(3):475–485

Thompson DD, Lingsma HF, Whiteley WN, Murray GD, Steyerberg EW (2015) Covariate adjustment had similar benefits in small and large randomized controlled trials. J Clin Epidemiol 68(9):1068–1075

Walker GA (2002) Common statistical methods for clinical research with SAS examples, 2nd edn. SAS Institute, Cary

Yu LM, Chan AW, Hopewell S, Deeks JJ, Altman DG (2010) Reporting on covariate adjustment in randomised controlled trials before and after revision of the 2001 CONSORT statement: a literature review. Trials 11(59)

Logistic Regression and Related Methods

91

Márcio A. Diniz and Tiago M. Magalhães

Contents

Introduction	1790
Binary Logistic Regression	1790
Estimation	1791
Bias Correction of the Maximum Likelihood Estimators	1792
Skewness of Maximum Likelihood Estimators	1792
Test Statistics	1793
Confidence Intervals	1794
Interpretation of the Model	1794
Multivariable Logistic Regression	1796
Sampling Design	1798
Assessing Model Fit	1798
Case Study	1804
Related Methods	1808
Conclusions	1809
Key Facts	1809
Cross-References	1809
References	1809

Abstract

Inference on binary outcomes is a common goal in clinical trials and case-control studies. Logistic regression is the usual approach to estimate treatment effect adjusted for categorical and continuous confounding variables. In this chapter,

M. A. Diniz (✉)
Biostatistics and Bioinfomatics Research Center, Samuel Oschin Cancer Center, Cedars Sinai Medical Center, Los Angeles, CA, USA
e-mail: Marcio.Diniz@cshs.org

T. M. Magalhães
Department of Statistics, Institute of Exact Sciences, Federal University of Juiz de Fora, Juiz de Fora, Minas Gerais, Brazil

© Springer Nature Switzerland AG 2022
S. Piantadosi, C. L. Meinert (eds.), *Principles and Practice of Clinical Trials*,
https://doi.org/10.1007/978-3-319-52636-2_122

model building, interpretation of parameters, diagnostics, and inference to small sample sizes are discussed. At last, a case study is presented applying the proposed analytic strategies.

Keywords

Binary response · Odds ratio · Case-control study · Cohort studies

Introduction

Categorical endpoints such as treatment response, disease stage, presence of disease, 30-day readmission, and death can be compared among groups using elementary tests for contingency tables. Nonetheless, tests for contingency tables have limitations when confounding variables are considered. For example, the comparison for presence of metastasis between control and treatment could be confounded by sex; therefore a solution would be to calculate a contingency table for each sex and test them separately. Unfortunately, this is a naive solution because multiple comparisons would inflate the type I error. If the investigators do not make any multiple comparison correction, they could state a false association between presence of metastasis and treatment for a given sex. If they do, they would decrease the power of the procedures, i.e., increasing the probability of missing a true association.

As alternative solution, one could use tests for stratified contingency tables, but they are also well-known for their lack of power in the presence of a qualitative interaction (Agresti 2003). Ultimately, tables of contingency would be unfeasible and populated by zeros when several confounding factors are considered such as sex, ethnicity, comorbidities, etc. Furthermore, the use of contingency tables with a continuous variable as age would require that arbitrary cutoffs be chosen by the investigators, which is not advised due to the loss of information.

The logistic regression is a regression model for binary categorical endpoints that allows the use of continuous variables without cutoffs and handles more than two confounding variables. The earliest applications of the logistic regression were introduced by Verhulst in population growth and later in bioassay by Wilson and Worcester (1943). It was strongly advocated as an alternative to the probit regression by Berkson (1944, 1951). Cox (1969) became one of the main responsibles for the broad use after exploiting several statistical applications, beyond bioassay: it can be linked with discriminant analysis, it leads to log-linear models, and it can be used in retrospective samples as in case-control studies. A more detailed history of the logistic regression can be found in Cramer (2002). Nowadays, it is often used as a predictive model in precise medicine.

Binary Logistic Regression

The randomness underlying binary endpoints is usually described by the Bernoulli distribution, with p defined as the probability of the event of interest. As an example of bioassay, a random variable indicating toxicity assumes only two categories (No/

Yes), and investigators are interested in the probability of toxicity as function of a drug dose, which is a continuous covariable.

Let Y be a binary random variable assuming 0 or 1, with $Y = 1$ indicating the occurrence of toxicity and $p = \mathbb{P}(Y = 1|X)$, where X is the dose received by a patient. Notice that X is assumed to be nonrandom, differently of Y. In a first attempt at modeling the binary response, an investigator might use the linear regression model with normal errors, $E(y|X = x) = p = \beta_0 + \beta_1 x$, where β_0 and β_1 are parameters in the real line. Nonetheless, there is not any constraint on the parameter space for (β_0, β_1) that restricts the estimation of p between 0 and 1.

A desirable solution is to model p using a function with the image set given by the interval (0, 1), which is an important property because p is a probability. A large number of functions satisfy this restriction: one of them is the logistic function, $p = \exp(\beta_0 + \beta_1 x)/[1 + \exp(\beta_0 + \beta_1 x)]$, which produces a sigmoid-shaped curve with values in (0, 1) for any value of x. It is helpful for some applications to rewrite the logistic model as a linear function in x,

$$\text{logit}(p) = \beta_0 + \beta_1 x, \tag{1}$$

where $\text{logit}(p) = \log\left(\frac{p}{1-p}\right)$ is the logarithm of the odds $\frac{p}{1-p}$ or log-odds.

The logistic model is a member of the model family known as generalized linear models (GLM), with the logit as the natural link function between $p = E(y|X = x)$ and the covariable x. There are several other link functions in the statistical literature such as probit, log-log complementary, and others in addition to the logistic regression in bioassay studies. They will not be discussed here, though. See more details in Sand et al. (2008).

Estimation

Let Y_i be the response of the *ith* subject, with Y_i independent and identically distributed random variables Bernoulli (p_i) for $i = 1,\ldots, n$. Then, a logistic model for a sample follows:

$$\log\left(\frac{p_i}{1-p_i}\right) = \beta_0 + \beta_1 x_i \Rightarrow p_i = \frac{\exp(\beta_0 + \beta_1 x_i)}{1 + \exp(\beta_0 + \beta_1 x_i)}. \tag{2}$$

The parameters (β_0, β_1) are unknown and will be estimated based on the available data. The most common estimation method is the maximum likelihood (ML). The likelihood of the observed response variables $y_1,\ldots, y_n$ given covariables $x_1,\ldots, x_n$ and the unknown parameters β_0 and β_1, assuming independence among n observations, is

$$L(\beta_0, \beta_1|\mathbf{y}, \mathbf{x}) = \prod_{i=1}^{n} L_i(\beta_0, \beta_1|y_i, x_i) = \prod_{i=1}^{n} p_i^{y_i}(1-p_i)^{1-y_i} \tag{3}$$

where p_i is given by (2), $\mathbf{y} = (y_1, \ldots, y_n)^\top$ is a vector with observed responses, and $\mathbf{x} = (x_1, \ldots, x_n)^\top$ is a vector with the covariables.

The parameters (β_0, β_1) are chosen to maximize the likelihood, which is mathematically equivalent to maximize the logarithm of the likelihood (log-likelihood) function

$$l(\boldsymbol{\beta}) = l(\boldsymbol{\beta}|\mathbf{y}, \mathbf{x}) = \sum_{i=1}^{n} \{y_i \log(p_i) + (1 - y_i) \log(1 - p_i)\}, \qquad (4)$$

with $\boldsymbol{\beta} = (\beta_0, \beta_1)^\top$, the parameter vector.

In order to maximize the log-likelihood, the score functions $\mathbf{U}(\boldsymbol{\beta}) = (U(\beta_0), U(\beta_1))$ which are the first derivatives of (4) with respect to β_0 and β_1 are calculated and set to zero. Unfortunately, the score function is nonlinear in $\boldsymbol{\beta}$ and requires a numerical method to obtain a solution for β_0 and β_1 such as Newton-Raphson. Furthermore, the Fisher information can also be calculated as a matrix of second derivatives of (4).

The maximum likelihood estimators (MLE) are denoted by $\widehat{\beta}_0$ and $\widehat{\beta}_1$. Under the usual regularity conditions for maximum likelihood (ML) estimation, it follows for large sample sizes that $\widehat{\boldsymbol{\beta}} \sim N(\boldsymbol{\beta}, \mathbf{K}^{-1})$, where $\widehat{\boldsymbol{\beta}} = \left(\widehat{\beta}_0, \widehat{\beta}_1\right)^\top$ and $\mathbf{K}^{-1}$ are the inverse of the Fisher information matrix.

Bias Correction of the Maximum Likelihood Estimators

Inferences based on maximum likelihood method depend strongly on asymptotic properties. Therefore, the estimators for regression coefficients could be biased resulting into not reliable confidence intervals and test of hypotheses when sample sizes are small or moderate. Fortunately, two approaches are available to correct the ML estimators: the corrective and the preventive.

In the corrective approach denoted by BCEc which was proposed by Cox and Snell (1968), the bias is corrected after the MLE calculation. As an alternative approach to BCEc, Firth (1993) proposed a preventive approach, denoted by BCEp, which is a modification in the score function $\mathbf{U}(\boldsymbol{\beta})$, such that the procedure already computes a less biased estimator than the regular maximum likelihood estimator.

Both methods are comparable, although Firth's approach is implemented in the main statistical softwares, and also can handle the phenomenon known as (complete or quasi) separation, i.e., when the frequency of the event of interest is too low (or high) for some covariable profiles resulting into estimated coefficients with high standard deviations. For more details of bias correction in logistic regression, see Anderson and Richardson (1979) and Schaefer (1983).

Skewness of Maximum Likelihood Estimators

Another important property of MLE is that $\widehat{\boldsymbol{\beta}}$ is approximately normally distributed. Again, this assumption can be questionable when the sample size is not large. The evaluation of the skewness coefficient is a simple way to verify whether this approximation is satisfied. The most well-known measure of skewness is Pearson's standardized third cumulant, $S(\widehat{\beta})$. A value of $S(\widehat{\beta})$ far from zero indicates departure from the normal distribution. In many models, there is not closed formula for $S(\widehat{\beta})$.

Bowman and Shenton (1998) proposed an approximation of the skewness coefficient for the logistic regression model. Additionally, Magalhães et al. (2019) proposed the following rule of thumb: when the absolute skewness value is greater than 0.3, the distribution is considered moderately asymmetric, and the normal approximation for the MLE should be adopted with caution. The use of the normal approximation for the MLE must be avoided when the absolute skewness value is greater than one.

Test Statistics

Investigators often are interested in testing whether a regression coefficient is different from zero. If so, they can state that the covariable is associated with the response variable because the regression coefficient in question has a non-zero effect on the response variable. A test of hypotheses and, consequently, a calculation of a p-value is performed based on a decision rule, which is defined based on a test statistic.

There are different approaches for the same test of hypotheses. The Wald statistic is the simplest statistic when the hypotheses are statements about a single regression coefficient; a particular case is the t-test. The likelihood ratio statistic is usually used when hypotheses involving several parameters are being tested, for example, an interaction effect. There are also the score statistic and more recently the gradient statistic as alternatives to the Wald statistic. An advantage of the gradient statistic over the Wald and the score statistics is that it does not involve knowledge of the information matrix, neither expected nor observed. Nonetheless their applications are not well spread due to software availability.

Under the null hypothesis $\mathcal{H}$ and when the sample size is large, the four statistics are chi-squared distributed with q degrees of freedom $\left(\chi_q^2\right)$ when the null hypothesis is true even though they have different mathematical expressions. If the null hypothesis is false, they may assume very different values. In this case, all the test statistics will be large, the p-values will be essentially zero, and they will all lead to reject $\mathcal{H}$.

Let S_* one of the four statistics, and s_* the value S_* after a sample is collected. A decision rule to reject the null hypothesis is $s_* > \chi_q^2(1-\alpha)$, where $\chi_q^2(1-\alpha)$ is the $1-\alpha$ quantile of the chi-squared distribution with q degrees of freedom and α is the significance level. Alternatively, $p\text{-value} = \mathbb{P}(S_* > s_* | \mathcal{H}) < \alpha$.

As discussed in the case of the MLE distribution, the approximation depends strongly on the sample size, i.e., the approximation of the true distributions of the statistics by their χ_q^2 asymptotic distribution may lead to considerable size distortions in the type I error probability of the tests in small- and moderate-sized samples. For instance, a test performed at 5% significance level in a small sample will have an actual percentage of incorrectly rejecting the null hypothesis greater than 5%. As alternative for small sample size, Bartlett or Bartlett-type corrections were suggested, making the chi-squared distribution approximation more reliable.

Confidence Intervals

The $100(1-\alpha)\%$ confidence interval for any regression coefficient β_i based on the Wald statistic is $\widehat{\beta}_i \mp t_{n-p,\alpha/2} \times \sqrt{\text{Var}(\widehat{\beta}_i)/n}$. The likelihood-based $100(1-\alpha)\%$ confidence interval can be written as $\left[l(\widehat{\beta}_i,\widehat{\boldsymbol{\beta}}_{-i}) - l(\beta_i^{(0)},\widetilde{\boldsymbol{\beta}}_{-i}) \leq \frac{1}{2}\chi_1^2(1-\alpha)\right]$, where $\beta_i^{(0)}$ is the value under the null hypothesis and $\widehat{\boldsymbol{\beta}}_{-i}$ is the restricted maximum likelihood estimation of $\boldsymbol{\beta}$ under $\mathcal{H}$. Both confidence intervals are invariant under transformation, but the latter does not require to estimate the variance of the estimator, and it does not necessarily produce symmetric intervals.

Interpretation of the Model

The next step after fitting a model and assessing the statistical significance of the estimated coefficients is to interpret such parameters. At a first glance, the interpretation of the regression coefficients in the logistic regression is not clear as it is in the linear regression with normal errors.

For example, let the response variable be the classification of patients into distressed ($Y = 0$) and non-distressed ($Y = 1$) using a quality of life score, then a logistic model can be applied. The link function between the probability of being non-distressed p and the strategy proposed by investigators to mitigate distress as an indicator covariable X is the logit. Therefore, β_1 represents the change on logit(p) because of the treatment as follows, logit($p_{X=1}$)– logit($p_{X=0}$) = $\beta_0 + \beta_1 \times 1 - \beta_0 - \beta_1 \times 0 = \beta_1$. For example, given $\beta_1 = 0.8$, the investigators will conclude that the treatment increases 0.8 of the log-odds of non-distress.

The interpretation of the parameters could be more clinically meaningful when the concept of odds is adopted. The odds of patient to be non-distressed when the patient received treatment ($X = 1$) and did not ($X = 0$) are given by

$$\text{odds}_{X=1} = \frac{p_{X=1}}{1 - p_{X=1}} = \exp(\beta_0 + \beta_1) \text{ and odds}_{X=0} = \frac{p_{X=0}}{1 - p_{X=0}} = \exp(\beta_0). \quad (5)$$

Then, the odds ratio between $X = 1$ and $X = 0$ is calculated as follows:

$$\text{OR}_{X=1/X=0} = \frac{\text{odds}_{X=1}}{\text{odds}_{X=0}} = \frac{\exp(\beta_0 + \beta_1)}{\exp(\beta_0)} = \exp(\beta_1). \quad (6)$$

Therefore, a non-distressed patient is $\exp(\beta_1) = 2.22$ as likely to be observed in patients who received the treatment than who did not. If X is a nominal polychotomous covariable such as ethnicity or marital status, then a series of mutually exclusive binary covariables are created with a common reference category, and the procedure described above is replicated for each new binary covariable. If X is continuous like age, an additional assumption about the functional form of X in the logistic model is required. The simplest choice is a linear function as it is assumed in model (1). In this way, the odds ratio between $X = x + 1$ and $X = x$ is given by

$$\begin{aligned} \mathrm{OR}_{X=(x+1)/X=x} &= \frac{\mathrm{odds}_{X=x+1}}{\mathrm{odds}_{X=x}} = \frac{\exp(\beta_0 + \beta_1(x+1))}{\exp(\beta_0 + \beta_1 x)} \\ &= \exp(\beta_1(x+1) - \beta_1 x) = \exp(\beta_1). \end{aligned} \quad (7)$$

Thus, the increase of 1 unit of x corresponds to the increase the odds by a factor of $\exp(\beta_1)$. The value of 1 unit of x might not be clinical meaningful, though. For example, a 1-year increase in age may be too small to be considered important. On the other hand, a change of 1 g/dL in albumin is too large because its normal range is between 3.5 and 5.5 g/dL. A change of 10 years in age and 0.01 in albumin may be more realistic, $\mathrm{OR}_{X=(x+10)/X=x} = \exp(10\beta_1) = \exp(\beta_1)^{10}$ and $\mathrm{OR}_{X=(x+0.01)/X=x} = \exp(0.01\beta_1) = \exp(\beta_1)^{0.01}$.

Confidence Intervals

Confidence intervals for odds ratios are calculated using the functional invariance property of the maximum likelihood estimators. For example, a 95% confidence interval for β_1 given by $[L_\beta, U_\beta]$ is transformed into a 95% confidence interval for $\exp(\beta_1)$ resulting into $[\exp(L_\beta), \exp(U_\beta)]$.

Nonlinear Forms

In case the linearity assumption for a continuous covariable is not reasonable, then nonlinear forms such as splines and fractional polynomials can be assumed as showed by Kahan et al. (2016). Categorizing a continuous covariable is a common solution, although it is not recommended as discussed by several authors like Becher (1992), Buettner et al. (1997), and Royston et al. (2006).

When more complex forms are assumed, the interpretation and inference for the regression coefficients become more sophisticated. For example, consider a logistic model with a quadratic functional form for X:

$$\mathrm{logit}(p_x) = \beta_0 + \beta_1 x + \beta_2 x^2, \quad (8)$$

The increase of 1 unit of X is quantified by β_1 and β_2, which is different from (7) as follows:

$$\begin{aligned} \mathrm{logit}(p_{X=x+1}) - \mathrm{logit}(p_{X=x}) &= \left[\beta_1(x+1) + \beta_2(x+1)^2\right] - \left[\beta_1 x + \beta_2 x^2\right] \\ &= \beta_1(x+1-x) + \beta_2\left[(x+1)^2 - x^2\right] \\ &= \beta_1 + \beta_2(2x+1). \end{aligned} \quad (9)$$

Then, the odds ratio between $X = x + 1$ and $X = 1$ is given by

$$\text{OR}_{X=(x+1)/X=x} = \exp\{\beta_1 + \beta_2(2x+1)\}. \tag{10}$$

Thus, either β_1 or β_2 do not have a clinical interpretation separately, and the OR also depends on the value of x. Moreover, confidence intervals for the odds ratio require the joint distribution of $(\beta_0, \beta_1, \beta_2)$ and a contrast matrix $\mathbf{C}$.

The matrix $\mathbf{C}$ has dimensions 1×3 because there are only one quantity of interest, $\text{OR}_{X=(x+1)/X=x}$, and the multivariate normal distribution has three components.

In this way, $\mathbf{C}$ should be defined such that

$$\beta_1 + \beta_2(2x+1) = \mathbf{C}\boldsymbol{\beta} = [c_0 \ c_1 \ c_2]\begin{bmatrix}\beta_0\\\beta_1\\\beta_2\end{bmatrix} = c_0\beta_0 + c_1\beta_1 + c_2\beta_2, \tag{11}$$

which results to $\mathbf{C} = (0, 1, 2x + 1)$. Therefore, $\mathbf{C}\hat{\boldsymbol{\beta}} \sim N(\mathbf{C}\boldsymbol{\beta}, \mathbf{C}\mathbf{K}^{-1}\mathbf{C}^T)$, where $\hat{\boldsymbol{\beta}} = (\hat{\beta}_0, \hat{\beta}_1, \hat{\beta}_2)^T$ and $\mathbf{K}^{-1}$ is the inverse of the Fisher information matrix.

The distribution of $\mathbf{C}\hat{\boldsymbol{\beta}}$ is univariate; therefore a confidence interval for $\mathbf{C}\boldsymbol{\beta}$ based on the Wald statistic can be calculated. Then, the same procedures used previously for β_i can be applied to obtain a confidence interval for $\text{OR}_{X=(x+1)/X=x}$ defined in (10) using the functional invariance property.

Multivariable Logistic Regression

Investigators often collect a large list of patients' characteristics in clinical trials and observational studies in order to demonstrate that treatment groups are balanced regarding to patients' covariables.

Therefore, covariables can be included into a univariable (or simple) logistic model (1) to adjust the treatment effect resulting into a multivariable (or multiple) logistic model as follows:

$$\log\left(\frac{p}{1-p}\right) = \beta_0 + \beta_1 x_1 + \ldots + \beta_p x_p \tag{12}$$

where $\beta_i \in \Re \ \forall \ i$. The interpretation of each regression coefficient is similar to the univariable regression, with the additional assumption that other covariable effects are additive and fixed:

$$\begin{aligned}\text{OR}_{X_i=(x_i+1)/X_i=x_i} &= \frac{\text{odds}_{X_i=x_i+1}}{\text{odds}_{X_i=x_i}}\\ &= \frac{\exp\{\beta_0 + \beta_1 + \cdots + \beta_i(x_i+1) + \cdots + \beta_p x_p\}}{\exp(\beta_0 + \beta_1 + \cdots + \beta_i x_i + \cdots + \beta_p x_p)} \\ &= \exp(\beta_i).\end{aligned} \tag{13}$$

Hence, $\exp(\beta_i)$ is interpreted as the odds ratio discussed for the univariable logistic regression at any other fixed values of the covariables $X_j = x_j$ for $j \neq i$.

While the need of a multivariable model in an observational study is often justified because of the lack of randomization, one could argue that the adjustment by covariables is dispensable in clinical trials because randomization leads to balanced groups. However, several authors support the adjustment for covariables even in clinical trials. Gail et al. (1984) showed that the treatment effect estimate is biased when covariables related to the response variable are omitted for logistic regression; Robinson and Jewell (1991) discussed that standard errors for regression coefficients increase after adjusting for covariables in the logistic regression, but it is always as or more efficient in testing the null hypothesis of no treatment effect. On the other hand, Gail et al. (1988) demonstrated that score tests from logistic regression maintain nominal size under omission of covariables; Hernández et al. (2004) and Jiang et al. (2017) presented simulations illustrating these theoretical results.

Another common interest of investigators is to find subgroups in which the treatment effect is heterogeneous, i.e., the treatment effect can be considered a function of the levels of some baseline covariable. In this scenario, the assumption of additive effects is no longer reasonable. For $p = 2$ in (12), an interaction term could be added into the model to describe such heterogeneity:

$$\log\left(\frac{p}{1-p}\right) = \beta_0 + \beta_1 x_1 + \beta_2 x_2 + \beta_3 x_1 x_2 \tag{14}$$

In this way, the main effects (β_1, β_2) cannot be interpreted separately as previously, but they should be interpreted jointly with the interaction effect, β_3. If both covariables X_1 and X_2 are continuous, then the odds ratio for $X_1 = x_1 + 1$ and $X_1 = x_1$ at $X_2 = x_2$ can be calculated:

$$\begin{aligned} \mathrm{OR}_{X_1=(x_1+1)/X_1=x_1} &= \frac{\mathrm{odds}_{X_1=x_1+1}}{\mathrm{odds}_{X_1=x_1}} \\ &= \frac{\exp\{\beta_0 + \beta_1(x_1+1) + \beta_2 x_2 + \beta_3(x_1+1)x_2\}}{\exp(\beta_0 + \beta_1 x_1 + \beta_2 x_2 + \beta_3 x_1 x_2)} \\ &= \exp(\beta_1 + \beta_3 x_2) \end{aligned} \tag{15}$$

Notice that $\mathrm{OR}_{X_1=(x_1+1)/X_1=x_1}$ is specific for a given value of X_2, contrasting to the odds ratio (13) that is constant for any fixed value of X_2 in the model (12). Similar rationale can be performed for $\mathrm{OR}_{X_2=(x_2+1)/X_2=x_2}$ at $X_1 = x_1$,

$$\mathrm{OR}_{X_2=(x_2+1)/X_2=x_2} = \exp(\beta_2 + \beta_3 x_1). \tag{16}$$

In addition, other functional forms can be used for either X_1 and X_2 besides the linear form, such that the additional terms will also be considered in the interaction. If X_1 is continuous and X_2 is binary, $\mathrm{OR}_{X_1=(x_1+1)/X_1=x_1}$ is given by (15) at $X_2 = 1, 0$, while $\mathrm{OR}_{X_2=1/X_2=0}$ at $X_1 = x_1$ follows from (16). For both X_1 and X_2 binary, $\mathrm{OR}_{X_1=1/X_1=0}$ at $X_2 = 0, 1$ is given by (15), and $\mathrm{OR}_{X_2=1/X_2=0}$ at $X_1 = 0, 1$ is given by (16).

The interaction plays an important role in an clinical trial because the analysis of subgroups is only appropriate if the interaction term is statistically significant. Brookes et al. (2004) demonstrated that often clinical trials are not powered to evaluate interactions; therefore they lack power to reject the null hypothesis that there is no heterogeneity on the treatment effect.

Pocock et al. (2002) and Wang et al. (2007) discussed that investigators commonly claim heterogeneity using separate tests of treatment effects within each of the levels of the baseline covariable or calculating treatment effect sizes within each subgroup. The first one inflates type I error and do not address the question whether the magnitude of the treatment effect depends on the levels of a baseline covariable, while the latter ignores the uncertainty around the estimates.

Rothwell (2005) recommended that subgroup analysis should be planned with few baseline covariables following a biological rationale. The p-value for the interaction term should be always adjusted when multiple subgroup analyses are performed, and post hoc interactions should be interpreted only as exploratory.

Sampling Design

The earliest applications of logistic regression were in cohort studies, in which the investigators would follow patients with a fixed vector of covariables $\mathbf{X}$ to observe a random response variable Y. Nonetheless, logistic regression is often applied in case-control studies, in which the investigators select patients based on their response variable Y; then a set of random covariables $\mathbf{X}$ is observed.

The widespread use of logistic regression is mostly due to the interest of investigators to estimate odds ratios for case-control studies. However, the definition of logistic regression requires that the response variable Y is random and the vector of covariables $\mathbf{X}$ is fixed, which matches a description of a cohort study. This apparent controversy was mathematically solved by Farewell (1979) and Prentice and Pyke (1979) showing that the likelihood of both models are proportional if the marginal distribution of $\mathbf{X}$ does not contain information about the coefficients β, which is a reasonable assumption.

Assessing Model Fit

Logistic regression does not have distribution assumptions unlike the linear regression with normal errors, except the independence of observations. On the other hand, two properties are expected from a fitted logistic model depending on the goal of the analysis: calibration and discrimination.

Calibration, also known as goodness-of-fit, is the ability to make unbiased estimates for the probability of the event of interest. Discrimination, also known as predictive performance, is the ability to separate different responses. These two properties are linked to the assumptions made in the model building process that need to be verified: linearity and additivity of the effects, in addition to the inclusion

Logistic Regression and Related Methods

of important covariables. This section will be focused only on calibration because the goal is not looking for prognostic factors.

An Illustration

Throughout this section, graphical methods will be illustrated using simulated data with sample size equal to 100 patients. A logistic model (1) with a linear functional form of X is fitted. The fitted model is considered corrected specified if the data is generated such that $Y_i \sim B(p_i)$, with p_i as function of a linear effect of X such as

$$\text{logit}(p_i) = -1 + 1.5x_i, \qquad (17)$$

where $X \sim U(-4, 4)$, for $i = 1, \ldots, 100$. On the other hand, if the data is generated with p_i as function of a quadratic effect of X such as

$$\text{logit}(p_i) = -1 + x + 0.5x_i^2, \qquad (18)$$

then the fitted model will be misspecified. Usually, goodness-of-fit is quantified as the difference between the observed $\mathbf{y}$ and fitted $\widehat{\mathbf{y}} = (\widehat{y}_1, \ldots, \widehat{y}_n)$ values, the so called residuals. One can say that a model is well fitted if a summary of the residuals is small, such that the contribution of each pair $(y_i, \widehat{y}_i)$ for $i = 1, \ldots, n$ does not show any nonrandom patterns. There are more than one definition of residuals for the logistic model.

Pearson and Deviance Residuals

The residuals are usually calculated to each pattern of covariables $\mathbf{X}_j$, instead of each observation $\mathbf{X}_i$, where m_j is the total number of subjects with $\mathbf{X} = \mathbf{x}_j$ for $j = 1, \ldots, J$. The most common are the Pearson and Deviance residuals such that their squared sum yields two summary statistics, χ^2 and D, respectively.

Evidence of lack of fit occurs when the values of these statistics are large. Under the null hypothesis that the fitted model with $p + 1$ parameters is correct, the asymptotic distribution of these statistics is supposed to be chi-squared with $J - (p + 1)$ degrees-of-freedom (d.f.), although the asymptotic null distribution does not hold when $J \approx n$, which is a common scenario when there is at least one continuous covariable. The calculated p-values following the chi-squared distribution will not be valid. Several alternative approaches overcame this limitation proposing to group the covariable patterns $\mathbf{X}_j$ such that $J < n$.

Hosmer-Lemeshow Test

Hosmer and Lemeshow (1980) proposed a test based on grouping the estimated probabilities. The estimated probabilities are grouping into percentiles, creating g groups such that usually $g = 10$. Then, a chi-squared statistic is calculated which follows an approximated chi-squared distribution with $g - 2$ d.f. under the null hypothesis that the fitted model is adequate.

Although the Hosmer-Lemeshow test is widely used, other authors like Tsiatis (1980), le Cessie and van Houwelingen (1991), and Royston (1992) described it as sensitive to the choice of grouping and lacking power to detect departures from the model in regions of the covariable patterns **X** that results into the same estimated probabilities.

Hosmer et al. (1997) compared the power of several goodness-of-fit tests to detect three different deviations from the correct model: (1) omission of a quadratic term of a continuous covariable; (2) omission of a binary covariable and its interaction with a continuous covariable; and (3) misspecified link function.

They showed that all tests discussed present power greater than 80% only when there is strong nonlinearity for sample size of 100 subjects and moderate nonlinearity for sample size of 500 subjects. Furthermore, all tests show low power to detect an omitted interaction between binary and continuous covariables, even with a large magnitude. Graphical methods can be applied as alternative.

LOWESS Scatterplot

In the linear regression with normal errors, a simple scatterplot between the response variable Y and a covariable X is helpful to show how Y depends on X. Unfortunately, the same cannot be said about the logistic regression. Figure 1 shows a scatterplot between Y and X for data generated from (17), which does not bring any information about their relationship, due to the binary nature of Y.

A simple alternative is creating intervals on X using its quantiles and calculate the average of Y for each of these intervals. Figure 2 shows the relationship when plotting $\overline{Y}$ and $\text{logit}(\overline{Y})$ against the midpoint of the intervals for X, with ten observations for each interval. The expected shapes are a sigmoid and a linear relationship, respectively.

The expected relationships are not observed clearly because the sample size is small (n = 10) for each interval. Copas (1983) suggested to smooth the values Y using nonparametric methods avoiding to create intervals. A very simple smoother

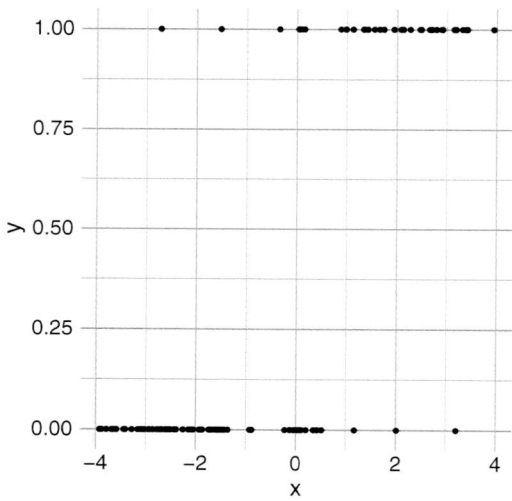

Fig. 1 Scatterplot of (X, Y) values

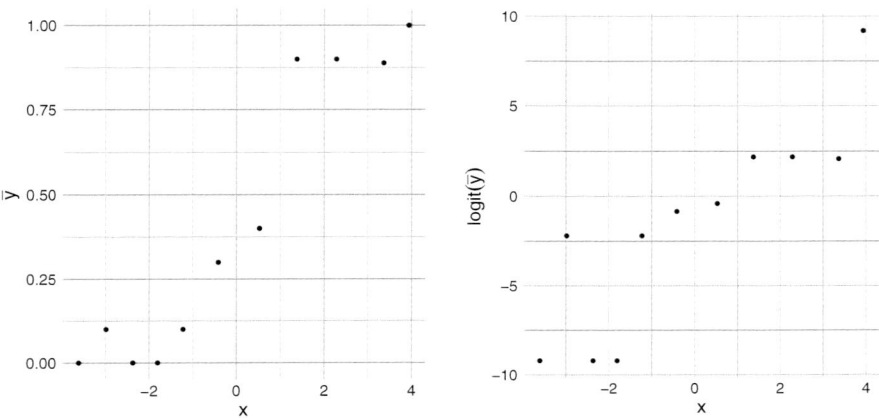

Fig. 2 Y (left panel) and $\text{logit}(\overline{Y})$ (right panel) versus midpoints of quantile intervals of X

can be defined calculating a weighted average of Y values within bins created around $X = x$, with weights decreasing for X values further away from $X = x$. The weighted average values of Y at each value of X generate a smoothed line. The amount of smoothing is controlled by the bin width and weights.

A more sophisticated smoother was proposed by Cleveland (1979), the locally weighted scatterplot smoothing (LOWESS) fits a linear regression to the data within a bin created around $X = x$. The underlying assumption is that the relationship between Y and X is locally linear, but without assuming that it is globally linear. The linear regression is fitted using weighted least squares, giving less weight to observations with X values further away from $X = x$.

Figure 3 shows the relationships when plotting the predicted values $\tilde{Y}$ and $\text{logit}(\tilde{Y})$ against X using LOWESS. It resembles more the expected patterns than Fig. 2. For data generated from (18), the relationships when plotting $\tilde{Y}$ and $\text{logit}(\tilde{Y})$ against X using LOWESS are displayed in Fig. 4, which resembles a nonlinear pattern.

The smoothed scatterplot should be interpreted carefully. With small data sets, there will not be enough information to estimate the relationship between Y and X, while with large data sets, the suggested functional form in the scatterplot could be not clear because of the small number of observations in certain parts of the support of X. Consequently, it is important to analyze the plots taking into account the distribution of X.

Similar approach can be applied to assess the presence of interaction between continuous and binary covariables. Specific smoothed curves of $\tilde{Y}$ and $\text{logit}(\tilde{Y})$ against X can be plotted for each category of the binary variable. If there is no interaction between them, it is expected to observe parallel curves. Furthermore, nonlinear forms and multiplicative effects can be evaluated in a more objective procedure when are incorporated into the model and tested using likelihood ratio tests.

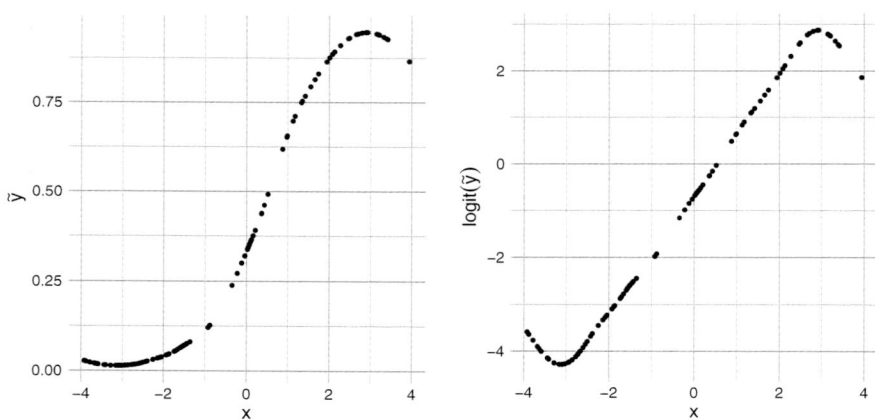

Fig. 3 $\tilde{Y}$ (left panel) and $\text{logit}(\tilde{Y})$ (right panel) versus X using LOWESS showing a linear effect of X on Y

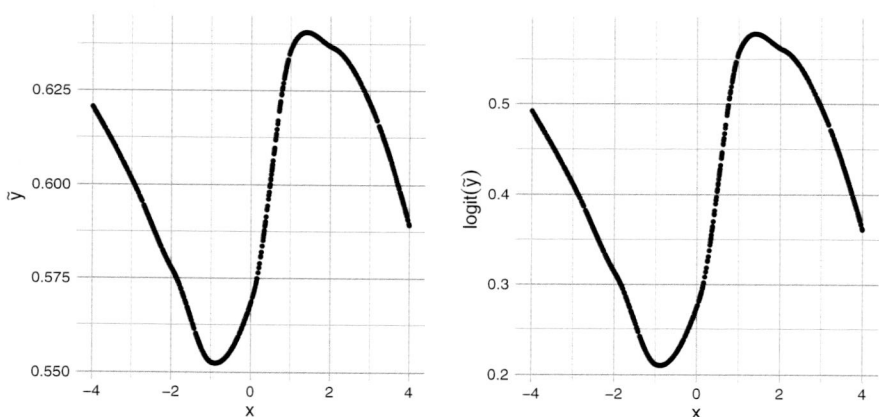

Fig. 4 $\tilde{Y}$ (left panel) and $\text{logit}(\tilde{Y})$ (right panel) versus X using LOWESS showing a quadratic effect of X on Y

Diagnostics

Summary statistics and LOWESS scatterplots can be helpful to identify lack of goodness-of-fit, but they do not allow to identify which covariable patterns might not be adequately modeled. Pregibon et al. (1981) extended the regression diagnostic framework of linear regression to logistic regression, discussing the change on the estimated coefficients β, the Pearson chi-squared (χ^2) and deviance statistics (**D**), when one particular covariable pattern is deleted from the data set. Hosmer and Lemeshow (2000) recommended to plot $\Delta\widehat{\beta}_j, \Delta\chi^2_j, \Delta D_j$ versus the estimated responses $\widehat{y}_j$ for $j = 1,\ldots, J$. In addition, they also suggested to plot $\Delta\chi^2$ versus the estimated responses with $\Delta\beta$ as the point size.

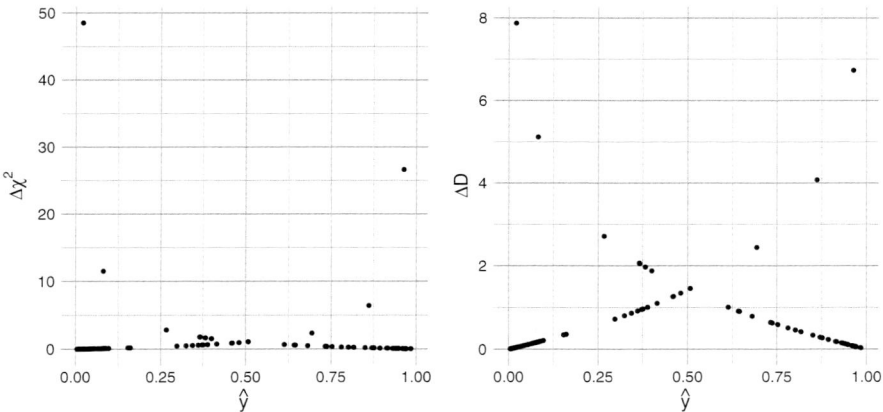

Fig. 5 $\Delta\chi^2$ (left panel) and ΔD (right panel) versus the estimated response $\hat{y}$

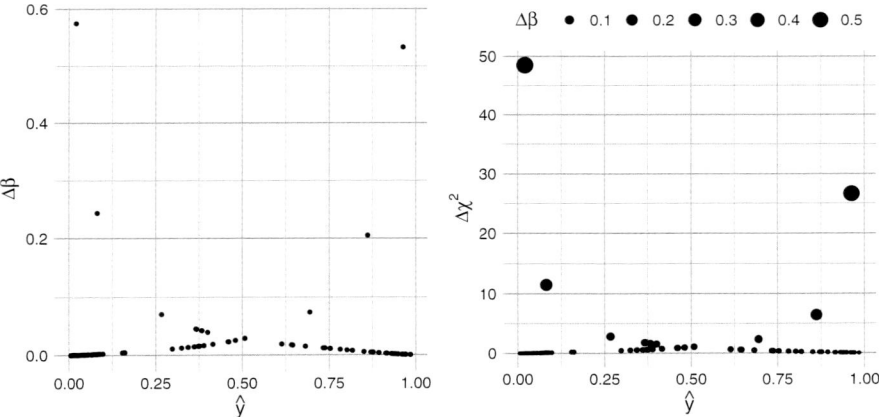

Fig. 6 $\Delta\beta$ (left panel) and $\Delta\chi^2$ (right panel) versus the estimated response $\hat{y}$, with point size proportional to $\Delta\beta$ (right panel)

Figure 5 shows $\Delta\chi^2$ and ΔD versus the estimated probabilities for data generated from (17). There are two curves with quadratic pattern: the points on the curve from the top left to bottom right correspond to the covariable patterns with $y_j = m_j$; the points on the curve from the bottom left to top right correspond to the covariable pattern with $y_j = 0$. Moreover, Fig. 6 shows $\Delta\beta$ versus the estimated probabilities, and $\Delta\chi^2$ versus the estimated probabilities with the point size proportional to $\Delta\beta$.

There is no clear threshold as in linear regression for $\Delta\chi^2$ and ΔD to identify them as a poorly fitted covariable pattern. Large values of $\Delta\chi^2$ and ΔD for a given pattern j in comparison to the other patterns are indicative that the covariable pattern j is poorly fitted by the regression model, while large values of $\Delta\beta$ are indicative that these covariable patterns are influential to the estimated parameters $\hat{\beta}$.

Diagnostic plots should also be interpreted carefully similar to LOWESS scatterplots. Notice that Fig. 5 shows large values of $\Delta\chi^2$ for a covariable pattern, even though the fitted model is correctly specified. Covariable patterns should not be removed from the data set only because diagnostic measures indicating the fitted model do not accommodate well some covariable patterns. Investigators need to be aware that such covariable patterns are not well described by the fitted model, and sensitivity analysis should be performed.

Case Study

Nastri et al. (2016) applied logistic regression to study the association between some single-nucleotide polymorphisms (SNPs) in the genes IFNL3 and IFNL4 and the response of hepatitis C patients to the standard treatment, consisted of pegylated interferon and ribavirin (PEG-IFN + RBV). The patients were divided into three groups based on their clinical outcome: spontaneous clearance (SC), sustained virological response (SVR), and non-responder (NR). In particular, investigators were interested in differences between SC and chronic hepatitis C (CHC = SVR + NR) patients. Three SNPs rs8099917 (TT, GT, GG), rs12979860 (CC, CT, TT), and rs368234815 (TT/TT, TT/ΔG, ΔG/AG) were examined. For the sake of brevity, only rs12979860 is discussed here. There was no missing data.

The initial step is to summarize the distribution of the risk factor (SNP) by treatment response using a contingency table as showed in Table 1. A two-sided chi-square test is applied because the expected frequencies are greater than 5, resulting into a p-value of 4.47e-05. Therefore, there is enough evidence to reject the null hypothesis of no association between rs12979860 and treatment response. The odds ratios of CHC are $OR_{CC:CT} = 5.11$, $OR_{CC:TT} = 4.55$, i.e., patients with the polymorphism CT and TT are 5.11 and 4.55 more likely to be CHC patients than patients with the polymorphism CC, respectively.

Investigators also collected age and sex of the patients because these covariables could be considered confounding factors in the association between SNPs and treatment response. Consequently, a logistic regression model is desirable to incorporate these covariables in the analysis. Let $Y \sim$ Bernoulli (p), where p is the probability of a patient be a CHC patient. First, a univariable logistic regression is proposed containing only the SNP rs12979860, with two dummy covariables with the polymorphism CC as reference:

Table 1 :rs12979860 distribution by treatment response

rs12979860	Response		
	CHC	SC	Total
CC	25	33	58
CT	55	14	69
TT	14	4	18
Total	94	51	145

$$\text{logit}(p) = \beta_0 + \beta_1 \text{rs12979860} : \text{CT} + \beta_2 \text{rs12979860} : \text{TT}. \quad (19)$$

The fitted model is presented in Table 2. The z value is the Wald statistic, such that under the null hypothesis that the regression coefficient is equal zero follows a t-student distribution with 142 d.f. In particular, the Wald test for the covariable rs12979860 is not appropriate to test the association between the SNP and treatment response because rs12979860 is represented by two dummy covariables. The Wald test allows the investigators to compare specific (TT, CT) polymorphisms versus the polymorphism reference (CC).

The likelihood ratio test is applied to test the null hypothesis that both regression coefficients (β_1, β_2) are zero. The *LR* statistic is calculated between the null model containing only the intercept (β_0) and the fitted model (19), which follows a chi-squared distribution with 2 d.f. under the null hypothesis. In this way, $LR = -20.093$ with p-value of 4.33331e-05 indicating association between rs12979860 and treatment as already observed in the contingency table. Odds ratios can also be calculated based on (β_1, β_2), and they are as showed in Table 3.

Hence, patients with genotype CT for SNP rs12979860 are 5.19 more likely to be HCC than patients with polymorphism CC. Similar conclusions can be done for polymorphism TT. These values are fairly close to the ones obtained using a contingency table. In order to adjust by age, which is a continuous covariable, the LOWESS scatterplot displayed in Fig. 7 is useful to study the linear effect of age on treatment response. The LOWESS scatterplot does not show a linear form for age, which led the investigators to use restricted cubic splines with *m* knots,

$$\text{RCS}(\text{age}) = \beta_1 \text{age}$$
$$+ \sum_{j=i}^{m-1} \beta_j \left[(\text{age} - k_j)_+^3 - \lambda_j (\text{age} - k_{\min})_+^3 - (1 - \lambda_j)(\text{age} - k_{\max})_+^3 \right],$$

where

Table 2 Fitted univariable logistic regression for treatment response as function of recessive model of rs12979860

Parameter	Estimate	Standard error	z value	p-value
β_0	−0.2776	0.2651	−1.047	0.2951
β_1	1.6459	0.3999	4.116	3.86e-05
β_2	1.5304	0.6259	2.445	0.0145

Table 3 Odds ratio for fitted univariable logistic regression model (19)

Comparison	OR	95% CI Wald	LR
CC:CT	5.19	[2.37; 11.36]	[2.41; 11.65]
CC:TT	4.62	[1.35; 15.76]	[1.46; 17.87]

Fig. 7 LOWESS scatterplot between smoothed observed probability of response to treatment and age

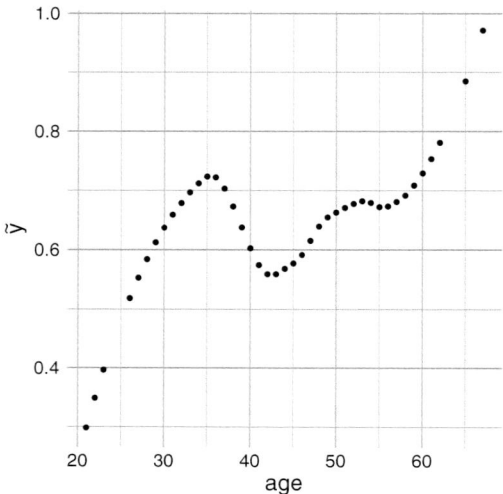

$$(\text{age} - k_j)_+^3 = \begin{cases} (\text{age} - k_j)^3 & \text{if age} \geq k_j \\ 0 & \text{if age} < k_j \end{cases} \text{ and } \lambda_j \frac{k_{\max} - k_j}{k_{\max} - k_{\min}}.$$

The recommended number of knots is three to five depending on the sample size and importance of the covariable in the study, with pre-specified locations based on the percentiles of age as suggested by Harrell (2015). In particular, five knots can be used since the sample size is greater than 100. Interactions between age and sex or SNP are not studied because of limitations of the sample size, though. Thus, a multivariable logistic regression given by (20) is fitted, and estimates of regression coefficients are presented in Table 4:

$$\text{logit}(p) = \beta_0 + \text{RCS}(\text{age}) + \beta_5 \text{sex} : M + \beta_6 \text{rs}12979860 : TG + \beta_7 \text{rs}12979860 : TT. \tag{20}$$

The Wald test is meaningless for age because it is testing whether each coefficient related to age is zero. The *LR* statistic is applied to test whether the effect of age represented by testing whether $(\beta_1, \beta_2, \beta_3, \beta_4)$ are zero. Furthermore, testing whether $(\beta_2, \beta_3, \beta_4)$ are zero is equivalent to test the assumption of linearity for age. In this way, a multivariable logistic regression with linear effect for age is fitted to calculate the *LR* ratio:

$$\text{logit}(p) = \beta_0 + \beta_1 \text{age} + \beta_2 \text{sex} : M + \beta_3 \text{rs}12979860 : TG + \beta_4 \text{rs}12979860 : TT. \tag{21}$$

Then, the *LR* statistic between (20) and (21) is 6.0001 with 3 d.f., resulting into a p-value of 0.11. At the end, the final fitted model will have age as a linear effect.

Table 4 Fitted multivariable logistic regression for treatment response as function of rs12979860 with age described using restricted cubic splines with five knots

Parameter	Estimate	Standard error	t value	p-value
β_0	−6.20792	3.03689	−2.044	0.0409
β_1	0.19557	0.09854	1.985	0.0472
β_2	−0.93706	0.48335	−1.939	0.0525
β_3	2.90649	1.72718	1.683	0.0924
β_4	−3.28687	3.30669	−0.994	0.3202
β_5	0.01822	0.39277	0.046	0.9630
β_6	1.78856	0.42329	4.225	2.39e-05
β_7	1.76747	0.67268	2.628	0.0086

Table 5 Fitted multivariable logistic regression for treatment response as function of rs12979860 with age described as linear

Parameter	Estimate	Standard error	t value	p-value	Skewness
β_0	−1.00950	0.85358	−1.183	0.237	−0.0862
β_1	0.01600	0.01739	0.920	0.357	0.0497
β_2	0.04807	0.38361	0.125	0.900	0.0459
β_3	1.61933	0.40237	4.024	5.71e-05	0.166
β_4	1.59246	0.63354	2.514	0.012	0.472

Table 6 Odds ratio for fitted multivariable logistic regression model (21)

OR	Estimate [95% CI]			
	LR	MLE Wald	BCEp Wald	BCEc Wald
CC:CT	5.05 [2.29; 11.11]	5.05 [2.67; 14.17]	4.79 [2.18; 10.47]	4.78 [2.17; 10.52]
CC:TT	4.91 [1.42; 17.02]	4.91 [1.71; 25.18]	4.38 [1.30; 14.76]	4.34 [1.25; 15.03]

Table 5 shows the estimated regression coefficients for model (21). The covariables age and sex are not statistically significant different from zero, but they will not be removed from the model to avoid the disadvantages of data-driven variable selection methods. Analogous tables for the bias-corrected estimated regression coefficients can also be presented.

Clinical interpretations of the parameters are based on Table 6. Notice that MLE presents higher values than BCEp and BCEc estimates. Based on the BCEp estimates, the patients with polymorphism CT are 4.79 more likely to be CHC than patients with polymorphism CC; patients with polymorphism TT are 4.38 more likely to be CHC than patients with polymorphism CC for a given age and sex. Confidence intervals are similar for a given odds ratio, such that $OR_{CC:TT}$ has a larger confidence interval than $OR_{CC:CT}$ due the smaller sample size of the polymorphism TT when compared to polymorphism CT. Furthermore, the skewness for β_4 is greater than 0.3 based on Table 5, leading the investigators to be careful with the inferences associated to the polymorphism TT.

Fig. 8 $\Delta\chi^2$ versus the estimated response $\hat{y}$, with point size proportional to $\Delta\beta$ for model (21)

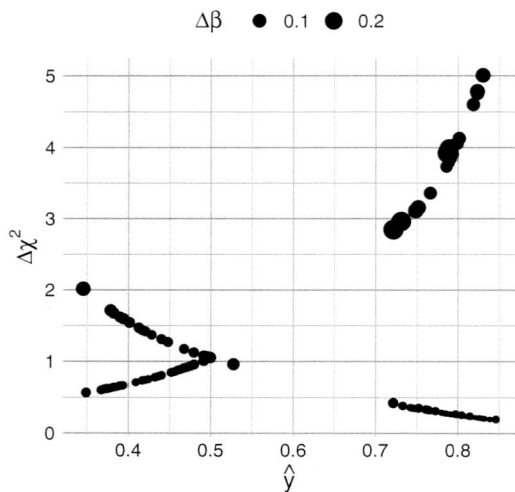

The model fit is assessed for different covariable patterns in Fig. 8, which does not show any compelling high value either of $\Delta\chi^2$ or $\Delta\beta$.

Related Methods

Statisticians have studied alternative models when categorical response variables are not binary or are ordinal. Hosmer and Lemeshow (2000) and Agresti (2003) discuss them further.

For categorical response variables with three or more categories, a multinomial logistic model can be applied instead to concatenate categories to transform the response into a binary variable. If there is an ordinal relationship among the response categories for the multinomial response, then an ordinal logistic regression could be appropriate. Both models have specific assumptions that must be checked in addition to the ones presented for logistic regression.

A second extension is when the observations are not independent. For example, when patients were matched in a case-control study, patients have repeated measures over time or space, and patients were correlated because they were from the same center in a multicenter study. Conditional logistic regression is a simple option for matched case-control studies; mixed logistic regression and general estimating equations (GEE) for logistic regression are more general methods that can be applied for all scenarios. The former allows the investigators to estimate individual-specific odd ratios, while the latter allows the investigators to estimate population-average odds ratios.

Furthermore, the logistic regression under a Bayesian framework has become as accessible as the frequentist approach because of the work of Polson et al. (2013), which is not so well disseminated yet. The Bayesian approach does not require asymptotic assumptions, and the investigators are able to incorporate historical data as prior information.

Conclusions

The widespread use of logistic regression is due to the meaningful interpretation of the parameters using odds ratio, which is appropriate for case-control studies. It also can be applied to cohort studies when the odds ratio is similar to the risk ratio. Nevertheless, a few technical aspects for the application of logistic regression have been neglected because of the lack of familiarity and accessible computational tools for non-statisticians.

Key Facts

- Logistic regression can be applied to case-control and cohort studies.
- Treatment effect should always be adjusted by confounding covariables even in randomized clinical trials.
- Bias-corrected estimates should be adopted when small sample sizes are considered.
- Subgroup analysis is performed only after a statistically significant interaction term.
- A covariable effect with more than two factors should be tested using a likelihood ratio test, unless comparisons with the reference level are the goal.
- Inferences should be interpreted carefully when samples are small or medium sizes.
- Additivity and linearity assumptions need to be checked.

Cross-References

▶ Confident Statistical Inference with Multiple Outcomes, Subgroups, and Other Issues of Multiplicity
▶ Essential Statistical Tests
▶ Missing Data
▶ Prognostic Factor Analyses

References

Agresti A (2003) Categorical data analysis. Wiley, Hoboken
Anderson JA, Richardson SC (1979) Logistic discrimination and bias correction in maximum likelihood estimation. Technometrics 21(1):71–78
Becher H (1992) The concept of residual confounding in regression models and some applications. Stat Med 11(13):1747–1758
Berkson J (1944) Application of the logistic function to bio-assay. J Am Stat Assoc 39(227):357–365
Berkson J (1951) Why I prefer logits to probits. Biometrics 7(4):327–339
Bowman KO, Shenton LR (1998) Asymptotic skewness and the distribution of maximum likelihood estimators. Commun Stat Theory Methods 27(11):2743–2760

Brookes ST, Whitely E, Egger M, Smith GD, Mulheran PA, Peters TJ (2004) Subgroup analyses in randomized trials: risks of subgroup-specific analyses: power and sample size for the interaction test. J Clin Epidemiol 57(3):229–236

Buettner P, Garbe c, Guggenmoos-Holzmann I (1997) Problems in defining cutoff points of continuous prognostic factors: example of tumor thickness in primary cutaneous melanoma. J Clin Epidemiol 50(11):1201–1210

Cleveland WS (1979) Robust locally weighted regression and smoothing scatterplots. J Am Stat Assoc 74(368):829–836

Copas JB (1983) Plotting p against x. Appl Stat 32(1):25–31

Cox DR (1969) Analysis of binary data. Chapman and Hall, London

Cox DR, Snell EJ (1968) A general definition of residuals. J Royal Statistical Soc Ser B (Methodological) 30(2):248–275

Cramer JS (2002) The origins of logistic regression. Technical Report 2002-119/4, Tinbergen Institute Working Paper. Available at SSRN: https://ssrn.com/abstract=360300 or https://doi.org/10.2139/ssrn.360300

Farewell V (1979) Some results on the estimation of logistic models based on retrospective data. Biometrika 66(1):27–32

Firth D (1993) Bias reduction of maximum likelihood estimates. Biometrika 80(1):27–38

Gail M, Wieand S, Piantadosi S (1984) Biased estimates of treatment effect in randomized trials. Control Clin Trials 5(3):303

Gail M, Tan W-Y, Piantadosi S (1988) Tests for no treatment effect in randomized clinical trials. Biometrika 75(1):57–64

Harrell F (2015) Regression modeling strategies: with applications to linear models, logistic and ordinal regression, and survival analysis. Springer series in statistics. Springer International Publishing, Cham

Hernández AV, Steyerberg EW, Habbema JDF (2004) Covariate adjustment in randomized controlled trials with dichotomous outcomes increases statistical power and reduces sample size requirements. J Clin Epidemiol 57(5):454–460

Hosmer DW, Lemesbow S (1980) Goodness of fit tests for the multiple logistic regression model. Commun Stat Theory Methods 9(10):1043–1069

Hosmer D, Lemeshow S (2000) Applied logistic regression, 2nd edn. Wiley, New York

Hosmer DW, Hosmer T, Le Cessie S, Lemeshow S (1997) A comparison of goodness-of-fit tests for the logistic regression model. Stat Med 16(9):965–980

Jiang H, Kulkarni PM, Mallinckrodt CH, Shurzinske L, Molenberghs G, Lipkovich I (2017) Covariate adjustment for logistic regression analysis of binary clinical trial data. Stat Biopharm Res 9(1):126–134

Kahan BC, Rushton H, Morris TP, Daniel RM (2016) A comparison of methods to adjust for continuous covariates in the analysis of randomised trials. BMC Med Res Methodol 16(1):42

le Cessie S, van Houwelingen JC (1991) A goodness-of-fit test for binary regression models, based on smoothing methods. Biometrics 47(4):1267–1282

Magalhães TM, Botter DA, Sandoval MC, Pereira GHA, Cordeiro GM (2019) Skewness of maximum likelihood estimators in the varying dispersion beta regression model. Commun Stat Theory Methods 48(17):4250–4260

Nastri AC d SS, de Mello Malta F, Diniz MA, Yoshino A, Abe-Sandes K, dos Santos SEB, de Castro Lyra A, Carrilho FJ, Pinho JRR (2016) Association of ifnl3 and ifnl4 polymorphisms with hepatitis c virus infection in a population from southeastern Brazil. Arch Virol 161(6):1477–1484

Pocock SJ, Assmann SE, Enos LE, Kasten LE (2002) Subgroup analysis, covariate adjustment and baseline comparisons in clinical trial reporting: current practice and problems. Stat Med 21(19):2917–2930

Polson NG, Scott JG, Windle J (2013) Bayesian inference for logistic models using pólya–gamma latent variables. J Am Stat Assoc 108(504):1339–1349

Pregibon D et al (1981) Logistic regression diagnostics. Ann Stat 9(4):705–724

Prentice RL, Pyke R (1979) Logistic disease incidence models and case-control studies. Biometrika 66(3):403–411

Robinson LD, Jewell NP (1991) Some surprising results about covariate adjustment in logistic regression models. Int Stat Rev/Revue Int Stat 59(2):227–240

Rothwell PM (2005) Subgroup analysis in randomised controlled trials: importance, indications, and interpretation. Lancet 365(9454):176–186

Royston P (1992) The use of cusums and other techniques in modelling continuous covariates in logistic regression. Stat Med 11(8):1115–1129

Royston P, Altman DG, Sauerbrei W (2006) Dichotomizing continuous predictors in multiple regression: a bad idea. Stat Med 25(1):127–141

Sand S, Victorin K, Filipsson AF (2008) The current state of knowledge on the use of the benchmark dose concept in risk assessment. J Appl Toxicol 28(4):405–421

Schaefer RL (1983) Bias correction in maximum likelihood logistic regression. Stat Med 2(1):71–78

Tsiatis AA (1980) A note on a goodness-of-fit test for the logistic regression model. Biometrika 67(1):250–251

Wang R, Lagakos SW, Ware JH, Hunter DJ, Drazen JM (2007) Statistics in medicine – reporting of subgroup analyses in clinical trials. N Engl J Med 357(21):2189–2194

Wilson EB, Worcester J (1943) The determination of ld 50 and its sampling error in bio-assay. Proc Natl Acad Sci 29(2):79–85

Statistical Analysis of Patient-Reported Outcomes in Clinical Trials

92

Gina L. Mazza and Amylou C. Dueck

Contents

Introduction	1814
Measurement	1815
Intent-to-Treat and Treatment Nonadherence	1815
Cross-Sectional Treatment Comparisons	1816
Responder Analysis	1817
Longitudinal Treatment Comparisons	1818
General Linear Mixed Modeling	1818
Area Under the Curve	1820
Time-to-Event Analysis	1821
Moderation	1821
Quality-Adjusted Life Years and Quality-Adjusted Time Without Symptoms or Toxicity	1822
Multiplicity	1823
Missing Data	1823
Missing Items	1824
Missing Scale Scores	1824
Data Visualization	1826
Summary and Conclusion	1826
Key Facts	1829
Cross-References	1829
References	1829

Abstract

Clinicians, researchers, funding agencies, regulatory agencies, and patients have long acknowledged the importance of patient-reported outcomes (PROs) in clinical trials. PROs refer to data provided directly by patients regarding their perceived health; presence, frequency, or severity of symptoms; health-related

---

G. L. Mazza (✉) · A. C. Dueck
Division of Biomedical Statistics and Informatics, Department of Health Sciences Research, Mayo Clinic, Scottsdale, AZ, USA
e-mail: Mazza.Gina@mayo.edu; Dueck.Amylou@mayo.edu

© Springer Nature Switzerland AG 2022
S. Piantadosi, C. L. Meinert (eds.), *Principles and Practice of Clinical Trials*,
https://doi.org/10.1007/978-3-319-52636-2_123

quality of life (HRQoL); or treatment satisfaction. Although definitional differences exist in the literature, HRQoL generally refers to the impact of disease, treatment, or perceived health on daily functioning. HRQoL and other PROs are measured by a single item or multiple items on questionnaires administered during clinic visits or completed by patients between clinic visits via various modes of administration including by paper, Internet-based survey, handheld device, mobile device application, automated telephone system, or interviewer (in-person or over the phone). PROs enhance clinicians' and researchers' understanding of patients' experiences before, during, and after treatment, particularly when these experiences are difficult or impossible to observe. When designing clinical trials, researchers should select PROs that are appropriate for the patient population of interest and that have established and acceptable psychometric (i.e., measurement) properties. When carrying out clinical trials, missing data should be prospectively minimized. Although this chapter describes some considerations specific to PROs, most analysis principles that apply to other endpoints also apply to PROs. As with other endpoints, researchers should select analyses that match their hypotheses and data characteristics, consider multiplicity issues, and properly handle missing data. Clinicians and researchers should also assess the clinical significance of the results.

Keywords

Patient-reported outcome · Quality of life · Questionnaire · Clinical trial · Patient-centered care · Treatment satisfaction · Clinical significance · Quality-adjusted life years · Multiplicity · Missing data

Introduction

Patient-reported outcomes (PROs) refer to data provided directly by patients regarding their perceived health; presence, frequency, or severity of symptoms; health-related quality of life (HRQoL); or treatment satisfaction (Cappelleri et al. 2014). Although definitional differences exist in the literature, HRQoL generally refers to the impact of disease, treatment, or perceived health on daily functioning (Mayo 2015). HRQoL and other PROs are important endpoints alongside survival and disease progression in clinical trials. PROs enhance clinicians' and researchers' understanding of patients' experiences before, during, and after treatment, particularly when these experiences are difficult or impossible to observe. During clinical trials, collection of PROs can improve safety monitoring as well as symptom detection and management (Pakhomov et al. 2008; Basch 2010). Following clinical trials, inclusion of PROs on product labels and consideration of PROs during treatment decisions can promote patient-centered care.

The purpose of this chapter is to review analyses relevant to clinical trials with PROs collected at a single time point or multiple time points. In general, analysis principles that apply to other endpoints also apply to PROs. However, considerations specific to PROs are described throughout this chapter. Key references for additional reading are provided.

Measurement

PROs are measured by a single item or multiple items on questionnaires administered during clinic visits or completed by patients between clinic visits via various modes of administration including by paper, Internet-based survey, handheld device, mobile device application, automated telephone system, or interviewer (in-person or over the phone). When an interviewer administers a PRO, the patients' responses are recorded without interpretation by the interviewer. Typically one or more scales are computed by summing or averaging the items that measure a single construct. For example, the Brief Pain Inventory consists of four items measuring severity on a 0 (no pain) to 10 (pain as bad as you can imagine) scale and seven items measuring interference with daily functioning on a 0 (does not interfere) to 10 (completely interferes) scale (Cleeland and Ryan 1994). Pain severity and interference scale scores are computed as means of these items. In the structural equation modeling framework, defining latent variables serves as an alternative to summing or averaging items (Hoyle 2012).

When designing clinical trials, researchers should select PROs that are appropriate for the patient population of interest. For example, if a clinical trial enrolls pediatric patients, then the PRO must be suitable for the intended age range. Other considerations include the patients' disease type, expected disease- or treatment-related symptoms, preferred languages, and cognitive abilities. Researchers should also select PROs that have established and acceptable psychometric (i.e., measurement) properties, including high reliability, high validity, responsiveness to change, measurement invariance across relevant subgroups, and measurement invariance across time (Reeve et al. 2007).

Intent-to-Treat and Treatment Nonadherence

In clinical trials, randomly assigning patients to treatment arms creates the strongest basis for causal inferences. Successful randomization provides strong ignorability, meaning patients in the treatment arms are equivalent, on average, at baseline and should thus only differ based on application of the treatments under investigation. An intent-to-treat analysis compares the endpoints of patients assigned to one treatment to those of patients assigned to another treatment, regardless of actual treatment received. For example, researchers may conduct an intent-to-treat analysis to examine whether, on average, patients assigned to one treatment experience greater HRQoL at a given post-baseline time point relative to patients assigned to another treatment.

An intent-to-treat analysis does not involve post-randomization exclusions due to treatment nonadherence or missing data. Post-randomization exclusions subvert the randomization and often produce selection bias. That is, patients who fully adhere to the treatment protocol may systematically differ from those who do not, and patients who provide complete data may systematically differ from those who do not. Consequently, post-randomization exclusions may lead to invalid causal inferences and limited generalizability of the results. In the PRO setting where at least some missing data are expected in virtually all clinical trials, an intent-to-treat analysis can still be conducted through strategies described by Altman (2009) and White et al. (2011). These strategies are consistent with the general approach to missing data described later in this chapter (see final paragraph of "Missing Data").

In clinical trials with treatment nonadherence, researchers can supplement an intent-to-treat analysis with one or more alternatives (e.g., per-protocol analysis, treatment effect bounding) (Sagarin et al. 2014). Researchers must consider whether the underlying assumptions of these alternatives are plausible. For example, a per-protocol analysis compares the endpoints of adherent patients assigned to one treatment to those of adherent patients assigned to another treatment. By excluding patients who do not adhere to their assigned treatment, a per-protocol analysis often produces nonequivalent groups and selection bias. That is, a per-protocol analysis yields biased estimates of the treatment effect unless adherence is ignorable (or conditionally ignorable), which is often implausible. The results of a per-protocol analysis should be interpreted with caution if a per-protocol analysis is conducted at all.

Cross-Sectional Treatment Comparisons

To assess treatment effects on continuous PROs at a given time point, parametric (e.g., two-sample t-test, analysis of covariance) or nonparametric (e.g., Mann-Whitney-Wilcoxon test, Kruskal-Wallis test) approaches can be used. Conditioning on patients' baseline status (as in an analysis of covariance) adjusts for potential imbalances across treatment arms at baseline and typically improves power (Vickers 2001). Parametric approaches rely on distributional assumptions about the endpoint (e.g., normality for the two-sample t-test and analysis of covariance), whereas nonparametric approaches do not. However, parametric approaches that assume normality are largely robust to violations of this assumption and provide greater power to detect treatment effects relative to nonparametric approaches. As such, parametric approaches are generally recommended unless the endpoint's distribution extremely departs from normality. Although ordinal PROs are non-normally distributed by definition, parametric approaches that assume normality are often still appropriate (Norman 2010; Sullivan and D'Agostino 2003). However, other parametric approaches (e.g., ordinal logistic regression) or nonparametric approaches can be used for ordinal PROs (e.g., symptom severity rated on a five-point scale). Similarly, parametric approaches (e.g., Poisson logistic regression) or nonparametric approaches can be used for count PROs (e.g., number of cigarettes smoked daily). Fisher's exact test, χ^2 test, Cochran-Mantel-Haenszel test, or logistic regression can be used for binary PROs (e.g., symptom presence or absence). Finally, multinomial logistic regression can be used for nominal PROs. Whereas these parametric and nonparametric approaches assume independence of observations, alternatives exist for clustered observations. For example, clustering occurs in cluster randomized designs where sites rather than patients are randomized to treatment arms. Analyses involving these data must account for clustering to avoid Type I error rate inflation. Mixed models for repeated measures (a common form of clustering) are described later in this chapter.

A treatment effect's clinical significance should be considered in addition to its statistical significance. Clinical significance broadly refers to whether a treatment effect has implications for patient management. Researchers should define clinical significance a priori in the statistical analysis plan. Anchor-based and distribution-based methods exist for defining clinical significance (Wyrwich et al. 2013). Anchor-based methods examine the association between a PRO and a clinically relevant comparator (referred to as an anchor), whereas distribution-based methods rely on measures of variability. One common distribution-based method is effect size calculation. Whereas significance tests assess the *existence* of a treatment effect, effect sizes assess the *magnitude* of a treatment effect. For example, Cohen's d defines the standardized difference between two means (i.e., mean difference across treatment arms divided by the pooled standard deviation). In general, standardized mean differences of $d = 0.20, 0.50$, and 0.80 represent small, medium, and large treatment effects (Cohen 1988). For example, $d = 0.50$ indicates that two treatment arms' means on a given PRO are half of a standard deviation apart. Whenever possible, researchers should rely on their expertise and guidelines in the literature rather than these conventions for small, medium, and large effect sizes. Because a clinically significant mean difference across treatment arms may be due to a few patients experiencing a dramatic improvement while the remaining patients experience little to no improvement, researchers can supplement effect size calculation with a responder analysis.

Responder Analysis

A responder analysis compares the proportion of patients who experience a clinically significant improvement since baseline across treatment arms (e.g., using Fisher's exact test, χ^2 test, or logistic regression). Researchers should define the threshold for clinically significant improvement a priori in the statistical analysis plan. Patients who meet or exceed this threshold are termed responders, while the remaining patients are termed nonresponders. For example, in the COMFORT-I trial, a patient was deemed a responder if he or she experienced a 50% or more reduction in symptom burden from baseline to Week 24, as assessed by the Myelofibrosis Symptom Assessment Form (MFSAF) version 2.0 (Verstovsek et al. 2012).

A responder analysis is useful for investigating whether a statistically significant treatment effect represents a clinically significant improvement for a meaningful proportion of patients. However, a responder analysis suffers from issues associated with dichotomizing ordinal or continuous measures (e.g., lower reliability) (MacCallum et al. 2002). A responder analysis can also suffer from loss of sample size (and thus power) if not all patients are eligible to experience a clinically significant improvement. For example, pain reduction may serve as a secondary endpoint in a clinical trial enrolling patients of all pain levels rated on a 0–10 scale. A

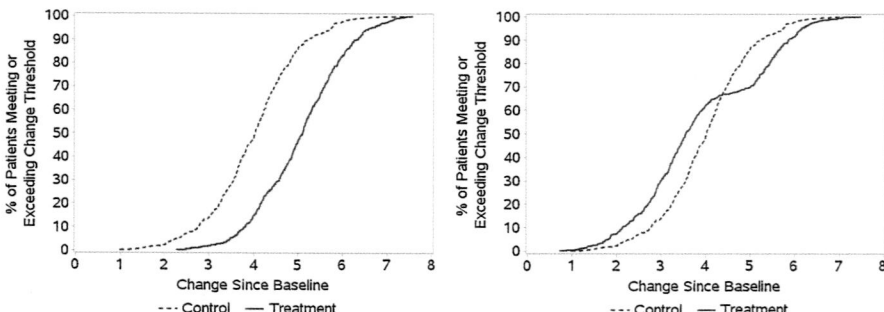

Fig. 1 Cumulative distribution function by treatment arm. Separation between the treatment arms' cumulative distribution functions (left) indicates that the responder analysis' conclusions would be consistent across the entire range of thresholds, whereas cumulative distribution functions that overlap or cross (right) suggest that the responder analysis' conclusions would differ across the range of thresholds

two-point reduction in pain is impossible for patients who reported no pain at baseline. If clinically significant improvement on a PRO serves as a primary endpoint, inclusion criteria for the clinical trial should consider patients' baseline status and ability to experience a clinically significant improvement. Researchers should base power calculations for a responder analysis on the expected number of patients with the ability to experience a clinically significant improvement.

Because setting a threshold for clinically significant improvement is sometimes arbitrary or subjective, researchers can supplement a responder analysis with a plot of the cumulative distribution function by treatment arm (see Fig. 1). For this plot, change since baseline is on the horizontal axis, and cumulative percentage of patients meeting or exceeding each threshold is on the vertical axis. Patients with missing change scores are typically considered nonresponders for all possible thresholds. Visually comparing the treatment arms' cumulative distribution functions allows researchers to assess whether the conclusions of a responder analysis would differ if another threshold representing clinically significant improvement were chosen. Separation between the treatment arms' cumulative distribution functions indicates that the responder analysis' conclusions would be consistent across the entire range of thresholds (see the left panel of Fig. 1). Cumulative distribution functions that overlap or cross suggest that the responder analysis' conclusions would differ across the range of thresholds (see the right panel of Fig. 1).

Longitudinal Treatment Comparisons

General Linear Mixed Modeling

In clinical trials with repeated measures, one commonly used general linear mixed model includes a fixed intercept; fixed effect for time, treatment arm, and treatment arm by time interaction; and residual covariance matrix that accounts for repeated measures within patients. An unstructured residual covariance matrix freely estimates the variance of patients' scores at each time point and freely estimates the covariance of patients' scores across each pair of time points, though at a cost of estimating a potentially large number of variances and covariances. Time is treated as nominal, meaning the order and spacing of assessments (e.g., baseline, post-surgery, post-radiation therapy following surgery) are not considered (Brahmer et al. 2017). This mixed model is conceptually similar to a repeated measures analysis of variance but allows for a non-normally distributed endpoint, unstructured residual covariance matrix, and imbalance on the number of assessments across patients. Researchers can specify contrasts to evaluate change within or between treatment arms. Longitudinal growth modeling, which is described next, does not treat time as nominal and can also be implemented in the mixed modeling framework.

Longitudinal growth modeling. Longitudinal growth modeling allows researchers to investigate both within-patient and between-patient change across time by modeling each patient's trajectory across time. Before estimating longitudinal growth models, researchers should plot patients' data to identify typical trajectories, calculate univariate descriptive statistics (e.g., mean, standard deviation, skew, kurtosis) for the full sample and by treatment arm at each time point, and calculate bivariate associations across time points (e.g., correlations). Plotting patients' data and examining descriptive statistics assist with understanding within-patient and between-patient change across time and across treatment arms. Selecting an appropriate time metric is important when plotting and modeling longitudinal data. For example, with unequal spacing between assessments, the first four waves of data collection may be represented as Waves 1, 2, 3, and 4 or as Weeks 0, 2, 6, and 12. A one-unit increase in time has different meanings with these two time metrics.

Longitudinal growth modeling can be conducted in the mixed modeling and structural equation modeling frameworks (Grimm et al. 2017). In the mixed modeling framework, longitudinal growth models are specified as random coefficient mixed models. Linear or nonlinear change across time may be modeled (Unger et al. 2017). When assuming linear change across time, a random intercept mixed model allows patients to differ in level but assumes that all patients change at the same rate (i.e., all patients improve at the same rate or all patients worsen at the same rate; see the left panel of Fig. 2). For example, when modeling patients' HRQoL across time, a random intercept mixed model allows patients to differ in their HRQoL means (i.e., on average, some patients experience higher HRQoL than others) but assumes that all patients change at the same rate (i.e., all patients improve [worsen] at the same rate). A random slope mixed model allows patients to change at different rates (i.e., some patients may improve [worsen] more quickly than others) and in different directions (i.e., some patients may improve while others may worsen; see the right panel of Fig. 2). Because the random slope mixed model includes both a random intercept and a random slope, researchers can examine the intercept-slope covariance. If the intercept represents patients' baseline status, then the intercept-slope covariance represents the association between patients' baseline status and their rate of change. For example, we may expect patients with lower HRQoL at baseline to worsen more quickly than patients with higher HRQoL at baseline.

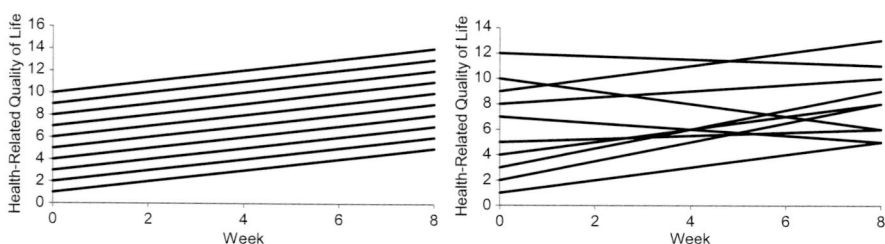

Fig. 2 Patient trajectories for a random intercept mixed model (left) and for a random slope mixed model (right)

Longitudinal growth models may include time-invariant and time-varying covariates. Time-invariant covariates remain constant across time, whereas time-varying covariates change across time. For example, researchers may hypothesize that patients' HRQoL across time depends on time-invariant covariates (e.g., treatment arm) as well as time-varying covariates (e.g., presence, frequency, or severity of symptoms) in clinical trials.

Area Under the Curve

For PROs collected longitudinally, area under the curve can be calculated as either a summary measure or statistic. As a summary measure, area under the curve is calculated for each patient by connecting a patient's observed scores across a fixed time period (e.g., 8 weeks), calculating the area of each resulting trapezoid, and summing the trapezoids' areas. For example, Fig. 3 shows a single patient's area under the curve, which summarizes his or her reported fatigue across 8 weeks. Area under the curve is then compared across treatment arms using one of the parametric or nonparametric approaches described earlier in this chapter (e.g., two-sample t-test or analysis of covariance adjusting for patients' baseline status). As a summary statistic, area under the curve is calculated for each treatment arm using parameter estimates from a mixed model. Area under the curve is then compared across treatment arms using a contrast.

When computing area under the curve as a summary measure, researchers often exclude patients with missing scores or perform single imputation such as last observation carried forward (replacing a patient's missing scores with his or her last observed score), patient mean imputation (replacing a patient's missing scores with the mean of his or her observed scores), extrapolation (imputing a patient's missing scores at later time points by linearly extrapolating from his or her observed scores), or interpolation (imputing a patient's missing scores at intermediate time points by linearly interpolating from his or her observed scores). However, Monte Carlo simulations conducted by Bell et al. (2014) indicated that excluding patients with missing scores or performing single imputation leads to substantial bias. Instead, they recommended computing area under the curve as a summary statistic in clinical trials with attrition (Bell et al. 2014).

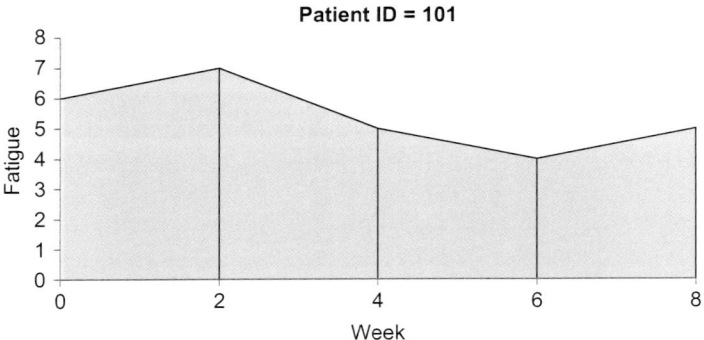

Fig. 3 Area under the curve for a patient who reported fatigue at Weeks 0, 2, 4, 6, and 8

Time-to-Event Analysis

A time-to-event analysis examines if and when patients experience a clinically significant improvement (or worsening) during a given time period (i.e., the duration of a clinical trial). Time-to-event is then compared across treatment arms using a Kaplan-Meier plot with log-rank tests or Cox proportional hazards regression. Right censoring occurs when patients do not experience a clinically significant change by the end of the clinical trial or by their last completed assessment. As with a responder analysis, researchers should define the threshold for clinically significant change a priori in the statistical analysis plan. Patients who cannot experience a clinically significant change should be excluded. If time to clinically significant change on a PRO serves as a primary endpoint, inclusion criteria for the clinical trial should consider patients' baseline status and ability to experience a clinically significant change. Researchers should base power calculations for a time-to-event analysis on the expected number of patients with the ability to experience a clinically significant change. In palliative care or advanced cancer settings, disease progression and/or death may be included along with PRO worsening as events in a time-to-event analysis. Interpreting differences between treatment arms in the combined endpoint (e.g., time to first occurrence of PRO worsening, progression, or death) may require subsequent analyses in which each endpoint is considered separately (Benzo et al. 2009).

Moderation

When conducting clinical trials, researchers may hypothesize that the treatment effect varies across levels of a so-called moderator. A moderator affects the strength and/or direction of the treatment effect. For example, Barton et al. (2013) examined whether the effect of ginseng on patient-reported fatigue at 8 weeks differed for patients who were currently receiving cancer treatment versus those who had completed cancer treatment. Simple main effects can be calculated at each level of a binary or nominal moderator, as in this example. That is, simple main effects can be calculated separately for these two subgroups (i.e., current versus previous receipt of cancer treatment) to examine the strength and direction of the effect of ginseng on 8-week fatigue in each subgroup. For an ordinal or continuous moderator, simple main effects can be calculated at a few clinically meaningful values or sample-based values (e.g., mean and one standard deviation above/below the mean) (Aiken and West 1991). For example, suppose that baseline fatigue significantly moderated the effect of ginseng on 8-week fatigue. Simple main effects can be calculated for patients who were at the mean of baseline fatigue, one standard deviation below the mean of baseline fatigue, and one standard deviation above the mean of baseline fatigue. Because clinical trials are often underpowered to detect these interactions, researchers should consider important subgroups or moderators in their power calculations (Aiken and West 1991).

Quality-Adjusted Life Years and Quality-Adjusted Time Without Symptoms or Toxicity

Quality-adjusted life years (QALYs) and quality-adjusted time without symptoms or toxicity (Q-TWiST) are often used to evaluate the utility of medical costs. QALYs combine survival time with HRQoL by discounting periods of survival when patients experience suboptimal HRQoL. Each patient's QALYs are calculated by multiplying time spent in a given health state by the HRQoL weight (i.e., utility) associated with that health state. HRQoL weights may range from 0 (death) to 1 (perfect health) or may include negative values to represent health states worse than death. Researchers often base HRQoL weights on EuroQol's EQ-5D, which assesses patients' problems with mobility, self-care, usual activities, pain/discomfort, and anxiety/depression (Herdman et al. 2011). Patients' responses to these five items are then used to calculate a single index representing the HRQoL weight. For example, suppose that a patient's HRQoL weight equaled 0.80, 0.75, 0.65, and 0.70 across 4 years. These 4 years of survival would correspond to $(0.80 \times 1 \text{ year}) + (0.75 \times 1 \text{ year}) + (0.65 \times 1 \text{ year}) + (0.70 \times 1 \text{ year}) = 2.90$ QALYs (though other possible calculations exist (Billingham et al. 1999)). If survival time is observed for all patients, QALYs can be compared across treatment arms using one of the parametric or nonparametric approaches described earlier in this chapter (e.g., two-sample t-test). If survival time is censored for some patients, QALYs can be computed for each treatment arm (rather than for each patient) using a model-based approach (Billingham et al. 1999).

Q-TWiST partitions survival time into time without symptoms or toxicity, time with symptoms or toxicity, and time with disease relapse (Gelber and Goldhirsch 1986). Similar to the calculation of each patient's QALYs, each patient's Q-TWiST is calculated as a weighted sum of time spent in each health state. That is, Q-TWiST discounts periods of survival when patients experience symptoms or toxicity as well as periods of survival following disease relapse.

Multiplicity

Multiplicity issues arise when researchers conduct multiple significance tests for a single clinical trial due to comparing three or more treatment arms, investigating multiple endpoints (e.g., multiple scales, multiple thresholds for clinically significant change), evaluating a single endpoint at multiple time points, or examining moderators (see other chapters in this book for detailed recommendations on multiplicity issues). For example, the European Organisation for the Research and Treatment of Cancer (EORTC) Core Quality of Life Questionnaire (QLQ-C30) includes a global health status and quality of life scale, five functioning scales (physical, role, emotional, cognitive, social), and nine symptom scales or items (Fayers et al. 2001). Conducting multiple significance tests (e.g., on each EORTC QLQ-C30 scale at multiple time points) leads to a familywise Type I error rate that is substantially higher than the nominal Type I error rate for a single significance test (typically $\alpha = 0.05$). With multidimensional PROs, researchers should focus on the most relevant scales and clearly indicate which scales serve as primary, secondary, or exploratory endpoints when outlining their hypotheses and statistical analysis plan in the protocol. Researchers should also justify any subgroups or moderators of interest. Where appropriate, researchers may sequence significance tests (i.e., use gatekeeping strategies) or calculate summary measures or statistics such as patients' minimum, maximum, or mean score across scales or time points; area under the curve; or time-to-event. Summary measures and statistics reduce the number of significance tests conducted by aggregating patients' scores across scales or time points. Extreme care should be taken when using summary measures and statistics as the impact of missing data may be difficult to assess, and aggregation of treatment effects in opposite directions may be interpreted as a combined nil treatment effect. Finally, researchers may apply p-value adjustments that control the familywise Type I error rate (e.g., Bonferroni, Hochberg's step-up, Bonferroni-Holm's step-down, and resampling methods) or false discovery rate.

Missing Data

As with other endpoints, noncompletion of PROs may result from missed clinic visits, attrition, or administrative errors. Noncompletion of PROs may also result from patient refusal. For example, patients may refuse due to illness, unease regarding the content of the questionnaire, or response burden. Patients may also forget to complete questionnaires administered at home. To reduce bias and power loss, researchers should prevent missing data as much as possible. Limiting administration time and response burden is essential and has motivated the development of abbreviated questionnaires. Staff training and careful development of the protocol can promote PRO completion during clinic visits, and automated reminders can promote PRO completion at home. Based on a systematic review, Mercieca-Bebber et al. (2016) provided additional design and methodological strategies for reducing rates of missing data on PROs. Nevertheless, researchers should anticipate missing data and prospectively collect reasons for noncompletion as well as auxiliary data related to the incomplete PRO (e.g., baseline covariates for a mixed model or multiple imputation) (Bell and Fairclough 2014).

Missing Items

Unlike other endpoints in clinical trials, item nonresponse must be considered with PROs. Item nonresponse refers to patients completing some, but not all, of the items measuring a single construct. Patients may inadvertently skip items, skip later items on a questionnaire, skip items considered not applicable, or skip sensitive items. Protocols should instruct staff to check paper forms for completeness, and online forms should prompt patients to complete or refuse items. To handle missing items on a questionnaire, researchers should generally follow the user manual or published scoring algorithm. User manuals and key publications for questionnaires often recommend proration, which refers to averaging the available items for each patient. For example, if a patient answers seven out of ten items, the prorated scale score is the average of the seven responses. Proration is equivalent to imputing each patient's missing scores with the mean of his or her observed scores. Typically, proration is only applied when patients complete at least half of the items. However, methodologists have raised serious concerns about proration. Notably, proration redefines a scale such that it is no longer the sum or average of the k items comprising the scale; its definition now varies across patients and depends on the missing data patterns and rates in the sample (Schafer and Graham 2002). Monte Carlo simulations conducted by Mazza et al. (2015) demonstrated that proration can produce bias even under a missing completely at random (MCAR) mechanism. In theory, proration yields biased parameter estimates unless the imputed items have the same properties as the remaining items on the scale. In practice, however, bias resulting from proration may be negligible if the item missing data rates are low (Mazza et al. 2019).

Missing Scale Scores

When patients skip an entire questionnaire or skip too many items to compute the scale score, missing data handling recommendations that apply to other endpoints also apply to PROs. Although easy to implement, excluding patients with missing scores or performing single imputation is not recommended (Schafer and Graham 2002; Enders 2010). Bias resulting from single imputation depends on how closely patients' imputed scores correspond to their would-be scores. For example, by replacing a patient's missing scores with his or her last observed score, last observation carried forward assumes that the patient's scores do not change over time. However, researchers typically collect PROs longitudinally because they expect patients' scores to change over time. As another example, replacing patients' missing scores with the sample mean (i.e., mean imputation) attenuates estimates of variability and association by adding scores to the center of a PRO's distribution. Single imputation also yields standard errors that are too small because the imputed scores are treated as observed scores. That is, single imputation does not account for the imputed scores being just one set of plausible replacement scores.

Appropriately addressing missing data requires an understanding of missing data mechanisms. Rubin's (1976) three mechanisms – MCAR, missing at random (MAR), and missing not at random (MNAR) – describe how the probability of missingness relates to the observed and missing scores on a set of analysis variables. These missing data mechanisms serve as untestable (or only partially testable) assumptions underlying analyses such as between-arm treatment comparisons. An MCAR mechanism states that the probability of missingness is unrelated to the observed and missing scores. An MCAR mechanism may hold when patients inadvertently miss questionnaires (e.g., due to missing a page of the questionnaire booklet) but not when patients miss questionnaires due to illness. Because the observed scores can be regarded as a random subsample of the hypothetical complete scores under an MCAR mechanism, excluding patients with missing scores (i.e., available-case analysis) yields unbiased parameter estimates under an MCAR mechanism but not under an MAR or MNAR mechanism. MCAR-based methods such as available-case analysis should be avoided.

An MAR mechanism states that the probability of missingness is unrelated to the missing scores after conditioning on the observed scores, while an MNAR mechanism states that the probability of missingness is related to the missing scores even after conditioning on the observed scores. Although MNAR-based analyses are intuitively appealing, they rely on other strict, untestable assumptions. Because even slight violations of these assumptions can produce parameter estimates that are even more biased than those from MAR-based analyses under an MNAR mechanism (Enders 2010), MAR-based analyses such as maximum likelihood estimation and multiple imputation are generally recommended.

Maximum likelihood estimation uses an iterative optimization algorithm to identify the set of parameter values that maximize the probability of the observed data. Multiple imputation involves creating multiple copies of the data set with different imputed scores (imputation phase), analyzing the imputed data sets as though they were complete data sets (analysis phase), and pooling the parameter estimates and standard errors across the imputed data sets to yield a single set of results (pooling phase). Unlike single imputation, multiple imputation accounts for imputation uncertainty. With maximum likelihood estimation and multiple imputation, both within-patient and between-patient data provide information about the missing scores. The baseline assessment is extremely important for missing data handling because typically all (or almost all) patients complete the baseline assessment, and patients' scores at later time points often moderately or highly correlate with their scores at earlier time points. Utilizing variables that highly correlate with an incomplete PRO and/or predict missingness (e.g., baseline status, clinician reports, medical records) reduces bias and power loss when conducting between-arm treatment comparisons (Donaldson and Moinpour 2005).

Researchers should examine the proportions of and reasons for missing data by time point and treatment arm. Researchers should also compare patients with and without missing data on baseline characteristics using parametric or nonparametric approaches (e.g., two-sample t-test to compare age between patients who did and did not complete the PRO at a given time point). The primary analysis should use all available data (e.g., should include all patients regardless of whether they completed one, some, or all PRO assessments) and assume an MAR mechanism holds. Because the missing data mechanisms serve as untestable (or only partially testable) assumptions, the primary analysis should be supplemented by sensitivity analyses to assess the robustness of the results across various sets of assumptions. Sensitivity analyses could include multiple imputation; selection, shared parameter, or pattern mixture modeling; or tipping point analyses (Fairclough 2010; Ratitch et al. 2013; Mallinckrodt et al. 2013).

Data Visualization

Results of hypothesis testing and tabular presentations of PROs can often be complemented by graphical presentations. A variety of graphical presentations have appeared in the literature (see Fig. 4). The ability of clinicians, researchers, and patients to accurately interpret PRO results varies across graphical presentations (Brundage et al. 2018), suggesting that care should be taken to ensure clarity. For example, suggested techniques in longitudinal line plots include consistently displaying higher scores to indicate "better" outcomes and providing threshold lines to indicate normal versus concerning scores (Snyder et al. 2017).

Summary and Conclusion

Clinicians, researchers, funding agencies, regulatory agencies, and patients have long acknowledged the importance of PROs in clinical trials. Given the growing utility of PROs for setting clinical guidelines and health policies including regulatory and reimbursement decisions, ongoing efforts exist to help researchers develop, select, and analyze PROs. For example, the National Institutes of Health funded the Patient-Reported Outcomes Measurement Information System (PROMIS) initiative to develop PROs with strong psychometric properties and promote standardization across projects (Reeve et al. 2007). The US Food and Drug Administration released a guide for using PROs to support product labeling claims (Food and Drug Administration 2009), and the European Medicines Agency released a related commentary (European Medicines Agency 2005). The National Cancer Institute developed the PRO version of the Common Terminology Criteria for Adverse Events (PRO-CTCAE) to incorporate the patient voice into symptomatic adverse event assessments in cancer clinical trials (Basch et al. 2014). Calvert et al. (2013) developed recommendations for reporting PROs in randomized clinical trials via the PRO extension to the Consolidated Standards of Reporting Trials (CONSORT-PRO) statement. Subsequently, Calvert et al. (2018) developed recommendations for writing protocols with PROs as primary or key secondary endpoints through a PRO extension to the Standard Protocol Items: Recommendations for Interventional Trials statement (SPIRIT-PRO). Finally, the EORTC convened the Setting International Standards in Analyzing Patient-Reported Outcomes and Quality of Life Endpoints Data (SISAQOL) Consortium to develop international standards for analyzing PROs in cancer clinical trials (Bottomley et al. 2016).

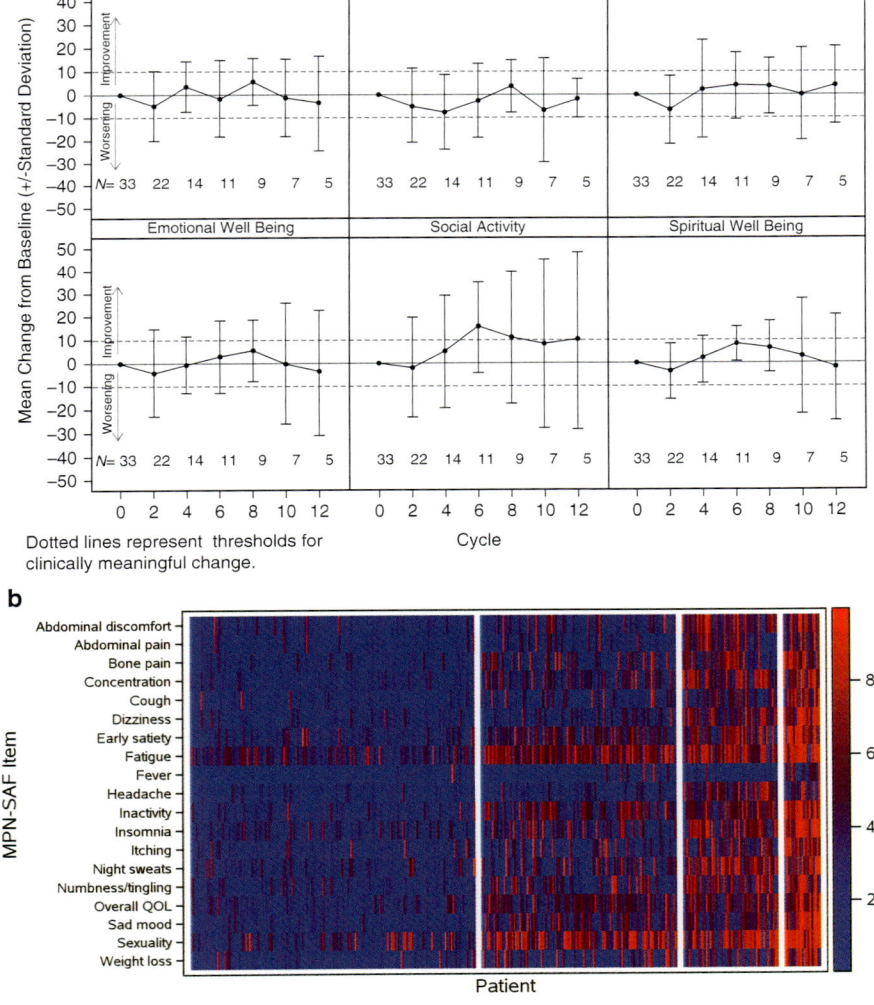

Fig. 4 (continued)

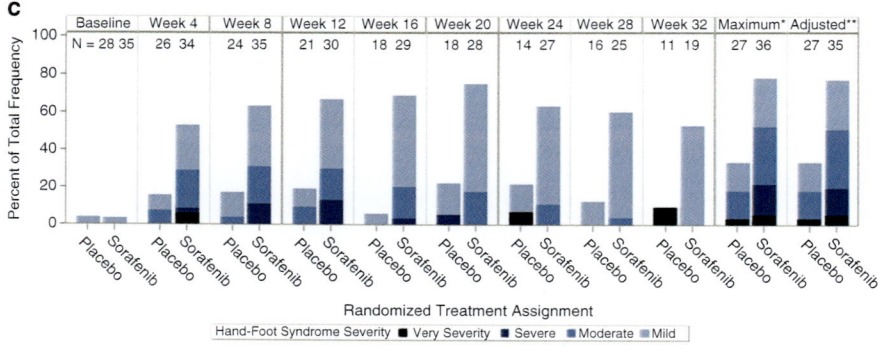

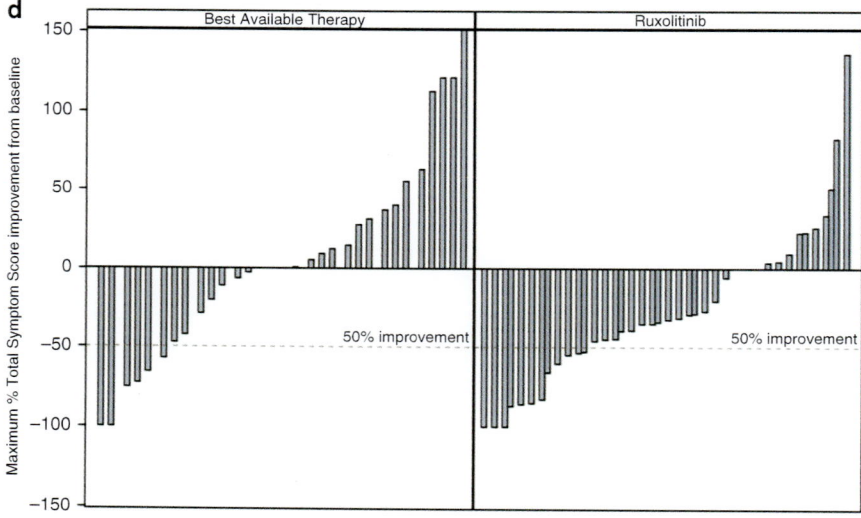

Fig. 4 Graphical representations of patient-reported outcomes: (**a**) line plot of mean quality of life as measured by the Linear Analogue Self-Assessment adapted from Tan et al. (2013); (**b**) heat map of individual patient symptom scores as measured by the Myeloproliferative Neoplasm Symptom Assessment Form adapted from Geyer et al. (2014); (**c**) relative frequency bar chart of Hand-Foot Syndrome Severity as measured by the Patient-Reported Outcomes version of the Common Terminology Criteria for Adverse Events adapted from Gounder et al. (2018); and (**d**) waterfall plot of maximum percentage reduction in Total Symptom Score computed from the Myeloproliferative Neoplasm Symptom Assessment Form adapted from Harrison et al. (2017)

Although this chapter described some considerations specific to PROs, most analysis principles that apply to other clinical trial endpoints also apply to PROs. As with other endpoints, researchers should select analyses that match their hypotheses and data characteristics (e.g., distribution of the endpoint being compared across treatment arms). The statistical analysis plan should address multiplicity as well as missing data. Every effort should be made to minimize missing data prospectively through careful clinical trial design and monitoring. The primary analysis should use all available data and assume an MAR mechanism holds. To supplement the primary analysis, sensitivity analyses can assess the robustness of the results across various sets of assumptions about the missing data. In general, regression-based analyses for longitudinal data are preferred over summary measures and statistics including responder analyses, though such analyses can be effective supplements for investigating or communicating clinical significance. Importantly, clinicians and researchers should evaluate a treatment effect based on its implications for patient management. Finally, standardized PRO tools, guidelines, and recommendations should be employed when available.

Key Facts

1. Patient-reported outcomes refer to data provided directly by patients regarding their perceived health; presence, frequency, or severity of symptoms; health-related quality of life; or treatment satisfaction.
2. When designing clinical trials, researchers should select patient-reported outcomes that are appropriate for the patient population of interest and that have established and acceptable psychometric (i.e., measurement) properties.
3. Most analysis principles that apply to other clinical trial endpoints also apply to patient-reported outcomes. As with other endpoints, researchers should select analyses that match their hypotheses and data characteristics. Multiplicity and missing data should be addressed. Statistical and clinical significance should be incorporated into interpretation of results.
4. Every effort should be made to minimize missing data prospectively through careful clinical trial design and monitoring. The primary analysis should use all available data and assume a missing at random mechanism holds. To supplement the primary analysis, sensitivity analyses can assess the robustness of the results across various sets of assumptions about the missing data.

Cross-References

▶ Confident Statistical Inference with Multiple Outcomes, Subgroups, and Other Issues of Multiplicity
▶ Essential Statistical Tests
▶ Missing Data
▶ Patient-Reported Outcomes

References

Aiken LS, West SG (1991) Multiple regression: testing and interpreting interactions. SAGE, Newbury Park

Altman DG (2009) Missing outcomes in randomized trials: addressing the dilemma. Open Med 3: e51–e53

Barton DL, Liu H, Dakhil SR et al (2013) Wisconsin ginseng (*Panax quinquefolius*) to improve cancer-related fatigue: a randomized, double-blind trial, N07C2. J Natl Cancer Inst 105:1230–1238

Basch E (2010) The missing voice of patients in drug-safety reporting. N Engl J Med 362:865–869

Basch E, Reeve BB, Mitchell SA et al (2014) Development of the National Cancer Institute's Patient-Reported Outcomes version of the Common Terminology Criteria for Adverse Events (PRO-CTCAE). J Natl Cancer Inst 106:dju244

Bell ML, Fairclough DL (2014) Practical and statistical issues in missing data for longitudinal patient-reported outcomes. Stat Methods Med Res 23:440–459

Bell ML, King MT, Fairclough DL (2014) Bias in area under the curve for longitudinal clinical trials with missing patient reported outcome data: summary measures versus summary statistics. SAGE Open 4:1–12

Benzo R, Farrell MH, Chang CC et al (2009) Integrating health status and survival data: the palliative effect of lung volume reduction surgery. Am J Respir Crit Care Med 180:239–246

Billingham LJ, Abrams KR, Jones DR (1999) Methods for the analysis of quality-of-life and survival data in health technology assessment. Health Technol Assess 3:1–146

Bottomley A, Pe M, Sloan J et al (2016) Analysing data from patient-reported outcome and quality of life endpoints for cancer clinical trials: a start in setting international standards. Lancet 17:510–514

Brahmer JR, Rodríguez-Abreu D, Robinson AG et al (2017) Health-related quality-of-life results for pembrolizumab versus chemotherapy in advanced, PD-L1-positive NSCLC (KEYNOTE-024): a multicentre, international, randomised, open-label phase 3 trial. Lancet Oncol 18:1600–1609

Brundage M, Blackford A, Tolbert E et al (2018) Presenting comparative study PRO results to clinicians and researchers: beyond the eye of the beholder. Qual Life Res 27:75–90

Calvert M, Blazeby J, Altman DG et al (2013) Reporting of patient-reported outcomes in randomized trials: the CONSORT PRO extension. JAMA 309:814–822

Calvert M, Kyte D, Mercieca-Bebber R et al (2018) Guidelines for inclusion of patient-reported outcomes in clinical trial protocols: the SPIRIT-PRO extension. JAMA 319:483–494

Cappelleri JC, Zou KH, Bushmakin AG, Alvir JMJ, Alemayehu D, Symonds T (2014) Patient-reported outcomes: measurement, implementation, and interpretation. CRC Press, Boca Raton

Cleeland CS, Ryan KM (1994) Pain assessment: global use of the Brief Pain Inventory. Ann Acad Med Singap 23:129–138

Cohen J (1988) Statistical power analysis for the behavioral sciences, 2nd edn. Lawrence Erlbaum Associates, Hillsdale

Donaldson GW, Moinpour CM (2005) Learning to live with missing quality-of-life data in advanced-stage disease trials. J Clin Oncol 23:7380–7384

Enders CK (2010) Applied missing data analysis. Guilford Press, New York

Committee for Medicinal Products for Human Use (2005) Reflection paper on the regulatory guidance for the use of health-related quality of life (HRQL) measures in the evaluation of medicinal products. European Medicines Agency, London

Fairclough DL (2010) Design and analysis of quality of life studies in clinical trials, 2nd edn. Chapman & Hall/CRC, Boca Raton

Fayers PM, Aaronson NK, Bjordal K, Groenvold M, Curran D, Bottomley A (2001) The EORTC QLQ-C30 scoring manual, 3rd edn. European Organisation for Research and Treatment of Cancer, Brussels

Food and Drug Administration (2009) Guidance for industry patient-reported outcome measures: use in medical product development to support labeling claims. Food and Drug Administration, Silver Spring

Gelber RD, Goldhirsch A (1986) A new endpoint for the assessment of adjuvant therapy in postmenopausal women with operable breast cancer. J Clin Oncol 4:1772–1779

Geyer HL, Scherber RM, Dueck AC et al (2014) Distinct clustering of symptomatic burden among myeloproliferative neoplasm patients: retrospective assessment in 1470 patients. Blood 123:3803–3810

Gounder M, Mahoney M, Van Tine B et al (2018) Sorafenib in advanced and refractory desmoid tumors. New Eng J Med 379:2417–2428

Grimm KJ, Ram N, Estabrook R (2017) Growth modeling: structural equation and multilevel modeling approaches. Guilford Press, New York

Harrison CN, Mead AJ, Panchal A et al (2017) Ruxolitinib vs best available therapy for ET intolerant or resistant to hydroxycarbamide. Blood 130:1889–1897

Herdman M, Gudex C, Lloyd A et al (2011) Development and preliminary testing of the new five-level version of EQ-5D (EQ-5D-5L). Qual Life Res 20:1727–1736

Hoyle RH (ed) (2012) Handbook of structural equation modeling. Guilford Press, New York

MacCallum RC, Zhang S, Preacher KJ, Rucker DD (2002) On the practice of dichotomization of quantitative variables. Psychol Methods 7:19–40

Mallinckrodt C, Roger J, Chuang-Stein C et al (2013) Missing data: turning guidance into action. Stat Biopharm Res 5:369–382

Mayo NE (ed) (2015) ISOQOL dictionary of quality of life and health outcomes measurement. International Society for Quality of Life Research, Milwaukee

Mazza GL, Enders CK, Ruehlman LS (2015) Addressing item-level missing data: a comparison of proration and full information maximum likelihood estimation. Multivar Behav Res 50:504–519

Mazza GL, Kunze KL, Langlais BT, et al. (2019) Item nonresponse on the Myeloproliferative Neoplasms Symptom Assessment Form (MPN-SAF): a comparison of missing data strategies. Leuk Lymphoma 60:1789–1795

Mercieca-Bebber R, Palmer MJ, Brundage M, Calvert M, Stockler MR, King MT (2016) Design, implementation and reporting strategies to reduce the instance and impact of missing patient-reported outcome (PRO) data: a systematic review. BMJ Open 6:e010938

Norman G (2010) Likert scales, levels of measurement and the "laws" of statistics. Adv Health Sci Educ Theory Pract 15:625–632

Pakhomov S, Jacobsen SJ, Chute CG, Roger VL (2008) Agreement between patient-reported symptoms and their documentation in the medical record. Am J Manag Care 14:530–539

Ratitch B, O'Kelly M, Tosiello R (2013) Missing data in clinical trials: from clinical assumptions to statistical analysis using pattern mixture models. Pharm Stat 12:337–347

Reeve BB, Hays RD, Bjorner JB et al (2007) Psychometric evaluation and calibration of health-related quality of life item banks: plans for the Patient-Reported Outcomes Measurement Information System (PROMIS). Med Care 45:S22–S31

Rubin DB (1976) Inference and missing data. Biometrika 63:581–592

Sagarin BJ, West SG, Ratnikov A, Homan WK, Ritchie TD, Hansen EJ (2014) Treatment non-compliance in randomized experiments: statistical approaches and design issues. Psychol Methods 19:317–333

Schafer JL, Graham JW (2002) Missing data: our view of the state of the art. Psychol Methods 7:147–177

Snyder CF, Smith KC, Bantug ET et al (2017) What do these scores mean? Presenting patient-reported outcomes data to patients and clinicians to improve interpretability. Cancer 123:1848–1859

Sullivan LM, D'Agostino RB (2003) Robustness and power of analysis of covariance applied to ordinal scaled data as arising in randomized controlled trials. Stat Med 22:1317–1334

Tan WW, Dueck AC, Flynn P et al (2013) N0539 phase II trial of fulvestrant and bevacizumab in patients with metastatic breast cancer previously treated with an aromatase inhibitor: a North Central Cancer Treatment Group (now Alliance) trial. Ann Oncol 24:2548–2554

Unger JM, Griffin K, Donaldson GW et al (2017) Patient-reported outcomes for patients with metastatic castration-resistant prostate cancer receiving docetaxel and Atrasentan versus docetaxel and placebo in a randomized phase III clinical trial (SWOG S0421). J Patient Rep Outcomes 2:27

Verstovsek S, Mesa RA, Gotlib J et al (2012) A double-blind, placebo-controlled trial of ruxolitinib for myelofibrosis. N Engl J Med 366:799–807

Vickers AJ (2001) The use of percentage change from baseline as an outcome in a controlled trial is statistically inefficient: a simulation study. BMC Med Res Methodol 1:6

White IR, Horton NJ, Carpenter J, Pocock SJ (2011) Strategy for intention to treat analysis in randomised trials with missing outcome data. BMJ 342:d40

Wyrwich KW, Norquist JM, Lenderking WR, Acaster S, Industry Advisory Committee of International Society for Quality of Life Research (2013) Methods for interpreting change over time in patient-reported outcome measures. Qual Life Res 22:475–483

Adherence Adjusted Estimates in Randomized Clinical Trials

93

Sreelatha Meleth

Contents

Introduction	1834
Potential Outcomes and Causal Models	1836
Neyman's Contribution	1836
Rubin's Causal Model	1837
Assumptions in the RCM	1838
Applications of Rubin's Causal Model	1840
Direct Application of RCM	1840
Structural Mean Model Approach	1841
CACE for Dichotomous Outcomes	1842
Software	1843
Maximum Likelihood (MLE) Method	1843
Estimating CACE for Longitudinal Outcomes	1844
Survival Outcomes	1845
Bayesian Models in Causal Inference	1846
Validity of Assumptions	1846
Limitations in the Literature	1848
Summary and Conclusion	1848
Key Facts	1848
Cross-References	1849
References	1849

Abstract

Randomized clinical trials (RCTs) are considered the gold standard for establishing the efficacy of an intervention. This is because randomizing patients to the different arms of an intervention ensures that the distributions of observed and unobserved confounders in the arms are the same. As a result, any differences in outcomes can be attributed to the difference in interventions. However, this

S. Meleth (✉)
RTI International, Atlanta, GA, USA
e-mail: smeleth@rti.org

© Springer Nature Switzerland AG 2022
S. Piantadosi, C. L. Meinert (eds.), *Principles and Practice of Clinical Trials*,
https://doi.org/10.1007/978-3-319-52636-2_124

advantage of randomization is lost when participants drop out, cross over to another treatment, or do not comply with the regimen. The traditional approach to the issue is to act as if randomization was maintained and analyze the data as intended in the design (intent to treat [ITT] analysis). However, the inference based on the ITT provides information on the prescription of the intervention rather than its use. Other approaches, such as looking at differences in outcome in those treated per protocol, are problematic because of the high risk of imbalance in measured and unmeasured confounders whose distribution cannot be assumed to be similar across arms because the randomization does not hold.

Using the potential outcome concept first published by Neyman, Rubin developed what has come to be known as Rubin's causal model (RCM) to address these issues. This chapter is a brief overview of the application of the RCM to the problem of poor adherence to treatment in RCTs. It provides existing solutions from the literature for most types of data that a researcher will encounter. It also looks at the validity of the assumptions of the RCM.

Keywords

RCTs · Noncompliance · CACE · Adherence adjusted estimates · Causal models · Rubin's causal models

Introduction

Is an intent to treat analysis always (ever) enough? Sheiner (2002) asked this question in a presentation he made at the Clinical Measurement and Drug Development meeting conducted by the Royal Society of Edinburgh.

After setting up the elements of the Rubin's causal model (described below), Sheiner discussed the difference between "method effectiveness" and "use effectiveness." The former he defines as the causal effect of a patient taking the drug and the latter as the causal effect of prescribing the drug. These terms are also often referred to as efficacy versus effectiveness (Fischer and White 2012), or biological efficacy versus programmatic effectiveness (Sommer and Zeger 1991). Because the stated purpose of a randomized clinical trial (RCT) that is testing a pharmacological agent is to determine the biological efficacy of a drug, Sheiner (2002) suggested that method effectiveness is a more important population attribute than use effectiveness.

The argument about which of these estimates is more relevant arises because for almost all RCTs, adherence to assigned treatment is never 100%. Participant noncompliance and dropout are common problems. This means that the distribution of measured and unmeasured confounders is not the same in both arms, and the very premise that everything in both arms being equal except for the pharmacological agent (or other intervention) is violated. The traditional response to this problem has been to maintain the randomization at baseline and – regardless of actual exposure – to measure the difference in outcomes as all participants had complied or as the original intention to treat. Lachin (2000) and Begg (2000) make forceful arguments about the primacy of intent to treat (ITT) analysis to avoid bias but also point out that noncompliance and dropout are study design issues that need to be addressed much earlier than during data analysis. However, the problem of not being able to get a good estimate of the efficacy of a treatment is a real-world issue, and most RCTs address this by supplementing the ITT analysis with a per protocol analysis in which the difference in outcomes based on the actual protocol followed is estimated. The issue with this estimate is that it is subject to selection bias because the two groups being compared are not equal in terms of known and unknown confounders as the random assignment is no longer valid.

The increasing cost of pharmacological trials, especially large phase 3 trials that are designed to provide a definitive answer about the efficacy of a drug, and the interest in maximizing the information obtained from an expensive RCT has resulted in a resurgence of interest in alternatives to ITT and per protocol estimates (Fischer and White 2012).

It is important to note that there is no suggestion in the relevant literature or in this chapter that ITT analysis should be replaced with the methods discussed. The effort is to supplement the ITT with estimates that maintain the advantages of randomization and provide additional information that can be used to develop policies. These methods move the focus from statistical inference to causal inference.

Traditionally, epidemiologists and statisticians have shied away from asserting causality especially based on a single study. Correlation does not equal causality is a mantra learned in the earliest courses on statistics with many examples that demonstrate the ridiculousness of attributing cause based purely on an association, for example, Pearl (2009) uses the fact that ice cream sales and murders both go up in the summer and therefore are correlated but clearly one cannot attribute increased murders to increased ice cream sales. The problem is that most of the time the discussion of causation typically ends with the discussion of situations where one cannot attribute cause and almost never crosses over to the discussion of how to assign cause.

RCTs are experiments in which all factors except the intervention under question are kept constant or equal across groups using techniques such as randomization. Therefore, changes in the outcome of interest can be causally attributed to the intervention. This is true even though the literature rarely uses the word "cause" in the context of the results from a single RCT. Attribution of cause and causal models' enter the discussion of adherence adjusted estimates because all the models used to estimate treatment effects from RCTs in the presence of noncompliance use the theory of causal models.

Causality is a topic that has been addressed by Hume in philosophy (Holland 1986), Hill in epidemiology (Hofler 2005), and many authors in statistics (Neyman 1923 [Dabrowska and Speed 1990]; Pearl 2009; Rubin 1990). Given the interest in obtaining effect estimates in the presence of nonadherence, the first section of this chapter focuses on the statistical literature on causal effects. This discussion of causal inference begins with Neyman's contribution (Dabrowska and Speed 1990); demonstrates how Rubin (1990) expanded it to what is now called the Rubin's causal model (RCM); and demonstrates through example how the RCM has been used to estimate adherence adjusted treatment effects. Validity of the assumptions and limitations in the existing approach are also discussed.

The chapter is not a comprehensive overview of adherence adjusted estimates. There is a burgeoning amount of literature in the area. In particular, Judea Pearl's approach to causal models is not discussed here. Pearl's (2009) theory of causal effects uses the structural causal model (SCM), which combines structural equation models, the potential outcome framework introduced by Neyman and developed by Rubin (1990), and Pearl's causal models to bring together the various models developed in the area of adherence adjusted estimates. His methods are particularly useful when designing an RCT to determine causal paths, confounders, identifiability of the estimates in the presence of noncompliance, and other factors. However, Pearl's theory involves a combination of SCMs and directed acrylic graphs and requires a fair amount of foundational explanations, putting it beyond the scope of this chapter.

Potential Outcomes and Causal Models

Neyman's Contribution

The concept of "potential outcomes" is core to the statistical development of causal models. Although other researchers had previously alluded to potential outcomes, Jerzy Neyman is credited with formalizing the notion of potential versus observed outcomes (Dabrowska and Speed 1990; Rubin 1990). He introduced the concept with respect to agricultural yield. He developed the notation U_{ik} to represent the agricultural yield from plot i when subject to seed/crop variety k. The set

$$U = \{U_{ik}; i = 1 \text{ to } v; k = 1 \text{ to } m\}$$

represents the potential yield (outcome) that is treated as a priori fixed but unknown. The best estimate of the yield from plot i, U_i is the average yield in plot U_i across all seed varieties or

$$a_i = \sum_{k=1}^{m} U_{ik}/m.$$

In reality, plot U_i will be exposed to a single variety. However, if it were exposed to all varieties and the researchers were interested in the differences in yield between variety k_i and k_j, the causal effect of changing from treatment k_i to treatment k_j would be estimated by the difference, $a_{k_i} - a_{k_j}$. Neyman (Dabrowska and Speed 1990) proved that in a completely randomized experiment with n_i units exposed to k_i and n_j units exposed to treatment k_j that the difference of averages in the two groups, $\overline{Y}_i - \overline{Y}_j$ is an unbiased estimate of the causal estimand, $a_{k_i} - a_{k_j}$. He also showed that the usual estimate of variance of the difference between two sample means is positively biased. The important conceptual difference in the interpretation of differences in mean outcomes between two treatment groups in an RCT is that when one is treating it as a causal estimate, it is an estimate of the average difference between the observed outcome and potential outcome for the same unit. In other words, it is the causal treatment effect for unit i even though in any experiment, the researcher can only observe one of those outcomes.

This inability to observe the outcomes of multiple treatments in the same unit is called the fundamental problem of causal inference (FPCI). While statistical inference can be improved by increased sample size, even an infinite sample will not resolve this issue of causal inference. Rubin resolves this problem in RCTs by treating the unobservability of the counterfactual outcomes for a unit as a missing data problem and assuming that compliance is a latent trait that is equally distributed across arms by virtue of randomization.

Rubin's Causal Model

Rubin extended Neyman's results to develop the Rubin's causal model of inference. The RCM has been used extensively in the literature that seeks to estimate treatment effects in the presence of noncompliance to treatment.

Little and Rubin (2000) provide a good overview of the thinking behind the causal model and its application to randomized experiments and observational studies. One factor not clearly addressed by Neyman, but clarified by the RCM, is the need to restrict the number of potential outcomes to be able to estimate the causal effect. If the potential outcome of one unit in a population could affect the potential outcome of other units, then even in experiments with just two units and two treatments, we are faced with four potential outcomes – $Y(11)$, $Y(12)$, $Y(21)$, and $Y(22)$ – where $Y(jk)$ is the outcome when the first individual receives treatment j and the second receives treatment k. As the number of subjects increases, this number will increase exponentially. To avoid this problem, Rubin stipulated that the causal effect for one individual cannot depend on the treatment assignments to other individuals. Therefore, if an experiment has two treatments, individual i has only two potential outcomes: the outcome with treatment i and the outcome with treatment j. Additionally, Rubin also said that to assign cause to the treatment of interest, one has to assume that there can be no hidden treatments affecting the outcome. These two assumptions form the stable unit treatment value assumption (SUTVA), though SUTVA cannot be verified from the data.

Randomization is the factor in RCTs that can help practitioners derive the causal effect of treatment. Random assignment implies that each unit has the same chance of receiving each possible treatment being tested and that the probability of one unit receiving a treatment is independent of the probability of any other unit receiving the treatment. Randomization means that the outcomes are not related to assignment. This independence of outcomes and assignment mechanism also allows researchers to assume that the average effect of the treatment $s = t$ over everyone in population U is the same as the average outcome of the people in U who were exposed to treatment s = t, where S(t, c) represents a treatment with (t = treatment, c = control). In other words,

$$E(Y_t) = E(Y_t \mid S = t)$$

This in turn allows the use of Neyman's derivation that the difference in average effects provides an unbiased estimate of the average treatment effect for unit u over all of U (Holland 1986). If randomization is maintained with no dropouts, crossovers, or other types of noncompliance during the conduct of the RCT, then the typical ITT estimate is an unbiased estimate of causal effect of treatment.

Before moving into the use of the RCM to estimate adherence adjusted estimates, it is useful to distinguish associational/statistical inference from causal inference. Holland (1986) distinguishes statistical models used to draw associational inference from statistical models used to draw causal inference. The table below summarizes the difference in the two approaches. Although, the difference in average effect in treatment groups is commonly estimated in most statistical models that estimate treatment effects in RCTs, as mentioned above, it is important to distinguish the two estimates conceptually.

Associational inference	Causal inference
Two observable variables, Y and A	Two observable variables, S and Y_s
A and Y are simply variables defined for all units in population U	S and Y_s are more complicated. S represents a cause (treatment) that is potentially exposable to all units in U, and S = t or c. Y_s is a post-exposure variable
Deals with joint conditional distributions of Y and A. A typical associational parameter is the regression of Y on A, i.e., the conditional expectation $E(Y \mid A = a)$	Concerned with $Y_t - Y_c$
Almost always involves statistical estimates that can be improved with larger sample sizes, and in the limit the estimate in an infinite population will be exact	Proceeds from observed values of treatment and outcomes and is based on assumptions that address the FPCI that are typically untestable. Increasing sample size cannot address the FPCI
	Need not involve statistical inference

Assumptions in the RCM

The RCM is based on the following four assumptions:

1. **SUTVA** (Rubin 1990) is a primary and essential assumption in the RCM. It consists of two sub-assumptions. First, there is no interference between unit

effects, that is, neither $Y_i(1)$ nor $Y_i(0)$ is affected by what action (treatment) any other unit received. Second, there are no hidden versions of treatments. In other words, the only effect observed is that of the treatment under observation no matter how unit i received treatment 1. The outcome that would be observed would be $Y_i(1)$, and the same is true for treatment 0.

2. **Constant effect** assumes that the effect of the treatment on any unit in the population is the same. This means if T is the treatment effect for unit u in population U, t is treatment, and c is control, then for all u in U,

$$T = Y_t(u) - Y_c(u)$$

3. **Exclusion restrictions** are often invoked to help derive causal estimates. Fischer and White (2012) describe the three levels of an exclusion restriction assumption. The most stringent is the strong exclusion restriction, which says that

$$P[(Y_u(t) = Y_u(c) \mid Z_i(t) = Z_i(c)] = 1$$

The Y here represents outcomes for unit i, and the Z represents actual exposure to treatment. This emphasizes the sub-assumption in SUTVA that there are no hidden causes. If the treatment exposure in the treatment arm and control arm is identical, then the outcomes are identical with probability of one. If there is no exposure to treatment, then the treatment effect is zero. A less stringent version, called the mean exclusion criterion, says that this would be true on average, that is, the average difference of outcomes would be zero given identical exposure levels and baseline covariates

$$E\left[(Y_u(t) - Y_u(c) \mid Z_u(t) = Z_u(c), X_u\right] = 0$$

The mean zero-exclusion criterion states that if there is zero exposure, then on average the treatment effect would be zero, given known exposure levels and baseline covariates

$$E\left[(Y_u(t) - Y_u(c) \mid Z_u(t) = Z_i(c) = 0, X_u\right] = 0$$

4. **Complier traits** describe four types of compliers in a population. As discussed above, the problem with noncompliance is that the assumption that every unit has the same probability of exposure to the same predetermined level of treatment is no longer justifiable and the ITT then becomes an estimate of prescribing a treatment rather than experiencing the treatment. Rubin resolved this issue by developing the notion of four compliance types in a population:

(a) **Always taker** will always opt for the active treatment whether assigned to it or not.
(b) **Never taker** never opts for the active treatment whether assigned to it or not.
(c) **Complier** always complies with the assigned treatment.
(d) **Defier** takes the control treatment if assigned to active and active treatment if assigned to control.

The characteristics of whether a person complies with the treatment is considered an unchangeable trait and therefore balanced across treatment groups by randomization. Although Rubin defined the defier as a possible compliance type, most RCM models assume that there are no defiers in the sample. This assumption is called the monotonicity assumption and ensures that the likelihood of getting treatment can only increase with treatment assignment, it will not decrease likelihood of receiving treatment. Based on these assumptions, the causal effect of treatment is estimated as the treatment effect in the subgroup of compliers. This effect is also called the complier average causal effect (CACE). The CACE is not meant to replace the ITT estimate. However, the CACE can give more information about the efficacy of the drug.

Applications of Rubin's Causal Model

This section describes several ways to estimate CACE. It also highlights some conditions in which the assumptions of the RCM may not be valid. The assumptions of RCM are primarily functions of design and cannot be tested with information from the data. Any inference from CACE should therefore be accompanied with a thorough discussion of whether the assumptions are valid.

Direct Application of RCM

In the simplest version of estimating CACE, let the frequency of never takers, compliers, and always takers in the population be w_n, w_c, and w_a. These proportions are estimated from the observed proportions as follows:

w_n = the proportion of participants in the active treatment arm who do not receive treatment.

w_a = the proportion of participants assigned to control who receive active treatment.

w_c = the proportion of participants in both arms that comply with assigned treatment = $1 - w_n - w_a$.

Never takers in both groups have mean outcome μ_n. Always takers in both groups have mean outcome μ_a. Compliers have means that depend on assignment, so μ_T or μ_C. The difference in means in the never takers group and the always takers group is zero and the difference between the average outcome in experimental and control groups; in other words, the ITT estimate then reduces to $w_c (\mu_T - \mu_C)$. The CACE, that is the difference in mean outcome between compliers $\mu_T - \mu_C$, can then be estimated as the ITT/w_c. Note that the randomization is maintained in this estimation. The instrumental variable (IV) approach described in Bloom (1984), Little and Yau (1998), Fischer and White (2012), and Maracy and Dunn (2011) all result in a similar estimate for CACE. There is a SAS macro (Houck and Mazumdar 2010) based on the IV method described by Maracy and Dunn. The Fischer and White (2012) approach is described below.

Structural Mean Model Approach

Fischer and White (2012) use structural mean models (SMM) to derive adherence adjusted ITT effects. They combine the randomization assumption and the exclusion restriction assumption to derive the estimate. The randomization assumption can be expressed as

$$Y_i(0), Y_i(1), Z_i(0), Z_i(1) \perp R_i \mid X_i$$

$Y_i(0)$, $Y_i(1)$ represent potential outcome for individual i when exposed to control and experimental treatment, respectively. Z represents exposure to experimental treatment. Thus, $Z_i(0)$ represents exposure to experimental treatment when assigned to control, and $Z_i(1)$ represents exposure to experimental treatment when assigned to the experimental treatment arm.

The equation above posits that randomization creates two comparable groups with respect to all observed and unobserved characteristics. As stated earlier, with noncompliance, the independence of outcomes to assignment cannot be assumed. However, one can use an SMM to define the adherence adjusted effect conditional on the compliance information and covariates, such as

$$E\left(Y_i(1) - Y_i(0) \mid Z_i(1), Z_i(0), X_i\right) = \gamma(Z_i(1), Z_i(0), X_i; \varphi)$$

The γ is a known function of the potential treatment exposures under the two assignments, baseline characteristics, and an unknown parameter vector φ. The aim of the analysis then, is to estimate the parameters in φ. A linear SMM could be expressed as

$$E\left(Y_i(1) - Y_i(0) \mid Z_i(1), Z_i(0), X_i\right) = \varphi^1 Z_i(1) - \varphi^0 Z_i(0)$$

The φ^1 and φ^0 here represent the treatment effect in the experimental treatment arm and effect of exposure to treatment in the control arm, respectively. This equation is consistent with the mean zero-exclusion restriction assumption, which states that the average treatment effect if there is no exposure to treatment is zero. In other words, that given assignment and covariates, the average difference in treatment effects is completely defined by the difference in exposure to experimental treatment in the two arms.

This can be simplified further so that the effect of treatment is the same for the same exposure, and then invoke the mean exclusion restriction, which states that identical exposure to the treatment in either arm results in identical treatment effect or that the average effect is zero for all subjects who receive the same dose of treatment. The equation above then simplifies to

$$E\left(Y_i(1) - Y_i(0) | Z_i(1), Z_i(0), X_i\right) = \varphi[(Z_i(1) - Z_i(0)]$$

Further simplification of this equation results in a single-parameter CACE estimate that is essentially the estimate derived above:

$$\varphi = \frac{\bar{y}_1 - \bar{y}_0}{\bar{z}_1 - \bar{z}_0}$$

They also describe a two-stage least squares approach to estimate φ. In the first stage, outcome and exposure variables are regressed on baseline covariates in each arm separately to get predicted values $\hat{Y}_i(0), \hat{Y}_i(1), \hat{Z}_i(0),$ and $\hat{Z}_i(1)$. In the second stage, $\hat{Y}_i(1) - \hat{Y}_i(0)$ is regressed on $\hat{Z}_i(1) - \hat{Z}_i(0)$ to get an estimate of φ.

Further, they derive a two-parameter model based on the mean zero-exclusion restriction. In this case $\varphi^0 = \partial + \varphi$; where $\varphi^1 = \varphi$. This is particularly relevant in trials that have two active treatments because in that case there is no zero effect due to zero treatment exposure. The equation then simplifies to

$$\frac{\bar{Y}_1 - \bar{Y}_0}{\bar{Z}_1 - \bar{Z}_0} = \varphi + \delta \frac{\bar{Z}_0}{\bar{Z}_1 - \bar{Z}_0}$$

For linear models, the difference in effect can also be estimated using a two-stage least squares procedure. Baseline covariates can be used in each arm as described above to get predicted values in stage one and in stage two. The difference $\hat{Y}_i(1) - \hat{Y}_0(0)$ is regressed on $\hat{Z}_i(1)$ and $\hat{Z}_i(0)$ without intercepts to estimate the parameters φ and $\varphi + \delta$. In a different publication, Fischer et al. (2011) show that the difference in the effect in the two arms with active treatment can be estimated without bias, even though the estimates of effects in the two arms may be biased.

CACE for Dichotomous Outcomes

Sommer and Zeger (1991) applied principles of the RCM to a community-based randomized trial in Indonesia that sought to establish the efficacy of vitamin A in reducing mortality in preschool children. The authors derived a relative risk

(RR) among compliers, which they called an efficacy RR that they argue is different from the program effectiveness RR derived using the ITT analysis. The program effectiveness suggested a 40% reduction in deaths in the group that received vitamin A. However, more than 20% of the villages randomized to receive vitamin A did not receive it. The mortality rate in the noncompliant villages was much lower than the rate in the placebo groups, so estimating biologic efficacy based on just those who received the treatment would overestimate the efficacy. Sommer and Zeger (1991) use the assumptions of RCM to derive the efficacy RR.

Specifically, they assume that (1) both groups have the same expected rate of compliance and (2) that the noncompliant groups in both arms would have the same mortality rate. The efficacy RR they derived was

$$\widetilde{R} = n_{11} \Big/ \left(m_1 \frac{M}{N} - n_{10} \right)$$

Where n_{11} represents the number of deaths in the treated compliers; n_{10} represents number of the deaths in the treated noncompliers; m_1 is the total number of deaths in the control group; M is the total of all controls; and N is the total of all treated. The efficacy estimate is a ratio of the observed to the expected mortality in the compliant groups. The variance is estimated using the delta method.

The typical RR if compliance were perfect would be

$$\widehat{R} = \frac{n_{11}}{n_{01}+n_{11}} \Big/ \frac{m_{11}}{m_{01}+m_{11}}$$

Software

The formula is easy to estimate using SAS or STATA. The variance is estimated using the delta methods for which there are multiple methods in SAS based on the model being used.

Maximum Likelihood (MLE) Method

The MLE version of CACE is derived using the assumptions of RCM and the three types of compliers and developing a likelihood equation for always takers, never takers, and compliers. The monotonicity assumption that is part of almost all RCM models means that there are no defiers in the likelihood equation. This results in a likelihood equation (Little and Yau 1998) that models the likelihood for each type of complier. The additional distributional assumption here is that the treatment effects are normally distributed, with different treatment effects but the same variance. This likelihood equation can also be used to extend CACE to models with other distributions.

MLE estimates are computed using the expectation-maximization (EM) algorithm (Dempster et al. 1977), treating compliance indicators C_i as missing data. CACE is then estimated as

$$\partial_c = \mu_{c1} - \mu_{c0}$$

The EM algorithm can be implemented in all the commonly used statistical software.

Little and Yau (1998) develops MLE models with and without covariates to estimate CACE for an intervention that tested the efficacy of a job training program in preventing the deterioration of mental health as a result of job loss and facilitating high-quality reemployment. The intervention arm was exposed to a 5-day workshop, and the control arm received brochures about the job search process. About 46% of the subjects who were randomized to the seminar did not show up and were treated as noncompliers. As the jobs seminar was only available to those randomized to the intervention, there were no always takers in this group by design. There were also no defiers.

The MLE model without covariates was

$$y_i = \beta_0 + \beta_c C_i + \beta_{CR} C_i R_i + \epsilon_i$$

β_0 is the estimated mean for never takers; $\beta_0 + \beta_c$ is the estimated treatment effect for the compliers in the control group; $\beta_0 + \beta_c + \beta_{CR}$ is the treatment effect for compliers in the treatment group; and β_{CR} is the CACE.

The corresponding model with covariates is

$$y_i = \beta_0 + \beta_c + \beta_c C_i + \beta_{CR} C_i R_i + \beta_X^T X_{Y_i} + (\beta_{CX}^T X_{Y_i}) C_i + (\beta_{CRX}^T X_{Y_i}) C_i R_i + \varepsilon_i$$

$\beta_0 + \beta_{CX}^T X_{Y_i}$ is the mean outcome for compliers with covariates X_y; $\beta_c + \beta_{CX}^T X_Y$ is the mean difference in outcome between control compliers and noncompliers; and $\beta_{CR} + \beta_{CRX}^T X_Y$ is the compliers averaged causal estimate. Compliance C_i is estimated using a logistic regression model that used baseline covariates to predict compliance. The EM algorithm is used to estimate unobserved compliance, estimate the parameters of the model above, and then iterating until convergence.

EM can be implemented in SAS and STATA.

Estimating CACE for Longitudinal Outcomes

Yau and Little (2001) extended the CACE model developed above to estimate CACE in the longitudinal setting using MLE. The model is an extension of a linear mixed model with $y_{i,t}$ the outcome for subject i at time t compliance C_i, random assignment R_i, and fixed baseline covariates X_{Y_i} that predict $y_{i.}$. The model is in the following form:

$$E(y_{it}) = \beta_{0,t} + \beta_{C,t}C_i + \beta_{CR,t}C_iR_i + \beta_{X,t}^T X_{Y_i} + \beta_{CX,t}^T C_i X_{Y_i} + \beta_{CRC,t}^T C_i R_i X_{Y_i}$$

Per this model, the CACE is $\beta_{CR,t} + \beta_{CRX,t}^T X_{Y_i}$.

Yau and Little (2001) have extensive directions in their appendix on implementing the EM algorithm to obtain these estimates. As in the cross-sectional model above, compliance is predicted with a logistic model using baseline predictors and the EM algorithm is applied. These models can be fit using standard statistical software in SAS, STATA, or R.

Survival Outcomes

Kim and White (2004) describe deriving compliance adjusted estimates for survival data using proportional hazards regressions. Individuals in the control arm are treated as compliers and noncompliers according to how they would have behaved if they had been randomized to treatment. The proportion of noncompliers α is the same in both arms per Rubin's definition. Let the probability of survival to time t be $S_{n0}(t)$ and $S_{c0}(t)$ for the noncompliers and compliers in the control group, respectively, and the probability of survival to time t as $S_{n1}(t)$ and $S_{c1}(t)$ for the noncompliers and compliers in the treatment group

$$S_j(t) = \alpha S_{nj} + (1 - \alpha) S_{cj}(t)$$

Given the exclusion restriction

$$S_{n0} = S_{n1}$$

The hazard ratio for compliers is ψ, so

$$S_{c0}(t) = S_{c1}(t)^{1/\psi}$$

Kaplan-Meier estimates of $S_{n1}(t)$ and $S_{c1}(t)$ are used to estimate CACE by solving for ψ in the equation. A value for ψ is one in which the survivor function below correctly predicts the observed number of events in the control arm

$$\widehat{S}_{c0}(t) = \widehat{\alpha}\widehat{S}_{n1} + (1 - \widehat{\alpha})\widehat{S}_{c1}(t)^{1/\psi}$$

STCOMPLY in STATA fits the proportional hazards regression (PHREG) model and estimates the CACE for the hazard.

Bayesian Models in Causal Inference

Imbens and Rubin (1997) developed Bayesian models to estimate CACE. The Bayesian approach to causal inference is framed in terms of the potential outcomes, in other words, responses to all treatments. The Bayesian approach (Imbens and Rubin 1997) uses parametric models to develop parametric inferences for causal estimates. The EM algorithm, data augmentation, or Markov chain processes are used to estimate posterior distributions. The assumptions and the concept of CACE are the same in these models as described above.

Besides CACE, compliance has also been used as a variable in models as a predictor of the outcome. An example of this is a paper by Efron and Feldman (1991). Using compliance as an explanatory variable, the authors proposed using the compliance measure to recover the "true dose-response" effect. They considered a patient's response to a placebo and a patient's compliance (measured as a proportion of the assigned dose) as an inherent property (trait) of a patient. In this sense, this approach is based on the RCM above that assumes that randomization would distribute compliance traits equally across the various arms in an RCT.

Efron and Feldman (1991) suggest that an individual's response to dose x for a drug equals the sum of the average response at dose x plus the individual's response to placebo plus the excess effect above placebo for the individual plus error. If there is no interaction between the dose and placebo effect, then the dose response will be the same as the compliance response.

The equation derived by Efron and Feldman (1991) is not strictly relevant to estimation treatment effects based on compliance; however, it is a good example of ways in which the assumptions of RCM have been used to utilize measured compliance to derive more information from an RCT. Standard regression software such as SAS, STATA, and others can be used to fit the Efron and Feldman (1991) model.

Validity of Assumptions

As mentioned earlier, the assumptions in the RCM are not verifiable from the data. This can only be done with knowledge of the science. The discussion below demonstrates cases in which the assumptions may be questionable and one example of a trial in which all the assumptions are met.

Sommer and Zeger (1991) point out two sources of bias in their CACE estimates for placebo-controlled trials. They both relate to the SUTVA assumption and its validity and to some extent the assumption of the compliance type as a trait that randomization distributes equally. The first is the potential that the placebo and experimental treatment may have different effect profiles, which in turn would affect compliance in the two arms differently, resulting in differing compliance profiles in the two arms. The second is that the causal effect of treatment is valid as a pure causal effect only if the assumption that there is no other cause that affects the outcome is valid. The latter is a violation of SUTVA, and the former questions the assumption that there are latent compliance traits in the population.

Little and Yau (1998) also discuss the validity of the SUTVA and the exclusion restriction assumption in an application of the models. They point out that SUTVA might be violated in this case if an influential member in the job training workshop group they studied affected how the others in the group feel and react; therefore, the potential outcomes in a group would be affected by this influencer. The exclusion restriction may also be violated here if randomization to the workshop group resulted in demoralization and therefore affected a participant's depression scores but randomization to the control group may not have. Once again, estimating CACE may be easy in these models, but assessing if the assumptions of CACE are valid is more difficult and one cannot correct for a violated assumption in an RCM.

As with the cross-sectional analysis of the job training data, for the reasons stated above, neither SUTVA nor independence of outcome from treatment assigned may be valid in the Yau and Little (2001) extension of the MLE approach to a longitudinal outcome.

Becque et al. (2015) extended Yau and Little's longitudinal models to incorporate time-varying treatment and transient treatment effects in a trial that randomized children with a condition called glue ear to surgery to insert ventilation tubes or nonsurgical management. The primary outcome was hearing loss. By the end of the trial, 54% of the children randomized to control had the surgery. The extension of the Little and Yau model to accommodate changing compliance over time is well developed in the paper and is not described here. It is however instructive to look at the validity of the assumptions of the RCM in this trial. SUTVA holds because the hearing loss of one participant does not affect the hearing loss of another; the exclusion restriction means that treatment assignment is unrelated to potential outcomes given treatment received. This is plausible in this study because outcome only depends on the time since receiving treatment and compliance. The no defiers assumption is also valid here because everyone who offered treatment took it. This study is thus an example of a study where all assumptions of the RCM are met.

Rubin questioned the assumption in Efron and Feldman's paper (1991) that the treatment response in excess of the expected placebo response could be considered a trait in this trial (Rubin 1991). His argument was that given the side effects of the treatment tested in the trial that Efron and Feldman (1991) used as the application for the method, the compliance to the treatment was most likely a function of multiple characteristics such as age, previous treatment, and others, and should not be assumed to be a trait. Thus, this example also illustrates the difficulty in knowing when the assumptions of the RCM are violated and more importantly that it is possible that the compliance types might vary based on the intervention being tested.

As in most models that apply concepts of the RCM, it is the interpretation of the effect based on the assumption of the model that is important.

Limitations in the Literature

It is important to note that compliance in these examples is assumed to be all or nothing. Although Sommer and Zeger (1991) discuss extending the model to continuous compliance measures, almost all the causal inference literature is based on all or nothing compliance.

Noncompliance in trials can also take multiple forms. A participant might drop out, cross over, be partially compliant, or be completely noncompliant. Rubin's four compliance types ignore this complexity. Conceptually, one could extend the four categories suggested by Rubin to different patterns of compliance, like different patterns of missing, and potentially define a causal effect for each pattern subpopulation, although this can become exponentially complicated quickly.

Summary and Conclusion

Noncompliance in RCTs is an issue that needs to be addressed. Ideally, it should be addressed at the design stage, but even the most thoughtfully designed RCT does not result in 100% compliance to the intervention. In an RCT that has cross over from one arm to the other, drop out, and poor adherence to treatment but also had a subgroup of individuals who were completely compliant, one could argue that the compliant group is qualitatively different from the rest of the sample and also that it is this group of participants that Rubin thinks of as compliers and that assumption that this quality of compliance is a trait is reasonable.

As the discussion about the validity of the assumptions of the RCM shows, these methods cannot be applied to every trial. There are several other researchers who have developed methods using potential outcomes. As mentioned above, Pearl (2009) is one of them. Robins (1994) has also contributed significantly to the concept of counterfactual (potential) outcomes and applied it to multiple trials.

As is evident, the area of adherence adjusted estimates is an active area of research with great potential.

Key Facts

- Although RCTs are considered the gold standard for research, poor compliance takes away this advantage.
- Typical approaches to the issue of noncompliance, such as per protocol analysis or as-treated analysis, are problematic because of the issue of selection bias, which nullifies the advantage of the randomization.
- The RCM is one way to estimate the causal effect of treatment without losing the advantage of randomization.
- The assumptions of the RCM may not be met in many interventions, and its application should be done judiciously.
- Several other approaches to estimating adherence adjusted estimates exist, but the RCM and its extensions are most frequently seen in the literature.

Cross-References

▶ Administration of Study Treatments and Participant Follow-Up
▶ Implementing the Trial Protocol
▶ Intention to Treat and Alternative Approaches

References

Becque T, White IR, Haggard M (2015) A causal model for longitudinal randomised trials with time-dependent non-compliance. Stat Med 34:2019–2034. https://doi.org/10.1002/sim.6468

Begg CB (2000) Ruminations on the intent-to-treat principle. Control Clin Trials 21:241–243

Bloom HS (1984) Accounting for no-shows in experimental evaluation designs. Eval Rev 8:225–246. https://doi.org/10.1177/0193841X8400800205

Dabrowska DM, Speed TP (translators) (1990) On the application of probability theory to agricultural experiments. Essay on principles. Section 9. Stat Sci 5:465–480. (original reference: Neyman, J [1923] Toczniki Nauk Rolniczych Tom X 1–51)

Dempster AP, Laird NM, Rubin DB (1977) Maximum likelihood from incomplete data via the EM algorithm. J R Stat Soc B (Methodol) 39:1–38

Efron B, Feldman D (1991) Compliance as an explanatory variable in clinical trials. J Am Stat Assoc 86:9–17

Fischer K, White IR (2012) Causal inference in clinical trials. In: Berzuini C, Dawid P, Bernardinelli L (eds) Causality: statistical perspectives and applications. Wiley, New York, pp 310–326

Fischer K, Goetghebeur E, Vrijens B, White IR (2011) A structural mean model to allow for noncompliance in a randomized trial comparing 2 active treatments. Biostatistics 12:247–257. https://doi.org/10.1093/biostatistics/kxq053

Hofler M (2005) The Bradford hill considerations on causality: a counterfactual perspective. Emerg Themes Epidemiol 2(11):11. https://doi.org/10.1186/1742-7622-2-11

Holland PW (1986) Statistics and causal inference. J Am Stat Assoc 81:945–960

Houck PR, Mazumdar S (2010) Macro for computing complier-average causal effect of treatment (CACE) using instrumental variable method. SAS. https://pdfs.semanticscholar.org/787b/8bb918a34667a435744a2c71517d39605a96.pdf?_ga=2.192472618.1643882847.1574720806-2081442218.1574720806

Imbens GW, Rubin DB (1997) Bayesian inference for causal effects in randomized experiments with noncompliance. Ann Stat 25:305–327

Kim LG, White IR (2004) Compliance-adjusted intervention effects in survival data. Stata J 4:257–264

Lachin JM (2000) Statistical considerations in the intent-to-treat principle. Control Clin Trials 21:167–189. https://doi.org/10.1016/s0197-2456(00)00046-5

Little RJ, Rubin DB (2000) Causal effects in clinical and epidemiological studies via potential outcomes: concepts and analytical approaches. Annu Rev Public Health 21:121–145. https://doi.org/10.1146/annurev.publhealth.21.1.121

Little RJ, Yau LHY (1998) Statistical techniques for analyzing data from prevention trials: treatment of no-shows using Rubin's causal model. Psychol Methods 3:147–159. https://doi.org/10.1037/1082-989x.3.2.147

Maracy M, Dunn G (2011) Estimating dose-response effects in psychological treatment trials: the role of instrumental variables. Stat Methods Med Res 20:191–215. https://doi.org/10.1177/0962280208097243

Pearl J (2009) Causal inference in statistics: an overview. Statist Surv 3:96–146. https://doi.org/10.1214/09-SS057

Robins JM (1994) Correcting for non-compliance in randomized trials using structural nested mean models. Commun Stat Theory Methods 23:2379–2412. https://doi.org/10.1080/03610929408831393

Rubin DB (1990) [On the application of probability theory to agricultural experiments. Essay on principles. Section 9.] Comment: Neyman (1923) and causal inference in experiments and observational studies. Stat Sci 5:472–480. https://pdfs.semanticscholar.org/26dc/e7587310c481da4d3a8a4625bdcc64a5fe46.pdf

Rubin DB (1991) Compliance as an explanatory variable in clinical trials: comment: dose-response estimands. J Am Stat Assoc 86:22–24

Sheiner LB (2002) Is intent-to-treat analysis always (ever) enough? Br J Clin Pharmacol 54:203–211

Sommer A, Zeger SL (1991) On estimating efficacy from clinical trials. Stat Med 10:45–52

Yau LHY, Little RJ (2001) Inference for the complier-average causal effect from longitudinal data subject to noncompliance and missing data, with application to a job training assessment for the unemployed. J Am Stat Assoc 96:1232–1244. https://doi.org/10.1198/016214501753381887

Randomization and Permutation Tests

94

Vance W. Berger, Patrick Onghena, and J. Rosser Matthews

Contents

Introduction	1852
Permutation Tests Defined and Contrasted with Parametric Tests	1854
Generalized Permutation Tests	1856
Path Dependence	1858
A New Beginning	1859
Parametric Analyses: Mere Approximations or of Inherent Interest?	1860
The Wisdom of Using Approximations When They Are Not Needed	1862
A Proposal	1864
Summary and Conclusions	1865
Cross-References	1866
References	1866

Abstract

This chapter will address the decision to use permutation tests as opposed to parametric analyses in the context of between-group analysis in randomized clinical trials designed to evaluate a medical intervention. It is important to understand at the outset that permutation tests represent a means to an end, rather than an end unto themselves. It is not so much that one seeks to use permutation tests just for the sake of doing so but, rather, that one recognizes the severe

V. W. Berger (✉)
Biometry Research Group, National Cancer Institute, Rockville, MD, USA
e-mail: vb78c@nih.gov

P. Onghena
Faculty of Psychology and Educational Sciences, KU Leuven, Leuven, Belgium
e-mail: patrick.onghena@kuleuven.be

J. R. Matthews
General Dynamics Health Solutions, Defense and Veterans Brain Injury Center, Silver Spring, MD, USA
e-mail: john.matthews2@gdit.com

© Springer Nature Switzerland AG 2022
S. Piantadosi, C. L. Meinert (eds.), *Principles and Practice of Clinical Trials*, https://doi.org/10.1007/978-3-319-52636-2_129

deficiencies of parametric analyses and wishes to use some other type of analysis that does not similarly suffer from these drawbacks. When viewed in this context, *properly conducted* permutation tests are the solution to the problem of how to compare treatments without having to rely on assumptions that cannot possibly be true. We argue that the default position would clearly be the use of exact analyses and that the burden of proof would fall to those who would argue that the approximate analyses are just as good or, as is sometimes argued, even better.

Keywords

Approximations · Normality · Parametric analyses · Precautionary principle

Introduction

Randomized clinical trials are considered, with good reason, to be the most reliable of all primary study designs used for the evaluation of medical interventions. The rationale for this preference is that many biases that plague observational studies can be controlled, meaning either minimized or eliminated altogether, in randomized trials. In other words, there is a recognition that (1) medical studies are sufficiently important that every effort should be made to obtain results that will come as close as possible to representing the underlying truth and (2) randomized trials represent our best chance of doing so.

And yet it is misleading to paint with an overly broad brush and group all randomized trials together and classify them as providing best evidence. Randomized trials have the potential to minimize or eliminate many biases, but this potential is rarely realized in practice. Almost all trials are randomized in an improper manner that invites selection bias (Berger 2005), and this drawback alone renders randomized trials *as actually conducted in practice* more similar to observational studies than they are to the upper limit of what randomized trials can ideally be. Beyond this, trials are ruined by the use of pre-randomization run-in periods, an overreliance on surrogate endpoints, improper handling of missing data, data suppression, changes to the primary endpoint on the fly, and other similar problems. Each of these problems warrants serious consideration, and remedial measures will need to be taken before trial results can be accepted at face value. But this chapter is limited to yet another problem often seen in randomized trials, namely, the use of approximate analyses rather than the very analyses they are trying to approximate, which themselves are readily available and can be obtained without the use of additional costs or resources.

For clarification, parametric analyses might be described more accurately as conditionally approximate (not to be confused with permutation tests which are conditional on the observed margins and often criticized on this basis), since they *would be* exact if all their assumptions held true. But distributional assumptions, such as normality, are at best incredibly implausible and at worst in direct conflict with the reality governing the data generation (Berger 2015).

For example, blood pressure measurements, weights, heights, and many other numerical variables measured in clinical trials cannot be negative; this alone precludes the possibility of their being normally distributed (Perlman et al. 2013). Although it may be difficult to specify a maximum attainable value for any of these variables, it is no great trick to specify a point beyond which these variables cannot go. Being bounded above is also a violation of normality, as is being discrete in nature (such as a Likert scale), rather than continuous. In fact, it is hard to imagine any actual medical variable, or residual, or sample mean, possessing the proper range for normality to be a possibility. But even if a continuous numerical variable *does* have an infinite range, and a bell shape, this in no way suggests that it possesses the *form* of an actual normal distribution, which is practically impossible to achieve and literally impossible to demonstrate, especially with a test that will generally lack power and will be set up in a backward manner that has normality specified as the null hypothesis and then claimed with failure to reject this null hypothesis. It is, in part, for this reason that Geary (1947) noted, correctly, that "Normality is a myth; there never was, and never will be, a normal distribution." In short, these data, which in a randomized clinical trial are almost never a random sample anyway, are *not* randomly drawn from a population which is normally distributed, even taking into consideration the central limit theorem.

Despite this unassailable fact, one often hears justifications for the use of normal-based models along the lines of normality being a useful model anyway, even if not technically and exactly describing the behavior of a variable that is close enough to being normally distributed, at least over the relevant range. But this justification is tantamount to an admission that an approximation is being used, which may or may not be accurate in any given case. To make matters worse, practitioners almost never check to see how good the approximation is, even though doing so would be straightforward, just by computing the exact p-value and comparing it to the approximate one. Berger (2017) did precisely this for a number of data sets chosen not to be representative but, rather, to make the point that, contrary to popular, and at times unstated, beliefs, the approximations are not, in fact, always close, even when the assumptions underlying their use appear to be valid. Berger (2000) noted the folly in assessing the discrepancy between the approximation and the true value indirectly, by assuming them to be true as a requirement for the approximation when we can just directly compute this discrepancy, with $\Delta = p1 - p2$ being the difference between the two p-values. The reality is that there is no check of an assumption that will ensure that Δ is small.

We will have more to say about the use of approximations in section "The Wisdom of Using Approximations When They Are Not Needed." First, in section "Permutation Tests Defined and Contrasted with Parametric Tests," we formally define permutation tests and contrast them with their more common parametric counterparts. In section "Generalized Permutation Tests" we introduce generalized permutation tests and distinguish them from the more traditional permutation tests which require a test statistic for their conduct. In section "Path Dependence" we discuss how we arrived at the perverse state we are in, with the approximation being preferred, almost uniformly, to the very quantity it is trying to approximate. In section "A New Beginning" we note that the conditions that initially favored the approximate analyses, namely, the inability to conduct exact analyses given the state of computing power when the approximations were developed and endorsed, no longer hold. In section "Parametric Analyses: Mere Approximations or of Inherent Interest?," we consider the question of whether parametric analyses are of inherent interest in their own right or if they serve only as approximations to exact permutation tests. In section "The Wisdom of Using Approximations When They Are Not Needed," we address whether there is, in fact, any wisdom in performing approximate analyses. In section "A Proposal" we offer a comprehensive proposal for improving clinical trials, the heart of which is using exact analyses whenever it is possible and feasible to do so and note, almost tautologically, that no great argument is needed to favor the exact test. The burden of proof is clearly on those who would argue the contrary position. We also note that it will almost always be the case, in a two-arm randomized trial, that permutation tests are both possible and feasible.

Permutation Tests Defined and Contrasted with Parametric Tests

A permutation test is a distribution-free significance test of the null hypothesis that samples are drawn from identical population distributions (Berry et al. 2016). If this null hypothesis is true, then any data from the observed samples are "exchangeable," or "permutable," hence the name for this type of test. This permutability under the assumption of a true null hypothesis enables the researcher to generate all possible data configurations without making any assumption about the shape of the population distribution.

For example, suppose that one wants to compare the number of adverse effects for US patients and the number of adverse effects for Canadian patients in a 1-year drug trial. For illustration purposes, suppose there is a sample of five patients from each population. For the US patients, the numbers are 13, 20, 25, 22, and 55. For the Canadian patients, the numbers are 16, 11, 12, 15, and 21. If the null hypothesis is true that the populations are identical, then these data arrangements are equally likely to, say, 11, 12, 13, 15, and 16 versus 20, 21, 22, 25, and 55 or also to any of the other possible data arrangements, $[10!/(5! \times 5!)] = 252$ in total.

A classical permutation test proceeds by calculating a p-value corresponding to a particular test statistic. This test statistic should be chosen judiciously to reflect the effect of interest. Suppose that this effect of interest is the difference between the average number of adverse effects in the two groups, and the expectation is that the average number of adverse effects for the US patients is larger than the average number of adverse effects for the Canadian patients. This difference of means can be taken directly as the test statistic for the permutation test, with an observed value of $27 - 15 = 12$. The p-value of the permutation test equals the proportion of test statistics computed for all the 252 data arrangements that have a difference between the average number of adverse effects of 12 or larger. It can be verified that there are 10 data arrangements that have a difference between the average number of adverse effects of 12 or larger. Consequently, the one-sided permutation test p-value equals $10/252 = 0.0397$.

A permutation test differs drastically from a parametric test in at least two respects:

1. No assumption is made about the shape of the population distribution.
2. The test has exact type I error rate control, even for small samples.

By contrast, parametric tests assume a particular distributional model and test one of the parameters of the model. Their validity is based on the plausibility of the theoretical model or on large-sample approximations. For example, the prototypical parametric test that would be used to test for a difference in the average number of adverse effects for the US patients versus the Canadian patients is the t-test. This test assumes a Gaussian population distribution and tests a null hypothesis about identical population means. Without an additional assumption of equal population variances, the result would be $t = 1.6036$, $df = 4.4672$, and one tailed p-value $= 0.0883$ (Welch approximation). Hence, the parametric test p-value is more than twice the permutation test p-value. Such a striking difference should come as no surprise because the assumptions and the null hypothesis tested are fundamentally different. The crucial question, however, is which technique is scientifically most interesting and relevant? Our position is that, in most applications, permutation tests are scientifically more interesting and relevant than the corresponding parametric tests because the former do not rely on untestable or implausible assumptions regarding the shape of the population distribution.

In the context of randomized clinical trials, a variant of permutation tests is even more relevant. This variant is called the "randomization test," and its validity is based on the random assignment as it was actually carried out in the trial (Edgington and Onghena 2007). Randomization tests are particularly relevant because no random sampling assumption is needed for their validity. This is convenient because randomized clinical trials almost never apply random sampling schemes (as used in surveys) but, by definition, implement random assignment. In fact, not all trials labeled as randomized even do that much, but it is important to bear in mind the distinction between random allocation, which is a trademark of properly conducted trials, and random sampling, which is not (Berger 2000).

Two remarks regarding the definition of randomization tests and permutation tests are in order here. First, the p-value of a randomization test or a permutation test for a small data set, as in the adverse effects example, can be calculated by hand easily, but for most applications and realistic data set sizes, the actual calculations depend on computer algorithms. In the most basic algorithm, only a random sample of all possible data arrangements is considered. Such a so-called Monte Carlo randomization test or Monte Carlo permutation test, if properly conducted, remains exactly valid (Edgington and Onghena 2007; Onghena and May 1995). Furthermore, the calculation of the p-value can be made as precise as needed, in terms of the number of significant digits, by increasing the number of data arrangements considered (Onghena and May 1995). Therefore, it is a false equivalence to claim that the p-value will be approximate either way, and, therefore, the parametric analysis is just as exact as the Monte Carlo permutation one.

Second, randomization tests and permutation tests are useful only for settings in which permutability is implied by the null hypothesis. For example, in a one-sample setting in which the researcher wants to test the null hypothesis that the population mean equals 25, permutations of the sample are to no avail. In such a setting, bootstrap tests are more appropriate. As Efron and Tibshirani (1993) phrased it:

> The bootstrap distribution was originally called the "combination distribution". It was designed to extend the virtues of permutation testing to the great majority of statistical problems where there is nothing to permute. When there is something to permute (...) it is a good idea to do so, even if other methods like the bootstrap are also brought to bear. (p. 218)

Randomized clinical trials are essentially comparative, and consequently "there is something to permute." In randomized clinical trials, it is "a good idea" to perform a permutation test or a randomization test (Berger 2000, 2017).

Generalized Permutation Tests

As discussed in section "Permutation Tests Defined and Contrasted with Parametric Tests," the construction of a permutation test relies on the use of a judiciously chosen test statistic, which must be made explicit prior to the initiation of data collection. But there are also approaches to constructing exact analyses that either use unorthodox test statistics or bypass the use of test statistics altogether. These types of analyses are categorized as generalized permutation tests, and three types will be developed here – starting with adaptive tests (Berger and Ivanova 2002). These tests allow for the test statistic to depend on the observed data, but in a valid manner that adjusts for this feature. Adaptive tests can be cast as standard permutation tests, but the test statistic would be the minimum among competing p-values, so this is not a standard test statistic. We then consider convex hull tests (Berger et al. 1998) and improved tests (Berger and Sackrowitz 1997), which do not use test statistics at all.

As noted in the Introduction, one of the major problems with how randomized clinical trials are conducted in practice is the tendency for researchers to change the primary endpoint on the fly. The change need not be from one endpoint to an entirely different one. For example, when considering an ordered categorical endpoint, such as objective tumor response (which may be graded as no response, partial response, or complete response), the primary analysis might be a binary analysis of just the complete response rate or a binary analysis of the overall response rate. For obvious reasons, neither of these is favored, but the appeal of binary endpoints can be understood, as can the temptation to switch if, after the data are in, the research team chose the wrong one. It would categorically *not* be valid to specify that the primary analysis compares the overall response rates and then, after the data are in, to switch to the complete response rate. However, it is possible to hedge, and in a valid manner no less, with adaptive tests that allow the choice of analysis to depend on the data. One could consider all possible permutations of the data and, for each one, both binary p-values, one for the complete response rata and one for the overall response rate. Obviously, the researchers would want to select the lower of these two p-values for the data set that actually obtained. This minimum p-value is not a valid p-value, but it *is* valid if it is used as a test statistic to be compared to a null reference distribution of other minimum p-values computed in exactly the same way, one for each permutation. This would be an adaptive test that essentially allows the data to determine whether the overall response rate or the complete response rate is considered. The adaptive test will, as one might expect, have a better overall power profile than either binary test.

A test statistic is generally understood to be a quantity that can be computed based on only the observed data, without reference to any other data sets that might have obtained. In the description of adaptive tests above, a test statistic that is the minimum of two binary p-values was used, but it was not specified whether these binary analyses would be chi-square or Fisher's exact test. If Fisher's exact test is used, then that would mean that the test statistic can in fact *not* be computed without considering the entire reference set. This would be fundamentally different from a standard test statistic, such as a rate, or a proportion, or a difference. This distinction is the key to understanding the convex hull test, whose test statistic is the directed data depth of the observed point among the entire reference set.

In other words, one would graph the entire reference set, as was done by Berger et al. (1998). Then, to this reference set, one would apply directional convex hull peeling. That is, one would wrap a rubber band around the set, and pick off the points of support, or the corners. It is not enough that a point touches the rubber band; to be included, its removal would need to alter the shape of the rubber band. These corner points comprise the set of outcomes that contain the most evidence against the null hypothesis, but with a directional one-sided alternative hypothesis, not all of them will go in the right direction. And only those that do will be picked off. This is the first level of data depth. These points are all assigned a value of 1 for the data depth test statistic. This directed convex hull peeling process is then applied to the set of remaining points, and the directed corners of that reduced reference set will then be assigned a value of 2, and so on. The convex hull test is a generalized permutation test based on this test statistic.

Improved tests also start with the graph of the reference set, and possibly with another test, defined here as a distribution of the available alpha level to a set of points, known as the rejection region, for which we would reject the null hypothesis. It is also possible to start with the "ignore the data" test, which replaces a rejection region with the value of alpha itself applied to each point. Either way, the test is then checked for admissibility (obviously the "ignore the data" test is not admissible). If the candidate test is already admissible, then it is used, but if not, then the improvement process is implemented so as to make the resulting improved test admissible. The precise specification of the null and alternative hypotheses will determine which alpha transfers result in improvements, meaning uniformly better power – see Berger and Sackrowitz (1997) for details. In general, there will be multiple alpha transfers that can be made, any one of which will result in uniformly better power. It has been shown that once no more, such transfers can be made, the final test is admissible.

The improved test process does represent an advance in the theory of hypothesis testing, but its use in randomized clinical trials must await some sort of objective algorithm that specifies precisely which alpha transfers to make and in which order. After all, the testing methodology used in randomized clinical trials must be objective and repeatable. Some vague description along the lines of "well, I really cannot recall what I did, but I improved the original test until I came up with an admissible test" will not suffice, especially considering that changing the order in which the alpha transfers are implemented will, in general, result in different final tests unless (unusually) a uniformly most powerful test exists, in which case the order will not matter, as all roads will then lead to Rome. But adaptive tests and convex hull tests are objective and in general offer much better global power profiles than the more standard linear rank tests. These should be considered for use right now.

Path Dependence

One way to explain the continued use of parametric rather than permutation tests is through path dependence. This is the idea that the precise manner in which the past unfolded, in conjunction with the ubiquitous resistance to change or inertia (Berger 2015), created the "path" that structured future decisions. But basing future decisions solely on past practice can cause one to gloss over important issues – as the history of statistical reasoning has repeatedly shown. Although Fisher pointed out a statistical error to Karl Pearson regarding the chi-square test, the statistician Austin Bradford Hill did not look to Fisher for theoretical inspiration when he introduced randomization into clinical trials (Magnello 2002). Instead, as one who had learned statistical methods by attending Pearson's lectures, Bradford Hill conceived of the clinical trial from within a Pearsonian framework.

The controversy between Fisher and Karl Pearson can be seen as a historical prelude to the issues of approximate versus exact analysis. Specifically, the issue was whether the cell probabilities can be used to compute an exact chi-square value or only an approximation. For Pearson, approximation was all that was possible. He wrote that "What we actually do is replace the accurate value of χ^2, which is unknown to us, and cannot be found, by an approximate value, and we do this with precisely the same justification as the astronomer claims, when he calculates his probable error on his observations, and not on the mean square error of an infinite population of errors which is unknown to him" (quoted in Baird, p. 112). This approach was a direct outgrowth of Pearson's overall philosophy of science. He accepted correlation as the organizing construct for inquiry in all fields of endeavor and viewed causation as *describing* the limit case of unitary correlation, i.e., something that may be achieved *in theory* but never *in fact* (Porter 1994). Given this view that all measurement was approximation, the pursuit of an "exact" solution would be seen as a futile endeavor.

In 1922, Fisher published an account showing that the cell frequencies are not simply approximations. Because the frequencies are a function of the data, an exact estimation is possible (Baird 1983). But Fisher's insight on this issue has not been widely appreciated by those who have designed clinical trials in the ensuing decades; rather, aspects of Fisher's work have been appropriated on an ad hoc basis.

Later controversies were similarly glossed over in the interest of achieving uniformity in statistical practice – even if this forged consensus was unwarranted. For instance, Fisher debated Neyman and Egon Pearson over the interpretation of significance tests. As discussed by Gigerenzer et al. (1989), the idea of expressing levels of significance prior to the test originated with Neyman-Pearson rather than Fisher, but the assertion that one should not draw conclusions from nonsignificant results derived from Fisher. Similarly, the distinction between type I and type II errors was more fully developed by Neyman and Pearson, but Neyman's behavioristic interpretation (we would only *behave* as if the result were true) did not become standard. However, in statistics textbooks written between the 1940s and 1960s, these differences were not addressed to present "the rules of statistics" to more pragmatically oriented consumers in various scientific disciplines.

At the time that this forced consensus was being achieved, the computer (in its modern form) was decades away. Consequently, approximate methods were more feasible, given the operational difficulties of computing exact results. When the first computers did become available (in the 1940s and 1950s), they were isolated to a few research centers, as well as being large, inefficient, and expensive (Berry et al. 2016, p. 4). The computing power of these now obsolete mainframe computers is easily surpassed by todays notebook computers – literally putting the capacity for exact computation "at one's fingertips." Frequently, one hears the power of computers discussed in terms of the size of the data set, the advent of "big data" (Efron and Hastie 2016), but the electronic computer has a much wider significance in that it can, among other things, also facilitate exact analysis based on permutation tests.

A New Beginning

If path dependence is a principal reason that approximate analyses are adopted, then it is time to reassess whether these methods should continue. This reassessment could be motivated by reviewing various models of conceptual change within the sciences. One historically famous model was developed by Thomas Kuhn (1962) and centered on the idea of a "paradigm." Although Kuhn was somewhat imprecise in his definition of the word "paradigm," the basic idea referred to a widely held framework for making sense of the world that was adopted by the scientific community. As long as the paradigm "worked" (i.e., explained the observed empirical regularities better than its alternatives), it was accepted as true. However, when disconfirming pieces of data – Kuhn called them "anomalies" – appeared, this would eventually induce a crisis within the scientific community, which would entail that the older paradigm be replaced with a newer one. For Kuhn, this process was what characterized a "scientific revolution," and he illustrated his model through classic examples from the history of science (e.g., the Copernican Revolution etc.).

Viewed through the lens of Kuhn's model of scientific change, the shift from approximate to exact analysis might be seen as one paradigm replacing another.

Specifically, given the computing capabilities in the early twentieth century, approximate analyses were "exact enough" for computation purposes when originally developed (i.e., the hybrid solution created by the statistical textbook writers produced results that satisfied everyone's needs). But this glossed over a more fundamental divide that has bedeviled biomedicine research since at least the middle decades of the nineteenth century – namely, the struggle between those who seek knowledge by understanding how the individual organism functions (i.e., in statistical parlance "$n = 1$") and those who have sought knowledge through patterns that emerge at the level of the population (Matthews 1995; Hanin 2017). Given that this struggle is ongoing, it is debatable whether we have risen to the level of a "crisis" as outlined by Kuhn; however, the contest does suggest that there may be "anomalies" that should no longer be ignored. In particular, approximate analyses may well be viewed as anomalous in that more exact analyses can now be easily obtained through advances in computing technology.

As an alternative to Kuhn, another widely discussed model of conceptual change has been developed by Peter Galison. According to Galison (2011), change does not happen *internal* to the scientific domain (as Kuhn argued). Rather, different disciplines cross-fertilize each other by creating hybrid languages that facilitate cross-disciplinary communication; they form intellectual "trading zones." As his prime example, Galison looked to the developing of computing technology to aid the physicists, chemists, mathematicians, and engineers who build the atomic bomb in World War II. For Galison, a consequence of this cross-fertilization is that tools developed in such trading zones (e.g., the computer) eventually came to be seen as characterizing reality more generally. What had been a "precise" mathematical description of reality in one era (e.g., a differential equation solvable by hand) became less so in another – when "machine readable" increasingly became the benchmark. As noted in section "Permutation Tests Defined and Contrasted with Parametric Tests," a similar type of dynamic has played itself out regarding randomization tests and permutation tests. While the p-value can be calculated directly for small data sets, computer algorithms are used for larger data sets; nevertheless, the p-value can be calculated "as precisely as needed" by increasing the number of data arrangements. In other words, following Galison, these types of transformations suggest that the computer is no longer merely a "tool"; it has become instrumental in helping us re-characterize what we mean by precision itself. Regardless of whether Kuhn or Galison is seen as more applicable to the issue of approximate versus exact analyses in the present context, there is sufficient congruence between these conceptual models and the empirical evidence at hand to suggest that new solutions should be considered.

Parametric Analyses: Mere Approximations or of Inherent Interest?

An argument for or against permutation tests would ideally be informed by the rationale for using parametric analyses. Therefore, a careful consideration must be given to the issue of whether parametric analyses are used because they are of inherent interest in their own right, or if they are used only as approximations to permutation tests. Berger (2000) considered this question and provided strong evidence in favor of the latter rationale. Namely, Berger (2000) questioned why there would be checks of assumptions otherwise. In other words, if the t-test (for example) was of inherent interest in its own right, and did not derive its utility exclusively as an approximation for a corresponding exact test, then why would we check for normality (one of the assumptions underlying the validity of the t-test) before conducting the t-test? Why would it matter?

One might respond to this question by appeal to the conditions under which any given test, for example, the t-test, would be valid, without any consideration of how it may or may not approximate an exact test. But therein lies the problem. If the t-test actually is valid, then it is also exact. That is the definition of validity in this context, namely, that it preserves the actual alpha level at the nominal level. It might be easier to understand this concept when stated in terms of its polar opposite. If 1000 different allocations of patients were randomized to the two treatment groups, and each of these 1000 possibilities has the same probability, 1/1000, then this fact can be used as the basis for inference, and the p-value of the t-test can be computed for each of the 1000 possibilities that might have occurred. A fair question would be how often is a p-value obtained that is less than the traditional alpha level of 0.05, or, ideally, a more principled alpha level. It may turn out that for some alpha levels, the null probability of a p-value lower than this alpha level exceeds alpha:

$$P\{p < \alpha\} > \alpha.$$

This is the definition of a lack of validity. By contrast, notice that this can be done directly. Just compute the p-value for each permutation of the data in accordance with how the trial was randomized, following Tukey's (1993) platinum standard. But in practice, this is done indirectly, by testing for normality. Note that the test for normality is generally going to be severely underpowered and will always be backward in terms of concluding normality by virtue of failing to reject the null hypothesis. Nevertheless, if this test of normality fails to find gross deviations from normality, then not only is normality concluded, but also validity. Then, researchers can bootstrap from a very questionable assertion of normality to an assertion also that for no alpha level is the null probability of a p-value under this alpha level greater than alpha.

This trick allows bypassing the actual computation of these null probabilities. But there is no practical difficulty in computing these null probabilities. The trick is used to cover up the reality that in many cases the t-test will in fact *not* be valid. This, too, provides evidence for the claim that parametric analyses are used only as approximations. If this were not the case, then their lack of validity would not be a concern and would not need to be covered up. But the primary rationale for asserting that parametric analyses are used only as approximations is the almost universal procedure of preliminary testing of assumptions. There would be no reason to do this if the parametric analyses were of inherent interest.

Furthermore, it is also useful to highlight the distinction between expectations and reality. To use an analogy, imagine if late night drivers felt that they did not need to look for oncoming traffic when merging onto the highway, because at this late hour, we do not expect there to be any traffic. It is not difficult to look to see if there are any cars coming, but this is not the action taken because of the belief that general patterns will also apply to this specific case. Likewise, pedestrians who have the right of way should feel free to cross the street without checking for cross traffic, because their right of way should mean that all motor vehicles will yield to them. Never mind that it would be a simple matter to actually look to see if, in this particular instance, it is or is not safe to cross the street. This flawed logic is at play when the specific (how different is the approximate p-value from the exact one?) is replaced with the general (we know from appeal to our test of normality that the two *should* be close). Making this mistake will not result in the researcher getting run over, but it may well result in distorted results informing future medical decisions, and when that happens, it is predictable that tangible harm will come to real patients. This is not benign.

Finally, it is worth mentioning the common criticism of exact analyses that they answer the wrong question, since they are conditional tests, akin to losing one's keys in the dark part of the parking lot, yet looking for them under the light only because of better visibility there. Better an approximate answer to the right question than an exact answer to the wrong question. But this criticism is predicated on the notion that parametric analyses do in fact address the right question. Clearly, there is a desire to know something about the population (of patients) at large, and not just the patients in the study (and a population generated by resampling of these same patients according to hypothetically repeating the randomization over and over again).

With a random sample from the target population, there would be a firm connection between the target population and the sample, and therefore the analysis of the sample would produce results applicable to the target population. But, as noted earlier, random sampling is not a feature of randomized trials, and therefore any connection between sample and target population is severed. It is no more than an illusion to suppose that statistical methods can draw a precise inference to a population, which has not been randomly sampled. At best, there is a sample of patients, which can be used in the manner already described to generate a population of pseudo data sets based on other outcomes of the randomization that might have obtained. Then other arguments are used to try to extend the results to the population at large, but it is not sound science to pretend that more precision is possible than the limitations imposed by the methods used to generate the data.

The Wisdom of Using Approximations When They Are Not Needed

Having concluded, in the previous section, that parametric analyses are, in fact, used only as approximations for permutation tests, we now turn our attention to the merit of using approximations. When would this be a good idea, and when would it not be? Though there is a technical distinction between an estimate and an approximation, the discussion might be illuminated by considering the merits of estimation, based on a sample, rather than using a census and obtaining the exact quantity being sought.

For example, the unemployment rate in a given population, perhaps a nation or a large city, might be desired. Once "unemployed" is defined (addressing whether or not to count students, women on maternity leave, consultants, part-time workers, and so on), the most direct way to obtain this to conduct a census of all individuals in the population, and find out, perhaps from tax records, if they are or are not employed. Alas, the resources required in following this approach would be prohibitive. It becomes more feasible to ask each participant if he or she is employed (rather than finding this out from official records) and to do this for only a sample rather than for the entire population. Obviously, there is a trade-off here: the desired perfect information would cost much more than the approximation.

Can this trade-off be used to justify the ongoing use of approximate analyses rather than their exact counterparts? As seen in section "Generalized Permutation Tests," this was the very reason that approximate analyses were developed and endorsed in the first place. But as seen in section "Path Dependence," computing power has caught up, and conducting exact analyses is no longer a burden, or at least not in most cases. When the exact p-value can be obtained just as easily as the approximate one (some software packages will even provide Fisher's exact test for 2×2 contingency tables as standard output with the chi-square test), then it becomes much more difficult to justify using the approximation.

Consider the inference to be drawn after the data are in, and have been analyzed, and (hopefully) provide a low p-value for comparing the treatment groups with respect to the primary efficacy end point. What can be concluded? If a parametric analysis is used that relies for validity on the normality assumption, then it must be concluded that either (1) the treatment works (the intended attribution) or (2) the data were not normally distributed. Given that the data were not normally distributed (misguided attempts to establish this notwithstanding), which of these two possibilities would Occam's razor prefer? On the other hand, if an exact analysis is used, then this problem disappears – although the possibility, or even inevitability, of other biases masquerading as treatment effects exists. If steps can be taken to minimize and/or eliminate these other biases, then Occam's razor would lead one to conclude that there is a treatment effect. In short, the raison d'être for the approximation no longer exists for multiple reasons:

1. It does not save money.
2. It does not save computing time.
3. It does not minimize the use of other resources.

In fact, the only savings that might be achieved with the use of parametric analyses would be smaller studies due to greater power. Alas, this greater power is an illusion, or pseudo power, attained at the cost of validity. If this were deemed to be a valid savings, then the same might be achieved by simply cutting the p-value in half or imagining that each patient had a twin or a clone and adding in one phantom patient for each real patient so as to double the sample size without increasing the costs. Or one could spare all costs and just make up data, without ever recruiting, treating, or monitoring any real patients. These steps would also increase the power, and, moreover, they would do so in a manner that is just as valid (which is to say, not at all) as gaining pseudo power from using a parametric analysis that is equally flawed.

The only legitimate argument in favor of a parametric analysis over an exact permutation test would be that the parametric analysis is uniformly more powerful *while also retaining validity*. But of course this is not possible. It is certainly possible that one permutation test is uniformly more powerful than another (Berger and Sackrowitz 1997), and in this case, the inadmissible one should not be used (Berger 1998). But the finding that a given permutation test lacks power serves as an indictment of only that particular permutation test; it is not simultaneously an indictment of permutation tests in general, and it certainly is not a call to replace them with approximate parametric analyses.

A Proposal

As already discussed, parametric analyses perversely make full use of the random sampling that was *not* performed and of the distributional form that does *not* describe the reality of the situation. This being the case, they bear little or no resemblance to reality and should not be considered for use for comparative analyses in randomized clinical trials. If the study is worth doing, and worth committing resources to, then it is also sufficiently important that only the best research methods should be used. This does not include parametric analyses, whose flaws are so readily apparent. When the exact solution is easily obtained, then there is no reason to consider using anything less than the best. And yet paradoxically, approximation is used in almost all situations, despite its known flaws and despite the ready availability of the exact tests.

Furthermore, the routine use of approximate parametric analyses represents not only bad science but also bad pedagogy. The reason that so many college students find statistics to be their most challenging and least comprehensible class is because much of what is taught actually does not make any sense, and it is a shame that students are drilled so as to see a naked emperor and recognize clothes that in fact do not exist. As one example, introductory classes may provide students with a set of heights and ask what proportion of these heights is above 6 ft. Any student not already indoctrinated will simply count the number of heights that exceed this threshold and divide by the total number given. No great trick to get the question right. But alas this answer, though correct, would be marked wrong, because this question appears in the chapter on the central limit theorem, and the student is supposed to recognize the Orwellian doublespeak, and know that what is called for here is to find the mean and variance of the data set, and then to use these to standardize the given height threshold of 6 ft (subtract the mean, divide by the standard deviation), and then refer this standardized height to the normal table in the back of the book to find the desired proportion. Is it any wonder that so many members of society think so little of the field of statistics?

Randomization and permutation tests will be adopted more broadly only if users and consumers of statistical inference become more aware of the issues involved in making implausible and untestable auxiliary assumptions about the populations sampled. As suggested by Onghena and May (1995), this awareness can be increased by teaching statistical hypothesis testing from the resampling perspective with a clear distinction between random sampling and random assignment models. Excellent early examples of introductory statistics courses taking this perspective are given by May et al. (1990) and Simon and Bruce (1991). More recently, influential statisticians have made convincing pleas for a "Ptolemaic" reform of all introductory statistics courses. Instead of putting the central limit theorem and the normal distribution at the center of the statistical universe, with all methods and techniques in an orbit around them, we should have randomization-based inference at the core:

> What we teach is largely the technical machinery of numerical approximations based on the normal distribution and its many subsidiary cogs. This machinery was once necessary, because the conceptually simpler alternative based on permutations was computationally beyond our reach. Before computers statisticians had no choice. These days we have no excuse. Randomization-based inference makes a direct connection between data production and the logic of inference that deserves to be at the core of every introductory course. Technology allows us to do more with less: more ideas, less technique. We need to recognize that the computer revolution in statistics education is far from over. (Cobb 2007, p. 1)

In 2011, at the United States Conference on Teaching Statistics, the consensus was that re-centering introductory courses around the core logic of inference, illustrated by randomization tests, was the next big thing in statistics education (Rossman 2015). Handbooks that put these ideas in practice are now widely available (e.g., Tintle et al. 2015). With all this available material, our proposal is that teachers of statistics, journal reviewers and editors, regulatory bodies, and funding agencies start to reconsider their courses, guidelines, and standards. The routine use of statistical methods and techniques based on Gaussian approximations is clearly a questionable research practice as defined by John et al. (2012) and may soon be widely recognized as such.

One possible argument against permutation tests is that they may not handle covariates easily, and so a researcher may wish to use, for example, Cox proportional hazards regression with survival data. In this case, one can still use a permutation test and get the best of both worlds. One would use the Cox p-value not as the final p-value per se but, rather, as the test statistic for use with a permutation test (just as with the adaptive tests discussed in section "Generalized Permutation Tests"). In this way, a p-value that may not have been valid is passed through the validation transformation where it is laundered (so to speak) so as to become valid. This approach can be used with any parametric analysis.

Summary and Conclusions

Although "randomization tests" appear in our title, this chapter is not about randomization per se other than how it provides a basis for inference. But it is naturally paired with permutation tests because this type of analysis exploits its potential. Furthermore, we have presented our case for why parametric analyses must now give way to the more exact and valid permutation tests that they are merely trying to approximate. It is hard to imagine a research team going before a funding agency and arguing that this proposed study is important enough to be funded, yet somehow just not important enough to merit the use of best research practices. It is even harder to imagine the research team making this case before the public or to the patient groups who rely on researchers to do valid research, rather than just doing whatever they feel like with no controls in place. Clearly, self-regulation has not worked very well. As we see, researchers left to their own devices will rarely opt for the best research methods. The need to do so must be imposed externally by somebody with the authority to offer both rewards for compliance and sufficient disincentives for persistence in conducting flawed research.

It is our hope that regulatory agencies, medical journals, and funding agencies will come together and finally insist that researchers do the right thing when doing the right thing as is easy as it is in this case. Indeed, one may wonder how far to trust researchers who cannot even get the easy ones right. Ultimately, however, it is the patients who are harmed by flawed medical research. When flawed studies are published, but then accepted as valid, the medical journals that decide to publish them do not suffer any adverse consequences. On the contrary, they can expect revenues from the sales of the reprints, plus possibly from advertising of the treatment that was "proven" safe and effective by these flawed studies. The funding agency considers it a feather in their cap to have funded so influential a study. The regulatory authority may eventually get around to seeing if the findings are actually valid. But they also may not. Phase IV (post marketing) commitments are often ignored with impunity. It is only when the patient groups take it upon themselves to mobilize and challenge accepted dogma and insist upon the routine use of best research methods that we will see studies conducted as well as they can be. We feel that this day cannot come soon enough.

Cross-References

▶ Intention to Treat and Alternative Approaches
▶ Principles of Clinical Trials: Bias and Precision Control

References

Baird D (1983) The fisher/Pearson chi-squared controversy: a turning point for inductive inference. Br J Philos Sci 34:105–118

Berger VW (1998) Admissibility of exact conditional tests of stochastic order. J Stat Plann Inference 66(1):39–50

Berger VW (2000) Pros and cons of permutation tests in clinical trials. Stat Med 19:1319–1328

Berger VW (2005) Selection bias and covariate imbalances in randomized clinical trials. Wiley, Chichester

Berger VW (2015) Conflicts of interest, selective inertia, and research malpractice in randomized clinical trials: an unholy trinity. Sci Eng Ethics 21(4):857–874

Berger VW (2017) An empirical demonstration of the need for exact tests. J Mod Appl Stat Methods 16(1):34–50

Berger VW, Ivanova A (2002) Adaptive tests for ordinal data. J Mod Appl Stat Methods 1(2):269–280

Berger V, Sackrowitz H (1997) Improving tests for superior treatment in contingency tables. J Am Stat Assoc 92(438):700–705

Berger VW, Permutt T, Ivanova A (1998) The convex hull test for ordered categorical data. Biometrics 54(4):1541–1550

Berry KJ, Mielke PW, Johnston JE (2016) Permutation statistical methods: an integrated approach. Cham, SW: Springer

Cobb GW (2007) The introductory statistics course: a Ptolemaic curriculum? Technol Innov Stat Educ 1(1). http://escholarship.org/uc/item/6hb3k0nz#main

Edgington ES, Onghena P (2007) Randomization tests, 4th edn. Chapman & Hall/CRC, Boca Raton

Efron B, Hastie T (2016) Computer age statistical inference: algorithms, evidence, and data science. Institute of mathematical statistics monographs. Cambridge University Press, Cambridge. https://doi.org/10.1017/CBO9781316576533

Efron B, Tibshirani RJ (1993) An introduction to the bootstrap. Chapman & Hall/CRC, Boca Raton

Galison P (2011) Computer simulations and the trading zone. In: Gramelsberger G (ed) From science to computational science. Diaphanes, Zürich, pp 118–157

Geary RC (1947) Testing for normality. Biometrika 34:209–242

Gigerenzer G, Swijtink Z, Porter T, Daston L, Beatty J, Kruger L (1989) The empire of chance: how probability changed science and everyday life. Cambridge University Press, Cambridge

Hanin L (2017) Why statistical inference from clinical trials is likely to generate false and irreproducible results. BMC Med Res Methodol 17:127. https://doi.org/10.1186/s12874-017-0399-0

John LK, Loewenstein G, Prelec D (2012) Measuring the prevalence of questionable research practices with incentives for truth telling. Psychol Sci 23:524–532

Kuhn TS (1962) The structure of scientific revolutions. University of Chicago Press, Chicago

Magnello E (2002) The introduction of mathematical statistics into medical research: the roles of Karl Pearson, Major Greenwood, and Austin Bradford Hill. In: Magnello E, Hardy A (eds) The road to medical statistics. Rodopi, Amsterdam

Matthews JR (1995) Quantification and the quest for medical certainty. Princeton University Press, Princeton

May RB, Masson MEJ, Hunter MA (1990) Applications of statistics in behavioral research. Harper & Row, New York

Onghena P, May RB (1995) Pitfalls in computing and interpreting randomization test p values: a commentary on Chen and Dunlap. Behav Res Methods Instrum Comput 27:408–411

Perlman P, Possen BH, Legat VD, Rubenacker AS, Bockiger U, Stieben-Emmerling L (2013) When will we see people of negative height. Significance 10(1):46–48

Porter T (1994) The death of the object: *Fin de siècle* philosophy of physics. In: Ross D (ed) Modernist impulses in the human sciences, 1870–1930. The Johns Hopkins University Press, Baltimore

Rossman A (2015) Interview with George Cobb. J Stat Educ 23(1). www.amstat.org/publications/jse/v23n1/rossmanint.pdf

Simon JL, Bruce P (1991) Resampling: a tool for everyday statistical work. Chance 4:22–32

Tintle N, Chance B, Cobb G, Rossman A, Roy S, Swanson T, Vanderstoep J (2015) Introduction to statistical investigations. Wiley, New York

Generalized Pairwise Comparisons for Prioritized Outcomes

95

Marc Buyse and Julien Peron

Contents

Introduction	1870
Pairwise Comparisons	1872
Generalization of the Wilcoxon-Mann-Whitney Test	1872
Measures of Treatment Effect	1873
Inference	1874
Stratification	1875
Single Outcome	1876
Binary Outcome	1876
Continuous Outcome	1876
Time-to-Event Outcome	1877
Multiple Outcomes	1878
Overall Pairwise Score	1878
Composite Pairwise Score	1878
Multiple Prioritized Outcomes	1879
Applications of Prioritized Outcomes for a Single Variable	1880
Thresholds of Clinical Relevance	1880
Repeated Observations	1884
Applications of Prioritized Outcomes for Several Variables	1884
Several Time-to-Event Outcomes	1884

M. Buyse (✉)
International Drug Development Institute (IDDI) Inc., San Francisco, CA, USA

CluePoints S.A., Louvain-la-Neuve, Belgium and I-BioStat, University of Hasselt, Louvain-la-Neuve, Belgium

Interuniversity Institute for Biostatistics and Statistical Bioinformatics (I-BioStat), Hasselt University, Hasselt, Belgium
e-mail: marc.buyse@iddi.com

J. Peron
CNRS, UMR 5558, Laboratoire de Biométrie et Biologie Evolutive, Université Lyon 1, France

Departments of Biostatistics and Medical Oncology, Centre Hospitalier Lyon-Sud, Institut de Cancérologie des Hospices Civils de Lyon, Lyon, France
e-mail: julien.peron@chu-lyon.fr

© Springer Nature Switzerland AG 2022
S. Piantadosi, C. L. Meinert (eds.), *Principles and Practice of Clinical Trials*,
https://doi.org/10.1007/978-3-319-52636-2_277

Benefit/Risk Assessment 1886
Conclusion 1889
Cross-References 1890
References 1891

Abstract

The Wilcoxon-Mann-Whitney U-statistic can be extended to perform generalized pairwise comparisons between two groups of observations. The observations are outcomes captured by a single variable, possibly repeatedly measured, or by several variables of any type (e.g., discrete, continuous, time to event). Generalized pairwise comparisons can include an arbitrary number of (possibly prioritized) outcomes and thresholds of clinical relevance. They extend standard nonparametric tests and lead to a general measure of the difference between the groups, the "Net Benefit," which is the probability that a patient randomly selected from the treatment group has a better outcome than a patient randomly selected from the control group, minus the probability of the opposite situation. One flexible approach to the analysis is to prioritize the outcomes from the most important to the least important. The order of priorities can be patient-dependent, and as such this approach paves the way to personalized medicine.

Keywords

Wilcoxon test · U-statistic · Generalized pairwise comparisons · Prioritized outcomes · Measure of treatment effect · Net Benefit · Win ratio

Introduction

In most clinical settings, and in particular in randomized clinical trials of experimental therapies, several outcomes (or "endpoints") are generally of interest. For example, in a cancer clinical trial comparing an experimental therapy for some advanced form of cancer to standard of care, interest may focus on the time to death from any cause (overall survival or "OS") and on the time to an increase in tumor size (time to progression or "TTP"), with the hope that the experimental therapy will prolong either or both of these times. Typically, one is also interested in showing that the experimental therapy does not cause undue harm because of treatment-related adverse events, so further outcomes such as serious toxicities also need to be compared between the randomized groups. Finally, there is increasing interest in capturing and analyzing patient-reported outcomes ("PROs"), which are arguably most relevant since they contribute to capturing "how patients feel, function or survive" (Biomarkers Definition Working Group 2001). All in all, in the vast majority of randomized clinical trials, multiple outcomes are of interest, some that may favor the experimental therapy, and some that may favor the standard of care.

Much statistical literature has been devoted to the problem of multiplicity in clinical trials (Moyé 2003). To put prioritized outcomes in perspective, it is useful to contrast the approaches available for the analysis of multiple outcomes

Table 1 Analysis methods for multiple outcomes

Analysis method	Major limitation
Multivariate analysis	Difficult to interpret when directions of effects differ
Single primary outcome	Predicates study interpretation on primary endpoint
Multiple testing procedure	Focuses on significance rather than effect size or relevance
Marginal benefit/risk analysis	Ignores associations between outcomes
Time to first event	Ignores subsequent events
Composite endpoint	Gives equal weight to all components
Weighted composite endpoint	Requires choice of weights
Prioritized outcomes	Requires choice of priority order
Prioritized weighted outcomes	Requires choice of priority order and weights

(Table 1). Multivariate analysis methods initially developed for several normally distributed variables have been extended to several times to event (Wei and Lachin 1984; Lachin and Bebu 2015) and to several variables of different types (Lachin 2014). While these methods gain power when all treatment effects are in the same direction, their use becomes problematic when treatment benefits and harms are simultaneously tested. In practice, the standard approach in the vast majority of trials is simply to designate one outcome as the "primary endpoint" of the trial, and all other outcomes as "secondary endpoints" that are tested for significance if, and only if, the analysis of the primary endpoint reaches statistical significance. One major limitation of this approach is that if the primary outcome of the trial fails to achieve significance, then no statistical claims can be made about secondary outcomes without inflating the type-I error, regardless of how impressive the treatment effects may be on secondary outcomes. Testing procedures that allow for multiple outcomes to be analyzed have become popular to address the limitation of a single primary outcome (Dmitrienko et al. 2010). These procedures can be quite complex and have the drawback of focusing on statistical significance rather than on the size of treatment effects and/or on the clinical relevance of the various outcomes considered. When a benefit/risk assessment is performed for a new therapy, for instance after approval of a new drug, the statistical significance of the treatment effect on the various outcomes is usually ignored and the benefits are weighed against the risks, using marginal treatment contrasts that ignore the correlation between the effects. Consider, for example, a therapy that causes substantial toxicity in a given proportion of patients, as is frequently the case in oncology. Two very different situations can occur: one in which the therapy induces both toxicity and better efficacy in some patients (e.g., severe skin rash in patients with solid tumors who respond to inhibitors of the epidermal growth factor receptor), vs. another in which the therapy causes toxicity in patients for whom it has no efficacy (e.g., cardiac toxicity in patients with *HER2-neu* amplified breast tumors treated with herceptin combined with anthracycline-based chemotherapy). Risk/benefit assessments should differ between these situations, yet marginal analyses of risks and benefits cannot differentiate between them, except in simple cases (e.g., when all outcomes are binary) (Evans and Follmann 2016; Giai et al. 2020).

To address the limitations of these analyses, composite endpoints have been suggested to combine several outcomes into a single analysis. For times to different types of events (e.g., myocardial infarction or stroke or death in cardiovascular disease trials), the time to first event is often used as the primary endpoint in the analysis. Events that occur after the first event are ignored in such an analysis, hence crucially important information may be lost because later events are often more important and patient-relevant than earlier events (e.g., time to death matters more than time to a non-disabling stroke). A different approach consists of using "generalized pairwise comparisons" (GPC) to compare patient pairs in terms of multiple outcomes (O'Brien 1984; Huang et al. 2008; Buyse 2010). One drawback of this approach is that all component outcomes are given the same importance, which does not reflect patient or physician preferences (Stolker et al. 2014). Weights can be used to reflect differences in clinical relevance of the various component outcomes (Rauch et al. 2014, 2018). The choice of weights is subjective and the clinical interpretation of the overall weighted treatment effect may be challenging. It may be more natural to prioritize the component outcomes rather than assigning them weights, an idea that was first proposed to augment a survival analysis with other clinical relevant data from patients still alive at the time of the analysis (Moyé et al. 1992; Finkelstein and Schoenfeld 1999). The concept was extended to several times to event in cardiology (Pocock et al. 2012), and in the most general case to multiple outcomes of any type (Buyse 2010). Defining the order of priority may be difficult because different physicians, let alone individual patients, may have markedly different views on the appropriate order for the various outcomes considered. For completeness, it is also possible to combine weighting based on clinical relevance *and* prioritizing outcomes (Rauch et al. 2018; Ramchandani et al. 2016), but interpretation may be challenging when both are used in the same analysis (Pocock et al. 2012).

Pairwise Comparisons

Generalization of the Wilcoxon-Mann-Whitney Test

The Wilcoxon-Mann-Whitney test can be used to compare two samples in terms of a continuous or ordered outcome. In clinical trials, for instance, the two samples are typically individuals randomly assigned to a treatment group (labeled "T") or to a control group (labeled "C"). Let the continuous or ordered outcome of these individuals be captured by a variable denoted X, taking values $X_1, \ldots, X_n$ in the treatment group and Y, taking values $Y_1, \ldots, Y_m$ in the control group. Consider all possible pairs (X_i, Y_j) consisting of one observation from group T and one from group C. The U-statistic for the Wilcoxon-Mann-Whitney test is

$$U = \frac{1}{n \cdot m} \sum_{i=1}^{n} \sum_{j=1}^{m} u_{ij} \qquad (1)$$

where

$$u_{ij} = \begin{cases} +1 & \text{if } X_i > Y_j \\ -1 & \text{if } X_i < Y_j \\ 0 & \text{if } X_i = Y_j \end{cases}$$

Generalized pairwise comparisons extend the idea behind the Wilcoxon-Mann-Whitney two-sample test. In the pairwise comparisons, the outcomes of the two individuals being compared need not be continuous or ordered, as long as there is a way to classify every pair as being "favorable," if the outcome of the individual in group T is better than the outcome of the individual in group C, "unfavorable," if the outcome of the individual in group T is worse than the outcome of the individual in group C, or "neutral," if there is no difference between the outcomes of the two individuals (Buyse 2010). Pocock et al. (2012) proposed to call favorable pairs "wins," unfavorable pairs "losses," and neutral pairs "ties" (Pocock et al. 2012).

Measures of Treatment Effect

Generalize the pairwise indicator u_{ij} to capture whether the pair of individuals formed by the ith individual ($i = 1, \ldots, n$) in group T and the jth individual ($j = 1, \ldots, m$) in group C is a win, a loss or a tie:

$$u_{ij} = \begin{cases} 1 & \text{if the pair is a win} \\ -1 & \text{if the pair is a loss} \\ 0 & \text{if the pair is a tie} \end{cases}$$

The "Net Benefit" Δ is defined as the difference between the number of wins and the number of losses (sometimes called the "win difference") divided by the total number of pairs. Δ is a generalization of the Wilcoxon-Mann-Whitney U-statistic (Eq. 1):

$$\Delta = U = \frac{1}{n \cdot m} \sum_{i=1}^{n} \sum_{j=1}^{m} u_{ij} \qquad (2)$$

The Net Benefit Δ was first named "proportion in favor of treatment" (Buyse 2010) and later "net chance of a better outcome" (Péron et al. 2016a). The Net Benefit can be interpreted as the probability that a patient randomly selected from the treatment group has a better outcome than a patient randomly selected from the control group, minus the probability of the opposite situation (Péron et al. 2016a). Δ is closely related to the "probabilistic index," $P(X > Y)$, defined as the probability that a patient randomly selected from the treatment group has a better outcome than an individual randomly selected from the control group (Acion et al. 2006; De Neve et al. 2013). The probabilistic index has also been called "probability of a superior outcome" (Grissom

1994), "individual exceedance probability" (Senn 1997), and "relative effect" (Brunner et al. 2001). It is closely related to the proportion of similar responses (Rom and Hwang 1996), the probability of overlap (Stine and Heyse 2001), the area under the ROC curve (Brumback et al. 2006), and the concordance index (Harrell 2001). Senn (2011) comments on some difficulties in interpreting the probabilistic index as a general measure of treatment effect (Senn 2011; Thas et al. 2012). He points out that the probabilistic index and related measures of effect such as the Net Benefit are only valid in a given sample of patients, and that they do not automatically generalize to other settings or different patient populations, where the variability of the outcome of interest could be quite different. Verbeeck et al. (2020) have studied the theoretical properties of the probabilistic index and the Net Benefit for a single continuous outcome variable. The Net Benefit extends traditional measures of benefit by incorporating thresholds of clinical relevance as well as multiple outcomes, as will be illustrated in sections "Applications of Prioritized Outcomes for a Single Variable" and "Applications of Prioritized Outcomes for Several Variables."

The Net Benefit is a linear transformation of the probabilistic index, $\Delta = 2 \cdot P(X > Y) - 1$, which results in the intuitive interpretation that positive values of Δ indicate treatment benefit while negative values indicate treatment harm. Δ is equal to 0 if there is no difference between the treatment groups, to 1 if the treatment group is uniformly better than the control group, that is, if all individuals in group T have a better outcome than those in group C, to -1 if the control group is uniformly better than the treatment group. This intuitive interpretation of the Net Benefit makes it attractive when multiple prioritized endpoints are considered in benefit/risk analyses, as will be illustrated in section "Applications of Prioritized Outcomes for Several Variables" of this chapter.

The "win ratio" Θ is defined as the ratio of the number of wins to the number of losses (Pocock et al. 2012):

$$\Theta = \frac{\sum_{i=1}^{n}\sum_{j=1}^{m}\mathbb{I}\{u_{ij} = 1\}}{\sum_{i=1}^{n}\sum_{j=1}^{m}\mathbb{I}\{u_{ij} = -1\}}, \qquad (3)$$

where $\mathbb{I}\{\cdot\}$ is the indicator function.

The win ratio Θ is a relative measure of treatment effect, with a value of 1 indicating no treatment effect, and values larger than 1 indicating treatment benefit. For time-to-event variables, Oakes (2016) points out that under proportional hazards, the reciprocal of Θ (the "loss ratio") is an estimate of the hazard ratio, with values smaller than 1 indicating treatment benefit.

Inference

The Net Benefit Δ has an asymptotically normal distribution. An approximate variance for Δ is obtained from the theory of U-statistics (Hoeffding 1948; Finkelstein and Schoenfeld 1999; Verbeeck et al. 2018):

$$Var(\Delta) = \frac{n+m}{(n \cdot m)^2} \left(\sum_{i=1}^{n} \sum_{j=1}^{m} \sum_{j' \neq j=1}^{m} u_{ij} u_{ij'} + \sum_{j=1}^{m} \sum_{i=1}^{n} \sum_{i' \neq i=1}^{n} u_{ij} u_{i'j} \right). \quad (4)$$

Inferences can be based on the asymptotically normal standardized test statistic

$$Z = \Delta / \sqrt{\frac{Var(\Delta)}{n+m}}. \quad (5)$$

If preferred, a randomization test can be used for the null hypotheses H_0: $\Delta = 0$. The randomization test requires simulation of a large number of experiments identical to the actual experiment being analyzed, with all individual data kept unchanged except treatment group (treatment or control), which is re-allocated at random. A potential advantage of this test, besides its validity for small sample sizes, is that the re-allocation process can use the same algorithm as in the original randomized experiment (e.g., simple randomization, permuted blocks within strata, minimization), thus generating the appropriate empirical distribution for Δ under the null hypothesis (Buyse 2010). The P-value can be calculated with arbitrary precision, but the approach is computer intensive, which can become an issue for large sample sizes (Rauch et al. 2018).

Asymptotic theory of U-statistics can also be used for estimation and testing of the win ratio (Luo et al. 2015; Bebu and Lachin 2016; Dong et al. 2016). Pocock et al. (2012) used bootstrapping to calculate confidence intervals for Θ (Pocock et al. 2012). Bootstrapping consists of generating an empirical distribution of Θ through repeated sampling with replacement from the original data. This approach too is computer intensive and therefore confidence intervals calculated from asymptotic theory may be preferred (Verbeeck et al. 2020).

Anderson and Verbeeck (2020) suggest to use exact bootstrap and permutation distributions as an alternative to either asymptotic methods (which may not be appropriate for small samples) or resampling approaches (which may be less precise or too onerous in terms of computer time). This approach is efficient and elegant, but it cannot be used in all situations, for example, if re-randomization is used instead of permutation to produce an empirical null distribution for the original treatment allocation algorithm, or if pairs are weighted to remove the dependence on censoring (Péron et al. 2018).

Stratification

In many experimental designs, stratification is used for important covariates such as gender, age, and stage of disease. In such designs, pairwise comparisons are naturally restricted to pairs of individuals within the same stratum. Assume there are S distinct strata (indexed by $s = 1, \ldots, S$), with $n = \sum_{s=1}^{S} n_s$, $m = \sum_{s=1}^{S} m_s$. Δ and Θ are defined similarly as above, with u_{ijs} a stratum-specific pairwise indicator of win, loss, or tie (Buyse 2010; Finkelstein and Schoenfeld 1999; Dong et al. 2018):

$$\Delta = \frac{\sum_{s=1}^{S}\sum_{i=1}^{n_s}\sum_{j=1}^{m_s} u_{ijs}}{\sum_{s=1}^{S} n_s \cdot m_s}, \tag{6}$$

and

$$\Theta = \frac{\sum_{s=1}^{S}\sum_{i=1}^{n_s}\sum_{j=1}^{m_s} \mathbb{I}\{u_{ijs}=1\}}{\sum_{s=1}^{S}\sum_{i=1}^{n_s}\sum_{j=1}^{m_s} \mathbb{I}\{u_{ijs}=-1\}}. \tag{7}$$

The number of pairs in all strata, $\sum_{s=1}^{S} n_s \cdot m_s$, is usually much smaller than $n \cdot m$, which offers computational advantages (Buyse 2010). More importantly, there can be an appreciable gain in precision of the estimates if the outcome has a large variance across the strata relative to the variance within the strata. While stratification may improve the estimate of the Net Benefit, interest may also focus on identifying covariates that have an impact on the Net Benefit. Thas et al. (2012) propose a semiparametric statistical model for the probabilistic index, a linear transformation of the Net Benefit (Thas et al. 2012). They use semiparametric theory to show asymptotic normality of the estimators and consistency of the covariance matrix of their model.

Single Outcome

Binary Outcome

If the outcome is binary, assume $X = 1$ (and $Y = 1$) indicate success, while $X = 0$ (and $Y = 0$) indicate failure. Pairs for which $X_i = 1$ and $Y_j = 0$ are wins, pairs for which $X_i = 0$ and $Y_j = 1$ are losses, and pairs for which $X_i = Y_j$ are ties. The randomization test for Δ is a Monte Carlo approximation to Fisher's exact test if the re-allocation to either treatment or control is constrained to keep the total number of individuals in each group fixed. If p_T and p_C denote the probabilities of success in the treatment and control groups, respectively, it is easy to see that, for binary outcomes, Δ is the absolute risk difference, $p_T - p_C$, while Θ is the odds ratio. Letting $\mathbb{P}\{\cdot\}$ denote the probability,

$$\begin{aligned}\Delta &= \mathbb{P}\{X=1, Y=0\} - \mathbb{P}\{X=0, Y=1\} = p_T(1-p_C) - (1-p_T)p_C \\ &= p_T - p_C.\end{aligned} \tag{8}$$

$$\Theta = \frac{\mathbb{P}\{X=1, Y=0\}}{\mathbb{P}\{X=0, Y=1\}} = \frac{p_T/(1-p_T)}{p_C/(1-p_C)}. \tag{9}$$

Continuous Outcome

If the outcome is continuous, the randomization test for Δ is a Monte Carlo approximation to the exact Wilcoxon test. If the outcome is normally distributed with common variance in the two groups, Δ is related to the standardized mean difference, also called Cohen's d or "effect size":

$$\Delta = 2 \cdot \Phi\left(d/\sqrt{2}\right) - 1, \tag{10}$$

where Φ is the cumulative density function of the standardized normal distribution.

In some applied settings, the difference between the values of the two patients in a pairwise comparison may have to exceed a prespecified threshold, denoted τ, to be considered meaningful (Buyse 2010; Thas et al. 2012). In clinical trials, the threshold can reflect a difference regarded as clinically relevant depending on the nature of the disease and the treatment under study. Assume without loss of generality that larger values of X (and Y) are preferable to smaller values of X (and Y). Pairs for which $X_i - Y_j > \tau$ are wins, pairs for which $X_i - Y_j < -\tau$ are losses, and pairs for which $|X_i - Y_j| \leq \tau$ are ties.

Time-to-Event Outcome

If the variable X (and Y) is possibly right censored, such as in time to event analyses, let variables ϵ and η denote censoring variables X and Y, respectively, with $\epsilon_i = 1$ (or $\eta_j = 1$) indicating that X_i (or Y_j) is a complete observation. Pairs for which $\{X_i - Y_j > \tau$ and $\eta_j = 1\}$ are wins, pairs for which $\{X_i - Y_j < -\tau$ and $\epsilon_i = 1\}$ are losses, and pairs for which $\{|X_i - Y_j| \leq \tau$ and $\epsilon_i = \eta_j = 1\}$ are ties. For all other pairs, it is not possible to determine which of the two individuals has a better outcome, and these pairs are called "uninformative." In the simplest analysis, these pairs do not contribute to the numerator of Eq. (2), in which case pairwise comparisons are equivalent, when $\tau = 0$, to Gehan-Gilbert's generalization of the Wilcoxon test.

Efron (1965) pointed out that the expectation of Gehan-Gilbert's U-statistic under the alternative hypothesis depends on the censoring distribution and the test is only valid if the censoring distributions are equal in the treatment and control groups. Moreover, the Gehan-Gilbert test is less efficient than the logrank test under the assumption of proportional hazards. Simple pairwise comparisons of times to event are subject to the same limitations, but pairs can be weighted using estimates of the survival function in order to remove the dependence on censoring (Péron et al. 2018) and improve the efficiency of the test (Luo et al. 2017). When the treatment effect is delayed and/or there is a cure rate, the efficiency of the test can also be improved by using a threshold of clinical relevance (Péron et al. 2016a).

Under proportional hazards, the win ratio Θ is equal to the inverse of the hazard ratio based on the Wilcoxon statistic (Oakes 2016). In this case, a simple relationship also exists between the Net Benefit Δ, the hazard ratio (HR), and the proportion of informative pairs f, which depends on censoring (Buyse 2008):

$$\Delta = f \cdot (1 - HR)/(1 + HR). \tag{11}$$

Multiple Outcomes

Overall Pairwise Score

O'Brien (1984) proposed a test for K outcomes, with pairwise comparisons counting the number of wins and losses across these outcomes (O'Brien 1984). Define pairwise indicators for each outcome ($k = 1, \ldots, K$):

$$u_{ij}(k) = \begin{cases} 1 & \text{if the pair is a win for the } k^{\text{th}} \text{ outcome} \\ -1 & \text{if the pair is a loss for the } k^{\text{th}} \text{ outcome} \\ 0 & \text{otherwise} \end{cases}$$

Note that $u_{ij}(k)$ can be set to 0 if the pairwise comparison is a tie or is uninformative for the kth outcome, in such a way that the pair can contribute to the analysis even if some of the K outcomes are missing. The (weighted) overall pairwise score is defined as

$$s_{ij} = \sum_{k=1}^{K} w_{ij}(k) u_{ij}(k). \tag{12}$$

where the weight $w_{ij}(k)$ reflects the relative clinical importance of the kth outcome. The (weighted) overall pairwise score leads to a U-statistic that can be used to test for an overall difference between the treatment groups:

$$U = \frac{1}{n \cdot m} \sum_{i=1}^{n} \sum_{j=1}^{m} s_{ij}. \tag{13}$$

This test may gain power as compared with a test for a single outcome. However, the U-statistic no longer has the simple probabilistic interpretation of the Net Benefit δ for a single outcome. In addition, when weights are used, the choice of weights is arbitrary and, as such, potentially debatable and/or patient-dependent. "Optimal" weights can also be chosen to maximize the power of the test for specific alternative hypotheses of interest (Ramchandani et al. 2016).

Composite Pairwise Score

Ramchandani et al. (2016) propose a general framework for pairwise comparisons of multiple outcomes. They define a composite pairwise score by applying a function ϕ to the vector of pairwise indicators $\boldsymbol{u}_{ij} = (u_{ij}(1), \ldots, u_{ij}(K))$ (Ramchandani et al. 2016). ϕ must satisfy some conditions for the test to be valid under the strong null hypothesis that the joint distributions of the outcomes are equal between the two treatment groups. The composite pairwise score leads to a U-statistic that can be used to test for a difference between the treatment groups:

$$U = \frac{1}{n \cdot m} \sum_{i=1}^{n} \sum_{j=1}^{m} \phi(u_{ij}). \qquad (14)$$

For O'Brien's overall pairwise score (O'Brien 1984; Ramchandani et al. 2016):

$$\phi(u_{ij}) = \sum_{k=1}^{K} w_{ij}(k) u_{ij}(k). \qquad (15)$$

Wittkowski et al. (2004) used a more complex composite pairwise score for several ordinal outcomes (Wittkowski et al. 2004; Ramchandani et al. 2016):

$$\phi(u_{ij}) = \mathbb{I}\{ \max_k \{u_{ij}(k) : k = 1, \cdots, K\} = 1\} \\ - \mathbb{I}\{ \min_k \{u_{ij}(k) : l = 1, \cdots, K\} = -1\}. \qquad (16)$$

This composite pairwise score declares a pair to be a win if all the outcomes of the treated patient are at least as good as the outcomes of the control patient, and at least one of these outcomes is better. Losses are defined similarly. Pairs for which some outcomes are better and some are worse are considered ties.

Multiple Prioritized Outcomes

A situation that deserves special attention is when the K outcomes can be prioritized. Assume they are numbered from 1 (highest priority level) to K (lowest priority level). Here (Buyse 2010; Ramchandani et al. 2016):

$$\phi(u_{ij}) = u_{ij}(1) + \mathbb{I}\{u_{ij}(1) = 0\} u_{ij}(2) + \cdots \\ + \mathbb{I}\{u_{ij}(1) = \cdots = u_{ij}(K-1) = 0\} u_{ij}(K). \qquad (17)$$

The composite pairwise score is calculated by performing pairwise comparisons in decreasing order of priority of the K outcomes, until the pair is a win or a loss. For pairs that are uninformative or neutral at priority level $k(k < K)$, the pairwise comparison is performed at level $k + 1$. Note that depending on the context and the nature of the outcomes, pairs that are neutral at level k can be considered informative (in which case the pairwise comparison declares a tie at level k) or uninformative (in which case the pairwise comparison is performed at level $k + 1$ if $k < K$).

Table 2 illustrates the simplest case of two prioritized outcomes, assuming ties are considered informative.

With prioritized outcomes, the Net Benefit can be decomposed into Net Benefits at all priority levels. The Net Benefit up to the kth prioritized outcome is calculated as

$$\Delta(k) = \frac{1}{n \cdot m} \sum_{l=1}^{k} \sum_{i=1}^{n} \sum_{j=1}^{m} u_{ij}(l). \qquad (18)$$

Table 2 Generalized pairwise comparisons for two prioritized outcomes

Prioritized outcome 1	Prioritized outcome 2	Pairwise comparison
Win	Ignored	Win
Loss	Ignored	Loss
Tie	Ignored	Tie
Uninformative	Win	Win
Uninformative	Loss	Loss
Uninformative	Tie	Tie
Uninformative	Uninformative	Uninformative

The Net Benefit up to the outcome of lowest priority, $\Delta(K)$, is the Net Benefit, denoted Δ as previously. The Net Benefit fraction is given by $\Delta(k)/\Delta$, which can be anywhere on the real line.

The information fraction IF up to the kth prioritized outcome is defined as the number of wins and losses up to the kth prioritized outcome divided by the total number of wins and losses. $IF(k)$ is a proportion bound between 0 and 1:

$$IF(k) = \frac{\sum_{l=1}^{k}\sum_{i=1}^{n}\sum_{j=1}^{m}\mathbb{I}\{u_{ij}(l) \neq 0\}}{\sum_{l=1}^{K}\sum_{i=1}^{n}\sum_{j=1}^{m}\mathbb{I}\{u_{ij}(l) \neq 0\}}. \tag{19}$$

The Net Benefits $\Delta(k)$ can be estimated and tested using asymptotic theory of U-statistics. No assumption of independence is required for the variables capturing the outcomes of interest. In order to preserve the overall significance level of a study, it is sufficient to observe that $\Delta(k)$ includes pairwise comparisons of the kth outcome and of all higher priority outcomes ($l = 1, \ldots, k - 1$). Hence significance testing of successive prioritized outcomes is akin to repeated significance testing in group sequential designs. The methods developed for group sequential testing can therefore be used for generalized pairwise comparisons, including flexible α-spending functions used with information fractions $IF(k)$ that are data-dependent rather than set by design (DeMets and Lan 1994). Mao (2018) and Luo et al. (2018) discuss the alternative hypotheses that are being tested when generalized pairwise comparisons are used for several time-to-event prioritized outcomes (Mao 2018; Luo et al. 2018).

Applications of Prioritized Outcomes for a Single Variable

Thresholds of Clinical Relevance

Prioritized outcomes can be defined flexibly. For example, decreasing thresholds of clinical relevance can be entertained in a single analysis. As a clinical example, consider patients with neovascular age-related macular degeneration (AMD), a disease that causes a progressive loss of vision over time. In clinical trials of therapies for AMD, the outcome of interest is the change in visual acuity from baseline to 12 months. Visual acuity is defined as the number of letters correctly read with one eye masked from a fixed distance on a standardized ophthalmic chart that comprises 14 lines of 5 letters each, with the size of the letters decreasing from the top line to the bottom line. A better outcome in pairwise comparisons could be defined as a difference in the change in visual acuity between two individuals of at least k letters, with k varying from more than 30 letters (a remarkable difference that reflects a highly relevant difference in vision) to less than 5 letters (a minor difference that could easily be due to measurement error, changes in reading conditions, or chance variation). In the regulatory setting of a new drug approval for AMD, a change in visual acuity of at least 15 letters is considered clinically relevant. In this example, thresholds representing decreasing differences in numbers of letters of visual acuity could be chosen as $k = 30, 25, 20$, and 15. Note that in this setting ties are considered uninformative, so that neutral pairs for higher priority thresholds can be categorized as wins or losses using lower priority thresholds.

The use of decreasing thresholds can be illustrated with data from a double-blind randomized clinical trial in 1186 patients with neovascular age-related macular degeneration (Gragoudas et al. 2004). Patients were randomized to receive intraocular injections of pegaptanib, an anti-vascular endothelial growth factor therapy, or sham injections with a syringe applied on the surface of the eye to simulate the pressure of an injection, every 6 weeks over a period of 1 year.

The "primary endpoint" of the trial was the proportion of patients losing at least 15 letters of visual acuity 1 year after starting therapy. The last available observation of visual acuity was carried forward for patients in whom the measurement at 1 year was unavailable. Such imputation would no longer be used today, as it can lead to biased estimates, but it was a regulatory standard at the time of this trial. The proportion of patients losing at least 15 letters of visual acuity was 35% for patients receiving a dose of 3 mg of pegaptanib vs. 45% for patients receiving sham injections (an absolute benefit of 10%, χ^2 test $P = 0.015$) (Gragoudas et al. 2004). Using GPC, changes in visual acuity at 1 year can be considered a continuous endpoint. The Net Benefit, considering a difference of at least 15 letters of visual acuity to be relevant, is 12.6% $(P = 0.0005)$ (row $l = 4$ in Table 3). The Net Benefit fractions indicate that half of the Net Benefit is due to pairwise comparisons showing a difference of at least 30 letters, which suggests that some patients enjoyed large benefits from pegaptanib (column "$\Delta(k)/\Delta$" of Table 3).

If any difference in visual acuity is considered clinically relevant (no threshold), the Net Benefit is 17.1% ($P = 0.0007$), about a third larger than when a threshold of 15 letters is used (last row of Table 4). In this case the GPC test is equivalent to a Wilcoxon test for the comparison of mean changes in visual acuity between the randomized groups. This example shows that a GPC test with a threshold of 15 letters is less sensitive than a GPC test without threshold (equivalent to a comparison of mean changes), but more sensitive than a comparison of proportions of patients losing at least 15 letters at 1 year. Importantly, the primary endpoint of this trial (proportion of patients losing at least 15 letters at 1 year) did not consider patients gaining vision, and as such could have missed truly important benefits of new drugs for this disease.

Table 3 Generalized pairwise comparisons in age-related macular degeneration trials ($\delta(k)$, Net Benefit due to kth prioritized outcome; $\Delta(k)$, Net Benefit up to kth prioritized outcome; $\Delta(k)/\Delta$, Net Benefit fraction up to kth prioritized outcome)

Prioritized outcome	Threshold	Wins (a)	Losses (b)	$\delta(k) = (a) - (b)$	$\Delta(k) = \sum_{i \leq k} \delta(i)$	$\Delta(k)/\Delta$	Information fraction
$k = 1$	≥30 letters	11.4%	4.9%	6.5%	6.5%	52%	39%
$k = 2$	≥25 letters	4.4%	2.6%	1.8%	8.3%	66%	56%
$k = 3$	≥20 letters	5.2%	3.1%	2.1%	10.4%	83%	76%
$k = 4$	≥15 letters	6.2%	4.0%	2.2%	12.6%	100%	100%
	No threshold	26.0%	21.5%	4.5%	17.1%		

Table 4 Generalized pairwise comparisons in age-related macular degeneration trials ($\delta(k)$, Net Benefit due to kth prioritized outcome; $\Delta(k)$, Net Benefit up to kth prioritized outcome; $\Delta(k)/\Delta$, Net Benefit fraction up to kth prioritized outcome)

Prioritized outcome	Threshold	Wins (a)	Losses (b)	$\delta(k)$ = (a) − (b)	$\Delta(k) = \sum_{i \leq k} \delta(i)$	$\Delta(k)/\Delta$	Information fraction
$k = 1$	Week 54	48.0%	35.0%	13.0%	13.0%	71%	84%
$k = 2$	Week 48	3.1%	1.0%	2.1%	15.1%	83%	88%
$k = 3$	Week 42	1.1%	0.8%	0.2%	15.3%	84%	90%
$k = 4$	Week 36	2.5%	1.0%	1.5%	16.8%	92%	94%
$k = 5$	Week 30	0.8%	1.0%	−0.2%	16.6%	91%	95%
$k = 6$	Week 24	0.9%	0.6%	0.3%	16.9%	92%	97%
$k = 7$	Week 18	0.8%	0.3%	0.5%	17.3%	95%	98%
$k = 8$	Week 12	1.2%	0.4%	0.8%	18.1%	99%	100%
$k = 9$	Week 6	0.3%	0.1%	0.2%	18.3%	100%	100%

Repeated Observations

Generalized pairwise comparisons are also useful to analyze repeated observations of an outcome of interest if the different occasions at which the outcome is measured are prioritized. For instance, when the variable is measured repeatedly over time (longitudinal data), as in the AMD clinical trial just discussed, a later difference between the groups may be more relevant than an earlier one in so far as it reflects a sustained effect of the intervention or treatment over time. In this case, a later difference will take priority over an earlier difference in pairwise comparisons. A win is defined in this situation by considering the latest occasion (at 1 year) first, and for any uninformative pair, occasions at earlier times. The advantage of such an approach is that for patients who miss later occasions, earlier occasions can be compared with similar occasions from other patients in the pairwise comparisons. Data imputation is thereby avoided, and all patients contribute their most relevant (in this case, latest) observations to the analysis.

In the AMD clinical trials, a GPC analysis could use the week 54 visual acuity for patients for whom the value was known, and earlier visual acuity for those who lacked it (Table 4). Using this approach, the Net Benefit was equal to 18.3% overall. The information fraction was over 80% at week 54 (last column of Table 4), which is useful information to quantify the potential impact of missing data at that time on the analysis. The impact of the missingness mechanism on the estimate of the Net Benefit is a matter for further investigation.

Applications of Prioritized Outcomes for Several Variables

Several Time-to-Event Outcomes

One of the initial motivations of generalized pairwise comparisons was to be able to perform an analysis of the time to the most important outcome, rather than the time to first outcome. The difference between these two analyses can be illustrated a randomized trial of 420 patients with advanced colorectal cancer (de Gramont et al. 2000). Patients were randomized to either a standard regimen of 5-fluorouracil and leucovorin, or to the same regimen plus the experimental drug oxaliplatin. Two time-to-event variables were of interest in this trial: progression-free survival (PFS), defined as the time from randomization to objective disease progression or death, whichever came first, and time to death or overall survival (OS). The trial showed a highly statistically significant benefit of the addition of oxaliplatin on PFS (hazard ratio $= 0.66$, logrank test $P = 0.0001$, Fig. 1), but it failed to reach conventional statistical significance for the benefit of oxaliplatin on OS (hazard ratio $= 0.83$, logrank test $P = 0.135$, Fig. 2). These results led to controversies in interpretation, and it took several years before oxaliplatin was granted marketing authorization.

Generalized pairwise comparisons provide additional insight to the standard analyses of these two endpoints. The Net Benefit of oxaliplatin on time to death (OS) was $\Delta = 10.1\%$ ($P = 0.05$, top panel of Table 5). Interestingly, 44% of the OS

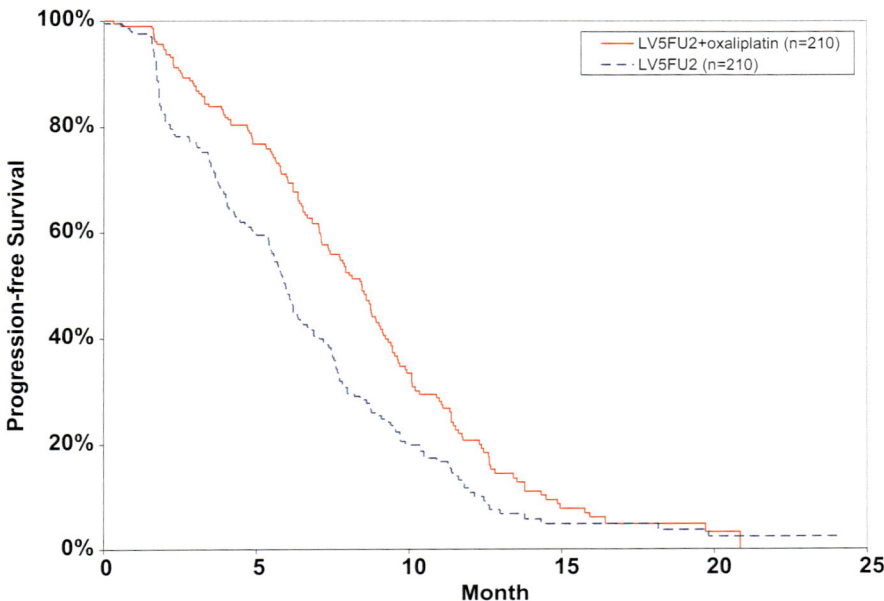

Fig. 1 Progression-free survival for patients with advanced colorectal cancer randomized to standard regimen of 5-fluorouracil and leucovorin (LVF5FU2), with or without the experimental drug oxaliplatin

Net Benefit was due to differences in excess of 12 months, which would probably be considered a worthwhile benefit by most patients. The Net Benefit may be a useful and intuitive measure of treatment benefit for patients: in this example, they could be told that there is a 10% probability (or 1 chance in 10) of a longer survival on the oxaliplatin treatment than on the control treatment, and a 4.4% probability (or 1 chance in 23) of a survival longer by at least 1 year on the oxaliplatin treatment than on the control treatment. These estimates may be more relevant to patients than hazard reductions or absolute risk reductions because they are expressed on the time scale.

The Net Benefit of oxaliplatin on PFS was $\Delta = 24.2\%$ ($P < 0.0001$, middle panel of Table 5), but only 6% of the Net Benefit on PFS was due to differences exceeding 12 months. A patient-oriented message would be that there is a 24% probability (or 1 chance in 4) of a longer progression-free survival on the oxaliplatin treatment than on the control treatment, but only a 1.5% probability (or 1 chance in 67) of a progression-free survival longer by at least 1 year on the oxaliplatin treatment than on the control treatment.

When using the two prioritized outcomes of death and progression, the Net Benefit of oxaliplatin was $\Delta = 10.1\%$ ($P = 0.0054$), with two-thirds of this Net Benefit due to differences in OS (bottom panel of Table 5). Generalized pairwise comparisons of the prioritized outcomes of death and progression are arguably more relevant than an

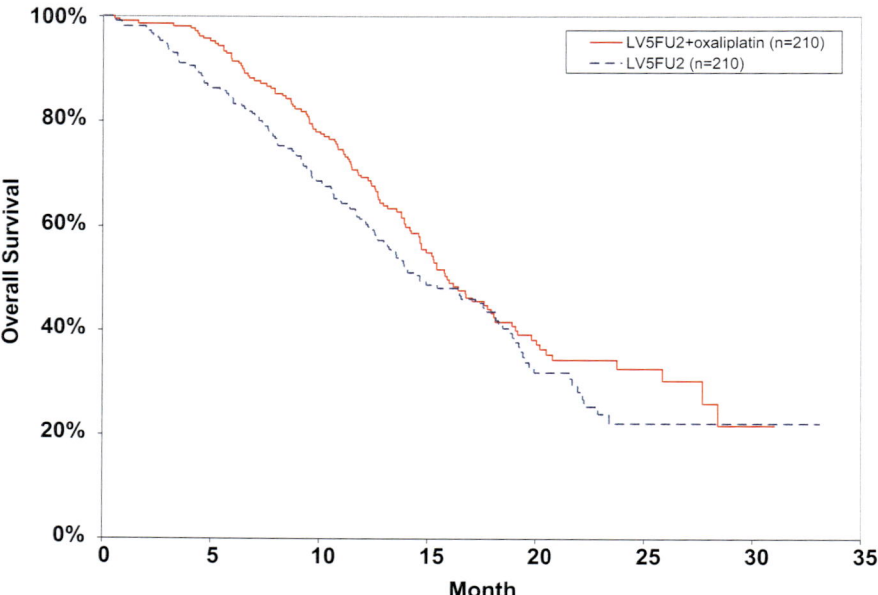

Fig. 2 Survival for patients with advanced colorectal cancer randomized to standard regimen of 5-fluorouracil and leucovorin (LVF5FU2), with or without the experimental drug oxaliplatin

analysis of either of these endpoints, since time to progression is only used for patients who have not yet died, and as such this analysis makes use of all the available information on the most important time-related events. A flexible and patient-relevant use of prioritized outcomes consists of defining thresholds of clinical relevance for both OS and PFS, so that times to progression are used only for pairwise comparisons of OS that do not reach the threshold of clinical relevance. Note that the GPC analysis crucially depends on the follow-up time, which may be viewed as a drawback since with a long enough follow-up, all patients will have died and the times to progression will be ignored in the analysis (except for tied survival times). Finkelstein and Schoenfeld (2018) propose to visually display the contribution of each component as a function of the follow-up time (Finkelstein and Schoenfeld 2018).

Benefit/Risk Assessment

Prioritized outcomes are frequently captured by variables of different types. In advanced cancer, for instance, in addition to time to death and time to disease progression, the achievement of a "tumor response," defined, for example, using the RECIST (Response Evaluation Criteria In Solid Tumors) criteria, is often a relevant indicator of treatment benefit, though the time to achieve such a response is generally unimportant since most responses are obtained soon after starting therapy. In

Table 5 Generalized pairwise comparisons in advanced colorectal cancer trial ($\delta(k)$, Net Benefit due to kth prioritized outcome; $\Delta(k)$, Net Benefit up to kth prioritized outcome; $\Delta(k)/\Delta$, Net Benefit fraction up to kth prioritized outcome)

	Wins (a)	Losses (b)	$\delta(k) = (a) - (b)$	$\Delta(k) = \sum_{i \leq k} \delta(i)$	$\Delta(k)/\Delta$	95% CI for $\Delta(k)$[a]	Test for $\Delta(k)$[a]
Thresholds for overall survival:							
≥12 months	10.8%	6.5%	4.4%	4.4%	44%	(0.1%, 8.5%)	$P = 0.043$
≥6 months	14.7%	10.8%	3.9%	8.3%	83%	(0.4%, 16.1%)	$P = 0.038$
No threshold	17.0%	15.2%	1.8%	10.1%	100%	(0.0%, 20.1%)	$P = 0.050$
Thresholds for progression-free survival:							
≥12 months	2.6%	1.1%	1.5%	1.5%	6%	(−0.2%, 3.3%)	$P = 0.090$
≥6 months	15.5%	5.4%	10.1%	11.6%	48%	(6.4%, 16.9%)	$P < 0.0001$
No threshold	35.5%	22.9%	12.6%	24.2%	100%	(14.1%, 34.4%)	$P < 0.0001$
Prioritized outcomes:							
Death	42.6%	32.5%	10.1%	10.1%	68%	(0.0%, 20.1%)	$P = 0.050$
Progression	9.1%	4.4%	4.7%	14.8%	100%	(4.4%, 25.2%)	$P = 0.0054$

[a]Unadjusted for multiplicity

generalized pairwise comparisons, tumor response could be a binary outcome with lowest priority, used only for those pairwise comparisons that are uninformative or neutral both for time to death and for time to disease progression. Note that GPC naturally take into account the correlation structure of the prioritized outcomes (Giai et al 2020). In the same spirit, Moyé et al. (1992) proposed a generalized Gehan-Wilcoxon test to combine time to death and, for patients still alive at the end of the study, a given decrease in ejection fraction in a post-myocardial infarction trial (Moyé et al. 1992). Finkelstein and Schoenfeld (1999) extended this idea to a test combining time to death with a longitudinally measured variable. They illustrated the versatility of their test in clinical trials for patients with acquired immune deficiency syndrome, in which various types of longitudinal data are relevant, such as repeated episodes of pneumonia, measurements of the head circumference in children, or quality of life assessments in adults (Finkelstein and Schoenfeld 1999).

GPC can be used to perform arbitrarily complex benefit/risk assessments. An illustrative example is provided by therapies currently approved for patients with advanced pancreatic cancer: erlotinib (Péron et al. 2015), FOLFORINOX (Péron et al. 2016b), and nab-paclitaxel + gemcitabine (Péron et al. 2019). Individual patient data were obtained from the randomized trials comparing each of these treatment regimens to gemcitabine alone. The data were analyzed using GPC, with two prioritized outcomes, overall survival (OS) using a threshold of x months, and occurrence of a toxicity of grade 3 of worse on the NCI/CTC (National Cancer Institute Common Toxicity Criteria) scale taking values 0 – no toxicity, 1 – mild, 2 – moderate, 3 – severe, 4 – life-threatening and 5 – death. The analysis was repeated for OS threshold ranging from 1 to 6 months. Table 6 shows how the pairwise comparisons proceeded for these two prioritized outcomes.

Figure 3 shows the Net Benefit for either OS or the prioritized outcomes of OS *and* grade ≥ 3 toxicity. The Net Benefit of erlotinib was much less than that of the other two treatment regimens, and when grade ≥ 3 toxicity was included in the analysis, the Net Benefit became negative for an OS threshold of about 3 months (Péron et al. 2015). In other words, if the purpose of giving another treatment than gemcitabine was to prolong OS by at least 3 months, then erlotinib would not be an effective alternative to gemcitabine. In fact, even though erlotinib was approved for the treatment of advanced pancreatic cancer, it is seldom used in the clinic because of insufficient efficacy and an unfavorable benefit/risk. At the other extreme, the Net Benefit of FOLFORINOX seemed greater than that of the other two treatment regimens, and remained positive for all OS thresholds even when grade ≥ 3 toxicity was included in the analysis (Péron et al. 2016b). The Net Benefit of nab-paclitaxel + gemcitabine was close to that of FOLFORINOX, but it decreased rapidly as a function of the OS threshold when grade ≥ 3 toxicity was included in the analysis (Péron et al. 2019). This was because the difference in toxicity between nab-paclitaxel + gemcitabine and gemcitabine alone was greater than between FOLFIRINOX and gemcitabine alone. Of note, nab-paclitaxel + gemcitabine was compared to gemcitabine in a pivotal trial for marketing authorization, whereas FOLFIRINOX was compared to gemcitabine alone in a clinical practice trial carried out by a cooperative group, so the reporting of toxicities may have been different in these two trials and may partly explain the contrasting risk/benefit assessments.

Table 6 Generalized pairwise comparisons for prioritized outcomes in advanced pancreatic cancer trials

Prioritized outcome 1 OS difference $\geq x$ months	Prioritized outcome 2 grade ≥ 3 toxicity	Pairwise comparison
Win	Ignored	Win
Loss	Ignored	Loss
Tie or uninformative	Win	Win
Tie or uninformative	Loss	Loss
Tie or uninformative	Tie or uninformative	Tie or uninformative

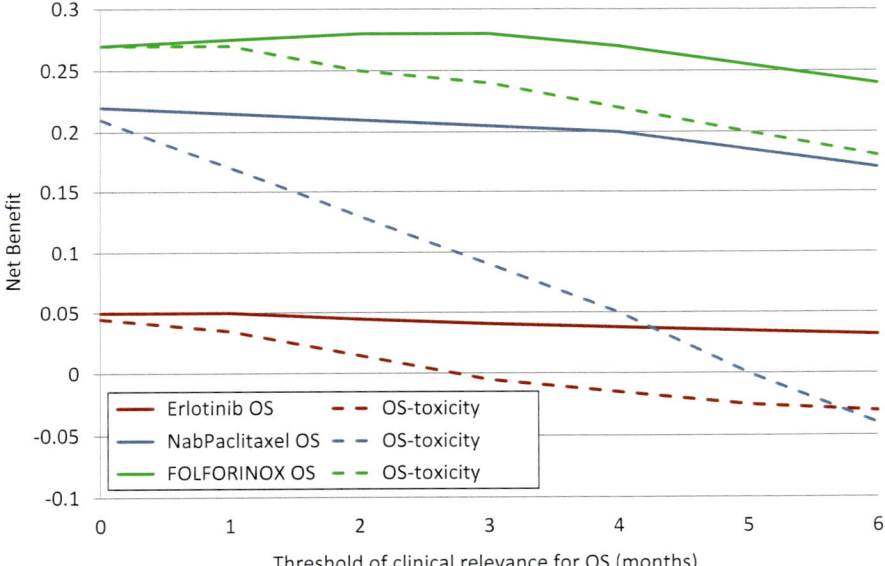

Fig. 3 Net Benefits of three treatments for advanced pancreatic cancer, erlotinib, nab-paclitaxel + gemcitabine and FOLFORINOX as compared to gemcitabine. Solid lines show the Net Benefit on OS for thresholds of increasing clinical relevance for OS (from 1 to 6 months). Dashed lines show the Net Benefit on OS *and* grade ≥ 3 toxicities for the same thresholds of clinical relevance for OS

Conclusion

GPC may serve various purposes: if a single outcome is of interest, defining thresholds of decreasing clinical relevance may provide valuable insight into the magnitude of treatment benefit, and for outcomes that are repeatedly measured over time, prioritized outcomes may eliminate the need for imputing missing data. If multiple outcomes are of interest, the power of the analysis of rare events (e.g., death) may be greatly enhanced by also considering other outcomes that have clinical relevance. If several outcomes are considered, it may be preferable to perform an analysis of time to most important outcome than an analysis of the conventional time to first outcome (regardless of importance). Finally, there may be a desire to offset the benefits of a toxic treatment or risky intervention with the harms caused by the intervention.

When several outcomes are considered, their respective priorities depend on the situation at hand, and may be a matter of debate or even personal preference. Deciding on the respective priorities of the different variables capturing all the outcomes of interest is a potential difficulty of GPC. When designing a prospective experiment, these priorities would have to be agreed upon such that the type I error of the experiment be controlled, and its power properly calculated (using simulations). When analyzing an experiment, different priorities could be given to the different variables and the analysis "personalized" to the preferences of an individual patient. This approach paves the way to truly personalized medicine, as opposed to "precision medicine" which requires a distinct statistical approach. The price to pay for such personalization is that there is no longer a population parameter that can be estimated to quantify the treatment effect (say, a shift in means). This is a major and somewhat unsettling departure from traditional statistical inference.

The Net Benefit, Δ, is a general measure of difference between the treatment groups being compared. When a single outcome measure is considered without threshold of clinical relevance, Δ is related to traditional measures of effect that depend on the type of variable considered. When prioritized outcomes are considered, the interpretation of the Net Benefit is less straightforward and is best interpreted as the net probability that a patient will do better in the treatment group than in the control group. Although this metric of treatment effect is unusual, it is arguably more patient relevant as well as being applicable to any number of prioritized outcome(s) regardless of their type.

GPC can shed additional light on traditional analyses of primary, secondary, and safety endpoints, as in the examples of sections "Applications of Prioritized Outcomes for a Single Variable" and "Applications of Prioritized Outcomes for Several Variables." Whether GPC can become the primary analysis of a trial requires further research. A range of problems remain to be addressed, including the control of multiplicity, the prespecification of priorities and thresholds of clinical relevance, the impact of missingness, and the computational burden of the method if trial design relies primarily on simulations.

Cross-References

- ▶ Estimation and Hypothesis Testing
- ▶ Randomization and Permutation Tests
- ▶ Safety and Risk Benefit Analyses

Acknowledgments The authors are grateful to Eyetech Inc., Pfizer Inc., and Sanofi–Aventis for permission to reanalyze data from clinical trials in age-related macular degeneration (Gragoudas et al. 2004) and advanced colorectal cancer (de Gramont et al. 2000). This research received funding from the Government of Wallonia (Biowin Consortium agreement no. 7979). R software (package BuyseTest) is available in CRAN to implement GPC.

References

Acion L, Peterson JJ, Temple S, Arndt S (2006) Probabilistic index: an intuitive non-parametric approach to measuring the size of treatment effects. Stat Med 25:591–602

Anderson WN, Verbeeck J (2020) Exact bootstrap and permutation distribution of wins and losses in a hierarchical trial. https://arxiv.org/abs/1901.10928

Bebu I, Lachin JM (2016) Large sample inference for a win ratio analysis of a composite outcome based on prioritized components. Biostatistics 17:178–187

Biomarkers Definition Working Group (2001) Biomarkers and surrogate endpoints: preferred definitions and conceptual framework. Clin Pharmacol Ther 69:89–95

Brumback L, Pepe M, Alonzo T (2006) Using the ROC curve for gauging treatment effect in clinical trials. Stat Med 25:575–590

Brunner E, Domhof S, Langer F (2001) Nonparametric analysis of longitudinal data in factorial experiments. Wiley, New York

Buyse M (2008) Reformulating the hazard ratio to enhance communication with clinical investigators (letter to the editor). Clin Trials 5:641–642

Buyse M (2010) Generalized pairwise comparisons for prioritized outcomes in the two-sample problem. Stat Med 29:3245–3257

de Gramont A, Figer A, Seymour M, Homerin M, Hmissi A, Cassidy J, Boni C, Cortes-Funes H, Cervantes A, Freyer G, Papamichael D, Le Bail N, Louvet C, Hendler D, de Braud F, Wilson C, Morvan F, Bonetti A (2000) Leucovorin and fluorouracil with or without oxaliplatin as first-line treatment in advanced colorectal cancer. J Clin Oncol 18:2938–2947

De Neve J, Thas O, Ottoy JP, Clement L (2013) An extension of the Wilcoxon–Mann–Whitney test for analyzing RT-qPCR data. Stat Appl Genet Mol Biol 12:333–346

DeMets DL, Lan KK (1994) Interim analysis: the alpha spending function approach. Stat Med 13:1341–1352

Dmitrienko A, Tamhane AC, Bretz F (2010) Multiple testing problems in pharmaceutical statistics. CRC Press, Boca Raton

Dong G, Li D, Ballerstedt S, Vandemeulebroecke M (2016) A generalized analytic solution to the win ratio to analyze a composite endpoint considering the clinical importance order among components. Pharm Stat 15:430–437

Dong G, Qiu J, Wang D, Vandemeulebroecke M (2018) The stratified win ratio. J Biopharm Stat 28:778–796

Efron B (1965) The two-sample problem with censored data. In: Proceedings of the fifth Berkeley symposium, vol 4. University of California Press, Berkeley, pp 831–853

Evans SR, Follmann D (2016) Using outcomes to analyze patients rather than patients to analyze outcomes: a step toward pragmatism in benefit:risk evaluation. Stat Biopharm Res 8:386–393

Finkelstein DM, Schoenfeld DA (1999) Combining mortality and longitudinal measures in clinical trials. Stat Med 18:1341–1354

Finkelstein DM, Schoenfeld DA (2018) Graphing the win ratio and its components over time. Stat Med 38:53–61

Giai J, Péron J, Ozenne B, Chiêm JC, Buyse M, Maucort-Boulch D (2020) Net benefit in the presence of correlated prioritized outcomes using generalized pairwise comparisons: a simulation study. Stat Med https://doi.org/10.1002/sim.8788

Gragoudas ES, Adamis AP, Cunningham ET, Feinsod M, Guyer DR, for the VEGF Inhibition Study in Ocular Neovascularization Clinical Trial Group (2004) Pegaptanib for neovascular age-related macular degeneration. N Engl J Med 351:2805–2816

Grissom R (1994) Probability of the superior outcome of one treatment over another. J Appl Psychol 79:314–316

Harrell F Jr (2001) Regression modeling strategies: with applications to linear models, logistic regression, and survival analysis. Springer, New York

Hoeffding W (1948) A class of statistics with asymptotically normal distribution. Ann Math Stat 19:293–325

Huang P, Woolson RF, O'Brien PC (2008) A rank-based sample size method for multiple outcomes in clinical trials. Stat Med 27:3084–3104

Lachin JM (2014) Applications of the Wei–Lachin multivariate one-sided test for multiple outcomes on possibly different scales. PLoS One 9:e108784

Lachin JM, Bebu I (2015) Application of the Wei–Lachin multivariate one-directional test to multiple event-time outcomes. Clin Trials 12:627–633

Luo XL, Tian H, Mohanty S, Tsai WY (2015) An alternative approach to confidence interval estimation for the win ratio statistic. Biometrics 71:139–145

Luo X, Qiu J, Bai S, Tian H (2017) Weighted win loss approach for analyzing prioritized outcomes. Stat Med 6:2452–2465

Luo XL, Tian H, Mohanty S, Tsai WY (2018) Rejoinder to "on the alternative hypotheses for the win ratio". Biometrics. https://doi.org/10.1111/biom.12953

Mao L (2018) On the alternative hypotheses for the win ratio. Biometrics. https://doi.org/10.1111/biom.12954

Moyé LA (2003) Multiple analyses in clinical trials. Fundamentals for investigators, 2nd edn. Springer, New York

Moyé LA, Davis BR, Hawkins CM (1992) Analysis of a clinical trial involving a combined mortality and adherence dependent interval censored endpoint. Stat Med 11:1705–1717

O'Brien PC (1984) Procedures for comparing samples with multiple endpoints. Biometrics 69:1079–1087

Oakes D (2016) On the win-ratio statistic in clinical trials with multiple types of event. Biometrika 103:742–745

Péron J, Roy P, Ding K, Parulekar W, Roche L, Buyse M (2015) Benefit-risk assessment of adding erlotinib to gemcitabine for the treatment of advanced pancreatic cancer. Br J Cancer 112:971–976

Péron J, Roy P, Ozenne B, Roche L, Buyse M (2016a) The net chance of a longer survival as a patient-oriented measure of benefit in randomized clinical trials. JAMA Oncol 2:901–905

Péron J, Roy P, Conroy T, Desseigne F, Ychou M, Gourgou-Bourgade S, Stanbury T, Roche L, Ozenne B, Buyse M (2016b) An assessment of the benefit-risk balance of FOLFORINOX in metastatic pancreatic adenocarcinoma. Oncotarget 7:82953–82960

Péron J, Buyse M, Ozenne B, Roche L, Roy P (2018) An extension of generalized pairwise comparisons for prioritized outcomes in the presence of censoring. Stat Methods Med Res 27:1230–1239

Péron J, Giai J, Maucort-Boulch D, Buyse M (2019) The benefit-risk balance of nab-paclitaxel in metastatic pancreatic adenocarcinoma. Pancreas 48:175–180

Pocock SJ, Ariti CA, Collier TJ, Wang D (2012) The win ratio: a new approach to the analysis of composite endpoints in clinical trials based on clinical priorities. Eur Heart J 33:176–182

Ramchandani R, Schoenfeld DA, Finkelstein DM (2016) Global rank tests for multiple, possibly censored, outcomes. Biometrics 72:926–935

Rauch G, Jahn-Eimermacher A, Brannath W, Kieser M (2014) Opportunities and challenges of combined effect measures based on prioritized outcomes. Stat Med 33:1104–1120

Rauch G, Kunzmann K, Kieser M, Wegscheider K, König J, Eulenburg C (2018) A weighted combined effect measure for the analysis of a composite time-to-first-event endpoint with components of different clinical relevance. Stat Med 37:749–767

Rom DM, Hwang E (1996) Testing for individual and population equivalence based on the proportion of similar responses. Stat Med 15:1489–1505

Senn SJ (1997) Testing for individual and population equivalence based on the proportion of similar responses. Stat Med 16:1303–1306

Senn S (2011) U is for unease: reasons to mistrust overlap measures in clinical trials. Stat Biopharm Res 3:302–309

Stine RA, Heyse JF (2001) Non-parametric estimates of overlap. Stat Med 20:215–236

Stolker JM, Spertus JA, Cohen DG, Jones PG, Jain KK, Bamberger E, Lonergan BB, Chan PS (2014) Rethinking composite end points in clinical trials: insights from patients and trialists. Circulation 130:1254–1261

Thas O, De Neve J, Clement L, Ottoy JP (2012) Probabilistic index models (with discussion). J R Stat Soc Ser B 74:623–671

Verbeeck J, Spitzer E, de Vries T, van Es GA, Anderson WN, Van Mieghem NM, Leon MB, Molenberghs G, Tijssen J (2018) Generalized pairwise comparison methods to analyze (non)-hierarchical composite endpoints. Stat Med 38:5641–5656

Verbeeck J, Ozenne B, Anderson WN (2020) Evaluation of inferential methods for the net benefit and win ratio statistics. J Biopharm Stat 30:765–82

Verbeeck J, Deltuvaite-Thomas V, Berckmoes B, Burzykowski T, Aerts M, Thas O, Buyse M, Molenberghs G (2020) Unbiasedness and efficiency of non-parametric and UMVUE estimators of the probabilistic index and related statistics. Stat Meth Med Res. https://doi.org/10.1177/0962280220966629

Wei LJ, Lachin JM (1984) Two-sample asymptotically distribution-free tests for incomplete multivariate observations. J Am Stat Assoc 79:653–661

Wittkowski KM, Lee E, Nussbaum R, Chamian FN, Krueger JG (2004) Combining several ordinal measures in clinical studies. Stat Med 23:1579–1592

Use of Resampling Procedures to Investigate Issues of Model Building and Its Stability

96

Willi Sauerbrei and Anne-Laure Boulesteix

Contents

Introduction	1896
Data and Possible Questions	1897
Glioma	1897
Breast Cancer	1898
Kidney Cancer	1899
General Issues in Building Regression Models	1899
Building Regression Models: Aims and Personal Preferences Play a Role	1899
Extract Information by Model Building in Resampling Replications	1900
Methods	1901
Traditional Variable Selection Procedures	1901
Candidate Variables and Their Effect on Variable Selection Stability	1901
Functional Form for Continuous Variables	1902
Treatment-Covariate Interaction in RCTs	1903
The Nonparametric Bootstrap to Assess Model Stability	1904
Results	1905
Model Selection in Bootstrap Replications	1905
Function Selection	1907
Treatment-Covariate Interaction	1909
Discussion	1910
Summary	1910
Some Issues in Identifying Influential Covariates and Deriving a Predictor	1911
Assumption of a Linear Effect of a Continuous Variable	1912
Interaction of Treatment with a Continuous Variable	1913

W. Sauerbrei (✉)
Institute of Medical Biometry and Statistics, Faculty of Medicine and Medical Center - University of Freiburg, Freiburg, Germany
e-mail: wfs@imbi.uni-freiburg.de

A.-L. Boulesteix
Institute for Medical Information Processing, Biometry, and Epidemiology, LMU Munich, Munich, Germany
e-mail: boulesteix@ibe.med.uni-muenchen.de

© Springer Nature Switzerland AG 2022
S. Piantadosi, C. L. Meinert (eds.), *Principles and Practice of Clinical Trials*,
https://doi.org/10.1007/978-3-319-52636-2_130

Which Resampling Technique? 1914
More Modelling Needed: Guidance Required 1914
Key Points 1915
Cross-References 1915
References 1916

Abstract

This chapter deals with issues in model building and the use of resampling procedures to assess model stability. Concentrating on the nonparametric bootstrap and taking material from five papers published between 1992 and 2015, procedures for variable selection, selection of the functional form for continuous variables, and treatment-covariate interactions are discussed. The methods are illustrated by using publicly available data from three randomized trials. General issues related to the selection of regression models as well as bootstrap procedures used as a pragmatic approach to gain further knowledge from clinical data are briefly outlined.

Keywords

Bootstrap · Continuous variables · Variable selection · Treatment interactions · Functional form · Stability investigations

Introduction

A decade ago, Sauerbrei and Royston (2007) argued that data-dependent modelling should become more popular in clinical trials. In a paper on some roles of the bootstrap, they argue in favor of making greater efforts to extract more information from large trials. It seems that possible information from many of the collected variables is hardly used. Well-known problems of multiplicity with increased type I error, biased estimates after data-dependent model building, and the restrictive role of regulators are possible reasons for this unfortunate situation. With increasing pressure to shorten the time for the development of new products, the pharmaceutical industry seems to be more open to innovative statistical methods.

Multivariable modelling can identify important prognostic information and may indicate treatment interactions and more. The results may be helpful to plan new studies and to generate new hypotheses for a treatment. In order to protect against erroneous conclusions from data-dependent modelling in a multivariable context, stability analyses and detailed checks of the results can be suitable instruments.

In this chapter, several stability issues in multivariable model building are illustrated by examples published in earlier papers. All data sets are publicly available and can be used for further investigations. Analyses of a large number of samples created using resampling procedures are intended as a pragmatic additional approach to extract further information which may otherwise go unnoticed and unused in the analysis of the original data.

Our discussion of the potential gain through complementary analyses of data from three randomized controlled trials (RCTs) aims at illustrating that data from many clinical trials contain a wealth of hidden relevant information and that further modelling can be a promising pathway to extract some of it. For many years, resampling procedures have been used as a suitable instrument to protect against overinterpretation and overoptimism. In the following examples, issues in model building and the use of resampling procedures to assess model stability are discussed. As in the early papers on model stability (Chen and George 1985; Altman and Andersen 1989), the nonparametric bootstrap is used. Alternative resampling approaches (e.g., subsampling) have been proposed, and many more modelling issues can be tackled. Some references discussing such issues in the context of model stability are given. Ideas and results are presented without referring to technical details. High-dimensional data and small sample sizes, scenarios in which stability investigations have become popular over the last decade, are not considered here (Meinshausen and Bühlmann 2010).

All analyses and some parts of the text are taken from earlier papers (Sauerbrei and Schumacher 1992; Sauerbrei 1999; Royston and Sauerbrei 2003; Sauerbrei and Royston 2007; Sauerbrei et al. 2015), all published by John Wiley & Sons Inc. The original text is often shortened and sometimes adapted. A reference to the original paper is given, and interested readers may find further information there.

In "Data and Possible Questions" three data sets are briefly introduced and potential research questions are considered. "General issues in building regression models" are discussed and methods used in this chapter are focused on in "Methods." Analyses and results of the three data sets are presented in "Results." A broader discussion of key issues surrounding this topic follows in "Discussion." Interested readers will find additional analyses and more details in the original papers.

Data and Possible Questions

Results from bootstrap analyses of three RCTs are presented. The following sections expand on the background of each study. All data sets are publicly available on the multivariable fractional polynomials website (http://mfp.imbi.uni-freiburg.de/).

Glioma

The data was collected in a randomized trial comparing two chemotherapy regimens including 447 patients with malignant glioma. At the time of the analysis, 293 patients had died, and the median survival time from the date of randomization was about 11 months. Besides therapy, 12 variables (age, three ordinal, and eight binary variables) which might influence survival time were considered. The three ordinal variables (the Karnofsky index, the type of surgical resection and the grade of malignancy) were each represented by two dummy variables, resulting in a total of

15 predictors denoted by $X_1, \ldots, X_{15}$. For these predictors complete data were available from 413 patients (274 events), used here in a complete case analysis. Two patients had follow-up time "0" and no event, therefore in later publications it may be stated that n = 411. For more details see Sauerbrei (1999) and references given.

In addition to therapy, the investigation of prognostic factors is of interest. For age, a linear effect was an acceptable assumption. Dummies for the three ordinal variables were handled like separate variables. This approach is acceptable here, although sometimes subject matter knowledge may be an important argument considering dummies representing one variable together. As none of the potential predictors exhibited a stronger effect with varying time, the standard Cox model was used. To select variables with influence on survival time, backward elimination with a significance level of 0.05 was used. Finally, model stability was investigated in bootstrap samples.

Breast Cancer

Between July 1984 and December 1989, the German Breast Cancer Study Group (GBSG) recruited 720 patients with primary node positive breast cancer into a factorial 2 × 2 trial investigating the effectiveness of three versus six cycles of chemotherapy and of additional hormonal treatment with tamoxifen. Tamoxifen had an effect on recurrence-free survival (RFS); however, there were no differences for the two chemotherapy groups. Several prognostic variables were available. Note that these data have been used to identify variables influencing RFS. As in earlier analyses (Sauerbrei and Royston 1999; Sauerbrei 1999), the recurrence-free survival time of 686 patients (299 events) will be considered with complete data for the standard factors: age, menopausal status, tumor size, tumor grade, number of positive lymph nodes, progesterone receptors, and estrogen receptors. Five of these seven factors are measured on a continuous scale. To handle continuous variables, the most popular approaches in the Cox model assume a linear effect or categorize the variable by using one or more cut points for each variable. Using the multivariable fractional polynomial (MFP, see 3.3) approach with a nominal significance level of 0.05 and adjusting for hormonal treatment, Sauerbrei and Royston (1999) derived a model (model III) which includes the number of positive nodes (transformed), an FP1 function for progesterone receptors, tumor grade, and an FP2 function for age. The nonlinear function selected for ages postulates that very young patients have a strongly increased risk, whereas the risk hardly changes for patients above 40 years. Obviously, this could not be detected when postulating a linear effect and was not detected with the categorized approach using pre-selected cut points 45 and 60. The variables menopausal status, tumor size, and estrogen receptor were not selected in the final MFP model. Using the nonparametric bootstrap, Royston and Sauerbrei (2003) investigated the stability of the selected MFP model. The focus, in this chapter, lies on the stability of the age effect; some dependencies of bootstrap inclusion fractions for correlated variables will also be illustrated.

Kidney Cancer

In the MRC RE01 randomized trial interferon-rx (IFN) was compared with medroxyprogesterone acetate (MPA) in patients with metastatic renal carcinoma. The study recruited 350 patients between 1992 and 1997. In the first paper based on 335 patients and 236 deaths, a 28% reduction in the risk of death in the IFN group was reported (MRCRCC 1999). To investigate potential interactions of treatment with a continuous covariate, Royston and Sauerbrei (2004) used updated data with 322 deaths in 347 patients. They found a significant interaction with white cell count (WCC) by using the multivariable fractional polynomial interaction (MFPI) procedure. These data will be used here for investigating the stability of the treatment effect function (TEF; see section "Treatment-Covariate Interaction") and compare model based with bootstrap-based TEFs and related confidence intervals. No interaction was found for another nine prognostic variables. More details are given in Sauerbrei and Royston (2007).

General Issues in Building Regression Models

Building Regression Models: Aims and Personal Preferences Play a Role

For most diseases, prognostic factors play a central role in clinical research, for example, in deriving prognostic models and predictors and aiding medical decision making. Consequently, many factors are routinely collected in clinical trials and data analysts are often faced with long lists of covariates that may influence an outcome. In fitting regression models, there is a consensus that subject matter knowledge should generally guide model building; however, this is often limited or at best fragile, making data-dependent model building necessary (Harrell 2001).

If the number of variables is large, a parsimonious model involving fewer than all of the available k variables is often preferable (Babu 2011). Issues and methods for variable selection are very similar among the three most popular models in the health sciences (linear regression model, logistic regression model, and Cox model). Usually, methods for variable selection and related issues have been developed and investigated for a linear regression model. However, the methods, or at least their basic ideas, are commonly transferred to generalized linear models and to models for survival data, although there are sometimes additional problems, such as definitions of residuals or equivalents of R^2 for censored data.

Despite the central importance of variable selection and more generally of model development issues in all areas of science in which data are analyzed, there is no widely accepted guidance concerning suitable methods. The literature is full of all types and also of conflicting criticism of selection strategies, but in practice a strategy has to be chosen. Whether a model is useful does not depend on the method used for selection but can be better judged by its appropriateness in helping to answer the subject matter question. As a consequence of the lack of generally accepted guidance, the decision for a specific modelling strategy often depends on personal preferences (Royston and Sauerbrei 2008).

Most analysts will agree that a good model should fit the data adequately, not be too complex, and should provide accurate predictions for new observations. Including variables without influence leads to the problem of overfitting and unnecessarily increases the variance of parameter estimates for correlated variables and the predictor. On the other hand, eliminating influential variables results in underfitting of the data with a worsening of the fit (increased residuals) and often in biased parameter estimates for other variables. As such, model selection criteria should balance the competing objectives of conformity to the data and parsimony. The effect of bias depends on the (multi)collinearity between the omitted and the selected variables (Sauerbrei 1999).

Depending on the aim of a particular study, the severity of the potential biases induced by model building may be considered in different ways. In the excellent paper entitled "To Explain or to Predict," Shmueli (2010) describes differences between three conceptual modelling approaches: descriptive, predictive, and explanatory modelling. A "complex" model including several covariates with "weak" effect may be tolerated if a suitable prediction is the only interest of a model. The situation is very different if a descriptive model with strong interest in identifying the influential covariates is the primary aim. Besides prediction performance, criteria such as generalizability, transportability, and practical usefulness are considered to be important. It is known that simpler models are more stable, an important argument for a useful explanatory model (Sauerbrei 1999).

Furthermore, recognizing covariates with differential subgroup treatment effects is a highly relevant issue of all RCTs. Several approaches for analysis are available, and the assessment of type I and type II errors and potential biases are key issues (Royston and Sauerbrei 2004; Donegan et al. 2015). Personal preferences play a role when weighting these biases.

Extract Information by Model Building in Resampling Replications

From a theoretical point of view, it would be preferable to prespecify a "main" model. This is often done in a statistical analysis plan for a clinical trial and helps to avoid various types of biases. However, it is to be expected that not all important information from clinical trials data will be extracted. For example, when exploring treatment by covariate interactions in RCTs, it seems still common practice to restrict investigations to a small number of prespecified variables and to dichotomize continuous variables. Several potentially relevant variables will never be considered and dichotomization introduces severe problems such as loss of power or assuming biologically unrealistic step functions (Royston et al. 2006). Therefore, Sauerbrei and Royston (2007) argue for more data-dependent modelling and discuss some roles of the bootstrap (Efron 1979) to assist in gaining information from larger trials. Resampling approaches can be used to check results of data-dependent modelling and conduct stability assessments to mention but a few. However, it is well-known that many resampling approaches exist and that for each type of application, careful consideration is needed to make sure that resampling works as expected (LePage and Billard 1992; Davison and Hinkley 1997). For some issues on the suitable use of bootstrap methods, see chapter 9 entitled "When Bootstrapping Fails Along with Remedies for Failures" in the monograph by Chernick (2008) and the discussion of pros and cons for various bootstrap methods for adjusting p-values in the context of multiple comparisons (Westfall 2011). Further general issues in building regression models are discussed in Sauerbrei et al. (2015).

Methods

Traditional Variable Selection Procedures

Besides the "full" model including all variables, many strategies are discussed in the literature and used in real data. When considering inclusion or exclusion of a variable as the only issue of multivariable model building for k candidate covariates, 2^k submodels have to be compared. Sequential strategies (such as forward selection, stepwise selection, or backward elimination) or all-subset selection with different optimization criteria (e.g., Mallows's Cp, Akaike information criterion (AIC), Bayesian information criterion (BIC)) seem to be the strategies used most often. The latter use penalties for every parameter in the model (2 for AIC, *ln(n)* for BIC) and select the model(s) with the minimal value(s). The BIC penalty is (much) larger, resulting in smaller models selected.

Information criteria are sometimes chosen as the stopping criteria for stepwise procedures, thus combining these approaches. The decision for the stop criterion is the key determinant of the complexity of a selected model. Adapted versions of AIC and BIC are popular information measures to compare and select models from the class of generalized linear models or models for survival data.

Candidate Variables and Their Effect on Variable Selection Stability

In all studies a decision is needed regarding candidate variables initially examined or considered for inclusion in models. Candidate variables may be selected based on background knowledge without any use of the data (e.g., in a prespecified statistical analysis plan), data dependently with or without inspecting correlation to the outcome or a combination thereof. Candidate variables may be defined as a result of initial data analysis with data cleaning, data screening, refining, and updating of initial variable definitions and thoughts expressed in the statistical analysis plan (Huebner et al. 2018) or as a result of preliminary investigations of the effect of specified variables on the outcome. In the latter case, a distinction needs to be made between univariable variable selection and more complex multivariable procedures.

All procedures used to define candidate variables influence the final model and its stability, but the potential problems related to post-selection inference introduced by those procedures that use the data are different. While the change of variable definitions may be an important consequence of initial data analysis (e.g., collapsing "very small" categories) without harming post-selection inference, the use of outcome data may result in biased estimates of the parameters from the final model. Candidate variables may also be selected by criteria referring to the measurement techniques such as reliability, simplicity, objectivity, or cost and on strength of correlations to other variables. Having stronger effects in a study often helps to stabilize the model selection process (Sauerbrei et al. 2015).

Regardless of the process that has taken place, it is important to list all candidate variables initially examined and to report relevant steps of the selection process (Altman et al. 2012).

Functional Form for Continuous Variables

For continuous covariates, a simple and popular approach is to assume a linear effect, but the linearity assumption may be questionable. To avoid this strong assumption, researchers often apply cut points to categorize the covariate, employing regression models with step functions. This simplifies the analysis and may or may not simplify the interpretation of results. It seems that the usual approach in clinical and psychological research is to dichotomize continuous covariates, whereas in epidemiological studies it is customary to create several categories, often four or five, allowing investigation of a crude dose-response relationship. However, categorization discards information and raises several critical issues such as how many cut points to use and where to place them (Altman et al. 1994; Royston et al. 2006). Sauerbrei (1999) illustrate several critical issues by investigating prognostic factors in patients with breast cancer. As a more suitable approach to analysis, they propose to model continuous covariates with fractional polynomials (FP).

FP functions are a flexible family of parametric models (Royston and Altman 1994). Here, one, two, or more power transformations of the form x^p are fitted, the exponent(s) p being chosen from a small, preselected set $S = \{-2, -1, -0.5, 0, 0.5, 1, 2, 3\}$ where x^0 denotes $\log x$. An FP function with two terms (FP2) is a model $\beta_1 x^{p_1} + \beta_2 x^{p_2}$ with exponents p_1 and p_2. For $p_1 = p_2 = p$ ('repeated powers'), FP2 is defined as $\beta_1 x^p + \beta_2 x^p \log x$. This gives eight FP1 functions (including linear) and 36 FP2 functions. The extension to functions with m terms (FPm) is straightforward.

To select a specific function, a closed test procedure was proposed (Royston and Sauerbrei 2008). The complexity of the finally chosen function is predicated on preliminary decisions as to the nominal p value (α) and the degree (m) of the most complex FP model allowed. In our type of applications, more than two terms are hardly needed. For $m = 2$ the function selection procedure (FSP) tests in up to three steps whether (1) the best FP2 function fits the data significantly better than the null, (2) the best FP2 fits better than the linear, and (3) the best FP2 fits better than the best FP1. Step (1) tests for an overall association of the outcome with X, step (2) examines the evidence for nonlinearity, and the last test chooses between a simpler or a more complex nonlinear model. See Royston and Sauerbrei (2008) for a monograph on this topic and related website: http://mfp.imbi.uni-freiburg.de. To assess the stability of individual functions, several measures were proposed (Royston and Sauerbrei 2003, 2009a).

Treatment-Covariate Interaction in RCTs

In RCTs, interactions between treatment and covariates are important because they are the basis of individualized treatment choices from a statistical point of view. Such covariates are often called predictive factors. When the covariate is continuous (such as age or white cell count), interactions are often sought by crude statistical methods, typically involving dichotomizing the continuous covariate. First, general issues regarding investigation of treatment-covariate interactions are briefly discussed followed by consideration of continuous covariates. For the latter, the multivariable fractional polynomial interaction (MFPI) approach is introduced (Royston and Sauerbrei 2004).

Some General Issues

The aim to determine a more individualized treatment for patients leads to the role of prognostic and predictive markers; in statistical terms, the latter are treatment-covariate interactions. Identifying a qualitative interaction in an RCT comparing treatment A with B is an indication that a subgroup of patients may benefit more from therapy A, whereas in the other subgroup B, a somewhat better or at least a comparable effect might be observed. Ideally, some important analyses of possible treatment-covariate interactions are prespecified in the protocol. This allows a sensible interpretation if a test for interaction is significant and treatment effects differ in two subgroups. However, subgroup analyses also introduce analytic challenges and can lead to overstated and misleading results. For example, unplanned subset analyses without a formal test for interaction are published. The report by Wang et al. (2007) outlines several challenges associated with conducting and reporting subgroup analyses.

Important issues raised are increased type I error because of repeated testing and the lack of power to detect differences of treatment effects in smaller subgroups. For a continuous covariate, it is necessary to either determine sensible cut point(s) to categorize the covariate or to choose an approach to model the dependency of the treatment effect on the value of the covariate. These critical issues are relevant, but it is also important to extract some of the "hidden" information from large randomized trials.

Interaction with a Continuous Covariate

The MFPI procedure is a method to detect and estimate interactions of treatment with a continuous covariate (Royston and Sauerbrei 2004). First, for each treatment group, MFPI estimates a fractional polynomial function representing the prognostic effect of the continuous covariate of interest, optionally adjusting for other covariates. Second, a significance test is conducted to investigate whether the continuous covariate has an influence on the treatment effect. The difference between the FP functions for the treatment groups is calculated and called "treatment-effect function." A plot of the difference (e.g., on the log hazard ratio scale) against the covariate, together with a 95% CI, is constructed and termed as "treatment-effect plot." The presence of interaction is indicated by a nonconstant line, often increasing or decreasing, whereas lack of interaction is indicated by a straight line parallel to the x-axis.

The Nonparametric Bootstrap to Assess Model Stability

There are many variations of resampling methods; however in this chapter only the nonparametric bootstrap is used (Efron 1979).

Irrespective of a specific model selection procedure, a critical issue is the selection of one specific model out of the set of candidate models, which usually consists of several thousand or even several millions of models. However, usually several competing models fit the data about equally well, and the particular model chosen by the selection procedure may depend on the characteristics of a small number of observations. If the data are slightly altered, a different model may be selected. Some variables with a "stronger effect" are selected with a high probability, whereas the selection of others may be a matter of chance. This issue has been known for a long time (Chen and George 1985; Altman and Andersen 1989) and seems to have been gaining more attention recently. See Sauerbrei et al. (2015) for further discussion.

Resampling procedures are well-suited to assess model stability. The "typical" bootstrap takes a random sample of size n with replacement from the original observations, which implies that on average 36.8% of the data is not included in a bootstrap replication, while some of the observations are included more than once. A large number of bootstrap replications, say M, are considered. Each of the M bootstrap samples is treated as an independent sample. The assumption is made that each replication, being based on a random sample of patients in the study, should reflect the underlying structure of the data. In each replication the analysis strategy is used to derive a model.

Already in the early papers, it was proposed that a larger number of bootstrap replications should be created and the percentage of variable inclusions in the model (often termed bootstrap inclusion fraction (BIF)) be used as a criterion for model selection (Chen and George 1985; Altman and Andersen 1989; Sauerbrei and Schumacher 1992). Unfortunately, this simple "summary" of the selected models in bootstrap replications may result in selecting a "bad" model if the inclusion of two (or more) variables depends on one another. One important reason is the correlation structure of the candidate variables, which can strongly influence BIFs of some variables. It is possible that one of two variables is included in each of the replications but, as the two BIFs are not much higher than 50%, neither of these two variables are considered as being highly relevant based on their BIF. To cope with such situations, Sauerbrei and Schumacher (1992) proposed considering dependencies among inclusion fractions and defined two bootstrap variable selection procedures, one aiming for a simpler model including strong factors only (strategy B) and one additionally including weaker factors (strategy A), which uses BIFs and their dependencies as criteria to select a final model. Stability investigations of models which select variables and the functional form for continuous variables can also be based on bootstrap investigations, but analyses of dependencies of results in bootstrap replications need substantial extensions. This is illustrated for the MFP model for the breast cancer data (Royston and Sauerbrei 2003, see section "Function Selection").

Results

Model Selection in Bootstrap Replications

Analysis of the glioma data with backward elimination ($\alpha = 0.05$) resulted in the selection of the five variables X_5, X_8, X_3, X_6, and X_{12}. Results from the first five bootstrap replications and BIFs for the number of bootstrap replications ranging from 50 to 1000 are given in Table 1b. It is important to note that this is a brief summary of the results presented in Tables V and IX in Sauerbrei and Schumacher (1992). When conducting this study, nearly 30 years ago, computer time was much longer and more expensive, and thus it was a relevant issue whether 50 replications were sufficient for an informative assessment of the importance of individual variables and of variable selection (in)stability.

Here $2^{15} = 32,768$ different models are considered. While results for single replications differ severely and clearly indicate that nearly every model selected is different, the conclusion drawn is that BIFs from 100 or more bootstrap replications give a good evaluation of the relevance of the 15 variables. The two variables X_8 and X_5 should be in the model and probably also X_3. X_6 entered in about two thirds of the models. With about 50% X_{11} and X_{12} are further candidates for a final model. Including one of these variables has an influence on the inclusion of the other. There are only 18 of 100 models where neither of these two variables are included and both are included in 19% (Table 4c in Sauerbrei and Schumacher 1992). Obviously, a suitable model should include one of the two but not both. All other variables seem to be less relevant. If selected, corresponding estimates of regression coefficients even have different signs, although in all cases one sign dominated noticeably. The model with five variables selected in the original data was observed in only two of the first 100 bootstrap replications, on which the analyses concentrated. Nevertheless, 26 of these 100 replications included all of these five variables and 84 replications included at least four of the five (Sauerbrei and Schumacher 1992). Results for backward elimination (BE) and stepwise selection (StS) with nominal significance levels 0.01, 0.05, 0.10, and 0.157 are given in Table 2 of Sauerbrei et al. (2007a). Furthermore, the all subsets procedure with the AIC criteria was used to derive a model. All nine models (BE and StS, each with 4 significance level and AIC) included a core set of four variables; more variables were added with larger significance levels. For a given significance level, models derived with BE and StS agreed, with the exception of 0.10. The AIC and the 0.157 models included nine

Table 1 Glioma. Bootstrap result matrix for the first five replications (using backward elimination, $\alpha = 0.05$; 0 – variable not included, 1 – variable included and bootstrap inclusion frequencies (BIF) for various numbers of replications. (Adapted from Sauerbrei and Schumacher (1992) with permission from Wiley & Sons Ltd.)

(a) Results for 5 replications

Bootstrap replication	X1	X2	X3	X4	X5	X6	X7	X8	X9	X10	X11	X12	X13	X14	X15
1	0	0	1	1	1	1	0	1	1	0	0	0	0	1	0
2	1	0	1	0	1	1	0	1	0	0	0	1	0	1	0
3	0	0	0	1	1	1	0	1	0	0	0	1	0	1	0
4	1	0	1	0	1	1	0	1	0	0	1	0	1	0	0
5	1	0	1	0	1	1	0	1	1	0	1	1	0	0	0

(b) BIF

Number of bootstrap replications	X1	X2	X3	X4	X5	X6	X7	X8	X9	X10	X11	X12	X13	X14	X15
50	18	12	88	46	100	76	6[a]	100	36	12[a]	64	38	14[a]	48[a]	12
100	33	19	88	38	100	66	13[a]	100	35[a]	19[a]	49	52	17[a]	56	23[a]
200	24	15	89	34[a]	99	74	7[a]	100	28	19[a]	51	39	13[a]	41	15
400	27[a]	18[a]	87	35	100	69	9[a]	100	35[a]	16	58	45	18[a]	39	16[a]
1000	22[a]	17[a]	87	37[a]	100	73	8[a]	100	35	14[a]	56	41	16[a]	43[a]	18[a]

[a]Different signs for the regression coefficients in the selected models. In all cases one sign dominated (more than 80%)

Table 2 Breast cancer. Selected powers in the first five bootstrap replications and percentages of selected powers from 5000 bootstrap replications. *X5 was transformed with a negative exponential function. (Adapted from Royston and Sauerbrei (2003) with permission from Wiley & Sons Ltd.)

Variable	Code	Power	Replication					Included	
			1	2	3	4	5	Number	Percentage
Age	X1	p1	−0:5	–	−2	−2	−2	4606	92.2
		p2	0	–	−1	−2	–	3810	76.2
Menopausal status	X2		–	–	–	–	1	985	19.7
Tumor size	X3	p1	3	–	−2	1	–	2008	40.2
		p2	3	–	–	–	–	315	6.3
Grade ≤ 2	X4a		1	1	–	–	–	2909	58.2
Grade 3	X4b		–	1	–	–	–	452	9
exp(−0:12 × lymph nodes)	X5*	p1	1	1	1	1	1	5000	100
Progesterone receptors	X6	p1	1	0	0	0.5	0	4941	98.8
		p2	–	–	–	–	–	213	4.3
Estrogen receptors	X7	p1	–	–	–	–	–	955	19.1
		p2	–	–	–	–	–	291	5.8

variables, eight of which were identical. This result confirms earlier experiences from real data and simulations that AIC usually selects very similar models compared to stepwise approaches using 0.157 as the stopping criterion.

Function Selection

Using the MFP algorithm to investigate the effect of age on RFS in the data from the German Breast Cancer Study Group, a nonlinear function for the prognostic effect of age was derived (Sauerbrei and Royston 1999).

The FP function selected postulates that very young patients have a strongly increased risk, whereas the risk hardly changes for patients above 40 years. This nonlinear effect could not be detected under the assumption of a linear effect of age and was not detected with the categorized approach because the preselected cutpoints 45 and 60 define a baseline category of patients younger than or equal to 45 years, which seems to be heterogeneous concerning the risk of an event.

When interpreting a selected model and postulated functions, it must be stressed that the MFP model was chosen from among several million candidates. Obviously, the stability of the model and the functional forms must be checked. The bootstrap is well suited for this task. Royston and Sauerbrei (2003) created 5000 bootstrap samples by sampling patients with replacement. Within each bootstrap sample, they used MFP to select a single model. Age was selected in 76.2% of the replications as a FP2 function and in a further 16.0% as a FP1 function (Table 2). A random sample from the FP2 functions is shown in Figure 1 (left). These bootstrap results confirm that the age function selected in the original data is not a result of mismodelling.

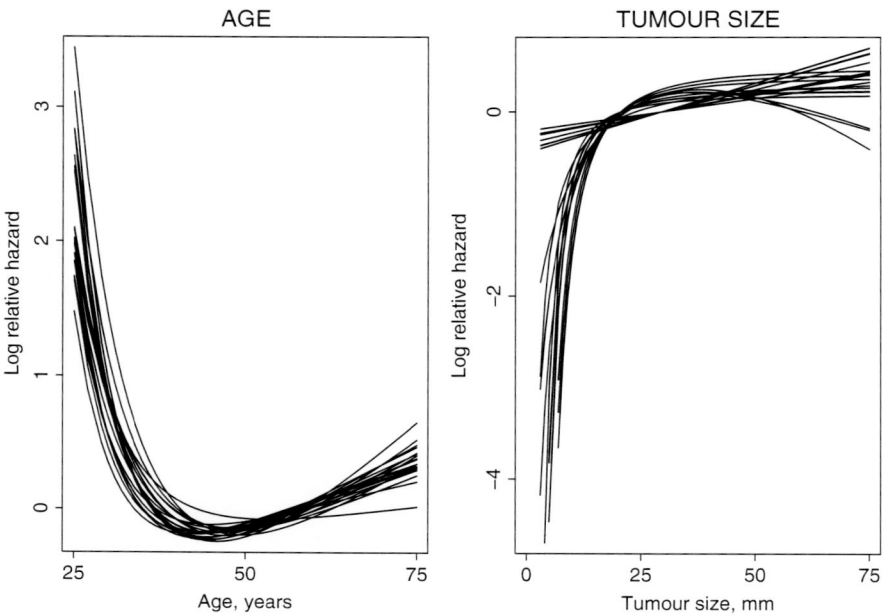

Fig. 1 Breast cancer. Functions selected with MFP in bootstrap replications (random sample of 20 curves); left: function for age; right: function for tumor size. (Reproduced from Sauerbrei and Royston (2007) with permission from Wiley & Sons Ltd.)

Figure 1 (right) shows selected functions for tumor size. This variable was eliminated in the original analysis but selected in 40.2% in the bootstrap replications (Table 2). If selected, Figure 1 shows that the estimated effect is either linear or strongly nonlinear (strong increase up to about 3 cm, hardly any further increase in risk for larger tumors). In 60% of the replications, the variable was not selected, in 16% a linear function (our default!) was chosen, and in 24% a similar nonlinear function was always selected. This result indicates that the power of the MFP procedure was insufficient to select the unknown "true" function which probably has a strong increase for small values and levels off for larger values. Such a functional type was also postulated in another very large study (Verschraegen et al. 2005). See Sauerbrei and Royston (2007) for more details.

Table 2 shows some dependencies between variables and simplified classifications (excluded, FP1, FP2) of functional forms selected in 5000 bootstrap replications. Using log-linear modelling to investigate dependencies in the bootstrap result matrix, Royston and Sauerbrei (2003) conducted a much more detailed investigation and determined a subset of the bootstrap replications (about 60%) with broadly similar results, calling it a stable subset.

Table 3a shows that menopausal status is hardly relevant (included in 19.7% of the replications), but if included it has a strong influence on the age function selected. A non-monotonic FP2 function as shown in Figure 1 is only chosen in a small number of replications (22.2%), whereas FP2 dominates if X_2 is excluded.

Table 3 Breast cancer. Relationship between inclusion frequencies of 5000 bootstrap replications. For continuous variables we restrict it to simplified classification of functions (excluded, FP1, FP2). Values in the tables are frequencies (and percentages of the relevant total). (**a**) Age and menopausal status (**b**) progesterone receptor and estrogen receptor. (Adapted from Royston and Sauerbrei (2003) with permission from Wiley & Sons Ltd.)

(a)

	X1 (age)			
X2 (menopausal status)	Excluded	FP(1)	FP(2)	Total
Excluded	357 (8.9)	67 (1.7)	3591 (89.4)	4015 (80.3)
Included	37 (3.8)	729 (74.0)	219 (22.2)	985 (19.7)
Total	394 (7.9)	796 (15.9)	3810 (76.2)	5000 (100)

(b)

	X6 (progesterone receptors)			
X7 (estrogen receptors)	Excluded	FP(1)	FP(2)	Total
Excluded	6 (0.2)	3864 (95.5)	175 (4.3)	4045 (80.9)
FP(1)	18 (2.7)	612 (92.2)	34 (5.1)	664 (13.3)
FP(2)	35 (12.0)	252 (86.6)	4 (1.4)	291 (5.8)
Total	59 (1.2)	4728 (94.6)	213 (4.3)	5000 (100)

Based on these results, X_2 is not a variable with a strong influence on the outcome, but its inclusion has a stronger effect on the selection of other variables and functions. Consequently, Sauerbrei et al. (2007) decided that replications with X_2 included give "unusual" results and exclusion of X_2 is one of the criteria to define the stable subset. For the two correlated receptor variables, the dependency of the function chosen is not that strong, but it is also clear that the inclusion of estrogen receptor has an influence on the function chosen for progesterone (Table 3b).

Treatment-Covariate Interaction

The kidney data is used to investigate the stability of the derived treatment effect function for white cell counts (WCC). Here, WCC is the only variable with a significant treatment-covariate interaction (Royston and Sauerbrei 2004). According to the model, patients with low WCC benefit from interferon, whereas those with higher WCC values do not. This result is confirmed by investigations in four subgroups defined by WCC values. While the estimated hazard ratio (95% confidence interval) in the overall population is 0.75 (0.60–0.93), the estimates in the four subgroups with increasing WCC values are 0.53 (0.34–0.83), 0.69 (0.44–1.07), 0.89 (0.57–1.37), and 1.32 (0.85–2.05). While the subgroup with lowest WCC values benefitted a lot from IFN treatment, patients with large WCC values seem to be harmed by IFN treatment.

The treatment effect function should have consequences for the treatment of patients if it is true. However, the postulated function may be a result of mismodelling the data with our flexible statistical approach or may be an obvious effect in this specific study caused by random variation. To check the latter, new data from an external validation study is required; the former can be assessed by internal validation and further checks of the treatment effect function. As in the prognostic factor

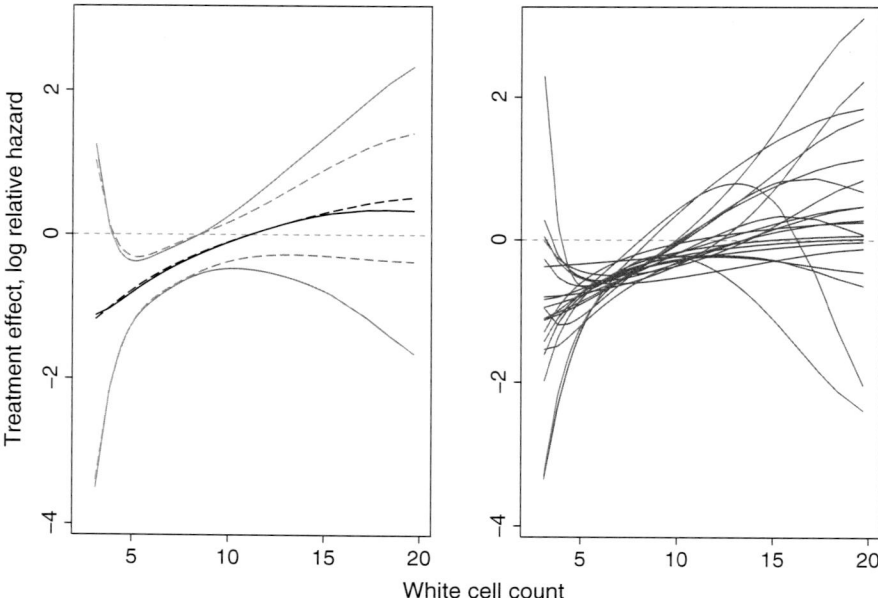

Fig. 2 Kidney cancer. Treatment effect function for WCC selected with MFPI in the original data and in 1000 bootstrap replications. The adjustment model is selected in each replication. Left: dashed lines, treatment effect with 95% pointwise confidence interval from the MFPI model on original data; solid lines, mean bootstrap with 95% pointwise confidence interval. Right: random sample of 20 bootstrap curves. (Reproduced from Sauerbrei and Royston (2007) with permission from Wiley & Sons Ltd.)

example, all parts of the MFPI analysis (step 1: select the adjustment model; step 2: estimate the treatment effect function) were repeated in 1000 bootstrap replications.

The right side of Fig. 2 shows a random sample of 20 treatment effect curves for WCC, illustrating that the stability of selected functions is high. Most of the curves agree well with the postulated curve from the original data; the corresponding mean curve in Fig. 2 (left, solid line) is nearly identical. As expected, the pointwise confidence interval from the bootstrap analysis is a bit wider than the interval from the original data, whose estimates ignore the uncertainty caused by the model selection process. See Sauerbrei and Royston (2007, section 3.2.2) for more details.

Discussion

Summary

In this chapter it has been demonstrated that resampling approaches are a valuable instrument to gain further knowledge in multivariable model building. Using three examples, it was illustrated that the selection of one final model that has been derived data dependently is partly a result of chance.

However, is that a surprise with "usual" sample sizes? For example, with 20 variables as many as $2^{20} = 1,048,576$ models are available if the "simple" problem of variable in- or exclusion is considered. With continuous variables there might be some concern around the assumption of a linear effect which was addressed by examining whether nonlinear functions increase the model fit. This resulted in a further increase in the number of potential models. Furthermore, it seems common practice to base inference on a "conditional model," as if the model had been given a priori. This ignores uncertainty of model predictions, estimates of effects, and variance caused by model selection. Breiman (1992) calls this a "quiet scandal."

Some Issues in Identifying Influential Covariates and Deriving a Predictor

In the examples, the identification of influential covariates, the identification of functional forms for continuous variables and the search for continuous variables interacting with treatment in an RCT are discussed. Related investigations on the development of a prediction model, derivation of a prediction model by incorporating model uncertainty, and checks for observations influencing a selected model and visualization of the model building process by using the stability path are presented in Sauerbrei et al. (2015). Obviously, the specific aim of a model has a strong influence on the choice of a suitable approach for analysis and on the appropriate type of investigation of model stability (Royston and Sauerbrei 2008; Heinze et al. 2018). However, it is important to stress that each type of investigation should be accompanied by investigation of the stability of the selected model. In practice, stability investigation needs to receive much more attention. In the following, some additional issues related to the examples are briefly discussed. Each could be a topic on its own. The focus will be on the research of the authors. Many additional relevant papers could be discussed and cited here, but for the sake of brevity and restrictions concerning the number of citations, a selection had to be made.

Using the bootstrap and inclusion frequencies from many runs was already proposed, in the 1980s, for the assessment of variable selection stability and identification of variables with an effect on the outcome and investigation of properties of predictions (Chen and George 1985; Altman and Andersen 1989). Sauerbrei and Schumacher (1992) extended this approach to handle the problem raised by co-dependence inclusions of two variables. They also proposed two strategies for variable selection. Strategy B aims to select a model in which only variables with a "stronger" influence are included, whereas Strategy A also allows the inclusion of variables with a weaker effect. Recently, De Bin and Sauerbrei (2017) compared the performance of the two approaches with those of the naïve strategy which ignores co-dependence inclusions and selects a model simply with respect to a threshold. They conclude 'All in all, we saw that strategies A and B have a positive effect in balancing the prediction ability and the sparsity of a model. As a general result from our paper, we note the advantages in using sparser models.' In principle, the main aims of the two strategies A and B relate to the important distinction "To explain or to predict" (Shmueli 2010). Investigations of co-dependence could be extended for three or more dimensions in a similar way or clustering approaches could be used to identify potential "classes of models" which are supported by different bootstrap samples (Hennig and Sauerbrei 2019). Further applications, for example, in the context of classification and regression trees, are presented in Schumacher et al. (2012).

It is an encouraging development that the use of resampling techniques and BIFs has become more popular as a tool to investigate model stability and related issues. The importance is clearly stressed in the explanation and elaboration paper of the TRIPOD guidelines for the reporting of a multivariate prediction model. Moons et al. (2015) state 'Studies developing new prediction models should therefore always include some form of internal validation to quantify any optimism in the predictive performance (for example, calibration and discrimination) of the developed model and adjust the model for overfitting. Internal validation techniques use only the original study sample and include such methods as bootstrapping or cross-validation. Internal validation is a necessary part of model development.'

However, it is also obvious that resampling methods must be used with care. Carpenter and Bithell (2000) discuss issues when deriving bootstrap confidence intervals, while Lusa et al. (2007) point to critical issues when assessing model performance. Missing values in the original data can cause various problems in resampling procedures, and using BIFs without considering co-dependencies can erroneously result in elimination of two variables, although one of them is included in each of the replications, as already outlined above. Furthermore, there is the key question about the cut point to use. Ariyaratne et al. (2011) selected four models based on BIFs (greater or equal to 80% (3 variables included), 70% (6 variables), 60% (8 variables), and 50% (10 variables)) as a predictor for early mortality and used external validation to select a final model. However, they ignored issues caused by co-dependence inclusions and the problem of missing values (number of patients decreases from 3527 (model with 3 variables) to 3232 (model with 10 variables)). More importantly, they did not even mention the variable selection procedure used. This is one of many papers whose interpretability is affected by insufficient reporting (Sekula et al. 2017).

Assumption of a Linear Effect of a Continuous Variable

In practice, it is common to have a mix of binary, categorical (ordinal or unordered), and continuous variables that may influence an outcome. Building a multivariable model for explanation, the main focus is on identification of variables with an influence on the outcome. Too often analysts do not put much thought into the choice of the functional forms for continuous variables.

Despite many well-known weaknesses (Altman et al. 1994; Royston et al. 2006), the method of categorizing continuous variables is still used often. Furthermore, assuming linear relationships with the outcome, possibly after a simple transformation (e.g., logarithmic or quadratic), is a popular choice. Often, however, the reasons for choosing such conventional representations of continuous variables are not discussed and the validity of the underlying assumptions is not assessed. Unfortunately, more flexible modelling based on various types of smoothers, including fractional polynomials (Royston and Sauerbrei 2008) and several "flavors" of splines (see Sauerbrei et al. 2014 for more details and references), are often still ignored.

In the breast cancer example, it was demonstrated that a fractional polynomial function of degree 2 gives a much better representation of the effect of age on RFS than a linear function and a step function based on two predefined cut points. Investigation of model stability is also possible for the joint problem of variable and function selection (Royston and Sauerbrei 2003; Binder and Sauerbrei 2009). In the earlier example, use of the bootstrap method provided interesting clinical insights into the effect of tumor size, which has a stronger nonlinear effect. Because of low power, it was not detected in the analysis of the original data. This example also illustrated that (appropriate) sample size is a critical issue in the MFP approach, whose results for the variable and function selection components depend on the nominal significance level to be chosen by the analyst.

Interaction of Treatment with a Continuous Variable

In RCTs, potential interactions between treatment and prognostic factors are important essential ingredients of stratified medicine, rather than assuming that "one size fits all." When a covariate is continuous (such as age or hormone receptor level), such interactions are often sought by crude and inadequate statistical methods, typically involving dichotomizing the continuous covariate (Royston et al. 2006). Sometimes, treatment effects are compared in derived subgroups; the results often depend on the cut-points chosen (Royston and Sauerbrei 2004). Methods that keep all the information in the covariate are considerably more powerful than dichotomization. The Subpopulation Treatment Effect Pattern Plot (STEPP) and the multivariable fractional polynomial interaction (MFPI) approach, an extension of the multivariable fractional polynomial (MFP) procedure, are two strategies proposed (Bonetti and Gelber 2004; Royston and Sauerbrei 2004; Sauerbrei et al. 2007b). In the latter paper, results from the two approaches are compared in the kidney cancer data; MFPI tests for an interaction between treatment and a continuous covariate and estimates a continuous treatment effect function. It also allows adjustment for other covariates. Several checks were proposed to reduce the problem of an increased type I error. This approach can also be used to improve investigation of prespecified treatment-covariate interactions if the covariate is measured on a continuous scale.

Regarding selection of the specific function, Royston and Sauerbrei (2009b) suggested four approaches with varying flexibility. In a large simulation study, Royston and Sauerbrei (2013, 2014) investigated these different variants of MFPI and compared them to strategies based on categorization or spline modelling. They conclude that the results provide sufficient evidence to recommend the MFPI procedure as a suitable approach to investigate interactions between treatment and a continuous variable.

Which Resampling Technique?

How to choose the most suitable resampling technique is an issue that has been discussed for a long time. For the investigation of model stability issues, the "usual" nonparametric bootstrap was the most popular approach, and it was used in all earlier investigations of the first author. In recent years, however, the research group of the second author conducted studies on the different behaviors of resampling without replacement (often denoted as "subsampling") and the commonly used resampling with replacement (often denoted as "bootstrap(ping)"). Very generally (and independently of model selection issues), it can be shown theoretically for several usual statistical tests that type I error is substantially larger than the nominal level if they are performed on a bootstrap sample drawn with replacement. Unsurprisingly, this increased type I error leads to too large inclusion frequencies for non-informative variables in the context of variable selection for regression models when bootstrapping is used as the resampling procedure (Janitza et al. 2016; De Bin et al. 2016). In contrast, subsampling does not suffer from this problem but has lower power than bootstrapping to include variables with true effects. Many authors (see De Bin et al. (2016) and references therein) used a subsampling fraction of 63.2% to ensure comparability with bootstrap samples that include an average of 63.2% of the observations from the original sample. More importantly, when global tests are used in the variable selection process to globally assess a multicategorical variable (coded as several binary variables), the increase of the type I error observed for bootstrap samples is more pronounced for tests with higher degrees of freedom, i.e., for variables with higher numbers of categories. This leads to a so-called variable selection bias: under the null hypothesis that all variables are non-informative, the variables with many categories are selected more often than the variables with fewer categories if bootstrap samples are used, and the difference in selection frequencies is substantial, as empirically assessed by Rospleszcz et al. (2016).

More Modelling Needed: Guidance Required

With the enormous power of technical equipment and recent developments of statistical approaches (machine learning techniques were not addressed here but for some tasks they are interesting alternatives) many more analyses are possible. It is likely that they would uncover much information "hidden" in the data. However, many of the methodological developments are ignored in practice. There are a variety of reasons for this unfortunate situation. In its introductory paper the STRengthening Analytical Thinking for Observational Studies (STRATOS) initiative wrote "[...] the increasing volume and complexity of data collected in medical studies, pose important conceptual and analytical challenges. In response, the ever-growing statistical research community continues to develop and refine new methods, each aimed at addressing specific problems encountered in real-life data analyses. The richness and the complexity of the new methodology being published, every month, in several dozen statistical journals makes it impossible for a single statistician, or even a group of collaborators or members of a given institution, to keep pace with these developments" (Sauerbrei et al. 2014).

Often important methodological achievements need a very long time before being used by analysts. Complexity of approaches and uncertainty about their properties, insufficient comparisons of competing approaches, shortage of experienced statisticians, and missing guidance for analysts with lower knowledge of statistical methodology are among the most important reasons for this unfortunate situation (Sauerbrei et al. 2014; Boulesteix et al. 2018).

Deriving accessible and accurate guidance in the design and analysis of observational studies is the over-arching objective of the STRATOS initiative. The guidance is intended for data analysts with varying levels of statistical education, experience, and interests.

Key Points

- Many clinical trials have hidden information and modelling is useful for extracting this information. Resampling approaches can be used to protect against overoptimism and potentially false claims caused by data-dependent modelling.
- Three important considerations in the modelling are variable selection of prognostic factors, the selection of a functional relationship between a continuous variable, and an outcome and the investigation of an interaction between treatment and a continuous variable.
- Flexible model building procedures can derive new information and resampling replications can provide important insight into model selection stability. Typically, many different models are selected across replications and inclusion frequencies and their dependencies can help extract relevant information not apparent from a "usual" analysis of the original data.
- The nonparametric bootstrap is used for illustration in this chapter. However, other resampling approaches are available and additional modelling issues can be tackled with resampling approaches.

Cross-References

▶ Biomarker-Driven Adaptive Phase III Clinical Trials
▶ Biomarker-Guided Trials
▶ Confident Statistical Inference with Multiple Outcomes, Subgroups, and Other Issues of Multiplicity
▶ Development and Validation of Risk Prediction Models
▶ Estimands and Sensitivity Analyses
▶ Prognostic Factor Analyses
▶ Survival Analysis II

Acknowledgment A special thanks to Harald Binder, Anika Buchholz, Patrick Royston, and Martin Schumacher, the co-authors of the papers which were used as cornerstones for this chapter. We also thank Georg Heinze and Christine Wallisch for comments on an earlier version, Alethea Charlton and Jenny Lee for linguistic improvements, and Tim Haeussler, Martin Haslberger, and Andreas Ott for administrative assistance. Finally, we thank the Deutsche Forschungsgemeinschaft who supported parts of the work with grants BO3139/4–3 to ALB and SA580/8–3 to WS and with grants to projects leading to some of the earlier papers.

References

Altman DG, Andersen PK (1989) Bootstrap investigation of the stability of a Cox regression model. Stat Med 8:771–783

Altman DG, Lausen B, Sauerbrei W, Schumacher M (1994) Dangers of using 'optimal' s in the evaluation of prognostic factors. J Natl Cancer Inst 86:829–835

Altman DG, McShane LM, Sauerbrei W, Taube SE (2012) Reporting recommendations for tumor marker prognostic studies (REMARK): explanation and elaboration. PLoS Med 9(5):e1001216

Ariyaratne TV, Billah B, Yap CH, Dinh D, Smith JA, Shardey GC, Reid CM (2011) An Australian risk prediction model for determining early mortality following aortic valve replacement. Eur J Cardiothorac Surg 38(6):815–821

Babu JG (2011) Resampling methods for model fitting and model selection. J Biopharm Stat 21:1177–1186

Binder H, Sauerbrei W (2009) Stability analysis of an additive spline model for respiratory health data by using knot removal. J R Stat Soc C 58:577–600

Bonetti M, Gelber RD (2004) Patterns of treatment effects in subsets of patients in clinical trials. Biostatistics 5:465–481

Boulesteix AL, Binder H, Abrahamowicz M, Sauerbrei W (2018) On the necessity and design of studies comparing statistical methods. Biom J 60(1):216–218

Breiman L (1992) The little bootstrap and other methods for dimensionality selection in regression: X-fixed prediction error. J Am Stat Assoc 87:738–754

Carpenter J, Bithell J (2000) Bootstrap confidence intervals: when, which, what? A practical guide for medical statisticians. Stat Med 19:1141–1164

Chen C, George SL (1985) The bootstrap and identification of prognostic factors via Cox's proportional hazards regression model. Stat Med 4:39–46

Chernick MR (2008) Bootstrap methods. A guide for practitioners and researchers. Wiley, Hoboken

Davison AC, Hinkley DV (1997) Bootstrap methods and their application. Cambridge University Press, Cambridge, MA

De Bin R, Sauerbrei W (2017) Handling co-dependence issues in resampling-based variable selection procedures: a simulation study. J Stat Comput Simul 88(1):28–55

De Bin R, Janitza S, Sauerbrei W, Boulesteix AL (2016) Subsampling versus bootstrapping in resampling-based model selection for multivariable regression. Biometrics 72(1):272–280

Donegan S, Williams L, Dias S, Tudur-Smith C, Welton N (2015) Exploring treatment by covariate interactions using subgroup analysis and meta-regression in cochrane reviews: a review of recent practice. PLoS one 10(6):e0128804

Efron B (1979) Bootstrap methods: another look at the jackknife. Ann Stat 7:1–26

Harrell FE (2001) Regression modelling strategies, with applications to linear models, logistic regression, and survival analysis. Springer, New York

Heinze G, Wallisch C, Dunkler D (2018) Variable selection – a review and recommendations for the practicing statistician. Biom J 60:431–449

Hennig C, Sauerbrei W (2019) Exploration of the variability of variable selection based on distances between bootstrap sample results. ADAC. To appear

Huebner M, Le Cessie S, Schmidt CO, Vach W (2018) A contemporary conceptual framework for initial data analysis. Obs Stud 4:171–192

Janitza S, Binder H, Boulesteix AL (2016) Pitfalls of hypothesis tests and model selection on bootstrap samples: causes and consequences in biometrical applications. Biom J 58:447–473

LePage R, Billard L (1992) Exploring the limits of bootstrap. Wiley, New York

Lusa L, McShane LM, Radmacher MD, Shih JH, Wright GW, Simon R (2007) Appropriateness of some resampling-based inference procedures for assessing performance of prognostic classifiers derived from microarray data. Stat Med 26(5):1102–1113

Medical Research Council Renal Cancer Collaborators (MRCRCC) (1999) Interferon-rx and survival in metastatic renal carcinoma: early results of a randomised controlled trial. Lancet 353:14–17

Meinshausen N, Bühlmann P (2010) Stability selection. J R Stat Soc B 72:417–473

Moons KG, Altman DG, Reitsma JB, Ioannidis JP, Macaskill P, Steyerberg EW, Vickers AJ, Ransohoff DF, Collins GS (2015) Transparent reporting of a multivariable prediction model for individual prognosis or diagnosis (TRIPOD): explanation and elaboration. Ann Intern Med 162(1):W1–W73

Rospleszcz S, Janitza S, Boulesteix AL (2016) Categorical variables with many categories are preferentially selected in bootstrap-based model selection procedures for multivariable regression models. Biom J 58:652–673

Royston P, Altman DG (1994) Regression using fractional polynomials of continuous covariates: parsimonious Parametic modelling. Appl Stat 43:429–467

Royston P, Sauerbrei W (2003) Stability of multivariable fractional polynomial models with selection of variables and transformations: a bootstrap investigation. Stat Med 22:639–659

Royston P, Sauerbrei W (2004) A new approach to modelling interactions between treatment and continuous covariates in clinical trials by using fractional polynomials. Statist. Med. 23:2509–2525

Royston P, Sauerbrei W (2008) Multivariable model-building—a pragmatic approach to regression analysis based on fractional polynomials for modelling continuous variables. Wiley, New York

Royston P, Sauerbrei W (2009a) Bootstrap assessment of the stability of multivariable models. Stata J 9:547–570

Royston P, Sauerbrei W (2009b) Two techniques for investigating interactions between treatment and continuous covariates in clinical trials. Stata J 9:230–251

Royston P, Sauerbrei W (2013) Interaction of treatment with a continuous variable: simulation study of significance level for several methods of analysis. Stat Med 32:3788–3803

Royston P, Sauerbrei W (2014) Interaction of treatment with a continuous variable: simulation study of power for several methods of analysis. Stat Med 33:4695–4708

Royston P, Altman DG, Sauerbrei W (2006) Dichotomizing continuous predictors in multiple regression: a bad idea. Stat Med 25:127–141

Sauerbrei W (1999) The use of resampling methods to simplify regression models in medical statistics. J R Stat Soc: Ser C: Appl Stat 48:313–329

Sauerbrei W, Royston P (1999) Building multivariable prognostic and diagnostic models: transformation of the predictors by using fractional polynomials. J R Stat Soc A Stat Soc 162:71–94

Sauerbrei W, Royston P (2007) Modelling to extract more information from clinical trials data: on some roles for the bootstrap. Stat Med 26:4989–5001

Sauerbrei W, Schumacher M (1992) A bootstrap resampling procedure for model building: application to the cox regression model. Stat Med 11:2093–2109

Sauerbrei W, Royston P, Binder H (2007a) Selection of important variables and determination of functional form for continuous predictors in multivariable model-building. Stat Med 26:5512–5528

Sauerbrei W, Royston P, Zapien K (2007b) Detecting an interaction between treatment and a continuous covariate: a comparison of two approaches. Comput Stat Data Anal 51:4054–4063

Sauerbrei W, Abrahamowicz M, Altman DG, le Cessie S, Carpenter J, on behalf of the STRATOS initiative (2014) STRengthening analytical thinking for observational studies: the STRATOS initiative. Stat Med 33:5413–5432

Sauerbrei W, Buchholz A, Boulesteix A, Binder H (2015) On stability issues in deriving multivariable regression models. Biom J 57:531–555

Schumacher M, Hollaender N, Schwarzer G, Binder H, Sauerbrei W (2012) Prognostic factor studies. In: Crowley J, Hoering A (eds) Handbook of statistics in clinical oncology, 3rd edn. Chapman and Hall/CRC, Boca Raton, pp 415–470

Sekula P, Mallett S, Altman DG, Sauerbrei W (2017) Did the reporting of prognostic studies of tumour markers improve since the introduction of REMARK guideline? A comparison of reporting in published articles. PLoS One 12(6):e0178531

Shmueli G (2010) To explain or to predict? Stat Sci 25:289–310

Verschraegen C, Vinh-Hung V, Cserni G, Gordon R, Royce ME, Vlastos G, Tai P, Storme G (2005) Modeling the effect of tumor size in early breast Cancer. Ann Surg 241:309–318

Wang R, Lagakos SW, Ware JH, Hunter DJ, Drazen JM (2007) Statistics in medicine—reporting of subgroup analyses in clinical trials. N Engl J Med 357(21):2189–2194

Westfall PH (2011) On using the bootstrap for multiple comparisons. J Biopharm Stat 21:1187–1205

Joint Analysis of Longitudinal and Time-to-Event Data

97

Zheng Lu, Emmanuel Chigutsa, and Xiao Tong

Contents

Introduction	1920
Joint Models of Longitudinal and Time-to-Event Data	1921
Model Specification and Estimation	1921
Joint Modeling of Longitudinal Biomarker and Time-to-Event Data from Clinical Trials	1923
Population Prediction Supporting Clinical Trial Design	1923
Individual Dynamic Prediction	1932
Summary and Conclusions	1933
Key Points	1933
Cross-References	1934
References	1934

Abstract

The longitudinal and time-to-event data are two kinds of common data generated from various clinical trials across different therapeutic areas. Joint modeling is appropriate to estimate unbiased effect of covariates that are measured longitudinally and are related to the event on the time to an event and then could be applied to predict the time to an event. An underlying random effects structure links the survival and longitudinal sub-models and allows for individual-specific predictions. This chapter provided the basic backgrounds of longitudinal and time-to-event data commonly generated from clinical trials and derivations of the joint likelihood function to be maximized when jointly modeling longitudinal and time-to-event data. In addition to these theoretical backgrounds, different

---

Z. Lu (✉)
Clinical Pharmacology and Exploratory Development, Astellas Pharma, Northbrook, IL, USA

E. Chigutsa
Pharmacometrics, Eli Lilly and Company, Zionsville, IN, USA
e-mail: chigutsa_emmanuel@lilly.com

X. Tong
Clinical Pharmacology, Biogen, Boston, MA, USA

© Springer Nature Switzerland AG 2022
S. Piantadosi, C. L. Meinert (eds.), *Principles and Practice of Clinical Trials*,
https://doi.org/10.1007/978-3-319-52636-2_131

applications of joint modeling of longitudinal and time-to-event data across different therapeutic areas and individual dynamic prediction were also extensively discussed.

Keywords

Longitudinal · Time-to-event · Joint

Introduction

Joint modeling of longitudinal and time-to-event data is a broad but not a new topic. The history of joint models can be tracked to the 1990s. The longitudinal data in clinical trials is generally comprised of the repeatedly measured endpoint of interest (drug's concentration, biomarker...), whether it is efficacy- or safety-related, across a specific scale (time, space, ...). The longitudinal data could be continuous without boundary, like drug concentration in the body, tumor size, prostate-specific antigen (PSA), blood pressure, circulating or residual (leukemic) cells (Wilbaux et al. 2015) at different time points. Although there is a lower boundary of 0 for this type of data, which cannot be negative, we seldom or never reach that boundary in reality; the longitudinal data could also be continuous with boundary and at boundary, like quality of life (QoL) questionnaire score treated as continuous by the sum of the answers to all questions, which define the specific domain or item (Song et al. 2017), variant allelic frequency (VAF) defined as the ratio of gene mutant reads to gene total reads with the unit interval [0, 1]. The longitudinal outcomes could be categorical (response [yes/no], bone fractures [yes/no]), ordered categorical (e.g., breast density in four levels (Armero et al. 2016), grades of adverse events [mild, moderate, severe]), count data (e.g., number of convulsions in a week). There are also additional considerations of multiple (≥ 2) longitudinal outcomes; both longitudinal number of $CD4^+$ T lymphocyte and amount of virus in the blood are widely used as biomarkers for progression to AIDS when studying the efficacy of drugs to treat HIV-infected patients (Martins et al. 2016).

For the time-to-event part, instead of the analysis of time-to-event from all causes, there may be a need to treat time-to-event as cause-specific by considering competing risks (Yu et al. 2008). The events could repeatedly occur like time to relapse instead of time to single event of death. By considering a proportion of patients may be cured and thus are no longer subject to risks of failure, a survival-cure model including a logistic regression model for cured status can be applied to time-to-event data and fraction of cured can also be estimated (Menggang Yu et al. 2008). With so many different types of longitudinal and time-to-event data, the link function between them could also be various, current true value, rate of change, area under the curve, baseline, change from baseline of longitudinal data could be considered as covariates having impacts on time-to-event. Although proportional hazards model is the model commonly used for the joint analysis of longitudinal and time-to-event data in most literatures, alterative accelerated failure time (AFT) model can also be considered for the time-to-event data by treating the effects of covariates on time to event instead of on the hazard where the proportional hazards assumption is violated.

Either two-stage (sequential) or one-stage (joint) approach (Zhang et al. 2003a, b) of analysis can be applied to the analysis of longitudinal and time-to-event data because both approaches are established for the purpose of modeling data of different types. In the analysis of longitudinal and time-to-event data, Desmée et al. (2015) compared the two-stage and joint sequential model with joint approach in the context of metastatic prostate cancer by simulation. With prespecified evaluation criteria, they found that the higher levels of bias of estimation with increasing effect of PSA on survival and systematical underestimation of the PSA effect on survival were corrected by using joint sequential models or joint models and the bias was largely reduced when using a joint model. They concluded that joint model provided unbiased parameters of both longitudinal and survival processes but also suggested that joint sequential model could be a relevant approach when joint model cannot be performed.

Joint Models of Longitudinal and Time-to-Event Data

Model Specification and Estimation

Since we are dealing with random variables in our analysis, from a probabilistic point of view, the model we are developing is a joint probability distribution. Even with only one type of data, longitudinal drug concentration data, the population model is dealing with the joint probability distribution of drug concentrations in plasma or blood (observations) and individual parameters across the individuals in the population because both of them are random variables in our model. When we deal with more than one type of data, longitudinal and time-to-event data, it is more intuitive to specify a joint probability distribution for this type of analysis and model parameters could be estimated by maximizing this joint likelihood function.

Let's assume $Y_{ij}(t) = Y_i(t_{ij})$ corresponds to the observations of the longitudinal data for individual i (i = 1, 2..., N) measured at time points t_{ij} (j = 1, 2..., ni). For the ith subject, let T_i^* and C_i be the event and censoring times, respectively. Rather than observing T_i^*, we observe only $T_i = \min(T_i^*, C_i)$ together with an indicator δ_i that equals 1 if $T_i^* \leq C_i$ and 0 otherwise, then the joint probability distribution of longitudinal and time-to-event data is $P(T_i, \delta_i, Y_i)$. For the shared random effects model of longitudinal and time-to-event data, we assume longitudinal data (Y_i) and time-to-event data (T_i, δ_i) are independent conditional on shared individual parameters (random effects η_i). Based on this assumption, $P(T_i, \delta_i, Y_i)$ can be simplified as

$$P(T_i, \delta_i, Y_i) = \int P(T_i, \delta_i, Y_i \mid \eta_i; \theta) P(\eta_i; \theta) d\eta_i$$
$$= \int P(T_i, \delta_i \mid \eta_i; \theta) P(Y_i \mid \eta_i; \theta) P(\eta_i; \theta) d\eta_i \quad (1)$$

Where θ is a vector of typical (population) model parameter, which is considered as fixed effects, η_i, which is assumed to have the normal distribution of mean 0 and covariance matrix Ω are the random variation across individuals in the population, then

$$P(\eta_i; \theta) = \frac{1}{\sqrt{2\pi|\Omega|}} \exp\left(-0.5\eta_i^T \Omega^{-1} \eta_i\right) \qquad (2)$$

If Y_i is the normally distributed continuous variables without boundary, which is the common situation, we have in the PKPD analysis, then

$$P(Y_i \mid \eta_i; \theta) = \prod_j^{n_i} \frac{1}{\sqrt{2\pi\Sigma}} \exp\left(-0.5(Y_i - Y_i^*)^T \Sigma^{-1}(Y_i - Y_i^*)\right) \qquad (3)$$

where $Y_i^* = f(g(\theta, \eta_i, x_i), X_i)$ is the true value of the observation by the model, Σ is the variance of the observation, x_i are fixed covariates (demography etc.), f(.) represent the pharmacokinetic or pharmacodynamic functions we choose, g(.) represent the function chosen for covariate model, X_i incorporate independent variables such as time (t_i), dose, etc. $\varepsilon_i(t_{ij}) = Y_i - Y_i^*$, within subject error which is assumed to have the normal distribution of mean 0 and covariance matrix of Σ often attributed to measurement error. There are three sets of parameters (θ, Ω, Σ) that need to be estimated and three types of vector-valued random variables (Y, η, ε) need to be predicted in the above model. If a parametric proportional hazards regression model is used to model the hazard of the event, then

$$P(T_i, \delta_i \mid \eta_i; \theta) = \left\{h_0(t)e^{\beta Y_i^*(t)+\gamma^T w_i(t)}\right\}^{\delta_i} e^{-\int_0^t h_0(x) e^{\beta Y_i^*(t)+\gamma^T w_i(t)} dx} \qquad (4)$$

where $h_0(t)$ is the baseline hazard function at time t, $w_i(t)$ is a row-vector of individual-specific baseline covariates (possibly time-dependent) with an associated vector of regression coefficients γ, the coefficient β is referred to as the association parameter since it quantifies the strength of the association between the longitudinal and event processes. So, based on (1), the joint likelihood function for the observed data, L_o, is

$$\int \left\{h_0(t)e^{\beta Y_i^*(t)+\gamma^T w_i(t)}\right\}^{\delta_i} e^{-\int_0^t h_0(x)e^{\beta Y_i^*(t)+\gamma^T w_i(t)} dx} \left\{\prod_j^{n_i} \frac{1}{\sqrt{2\pi\Sigma}} \exp\left(-0.5(Y_i - Y_i^*)^T \Sigma^{-1}(Y_i - Y_i^*)\right)\right\}$$
$$\frac{1}{\sqrt{2\pi|\Omega|}} \exp\left(-0.5\eta_i^T \Omega^{-1} \eta_i\right) d\eta_i$$

(5)

This is the joint likelihood function of longitudinal and time-to-event model and longitudinal data are normally distributed continuous data without boundary. This basic joint likelihood function could be extended when we deal with longitudinal proportional data ($0 < Y_i < 1$) or continuous proportional data with boundary and at boundary ($0 \leq Y_i \leq 1$).

For all joint likelihood functions based on types of data we model, depending on the dimension of η_i, the integral in the joint likelihood functions could be multidimensional and intractable to make computations difficult. Some numerical integration methods such as Gaussian quadrature, stochastic approximation expectation-maximization (SAEM), and approximate likelihood methods based on Laplace approximations have been proposed to make computations more efficient.

Joint Modeling of Longitudinal Biomarker and Time-to-Event Data from Clinical Trials

Population Prediction Supporting Clinical Trial Design

Data in some clinical trials can often involve multiple endpoints (e.g., primary and secondary endpoints). The primary endpoint can often be continuous and after a specific duration of treatment. A common way to analyze this kind of data is a comparison of the percent change from baseline in the endpoint of interest between the different study arms. These analyses are relatively straightforward and can include standard statistical tests such as a Wilcoxon rank sum test as was done in a trial investigating changes in cholesterol after 12 weeks or 52 weeks on treatment with a drug being tested as an antihyperlipidemic agent (Ridker et al. 2017). Clinical trials of antidiabetic drugs often involve analyses of percent change from baseline in fasting blood glucose and glycosylated hemoglobin (HbA1c) after 26 weeks and could be analyzed in a similar manner.

Sometimes the endpoint of interest can be categorical such as a clinical trial investigating conversion from a positive test for tuberculosis in sputum to a negative test result after 2 months of treatment with antitubercular drugs (Velayutham et al. 2014). Another example would be a trial investigating the proportion of patients with psoriatic arthritis who achieve at least 20% improvement in the American College of Rheumatology response criteria (ACR20) after 24 weeks of drug treatment (McInnes et al. 2015). In these cases, logistic regression would be a common method of analysis in which the probability of achieving one outcome or the other is calculated in each arm of treatment. The impact of drug treatment or other covariates of interest can be evaluated on this probability. In oncology, the endpoint is usually categorical and often is survival in nature. Survival data, also known as time-to-event data is data that has to do with the length of time it took until a particular event or outcome occurred. Survival data can be overall survival in which the data is comprised of how long each patient remained alive in the clinical trial (in other words, time until death). Or it can be termed "progression-free-survival" (PFS) in which case the definition is related to how long it took a patient to have progressive disease. Progressive disease in cancer is based on the Response Evaluation Criteria in Solid Tumors (RECIST) (Eisenhauer et al. 2009) and defined as having an increase of at least 20% in the sum of diameters of tumor lesions. Time-to-event data in clinical trials can also be found outside the oncology field, e.g., in cardiovascular outcome trials where the endpoint can be the time it took patients to have a heart attack or a stroke (Major Adverse Cardiac Events [MACE]). Analysis of time-to-event data (also known as survival analysis) can include Kaplan Meier curves, Cox proportional hazard models, accelerated failure time models, and other nonparametric and parametric methods covered in standard statistical books (Collett 2003) but this level of detail is outside the scope of this chapter.

Whether the endpoint of interest is continuous or categorical, it stands to reason that the outcome at a specific time point or landmark is a culmination of a trajectory that occurred from the time an intervention took place in a clinical trial (usually the randomization time or the baseline) up to the time point of interest. For example, a single MACE event such as a heart attack could be at least partially (if not mainly) driven by high blood pressure over a period. Clinical trials usually have patients visit the clinic for various assessments at frequent intervals (e.g., weekly or monthly depending on the trial). For continuous endpoints, it is possible that the measure of interest at the end of the trial (e.g., HbA1c or cholesterol, etc.) is also available from these prior visits. A variety of models could be used to describe the time course of drug action on the endpoint of interest, and these could be mechanistic or empiric in nature or something in between. A commonly used modeling approach to describing the time course of drug action on continuous endpoints is the indirect response model (Jusko and Ko 1994) although there are many others beyond the scope of this chapter. Similarly, it is possible for some categorical assessments to be available from prior study visits (e.g., attainment of ACR20). A commonly used approach for modeling this kind of data is the latent variable model (Hu et al. 2010), although there are several other approaches.

In both cases of longitudinal continuous or categorical data, it makes sense to use all available information in the analysis of data from a clinical trial and various methods of analyzing longitudinal data are at the disposal of the data analyst. Using all the information increases the robustness of the analysis and often increases the statistical power. This is where the utility of biomarkers comes in. In many instances, the endpoint of interest in a clinical trial is something that changes slowly (or something investigated at a single snapshot in time) while biomarkers may show more rapid changes. Biomarkers may be useful to inform clinical endpoints that change more slowly if it is established that the biomarker is predictive of the clinical endpoint. In tuberculosis, the endpoint can be 2-month sputum conversion status, or time to sputum culture conversion, but with weekly culture data being available. One could develop a time-to-event model describing the time to sputum conversion, but enrich the information using all the data from prior visits (Chigutsa et al. 2013) instead of focusing on the 2-month time point only. The underlying disease process and drug treatment in tuberculosis (and many other infectious diseases) dictates that one has a relatively high bacterial burden at baseline and would test positive for the bacteria of interest (e.g., *Mycobacterium tuberculosis*). With successful drug treatment, this bacterial load would decrease over time. This situation can be represented mathematically using a biexponential model (Davies et al. 2006):

$$N_t = A \times e^{-\alpha.t} + B \times e^{-\beta.t} \quad (6)$$

where N_t is the number of bacteria at time, t; A is the baseline amount of one bacterial population, killed at a rate α; B is the baseline amount of another bacterial subpopulation, killed at a rate, β.

In a tuberculosis trial where measurements of bacterial load are available (perhaps weekly) one could easily use the above model to describe the time course of this continuous longitudinal measurement. The categorical primary endpoint of sputum conversion (at 2 months or 6 months) can be analyzed through a time-to-event modeling approach [11] with the hazard of a positive tuberculosis test described by any of the parametric hazard equations below.

$$\frac{dHaz}{dt} = \lambda; constant\ hazard \quad (7)$$

$$\frac{dHaz}{dt} = \lambda \times e^{\theta \times t}; timevarying\ hazard\ with\ Gompertz\ distribution\ of\ event\ times \quad (8)$$

$$\frac{dHaz}{dt} = \lambda \times e^{\theta \times \log(t)}; timevarying\ hazard\ with\ Weibull\ distribution\ of\ event\ times \quad (9)$$

where Haz is the hazard of a positive test result; λ is the baseline hazard; θ is a shape parameter describing the time-varying nature of the hazard (if θ is positive it means the hazard increases with time, while a negative value indicates a hazard that decreases with time); t is time.

There are other hazard models that can be tested (e.g., log-logistic, log-normal, gamma distributions) (Collett 2003) and the data analyst should be guided by goodness-of-fit to see which model best fits the data.

The survival would be the probability of negative culture result at a certain time, which is the inverse of the exponent of the cumulative hazard. The cumulative hazard is the time integral of the hazard. Therefore:

$$Surv_t = e^{-\int_0^t Haz_t.dt} \quad (10)$$

where $Surv_t$ is the survival at time, t; Haz_t is the hazard at time, t.

The likelihood of a positive culture result at a certain time is the probability density function (pdf) calculated as:

$$pdf_t = Surv_t \times Haz_t \quad (11)$$

Up to this point, the sputum conversion time-to-event data and the kinetics of bacterial load have been described independently. This is often the way in which the data are analyzed, i.e., one or the other is the method of analysis. However, the two pieces of data can be modeled simultaneously in a joint model through testing the impact of the bacterial load on the hazard of sputum conversion. A simple example assuming a constant hazard is shown below.

$$\frac{dHaz}{dt} = \lambda \times e^{\kappa \times N_t} \qquad (12)$$

where N_t is the number of bacteria at time, t and κ is an estimated parameter that describes the extent to which bacterial load influences the hazard.

In oncology, if the primary endpoint is overall survival, death of a patient is something that could take years to happen. On the other hand, changes in tumor size could be detected monthly. It is likely that if the tumor size in increasing, the hazard of death increases, with the converse being true. Drug administration could therefore be modeled to impact the survival indirectly through a change in tumor size, or directly in a manner independent of measured tumor lesions or both. This framework can be illustrated in a joint tumor size and survival model (Fig. 1).

The pharmacokinetic (▶ Chap. 98, "Pharmacokinetic and Pharmacodynamic Modeling") (PK) model would describe the relationship between the administered dose and the time course of drug concentrations. The drug concentration would then influence the change in tumor size, which would subsequently influence the survival. The survival could be overall survival or PFS, whichever is of interest. The equations describing the time-to-event model for survival and the connection between that and the tumor size would be like those described above for sputum conversion (Eqs. 2–7). However, the models describing change in tumor size (which is the sum of tumor growth and tumor shrinkage) might differ. An empiric model for change in tumor size might include zero order growth and first order shrinkage (Wang et al. 2009):

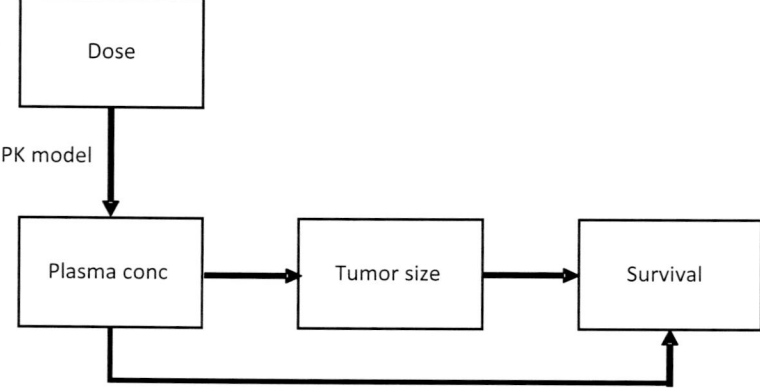

Fig. 1 Model diagram for joint tumor size – survival model with drug effect

$$\text{Tumor size}(t) = \text{Base} \times e^{-k_s \times t} + k_g \times t \qquad (13)$$

where Base is the baseline tumor size (before drug treatment); k_s is a first order tumor shrink rate constant; k_g is a zero-order tumor growth rate.

In Eq. 13, one could then have a measure of drug exposure (dose, area under the curve [AUC], steady-state concentration, trough concentration, etc.) influencing k_s. Various kinds of models could be investigated (linear, Emax or sigmoidal Emax, etc.)

While Eq. 13 can work well in many cases, a problem arises when one wants to use dynamic drug concentrations instead of the time-invariant summary PK metrics. In oncology clinical trials, dose reductions or drug holidays due to drug toxicity are a common occurrence. In such cases, the use of time-invariant summary PK metrics such as AUC or trough concentration could lead to inaccurate elucidation of the true exposure–response relationship. If dose reductions or drug holidays are a significant occurrence in a trial, it would be better to use dynamic PK concentrations driven by the actual administration of drug doses in the trial. However, it is readily apparent from Eq. 8 that a change in the drug concentration (and hence a change in k_s) results in an immediate change in the tumor size. This should not be the case as this does not happen. The tumor size changes after some delay in time. A common semi-mechanistic approach to appropriately characterize this delay is having a series of transit compartments as previously described by Simeoni *et al.* modeling xenograft experimental data (Simeoni et al. 2004) and shown in the figure below. The model describes the total measured tumor size (or tumor volume) as the sum of healthy proliferating tumor cells and tumor cells that are going through a series of damage until eventual death and disappearance from the tumor (Fig. 2).

A potential difference between the mouse xenograft data that Simeoni *et al.* used to develop their model and clinical data is that xenograft experimental data often involves early tumor growth when the tumor is growing exponentially, and then this growth switches to linear (zero order) growth as the tumor matures with time. On the other hand, by the time a patient presents in a clinical trial, the tumor(s) are already established and are likely in the linear growth phase. Therefore, the switch from exponential to linear growth incorporated by Simeoni *et al.* can be reduced to only include linear growth, leading to the following set of equations to be understood in the context of the figure above:

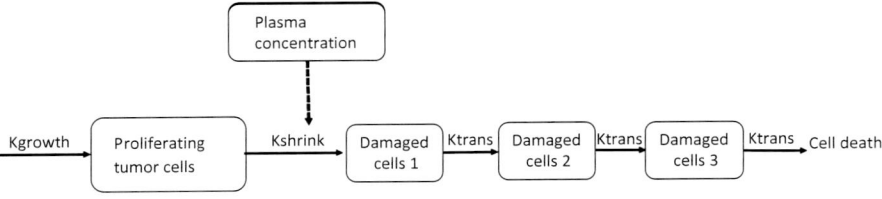

Fig. 2 Semi-mechanistic PK – change in tumor size model (Adapted from Simeoni et al. 2004)

$$\frac{dProliferating}{dt} = k_{growth} - k_{shrink} \times conc \times Proliferating \quad (14)$$

$$\frac{dDamaged1}{dt} = k_{shrink} \times conc \times Proliferating - k_{trans} \times Damaged1 \quad (15)$$

$$\frac{dDamaged2}{dt} = k_{trans} \times (Damaged1 - Damaged2) \quad (16)$$

$$\frac{dDamaged3}{dt} = k_{trans} \times (Damaged2 - Damaged3) \quad (17)$$

$$Tumor\ size\ (t) = Proliferating + Damaged1 + Damaged2 + Damaged3 \quad (18)$$

The drug concentration in Eq. 10 is a value that would be coming from a PK model and can change with time. The impact of this change in drug concentration is "dampened" and delayed by the series of transit compartments so that it will take long time for the change in concentration to translate to a change in the predicted size in Eq. (18).

The tumor size models described above would be good starting points for model development depending on the situation but could be modified depending on the available data. For example, if development of drug resistance is thought to occur, this could be incorporated in various ways including a time-dependent tumor shrink rate or a time-dependent drug effect, or a baseline tumor subpopulation that is resistant to the drug tumor shrink effect.

Upon adequate characterization of the tumor size, the predicted value can influence the hazard or death or the hazard of disease progression. This would be a joint tumor size – time-to-event modeling approach. A simple example assuming a constant hazard is shown below:

$$\frac{dHaz}{dt} = \lambda \times e^{\kappa \times TS_t} \quad (19)$$

where Haz is the hazard of the event of interest; TS_t is the tumor size at time, t; λ is the baseline hazard; κ is an estimated parameter that describes the extent to which tumor burden influences the hazard.

The extent to which the tumor size influences the hazard depends on the type of cancer, the type of tumor measurement, and the type of hazard. Since PFS is dependent upon tumor size measurements, tumor size would have a stronger influence on the hazard than if the hazard was to do with overall survival. In cases of metastatic cancers, tumor size would still be important, but it could be that metastases also have a significant impact on the hazard of death.

Apart from being better able to characterize the factors influencing the primary endpoint, the importance of joint tumor size – time-to-event modeling approach is also realized when changes in tumor size (which is available quite readily and early on in a clinical trial) can predict the primary endpoint. An example is a case where time to tumor regrowth determined using a tumor growth inhibition model was able to predict overall survival in patients with colorectal cancer. The median overall survival time was about 20 months, yet the median time to tumor regrowth was about 6 months (Claret et al. 2013). Another example is a case where PFS in renal cell carcinoma could be predicted from a model that used 8-week tumor size data (Claret et al. 2016). Therefore, early clinical trial data comprising tumor size-based metrics could be used to inform decisions about the primary endpoint, which could take years to realize.

The tumor size – time-to-event models can be further expanded if there is biomarker data available, which could be correlated with changes in tumor size. The biomarker could be an easily sampled blood measurement and the advantage then is that an even earlier or faster changing metric can be used to ultimately predict longer term outcomes such as survival.

A good example of a joint modeling approach of tumor dynamics and overall survival during treatment of lung cancer has been described in patients being treated with necitumumab. In this work, the PK of necitumumab was first described using a parallel first order and mixed order elimination model (Long et al. 2017). The PK model was used to obtain the average steady-state plasma concentration of necitumumab for each patient, which was then used as driver of tumor shrinkage according to the equations below:

$$\frac{dSize}{dt} = Size_0 \cdot e^{-shrink \cdot t} \cdot (-shrink) + growth \tag{20}$$

$$shrink = \theta \times \left(1 + \frac{Emax \times Css^{HILL}}{EC50^{HILL} + Css^{HILL}}\right) \tag{21}$$

where $Size_0$ is the baseline tumor size, $shrink$ is the first order exponential decrease in the size of the tumor, $growth$ is the tumor growth rate constant, θ is the baseline tumor shrink rate in the absence of treatment with necitumumab, $Emax$ is the maximum effect of necitumumab in increasing the tumor shrink rate, Css is average steady-state plasma concentration, EC_{50} is the concentration that results in half the maximum effect, and $HILL$ is the Hill coefficient of sigmoidicity.

Resistance is something that often occurs during treatment with anticancer drugs and it can be incorporated in modeling in various ways such as a time-dependent increase in the EC_{50} of a drug, or a time-dependent decrease in the shrink rate shown in the equation below.

$$Shrink_t = Shrink_0 \times e^{-resist \times t} \tag{22}$$

where $Shrink_t$ is the first order shrink rate of the tumor at time, t, $Shrink_0$ is the shrink rate at the beginning of treatment, and $resist$ is the rate of decline of the shrink rate.

For necitumumab, the tumor size at any time during treatment (predicted from Eq. 20) was then tested as a predictor of the hazard of death at the corresponding time in a model simultaneously describing overall survival and change in tumor size. The estimation of tumor size and survival parameters was done simultaneously, which has the advantage of using all the available data jointly.

$$\frac{dHaz}{dt} = \lambda \times e^{[Gomp \times t + Weib \times LOG(t)]} \times e^{\kappa \times Size(t)} \quad (23)$$

where λ is the baseline hazard at the beginning of the study, $Gomp$ is the shape parameter representing a Gompertz distribution of event times, $Weib$ is the shape parameter representing the Weibull distribution, κ is the estimated link between model predicted tumor size at time t and the hazard.

Equation 18 indicates a distribution of event times that follows a combination of Gompertz and Weibull distributions and this combination best described the survival profiles in the necitumumab study. Since the necitumumab drug concentration affects tumor size, it inherently influences the overall survival through Eq. 23. However, as described earlier, the target lesions are not necessarily the only determinant of overall survival. The limited number of tumor lesions measured in clinical trials is not 100% predictive of overall survival, and multiple factors (albeit related to the disease) outside of measured target lesions can contribute to a patient's death. The drug can influence these other factors (e.g., metastases), hence the need for an additional drug effect on survival. Therefore, drug effect was also added on the baseline hazard, λ, as follows:

$$\lambda = \theta \times \left(1 + \frac{Emax \times Css^{HILL}}{EC50^{HILL} + Css^{HILL}}\right) \quad (24)$$

The overall model structure is therefore like what is shown in Fig. 1 above. In the case of necitumumab, the tumor size data (continuous and measured at multiple clinic visits) and the survival data were modeled simultaneously, which increases the power of the analysis.

A common population modeling software tool is NONMEM (ICON Development Solutions; Hanover, MD). The necitumumab PKPD modeling was performed using NONMEM. Due to model complexity and the number of equations, the Stochastic Approximation Expectation-Maximization (SAEM) estimation algorithm was used, with mu-referencing of parameters. Goodness-of-fit plots and visual predictive checks indicated that the modeling described above adequately described both the tumor size and the survival data. Further details of this modeling and simulation and NONMEM code is described by Chigutsa et al. 2017.

The concepts described in this chapter, linking a continuous variable that is frequently measured, to a time-to-event model can be easily extended to other categorical endpoints such as response status (yes/no) at a specific time point in a clinical trial. These categorical endpoints are usually modeled using logistic regression where the probability of having a particular outcome would be determined as follows:

$$P_r = \frac{e^{lgtr}}{1 + e^{lgtr}} \quad (25)$$

where Pr is the probability of the outcome of interest; lgtr is an estimated logit parameter.

In the logistic regression model above, various biomarkers modeled using indirect response models or other methods as appropriate can be incorporated to influence the logit in a simple additive manner and thus constitute a joint longitudinal – categorical model. In the case of latent variable time course models (Hu et al. 2010), the latent variable could be driven by various variables including drug concentration and biomarkers.

The advantage of joint modeling of longitudinal and categorical data is that multiple kinds of data can speak to each other and this increases the robustness of the analysis. A simultaneous population modeling approach also has the advantage of being able to borrow information from one endpoint when a measurement from another is missing. Furthermore, when the connection between the more frequently sampled measure and the further out primary endpoint is reliably established, this enables prediction of the primary endpoint based upon earlier data. In other words, using biomarker data alone could predict clinical trial outcomes and potentially save time in screening multiple compounds in drug development. This requires a reliable biomarker–outcome relationship, which should be thoroughly evaluated during PKPD model development.

Joint modeling approach integrating the longitudinal tumor dynamic and time-to-event analysis for oncology drugs has gained increasingly interest in different therapeutic area. Vu et al. in 2012 first used joint model incorporating the time-dependent disease progress as a predictor of clinical events (survival, disability, cognitive impairment, and depression) in Parkinson's disease. In this model a nonlinear Parkinson disease progression model (Holford et al. 2006) was integrated as time-changing covariate to the parametric Gompertz hazard function for survival analysis. The hazard of dropout due to causes other than death was described by the sum of two Gompertz distributions based on time and a Weibull distribution function. By using the joint modeling approach, Vu et al. were able to differentiate the beneficial effects (i.e., symptomatic and/or disease modifying) and the adverse effects of anti-parkinsonian medications on the progression of Parkinson's disease and found a significant association between continued selegiline treatment and mortality.

In oncology, integrating tumor growth kinetics in response to antitumor drug effect as time-changing covariate in the parametric survival analysis has offered a better understanding of the relation among drug exposure, short-term tumor response, and long-term survival. Tong et al. (2018) presented a retrospectively analysis where the joint model developed with phase 2 data was used to predict the progression-free survival in phase 3 trial, based on early phase 3 tumor measurements. Phase 2 trial data of selumetinib in patient with non-small cell lung cancer (NSCLC) was first used to develop a joint model of tumor size dynamic and progression-free survival (PFS), where linear quadratic tumor size dynamic model was integrated as time-changing covariate in cox proportional hazard function. The model adequately captured the tumor size dynamic and PFS of the selumetinib phase 2 data. As an external validation, the final model developed with phase 2 data was further applied to selumetinib phase 3 data, to predict the selumetinib phase 3 PFS over 2 years period, based on only the first 4 months of phase 3 tumor size measurement. The predicted phase 3 PFS are well correlated with the observed phase 3 PFS and has confirmed with the clinical finding of selumetinib trials.

However, the capacity of joint model analysis based on tumor size kinetics for the longitudinal part can be limited due to the highly sparse nature of tumor size measurement in clinical setting. Other longitudinal biomarkers such as prostate-specific antigen (PSA) in prostate cancer patients, has gained increasing attention and has shown promising results. Desmée et al. developed a mechanistic joint model to characterize the kinetics of PSA described by ODEs and linked to the time-to-event survival in metastatic castration-resistant prostate cancer (mCRPC) patient. In Desmée's work, mathematical model for PSA kinetics was defined assuming that PSA was produced by two types of cells, namely, treatment-sensitive cells, and treatment-resistant cells. Nonlinear mixed-effect models (NLMEM) were used to analyze all the longitudinal PSA measurements before, during, and after treatment. The time-to-death was modeled using a parametric hazard described by Weibull function. The log-likelihood of the joint function was maximized using the SAEM algorithm implemented in Monolix 4.3.2. The developed joint model went through an internal validation where the individual trajectories for both PSA and the hazard function in a patient were calculated using only the observed PSA measurements.

Desmée's model allowed to capture a variety of patterns in PSA kinetics observed during and after anticancer therapy. The model further identified that two quantities, treatment-sensitive and resistant cancer cells, may have a large impact on long-term survival. However, the only observed quantity was the PSA value, which was assumed to be proportional to the total number of cancer cells, the portion of treatment resistant cells was not observed and only estimated by the joint model. Study shows that the kinetics of treatment-resistant cells had a larger impact on survival than the kinetics of treatment-sensitive cells. Since the kinetics of resistant cells drives the increase in PSA levels in the long run, prediction is consistent with the previous findings that the final tumor growth rate being highly predictive of the time-to-death (Stein et al. 2008). The external validation of Desmée's model shows that the model could be used to predict the survival curve of the patients of independent population that had not been used for model building. By only including the longitudinal information of PSA, the model prediction by simulation well matched with the observed survival in patients from the validation dataset. This approach sheds new light on the relationship between PSA and death in mCRPC patients and opens the way for the use of more complex and physiological models to improve treatment evaluation and survival prediction.

Individual Dynamic Prediction

Recent literature has explored the dynamic predictive ability of the longitudinal biomarker for the time-to-event outcome with the use of joint modeling framework

(Rizopoulos 2011). Given a joint model with a set of parameters estimated in a large dataset, now we are interested in estimating individual survival of a new subject i with longitudinal biomarker measurements available until a landmark time L and aim to predict the risk of death until time $L + t$ ($t > 0$). Desmée et al., in another study, extended the use of their nonlinear joint model developed previously to individual dynamic prediction, more specifically for predicting the long-term risk of death in mCRPC patients with early phase PSA measurements. By using the estimated population parameters of the developed joint model as priors, the a posteriori distribution of individual parameters was computed and the prediction interval for the individual risk of death was derived accordingly for a new patient knowing his PSA measurements until a given landmark time. The computation was done with Hamiltonian Monte Carlo algorithm implemented in Stan software (Desmee et al. 2017a, b). Time-dependent area under the ROC curve (AUC) and Brier score (BS) were derived to assess discrimination and calibration of the model predictions, on both simulated patients and real patients that are not included to build the model. According to Desmée's work, individual dynamic predictions provide good predictive performances for landmark time L larger than 12 months and t up to 18 months for both simulated and real data. The AUC and the BS both improved over the landmark time in the simulation study and tend to stagnate in the real data since in the real data PSA measurements become less frequent over time in patients after the end of treatment. The model has also shown potential to better distinguish patients of low and high risk of death in the long term. Beside this concrete application in patients with mCRPC, this approach can be exemplified to develop more biologically relevant models in various medical contexts.

Summary and Conclusions

The purpose of this chapter is to provide the basic knowledge of approach, methodology, and applications of joint modeling of longitudinal and time-to-event data in clinical trials. The joint model can reduce the bias of estimation of model parameters and systemic underestimation of effect of longitudinal data on time to an event. The jointly integrated model of longitudinal and time-to-event data enabled prediction of treatment outcome of time to an event based on dynamics of covariates longitudinally measured and potentially can serve as a novel quantitative tool to predict time to an event at early stage.

Key Points

- Types of longitudinal and time-to-event data.
- Joint likelihood function to be maximized when jointly modeling longitudinal and time-to-event data.

- Applications of jointly modeling longitudinal and time-to-event data in clinical trials.
- Individual dynamic predications.

Cross-References

▶ Pharmacokinetic and Pharmacodynamic Modeling

References

Armero C, Forné C, Rué M, Forte A, Perpiñán H, Gómez G, Baré M (2016) Bayesian joint ordinal and survival modeling for breast cancer risk assessment. Stat Med 35(28):5267–5282

Chigutsa E et al (2013) A time-to-event pharmacodynamic model describing treatment response in patients with pulmonary tuberculosis using days to positivity in automated liquid mycobacterial culture. Antimicrob Agents Chemother 57(2):789–795

Chigutsa E, Long AJ, Wallin JE (2017) Exposure-response analysis of necitumumab efficacy in squamous non-small cell lung cancer patients. CPT Pharmacometrics Syst Pharmacol 6(8):560–568

Claret L et al (2013) Evaluation of tumor-size response metrics to predict overall survival in Western and Chinese patients with first-line metastatic colorectal cancer. J Clin Oncol 31(17):2110–2114

Claret L et al (2016) Model-based prediction of progression-free survival in patients with first-line renal cell carcinoma using week 8 tumor size change from baseline. Cancer Chemother Pharmacol 78(3):605–610

Collett D (2003) Modelling survival data in medical research. Chapman & Hall/CRC texts in statistical science series, 2nd edn. Chapman & Hall/CRC, Boca Raton. 391 p

Davies GR et al (2006) Use of nonlinear mixed-effects analysis for improved precision of early pharmacodynamic measures in tuberculosis treatment. Antimicrob Agents Chemother 50(9):3154–3156

Desmée S, Mentré F, Veyrat-Follet C et al (2015) Nonlinear mixed-effect models for prostate-specific antigen kinetics and link with survival in the context of metastatic prostate cancer: a comparison by simulation of two-stage and joint approaches. AAPS J 17:691–699

Desmee S et al (2017a) Nonlinear joint models for individual dynamic prediction of risk of death using Hamiltonian Monte Carlo: application to metastatic prostate cancer. BMC Med Res Methodol 17(1):105

Desmee S et al (2017b) Using the SAEM algorithm for mechanistic joint models characterizing the relationship between nonlinear PSA kinetics and survival in prostate cancer patients. Biometrics 73(1):305–312

Eisenhauer EA et al (2009) New response evaluation criteria in solid tumours: revised RECIST guideline (version 1.1). Eur J Cancer 45(2):228–247

Holford NH et al (2006) Disease progression and pharmacodynamics in Parkinson disease – evidence for functional protection with levodopa and other treatments. J Pharmacokinet Pharmacodyn 33(3):281–311

Hu C et al (2010) A latent variable approach for modeling categorical endpoints among patients with rheumatoid arthritis treated with golimumab plus methotrexate. J Pharmacokinet Pharmacodyn 37(4):309–321

Jusko WJ, Ko HC (1994) Physiologic indirect response models characterize diverse types of pharmacodynamic effects. Clin Pharmacol Ther 56(4):406–419

Long A, Chigutsa E, Wallin J (2017) Population pharmacokinetics of Necitumumab in cancer patients. Clin Pharmacokinet 56(5):505–514

Martins R, Silva GL, Andreozzi V (2016) Bayesian joint modeling of longitudinaland spatial survival AIDS data. Stat Med 35:3368–3384

McInnes IB et al (2015) Secukinumab, a human anti-interleukin-17A monoclonal antibody, in patients with psoriatic arthritis (FUTURE 2): a randomised, double-blind, placebo-controlled, phase 3 trial. Lancet 386(9999):1137–1146

Ridker PM et al (2017) Lipid-reduction variability and antidrug-antibody formation with Bococizumab. N Engl J Med 376(16):1517–1526

Rizopoulos D (2011) Dynamic predictions and prospective accuracy in joint models for longitudinal and time-to-event data. Biometrics 67:819–829

Simeoni M et al (2004) Predictive pharmacokinetic-pharmacodynamic modeling of tumor growth kinetics in xenograft models after administration of anticancer agents. Cancer Res 64(3):1094–1101

Song H, Peng Y, Tu D (2017) Jointly modeling longitudinal proportional data and survival times with an application to the quality of life data in a breast cancer trial. Lifetime Data Anal 23:183–206

Stein WD et al (2008) Tumor growth rates derived from data for patients in a clinical trial correlate strongly with patient survival: a novel strategy for evaluation of clinical trial data. Oncologist 13(10):1046–1054

Tong X et al (2018) Abstract 4760: Joint modeling of longitudinal tumor dynamics and survival in non-small cell lung cancer (NSCLC) patients. Cancer Res 78(Suppl 13):4760

Velayutham BV et al (2014) Sputum culture conversion with moxifloxacin-containing regimens in the treatment of patients with newly diagnosed sputum-positive pulmonary tuberculosis in South India. Clin Infect Dis 59(10):e142–e149

Vu TC, Nutt JG, Holford NH (2012) Disease progress and response to treatment as predictors of survival, disability, cognitive impairment and depression in Parkinson's disease. Br J Clin Pharmacol 74(2):284–295

Wang Y et al (2009) Elucidation of relationship between tumor size and survival in non-small-cell lung cancer patients can aid early decision making in clinical drug development. Clin Pharmacol Ther 86(2):167–174

Wilbaux M et al (2015) A joint model for the kinetics of CTC count and PSA concentration during treatment in metastatic castration-resistant prostate cancer. CPT Pharmacometrics Syst Pharmacol 4:277–285

Yu M, Taylor JMG, Sandler HM (2008) Individual prediction in prostate cancer studies using a joint longitudinal survival-cure model. J Am Stat Assoc 103(481):178–187

Zhang L, Beal SL, Sheiner LB (2003a) Simultaneous vs. sequential analysis for population PK/PD data I: best-case performance. J Pharmacokinet Pharmacodyn 30:387–404

Zhang L, Beal SL, Sheiner LB (2003b) Simultaneous vs. sequential analysis for population PK/PD data II: robustness of methods. J Pharmacokinet Pharmacodyn 30:405–416

Pharmacokinetic and Pharmacodynamic Modeling

98

Shamir N. Kalaria, Hechuan Wang, and Jogarao V. Gobburu

Contents

Introduction	1938
Disease-Drug Trial Models	1940
Case: Use of a Disease-Drug-Trial Model to Influence Study Design	1943
PKPD Modeling for First in Human Studies	1945
Case: Applying Mechanistic Modeling to Enable Preclinical to Clinical Translation and Guide the FIH Trial Design of a Monoclonal Antibody	1946
PKPD Modeling for Proof of Concept Studies	1947
Case: An Integrated Mechanistic PK-PD Modeling of the Testosterone Suppression Effect of Degarelix Using Data in Healthy Male Subjects from Three Clinical Studies	1947
Case: PK-PD Modeling of the Antimalarial Effect of Actelion-451,840 in a Malaria Study in Eight Healthy Subjects from a Proof-of-Concept Study	1948
Dose Ranging Studies	1948
Case: Dose-Ranging Trial to Characterize and Confirm a Dose-Response Relationship	1951
Case: Evidence of Effectiveness Derived Using Dose-Response Relationship	1952
Case: Risk Mitigation Using an Exposure-Safety Relationship	1952
Case: Dose Optimization for Future Clinical Trials	1953
Use of PK-PD Modeling for Precision Medicine	1954
Case: Precision Medicine and Bayesian Forecasting to Improve Patient Outcomes	1955
Summary and Conclusions	1956
Key Facts	1957
Cross-References	1958
References	1958

S. N. Kalaria · H. Wang · J. V. Gobburu (✉)
Center for Translational Medicine, University of Maryland School of Pharmacy, Baltimore, MD, USA
e-mail: skalaria@umaryland.edu; hechuan.wang@umaryland.edu; jgobburu@rx.umaryland.edu

© Springer Nature Switzerland AG 2022
S. Piantadosi, C. L. Meinert (eds.), *Principles and Practice of Clinical Trials*,
https://doi.org/10.1007/978-3-319-52636-2_284

Abstract

Pharmacokinetic and pharmacodynamic (PKPD) concepts and approaches play a critical role by increasing the efficiency throughout the drug development process and optimizing clinical therapeutics. Innovative quantitative analysis that integrate PKPD and disease progression knowledge are pivotal in regulatory decision-making and have shown to provide supportive evidence of effectiveness. Objective approaches to dose-selection that are informed by exposure-response analyses can assist in visualizing benefit-risk profiles on an individual and population level. Clinical trial simulations using quantitative models that incorporate structural and stochastic components along with prior knowledge can allow for informing clinical trial design features, dose selection in unstudied patient populations, and regulatory policy development. This chapter presents various PKPD-based analyses throughout the drug development process and within precision medicine. Emphasis on the use of PKPD analysis for proof of concept, dose-ranging, and first in human dose studies are subsequently provided. Case studies are highlighted to better illustrate the impact of quantitative analyses for decision-making.

Keywords

Pharmacokinetics · Pharmacodynamics · Modeling and Simulation · Non-Linear Mixed Effect · Learn and Apply · Disease-Drug Trial Model · First in Human Dose Study · Proof of Concept Study · Dose Ranging Study

Introduction

Over the last century, a philosophical debate on different statistical approaches to justify causal inference has led statisticians, clinical pharmacologists, and clinicians to identify with one of the two prominent schools of thought: Bayesian and frequentist. For the purpose of this report, Bayesian approach is confined to analysis of clinical trial data using biologically plausible models ("Pharmacometrics approach"). Pure Bayesian inferential statistics is not the focus. The fundamental difference between frequentists versus pharmacometrics approaches is that frequentist approach rigidly relies on confirming the hypothesis for a known question. Whereas, the pharmacometrics approach relies on integrating the clinical trial observations and the current understanding of the pharmacology to generalize inferences. Further confirmation of these inferences is not necessarily required as they rely on pharmacologic principles.

The conventional frequentist approach is based on the concept that any given investigation can be considered a sample of an infinite number of repetitions of that same investigation (Senn 2003). Inferences are derived from a sampling distribution of sample means from these infinite numbers of repeated investigations. The concept of P value is deeply rooted into the frequentist approach that represents the proportion of times an observed outcome will occur in a series of repeated investigations given that the null hypothesis is true (e.g., H_0: Difference between treatment and placebo effect is equal to zero). Frequentist measures, such as p-values and confidence intervals dominate current clinical research and provide a sharp cut-off for decision-making. However, their interpretations are often misunderstood (Senn 2003; Bittl and Yulei 2017). Bayes' theorem predates the use of frequentist approaches by over a century. Due to the increasing availability of big data and powerful computers, a growing number of scientific disciplines such as engineering, physics, genetics, finance, and computer science have utilized Bayesian approaches for decision-making. Bayesian statistics provides the direct probability of an outcome based on prior knowledge of conditions related to that outcome. The power of Bayesian inference is that it is subject to change based on the availability of new knowledge (Senn 2003). A surge of newer Bayesian adaptive clinical trial designs have been used for the development drugs and devices. Clinical practice guidelines such as the American College of Cardiology and the American Heart Association have recently supported the use of Bayesian analysis to justify specific cardiovascular interventions (Bittl and Yulei 2017).

The Kefauver Harris Amendment of 1962 to the Food, Drug and Cosmetic Act introduced the requirement for drug manufacturers to provide proof of effectiveness and safety of drugs prior to regulatory approval following the well-known thalidomide tragedy. The amendment introduces the concept of "substantial evidence" which consist of "adequate and well-controlled investigations" to evaluate the effectiveness of a drug. Traditionally, frequentist statistical approaches have been used to analyze at least two confirmatory registration trials at a p-value ≤ 0.05. However, the entire drug development spectrum has relied on Bayesian principles, where knowledge gained from prior experiences can be leveraged to confirm the effect of a therapeutic intervention (Peck et al. 2003). Safety information gathered from preclinical animal studies allow for the justification for a first in human dose. Treatment effect sizes observed from earlier proof of concept studies allow developers to determine the required sample size for future registration trials. The passage of the Food and Drug Administration Modernization Act (FDAMA) of 1997 was a major piece of legislation that exemplified the use of Bayesian principles in drug development. The act allowed for a single "adequate and well controlled" trial with "confirmatory evidence" to conclude the presence of substantial evidence of effectiveness. FDAMA paved the way for streamlining drug development in various areas such as pediatrics, where previous experience in adults could be used to establish evidence of effectiveness. Approval of extended release formulations after the approval of immediate release products can also be supported with a single clinical trial.

Integration of knowledge is inherently a Bayesian principle, although analyses could be based on various statistical approaches. Drug development is a continuous process of multiple learning and confirming cycles (Sheiner 1997). Knowledge is accumulated from preclinical, PK-PD, and early proof of concept studies Meno-Tetang and Lowe (2005). Application of this knowledge to dosing finding studies and large multicenter clinical trials lead to updated benefit-risk profiles that assist in making informed decisions (Gobburu and Marroum 2001; Powell and Gobburu 2007). This chapter aims to provide an understanding how quantitative relationships can be utilized to support evidence of effectiveness, provide for informative dosing recommendations, and aid in efficient clinical trial design by harnessing data generated across drug development programs. Specific modeling strategies will be highlighted and case examples will be provided to showcase their impact on drug development and regulatory decision-making. Please go to the following chapters in this book if you are interested in learning more about this section (▶ Chaps. 59, "Interim Analysis in Clinical Trials," ▶ 60, "Bayesian Adaptive Designs for Phase I Trials," and ▶ 61, "Adaptive Phase II Trials").

Disease-Drug Trial Models

According to recent statistics, approximately 50% of all pivotal trials intended for regulatory approval fail. The major reason for trial failure centers on not being able to meet primary and secondary efficacy endpoints. Subfactors that may contribute to lack of efficacy include suboptimal dose selection, heterogeneous patient populations, study operations (e.g., dropouts), insufficient sample size, and high placebo response. Efforts to utilize knowledge gained from previous drug experience have shown to unequivocally increase the probability of success for future clinical trials. Accrual of information with regards to disease specific changes and exposure-response relationships can be integrated together to assist in designing larger clinical studies. Gobburu et al. first introduced the concept of disease-drug-trial models as a tool to improve the "predictability and productivity" throughout the drug development process (Gobburu and Lesko 2009). Conceptually, disease-drug-trial models are mathematical representations of the natural time course of a disease (e.g., clinical response in the absence of receiving placebo or drug treatment), placebo effects, drug effects, and clinical trial characteristics.

The disease submodel aims to quantify changes in the natural pathobiological system in the absence of any treatment intervention. Several components of the disease model include surrogate biomarkers, natural progression of clinical response, and placebo effects. Quantitative approaches to describe disease knowledge can be mechanistic, semi-mechanistic, or empirical. Mechanistic models that incorporate biological processes at a molecular level based on in-vitro or in-vivo experiments are referred to as systems biology or physiologically based models. On the other hand, semi-mechanistic and empirical models are heavily data-driven and simplify the biological aspects of the specific disease. Usually these models are narrow in scope and do not consider other interacting systems (Gobburu and Lesko 2009). Over the last decade, there has been an increase in the number of patient registries and data repositories that contain longitudinal natural history progression for several therapeutic areas. Utilization of real-world-evidence and natural history data in addition to clinical trial data could help develop robust disease models. However, clinical study design could limit the availability of disease progression data in patients. The use placebo arms to describe both the placebo effect and disease progression have commonly been reported when natural history data is not available. The placebo effect observed in clinical trials is a perceived effect that is confounded by factors such as: natural disease time course, external factors leading to fluctuations in symptoms, individual regression towards the mean natural state, and the use of additional medications or receiving psychological interventions outside of a clinical study (Weimer et al. 2015; Fava et al. 2003). One possible way to parse out disease progression from placebo effect would be to enroll subjects into an untreated arm and follow them throughout the duration of the study (Ernst and Resch 1995). The effect observed from the untreated group could be subtracted from the placebo group to obtain the "true placebo effect." Examples of disease models for diabetes, Alzheimer's disease, Parkinson's disease, bipolar disorder, and depression are currently available (Krudys et al. 2005; Holford and Peace 1992; Holford et al. 2006; Gomeni and Merlo-Pich 2007; Sun et al. 2013).

Drug effect models are synonymous to dose-response/exposure-response models that describe a drug's pharmacological effect on clinical response. Information for drug effect models is mostly gathered from well-designed dose-ranging studies. Please refer to the "Disease-Drug Trial Models" section for more information. Drug models can be used for appropriate dose selection for specific subgroup populations depending on the inclusion of certain prognostic factors. Differences in trial design used to develop the model also need to be taken into consideration. Even though a great emphasis is placed on exposure-response modeling with regards to efficacy, exposure-safety relationships can also be used to identify early safety markers that are predictive of long-term safety risks.

Clinical trial design and trial execution can be a major determinant for trial success. Trial characteristics such as inclusion/exclusion criteria, dropout rates, and protocol compliance can meaningfully influence trial outcomes. When conducting clinical trial simulations, it is important to understand the basis of our virtual patient population. Baseline characteristics of the enrolled patient population are often reported as mean with a standard deviation or a median with a range. Simply using univariate statistical distributions to simulate patient characteristics such as race, gender, age, weight, and height does not take into account the presence of an existing correlation. For example, weight, age, and sex are known to be highly correlated and quantitative relationships amongst these patient characteristics must be developed to adequately simulate pediatric clinical trials. The ability to describe trends in patient adherence to medication throughout a trial is important when simulating drug exposures that can ultimately impact safety and efficacy profiles. Often times, patients discontinue participating in a trial because of completely random reasons (missing completely at random) or for reasons related to lack of drug efficacy or increased toxicity (missing at random/missing not at random). Understanding reasons for patient withdrawal will not only assist in enriching future trials but also could be used to incorporate knowledge of dropout patterns during simulations. Parametric time to event models have been frequently used to model and simulate dropout trends. Please go to the following chapter in this book if you would like to learn more about this section.

Before discussing the use of the aforementioned techniques to describe changes in pharmacokinetic and pharmacodynamic data, it would be useful to understand the technical premise regarding the use of commonly used hierarchical model structures. Consider the Cockcroft-Graf formula for estimating creatinine clearance. All males or females with the same age, body weight, and creatinine will have the same estimated creatinine clearance. This value is called the fixed effect. However, the true creatinine clearance in each patient will be different from this fixed effect, due to a random effect (variability). A mixed effect model is a pharmaco-statistical model containing both fixed effects and random effects. The fixed effects reflect the mechanistic or pharmacologic features of the underlying system. The random effects reflect the unexplained features of the system. Mixed effects modeling of pharmacokinetic and pharmacodynamic data (referred to as PKPD models) has the advantage of using sparse data in a single subject, which is particularly useful for data analysis in therapeutic drug monitoring or large clinical efficacy and safety trials. The PK data includes drug concentration measurements in biofluids such as blood, plasma, urine, or other tissues. The PD data includes measurements related to the pharmacologic effect of the drug such as biomarkers (e.g., BP, BMD) or clinical endpoints (e.g., pain score, survival).

In the 1970s, mixed effect modeling methods were introduced by Sheiner et al. to the pharmacokinetic community (Sheiner et al. 1972). They recognized the nonlinear relationship between the PK data and parameters by analyzing routine clinical sparse data of warfarin and digoxin, and identified the potential use of nonlinear mixed effects modeling to optimize warfarin and digoxin therapeutic dosage regimens. In the subsequent two decades, PKPD based on NLME made a large impact on drug development by facilitating drug approvals. The Food and Drug Administration (FDA) issued their first Population PK guidance for the pharmaceutical industry in 1999. In the most recent 10 years, research has focused on Bayesian estimation of NLME modeling to develop individualized dosing regimens and their clinical applicability.

A key feature of mixed effect modeling is the use of two levels of effects in describing the model parameters: fixed and random effects. Fixed effects of the model parameters show how the mean response changes over time. The general form of the mean plasma concentration Cp_j at time j for a drug following one-compartment elimination kinetics administered as an intravenous (IV) bolus is:

$$Cp_j = \frac{Dose}{tvV} \cdot e^{-\frac{tvCL}{tvV} \cdot t_j}$$

where, Cp_j is the mean plasma drug concentration at time j, $Dose$ is the dose administered to a typical subject in the patient population, tvV is the typical value of the volume of distribution for the typical patient, $tvCL$ is the typical value of clearance, t_j is time j since the end of IV bolus. The $tvCL$ and tvV here are the fixed effects of the PK parameters.

Random effects include parameter variability from subject to subject and residual variability in the observation that accounts for the variability within the subject. If we assume that the population PK parameters (CL and V) vary among subjects, then we are interested in knowing the variability of the parameters from one subject to another in the population.

$$CL_i = tvCL \cdot e^{\eta_i}$$

where, CL_i is the individual clearance for patient i, η_i is the corresponding between subject variability for patient i which is assumed to follow normal distribution with mean 0 and variance of ω_i^2. Residual variability accounts for any variability that is unexplained including within subject variability, between-occasion variability, model misspecification, bioanalysis assay errors, and dosing history errors et cetera.

$$Cp_{ij} = \widehat{Cp}_{ij} + \varepsilon_{ij}$$

Where, Cp_{ij} and $\widehat{Cp}_{ij}$ are the observed and individual predicted plasma drug concentrations for patient i at time j, respectively, ε_{ij} is the corresponding additive residual error term for patient i at time j, which is assumed to follow a normal distribution with mean 0 and variance of σ^2. Randomness in the individual PK parameters can be explained by subject specific covariates; e.g., If V is dependent on weight, then weight can be built into the covariate model and the between-subject variability of V will decrease. Individualized dosing regimens can be developed based on significant covariate relationships in the model. Please go to the following chapter in this book if you would like to learn more about this section ("Model Building and Stability").

The commonly used mechanistic pharmacodynamic models were previously developed and presented with regard to their important features, operable equations, and representative profiles including the direct response model (Wagner 1968), the indirect response model (Dayneka et al. 1993), the effect compartment model (Sheiner et al. 1979), the signal transduction model (Sun and Jusko 1998), and the irreversible effect model (Jusko 1971).

Case: Use of a Disease-Drug-Trial Model to Influence Study Design

Background: There has been a heavy investment by the pharmaceutical industry in the development of drugs that intend to slow the progression of Parkinson's disease. To demonstrate symptomatic benefit, randomized double blind, placebo-controlled parallel study designs have been the norm. An alternative design to evaluate disease-modifying effects is the delayed start design, where patients are initially randomized to treatment or placebo for a prespecified duration (placebo control phase) and then patients that were randomized to placebo are switched to receiving the study drug (active control phase). Patients that were initially randomized to the study drug, continue to receive the drug. Evidence of disease modifying drug effects can be supported if (1) the slope of the change in the primary efficacy variable over time is shallower for the treatment group than the placebo group during the placebo control phase, (2) the patients that received treatment all throughout the trial experienced a greater clinical response at the end of the active control phase as compared to patients who started on placebo and switched to treatment, and (3) the slope of the primary efficacy variable over time is similar between the patients that started on placebo and patients who started on treatment during the active control phase. A database of 1,500 patients with Parkinson's disease was developed to characterize disease progression, treatment effects, and patient discontinuation patterns (Bhattaram et al. 2009).

Key Questions: What quantitative model best describes the progression of total Unified Parkinson's Disease Rating Scale (UPDRS) score and what approaches should be undertaken to evaluate disease-modifying effects of a drug in a delayed start design?

Impact: A disease-drug-trial model was developed to adequately describe the longitudinal time course of UPDRS scores in patients receiving treatment or placebo. Patient dropouts were taken into consideration based on the need for additional symptomatic therapy within 12 months of treatment initiation and treatment related adverse events between 12 and 20 weeks. Figure 1 illustrates the final quantitative model structure used for simulations. The model suggests that patients with Parkinson's disease experience deterioration at a rate of 8 points on the total UPDRS score per year. The data suggested that the change in total UPDRS scores after 12 weeks was reasonably linear. Sample size calculations derived from simulations concluded that to achieve 80% power of concluding a disease-modifying effect, a trial must enroll at least 600 patients in both drug and placebo groups under the assumption that the drug effect is at least 40%. Due to limited information from dose-ranging studies, information regarding the onset of drug effects could not be evaluated. Clinical trials simulations ultimately concluded that differences in slopes between placebo and treatment arms during the placebo-controlled phase and a constant difference between the two treatment arms during the active control phase could support a disease-modifying claim. Equation 1 represents a disease-drug model that describes the longitudinal change in total UPDRS score from baseline.

$$\Delta \text{ Total UPDRS Score} = \beta_0 + (\beta_1 \cdot Plb + \beta_2 \cdot TRT) \cdot \text{Time} + (\beta_3 \cdot Plb + \beta_4 \cdot TRT) \cdot (1 - e^{k \cdot \text{Time}}) \quad (1)$$

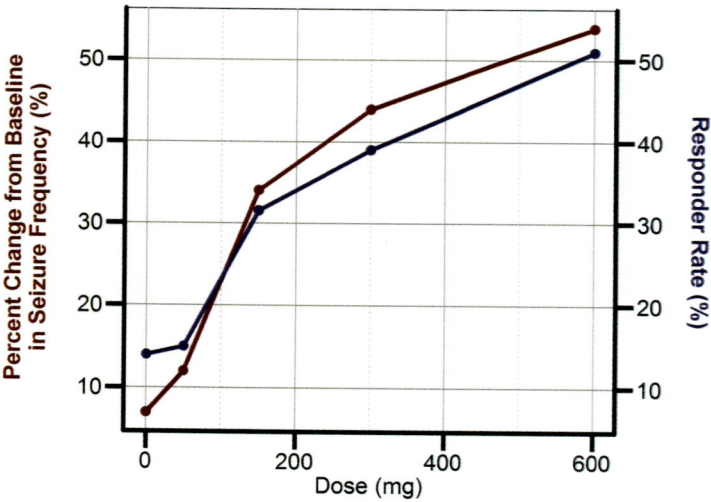

Fig. 1 Dose response curve in refractory patients receiving adjunctive pregabalin for the treatment of partial onset seizures. Red lines and dots represent percent change from baseline in seizure frequency and blue lines and dots represent percent responders. (Figure adapted from French et al. 2003)

Plb refers to placebo, Trt refers to treatment, β_0 to the intercept, β_1 to the disease progression slope of the placebo group, β_2 to the disease progression slope of the treatment group, β_3 to the symptomatic effect in the placebo group, β_4 to the symptomatic effect in the treatment group, and k to the rate constant which can be used to derive the time to reach the maximum symptomatic effect. When the difference between $(\beta_1 - \beta_2)$ is equal to zero, there is no disease-modifying benefits.

PKPD Modeling for First in Human Studies

Estimating the starting dose in a first in human (FIH) trial is the initial step in clinical drug development. A high starting dose in a FIH clinical trial may cause serious toxicity in subjects, while a low starting dose may prolong the dose escalation and optimization processes, thus leading to unnecessary delays in clinical drug development programs Lowe et al. (2007). In 2005, the US Food and Drug Administration (FDA) issued Guidance on estimating the maximum safe starting dose in initial clinical trials for therapeutics in healthy adult volunteers, which provided a framework for carrying out the calculation of the starting dose in FIH trials US Food and Drug Administration (2005). The guidance from the FDA is based on selecting a dose with minimal toxicity risk in humans. It outlines a process for deriving the maximum recommended starting dose (MRSD) in the initial clinical study. First, determine no observed adverse effect level (NOAEL) in preclinical toxicology studies. Then convert the NOAEL from the most appropriate species into human equivalent dose (HED) using appropriate scaling factors. Last, determine the maximum recommended starting dose (MRSD) for the initial clinical study by dividing the HED derived from the animal NOAEL by the default safety factor.

Recently, PK-PD modeling approaches started being used in deriving the starting dose in FIH studies. The starting dose estimated from PK-PD modeling approaches is based on PK properties rather than an empirical scaling factor, and it takes into consideration the interspecies differences in both PK and PD, reducing the reliance on empirical safety factors.

Human PK parameters can be predicted from preclinical data through population PK or PBPK approaches. The human exposure-response relationships can be simulated by PK-PD models developed using data from several animal species by the following steps designed by Lowe et al.:

Step 1: Predict Human PK Parameters

The PK parameters in humans and animals can be projected based on allometric scaling using the plasma drug concentration measurements in animal species. The NOAEL and corresponding PK exposure metrics, e.g., Cmax and AUC in animal species can be determined. The species that produces the lowest NOAEL is used as the index species for scaling into human doses, with the assumptions that only the parent compound is active, and the drug shows equal pharmacological activity or toxicity between human and nonhuman animal species at equal plasma drug concentration levels.

Step 2: Establish the Exposure-Response Relationships in Animal Species
The exposure-response relationships in animal species are developed with efficacy/toxicity data from preclinical studies and the established PopPK models from Step 1. The interspecies differences can be identified through the exposure-response profiles, for both efficacy and toxicity.

Step 3: Simulate the Exposure-Response Profiles in Humans
The predicted human PK parameters and the PD model from the selected animal species are integrated to predict human exposure-response profiles under different dosing regimens. The initial dose is determined based on the developed human PK-PD model, which can be refined later with initial human PK and PD data. Subsequent doses after the initial dose can be administered adaptively to mitigate the toxicities in subjects in the FIH study.

Case: Applying Mechanistic Modeling to Enable Preclinical to Clinical Translation and Guide the FIH Trial Design of a Monoclonal Antibody

Background: TAM-163 is an agonist monoclonal antibody targeting tyrosine receptor kinase-B (TrkB). It was in development as a potential body weight modulatory agent in humans. To support the selection of the dose range for the first-in-human trial, a target-mediated drug disposition (TMDD) model and an Emax PD model were developed with PK (TAM-163 concentration) and PD (body weight gain) data obtained in lean cynomolgus and obese rhesus monkeys following single doses ranging from 0.3 to 60 mg/kg. The model development was supported by the binding affinity constant (9.4 nM) and internalization rate of the drug-target complex (2.08/hour) from previous in-vitro studies Vugmeyster et al. (2013).

Key Question: What are the doses and regimens to be studied in the FIH trial?

Impact: The analysis results indicated that $\geq 38\%$ target coverage (averaged by time) was required to achieve significant body weight gain in monkeys. Assuming similar relationship between the target coverage and pharmacological activity between monkeys and human, 1 and 15 mg/kg were projected to be minimally and the fully pharmacologically active doses in human, respectively, based on the scaling of the PK model from monkeys to humans. A dose of 0.05 mg/kg was recommended as the starting dose for the FIH trial, at which dose level, $<10\%$ target coverage was predicted at Cmax. Dose levels ≥ 1 mg/kg were suggested to be included into the FIH trial to observe pharmacological activity. Additionally, doses greater than 15 mg/kg are unlikely to show improvement in the pharmacological activity because nearly maximal target coverage 97% is projected to be already achieved at this dose. Therefore, the top dose selection should be lower than 15 mg/kg and would require integration of safety and pharmacology data. We recommend the following chapters in this book for the readers who are interested in learning more about this section (▶ Chaps. 41, "Power and Sample Size" and ▶ 52, "Translational Clinical Trials").

PKPD Modeling for Proof of Concept Studies

In early clinical trials, the study drug is tested for the first time for its efficacy in patients with the disease or the condition targeted by the medication. This usually begins with early clinical trials, in which the goal is to obtain an initial proof of concept (POC). These small-scale studies are designed to detect a signal that the drug is active on a pathologically relevant mechanism, as well as preliminary evidence of efficacy for a clinically relevant endpoint.

Pharmacokinetic-Pharmacodynamic modeling is a fundamental tool to characterize exposure-response relationships Bonate (2011). It can be used to plan and design POC studies as well as analyze the results from POC studies to provide support for Go/No-Go decision-making in early clinical development. With prior information, e. g., effective concentrations from preclinical studies, PK characteristics, tolerability and biomarkers and data from the standard treatment in the therapeutic area, exposure-response analysis can be used to inform the dose selection in a POC study design Tett et al. (1998). The applicability of population PK modeling on plasma drug concentration measurements from POC studies can help researchers understand the PK characteristics in target populations and possibly reduce interindividual variability in exposure through identified significant covariates and reduce the signal/noise ratio. Exposure-response analysis for multiple endpoints including efficacy and safety can guide the next steps in drug development.

Case: An Integrated Mechanistic PK-PD Modeling of the Testosterone Suppression Effect of Degarelix Using Data in Healthy Male Subjects from Three Clinical Studies

Background: Degarelix (Firmagon) is a hormonal therapy used in the treatment of prostate cancer by binding to gonadotropin-releasing hormone (GnRH) receptors in the pituitary gland, which induces a fast reduction in luteinizing hormone (LH) and leads to testosterone (T) suppression. PK (degarelix concentrations) and PD (LH and T levels) data in healthy male subjects with normal serum T levels from three short-term clinical trials (degarelix administered intravenously or subcutaneously) were available. A mechanistic PKPD model explaining the interrelation between GnRH, LH, T, and degarelix concentration was developed. The proposed model reasonably described time course of drug effect and the observed rebound based on the short-term data. Simulations were conducted to predict long-term responses Jadhav et al. (2006).

Key Question: What's the relationship between GnRH, LH, and T levels after short-term IV administration of degarelix? What are the doses and regimens to be studied in future long-term trials?

Impact: The mechanistic PKPD model could explain the interrelation between GnRH, LH, T, and degarelix concentration. It allowed to predict the drug effects after both IV and SC of administration and can be extended to other GnRH agonists. After a novel modification to the precursor models, the reported model can be of general use for predicting long-term responses and suggest the doses and regimens to be studied in long-term trials. The integration of prior physiological knowledge from in-vitro and preclinical studies, PKPD data from early clinical studies, with population modeling approach could inform the future drug development.

Case: PK-PD Modeling of the Antimalarial Effect of Actelion-451,840 in a Malaria Study in Eight Healthy Subjects from a Proof-of-Concept Study

Background: Actelion-451840 is a new compound with potent activity against sensitive and resistant Plasmodium falciparum strains. Eight healthy male subjects were infected with blood stage P. falciparum. After 7 days, a single dose of 500 mg of Actelion-451,840 was administered under fed conditions. Parasite and drug concentrations were sampled frequently. Parasite growth and the relation to drug exposure were estimated using PK-PD modeling. Simulations were undertaken to derive estimates of the likelihood of achieving cure in different scenarios (Krause et al. 2016).

Key Questions: Does Actelion-451,840 have pharmacological activity that is effective against blood stage P. falciparum infection and if so, what dosing regimen will provide the desired target exposure?

Impact: Model-based predictions based on a large simulated population of patients allow estimation of curative doses or dosing regimens in patients with clinical malaria. Single dose treatment markedly reduced the level of P. falciparum parasitemia, with a weighted average parasite reduction rate of 73.6 (95% CI 56.1, 96.5) and parasite clearance half-life of 7.7 h (95% CI 7.3, 8.3). A two compartment PK/PD model with a steep concentration-kill effect predicted the maximum effect with a sustained drug concentration of 10–15 ng/ml. The model predicted that 90% of subjects would be cured with six daily doses of Actelion-451,840. Larger doses or more frequent dosing were not predicted to achieve more rapid cure. Thus, a small study coupled with population modeling provided sufficient information for dose and schedule selection for future studies. This information is also critical to convince regulatory authorities to agree with the drug development plans.

Dose Ranging Studies

Dose-ranging or exposure response studies serve as a vital tool that provides dosage and administration, and efficacy/safety information for product labeling. Knowledge regarding the relationship between drug exposures (e.g., dose, plasma concentrations) and therapeutic outcomes (e.g., clinical endpoints, biomarkers, and surrogate effects) relating to safety and efficacy can help identify optimal dosing strategies that can provide favorable clinical benefits and limit unacceptable side effects. Although relationships between doses and blood concentrations in diverse populations are critically evaluated a priori to recommend dose adjustments based on pharmacokinetic differences, historically, limited information regarding the relationship between drug exposure and clinical response (PK-PD) was available at the time of regulatory approval. Post-marketing experience for many drugs would later recognize that approved dosing regimens exhibited adverse consequences with no additional clinical benefit. For example, numerous cases of hypokalemia and metabolic changes were reported in patients receiving standard doses (100 mg) of chlorthalidone, a thiazide-type diuretic for hypertension. Retrospective analysis of dose-response demonstrated only 25 mg was adequate for full antihypertensive effects without severe hypokalemia. As a result, the ICH E4 guidelines (1994) strongly encouraged the use of dose-response analysis at every stage of drug development (International Conference on Harmonization 1994).

Characterizing an exposure-response relationship does not necessarily tell you what dose to pick. Factors such as urgency of need for effect, degree of separation between efficacy and safety, extent of individual variability in pharmacokinetic or pharmacodynamic response, and ability to titrate doses will assist in providing meaningful dosing instructions. For example, a high starting dose (on the plateau of the dose-response curve) might be used for a drug with a large separation between useful and undesirable effects or when there is an urgent need for intervention based on the disease. In most cases, decisions regarding dose selection are often guided by population average dose-response relationships. However, when dose-adjusting individual patients based on observed clinical response, characterization of individual dose-response information is most useful to select a more "individualized" dosing regimen. Pharmacokinetic differences due to disease (e.g., renal failure), concurrent medications, diet, patient characteristics (e.g., weight, age, gender, and race), and formulation (e.g., extended release) can lead to misinterpretations of dose-response. Therefore, blood concentrations can be collected to establish concentration-exposure relationships that can assist in evaluating the impact of different PK profiles.

Exposure response information can also be gathered from preclinical and early clinical studies to support drug discovery and development. Relationships between drug exposure and surrogate endpoints explored through in-vitro receptor occupancy and preliminary small animal studies can be used to support the hypothesized mechanism of action prior to first in human studies. Dose-response relationships evaluated in early proof of concept clinical studies may also serve as a benchmark and assist in dose selection for future pivotal clinical trials. Even though collecting drug concentrations should be considered as routine practice, it is highly encouraged in dose-response studies when: the investigated drug is known to have a high degree of inter-individual variability with respect to PK and clinical response, active metabolites are present, and the number of doses evaluated is limited.

According to the FDA Guidance for Industry on Exposure Response Relationships, exposure-response studies are in fact "adequate and well controlled trials" that can provide direct evidence of effectiveness to support regulatory approval (US Food and Drug Administration 2003). Convincing results from a dose-response study can support the notion of exhibiting internal consistency. These studies usually comprise of multiple comparisons between each dose level and a control arm. The presence of an increasing response with dose in addition to demonstrating statistical significance at several doses when compared to placebo suggests that the drug effect is not due to chance. Depending on the size and outcome studied, a single dose-response study can be relied upon to provide evidence of effectiveness. A PKPD relationship developed using exposure-response data can also be leveraged to determine clinical response for new doses or dosing regimens, different routes of administrations, and various formulations without the need for additional clinical studies. To support the use of a previously approved drug in a new target population, an established exposure-response relationship can also be utilized to bridge efficacy data between the studied and target population.

The study design in dose-response trials is dependent on the disease and the development stage. Life threatening or serious conditions with irreversible outcomes may warrant the use of higher doses rather than doses below the maximal tolerated threshold. Including diverse patient populations with different disease severities could also allow for the determination of important covariate relationships that could explain differences in response among patient subgroups. During drug discovery or early development stages, studies can be more exploratory in nature and may include nonrandomized approaches to develop mechanistic models to quantify the relationship between exposure and response. Studies intended to establish evidence of efficacy should consider randomization of patients to different exposure levels including a control group. The following study designs have been commonly used to assess dose-response and/or exposure-response relationships:

1. **Parallel Fixed Dosed Design**
   Subjects are randomized to parallel fixed dose groups that is considered to be the final or maintenance dose. Patients could directly receive the target dose or could be titrated gradually to the target dose to avoid safety concerns. The target dose should be maintained for a period of time based on clinical reasoning to allow for unbiased comparisons. The inclusion of a placebo group is needed if drug effect sizes are to be measured, however it is not necessary to demonstrate a positive dose-response relationship. Furthermore, the inclusion of a placebo group could salvage a study that included a narrow or high dose range by demonstrating statistical significance over placebo in pairwise comparisons in lieu of a flat dose-response relationship. This design provides a population average dose-response relationship and can be particularly useful for long-term, chronic disease states where response to an intervention may not be reversible. However, this study design requires a relatively large number of subjects since patients are randomized to one dose level. Adequate safety information can also be relatively captured.
2. **Cross-over Design**
   The implementation of a randomized cross-over study design could be beneficial for cases where patients have stable disease, the time of onset of drug effect is rapid, baseline conditions are reached after cessation of therapy, and drug effect is reversible. A major advantage of this design is that individual dose-response

information can be collect since patients receive several different doses. The population average dose-response can therefore be derived from the distribution of individual dose-response curves. Although fewer patients are needed as compared to parallel fixed dose designs, patient dropouts can extend the time to study completion and cause analytical issues. Cross-over trials are generally longer in duration than other designs due to multiple treatment periods and longer treatment washout periods to mitigate potential carry-over effects.

3. **Forced Titration Design**

    Forced titration studies are typically conducted as proof of concept studies where all subjects receiving rising doses of a drug throughout the duration of the study. Depending on the inclusion of a control group, the forced titration design can be used to compare all subjects randomized to drug, regardless of dose, with the concurrent control arm. For drugs that demonstrate a delayed drug effect, this design will not identify response to increase doses from a time-dependent response. In other words, a "time effect" would confound the relationship between dose and response or drugs for specific drugs. In the event that a delayed dose effect is not observed, this design can provide a distribution of individual dose-response relationships which can be used to derive population dose-response. Although this design may need fewer patients, several disease states are prone to spontaneous improvements resulting in lower observed effects at higher doses. Safety information may not be adequately related to dose since many adverse events share time-dependent characteristics.

4. **Optional Titration Design**

    This study design imitates real-world clinical practice where patients are titrated until a prespecified favorable or unfavorable clinical response is achieved. Disease states where response is an irreversible event may not benefit from this design. Because poor-responders are titrated to higher doses, a common "U-shaped" dose-response curve may provide misleading interpretations. Quantitative models could describe population and individual dose-response relationships. This study, similar to the forced titration design, may require lesser number of patients, but also runs the problem of confounding time and drug effects for both safety and efficacy response measures.

Case: Dose-Ranging Trial to Characterize and Confirm a Dose-Response Relationship

Background: Pregabalin, α_2-δ ligand that exhibits anticonvulsant activity, was investigated to establish a dose-response relationship and to characterize tolerability when adjunctively administered twice daily without dose-titration in patients with partial seizures. French et al. utilized a randomized fixed parallel fixed dose design that consisted of an 8-week baseline and 12-week double blind treatment period. Patients were randomized to placebo or 50, 150, 300, and 600 mg/day. Clinical response was based on percent seizure frequency reduction and responder analysis (French 2003).

Key Questions: What is the relationship between dose and clinical response in treatment refractory patients receiving pregabalin and could patients receive their target dose upon initiation without a titration period?

Impact: Dose-response analysis demonstrated that pregabalin was safe and effective between doses of 150–600 mg/day, administered twice daily without the need for dose titration. A linear dose-response relationship was identified and supported evidence of efficacy (Fig. 1). The highest dose of 600 mg/day was associated with the greatest number of discontinuations. The absence of a dose-response analysis may have led to an initial recommended dose of 50 mg/day. However, the results of this study led to an approved label that recommended a starting dose of 150 mg/day divided in two doses with a maximum dose of 600 mg/day based on individual tolerability.

Case: Evidence of Effectiveness Derived Using Dose-Response Relationship

Background: Tetrabenazine was evaluated for the treatment of Huntington's chorea, a disease state that did not have any treatment options available at the time of regulatory review. The drug applicant performed two double-blind, controlled clinical trials that randomized patients to placebo or tetrabenazine. Patients experienced weekly dose titrations for 7 weeks, followed by a maintenance period with no dose changes for an additional 5 weeks. One out of two trials was found to demonstrate a significant drug effect using change from baseline in chorea scores at 12 weeks as the study endpoint (US Food and Drug Administration 2001).

Key Question: Does the dose-response relationship for chorea scores provide confirmatory evidence of effectiveness for tetrabenazine?

Impact: Due to the short half-life of tetrabenazine (5 h), it was assumed that patients would achieve pharmacokinetic steady state by the end of each day. Exploratory analysis demonstrated that tetrabenazine elicits its effects on chorea scores within a single week after a dose change. Therefore, a time-effect did not confound dose-effect and chorea scores measured at weekly visits were related to the full effect of that dose level. A linear mixed effect model was used to describe the dose-response relationship that was consistent across different clinical trials (Fig. 2). It was concluded that the significant dose-response relationship provided substantial evidence of effectiveness which would ultimately lead to regulatory approval. If dose-response was ignored, investigators would need to conduct additional clinical trials to provide additional evidence of effectiveness.

Case: Risk Mitigation Using an Exposure-Safety Relationship

Background: After the initial regulatory approval of zoledronic acid, data from published post-marketing reports and clinical studies assessing efficacy and safety for the treatment of hypercalcemia of malignancy and for the treatment of osteolytic

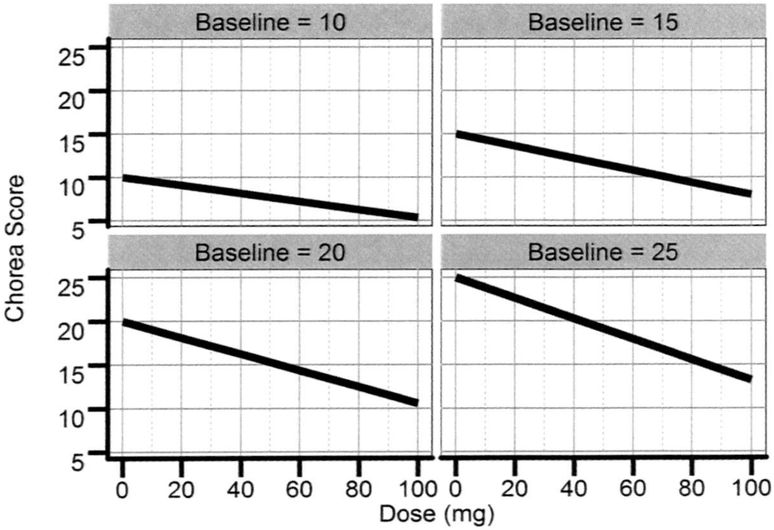

Fig. 2 Population average dose-response curve in patients with baseline total chorea scores of 10, 15, 20, or 25

bone metastases secondary to solid tumors and multiple myeloma indicated an increased risk for renal toxicity (Bhattaram et al. 2005).

Key Questions: Given that zoledronic acid is renally eliminated from the body and safety data further suggests drug-induced renal-toxicity, what dosing regimens should be recommended for renally impaired patients?

Impact: Although the pivotal clinical trials used to establish evidence of effectiveness lacked pharmacokinetic information, data from early phase pharmacokinetic studies were used to develop a pharmacokinetic model that described the concentration-time profile for zoledronic acid. The developed model was use to derive exposure metrics, such as AUC, in patients enrolled in the pivotal trials. Results from various approaches, including logistic regression, time to event analysis, and linear mixed effects modeling, consistently demonstrated that higher drug exposures were related to an increased risk of renal toxicity. PK/PD modeling suggested that the risk of renal deterioration was doubled in patients with a creatinine clearance of less than 10 ml/min and that dose adjustments are recommended for patients with a creatinine clearance of less than 60 ml/min (Bhattaram et al. 2005; US Food and Drug Administration 2002).

Case: Dose Optimization for Future Clinical Trials

Background: In the oncology setting, mortality plays a major role in evaluating efficacy and safety. Dosing regimens for one type of cancer is commonly based on prior knowledge in other cancers studied. Although, these empiric doses may be clinically effective, the benefit-risk profile may not be truly optimized. During the development of trastuzumab, a dosing regimen (loading dose of 8 mg/kg followed by a 6 mg/kg every 3 weeks) that was successfully approved for use in breast cancer patients was selected for the treatment of metastatic HER-2 positive gastric cancer when given with a fluoropyrimidine and cisplatin.

Key Question: Is the proposed dosing regimen found in HER-2 positive breast cancer patients optimal for patients with overexpressed HER-2 positive metastatic gastric cancer? If not, what would be the optimal dosing recommendation?

Impact: Population PK models were used to simulate trough concentrations at the end of cycle 1 for each patient in order to assess the relationship between trastuzumab exposures and overall survival. A case control analysis was further incorporated in order to reduce bias due to confounding risk factors (e.g., poor ECOG performance, no prior gastrectomy, non-Asian, and number of metastatic sites). Prior to the case control analysis, lower trough concentrations at the end of the cycle 1 was found to have a shorter median overall survival. However, after matching for confounding risk factors, the lowest exposure group still did not benefit from trastuzumab therapy, whereas patients with higher exposures experiences a median survival benefit of 3 months. The results of this analysis provided the rational for a post marketing study to assess dosing regiments that could lead to higher exposures in the identified subgroup. We recommend the readers to read the following chapter if you are interested in learning more about dose-ranging studies (▶ Chap. 53, "Dose-Finding and Dose-Ranging Studies").

Use of PK-PD Modeling for Precision Medicine

In 2015, President Obama launched the Precision Medicine Initiative with the intent to revolutionize healthcare by enabling health care providers to individualize treatment decisions based on patient specific characteristics (e.g., genetic, health history, lifestyle, and diet) Fact Sheet: President Obama's Precision Medicine Initiative (2015). Currently, a majority of treatments options and dosing recommendations are intended for the average patient. This "one size fits all" strategy may lead to a decrease in efficacy benefit or an increase in the risk of adverse effects in other clinical scenarios (e.g., organ impairment, pediatrics, obesity, and critical care). Over the last decade, advances in genetic testing, biomarker identification, diagnostic imaging, and basic research in combination with the evolving field of data science has given rise to newer targeted and innovative drugs. Due to an infinite number of patient characteristic combinations, numerous clinical studies would have to be conducted to determine individual dosing recommendations, making this process inefficient. The rise of precision medicine is correlated with the increase use of modeling and simulation in clinical research. Model-based approaches can assist in identifying patient factors that contribute to variability in drug exposure and clinical response. Informative data collected from electronic health records and clinical trials can provide further insight into different exposure and response targets for patient subgroups. This can ultimately allow for individual dose selection during treatment initiation or dosing adjustments throughout the course of therapy Yang et al. (2013).

In order to develop impactful individualized dosing recommendations, optimal experimental design must be utilized to design informative studies. During protocol development for pharmacokinetic studies, optimization decisions incorporate prior pharmacokinetic information to select study design factors including: required sample size, pharmacokinetic sampling time points, and the number of samples needed from each subject. Often times, practical restrictions such as the number of subjects, blood volume limitations, and financial burden can play a role in designing an optimal study. Advanced mathematical algorithms and simulations can be used to create an optimal study design that can increase the precision of parameter estimates when performing post-hoc model-based population PK-PD analysis. Optimal design strategies could result in exact designs that exhibit a fixed structure (e.g., number of groups, subjects per group, samples per subject, and sampling times are fixed) or statistical designs that can result in a flexible structure (e.g., staggered sampling time points, different number of subjects per group, and number of samples per subject).

The identification of patient covariates is a key objective when developing population PK-PD models to develop initial dosing strategies. Preliminary exploratory analysis should always be conducted prior to developing models in order to evaluate any differences in patient subgroups on drug exposures and clinical response. Even though various statistical methodologies are used to evaluate the inclusion of covariates, relationships between covariates and model parameters should be critically evaluated based on mechanistic understanding of the disease and drug behavior. For example, creatinine clearance could be valid covariate on drug clearance for a drug that is highly eliminated by the kidneys. The inclusion of covariates on model parameters should reduce the associated unexplained between subject variability and the uncertainty around individual model parameters when using a hierarchical model structure (Mould et al. 2014). In the example provided, since lower drug clearance is associated with higher drug exposure, lower doses would be required in patients with severe renal dysfunctions relative to patients with normal renal function.

Recently, the use of "Bayesian forecasting" has been utilized in the area of personalized medicine to adjust therapy based on prior exposure or response data collected within a patient. Bayesian forecasting uses Bayes Theorem to estimate new, "updated" model parameters using new data that arises and prior distributions of population parameter values. In Bayesian forecasting, a curve-fitting function is used to select various individual parameter estimates by minimizing the difference between model predicted response and observed data and the difference between population parameter values and current model estimates for individual parameters (Mould et al. 2014; Standing 2017). As a result, the updated individual parameter estimates could be used to forecast drug exposures and clinical outcomes under different dosing regimens.

Case: Precision Medicine and Bayesian Forecasting to Improve Patient Outcomes

Background: Acetaminophen (APAP) overdose is represented as a large population admitted to emergency departments and is one of the leading causes of acute liver injury in the United States. The mainstay of therapy is initial treatment with activated charcoal depending on the time of overdose and N-acetylcysteine (NAC). The Rumack-Matthew nomogram is used to make decisions regarding the administration of NAC based on plasma APAP concentration levels between 4 and 24 h post ingestion. However, failure to predict toxicity based on one APAP plasma concentration and the inability to use concentrations less than 4 h post ingestion has rendered the current approach impractical. Therefore, there is a need for tools to inform earlier NAC administration decisions for high risk patients and to improve patient outcomes and decrease healthcare-costs (Derrochers et al. 2017).

Key Questions: What patient prognostic factors influence the pharmacokinetics of APAP/NAC pharmacokinetics and how can APAP concentration levels guide personalized treatment decisions?

Impact: Population PK analysis demonstrated differences in drug absorption in patients who ingested different APAP products (e.g., extended release vs. immediate release, APAP monotherapy vs. opioid combination products). Administration of activated charcoal reduced the relative bioavailability of APAP. The developed model adequately predicted individual concentration-time profiles following APAP overdose when given at least one APAP plasma concentration. Bayesian forecasting demonstrated that decisions to treat with NAC could be based on only one APAP plasma concentration within 4 h of overdose. Subsequent analysis suggested high concordance with the current nomogram method. The implementation of this forecasting tool for clinical decision can reduce healthcare costs by shortening hospital length of stay. To make the population PK model and forecasting framework user friendly, dashboard systems that use specialized software can be used for clinical decision support.

Summary and Conclusions

PKPD modeling-based drug development is now widely accepted by regulatory agencies such as US FDA and European Medicines Agency (EMA). Population pharmacokinetic and exposure-response model-based analysis are now routinely conducted to influence drug development, regulatory or therapeutic decisions Pillai et al. (2005). Applications include the evaluation of various intrinsic (e.g., age, weight, sex, and race) and extrinsic patient factors (e.g., concomitant medications, smoking, and food effect), assessment of new doses and dosing regimens, dose selection in an unstudied population, informing clinical trial design, and providing supportive evidence of effectiveness (Fig. 3).

In recent days, physiologically based pharmacokinetic (PBPK) and quantitative system pharmacology (QSP) modeling started being used in drug discovery and development Visser et al. (2014). PBPK modeling is a compartment and flow-based type of PK modeling. In PBPK models, each compartment represents a physiologically discrete entity such as an organ or tissue, and the blood flow into and out of that organ Hahn et al. (2018). QSP models the pharmacodynamic effect of the drug on tissues and organs mechanistically. Mechanistic nature of PBPK and QSP models can increase the understanding of PK characteristics, efficacy, and adverse events in

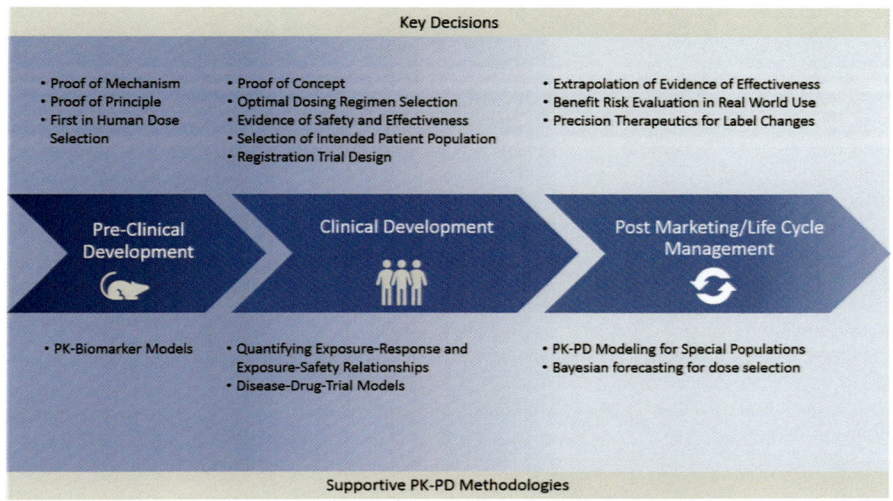

Fig. 3 Use of PK-PD modeling methodologies for informed decision-making throughout drug development

specific diseases and patient populations. In this way, the utilization of PBPK and QSP models can lead to enhanced decision-making by integrating knowledge from various studies Thiel et al. (2018). However, a limitation of PBPK and QSP models is that they are commonly very complex and that the parameters cannot be estimated using traditional statistical methods. Sometimes the parameters can be fixed to data collected in vitro or preclinically, but this requires the availability of such data (some of these data are not typically available during drug development) Vugmeyster et al. (2013). Continued efforts are required to maximize the potential benefit of more innovative, mechanistic modeling in drug discovery and development.

Key Facts

- Obtaining critical pharmacokinetic and pharmacodynamic observations from early informative clinical studies can be used to develop population exposure-response relationships, justify appropriate future trial designs, and increase the probability of trial success.
- PKPD-based analyses can be utilized to provide supportive evidence of effectiveness and safety, support new doses and dosing regiments in new target populations, and evaluate the impact of changes in dosage form or routes of administration.
- Analyzing real world data using various quantitative approaches can serve to reassess benefit-risk among subgroups in a more generalizable population.

- Innovative, mechanistic methodologies, such as PBPK and QSP, can increase the understanding of PK characteristics, efficacy and adverse events in specific diseases, and patient populations.

Cross-References

▶ Designs to Detect Disease Modification
▶ Dose Finding for Drug Combinations
▶ Dose-Finding and Dose-Ranging Studies
▶ Monte Carlo Simulation for Trial Design Tool
▶ Translational Clinical Trials

References

Bhattaram V, Booth BP, Ramachandani RP, Beasley N, Wang Y, Tandon V, Duan JZ, Baweja RK, Marroum PJ, Uppoor RS, Rahman NA, Sahajwalla CG, Powell JR, Mehta MU, Gobburu J (2005) Impact of pharmacometrics on drug approval and labeling decisions: a survey of 42 drug applications. AAPS 7:e503–e512

Bhattaram VA, Siddiqui O, Kapcala LP, Gobburu JV (2009) Endpoints and analyses to discern disease-modifying drug effects in early Parkinson's disease. AAPS 11:456–464

Bittl JA, Yulei H (2017) Bayesian analysis: a practical approach to interpret clinical trials and create clinical practice guidelines. Circ Cardiovasc Qual Outcomes 10:e003563

Bonate P (2011) Pharmacokinetic-Pharmacodynamic modeling and simulation. Springer Science & Business Media, Boston

Dayneka NL, Garg V, Jusko WJ (1993) Comparison of four basic models of indirect pharmacodynamic responses. J Pharmacokinet Biopharm 21:457–478

Derrochers J, Wojciechowski J, Klein-Schwartz W, Gobburu JV, Gopalakrishnan M (2017) Bayesian forecasting tool to predict the need for antidote in acute acetaminophen overdose. Pharmacotherapy 37:916–926

Ernst E, Resch K (1995) Concept of true and perceived placebo effects. BMJ 311:551–553

Fact Sheet: President Obama's Precision Medicine Initiative (2015) Whitehouse.gov. Retrieved 25 Dec 2018

Fava M, Evins AE, Dorer DJ (2003) The problem of the placebo response in clinical trials for psychiatric disorders: culprits, possible remedies, and a novel study design approach. Pscyhother Psychosom 72:115–127

French JA, Kugler AR, Robing JL, Knapp LE, Garofalo EA (2003) Dose-response trial of pregabalin adjunctive therapy in patients with partial seizures. Neurology 60:1631–1637

Gobburu JV, Lesko L (2009) Quantitative disease drug trial models. Ann Rev Pharmacol Toxicol 49:291–301

Gobburu JV, Marroum PJ (2001) Utilization of pharmacokinetic-pharmacodynamic modeling and simulations in regulatory decision making. Clin Pharmacokinet 40:883–892

Gomeni R, Merlo-Pich E (2007) Bayesian modeling and ROC analysis to predict placebo responders using clinical score measured in the initial weeks of treatment in depression trials. Br J Clin Pharmacol 63:595–613

Hahn D, Emoto C, Euteneuer JC, Mizuno T, Vinks AA, Fukuda T (2018) Influence of OCT 1 ontogeny and genetic variation on morphine disposition in critically ill neonates: lessons from PBPK modeling and clinical study. Clin Pharmacol Ther 122:49–53

Holford NH, Peace KE (1992) Methodologic aspects of a population pharmacodynamic model for cognitive effects in Alzheimer patients treated with tacrine. Proc Natl Acad Sci 89:11466–11470

Holford NH, Chan PL, Nutt JG, Kieburtz K, Shoulson I, Parkinson Study Group (2006) Disease progression and pharmacodynamics in Parkinson disease: evidence for function protection with levodopa and other treatments. J Pharmacokinet Pharmacodyn 22:281–311

International Conference on Harmonization (1994) Guidance on E4 dose response information to support drug registration; availability. Notice. Fed Regist 59:55972–55976

Jadhav PR, Agersø H, Tornøe CW, Gobburu JV (2006) Semi-mechanistic pharmacodynamic modeling for degarelix, a novel gonadotropin releasing hormone (GnRH) blocker. J Pharmacokinet Pharmacodyn 33(5):609–634

Jusko WJ (1971) Pharmacodynamics of chemotherapeutic effects: dose-time-response relationships for phase-nonspecific agents. J Pharm Sci 60:892–895

Krause A et al (2016) Pharmacokinetic/pharmacodynamic modelling of the antimalarial effect of Actelion-451840 in an induced blood stage malaria study in healthy subjects. Br J Clin Pharmacol 82(2):412–421

Krudys KM, Dodds MG, Nissen SM, Vicini P (2005) Integrated model of hepatic and peripheral glucose regulation for estimation of endogenous glucose production during the hot IVGTT. Am J Physiol Endocrinol Metab 288:1038–1046

Lowe PJ, Hijazi Y, Luttringer O, Yin H, Sarangapani R, Howard D (2007) On the anticipation of the human dose in first-in-man trials from preclinical and prior clinical information in early drug development. Xenobiotica 37:1331–1354

Meno-Tetang GM, Lowe PJ (2005) On the prediction of the human response: a recycled mechanistic pharmacokinetic/pharmacodynamic approach. Basic Clin Pharmacol Toxicol 96:182–192

Mould DR, Upton RN, Wojciechowski J (2014) Dashboard systems. Implementing pharmacometrics from the bench to the bedside. AAPS 16:925–937

Peck CC, Rubin DB, Sheiner LB (2003) Hypothesis: a single clinical trial plus casual evidence of effectiveness is sufficient for drug approval. Clin Pharmacol Ther 72:481–490

Pillai G, Mentré F, Steimer JL (2005) Non-linear mixed effects modeling – from methodology and software development to driving implementation in drug development science. J Pharmacokinet Pharmacodyn 32:161–183

Powell JR, Gobburu JV (2007) Pharmacometrics at FDA: evolution and impact on decisions. Clin Pharmacol Ther 82:97–102

Senn S (2003) Bayesian, likelihood, and frequentist approaches to statistics. Applied Clinical Trials 12:35–38

Sheiner LB (1997) Learning versus confirming in clinical drug development. Clin Pharmacol Ther 61:275–291

Sheiner LB, Rosenberg B, Melmon KL (1972) Modelling of individual pharmacokinetics for computer-aided drug dosage. Comput Biomed Res Int J 5:411–459

Sheiner LB, Stanski DR, Vozeh S, Miller RD, Ham J (1979) Simultaneous modeling of pharmacokinetics and pharmacodynamics: application to d-tubocurarine. Clin Pharmacol Ther 25:358–371

Standing J (2017) Understanding and applying pharmacometric modeling and simulation in clinical practice and research. Br J Clin Pharmacol 83:247–254

Sun YN, Jusko WJ (1998) Transit compartments versus gamma distribution function to model signal transduction processes in pharmacodynamics. J Pharm Sci 87:732–737

Sun W, Laughren TP, Zhu H, Hocchaus G, Wang Y (2013) Development of a placebo effect model combined with a dropout model for bipolar disorder. J Pharmacokinet Pharmacodyn 40:359–368

Tett SE, Holford NH, McLachlan AJ (1998) Population pharmacokinetics and pharmacodynamics: an underutilized resource. Drug Inf J 32:693–710

Thiel C, Smit I, Baier V, Cordes H, Fabry B, Blank LM, Kuepfer L (2018) Using quantitative systems pharmacology to evaluate the drug efficacy of COX-2 and 5-LOX inhibitors in therapeutic situations. NPJ Syst Biol Appl 4(1):28

US Food and Drug Administration (2001) Drug approval package: Xenazine (tetrabenazine) [FDA application no. (NDA) 021894; online]. Available from URL: https://www.accessdata.fda.gov/drugsatfda_docs/nda/2008/021894s000TOC.cfm. Accessed 19 Dec 2018

US Food and Drug Administration (2002) Drug approval package: Zometa (zoledronic acid) [FDA application no. (NDA) 021223; online]. https://www.accessdata.fda.gov/drugsatfda_docs/nda/2002/21-386_Zometa.cfm. Accessed 19 Dec 2018

US Food and Drug Administration (2003) Guidance for Industry: Exposure-response relationships-study design, data analysis and regulatory application. https://www.fda.gov/downloads/drugs/guidancecomplianceregulatoryinformation/guidances/ucm072109.pdf. Accessed 19 Dec 2018

US Food and Drug Administration (2005) Guidance for industry: estimating the maximum safe starting dose in initial clinical trials for therapeutics in adult healthy volunteers. https://www.fda.gov/downloads/Drugs/Guidances/UCM078932.pdf. Accessed 24 Dec 2018

Visser SAG, De Alwis DP, Kerbusch T, Stone JA, Allerheiligen SRB (2014) Implementation of quantitative and systems pharmacology in large pharma. CPT Pharmacometrics Syst Pharmacol 3(10):1–10

Vugmeyster Y, Rohde C, Perreault M, Gimeno RE, Singh P (2013) Agonistic TAM-163 antibody targeting tyrosine kinase receptor-B: applying mechanistic modeling to enable preclinical to clinical translation and guide clinical trial design. mabs 5(3):373–383. Taylor & Francis

Wagner JG (1968) Kinetics of pharmacologic response. I. Proposed relationships between response and drug concentration in the intact animal and man. J Theor Biol 20:173–201

Weimer K, Colloca L, Enck P (2015) Placebo effects in psychiatry: mediators and moderators. Lancet Psychiatry 2:246–257

Yang J, Zhao H, Garnett C, Rahman A, Gobburu JV, Pierce W, Schechter G, Summers J, Keegan P, Booth B, Wang Y (2013) The combination of exposure-response and case-control analyses in regulatory decision making. J Clin Pharmacol 53:160–166

Safety and Risk Benefit Analyses

99

Jeff Jianfei Guo

Contents

Introduction	1962
Pharmacovigilance	1963
Post-Marketing Surveillance	1963
Drug Safety Surveillance: Passive and Proactive Models	1964
Safety Signal Detections and Regulatory Interventions	1965
Signal Detection Algorithms	1966
Regulatory Interventions for Drug Safety	1968
Benefit and Risk Assessments	1969
Quantitative Framework for Benefit-Risk Assessment (QFBRA)	1971
Benefit-Less-Risk Analysis (BLRA)	1972
Quality-Adjusted Time Without Symptoms and Toxicity (Q-TWiST)	1973
Number Needed to Treat (NNT) and Number Needed to Harm (NNH)	1973
Minimum Clinical Efficacy (MCE)	1974
Incremental Net Health Benefit (INHB)	1975
Relative-Value-Adjusted Number Needed to Treat (RV-NNT) and RV-NNH	1975
Risk-Benefit Plane (RBP) and Risk-Benefit Acceptability Threshold (RBAT)	1975
Probabilistic Simulation Methods (PSM) and Monte Carlo Simulation (MCS)	1976
Multi-Criteria Decision Analysis (MCDA)	1976
Risk-Benefit Contour (RBC)	1976
Stated Preference Method (SPM) or Maximum Acceptable Risk (MAR)	1977
Conclusions	1977
Key Facts/Points	1977
Cross-References	1978
References	1978

J. J. Guo (✉)
Division of Pharmacy Practice and Administrative Sciences, University of Cincinnati College of Pharmacy, Cincinnati, OH, USA
e-mail: jeff.guo@uc.edu

© Springer Nature Switzerland AG 2022
S. Piantadosi, C. L. Meinert (eds.), *Principles and Practice of Clinical Trials*,
https://doi.org/10.1007/978-3-319-52636-2_136

Abstract

In the past two decades more than 20 high-profile brand-name drugs including rofecoxib, troglitazone, cisapride, cerivastatin, natalizumab, gemtuzumab, and sibutramine were withdrawn from the market due to drug safety concerns related to severe adverse events. In 2005, the Food and Drug Administration (FDA) issued risk management guidance for the pharmaceutical industry. Subsequently the FDA Amendments Act in 2007 gave the FDA the authority to require pharmaceutical companies to develop and implement a Risk Evaluation and Mitigation Strategy (REMS) for specified prescription drugs and initiated the FDA Sentinel safety surveillance program in order to enhance the benefit-risk balance for pharmaceutical products. This chapter describes some basic concepts of drug safety, post-marketing surveillance, pharmacovigilance, and risk management. The safety signal detection algorithms and regulatory interventions will be also discussed. Finally some commonly used benefit-risk assessments (BRA) will be reviewed and discussed briefly in this chapter since the BRA methods are becoming critical tools for the life cycle of drug development and enhancing decision-making and regulatory interventions. The BRA is only one of unique analyses for clinical trials. Some concepts and methods of BRA may crossover with other analyses discussed in other chapters like "Intention to treat and alternative approaches," "Cost effectiveness analyses," and "Development and validation of risk prediction models" Bayesian adaptive designs.

Keywords

Drug safety · Pharmacovigilance · Post-marketing surveillance · Risk management · Risk evaluation and mitigation strategy · Signal detection · Regulatory intervention · Benefit-risk assessments

Introduction

In response to 1937 drug safety tragedy of sulfanilimide elixir, the US Food Drug and Cosmetic Act was established in 1938 (FDA 2019). Due to the infamous thalidomide birth defect disaster in 1961, the Kefauver-Harris Amendment Act was passed in 1962 (FDA 2019). Both safety and efficacy have been two primary considerations for any new drug approval. Since the mid-1990s more than 20 high-profile brand-name drugs, including rofecoxib (Vioxx®), troglitazone (Rezulin®), cisapride (Propulsid®), cerivastatin (Baycol®), pemoline (Cylert®), natalizumab (Tysabri®), gemtuzumab (Mylotarg®), sibutramine (Reductil®), trovafloxacin (Trovan®), and propoxyphene (Darvocet/Darvon®), were withdrawn from the market (FDA 2005; Guo et al. 2010; Lis et al. 2012). In March 2005, the FDA issued risk management guidance for the pharmaceutical industry, which included three separate guidelines: Premarketing Risk Assessment, Development and Use of Risk Minimization Action Plans, and Good Pharmacovigilance Practices and

Pharmacoepidemiologic Assessment (FDA 2005). Subsequently Title IX of the FDA Amendments Act in 2007 gave the FDA the authority to require pharmaceutical companies to develop and implement a Risk Evaluation and Mitigation Strategy (REMS) for specified prescription drugs (Lis et al. 2012).

Regarding drug safety, some concepts and regulation requirements may crossover with this textbook Part 3, "Regulation and Oversight," ► Chap. 37, "Data and Safety Monitoring and Reporting" Below let us discuss briefly about pharmacovigilance, drug safety surveillance, and post-marketing surveillance.

Pharmacovigilance

The FDA Good Pharmacovigilance Practices and Pharmacoepidemiologic Assessment guideline defined pharmacovigilance as "generally regarded as all post-marketing scientific and data gathering activities relating to the detection, assessment, understanding, and prevention of adverse events or any other product-related problems" (FDA 2005). "Pharmaco-" refers to pharmacology for pharmaceutical products. "Vigilance" is watchfulness in guarding against danger or providing for safety. The International Conference on Harmonization recommended similar pharmacovigilance planning E2E guideline (ICH 2004). The EU European Medicines Agency (EMA) provided guidelines for risk management plan (RMP) and good pharmacovigilance practices for pharma industry (Lis et al. 2012).

The scope of pharmacovigilance is focused on post-marketing activities. It applies pharmacoepidemiology theory and methodology to guide its related research or evaluation and plan for intervention. It also covers research activities related to drug utilization, spontaneous reporting system like FDA adverse event reporting systems, clinical pharmacology, pharmacogenetics, and regulatory sciences.

Post-Marketing Surveillance

Similar to pharmacovigilance, post-marketing surveillance is also a practice of monitoring the safety of pharmaceutical products and medical device after the product is approved by FDA. From clinical perspective, many effects of pharmaceutical products are usually not clear or unknown at the market entry. It is important to conduct post-marketing surveillance in general or specific population. Here are four major reasons for post-marketing surveillance.

1. During the clinical trials phases I, II, and III, there are usually relatively small numbers of study subjects involved in clinical trials. It will be impossible to capture or confirm many clinical effects or adverse events occurring in less than 1/500 due to limited sample size and statistical power.
2. Usually clinical trials have restricted study population. There are many inclusion and exclusion criteria for trials. Recruited study subjects or patients usually do not include elderly patients, pregnant women, or children.

3. Clinical trials are usually conducted during relatively short durations of exposure. Trials cannot detect long-term or delayed effects, for example, hepatotoxicity effects.
4. Clinical trials are usually involved in rigorous controlled drug use and lack of drug interaction information.

During the post-marketing phase, large numbers of patients may be exposed to medication therapy. Many elderly, children, and even pregnant women are likely involved in these medication exposures. It will be possible to measure the drug use and effects in large population. Post-marketing surveillance becomes a useful approach to monitor drug safety using real-world data like FDA Adverse Event Reporting Systems (FAERS) data, health insurance claims, electronic medical records, patient registries, and other electronic device or application collected health records. Post-marketing surveillance is essential to detect and confirm the rare adverse event or specific effects.

Drug Safety Surveillance: Passive and Proactive Models

Unlike post-marketing surveillance, the modern drug safety surveillance involves multidisciplinary methods to document, monitor, and evaluate adverse drug events or adverse drug reactions, and plan effective interventions using risk management tools. It applies to the life cycle of a drug development including investigational new drug, clinical trials phases I, II, III, new drug application, post-marketing (phase IV), and even removal from market. Drug safety surveillance incorporates epidemiologic methodology to monitor drug use and effects in large population using real-world data and modern risk management tools. Real-world data often include spontaneous reporting systems (e.g., FDA FAERS, WHO ADR), product and disease registries, electronic medical records, health survey data, computerized medical insurance claims, data collected from social media or special applications or devices, even pragmatic clinical trial data, and other public health records like national death index.

Figure 1 describes the traditional time line for drug development life cycle from preclinical animal and cell studies to clinical trials, to FDA new drug application, and to post-marketing Phase IV studies. Both pharmacovigilance and post-marketing surveillance are focused on Phase IV after products are approved with a small circle or scope. Drug safety surveillance, however, is involved in the life cycle of drug development with a large circle or scope.

Traditionally the pharmaceutical industry relied on the passive model of safety surveillance for several decades, which is to use FDA spontaneous reporting system (SRS) to identify any adverse event signals or cases of suspected drug-induced disease/condition and plan for interventions. All adverse cases are voluntary based. No specific efforts are made to make sure more or all cases are reported. Passive surveillance is integrated to routine health-care delivery system.

In contrast, proactive safety surveillance involves "a systematic process for analyzing multiple observational health care data sources to better understand the effects of medical products" (Stang et al. 2010). Based on the proactive safety surveillance, there is a periodic solicitation of adverse event case reports, such as: (1) the FDA

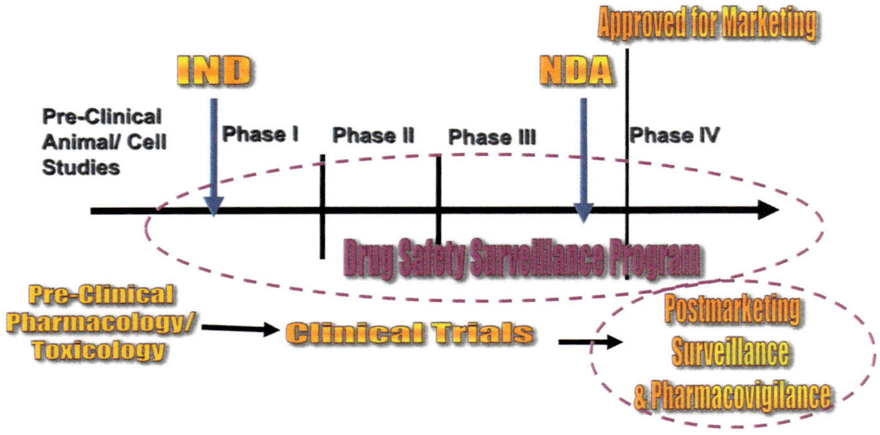

Fig. 1 Drug safety surveillance vs. post-marketing surveillance

adverse event surveillance system; (2) acute severe hepatotoxicity surveillance program; (3) active post-marketing surveillance among the US hospitals; and (4) the US death certificate surveillance project. In 2008, the FDA launched the Sentinel Initiative which enhances the FDA's ability to proactively monitor the safety of drug, biologic and medical device products, which is a complement of existing FDA adverse event reporting system (Stang et al. 2010). With the Sentinel Initiative, the FDA can rapidly access medication use and effect at the patient level in large population using electronic health-care data. Based on a series of FDA-developed, standardized computer codes, all Sentinel partners (hospitals or health insurance companies) will generate a set of patient-level data accordingly. The large observational data allows one to identify potential cases actively through screening of hospital admission records, emergency department logs, medical wards, intensive care units, outpatient care, and medication use and effect. Appropriate screening terms and rigorous standardized procedures are necessary to minimize the number of missing cases.

The current practice involves a combination of active and passive systems using multiple resources and data, including: (1) real-world data from general population and special population; (2) disease history data of disease incidence and prevalence; (3) diagnosis and drug utilization data from outpatient and inpatient records. This kind of combination practice requires coordination and collaboration among various programs, clinicians, pharmacists, health-care providers, epidemiologists, information system specialists, research design efforts, and other health-care stakeholders.

Safety Signal Detections and Regulatory Interventions

All adverse events collected from clinical trials or post-marketing phase are required to document and evaluate accordingly. When relationship between drug and adverse event is established, a potential safety signal is created. The relevant adverse events are treated as signals that may involve in some suspicious adverse event or reaction.

Commonly used safety signal detection algorithms and common regulatory interventions for drug safety surveillance are discussed below.

Signal Detection Algorithms

Compared to clinical trials and traditional epidemiologic studies like case-control and cohort study, the computerized drug safety signal detection algorithms or data mining algorithms are relatively new and characterized by providing a fast and efficient way of detecting possible adverse safety signals. Many large SRS databases have been developed in different countries and World Health Organization (WHO), which can be used for early safety detection using signal detection algorithms. Commonly used SRS available to the public access include the FAERS, the UK Yellow Card System, Canadian Adverse Drug Reaction Monitoring Program, WHO Uppsala ADR Center, etc.

Several signal detection algorithms have been described in literature, mainly including the reporting odds ratio (ROR) introduced by the Netherlands Pharmacovigilance Center Lareb, the proportional reporting ratio (PRR) introduced by the UK Yellow Card Scheme, the Multi-item Gamma Passion Shrinker (MGPS) adopted by the US FDA, and the information component (IC) introduced by WHO Uppsala ADR center (Chen et al. 2008b). Other algorithms including the Yule's Q and the Chi-square have been also introduced, but they are rarely used. Screening the adverse event reports based on safety signal detection algorithms could often save time and prevent some unnecessary efforts.

ROR is a measure of disproportionality. Compared to other algorithms, ROR is relatively easy to calculate. Like the traditional odds ratio in epidemiology, the ROR is an estimate of incidence rate ratio, calculating the odds of the exposure of suspected drug in those who had adverse events divided by the odds of the exposure of suspected drug in those without adverse events (Almenoff et al. 2005). The ROR with 95% confidence interval is computed using a 2 x 2 table: ROR = (A/B)/(C/D) = AD/BC. See Table 1 below.

Table 1 The 2 x 2 table for the calculation of adverse event (AE) safety signals

	AE reports with the suspected drug	AE reports with all other drugs	Total
Reporting with suspected AEs	A	B	(A + B)
Reporting with other AEs	C	D	(C + D)
Total	(A + C)	(B + D)	N = A + B + C + D

Notes: A = the number of reports containing both suspected drug and suspected AE; B = the number of reports containing other drug use but with other AE; C = the number of reports containing the suspected AE but with other medications; D = the number of reports concerning other medications and other AEs

The PRR is another early attempt of quantitative analysis of adverse drug reaction reports. It measures the strength of association between the suspected events and suspected drugs, using the similar calculation of the relative risk (RR). The higher value of PRR is the stronger strength of the safety signal appears to be. Literature suggests that criteria for the PRR consisting of PRR greater than 2, Chi-square greater than 4, and three or more reported cases are often used to identify the possible safety signals (Evans et al. 2001). In practice, the PRR with a value of more than 3 may highlight a need for evaluation of cases and further investigation. The computation of PRR is same as the RR estimated in epidemiology and can be calculated using the 2x2 table.

$$PRR = [A/(A+C)]/[B/(B+D)] = A(B+D)/B(A+C).$$

Incorporating Bayesian approaches into data mining is a major initiative in the safety signal detection. Two slightly different Bayesian algorithms have been developed and applied in the post-marketing surveillance. One is IC of Bayesian Confidence Propagation Neural Network (BCPNN) (Bate et al. 2002). The other is the MGPS (DuMouchel 1999).

The WHO Uppsala Monitoring Center (UMC) has been applying the IC/BCPNN to detect drug safety signals using the WHO adverse drug reaction (ADR) database. The UMC collects ADR reporting data from more than 160 member countries, including the USA, the UK, German, France, Span, Italy, Japan, China, India, Canada, Mexico, Brazil, South Africa, etc. The computation for the IC/BCPNN basically includes two steps: (1) making an estimation of a prior probability (i.e., constructing a prior and a likelihood function); and (2) improving the estimation in light of incoming new information (i.e., updating the posterior mean) (Bate et al. 2002).

The MGPS is another approach that applies the Bayes' law into the adverse event signal detection. It was initially developed and applied to the FAERS database. This method assumes that the expected number of reports containing both the suspected drug and the suspected adverse event is fixed known, and could be computed after stratifying the reports based on the age, sex, or other factors that may influence the reports of drug and events (DuMouchel 1999).

The basic concepts involved in the AE signal detection or data mining algorithms are related to the 2 x 2 table presented in Table 1. They are related to analytical approaches of disproportionality analysis. Both ROR and PRR are relatively easy to understand. The computation is relatively inexpensive compared to IC/BCPNN and MGPS. Both IC and MGPS apply the Bayesian inference with slightly different models. Based on limited literature comparing the performance and sensitivity of these signal detections, Hauben and Reich study (2004) indicated PRR could signal almost twice as many drug-event combinations as the MGPS did. Chen et al. (2008a, b) showed that ROR has better performance compared to PRR, IC, and MGPS. Both IC and MGPS require a set of mathematical knowledge and complicated calculations but often believed to provide more stable estimation compared to the ROR and PRR, especially with small frequency of drug-event combinations.

Regulatory Interventions for Drug Safety

Every pharmaceutical product has its unique experience of safety surveillance and government intervention story. Figure 2 illustrates a typical workflow of drug safety surveillance in post-marketing phase in the USA. After new drug application approval, FDA will actively document and evaluate the adverse drug events based on FAERS database. FAERS documented five key components including suspected drug and concomitant medication, suspected adverse event and outcomes, patient information, pharmaceutical information, and reporter's information which is confidential only use for FDA internal review. Once a safety signal is detected from an SRS, case review will be performed based on clinical information. For any significant case, pharmaceutical industry or government agency or academic institution would like to conduct pharmacoepidemiologic study using large real-world data, such as electronic health records, insurance claims database, or disease or drug registry data.

When the risk of drug adverse event is confirmed, FDA and pharmaceutical industry will plan for regulatory interventions, including label change or black box warning. Usually "Dear Doctor" and/or "Dear Pharmacist" "Dear Health Practitioner" letters will be sent out to relevant prescribers and health practitioners like pharmacists and nurse practitioners. Continue educations for relevant medical doctors and pharmacists/nurses will be conducted to inform the product risk and benefit. For some specific products, the restricted use may be applied for its distribution. Meanwhile government, pharmaceutical industry and academic institute will continue to assess the risk-event combinations and effectiveness of planned interventions. If the intervention is proved ineffective or risk remains high, the product will be withdrawn from the market either by FDA or by pharmaceutical industry voluntarily.

From the above discussion, the traditional common interventions include (1) labeling changes; (2) general warning or black-box warnings; (3) continue educations among medical doctors, pharmacists, and nursing communities; (4) "Dear Doctor Letter," or "Dear Health Practitioner (Pharmacist) Letter"; (5) restricted distribution; and (6) withdrawal (Guo et al. 2003, 2008).

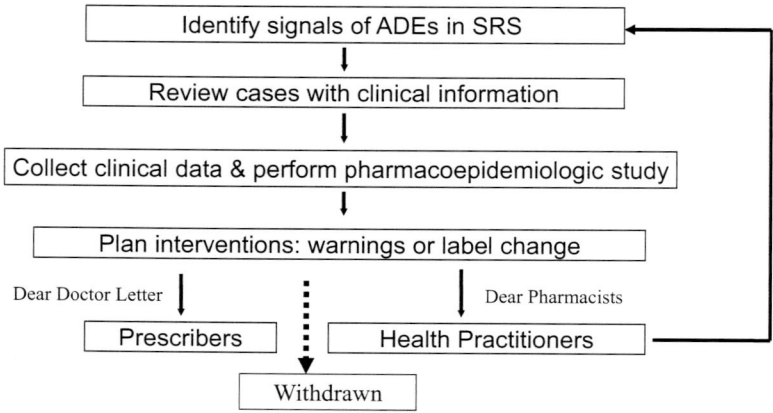

Fig. 2 Drug safety workflow for post-marketing surveillance

In the recent years, other interventions have been practiced in the USA. These include: the third class or behind the counter of drug, modifying standards of new drug approval, new labeling models, patient package inserts (patient labeling), Medication Guides, special advertising campaign for product risk and benefit information, formal risk management plan with relevant informed consent and restrictions, and mandatory monitoring registries (e.g., isotretinoin, thalidomide).

The third class of drug refers to some certain pharmaceutical products to be used only under the supervision of a physician or dentist or pharmacist (Pray and Pray 2011). The other two classes of pharmaceutical products are related to prescription and over-the-counter medications. Some states have created a third class of medications including certain codeine-containing syrups, methamphetamine (meth), and pseudoephedrine due to overdose pain medication use.

For the need of safety assessment in post-marketing surveillance, some safety monitoring registries have been utilized for some specific products like isotrotenoin (Accutane®), thalidomide (Thalomid®), alosetron (Lotronex®), etc. The System for Thalidomide Education and Prescribing Safety (STEPS) is a good example of this kind of registry to prevent exposure to thalidomide during pregnancy (Zeldis et al. 1999). As a comprehensive program to control prescribing, dispensing, and use of the drug, the STEPS registry achieves the goals of controlling access to thalidomide; educating prescribers, pharmacists, and patients about risk and benefits of the product; and monitoring compliance of thalidomide use. Prescribing physicians need to ensure patient eligibility criteria and monitoring procedures. Pharmacies must also agree to comply with patient identification and monitoring criteria. Patients receive visual aids, written material, and verbal counseling about the benefit and risk of thalidomide therapy.

The iPLEDGE® program is a computer-based risk management registry designed to eliminate fetal exposure to isotretinoin during pregnancy through a special restricted distribution program. The brand-name was withdrawn from the US market in 2009. The iPLEDGE® is used for both prescribing and dispensing all isotretinoin with two goals: (1) no female patient starts isotretinoin therapy if pregnant; (2) no female patient on isotretinoin therapy becomes pregnant (see Website page: https://www.ipledgeprogram.com/iPledgeUI/home.u).

The Prescribing Program for Lotronex (alosetron) is another registry used for providers, pharmacists, and patients to reduce the risk of severe gastrointestinal adverse events. Alosetron prescribing doctors have to sign up online and confirm that they can understand and diagnose irritable bowel syndrome with diarrhea and the possible side effects like constipation. (See Website page: https://www.lotronex.com/PrescribingProgramForLotronex.aspx.)

Benefit and Risk Assessments

From the public health perspective, the FDA evaluates the risks and benefits for the population perspective. For any approved medication, the prescriber serves as agent to manage risks and benefits for the individual patient. Meanwhile patients make their own decisions about treatment choices based on their personal valuation of benefits and risks. While the government agency cannot involve in any individual treatment decision, FDA's role is to ensure that accurate, substantiated, and balanced information about any approved drug and biologic product is available to the prescriber and the patient.

For ensuring drug safety, FDA issued risk management guidance for industry in 2005, including pre-marketing risk assessments, good pharmacovigilance and pharmacoepidemiological assessment, and risk minimization action plan (FDA 2005a, 2005b, 2005c). The risk management was defined as an iterative process designed to optimize the benefit-risk balance regulated products, which involves in assessing a product's risk-benefit balance, developing tools to minimize risk while preserving benefits, evaluating tools' effectiveness and reassessment risk-benefit balance, and making adjustments to risk management tools further to improve risk-benefit balance. (FDA 2005b). Incorporating with risk management guidance, the 2007 FDA Amendment Act gave the FDA the authority to require pharmaceutical companies to develop and implement an REMS for specified pharmaceutical products.

In March 2018, the US FDA published "benefit-risk assessment (BRA) in drug regulatory decision-making" which provides the general benefit-risk framework and calls for more creative approaches to conceptualizing, measuring, and applying BRA throughout the life cycle of a drug and biologic product (FDA 2018). The benefit-risk framework (BRF) is defined as "a structured, qualitative approach focused on identifying and clearly communicating key issues, evidence, and uncertainties in FDA's BRA and how those considerations inform regulatory decision." BRF should include four dimensions: analysis of condition, current treatment options, benefit, and risk management. For each dimension, two aspects of consideration need to be specified: (1) The detailed treatment of evidence and uncertainties about a drug's benefits and risks are considered in the context of the severity of the condition and the current medical needs for patients. (2) The conclusion and reasons about the drug benefit and risk in each dimension should be also documented.

Similarly, for the European Union, the Committee for Medicinal Products for Human Use is responsible to provide guidance for industry how to assess risks and benefits of authorized medicines on behalf of the EMA. The EMA also created the European Network of Centres for Pharmacoepidemiology and Pharmacovigilance to develop an algorithm to articulate risks and benefit profiles for pharmaceutical products.

Appropriate BRA can provide useful information for proactive intervention in health-care settings, which could save lives, reduce litigation, and lead to improved patient safety, better health outcomes, and lower overall health-care costs (Guo et al. 2010). Guo et al. (2010) systematically reviewed literature and summarized some common used quantitative BRA including:

- Quantitative framework for risk-benefit assessment (QFRBA)
- Benefit-less risk analysis (BLRA)
- Quality-adjusted time without symptoms and toxicity (Q-TWiST)
- Number needed to treat (NNT) versus number needed to harm (NNH)

- Relative value adjusted number needed to treat (RV-NNT)
- Minimum clinical efficacy (MCE)
- Incremental net health benefit (INHB)
- Risk-benefit plane (BRP) and risk-benefit acceptability threshold (RBAT)
- Probabilistic simulation methods (PSM) and Monte Carlo simulation (MCS)
- Multi-criteria decision analysis (MCDA)
- Risk-benefit contour (RBC)
- Stated preference method (SPM) or maximum acceptable risk (MAR)

In addition, other BRAs were found in the literature such as net efficacy adjusted for risk, net clinical benefit analysis, the principle of threes, and net-benefit-adjusted-for-utility analysis. Due to the uniqueness and complexity of each assessment, some commonly used BRA methods are discussed below.

Quantitative Framework for Benefit-Risk Assessment (QFBRA)

The QFBRA is widely used in drug safety surveillance by regulatory agencies and by the pharmaceutical industry, although it cannot combine risks and benefits into a single value. It includes all commonly used epidemiologic assessments such as incidence, relative risk, odds ratios, attributable risk, risk difference, relative risk reduction, and absolute risk reduction (Guo et al. 2010).

The Risk refers to a comprehensive set of all possible adverse drug events (ADEs) and a set of probabilities associated with these adverse outcomes. The basic expression of risk for pharmaceutical products is the **incidence** of an ADE, which can be defined as the number of new adverse drug events occurred in a defined population over a specific period of time divided by the population at risk over a specific period of time. There are two types of incidence measures: cumulative incidence and incidence density rate. The cumulative incidence is calculated as the number of new cases of ADE during a specified period divided by the total number of persons at risk for developing the ADE during the period. The incidence density rate is calculated as the number of new cases of ADEs during a specified period divided by the total number of person-time observed in population at risk during that period. For example, 77 new cases of acute pancreatitis were identified among 1838 newly diagnosed patients receiving HIV treatment. These newly diagnosed patients had a total of 3943 treatment follow-up person-years. The incidence density rate was calculated as $77 / 3943 = 1.95$ per 100 person-years (Guo 2005).

Relative risk (RR) or risk ratio can be calculated as probability of developing the ADEs with a risk factor divided by probability of developing the ADE without a risk factor. Using Table 1 2x2 table, $RR = [A/(A + B)] / [C/(C + D)]$. Confidence intervals (CI 95%) and p values are then calculated to answer the question as to whether there is a statistically significant risk. A relative risk without these parameters is of no value to the clinician. A relative risk of 1, of course, is the null or "no difference" relative risk. It is important to note that the relative risk does not indicate the magnitude of absolute risk. In other words, it reveals nothing about the incidence of the adverse events in either group. Similarly to RR, the odds ratios (OR) is often an estimate of RR and calculated as odds of exposed to risk factor divided by odds of no exposed to risk factor

$$OR = (A/B)/(C/D).$$

Attributable Risk (AR) otherwise known as **Risk Difference (RD)** is useful to measure absolute risk differences which can calculate the additional risk (incidence, probability) of ADEs in individual patient taking a new drug over or above that experienced by patients who are taking conventional drug therapy. Attributable risk is the additional incidence of an ADE related to exposure to either drug, taking into account the background incidence of ADEs, presumably from other causes that could include other drugs. AR or RD = probability of exposed to risk factor − probability of not exposed to risk factor. The population-based attributable risk is an extension of AR that uses total population data.

The *benefit* associated with a medication can measure how much risk reduced for adverse events associated with the disease. The **relative risk reduction (RRR)** is useful to calculate the ratio between the proportion of exposed individuals who experience a decline in adverse events divided by the proportion of unexposed individuals who experience such a benefit. Similarly, **attributable risk reduction or *absolute risk reduction* (ARR)** represents the decline in adverse events between exposed and unexposed groups. The main disadvantage of using the relative risk reduction in clinical decision-making is that it does not reflect the magnitude of the benefit over no therapy (e.g., the control group). Therefore, it will overestimate or underestimate the absolute impact of therapy when the outcome event incidence is very rare or very common, respectively. From clinical trials, benefit measurements might include clinically relevant efficacy parameters such as specific biomarkers, surrogates, and putative surrogate endpoints. For a safety surveillance study, benefit can be measured as medication adherence rate or treatment effectiveness.

Benefit-Less-Risk Analysis (BLRA)

The BLRA is a ratio combing both benefit and risk into one measurement. The benefit is measured by the response rate and risk is determined by the incidence of a serious side effect. Considering BRA only when there are serious side effects is not good enough because there are many situations when a treatment has a better efficacy outcome at the cost of more side effects even though none of the side effects are considered to be serious. In the latter case, it is often important to take into consideration the increased side effects when evaluating the benefit of the treatment. This approach of BR evaluation discounts the observed benefit of a treatment by the observed risk, and hence the name "benefit-less-risk." The discounting, applied to each individual in a trial, utilizes a method proposed by Chuang-Stein (Chuang-Stein 1994) to consolidate the safety data collected in a clinical trial. The collating of the safety information allows one to estimate quantitatively the risk experienced by each individual, and therefore enables the construction of a risk-adjusted benefit measure for the same individual.

Each patient's efficacy experience (benefit) of a therapy is represented by a binary response variable; "1" signifies that a therapy response is obtained, and "0" means that no response is achieved. The patient's side-effect experience (risk) from five different body functions is represented by a value ranging from 0.0 to 1.0, where the value of 1.0 represents the worst safety experience and 0.0 means no safety concern (Chuang-Stein 1994). If a pretreatment ordinal response is also available, the change in the response variable will serve as an estimate for the benefit; otherwise, the post-treatment response will be used for E_i. To construct a risk-adjusted benefit measure E^*_i for individual i, E_i has to be discounted by a suitable multiple of the R_i, as: $E^*_i = E_i - F * R_i$, where F is a proportionality constant which determines how much penalty the side effects exert on the original benefit measure. The quantity E^*_i is the risk-adjusted benefit, or the estimated net benefit, for individual i. The choice of F may depend on many factors (Chuang-Stein 1994).

Quality-Adjusted Time Without Symptoms and Toxicity (Q-TWiST)

Q-TWiST considers the importance of time without symptoms of disease and toxicity effects and adjusted the relevant quality (Gelber and Goldhirsch 1986; Gelber et al. 1996). This is known as quality-adjusted TWiST. The Q-TWiST is like a revised version of the quantitative comparisons of BLRA. The benefit is measured by drug attributed gain of quality-adjusted life years (QALY). Cumulative risks of toxicities and disease progression are calculated for drug attributed loss of QALY. Q-TWiST compares the relative therapeutic value of treatments based on the patient experience within the context of clinical outcomes related to cancer and its treatment (Gelber et al. 1996). This method assumes that cancer patients progress through a set of health states of varying utility value for the individual patient. This Q-TWiST has been used for risk-benefit of cancer treatment. By weighting the durations of health states according to their quality of life, patient arrives at a single end point reflecting the duration of survival and the quality of life. Using survival analysis methods, the mean duration of each disease state and mean quality-adjusted survival time are estimated.

Number Needed to Treat (NNT) and Number Needed to Harm (NNH)

The number needed to treat NNT is defined as the number of patients who need to be treated to prevent or eliminate the occurrence of one additional event of disease of interest. NNT can be calculated by taking the reciprocal of the absolute risk reduction. NNT $= \frac{1}{(P_1 - P_2)} = \frac{1}{Absolute\_Risk\_Reduction}$, where P_1 and P_2 are proportions of the disease of interest in the control group and treatment group, respectively (Holden et al. 2003). In epidemiologic terms, P_1 and P_2 are risks associated with treatments and their difference is the absolute risk reduction, which can also be considered as the difference in outcome event incidence between the control and treatment groups. For example, patients with severe hyperlipidemia may receive a statin medication for a year and 8.2% mortality rate is observed compared to 11.5% mortality rate is observed for patients without receiving any statin. The absolute risk reduction is equal to (11.5% − 8.2% = 3.3%). The NNT = 1/0.033 = 30, which means 30 patients with hyperlipidemia needed to treat in order to avoid one death.

While the NNT is to measure the therapy benefit effect with a specific number of treated patients, the number needed to harm (NNH) can be calculated for adverse effects related to a specific therapy treatment. NNH can be calculated as follows: NNH = $1 / (Q_2 - Q_1)$, where Q_1 and Q_2 are the risks of AE of interest in the untreated and treated groups, respectively, and it is assumed that $Q_1 < Q_2$ because treated group has higher risk than untreated group.

Both NNT and NNH have been used widely for BRA across different therapeutic areas. A comparison between NNT and NNH can be used as a very basic comparison of benefit versus risk for a population of patients who may benefit from the treatment. Indeed, a *risk-benefit ratio* equal to NNH/NNT can be calculated between treatment and control groups. If the ratio is greater than 1 (i.e., NNH/NNT > 1 or NNT < NNH), then fewer patients need to be treated in order to achieve benefit than will be treated to have one additional occurrence of an ADE.

Minimum Clinical Efficacy (MCE)

For a new treatment, MCE can be defined as the minimal clinical efficacy needed for it to be worth considering as an alternative treatment after taking into account, including the efficacy of the standard treatment, the adverse event profiles associated with standard treatment, new treatment, and the risk of disease of interest associated with no treatment (Djulbegovic et al. 1998). MCE seeks to improve clinical care by a quantitative comparison of the potential benefit against the potential risk of a particular treatment. It seeks to find the minimal therapeutic benefit at which a treatment is still worth administering. MCE takes into account not only the benefits and harms of the new and standard treatments but also the natural characteristics of the disease in the general population, represented by untreated group.

The relative efficacy of the new treatment as compared to the conventional treatment should be at least the same as the relative efficacy of the conventional treatment plus the difference in risk of the AE divided by the risk of the disease of interest in the untreated group. The MCE method seeks to find the minimal therapeutic benefit at which a treatment is worth administering, which can be used as a yardstick for acceptance of a new treatment alternative. The details required to balance the ADE profiles as well as efficacy impact can be extensive.

Incremental Net Health Benefit (INHB)

The incremental net health benefit (INHB) of new Drug 2 versus current therapy Drug 1 can be expressed as: **INHB = $(E_2 - E_1) - (R_2 - R_1)$**, where effectiveness (E) is measured in quality-adjusted life years (QALYs) and risk (R) can also be measured in QALYs (Garrison et al. 2007). When $(E_2-E_1) > (R_2-R_1)$, a favorable risk-benefit balance is achieved. That is, the expected QALYs gains as a result of efficacy exceed the expected losses to safety problems. The QALY represents an adjustment to length of life for the quality of life experienced. Quality of life is measured with a preference scale or index, where 0 represents the value for death and 1 represents normal health. This measure can be adapted to BRA by separating the outcomes into expected health improvements with positive QALYs (benefits) and adverse health impacts with negative QALYs (risks). Some of the literature mentioned that the benefits and risks for INHB could be measured using value-adjusted life years as opposed to QALYs (Garrison et al. 2007). The INHB approach is a theoretically sound modeling method with strong potential for usefulness in clinical and regulatory decision making.

Relative-Value-Adjusted Number Needed to Treat (RV-NNT) and RV-NNH

In order to account for patient preferences, both the NNT and NNH measures have been revised to incorporate patients' relative utility values. Relative utility values are obtained using either the standard-gamble method or the time-trade-off approach. The relative value (RV) is calculated from a numeric representation of patients' preferences for specific outcomes. Hence RV-NNT and RV-NNH can be calculated between treatment and control comparison groups. A favorable BRA outcome is obtained when RV-NNH /NNT > 1 (Holden et al. 2003).

Risk-Benefit Plane (RBP) and Risk-Benefit Acceptability Threshold (RBAT)

A hypothetical model of the risk–benefit plane (RBP) is a two-dimensional plot with benefit and risk on the two axes, including four quadrants NE, SE, NW, and SW (Lynd and O'Brien 2004). The risk measurement can be incidence of ADEs or frequency of ADE. If the risk is on X-axis, the risk for the new therapy increases from left to right. The benefit measurement can be incidence of benefit or product of efficacy and responder rate. The benefit on Y-axis increases from bottom to top. Hence, risk-benefit ratios in NW depicts that experimental therapy dominates due to this treatment option with low risk and high benefit. In the SE quadrant, the active treatment option has higher risks and lower benefits (with a high benefit-risk ratio), and the control therapy is said to dominate. The remaining two quadrants involve high risk and more benefit in SW, and less risk and less benefit in NE. An appropriate risk-benefit acceptability threshold (RBAT) will be determined in BRP plot, which is indicated by a slope of line that crosses over the SW and NE quadrants (Lynd and O'Brien 2004).

Probabilistic Simulation Methods (PSM) and Monte Carlo Simulation (MCS)

Similar to the above RBP model, the average difference in the probability of achieving a benefit with the new therapy relative to conventional therapy can be plotted on the X-axis (ΔB) and the average difference in the probability of risk for the new therapy can be plotted on the Y-axis (ΔR). Both axes therefore range from -1 to 1, with 0 at the origin (Lynd and O'Brien 2004). Then, four quadrants are labeled with points of the compass NE, SE, NW, and SW. For a hypothetical model of **PSM,** using differences in the probability of achieving benefit and risk, the incremental risk-benefit ratio (IRBR) related to the new therapy can be defined as the incremental probability of an ADE (ΔR) with a new therapy relative to conventional treatment divided by the incremental probability of a beneficial effect (ΔB). The Y-axis represents average difference in the probability of risk for the new therapy versus conventional treatment. In a clinical study, an **MCS** was applied to compare the efficacy and safety of administering anticoagulants to trauma patients who are already at an elevated risk of bleeding (Lynd and O'Brien 2004).

Multi-Criteria Decision Analysis (MCDA)

MCDA is a decision tool aimed at supporting decision makers who are faced with making numerous risk and benefit evaluations. The risk can be measured by incidence of ADEs, discontinuation rate due to ADEs, and other risk factors such as potential drug interactions, off-label use leading to safety hazards, and safety issues observed in preclinical safety studies. The benefit involves clinical relevant end-points from clinical trials and other benefit criteria. Using a decision value tree, a risk-benefit ratio for a specific drug therapy can be evaluated systematically. Both benefit and risk criteria can be split into multiple criteria in case of different primary endpoints, relevant subgroups, and relevant interactions. Although the MCDA model can be customized by adding or changing benefit and risk criteria, data extraction from clinical trials is critical for the internal validity assessment of the MCDA technique (Mussen et al. 2007).

Risk-Benefit Contour (RBC)

The RBC is to provide a two-dimensional graph showing both the probability of benefit from treatment, based, for example, on the survival rate, and the probability of drug toxicity or ADEs (the risk). The degree of drug benefit is captured along the X-axis, and the degree of drug risk is measured along the Y-axis. By finding out from each patient the amount of risk he or she is willing to accept to obtain a certain benefit, a set of individual risk-benefit contours can be determined (Shakespeare et al. 2001).

Stated Preference Method (SPM) or Maximum Acceptable Risk (MAR)

SPM or MAR is based on hedonic-utility principles, and therapeutic treatment options (commodities) over which consumers make choices. Consumer choices can be considered as a random utility function specified as $U_j = V_j + \varepsilon_j$ with $V_j = X_j\beta$ (Hauber et al. 2009), where V_j is the determinate part of the utility function for treatment j; X_j is a vector of attribute levels for treatment j; β is a vector of attribute parameters; and ε_j is a random error. Benefit-risk trade-off preferences can be estimated based on consumer experience or probability of AEs. Patient's preferences can be collected from survey questionnaires and interview techniques such as contingent valuation techniques. The current best practice standard requires participants to make trade-offs between choices using discrete choice experiments. Best-worst scaling methods are also being developed and may become more wisely used in the future. Using SPM or MAR, the risk-benefit trade-off can be calculated as the increase in risk of AEs that reduces the patients' satisfaction scores between two treatment options.

Conclusions

In summary, multiple BRAs are available for drug safety surveillance during new drug development. Various BRA methods have been utilized for clinical decision-making in different therapeutic areas, including oral contraceptives, antipsychotics, antihyperlipidaemia medications, cancer chemotherapy, iron-chelation, and antihypertensives. Above BRA methods discussed should cover mainstream BRA methods, but may not cover all available methods due to the limited effort for literature review. All BRA methods can be utilized for safety surveillance not only in pharmaceutical and biologics but also in medical devices and other products. There are increasing safety considerations about medical devices such as implantable "Essure" device for sterilization (Johal et al. 2018), implantable metal device containing cobalt, and Davinci robotic system. Although all BRA methods have their limitations related to data requirements, statistical properties, and availability of patient preference (utility) measurement, the BRA methods are becoming more visible and useful supplemental tools for informed decision-making and regulatory interventions.

Key Facts/Points

- **Drug safety surveillance** is a multidisciplinary method to document, monitor, and evaluate adverse drug events, and plan effective interventions. It applies to the life cycle of a drug development.

- **Pharmacovigilance** is generally regarded as all post-marketing scientific and data gathering activities relating to the detection, assessment, understanding, and prevention of adverse events. It is often referred to **post-marketing surveillance**.
- **Risk management** is an iterative process designed to optimize the benefit-risk balance regulated products including assessment, development, evaluation, reassessment, and adjustment for risk-benefit balance.
- There are four key **safety signal detection algorithms** like reporting odds ratio (ROR), proportional reporting ratio (PRR), Multi-item Gamma Passion Shrinker (MGPS), and information component (IC).
- Many traditional and innovative regulatory are commonly used in USA, such as labeling changes, black-box warnings, continue educations, "Dear Doctor Letter," "Dear Health Practitioner Letter," restricted distribution, medication guides, withdrawal, etc.
- Common quantitative **benefit-risk assessments (BRAs)** include quantitative framework for risk-benefit assessment (QFRBA), benefit-less risk analysis (BLRA), quality-adjusted time without symptoms and toxicity (Q-TWiST), number needed to treat (NNT) versus number needed to harm (NNH), relative value adjusted number needed to treat (RV-NNT), minimum clinical efficacy (MCE), incremental net health benefit (INHB), risk-benefit plane (BRP) and risk-benefit acceptability threshold (RBAT), probabilistic simulation methods (PSM) and Monte Carlo simulation (MCS), multi-criteria decision analysis (MCDA), risk-benefit contour (RBC), and stated preference method (SPM) or maximum acceptable risk (MAR).
- This chapter review is based on the author's previous research work and expertise. A recent formal literature search for this review was not performed. The author is indebted to current and past graduate students and colleagues who worked together with the author for the related research subjects in drug safety and benefit-risk analysis.

Cross-References

▶ Bayesian Adaptive Designs for Phase I Trials

References

Almenoff JS, Tonning JM, Gould AL et al (2005) Perspectives on the use of data Mining in Pharmacovigilance. Drug Saf 28:981–1007

Bate A, Lindquist M, Edwards IR, Orre R (2002) A data mining approach for signal detection and analysis. Drug Saf 25:393–397

DuMouchel W (1999) Bayesian data mining in large frequency tables, with an application to FDA spontaneous reporting system. Am Stats 53:177–190

Chen Y, Guo JJ, Healy D, Lin X, Patel NC (2008a) Risk of hepatotoxicity associated with the use of Telithromycin: signal detection based upon the FDA's spontaneous reporting system. Annals Pharmacotherapy 42(12):1791–1796

Chen Y, Guo JJ, Steinbuck M, Lin XD, Buncher CR, Patel C (2008b) Comparisons of data mining algorithms for adverse drug reactions: an empirical study based on the adverse event reporting system of the Food and Drug Administration. J Pharm Med 22(6):359–365

Chuang-Stein C (1994) A New Proposal for Benefit-Less-Risk Analysis in Clinical Trials. *Controlled Clinical Trials* 15:30–43

Djulbegovic B, Hozo I, Fields K, Sullivan D (1998) High-dose chemotherapy in the adjuvant treatment of breast cancer: benefit/risk analysis. Cancer Control 5:394–405

Evans SJV, Waller PC, Davis S (2001) Use of proportional reporting ratios (PRRs) for signal generation from spontaneous adverse drug reaction reports. Pharmacoepidemiol Drug Saf 10:483–486

Food and Drug Administration (FDA) (2005) FDA Guidance for industry: Premarketing risk assessment. Good Pharmacovigilance Practices and Pharmacoepidemiologic Assessment. Development and use of risk minimization action plans (RiskMAP). Online available at: https://www.fda.gov/downloads/drugs/guidancecomplianceregulatoryinformation/guidances/ucm071696.pdf

Food and Drug Administration (FDA) (2018) Benefit-risk assessment in drug regulatory decision-making. Online available at: https://www.fda.gov/files/about%20fda/published/Benefit-Risk-Assessment-in-Drug-Regulatory-Decision-Making.pdf

FDA. (2019) Federal Food, Drug, and Cosmetic Act (FD&C Act). Kefauver-Harris Amendments revolutionized drug development. U.S. Department of Health and Human Services. Online available at: https://www.fda.gov/ForConsumers/ConsumerUpdates/ucm322856.htm.https://www.fda.gov/regulatoryinformation/lawsenforcedbyfda/federalfooddrugandcosmeticactfdcact/default.htm. Accessed on January 22, 2019

Garrison LP, Towse A, Bresnahan BW (2007) Assessing a structured, quantitative health outcomes approach to drug risk-benefit analysis. Health Aff 26(3):684–695

Gelber RD, Goldhirsh A (1986) A new endpoint for the assessment of adjuvant therapy in postmenopausal women with operable breast cancer. J Clin Oncol 4:1772–1779

Gelber RD, Goldhirsch A, Cole BF, Wieand HS, Schroeder G, Krook JE (1996) A quality-adjusted time without symptoms or toxicity (Q-TWiST) analysis of adjuvant radiation therapy and chemotherapy for resectable rectal cancer. J Natl Cancer Inst 88(15):1039–1045

Guo JJ, Curkendall S, Jones J, Fife D, Goehring E, She DW (2003) The impact of cisapride label change on codispending of contraindicated medications. J Pharmacoepidemiology Drug Safety 12:295–301

Guo JJ, Jang R, Louder A, Cluxton RJ (2005) Acute pancreatitis associated with different drug therapies among HIV-infected patients. Pharmacotherapy 25(8):1044–1054

Guo JJ, Goehring E, Jones JK (2008) The story of cisapride and its withdraw from market: a case study [book chapter 29]. In: Hartzema AG, Tilson HH, Chan AK (eds) Pharmacoepidemiology and therapeutic risk management. Harvey Whitney Books, Cincinnati, pp 727–738

Guo JJ, Pandey S, Doyle J, Bian B, Raisch D (2010) A review of current risk-benefit assessments for drug safety: report of ISPOR risk-benefit management working group. Value Health 13(5):657–666

Hauben M, Reich L (2004) Safety related drug-labeling changes: findings from two data mining algorithms. Drug Saf 27:735–744

Hauber AB, Mohamed AF, Johnson FR, Falvey H (2009) Treatment preferences and medication adherence of people with type 2 diabetes using oral glucose-lowering agents. Diabet Med 26:416–424

Holden WL, Juhaeri J, Dai W (2003) Benefit-risk analysis: a proposal using quantitative methods. Pharmacoepidemiol Drug Saf 12:611–616

International conference on harmonization (ICH) technical requirements for registration of pharmaceuticals for human use. (2004) ICH harmonized tripartite guideline pharmacovigilance planning E2E. November 2004. Online available at: https://www.ich.org/fileadmin/Public_Web_Site/ICH_Products/Guidelines/Efficacy/E2E/Step4/E2E_Guideline.pdf. Accessed on Jan 22, 2019

Johal T, Kuruba N, Sule M, Mukhopadhyay S, Raje G (2018) Laparoscopic salpingectomy and removal of Essure hysteroscopic sterilization device: a case series. Eur J Contracept Reprod Health Care 23(3):227–230

Lis Y, Roberts MH, Kamble S, Guo JJ, Raisch DW (2012) Comparison of FDA and EMA risk management implementation for recent pharmaceutical approvals: report of the International Society for Pharmacoeconomics & outcomes research risk management working group. Value Health 15(8):1108–1118

Lynd LD, O'Brien BJ (2004) Advances in risk-benefit evaluation using probabilistic simulation methods: an application to the prophylaxis of deep vein thrombosis. J Clin Epidemiol 57:795–803

Mussen F, Salek S, Walker S (2007) A quantitative approach to benefit-risk assessment of medicines – part 1: the development of a new model using multi-criteria decision analysis. Pharmacoepidemiol Drug Saf 16:S2–S15

Pray WS, Pray GE (2011) Behind-the-counter products: a third class of drugs. US Pharmacist 36(9):11–15

Shakespeare TP, Gebski VJ, Veness MJ, Simes J (2001) Improving interpretation of clinical studies by use of confidence levels, clinical significance curves, and risk-benefit contours. Lancet 357:1349–1353

Stang PE, Ryan PB, Meng R, Racoosin JA, Overhage JM, Hartzema AG et al (2010) Advancing the science for active surveillance: rationale and design for the observational medical outcomes partnership. Ann Int Med 153:600–606

Zeldis JB, William BA, Thomas SD, Elsayed ME (1999) S.T.E.P.S. a comprehensive program for controlling and monitoring access to thalidomide. Clin Therap 21(2):319–330

Causal Inference: Efficacy and Mechanism Evaluation

100

Sabine Landau and Richard Emsley

Contents

Introduction	1982
Evaluating Efficacy under Nonadherence with Allocated Treatments	1984
Assessing Treatment Effect Modification by Process Variables	1989
Assessing Treatment Effect Mediation	1993
Assessing Treatment Effectiveness in Populations Defined by the Value of an Intermediate Outcome	1996
Summary and Conclusion	1999
Keyfacts	1999
Cross-References	1999
References	2000

Abstract

In randomized trials, the primary analysis is usually based on an intention-to-treat approach which answers the question "What is the effect of offering treatment?" There are many other questions that investigators could pose such as "Does this treatment work if it is received?" "What factors make the treatment work better?" and "How does the treatment work?" These questions require alternative analysis approaches based on statistical methods drawn from the causal inference literature, including instrumental variables and causal mediation analysis. This chapter will define relevant causal estimands and describe methods that can be used to estimate them, their underlying assumptions, and the estimation procedures. The methods will be illustrated using examples drawn from the literature.

S. Landau (✉) · R. Emsley
Department of Biostatistics and Health Informatics, King's College London, London, UK
e-mail: sabine.landau@kcl.ac.uk; richard.emsley@kcl.ac.uk

> **Keywords**
>
> Confounding · Controlled direct effect · Efficacy · Estimand · Instrumental variables methods · Mechanism · Mediation analysis · Nonadherence · Process variable · Treatment effect modification

Introduction

The evaluation of causal treatment effects is the overriding aim of the randomized controlled trial (RCT). Experimental design, that is the existence of a control group and random allocation of study participants to trial arms, combined with intention-to-treat (ITT) analysis, ensures that the causal effect of the intervention under investigation can be estimated without bias. ITT analysis addresses the question "Is there a difference between the randomized trial arms in terms of a clinical outcome?" It estimates the so-called *ITT effect:* the difference in outcome between patients who were offered the control treatment and those who were offered the comparator treatment, with randomization ensuring that both these populations are representative of the trial's target population.

Whether ITT analysis is all that is needed in an RCT depends on the research questions being asked. Most trials target ITT effects. In particular, pragmatic trials such as those funded by the National Institutes of Health Research (NIHR) Health Technology Assessment (HTA) programme in the UK seek to evaluate the effectiveness of interventions and typically target the causal effect of the treatment policy. In contrast, explanatory trials such as those funded by the UK NIHR/Medical Research Council (MRC) Efficacy and Mechanism programme seek to evaluate the efficacy of the intervention and the mechanism by which the intervention is efficacious. ITT analysis can address the former but is not sufficient to answer the latter research questions.

In order to identify appropriate analysis methods, clinical investigators need to translate trial objectives into target population quantities which they wish to estimate. The statistical literature refers to such quantities as "estimands" or "target parameters." The term *estimand* is more generic in that it does not require the existence of a parametric model and is adopted here. Trials focus on estimands that describe the causal effects of treatments. As will be shown below, these can be defined in different ways to quantify the efficacy or effectiveness of treatments. The addendum to the "Statistical Principles for Clinical Trials" on estimands and sensitivity analysis in clinical trials recently released by the International Council for Harmonisation of Technical Requirements for Pharmaceuticals for Human Use (ICH E9) also emphasizes the need to elaborate on the choice of the estimand (EMA 2017).

When estimands other than the ITT effect are of interest, more complex analysis approaches might be needed. The field of causal inference is concerned with principled approaches for estimating estimands that have a causal interpretation, that is, methods that can provide unbiased assessments under clearly specified assumptions.

In this chapter, we describe causal inference methods for addressing non-ITT research questions in trials. The following are typical questions considered in phase 2 explanatory trials:

Does the Treatment Work, i.e., Is It Efficacious?
As an example consider the Outcomes of Depression International Network (ODIN) trial (Dowrick et al. 2000). This trial evaluated the effect of two psychological interventions (psycho-education and problem solving) for the treatment of depression in primary care. The primary outcome was depression measured by the Beck Depression Inventory (BDI). Only about half of the patients in the therapy arms adhered to the treatment, while all the control patients received the control condition prompting the question "What was the effect of therapy in those patients who actually received it?" (Dunn et al. 2003).

Does the Efficacy of the Treatment Depend on Aspects of the patient's Treatment Experience?
Aspects of the treatment experience may modify the efficacy of the treatment. Such research questions are often asked in therapy trials with clinical psychologists suggesting that the success of therapy is contingent on factors such as the amount of therapy patients are able to take part in or the ability to build an alliance with the therapist. As an example consider the multicenter Study of the Cognitive Realignment Theory in Early Schizophrenia (SoCRATES) which investigated the effect of cognitive behavioral therapy (CBT) or supportive counseling in addition to treatment as usual (TAU) for acutely ill patients with recent onset schizophrenia. Primary outcomes included symptom measures at 18 months follow-up (Positive and Negative Syndrome Scale, PANSS). The original ITT analysis detected a treatment by center interaction which was interpreted as psychological therapies having beneficial long-term effects for some patients (Tarrier et al. 2004). Subsequently secondary analyses sought to disentangle this finding and investigated whether the perceived alliance of the patients with their therapists (measured using the short 12-item patient-completed version of the California Therapeutic Alliance Scale, CALPAS) affected how the treatment effect varies with the number of therapy sessions received with some intriguing results (Dunn and Bentall 2007; Emsley et al. 2010; Goldsmith et al. 2015).

How Does the Treatment Work?
Investigators are often interested in understanding how treatments achieve their effects, if they are present. The treatment may be based on a theoretical model and it is of interest to show empirically that this is the mechanism through which it works. Similarly, the treatment might be designed to target a specific mechanism and investigators wish to test if changing that mechanism leads to an improvement in some distal outcome such as symptoms. Addressing such questions involves checking whether treatment-induced changes in the hypothesized mechanism can explain an observed treatment effect on the outcome. This can be done using statistical methods known as mediation analysis and which we will discuss in detail in a later section. We consider the example of a trial testing the effect of a digital psychological intervention for sleep. The intervention has previously been shown to successfully improve sleep, and the question of interest was whether improving

sleep would lead to an improvement in other aspects of mental health and well-being. In the Oxford Access for Students Improving Sleep (OASIS) trial (Freeman et al. 2017), this hypothesis was tested in a sample of university students. The trial was designed to assess whether the sleep intervention would reduce nonclinical levels of paranoia and hallucinations.

What Would Be the Effectiveness of the Treatment for a Population with Fixed Value of an Intermediate Trial Outcome?
It is possible that participants in trials can access alternative treatments to those under investigation, for an example from surgery see (Sharples et al. 2020). Similarly, one component of an intervention might be to encourage or discourage the use of additional interventions. Consider the example of the Methods for Improving Reproductive Health in Africa (MIRA) trial that investigated the effect of diaphragm and lubricant gel use in the reduction of HIV infection among susceptible southern African women (Padian et al. 2007). One alternative that affects HIV infection is use of condoms, and this might itself be influenced by receiving the trial interventions. Here, the question of interest is how effective the trial interventions are in the presence or absence of condom use, rather than whether the effect of the interventions is acting through condom use.

The scope of this chapter is limited to parallel group trial designs comparing a control (placebo or "treatment as usual" condition) with an added active intervention and focuses on continuous outcome measures. Extension to other designs and outcomes are possible and some suggestions will be made at the end of each section.

Evaluating Efficacy under Nonadherence with Allocated Treatments

This section is concerned with treatment effect evaluation when participants depart from their random allocation. The simpler all-or-nothing compliance scenario is considered here, that is those not adhering to treatment in the active trial arm receive the control condition and those not adhering in the control arm receive the active treatment.

Potential Outcomes and Efficacy Estimands
The following variables are observed for trial participants $i \in \{1, \ldots, n\}$

- R_i is the treatment offered to participant i with possible values $r = 0$ for being allocated to the control arm and $r = 1$ for the active arm.
- D_i is the binary treatment received by participant i with possible values $d = 0$ when receiving control and $d = 1$ when receiving the active treatment.
- $Y_{i,\,pre}$ and $Y_{i,\,post}$ are the values measured on a continuous clinical outcome variable for participant i at baseline (prerandomization) and postrandomization, respectively.

Two potential outcomes (Rubin 1974) can be defined for individuals from the target population:

- $Y_{i,\,\text{post}}(D=d) = Y_{i,\,\text{post}}(d)$ the clinical outcome that would have been observed if individual i had received treatment $d = 0, 1$. It follows that

$$Y_{i,\,\text{post}} = \begin{cases} Y_{i,\,\text{post}}(D=1) \text{ if } D_i = 1 \\ Y_{i,\,\text{post}}(D=0) \text{ if } D_i = 0 \end{cases}$$

An individual causal treatment effect on the clinical outcome can be defined as the contrast

$$\Delta_i := Y_{i,\,\text{post}}(D=1) - Y_{i,\,\text{post}}(D=0).$$

Importantly the individual treatment effects can vary between patients and so this definition allows for treatment effect heterogeneity.

An efficacy estimand is given by the *Average Treatment Effect* in the target population:

$$\text{ATE} := E_\Delta(\Delta_i).$$

It is possible to restrict attention to those patients who would ultimately receive the treatment by focusing on the *Average Treatment effect in the Treated*:

$$\text{ATT} := E_\Delta(\Delta_i | D_i = 1).$$

Finally, attention can be restricted to the subgroup of compliers. We define a *Complier* to be an individual who receives the treatment that they are offered, that is, for whom $D_i(R=1) - D_i(R=0) = 1$. Note that the subgroup of compliers is a latent class or stratum defined at baseline. A third efficacy estimand is then given by the *Complier Average Causal Effect*:

$$\text{CACE} := E_\Delta[\Delta_i | D_i(R=1) - D_i(R=0) = 1].$$

Figure 1 shows a structural equation diagram for the ODIN trial. In such diagrams, arrows imply causal effects and importantly, the absence of a directed path from one variable to another implies the conditional independence of the variables. In ODIN the clinical outcome was depression 6 months after randomization (BDI6). For simplicity the two trial arms allocated psychological interventions were combined into a single arm (variable Therapy offer). Therapy receipt was categorized as "yes" or "no" (Dunn et al. 2003). The efficacy estimand of interest is represented by the coefficient β of the causal path from Therapy receipt to BDI6.

Standard Approaches and Confounding Problem

ITT analysis estimates the effect of the treatment offer in the target population and underestimates the causal effect of treatment receipt (ATE) under nonadherence with allocated treatments. Clinicians have long been concerned about this and have put forward per protocol (PP, an attempt to estimate ATT) and as-treated (AsT) analyses as alternatives for estimating efficacy. However, both these approaches suffer from

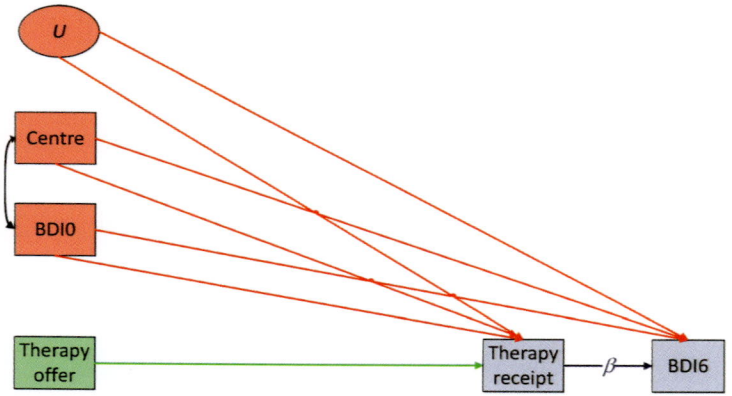

Fig. 1 Causal diagram for ODIN trial (blue = causal efficacy estimand, red = confounding paths, green = instrumental variable)

confounding biases when there are unobserved variables that are common causes of both the outcome and the adherence with allocated treatment (Sheiner and Rubin 1995).

For example, in the ODIN trial two such potential confounding variables were observed, depression at baseline (BDI0) and Study center (Fig. 1). Further common causes may exist but have not been measured. These are represented by the latent variable U. Thus, observed and unobserved baseline variables open up a so-called "unblocked backdoor paths" connecting Therapy receipt and BDI6. The existence of these paths leads to bias when β is estimated based on Therapy receipt and BDI6 alone. Conditioning on observed covariates BDI0 and Centre in the analysis can "block" some of the confounding paths, but some residual confounding will remain since latent U cannot be conditioned on.

Instrumental Variables Estimators for Assessing Efficacy and their Assumptions
Instrumental variables methods can be used to assess the efficacy of treatments in the presence of hidden confounding in trials (latent variable U). IV methods provide a consistent estimator of the CACE efficacy estimand provided the following assumptions hold:

- **SUTVA:** The *Stable Unit Treatment Assumptions* states that a patient's response to a treatment will be the same regardless of the treatment(s) received by other patients.
- **Monotonicity:** The target population does not include individuals who receive the opposite to what they are offered (known as *Defiers*).
- **Exclusion restriction**: For those who never (always) receive the active treatment irrespective of offer (knowns as *Never-takers* or *Always-takers,* respectively), the offer of treatment does not influence average clinical outcome.

As the name suggests, such methods rely on the existence of relevant *Instrumental Variables* (IVs). The explanatory variables of a linear structural model for the clinical outcome can be categorized as *endogenous* or *exogenous* variables: An explanatory variable that is correlated with the model's error term is endogenous. Conversely exogenous variables are independent of the model's error term. The effects of endogenous variables cannot be estimated without biases by standard methods such as the ordinary least squares estimator. IVs are additional variables – not part of the linear model – which can help avoid such biases. To do so, IVs need to fulfill two conditions:

- **Relevance condition:** The set of IVs must be predictive of the set of endogenous variables.
- **Instrumental variables condition:** The IVs are not correlated with the linear model's error term.

In trials subject to nonadherence with allocated treatments and a single endogenous explanatory variable "treatment receipt," at least one instrumental variable is required. For example, in ODIN Therapy receipt is the single endogenous variable as it is correlated with the latent confounder U which forms part of the error term of the linear model for BDI6. Random treatment offer provides a potential instrumental variable as it predicts treatment receipt and due to randomization there are no variables that drive both treatment offer and outcome. However, for the instrumental variables condition to be fulfilled in trials we still require the exclusion restriction assumption to hold. So for Therapy offer to provide an instrumental variable for ODIN we need to assume the absence of a directed path from Therapy offer to BDI6 other than via Therapy receipt (Fig. 1).

Two-Stage Least Squares Estimator of CACE

Instrumental variables estimators are consistent for the causal effect of the endogenous variable. In the trial context, this is the causal effect of treatment receipt. IV methods were originally developed within the econometrics literature assuming effect homogeneity; for details see for example Wooldridge (2010). Work from the causal inference field subsequently showed that IV estimators in trials with all-or-nothing compliance can allow for treatment effect heterogeneity and estimate CACE under monotonicity (Angrist et al. 1996).

The most commonly used instrumental variables estimator is the two-stage least squares estimator (2SLS). It derives its name from the fact that it can be calculated by a two-stage procedure: First regress the endogenous variable on the instrument(s) and exogenous explanatory variables and derive a prediction of the endogenous variable. Second regress the clinical outcome on the prediction of the endogenous variable and the exogenous covariates. The estimated regression coefficient of the predicted variable is the CACE estimate. Most general purpose statistical software packages implement a 2SLS estimator based on matrix algebra which enables generation of model-based standard errors (e.g., STATA's **ivregress 2sls** command, SAS's **PROC SYSLIN** or R's **ivreg** function).

Table 1 shows the results of applying the various estimators to the ODIN trial data. The ITT approach estimates the effect of offering psychological therapy (effectiveness) and shows a significant reduction in depression. Surprisingly PP

Table 1 Estimates of the efficacy of psychological intervention from the ODIN trial (N = 427)

Estimator[a]	Estimated trial arm difference (psychological intervention – control) in BDI6	95% confidence interval
ITT	−2.52	−4.44 to −0.61
AsT	−1.04	−2.94 to 0.86
PP (N = 319)	−1.77	−3.87 to 0.32
2SLS	−4.60	−8.12 to −1.08

[a]Using inverse probability weighting based on trial arm and non-adherence within the active arm to accommodate a missing at random (MAR) missing data generating process whereby non-adherence to psychological therapy can also predict missing BDI6 values. The analyses were conditioned on BDI0 and Centre

and AsT estimators which target the efficacy of the psychological intervention result in smaller effect sizes and leading the authors to suspect that residual confounding is at play here (Dunn et al. 2003). In contrast, the 2SLS estimate of CACE is larger in absolute size than the ITT estimate.

Interpretation

Choosing between an AsT (or PP) and an IV efficacy estimator in a trial subject to nonadherence is an assumptions trade-off. If relevant confounding variables have been measured and conditioned on in the analysis model then the "no hidden confounding" assumption underlying the AsT and PP approaches might be realistic. In contrast, when the presence of unmeasured confounders is suspected then the exclusion restriction might be the better assumption to make. How defensible the exclusion restriction is will depend on the trial context. While there is no reason why the offer of treatment should affect outcome in the Never-takers or Always-takers in a double-blind placebo controlled trial, there could be processes that lead to such effects in an open label trial where participants are aware of their treatment allocation and it differs from their desired allocation.

When effect heterogeneity is allowed, the 2SLS estimator estimates CACE, that is, it targets the average treatment effect in the subpopulation of compliers. It is important to appreciate that an IV estimator evaluates the treatment effect for compliers in the context of the trial setting. A patient may comply with treatment offer in a trial setting but not when the treatment is rolled out in routine clinical practice. Conversely, a patient may not comply with a novel treatment offer in a trial but may be willing to take the treatment once it has been shown to be efficacious.

Extensions

It has been shown that CACE estimation by 2SLS is equivalent to fitting structural mean models, see for example Fischer-Lapp and Goetghebeur (1999), (Dunn and Bentall 2007). In addition, the semiparametric 2SLS/structural mean model approach is not the only way of generating a consistent CACE estimator. Alternative IV approaches for fully parametric models include full (FIML) and limited information maximum likelihood (LIML). Furthermore extensions of the 2SLS method to nonlinear models exist including for binary (Clarke and Windmeijer 2012) or censored survival outcomes (Tchetgen et al. 2015).

A CACE estimator for continuous or binary outcomes can also be constructed by fitting a structural equation model that contains the Complier, Never-taker and Always-taker strata as latent classes (known as *principal stratification* (Frangakis and Rubin 2002)). The latter has the advantage that missing data assumptions can be relaxed to allow compliance status to drive missingness of outcome (so-called *latent ignorability* Pickles and Croudace 2010).

Finally, for longitudinal studies where the mechanism which leads to non-adherence with allocated treatments is known and relevant time-varying covariates driving the treatment decision are observed (typically side effects and earlier treatment response), it is possible to estimate ATE using inverse probability of censoring weights (Dodd et al. 2017a, b).

Assessing Treatment Effect Modification by Process Variables

This section is concerned with assessing treatment effect modification by variables that measure an aspect of the patient's treatment experience. For simplicity, it is assumed that there is no treatment contamination, that is, participants allocated to the control condition cannot access the active treatment. For continuous modifier variables, it is further assumed that the size of the treatment effect changes at a constant rate with increasing values (linear dose response relationships).

Process Variables and Treatment Effect Modification Estimands
A *process variable* is a variable that measures an aspect of the patient's treatment experience. Its definition is specific to the treatment investigated, and in a trial the variable can only be observed for patients who have been offered this treatment. For example, for psychological therapies variables such as the number of therapy sessions attended or the alliance built with their therapist characterize the patient's therapy experience. Formally, a process variable is defined as another potential outcome:

- $A_i(R = 1)$ is the aspect of treatment that would have been experienced if individual i had been allocated to the active trial arm.

An interesting research question might be whether an aspect of the treatment experience modifies the treatment effect, that is, whether the size of the causal effect of the treatment offer varies with the level of the respective process variable.

- The individual causal effect of the treatment offer is measured by the contrast $\nabla_i := Y_{i,\text{post}}(R = 1) - Y_{i,\text{post}}(R = 0)$ and the intention-to-treat effect is ITT $= E_\nabla(\nabla_i)$.
- In addition, the *Local Average Treatment Effect* for those with process variable value a is given by LATE$(a) := E_\nabla(\nabla_i| A_i(R = 1) = a)$.

Treatment effect modification can then be quantified by the modification estimand

$$\beta := \text{LATE}(a+1) - \text{LATE}(a)$$

with $\text{LATE}(1) = \beta$ if $\text{LATE}(0) = 0$.

Figure 2 shows a structural equation diagram for the SoCRATES trial. The clinical outcome was schizophrenia symptoms 18 months after randomization (PANSS18). The CBT and supportive counseling arms were again combined into a single arm (Therapy offer). Psychological therapy experience was characterized by two process variables: the number of sessions received if offered therapy (Sessions process variable) and the alliance built with the therapist if offered therapy (Alliance process variable, CALPAS scores rescaled such that scores ranged from −6 to 0, with higher scores indicating greater psychotherapeutic alliance and a value of zero the best therapeutic alliance achieved in this trial). The SoCRATES re-analyses (Dunn and Bentall 2007; Emsley et al. 2010; Goldsmith et al. 2015) interrogated two effect modification estimands: The first measured the change in treatment effect as patients, who had the best possible alliance with their therapist, took part in an increasing number of sessions. The second estimand quantified how this dose response relationship changed as the alliance rating worsened. These estimands are reflected in the causal diagram by the path coefficients β_1 and β_2 of respective interaction product terms. The first interaction term (product of Therapy offer and Sessions process) is simply the number of therapy sessions attended by a patient (referred to as Sessions). The second interaction term is Sessions multiplied by observable alliance (the interaction term is zero for controls and those not attending any sessions in the active arm), here referred to as SessionsxAlliance. Importantly these product terms can be observed despite the process variables being

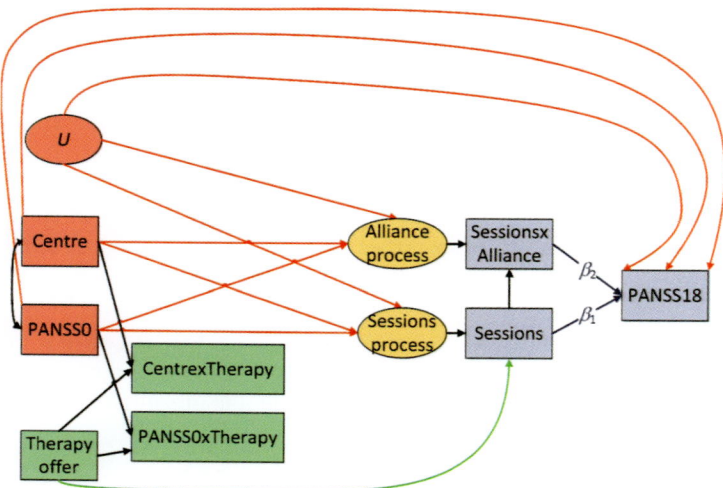

Fig. 2 Causal diagram for SoCRATES trial (blue = effect modification estimand, orange = process variables, red = confounding paths, green = instrumental variables)

unobservable for patients randomized to the control arm. Figure 2 does not include direct causal effects of the process variables, nor of the product of Therapy offer and Alliance process. These variables are counterfactual in the control arm and hence cannot impact on PANSS18 directly.

Standard Approaches and Confounding Problem

Clinical investigators often assess the relationship between the process variable and the clinical outcome within the active arm. If detected, such a relationship is typically interpreted as treatment effect modification by the process variable. For example, the outcome improving with increasing number of therapy sessions in the therapy arm is frequently interpreted as the therapy becoming more beneficial the more sessions the patient receives. However, there are two mechanisms that can lead to an observed association between the process variable and the outcome in the treated: (i) prognostic effects of the process variable or (ii) treatment effect modification by the process variable. It is not possible to disentangle these two mechanisms without using outcome data from the control group, and thus such effect modification assessments are biased unless prognostic effects can be ruled out (Dunn et al. 2015).

The existence of prognostic effects is equivalent to the presence of a confounding path connecting the relevant interactions term with clinical outcome. Figure 2 illustrates this for the SoCRATES trial. Some baseline variables which drive both the process variables and PANSS18 were observed, including symptoms at baseline (PANSS0) and Centre. Further unobserved common causes may exist. These are represented by latent variable U.

Instrumental Variables Estimators for Assessing Effect Modification by Process Variables

Instrumental variables estimators can be used to assess treatment effect modification by process variables in the presence of hidden confounding in trials. Such methods provide consistent estimators of modification estimands provided the following assumptions hold (Ginestet et al. 2017):

- **SUTVA**
- **No unaccounted variability in average treatment effects:** The linear model fully explains the variability in average treatment effects, that is, LATE$(a) = \beta a$ for all $a \neq 0$.
- **Exclusion restriction**: R provides an IV if the offer of treatment does not influence the average clinical outcome in the subpopulation where the process is absent, that is, LATE$(0) = 0$.
- **Instrumental variables condition**: For example, for an observed baseline variable B, the interaction term $B \times R$ provides an IV if B is predictive of the process variables and the interaction term does not have a direct effect on the outcome.

In the presence of hidden confounding, all treatment offers by process variable interaction terms in linear models for treatment effect modification are endogenous. To estimate their effects without bias at least as many IVs as endogenous variables are needed. One of these IVs is provided by random treatment offer itself if the exclusion restriction holds. If the exclusion restriction does not hold, or more than one IV are needed, interactions between observed baseline variables that predict the process variable and treatment offer hold the most promise. Such interaction terms meet the relevance condition as they predict the endogenous interaction term. They meet the instrumental variables condition provided they do not have a direct effect on the clinical outcome. This is because there are no unblocked backdoor paths connecting the putative interaction IV and the model's error term due to randomization. Figure 2 shows two extra IVs in addition to random Therapy offer – PANSS0xTherapy offer and CentrexTherapy offer. These three baseline variables predict the two endogenous interaction terms Sessions and SessionxAlliance. The instrumental variables assumptions are represented by the absence of direct paths from these three variables to PANSS18.

Two Stage Least Squares Estimator for Assessing Effect Modification by Process Variables

IV estimators including the 2SLS estimator can handle multiple endogenous variables provided a sufficient number of instruments are available. Ginestet et al. (2017) estimated the regression coefficients of a linear model for PANSS18 with endogenous explanatory variables Sessions, and SessionsxAlliance and a set of exogenous baseline covariates (including PANSS0 and Centre). 2SLS estimation was used with IVs treatment offer and interactions with treatment offer (including PANSS0xTherapy and CentrexTherapy). Figure 3 illustrates the predicted change in PANSS18 in the therapy arm with increasing number of therapy sessions and for different levels of therapeutic alliance. Note that due to the exclusion restriction the PANSS18 score predicted for zero sessions in the therapy arm is the same as that predicted for the control arm. For patients who can build a maximum alliance with the therapist (rescaled score zero), symptoms decrease as they receive more sessions. However, this relationship changes as the alliance rating worsens, with patients who have the most difficulty relating to their therapist (rescaled score -6) showing increased symptoms when attending more sessions.

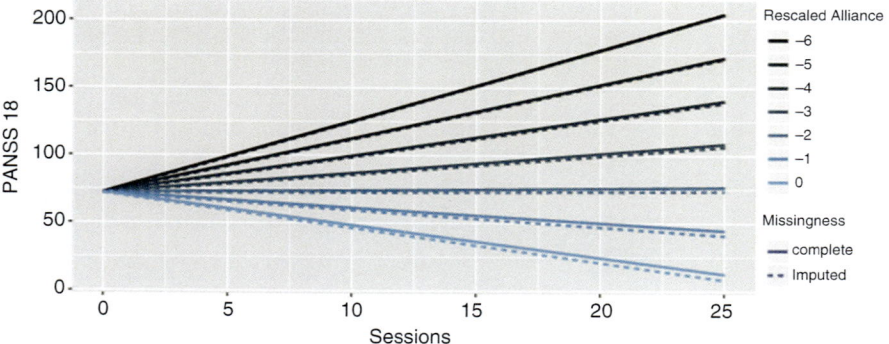

Fig. 3 Predicted PANSS18 scores for SoCRATES psychological therapies arm from 2SLS analysis* by sessions and alliance rating (Ginestet et al. 2017). (* Two methods were used to deal with missing data: Complete case analysis and multiple imputation)

Extensions

The assessment of treatment effect modification by process variables as described here has assumed that the relationship between treatment effect and a continuous "dose" variable such as the number of therapy sessions is linear (Maracy and Dunn 2011). Provided the data set is large enough, it also possible to allow for nonlinear dose-response relationships (Burgess et al. 2014, 2017).

IV estimators can remove bias at the cost of inflated variances, with the variance inflation depending on the strength of the IVs. An alternative approach is given by the Stein estimator which seeks to minimize the mean square error of the estimator and thus can accommodate small amounts of bias in order to avoid large variance increases; a demonstration using SoCRATES is provided by Ginestet et al. (2017).

Assessing Treatment Effect Mediation

This section is concerned with assessing how a treatment works through the application of mediation analysis. A *mediator* (M) is a variable that occurs in the causal pathway from an exposure (R) to an outcome variable (Y). It causes variation in the outcome and itself is caused to vary by the exposure variable. This causal chain implies a temporal relation in that R occurs before M and M occurs before Y. For simplicity, we consider the setting where both M and Y are continuous variables. Note that by definition the mediators are different to the process variables in the previous section, since mediators can be fully observed in all participants.

Figure 4 describes a linear structural equation model of mediation for the OASIS trial introduced previously. In general, random allocation of treatment R (therapy offer) has an effect (α) on an intermediate outcome M (insomnia). The intermediate outcome, in turn, has an effect (β) on the final outcome Y (paranoia). There is also a

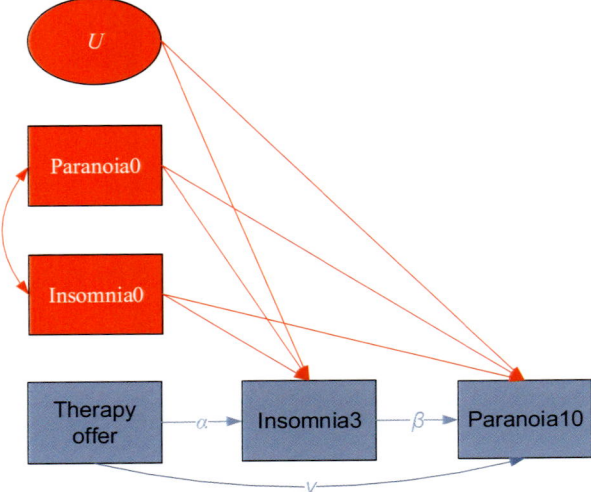

Fig. 4 Mediation model for the OASIS trial. (blue = causal mediation estimands, red = confounding paths)

possible "direct" effect of R on Y (γ), which represents any other pathway from R to Y not acting through M. The part of the influence of R on Y that is explained through the effect of R on M, and of M on Y is an "indirect" or mediated effect; and the intermediate variable, M, is a treatment effect mediator. Covariates could predict the mediator and/or the outcome, for example, the baseline measures of insomnia and paranoia. The U represents unmeasured confounders of the effect of M on Y, a critical point expanded on below; it is shown as a latent variable in this diagram. When M and Y are continuous, the total causal effect of R on Y, the ITT effect, can be decomposed into the sum of the direct and indirect effects, that is, ITT=$\gamma + \alpha\beta$.

Mediator Variables and Treatment Effect Mediation Estimands

To investigate a mediation hypothesis, the intermediate and the distal clinical outcome need to be observed for trial participants $i \in \{1, \ldots, n\}$

- $M_{i,\,\text{pre}}$ and $M_{i,\,\text{post}}$ are the values measured on a continuous mediator variable for participant i at baseline (pre-randomization) and post-randomization, respectively.
- $\mathbf{X}_i$ are a set of baseline variables measured pre-randomization, potentially including $M_{i,\,\text{pre}}$ and $Y_{i,\,\text{pre}}$.

Similarly to the clinical outcome, the following potential outcomes of the intermediate variable with respect to the randomization variable R can be defined as:

- $M_{i,\,\text{post}}(R = r) = M_{i,\,\text{post}}(r)$ the mediator outcome that would have been observed if individual i had been randomized to $r = 0,1$.

In order to formalize the notion that the outcome Y is caused by both R and M, the definition of the potential outcomes of the clinical outcome can be extended to $Y_{i,\,\text{post}}(R = r_1, M_{i,\,\text{post}} = M_{i,\,\text{post}}(r_2))$, the clinical outcome with treatment offer set to level r_1 and mediator variable $M_{i,\,\text{post}}$ set to level r_2 (which could be a different level to r_1). Using this nested potential outcomes notation, $Y_{i,\,\text{post}}(0, M_{i,\,\text{post}}(0))$ is the clinical outcome for a participant i when randomized to the control condition, and $Y_{i,\,\text{post}}(1, M_{i,\,\text{post}}(1))$ is the clinical outcome when randomized to the treatment.

This enables partitioning the (total) causal effect of the treatment offer for participant i as follows:

$$\nabla_i := Y_{i,\text{post}}(R = 1) - Y_{i,\text{post}}(R = 0)$$
$$= \{Y_{i,\text{post}}(1, M_{i,\text{post}}(0)) - Y_{i,\text{post}}(0, M_{i,\text{post}}(0))\}$$
$$+ \{Y_{i,\text{post}}(1, M_{i,\text{post}}(1)) - Y_{i,\text{post}}(1, M_{i,\text{post}}(0))\}$$

The first term of this decomposition is the *direct effect* of random allocation given the mediator was held at the level $M_{i,\,\text{post}}(0)$ that it takes under control offer. The second term is the effect of the change in the mediator values if the participant were allocated to the intervention arm (i.e., $R = 1$). The expected value of the first term is referred to as the *natural direct effect* (NDE), and that of the second term as the *natural indirect effect* (NIE) (Robins and Greenland 1992).

Regression Approach and Confounding Problem

One approach to estimating these mediation estimands would use two linear regression models allowing for an interaction between treatment offer and the mediator, with expectation over all participants:

$$\text{Mediator model}: \text{E}\left[M_{i,\,\text{post}}|R_i = r, \mathbf{X}_i = \mathbf{x}\right] = \mu + \alpha r + \delta'\mathbf{x}$$

$$\text{Outcome model}: \text{E}[Y_{i,\text{post}}|R_i = r, M_i = m, \mathbf{X}_i = \mathbf{x}] = \tau + \gamma r + \beta m + \lambda rm + \varphi'\mathbf{x}$$

In the absence of an $R \times M$ interaction, the NIE is estimated from the multiplication of the (estimated) effect of R on M and the effect of M on Y ($\alpha\beta$). The NDE is estimated by the effect of R on Y in the model for Y which also contains M (γ). In the presence of the $R \times M$ interaction, VanderWeele and Vansteelandt (2009) extend these formulas for the NIE and NDE and corresponding standard errors and also derive these for nonlinear models for M and Y. These have been fully implemented in standard statistical packages such as Stata, SAS, SPSS, and R (Valeri and VanderWeele 2013).

The parametric regression modeling approach provides consistent estimates of NDE and NIE provided the following assumptions hold:

- (A1) **No unmeasured treatment-outcome confounding given X**.
- (A2) **No unmeasured mediator-outcome confounding given X**.
- (A3) **No unmeasured treatment-mediator confounding given X**.
- (A4) Either **no effect of exposure that confounds the mediator-outcome relationship**, or **absence of an** $R \times M$ **interaction**.

Assumption (A1) is required to estimate total (ITT) effects and is satisfied by randomization in a trial, as is (A3). No unmeasured mediator-outcome confounding (A2) is possibly the most difficult to satisfy, as investigators can never rule out the presence of some factors which influence both the mediator and the outcome. If these are measured, then they can be incorporated into the statistical models as elements of $\mathbf{X}$. However, if these are not measured or modeled, then the estimate of β will be biased. As this contributes directly to the calculation of the NIE, this estimate will also be biased. Furthermore, since β is estimated by fitting the outcome model, estimates of other coefficients in this model will also be subject to bias including the estimate of NDE (γ) (Emsley et al. 2010). A similar issue arises with the presence of measurement error in the mediator, which will attenuate the size of β and lead to underestimation of the NIE. Some solutions to the problem of measurement error are provided by Pickles et al. (2015) and Goldsmith et al. (2018a).

One particular issue is the appropriate treatment of variables $M_{i,\,\text{pre}}$ and $Y_{i,\,\text{pre}}$ in the outcome and mediator models, since both are likely to be predictive of both $M_{i,\,\text{post}}$ and $Y_{i,\,\text{post}}$. In a total effects analysis, inclusion of baseline variables in the statistical model increases precision of the ITT estimate but is not required for bias reduction. However, in the mediation context, they are confounders of the $M - Y$

Table 2 Mediation analyses results in OASIS trial. Mediator is insomnia at week 3. Paranoia was measured at week 10. All effect estimates are statistically significant at $p < 0.001$

Outcome	Total effect* (95% CI)	Direct effect (95% CI)	Indirect effect (95% CI)	Percent mediated
Paranoia	−2.27 (−3.03; −1.51)	−0.97 (−1.80; −0.14)	−1.31 (−1.60; −1.02)	57.8%

relationship and so need to be adjusted for in order to prevent bias in the estimation of the NIE (Landau et al. 2018).

Linear Regression Approach for Assessing Treatment Effect Mediation
Now consider the OASIS trial from Fig. 4. In total, 3,755 University students were recruited and the study was conducted entirely online. Students were randomized to receive either digital cognitive behavior therapy for insomnia (Sleepio) or usual practice (then offered Sleepio after the end of follow-up). The outcomes of insomnia and paranoia were measured at 0, 3, 10, and 22 weeks; for this illustration, we will focus on 3 and 10 week timepoints. Insomnia was measured using the Sleep Condition Indicator 8-item version (variable Insomnia3) and paranoia using the Green et al. Paranoid Thought Scales (Paranoia10).

A full description of the trial and the measures is provided in (Freeman et al. 2015) and the results in (Freeman et al. 2017).

The intervention improved the insomnia score compared to control at 3 weeks (adjusted mean difference 2.62 (95% CI: 2.19; 3.06), Cohen's d effect size 0.61) and smaller but significant reductions in paranoia at 10 weeks (−2.22 (−2.98; −1.45), $d = 0.19$). Considering that this intervention only targets sleep, and not paranoia directly, the theoretical model is that sleep is on the causal pathway from the intervention to paranoia. This needs to be demonstrated empirically by testing whether sleep at week 3 mediates the effect of the intervention on clinical outcomes at week 10, adjusting for baseline levels of insomnia and the respective outcome being considered.

Table 2 shows the results of the mediation analyses. It demonstrates that nearly 60% of the effect on paranoia is mediated through an indirect effect on reducing insomnia. The 95% confidence intervals for both NDE and NIE excluded 0. Since the intervention specifically targeted sleep, the significance of the NDEs can be interpreted as representing the effect of the intervention through other mechanisms, including possibly aspects of sleep not captured by the measure of insomnia used.

Assessing Treatment Effectiveness in Populations Defined by the Value of an Intermediate Outcome

In the previous section, the question of interest was whether the treatment was acting on the clinical outcome through a specified target mechanism. In this section, the question is how to deal with variables on the causal pathway from treatment to clinical outcome that might be considered a "nuisance" factor; that is, the treatment is not designed to act through these factors but they do affect the effectiveness of the treatment itself.

As an example, consider again the MIRA trial, and the role of condom use as a secondary intervention. Here, the question of interest is how effective the trial interventions are in the presence or absence of condom use, rather than whether the effect of the interventions is acting through condom use. Note that while condom use is a post-randomization variable, this scenario is different to that considering process variables such as therapeutic alliance earlier in the chapter. For process variables, interest centers on assessing the effect of treatment within subpopulations defined by aspects of their experience of the active intervention, for example, whether the alliance that a patient would be able to build with their therapist if offered therapy affects the size of the treatment effect. In the current context, the research question addressed is whether the treatment effect varies in the hypothetical populations where the value of a mediator variable is set at a fixed value for everybody.

Effectiveness Estimands for Hypothetical Populations Defined by an Intermediate Variable

The *controlled direct effect* (CDE) of treatment offer on outcome at mediator level m is defined as:

$$\mathrm{E}\left[Y_{i,\,\mathrm{post}}(R=1, M_{i,\,\mathrm{post}}=m) - Y_{i,\,post}(R=0, M_{i,\,\mathrm{post}}=m)\right].$$

It measures the average effect of the treatment offer for patients for whom the value of the intermediate outcome is set to fixed value m. This effect may be of interest for several hypothetical populations defined by suitable settings m. In the condom use example, m might take the value 0 for no condom use, and 1 for condom use. Therefore, we might wish to know the effectiveness of the diaphragm and lubricant gel (i.e., the offer of these) in both the presence ($M=1$) and absence ($M=0$) of condom use at the population level. These estimands would be defined as:

$$\mathrm{CDE}(1) = \mathrm{E}\left[Y_{i,\,\mathrm{post}}(R=1, M_{i,\,\mathrm{post}}=1) - Y_{i,\,\mathrm{post}}(R=0, M_{i,\,\mathrm{post}}=1)\right]$$

$$\mathrm{CDE}(0) = \mathrm{E}\left[Y_{i,\,\mathrm{post}}(R=1, M_{i,\,\mathrm{post}}=0) - Y_{i,\,\mathrm{post}}(R=0, M_{i,\,\mathrm{post}}=0)\right]$$

There are two important points to note here. The first is that these estimands are population level summaries and not conditional or within subgroups. In the example, it is not the effectiveness of the treatment in the subgroup of participants who used condoms that is assessed, but the effectiveness if everyone in the population used condoms. The second point is that the CDEs will only be different in the presence of an $R \times M$ interaction on Y. If this interaction is not present, then the level of $M_{i,\,\mathrm{post}}$ does not affect the effect of R on Y, and so $\mathrm{CDE}(1) = \mathrm{CDE}(0) = \mathrm{NDE}$.

Estimating a Controlled Direct Effect

The same parametric regression modeling approach outlined previously can be used to estimate the CDE and requires both the "no unmeasured treatment-outcome confounding (A1)" and the "no unmeasured mediator-outcome confounding (A2)" assumptions to hold.

Returning to the MIRA example, 5045 HIV-free women were randomized (2523 to the intervention, 2522 to control) and overall HIV incidence was 4.0% per 100 woman-years: 4.1% in the intervention group (n = 2472) and 3.9% in the control group (n = 2476), corresponding to a relative risk of 1.05 for the intention-to-treat effect (95% CI 0.84-1.30). However, the proportion of women using condoms at their last sexual encounter was significantly lower in the intervention than in the control group (54% vs. 85% of measurement visits, $p < 0.0001$). This posed the question as to how the groups had similar incidence of HIV given that condom use, a known preventative measure for HIV, was significantly higher in the control group. In particular, it poses the question as to whether the lack of a difference between the groups is because the control group are taking alternative preventative measures outside of the trial treatments, and the CDE(1) and CDE(0) estimands then naturally become of interest.

For CDE(1), the estimated relative risk by visit 8 of HIV infection for assignment to the intervention versus control group, had all participants been constrained to always use condoms at all visits, was 0.96 (95% CI 0.61-1.48). By contrast, for CDE (0) the estimated analogous relative risk by visit 8 of HIV infection had all participants never used condoms at all visits was 0.59 (0.23-3.17). Full details of the analysis are reported in Rosenblum et al. (2009).

Extensions

The parametric regression model approach does not allow for unobserved confounders between mediator and outcome, and it is incumbent on the analyst to carefully measure and adjust for important predictors of the exposure, mediator, and outcome.

There are two alternative approaches which either relax or test sensitivity to this assumption. The first is the instrumental variables method described in the first two sections of this chapter. In the mediation context, randomization is no longer suitable as an instrument for the endogenous variable M since we are trying to estimate the effect of R on M and Y (as seen in Fig. 4). Instead we require additional exogenous variables to act as instruments. Emsley et al. (2010) discuss the necessary identifying assumptions to use baseline by treatment offer interactions as instruments and Dunn et al. (2013) discuss how this can be built into a trial design. Ginestet et al. (2020) present a Stein estimator approach combining the IV approach with the parametric regression approach to produce estimators with the lowest mean square error.

The second approach is to conduct sensitivity analysis on the strength of any unmeasured confounding, and the impact these have on estimates of the NIE and NDE. The various sensitivity approaches for single parameters are summarized in VanderWeele (2015), while (McCandless and Somers n.d.) present a Bayesian sensitivity analysis for all relationships simultaneously.

The presentation in this chapter has focused on defining mediated effects under a single mediator measured once post-randomization. More realistically, there are likely to be repeated measures of a single mediator (and outcome), and this relationship can be estimated using a variety of longitudinal approaches (Goldsmith et al. 2018b). Similarly, there could be multiple mediators which require extending the definitions of a natural indirect effect if the mediators are sequentially ordered

(Daniel et al. 2015; Albert and Nelson 2011), etc.) or using so-called "interventional (in)direct effects" if the structural dependence between the multiple mediators is unknown (Vansteelandt and Daniel 2017).

Summary and Conclusion

The approaches considered here are of a confirmatory nature. They assume that the investigator has a theory regarding the mechanisms by which the treatment works. Such theories can then be translated into statistical hypotheses regarding treatment effect modification by process variables or treatment effect mediation by intermediate outcomes. Mechanistic theories often exist. Thus, the causal methods discussed in this chapter can be used to confirm such theories and/or inform the development of new interventions.

Keyfacts

- When estimands other than ITT are of interest in an RCT confounding can be an issue.
- Methods from the causal inference field can help to define relevant causal estimands.
- Instrumental variables methods can be used to assess the complier average causal effect under nonadherence with randomized treatments and to examine treatment effect modification by process variables.
- Parametric regression models can be used to assess how a treatment works by estimating natural direct and indirect effects.

Cross-References

- ▶ Adherence Adjusted Estimates in Randomized Clinical Trials
- ▶ Cluster Randomized Trials
- ▶ Complex Intervention Trials
- ▶ Controlling Bias in Randomized Clinical Trials
- ▶ Estimands and Sensitivity Analyses
- ▶ Intention to Treat and Alternative Approaches
- ▶ Reading and Interpreting the Literature on Randomized Controlled Trials

Acknowledgments This work was supported by a grant from the UK Medical Research Council (MRC) (project Grants MR/K006185/1). R.E. was further supported by the MRC North West Hub for Trials Methodology Research (MR/K025635/1). S.L. and R.E are part-funded by the National Institute for Health Research (NIHR) Biomedical Research Centre at South London and Maudsley NHS Foundation Trust and King's College London. S.L. is also supported by the NIHR Applied Research Collaboration South London (NIHR ARC South London) at King's College Hospital

NHS Foundation Trust. The views expressed are those of the authors and not necessarily those of the NIHR or the Department of Health and Social Care.

The work described here is the result of many years of collaborative research. The authors would like to thank Cedric Ginestet, Kim Goldsmith, Andrew Pickles, and Ian White for their contributions and suggestions. The authors dedicate this chapter to their late friend, colleague and mentor Graham Dunn, with whom these ideas were developed through many years of work.

References

Albert JM, Nelson S (2011) Generalized causal mediation analysis. Biometrics 67:1028–1038

Angrist JD, Imbens GW, Rubin DB (1996) Identification of causal effects using instrumental variables. J Am Stat Assoc 91:444–455

Burgess S, Davies NM, Thompson SG, E. PIC-InterAct Consortium (2014) Instrumental variable analysis with a nonlinear exposure-outcome relationship. Epidemiology 25:877–885

Burgess S, Small DS, Thompson SG (2017) A review of instrumental variable estimators for Mendelian randomization. Stat Methods Med Res 26:2333–2355

Clarke PS, Windmeijer F (2012) Instrumental variable estimators for binary outcomes. J Am Stat Assoc 107:1638–1652

Daniel RM, De Stavola BL, Cousens SN, Vansteelandt S (2015) Causal mediation analysis with multiple mediators. Biometrics 71:1–14

Dodd S, White IR, Williamson P (2017a) A framework for the design, conduct and interpretation of randomised controlled trials in the presence of treatment changes. Trials 18

Dodd S, Williamson P, White IR (2017b) Adjustment for treatment changes in epilepsy trials: a comparison of causal methods for time-to-event outcomes. Stat Methods Med Res 0:1–17

Dowrick C, Dunn G, Ayuso-Mateos JL, Dalgard OS, Page H, Lehtinen V, Casey P, Wilkinson C, Vazquez-Barquero JL, Wilkinson G, Grp O (2000) Problem solving treatment and group psychoeducation for depression: multicentre randomised controlled trial. Br Med J 321:1450–1454

Dunn G, Bentall R (2007) Modelling treatment-effect heterogeneity in randomized controlled trials of complex interventions (psychological treatments). Stat Med 26:4719–4745

Dunn G, Maracy M, Dowrick C, Ayuso-Mateos JL, Dalgard OS, Page H, Lehtinen V, Casey P, Wilkinson C, Vazquez-Barquero JL, Wilkinson G, Grp O (2003) Estimating psychological treatment effects from a randomised controlled trial with both non-compliance and loss to follow-up. Br J Psychiatry 183:323–331

Dunn G, Emsley R, Liu HH, Landau S (2013) Integrating biomarker information within trials to evaluate treatment mechanisms and efficacy for personalised medicine. Clin Trials 10:709–719

Dunn G, Emsley R, Liu HH, Landau S, Green J, White I, Pickles A (2015) Evaluation and validation of social and psychological markers in randomised trials of complex interventions in mental health: a methodological research programme. Health Technol Assess 19

EMA (2017) ICH E9 (R1) addendum on estimands and sensitivity analysis in clinical trials to the guideline on statistical principles for clinical trials. In: European Medicines Agency

Emsley R, Dunn G, White IR (2010) Mediation and moderation of treatment effects in randomised controlled trials of complex interventions. Stat Methods Med Res 19:237–270

Fischer-Lapp K, Goetghebeur E (1999) Practical properties of some structural mean analyses of the effect of compliance in randomized trials. Control Clin Trials 20:531–546

Frangakis CE, Rubin DB (2002) Principal stratification in causal inference. Biometrics 58:21–29

Freeman D, Sheaves B, Goodwin GM, Yu LM, Harrison PJ, Emsley R, Bostock S, Foster RG, Wadekar V, Hinds C, Espie CA (2015) Effects of cognitive behavioural therapy for insomnia on the mental health of university students: study protocol for a randomized controlled trial. Trials 16(8)

Freeman D, Sheaves B, Goodwin GM, Yu LM, Nickless A, Harrison PJ, Emsley R, Luik AI, Foster RG, Wadekar V, Hinds C, Gumley A, Jones R, Lightman S, Jones S, Bentall R, Kinderman P, Rowse G, Brugha T, Blagrove M, Gregory AM, Fleming L, Walklet E, Glazebrook C, Davies EB, Hollis C, Haddock G, John B, Coulson M, Fowler D, Pugh K, Cape J, Moseley P, Brown G, Hughes C, Obonsawin M, Coker S, Watkins E, Schwannauer M, MacMahon K, Siriwardena AN, Espie CA (2017) The effects of improving sleep on mental health (OASIS): a randomised controlled trial with mediation analysis. Lancet Psychiatry 4:749–758

Ginestet CE, Emsley R, Landau S (2017) Dose-response modeling in mental health using stein-like estimators with instrumental variables. Stat Med 36:1696–1714

Ginestet CE, Emsley R, Landau S (2020) Stein-like estimators for causal mediation analysis in randomized trials. Stat Methods Med Res 29:1129–1148

Goldsmith LP, Lewis SW, Dunn G, Bentall RP (2015) Psychological treatments for early psychosis can be beneficial or harmful, depending on the therapeutic alliance: an instrumental variable analysis. Psychol Med 45:2365–2373

Goldsmith KA, Chalder T, White PD, Sharpe M, Pickles A (2018a) Measurement error, time lag, unmeasured confounding: considerations for longitudinal estimation of the effect of a mediator in randomised clinical trials. Stat Methods Med Res 27:1615–1633

Goldsmith KA, MacKinnon DP, Chalder T, White PD, Sharpe M, Pickles A (2018b) Tutorial: the practical application of longitudinal structural equation mediation models in clinical trials. Psychol Methods 23:191–207

Landau S, Emsley R, Dunn G (2018) Beyond total treatment effects in randomised controlled trials: baseline measurement of intermediate outcomes needed to reduce confounding in mediation investigations. Clin Trials 15:247–256

Maracy M, Dunn G (2011) Estimating dose-response effects in psychological treatment trials: the role of instrumental variables. Stat Methods Med Res 20:191–215

McCandless LC, Somers JM (n.d.) Bayesian sensitivity analysis for unmeasured confounding in causal mediation analysis. Stat Methods Med Res 0:0962280217729844

Padian NS, van der Straten A, Ramjee G, Chipato T, de Bruyn G, Blanchard K, Shiboski S, Montgomery ET, Fancher H, Cheng H, Rosenblum M, van der Laan M, Jewell N, McIntyre J, Team M (2007) Diaphragm and lubricant gel for prevention of HIV acquisition in southern African women: a randomised controlled trial. Lancet 370:251–261

Pickles A, Croudace T (2010) Latent mixture models for multivariate and longitudinal outcomes. Stat Methods Med Res 19:271–289

Pickles A, Harris V, Green J, Aldred C, McConachie H, Slonims V, Le Couteur A, Hudry K, Charman T, PACT Consortium (2015) Treatment mechanism in the MRC preschool autism communication trial: implications for study design and parent-focussed therapy for children. J Child Psychol Psychiatry 56:162–170

Robins JM, Greenland S (1992) Identifiability and exchangeability for direct adn indirect effects. Epidemiology 3:143–155

Rosenblum M, Jewell NP, van der Laan M, Shiboski S, van der Straten A, Padian N (2009) Analysing direct effects in randomized trials with secondary interventions: an application to human immunodeficiency virus prevention trials. J R Stat SocA Stat Soc 172:443–465

Rubin DB (1974) Estimating causal effects of treatmets in randomized and nonrandomized studies. J Educ Psychol 66:688–701

Sharples L, Papachristofi O, Rex S, Landau S (2020) Exploring mechanisms of action in trials of complex surgical interventions using mediation. Clin Trials. in press

Sheiner LB, Rubin DB (1995) Intention-to-treat analysis and goals of clinical trials. Clin Pharmacol Ther 57:6–15

Tarrier N, Lewis S, Haddock G, Bentall R, Drake R, Kinderman P, Kingdon D, Siddle R, Everitt J, Leadley K, Benn A, Grazebrook K, Haley C, Akhtar S, Davies L, Palmer S, Dunn G (2004) Cognitive-behavioural therapy in first-episode and early schizophrenia – 18-month follow-up of a randomised controlled trial. Br J Psychiatry 184:231–239

Tchetgen EJT, Walter S, Vansteelandt S, Martinussen T, Glymour M (2015) Instrumental variable estimation in a survival context. Epidemiol 26:402–410

Valeri L, VanderWeele TJ (2013) Mediation analysis allowing for exposure-mediator interactions and causal interpretation: theoretical assumptions and implementation with SAS and SPSS macros. Psychol Methods 18:137–150

VanderWeele TJ (2015) Explanation in causal inference: methods for mediation and interaction. Chapman Hall CRC, New York

VanderWeele TJ, Vansteelandt S (2009) Conceptual issues concerning mediation, interventions and composition. Stat Interface 2:457–468

Vansteelandt S, Daniel RM (2017) Interventional effects for mediation analysis with multiple mediators. Epidemiology 28:258–265

Wooldridge JM (2010) Econometric analysis of cross section and panel data. MIT Press

Development and Validation of Risk Prediction Models

101

Damien Drubay, Ben Van Calster, and Stefan Michiels

Contents

Introduction	2004
Different Types of Risk Prediction Models	2005
Developing a Risk Prediction Model	2006
Main Objective and Study Design	2006
Sample Size	2007
Data Collection	2007
Missing Data	2008
Variable Selection	2008
Modeling of Continuous Predictors	2009
Interaction Effects	2009
Using High-Dimensional Data	2010
Flexible Machine Learning Algorithms	2011
Model Validation	2011
Metrics of Model Performance	2011
Apparent Validation	2017
Internal Validation	2017
External Model Validation	2019
Model Reporting	2020
Demonstrating Clinical Impact	2020
Conclusion	2021
Key Points	2021
References	2022

D. Drubay · S. Michiels (✉)
INSERM U1018, CESP, Paris-Saclay University, UVSQ, Villejuif, France

Gustave Roussy, Service de Biostatistique et d'Epidémiologie, Villejuif, France
e-mail: damien.drubay@gustaveroussy.fr; stefan.michiels@gustaveroussy.fr

B. Van Calster
Department of Development and Regeneration, KU Leuven, Leuven, Belgium

Department of Biomedical Data Sciences, Leiden University Medical Center, Leiden, The Netherlands
e-mail: ben.vancalster@kuleuven.be

© Springer Nature Switzerland AG 2022
S. Piantadosi, C. L. Meinert (eds.), *Principles and Practice of Clinical Trials*,
https://doi.org/10.1007/978-3-319-52636-2_138

Abstract

There has been increased interest in the use of clinical risk prediction models for decision-making in medicine for patient care. This has been accelerated through the focus on precision medicine, the revolution in omics data, and increasing use of randomized controlled trial and electronic health record databases. These models are expected to assist diagnostic assessment, prognostication, and therapeutic decision-making. Randomized controlled trial data are highly relevant for modeling treatment benefit and treatment effect heterogeneity. The development and validation of prediction models requires careful methodology and reporting, and an evidence-based approach is needed to bring risk prediction models to clinical practice. This chapter provides an overview of the key steps and considerations to develop and validate risk prediction models. We comment on the role of clinical trials throughout the process. A risk prediction model for the occurrence of breast cancer is used as an example.

Keywords

Prediction models · Diagnostic · Prognostic · Treatment effect · Precision medicine · Development · Predictors · Validation · Calibration · Discrimination · Utility

Introduction

Risk prediction models are becoming increasingly important for personalized clinical decision-making. Such models aim to provide patient-specific risk estimates of a clinical event, conditional on a set of measurements for an individual patient (Steyerberg 2008). Such risk estimates should be seen as an assumed likelihood of the event for individuals with similar measurements. It is important to underscore that prediction models are not primarily interested in causal effects but rather in providing reasonable event likelihoods that can be used to counsel patients or support clinical decisions.

Some examples are the Framingham risk score to predict the risk of coronary heart disease (Damen et al. 2016), the Tyrer-Cuzick model to predict the risk of developing breast cancer in the general population (Tyrer et al. 2004), the prognosTILs model to predict survival in early-stage triple-negative breast cancer patients (Loi et al. 2019), and the SYNTAX score II to predict mortality in patients treated for complex coronary artery disease using coronary artery bypass graft surgery or percutaneous coronary intervention (Farooq et al. 2013).

This chapter provides an overview of the key steps and considerations when developing and validating risk prediction models. This overview focuses on the use of classical statistical models (e.g., logistic regression or Cox proportional hazard regression). Where appropriate, comments on more flexible machine learning algorithms are provided.

Different Types of Risk Prediction Models

Risk prediction models can focus on a wide variety of clinical outcomes. We discern diagnostic, prognostic, and treatment effect prediction models. First, diagnostic prediction models estimate the probability that a patient has an event or disease at the time of examination. A typical outcome is, for example, whether a tumor is benign or malignant in order to decide how to manage the patient. The predicted outcome for diagnostic models is typically categorical in nature (i.e., binary or multinomial). Logistic regression techniques are commonly used statistical approaches to develop diagnostic prediction models. A high predicted probability can be used to refer a patient to further testing or to start treatment. Diagnostic models are commonly derived from cross-sectional data.

Second, prognostic models estimate the risk that a clinically relevant endpoint will happen in the future. In this case, the outcome is often the time to event and modeled using survival techniques such as the Cox proportional hazard regression model. If the time horizon is fixed and clearly defined, the outcome may also be categorical. A typical outcome for prognostic models is mortality. For example, prognostic risk prediction models (Steyerberg et al. 2013) may aim to predict the development of the disease in order to assist clinicians with therapeutic decision-making. Prognostic models are typically derived on cohort data, including electronic health records (EHR), or on data from randomized controlled trials.

Third, treatment effect models estimate the probability of a clinically relevant outcome conditional on having received particular treatments (Kent et al. 2018). Such risk prediction models integrate one or more treatment modifiers. In the context of precision medicine, in which medical decision-making is tailored to characteristics of individual patients, these risk prediction models aim to predict which patients benefit most from interventions (Hingorani et al. 2013). The predicted outcome for such models is usually of prognostic nature. The most appropriate way to develop a risk prediction model for treatment benefit is using data from a randomized clinical trial (Pajouheshnia et al. 2019) in which the treatments have been randomly allocated to patients, by using interaction effects of treatment with baseline characteristics (Michiels et al. 2016). However, treatment effect models may also result from the integration of absolute risk predictions from cohort data with relative treatment effects from randomized controlled trials. An example of such a strategy is the Adjuvant!Online model for prognosis of early breast cancer patients.

Depending on the type of model and the clinical context, predictors can be demographic variables, medical history assessments, clinicopathological characteristics, environmental exposures, biomarkers (De Bin et al. 2014), imaging (Bi et al. 2019) parameters, and others.

In this chapter, some concepts will be illustrated by the comparison of prognostic models using a data set of 2,392,998 observations to predict the 1-year probability of invasive or ductal cancer (11,638 events) obtained from the Breast Cancer Surveillance Consortium (BCSC) (Barlow et al. 2006). A logistic regression prediction model based only on patient age in 10 categories, the factor that is used for breast cancer screening guidelines, will be compared to a prediction model using the predictors from the BCSC model (Vachon et al. 2015): age in ten categories, race/Hispanic ethnicity, family history of breast in a first-degree relatives, history of a breast biopsy, and BI-RADS® breast density. Age was not available as continuous variable in the data set. The part of the dataset previously used as training set for the original BCSC model (Vachon et al. 2015) (75% = 1,795,139 observations, 8767 events) was used to train the two models. The remaining part (25% = 597,859 observations, 2871 events) was used as a test set.

Developing a Risk Prediction Model

Main Objective and Study Design

The first step is to evaluate the context. For which clinical application should we predict which outcome event in which target population? It is important to know what risk prediction models already exist for the same context and whether a new model is really necessary. The literature is abound with prediction models, so often it is better to use, update, or validate an existing model rather than to add a new model to the collection.

Next, we should be clear about the moment at which the prediction is needed in clinical practice, to determine which type of data we need to develop a model to make these predictions. Usually, prospective data are preferred because there are more opportunities to tailor the study data to the prediction modeling context, for example, by collecting and standardizing the important predictors and clinical outcome. Retrospective data are to be used as is, even though important predictors may not be available, largely missing, or not measured in an optimal way. Currently, EHR are an increasingly popular source of data for developing prognostic risk prediction models for use in routine clinical practice, with the argument that EHR consists of information exactly from routine clinical practice. However, such data carry many disadvantages in terms of quality and standardization that will compromise optimal predictions. The opposite is also important: routine clinical practice should evolve over time such that it better captures the key measurements for making optimally clinically relevant predictions. Developing risk models on data from randomized clinical trials has many advantages (Pajouheshnia et al. 2019) with respect to standardization but always carries the limitation of lack of generalizability depending on the stringency of the inclusion and exclusion criteria. The use of data from case-cohort or (nested) case-control designs is less efficient, but they may be used in the case of rare outcomes or expensive candidate predictor measurements. Such designs artificially change the outcome event prevalence/incidence. The resulting risk model should be corrected accordingly, in order to avoid predicted risks that are systematically too low or high.

The study should include individuals who are representative of the target population. For example, the study data should not include (only) adults if the model is intended to be used in children. To enhance model generalizability and transportability, it is recommended to use multicenter data or to combine individual patient data from multiple studies. In this case, the study should devote appropriate attention to heterogeneity between centers or studies (Riley et al. 2016).

Sample Size

Sample size is one of the main building blocks of the study design. In the context of risk prediction models, sample size considerations should not be based on power but rather on whether we can develop a model that produces reliable risk estimates. When developing a prediction model, we should avoid overfitting, which refers to the situation where the model captures too much idiosyncrasies ("noise") of the development data. The more a prediction model captures noise, the less well the model will generalize to new data. In practice, the result is that risk predictions are too extreme: high risks are overestimated, whereas low risks are underestimated. Overfitting is typically the result of fitting a model that is too complex for the available data. For binary or survival outcomes, a well-known rule of thumb has been to include ten events per variable (Peduzzi et al. 1996). Notice that this refers to variables that are considered for inclusion, not just to variables that end up in the final prediction model. This refers to model development without the use of data-driven variable selection (e.g., stepwise procedures). Recent research has indicated that this rule of thumb is too general and is usually insufficient (Van Smeden et al. 2018). Several propositions of more theoretically justified criteria were recently proposed for continuous, binary, or survival outcomes (Riley et al. 2019).

A large proportion of clinical risk prediction models have been developed as a secondary analysis of data from an observational or interventional study. In these cases, the sample size was usually based on the primary objective of the study. In order to avoid overfitting, the modeling strategy for the prediction model may have to be simplified to the available sample size. Possible simplifications include that less predictors and/or less nonlinear and interaction effects (cf. supra) are considered. If too much simplification is required, perhaps the data are insufficient for developing a prediction model.

When sample size is low, penalized regression methods have been recommended. These methods aim to keep the model coefficients low in order to keep overfitting under control. It has been suggested that penalization is useful up to 20 events per variable (Steyerberg et al. 2001). The most common methods are ridge (or L2), lasso (or L1), and elastic net (combination of ridge and lasso). The key difference between ridge and lasso is that the latter also performs variable selection by penalizing some coefficients to 0.

Data Collection

It is important to carefully identify the candidate predictor variables. These variables should be available at the very moment the prediction is to be made in clinical practice. The identification of candidate predictors should maximally rely on a priori domain knowledge, in order to limit further data-driven variable selection to a minimum. In addition to domain knowledge, it makes sense to prioritize variables that are easy/cheap to collect. To the extent that this is possible, variable and outcome definitions should be clear and standardized in advance, in order to control the consequences of measurement error (Luijken et al. 2019). When using retrospective observational data, this is often problematic. In a similar vein, when possible the amount of missing data should be minimized.

Missing Data

Even with the best design and data collection procedure, missing data is unavoidable (Janssen et al. 2009). It is good practice to consider plausible "missingness mechanisms," i.e., reasons that lead to the unavailability of certain measurements. Missing values may be caused by non-compliance to treatment, dropout, measurement errors, and lack of clinical need to perform the measurement, among others. It is safe to assume that missing values are not "missing completely at random," unless there are very convincing arguments for believing they are. Hence, ignoring patients with missing values is likely to induce selection bias and poor generalizability of the resulting risk predictions (Sterne et al. 2009). A complete case approach is therefore discouraged as a default approach. There are many approaches to deal with missing values. Simple ad hoc methods such as mean imputation or last observation carried forward are known to induce bias and should be avoided. Multiple imputation of missing values is the most commonly used and recommended approach. Multiple imputation can be readily implemented using methods such as multivariate imputation by chained equations (MICE) (White et al. 2011). Nevertheless, it is important to note that the imputation model in MICE be carefully set up and that the outcome to be predicted is included in the imputation process (Vergouwe et al. 2010). When the proportion of missing values per variable is very low, single stochastic imputation (which can also be done using MICE) may be a solution that avoids complicated analyses of multiple imputed data. On the contrary, a high proportion of missing data (e.g., more than 20%) may suggest that the predictor is difficult to collect, limiting its use in practice. In these cases, consider exclusion of the variable from the prediction model.

Variable Selection

Due to the trade-off between interpretability, user friendliness, and predictive accuracy, the selection of predictors is essential. It is well known that data-driven variable selection procedures such as stepwise selection or backward elimination lead to exaggerated coefficients and hence overfitting (Steyerberg 2008; Steyerberg et al. 2018). The consequences are less serious when the number of events per variable is very high (e.g., 50 or more), or when the criteria for including or eliminating variables are very lenient in order to have weaker data-driven selection. The issue is that model selection and coefficient estimation are done on the same data, leading to "testimation bias." Therefore, the recommendation is to rely on a priori selection as much as possible. Such a priori selection may still be followed by a limited data-driven procedure. A candidate predictor could also be of interest if it provides a more reproducible, cheaper, or more accurate measurement of an already existing predictor that has proven clinical utility so that the clinical prediction rule could be updated (Michiels et al. 2011).

Modeling of Continuous Predictors

Although it is common practice to dichotomize continuous predictors when adding them to a risk prediction model, this should be avoided (Royston et al. 2006). It leads to a loss of information, and such modeling is biologically implausible. Sometimes, researchers categorize continuous predictors into, say, 10 groups, which was unfortunately done in the publicly available BCSC data set we used for illustration. Such an approach will capture some of the nonlinearity, if present, but should nevertheless be avoided for the same reasons that dichotomization should be avoided. Rather, continuous variables should be modeled continuously. Ideally, the existence of a nonlinear relationship with the outcome should be taken into account. Common approaches for allowing nonlinear relationships are the use of a transformation, the use of fractional polynomials, or the use of spline functions. The logarithmic transformation is very popular, but such a transformation should not simply be considered when a variable is far from normally distributed, although positively skewed predictors such as biomarkers often appear to have a log-linear relationship with the outcome.

Nowadays, the use of smooth functions such as splines or fractional polynomials can be easily implemented using standard statistical software such as R, Stata, or SAS. Modeling nonlinear associations adds complexity (degrees of freedom) to the model. Therefore, when sample size is modest, it may still be a reasonable strategy to assume linearity upfront.

Interaction Effects

An interaction effect means that the association of a predictor with the outcome depends on the value of another predictor. This is typically modeled by adding the product of both predictors as an additional term in the model. In clinical prediction problems, the addition of interaction effects will usually not strongly improve predictive performance relative to a main effect model. Of course, there are notable exceptions, usually when interaction effects are qualitative. For example, to predict early pregnancy loss, size of the gestational sac interacts with the presence of a fetal heartbeat (Bottomley et al. 2013). When a heartbeat is present, small gestational sacs increase the risk of early pregnancy loss. When a heartbeat is not present, large gestational sacs increase the risk of early pregnancy loss.

Considering interaction effects again adds complexity to the modeling strategy. It is recommended to prespecify a limited number of interaction terms of potential interest, if any. Also, if sample size is limited, consider to assume additivity of the main effects (unless there is a priori knowledge of the existence of an indispensable interaction effect). Finally, assessment of nonlinearity should typically precede any assessment of interaction effects. Inappropriate modeling of continuous variables may lead to the detection of spurious interactions.

For treatment effect models, the situation is different. Here, the very aim of the model is to assess the outcome risk depending on the received treatment. Consequently, the addition of interaction terms of baseline predictions with treatment is a key aspect in this situation (Kent et al. 2018). This approach has a serious risk of overfitting. To control this risk, a reasonable recommendation is to only include interaction terms that are considered important or plausible a priori and to fit the model using penalized regression (Van Klaveren et al. 2019). Even then, robust modeling of interaction terms requires much more data than robust modeling of main effects.

Using High-Dimensional Data

High-dimensional data like genomic or genetic data and imaging are expected to increase the performance of risk prediction models. However, their development is difficult, and their superiority against more simple models including only standard clinical factors is still not clearly demonstrated. Indeed, there are several caveats due to the curse of dimensionality. Sample size is often small relatively to the number of variables. When the number of variables increases, the number of candidate models increases exponentially with the number of predictors (2^p, ignoring interactions and nonlinear effects). The comparison of all these models becomes rapidly computationally difficult, especially if the candidate models are complex or include random effects. Beyond the computational issues, in the high-dimensional data setting (number of individuals < number of variables), maximum likelihood estimation fails because there is no unique solution, i.e., different combinations of parameter values correspond to the same likelihood. In these settings, the parameters are non-identifiable, and the model is singular (in opposition to regular model). Several methods have been developed to build high-dimensional regression models. Sparse methods based on shrinkage methods such as the LASSO can lead to acceptable prediction accuracy of models but provide biased estimates of model coefficients and their variances. More research is needed regarding calibration performance of these models. For the development of treatment effect models with high-dimensional data, the use of shrinkage methods has also been advocated (Ternès et al. 2017).

An interesting compromise when faced with high-dimensional data is to force clinically pertinent variables into the model and then perform variable selection for the additional candidate biomarkers (De Bin et al. 2014). De Bin et al. (2014) illustrated that the advantage of the addition of high-dimensional data to low-dimensional clinical data may be counteracted by the overfitting due to the addition of the corresponding parameters, even with the state-of-the-art methods for this type of data (penalized regression or boosting). This illustrates the trade-off between explanation and prediction, as high-dimensional genomic data could be informative to explain the biological process, but may not add a lot of prediction accuracy to standard low-dimensional factors.

Flexible Machine Learning Algorithms

The use of more flexible machine learning methods is increasing. Popular algorithms include neural networks (including deep learning), random forests, support vector machines, and gradient boosting machines. The main difference from traditional statistical techniques is that flexible algorithms learn the model structure automatically based on the data. This implies that researchers do not have to decide upon a strategy for modeling nonlinear associations or interaction effects. The enormous flexibility of this approach comes with a downside, which is that such algorithms easily overfit, inducing non-reproducible results. As a result, there are mechanisms to control the complexity of the models. These often take the form of hyperparameters, such as the C regularization parameter for support vector machines, the number of hidden neurons in a neural network, or the penalization parameter (s) in penalized regression, which have to be tuned. This should be done during the model development (cf below).

Due to the difficulty of parameter identifiability in high-dimensional space and the complex tuning of the hyperparameters, it is not guaranteed that these algorithms lead to better performance than more standard risk prediction models (Christodoulou et al. 2019).

Model Validation

This section first provides an overview of key elements of performance of risk prediction models. The difference between apparent, internal, and external validation of performance is described.

Metrics of Model Performance

While checking regression model assumptions and influential observations is to be recommended, this is not the ultimate check of a model's value. Also, traditional statistical measures such as odds ratios or statistical significance are not synonyms of good prediction accuracy (Pepe et al. 2004). For risk prediction models, key issues are whether the predicted risks are accurate (calibration), whether the model discriminates between patients with and without the outcome event (discrimination), and whether the use of a model leads to good decision-making (utility).

Predicted Risk Distribution

A histogram of the predicted risk values from a model may give some information about its performances (see Fig. 1 for predicted values obtained by the two models on the breast cancer example). The model adjusted for age had a smaller range of predicted risk as compared to the model adjusted for the predictors in the BCSC model.

Model Calibration

Risk prediction models should provide risk estimates that are accurate. Model calibration is related to model goodness-of-fit. Although there are several levels of

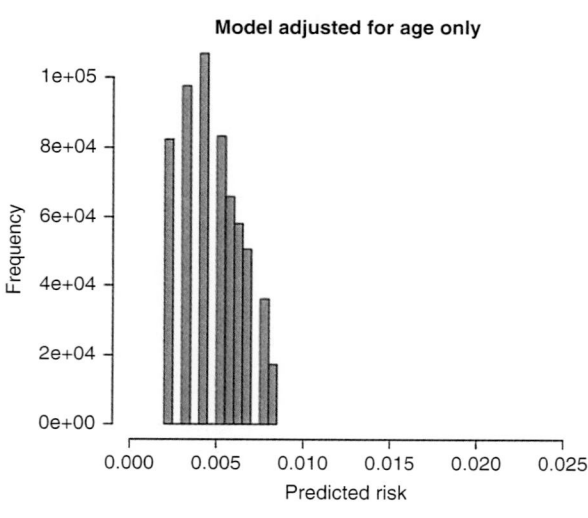

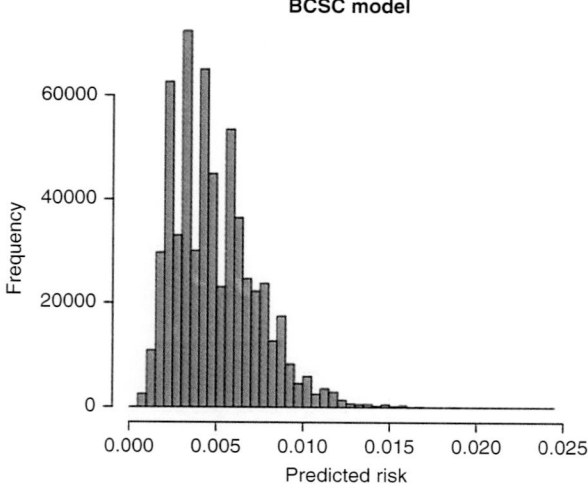

Fig. 1 Distribution of the predicted risk values on the test set for the logistic models adjusted for the age only (top) and the BCSC model (bottom) of 1-year breast cancer occurrence

calibration, it is most common to refer to the level of "moderate calibration": among patients with an estimated risk of the event of X%, is the event really observed in X out of 100 (Van Calster et al. 2016)? A simplified assessment, labeled "weak calibration," quantifies the calibration intercept and slope. To estimate the slope for prediction models based on logistic regression, one predicts the outcome using the linear predictor (i.e., the regression formula, which equals the logit of the predicted risk) using logistic regression. The slope is the resulting coefficient for the linear predictor. When the slope is below the target value of 1, it means that predicted risks are too extreme: high risks tend to be overestimated, while low risks tend to be underestimated. If the slope is above 1, the opposite holds. The calibration intercept is obtained by predicting the outcome in a logistic regression analysis where the linear predictor is used as an offset term (i.e., fixing the coefficient at 1). The calibration intercept is the intercept from this logistic regression analysis. If it is above the target value of 0, it means that predicted risks are on average too low. The opposite holds when the calibration intercept is below 0.

The construction of calibration curves is more interesting, in particular for external validation (see below). Often, grouped curves are constructed. To do so, observations are stratified in groups according to the predicted risk, and then a scatter plot is created with mean predicted risk on the x-axis and estimated observed frequencies of the outcome event on the y-axis. Usually, stratification into deciles is used. Ideally, the points in the scatter plot should fall on the diagonal. A more advanced calibration plot is based on the logistic analysis to estimate the calibration slope, where the association of the linear predictor with the outcome is assessed using smooth functions such as splines or loess (Van Calster et al. 2016). Figure 2 presents such calibration curves for the two models of the breast cancer case study, based on the test set. Both curves are very close to the diagonal.

The Hosmer-Lemeshow test is frequently used to evaluate the calibration, but its use is discouraged because it does not assess either the direction or magnitude of calibration and suffers from low statistical power.

Model Discrimination

Model *discrimination* assesses the ability of the model to distinguish patients with the event (cases) from patients without the event (non-cases). A commonly used metric is the concordance (c) statistic, which equals the area under the ROC curve (AUC) for binary outcomes. When a probability cutoff to classify patients as high vs low risk for the event is defined, sensitivity (true positive rate) and specificity (1 minus false-positive rate) can be calculated. The ROC curve presents the sensitivity versus 1 minus specificity of a model when varying the probability cutoff between 0 and 1. A ROC curve of a nearly perfect prediction model would reach the top-left corner of the plot, inducing a large AUC. The AUC equals the c-statistic and estimates the probability that a random case has a higher risk estimate than a random non-case. The higher the c-statistic, the better the model discriminates. Models with random predictions have a c-statistic of 0.5. Returning to the breast cancer example, in many countries, organized screening for breast cancer is driven by age alone. In Fig. 3, the ROC curve of a model with age alone and the abovementioned BCSC

Fig. 2 Calibration plot using a spline function for the logistic models adjusted for age only (top) and the BCSC model (bottom) of 1-year breast cancer occurrence, using stratification based on the decile of the predicted cancer probabilities on the test set

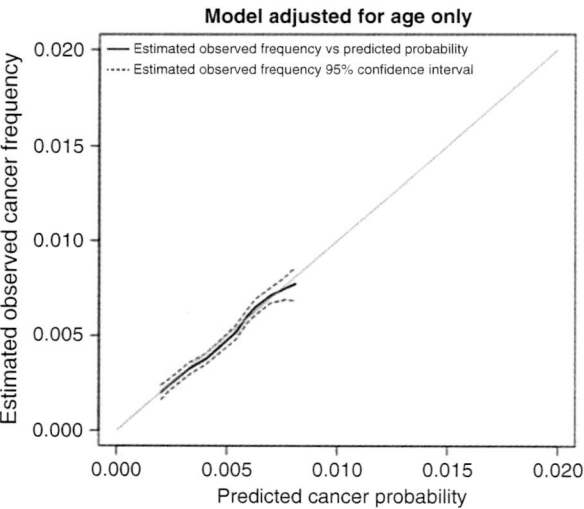

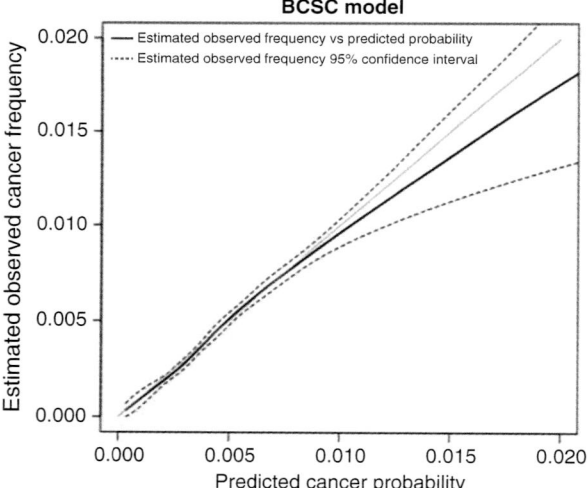

model are shown. AUCs on the test set were 0.604 and 0.639, respectively (ΔAUC = 0.035, 95% bootstrap confidence interval 0.027–0.042). Classifying women with a predicted 1-year risk of 0.33% or higher as "high risk" (i.e., the 5-year risk threshold of the FDA guideline, 1.67% at 5 years, to treat women with risk-lowering drugs (tamoxifen or raloxifene), divided by 5), the specificity of the two compared models is similar (0.30), but the prediction model using the predictors from the BCSC model should be favored due to its higher sensitivity (0.86) than the one of the model based only on patient age (0.82).

While the c-statistic is a global indicator of discrimination, for decision-making a suitable cutoff is needed to identify patients who could benefit from further testing or

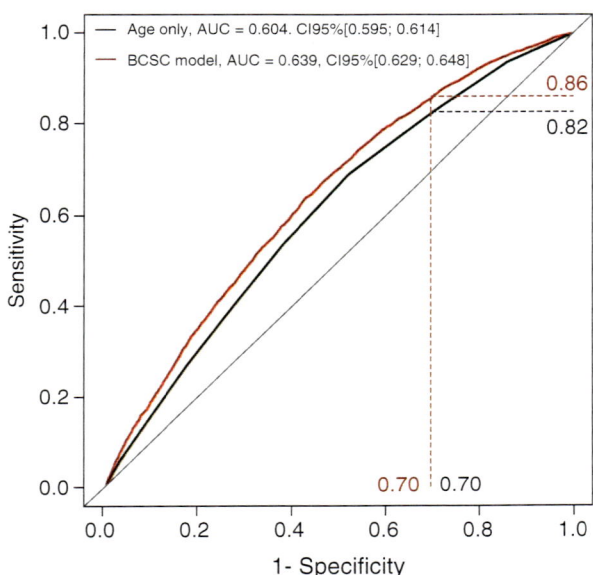

Fig. 3 ROC curve for the logistic models adjusted for the age only (black) and the BCSC model (red) for the 1-year breast cancer occurrence risk in the test set. Dashed lines indicate the sensitivity and the false-positive rate (1-specificity) for a cutoff of 0.33% of predicted 1-year breast cancer occurrence

undergoing an intervention. Often, statistical considerations are used to determine the "optimal" cutoff, although this will often not provide an optimal cutoff for clinical practice. For example, in the context of disease screening, the aim is typically to avoid classifying non-cases as at high risk. This would correspond to a high probability cutoff. On the contrary, when the aim is the diagnosis of a serious disease for which a straightforward treatment exists with little side effects, low-risk cutoffs would be preferred. More generally, decision theory states that the probability cutoff relates to the risk at which we are indifferent about applying the intervention for which the model was used as decision support (Pauker and Kassirer 1980). More details are provided in the section on clinical utility.

Overall Performance Measures

The overall performance of a model may be measured in terms of prediction error (distance between predicted and observed outcome). Typical examples are the Brier score or measures of explained variation (Schemper 2003). These measures capture aspects of discrimination and calibration.

Clinical Utility

Discrimination and calibration assess predictive performance from a statistical perspective, and hence do not include consequences of using a model for clinical decision-making. Full-scale cost-effectiveness studies or impact studies may be performed, but these are complicated and location-dependent. A useful compromise is the decision curve analysis, which plots "Net Benefit" conditional on the adopted probability cutoff. Net Benefit incorporates the relative importance of true positives (TP) vs false positives (FP) into a single number. According to decision theory, the adopted probability cutoff informs on the relative importance of TP vs FP: the odds of the cutoff equals the ratio of the overall harm of a FP and the overall benefit of a TP. Net Benefit equals (#TP − (r/1-r)∗#FP)/n, where r is the cutoff and n the sample size. By correcting the proportion of TPs (higher is better) for the proportion of FPs (higher is worse), Net Benefit gives the "net" proportion of TPs. For a given cutoff, the Net Benefit of using the model to selection patients for an intervention can be compared to the Net Benefit of giving the intervention to everyone ("treat all") or no one ("treat none") by default. Usually, there is no single probability cutoff that is agreed upon by everyone. Then, the decision curve plots Net Benefit over a reasonable range of cutoffs (Van Calster et al. 2018).

Clinical utility is affected by discrimination and calibration. Higher levels of discrimination will tend to increase Net Benefit. Likewise, poor calibration will tend to decrease Net Benefit. For example, if a model systematically underestimates risk, then taking decisions based on a target probability cutoff will lead to wrong decisions: the number of TPs and FPs will be lower than they should be if risks were accurately estimated, leading to less good clinical decisions. Poor calibration may even lead to decisions that are worse than treat all or treat none, even when the model has discriminatory ability (Van Calster et al. 2018).

For the breast cancer example, considering as previously the predicted risk threshold of 0.33% to propose breast cancer risk-lowering drugs to women, the model using the logistic model using the BCSC predictors had numerically higher Net Benefit than the model using age only, and its Net Benefit was also higher than that for treat all (gray line) or treat none (black line) (Fig. 4).

Using this risk threshold of 0.33% for therapeutic intervention by tamoxifen or raloxifene implies that about 300 FPs per TP are acceptable (odds of $0.33 = 0.33/99.67 \approx 1/300$). When a threshold of 1% is preferred, i.e. at most 99 FPs per TP would be acceptable, the model has similar Net Benefit to treat all and treat none. This means that, treatment decisions based on this model have almost no utility. Decision curve analysis can be extended to also account for the cost or invasive nature of the intervention (Van Calster et al. 2018).

Models for a Time-to-Event Outcome

When a time-to-event clinical outcome is predicted, for example, using Cox proportional hazard regression, performance evaluation becomes more complicated because of the time factor. Methods for assessing calibration, discrimination, overall performance, and utility have been proposed (Royston and Altman 2013). For example, c-statistics for censored data exist, such as the Uno c-statistic, as well as c-statistics that also take time-dependent markers or competing risks into account (Vickers et al. 2008; Royston and Altman 2013; Blanche et al. 2013).

Treatment Effect Modeling

For treatment effect models, the aim is to evaluate how well the model predicts benefit for individual patients, which is quantified as the difference in risk of the outcome between the alternative treatment strategies. Standard discrimination and calibration assessments are of limited value in this specific setting. Recently, a "c-statistic for benefit" has been suggested for this purpose (Van Klaveren et al. 2018).

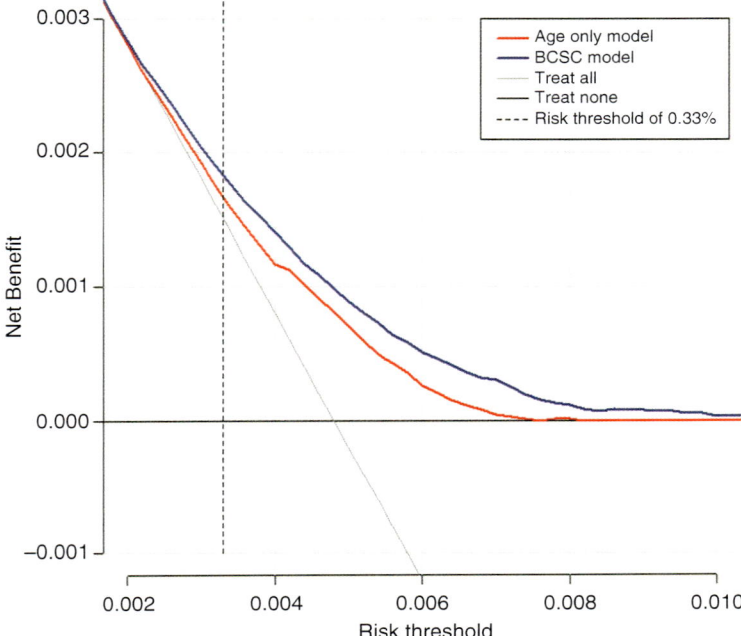

Fig. 4 Decision curve for the logistic models adjusted for age only and the BCSC model. The blue line represents the Net Benefit of the BCSC model to assist decision-making by using a risk threshold to select patients for treatment and the red line of the model adjusted for age only. The grey line represents the Net Benefit of giving the intervention to all individuals ("treat all"). The horizontal black line at zero represents the Net Benefit of withholding the intervention to all individuals ("treat none")

Likewise, extensions of calibration and decision curve analysis to this setting have been proposed (Vickers et al. 2007).

Apparent Validation

The assessment of performance on the same data that were used to develop the model is called apparent validation. Obviously, model performance is too optimistic on apparent validation. The level of discrimination in terms of the c-statistic, sensitivity, and specificity will be too high. When developing a model using standard (i.e., non-penalized) regression models, calibration in terms of the intercept and slope will be perfect by definition. A calibration curve may deviate from the diagonal, however, if important nonlinear associations or interaction effects are omitted.

Internal Validation

Internal validation refers to the validation of the model on test data that are independent from the model development data but that come from the same dataset, such that the underlying populations of the development and test data are fully identical. Internal validation will address the issue of statistical overfitting, because of the use of different dataset for training and testing, but not the issue of generalizability to other settings, because of the issue of identical populations. An estimate of the calibration slope is sufficient in order to assess whether overfitting leads to overly extreme risk estimates on new data from the same population. If a calibration curve is constructed, slopes of less than 1 are reflected in curves that are more horizontal than the ideal diagonal line. Key approaches for internal validation are the use of a holdout sample, cross-validation, and bootstrapping.

Holdout or Split-Sample Method

The most straightforward internal validation approach is to randomly "hold out" a part of the dataset, develop the model on the remaining data (training set), and validate them on the held-out data (test set). The test set is usually smaller to maximize the information, and statistical power, for model training.

The key limitation of this approach is its inefficiency: the dataset is randomly divided into two smaller parts, hence making the development as well as the internal validation unstable. Moreover, due to the single random draw that underlies the holdout approach, in studies with limited overall sample size, the results are dependent on the specific draw that was used. It is therefore an option to repeat the holdout many times. In this scenario, model development is first done on the entire dataset. Then, k train-test splits are created. On each of the k train sets, the full modeling strategy is repeated (instead of only fitting the final model), and the performance is assessed on the accompanying test sets. Finally, test set performances are averaged.

Cross-Validation

An alternative is k-fold cross-validation (CV). First, the model is developed on the entire dataset. Then, the principle of CV for internal validation is to randomly split the full dataset in k subsamples, using each one in turn as a test dataset (the training dataset including the remaining $k-1$ subsamples). Unlike the repeated holdout procedures, CV ensures that each observation serves as a test observation exactly one time. In each of the k splits, the modeling strategy is applied to the training set, and the resulting model is validated on the test set. The performance metrics are averaged over the k iterations. Still, to minimize the effect of randomly allocating the data to folds, it is advisable to repeat the CV process multiple times to increase model stability (Roberts and Nowak 2014). For example, often internal validation is done using ten repetitions of tenfold CV.

In the case of multicenter study, a leave-center-out CV can be used for model validation (Loi et al. 2019). This has also been called internal-external CV, because centers do not have identical populations (Royston et al. 2004). In this way, heterogeneity of performance across centers can be addressed.

Bootstrapping

Here, too, the model is first developed on the entire dataset, and apparent performance can be calculated. For internal validation, a bootstrap sample is drawn from the full dataset. On this bootstrap sample, the full modeling strategy is applied. Then model performance of this model is calculated on the bootstrap sample itself and on the original dataset. The difference in performance provides an estimate of optimism. This procedure is repeated b times, usually at least 200. The average optimism over the b repetition is then subtracted from the apparent performance, in order to provide an internally validated (optimism-correct) estimate of performance (Steyerberg 2008).

Flexible Machine Learning Models

Flexible algorithms, including penalized regression, neural networks, or random forests, require tuning of hyperparameters. Studies focusing on developing machine learning prediction models often tune hyperparameters. Often, tuning is based on a grid search algorithm using CV. If the holdout method is used for internal validation, the CV for hyperparameter tuning is performed on the training set. When optimal values for the hyperparameters are determined, the model is fitted with these optimal values on the entire training set. This final model is then validated on the test set. This has the same limitations as the simple holdout method for model validation. A double CV could be used as alternative. The first CV is used for internal validation. On each training set, a second CV is performed to tune hyperparameters. This does not dispense the need for external validation before to draw definitive conclusion on the model performance, due to the homogeneity of the data used for the model selection.

External Model Validation

External validation is the checking of model performance on a completely new dataset. The external study can be collected at a later point in time from the same center(s) (temporal validation) or at different centers in a multicenter study (geographical validation) (Justice et al. 1999). The key issue is that the underlying population of the external validation dataset is different from that of the development dataset. This is also the case for temporal validation, because the populations evolve over time. At external validation, model performance may reflect both statistical overfitting and also the impact of population differences. Generally, it is to be expected that model performance is lower on external validation (Siontis et al. 2015).

Criteria for sample size calculation for external validation studies have been established. Generally, these are based on achieving reasonable precision in the estimated c-statistic, calibration slope, or calibration curve. At least 100 but preferably 200 cases and non-cases are required (Van Calster et al. 2016). For prediction models, it is possible but typically less interesting to base sample size on statistical tests to compare the c-statistic to an expected value, current gold standard, or that of a competing model. Such calculations are focused on statistical significance, although the key issue is to have a precise estimate.

It is to be recommended, where possible and appropriate, to compare model performance to that of other – perhaps established or clinically implemented –

models (Collins and Moons 2012). This maximizes the value of external validation studies. In addition, models should be externally validated in many centers in order to assess heterogeneity in model performance (Riley et al. 2016). If the aim of the model is to predict the magnitude of treatment effect, model validation may be performed using data from another randomized trial.

Model Reporting

In order to maximize the value from a prediction model development study, it is vital that reporting is complete, honest, and transparent. To this end, the "transparent reporting of a multivariable prediction model for individual prognosis or diagnosis" (TRIPOD) guidelines have been established (Collins et al. 2015). It is strongly recommended to adhere to these guidelines. It is clear from systematic reviews that model reporting is often incomplete and unclear (Christodoulou et al. 2019). Then, it is unclear what was exactly done. Reports sometimes fail to provide the full model equation, such that the model cannot be validated. For logistic regression models, the intercept should always be reported. For Cox proportional hazard models, the baseline hazard at one or more timepoints should be reported, such that predictions for that time horizon can be calculated. Flexible machine learning algorithms cannot be represented by a simple formula. In these cases, more work is needed to make such models readily available for validation.

Nowadays, new models are often implemented on online calculators or apps for mobile devices. This may help in getting more models externally validated, but it is important to provide clear information about the status of the model in terms of validation studies, as well as about necessary information to use the model (e.g., target population, clear definitions of variable, and outcomes).

Demonstrating Clinical Impact

In order to assess the readiness of risk prediction models for guiding patient care, clinical impact should be demonstrated ideally through prospective studies. Clinical impact of a risk prediction model can be defined as evidence of improved clinical outcomes, and its clinical usefulness and added value to patient decision-making, compared with management without the risk prediction model. Several trial designs have been proposed for impact studies. Ideally, randomized designs are needed, such as cluster randomized trials or randomization of discordant cases (Bossuyt et al. 2000). For example, in the MINDACT study (Cardoso et al. 2016), a randomized trial was set up in the discordant risk population – based on a standard-of-care risk prediction model and a genomic risk prediction model – to evaluate the capacity of the genomic model to identify patients in whom chemotherapy can be avoided when the standard model says otherwise. A Biomarker-based strategy trial design (Buyse et al. 2011) was chosen in the MyPeBS study (mypebs.eu), in which patients are randomized to either a breast cancer screening strategy based on a risk prediction model for breast cancer occurrence integrating clinicopathological and genetic predictors to a standard screening strategy in five European countries.

A final step consists of a cost-effectiveness analysis (Janssen et al. 2009; Steyerberg et al. 2013) according to clinical care parameters, such as length of hospitalization, number of unnecessary medical interventions, days off work, time to diagnosis, morbidity, or quality of life. Review of the medical literature suggests that few risk prediction models reach this stage of investigation (Steyerberg et al. 2013).

Conclusion

There is a growing interest for risk prediction models based on regression methods or more flexible machine learning algorithms in the context of precision medicine. Recent work focuses on prediction modeling for treatment effect heterogeneity based on RCT data. The development and validation of a robust model is not straightforward, with several pitfalls (Steyerberg et al. 2018). It should be appropriately planned, conducted, presented, and reported, adhering to current methodological standards. More attention should be given to external validation and impact studies than to the development of new models, to increase their clinical usefulness in medical practice.

Key Points

- There is growing interest in risk prediction models for clinical decision-making in the context of precision medicine.
- Treatment benefit and treatment effect heterogeneity can be sensibly studied using prediction modeling approaches on data from randomized controlled trials.
- Specific metrics for prediction model performance should be used, focusing on discrimination, calibration, and clinical utility.
- When several prediction models exist for a clinical application, it is often better to use, update, or validate an existing model rather than to add a new one to the collection.
- In order to implement risk prediction models in clinical care, it is essential to externally validate in different populations, design prospective impact studies, and perform cost-effectiveness analyses.

Acknowledgments Data collection and sharing was supported by the National Cancer Institute-funded Breast Cancer Surveillance Consortium (HHSN261201100031C). You can learn more about the BCSC at http://www.bcsc-research.org/. We thank the BCSC participants, investigators, mammography facilities, and radiologists for the data they have provided for this study.

This project has received funding from the European Union's Horizon 2020 research and innovation programme under grant agreement No 755394. (MyPeBS study), and from the Research Foundation – Flanders (FWO) grant G0B4716N; Internal Funds KU Leuven grant C24/15/037.

References

Barlow WE, White E, Ballard-Barbash R et al (2006) Prospective breast Cancer risk prediction model for women undergoing screening mammography. JNCI J Natl Cancer Inst 98:1204–1214. https://doi.org/10.1093/jnci/djj331

Bi WL, Hosny A, Schabath MB et al (2019) Artificial intelligence in cancer imaging: Clinical challenges and applications. CA Cancer J Clin 69:caac.21552. https://doi.org/10.3322/caac.21552

Blanche P, Dartigues J-F, Jacqmin-Gadda H (2013) Estimating and comparing time-dependent areas under receiver operating characteristic curves for censored event times with competing risks. Stat Med 32:5381–5397. https://doi.org/10.1002/sim.5958

Bossuyt PM, Lijmer JG, Mol BW (2000) Randomised comparisons of medical tests: sometimes invalid, not always efficient. Lancet (London, England) 356:1844–1847. https://doi.org/10.1016/S0140-6736(00)03246-3

Bottomley C, Van Belle V, Kirk E et al (2013) Accurate prediction of pregnancy viability by means of a simple scoring system. Hum Reprod 28:68–76. https://doi.org/10.1093/humrep/des352

Buyse M, Michiels S, Sargent DJ et al (2011) Integrating biomarkers in clinical trials. Expert Rev Mol Diagn 11:171–182. https://doi.org/10.1586/erm.10.120

Cardoso F, van't Veer LJ, Bogaerts J et al (2016) 70-gene signature as an aid to treatment decisions in early-stage breast Cancer. N Engl J Med 375:717–729. https://doi.org/10.1056/NEJMoa1602253

Christodoulou E, Ma J, Collins GS et al (2019) A systematic review shows no performance benefit of machine learning over logistic regression for clinical prediction models. J Clin Epidemiol 110:12–22. https://doi.org/10.1016/j.jclinepi.2019.02.004

Collins GS, Moons KGM (2012) Comparing risk prediction models. BMJ 344:e3186. https://doi.org/10.1136/bmj.e3186

Collins GS, Reitsma JB, Altman DG, Moons KGM (2015) Transparent reporting of a multivariable prediction model for individual prognosis or diagnosis (TRIPOD): the TRIPOD statement. BMJ 350:g7594

Damen JAAG, Hooft L, Schuit E et al (2016) Prediction models for cardiovascular disease risk in the general population: systematic review. BMJ 353:i2416. https://doi.org/10.1136/bmj.i2416

De Bin R, Sauerbrei W, Boulesteix A-L (2014) Investigating the prediction ability of survival models based on both clinical and omics data: two case studies. Stat Med 33:5310–5329. https://doi.org/10.1002/sim.6246

Farooq V, van Klaveren D, Steyerberg EW et al (2013) Anatomical and clinical characteristics to guide decision making between coronary artery bypass surgery and percutaneous coronary intervention for individual patients: development and validation of SYNTAX score II. Lancet 381:639–650. https://doi.org/10.1016/S0140-6736(13)60108-7

Hingorani AD, van der WDA, Riley RD et al (2013) Prognosis research strategy (PROGRESS) 4: stratified medicine research. BMJ 346:e5793. https://doi.org/10.1136/bmj.e5793

Janssen KJM, Vergouwe Y, Donders ART et al (2009) Dealing with missing predictor values when applying clinical prediction models. Clin Chem 55:994–1001. https://doi.org/10.1373/clinchem.2008.115345

Justice AC, Covinsky KE, Berlin JA (1999) Assessing the generalizability of prognostic information. Ann Intern Med 130:515–524

Kent DM, Steyerberg E, van Klaveren D (2018) Personalized evidence based medicine: predictive approaches to heterogeneous treatment effects. BMJ 363:k4245. https://doi.org/10.1136/bmj.k4245

Loi S, Drubay D, Adams S et al (2019) Tumor-infiltrating lymphocytes and prognosis: a pooled individual patient analysis of early-stage triple-negative breast cancers. J Clin Oncol 37:559. https://doi.org/10.1200/jco.18.01010

Luijken K, Groenwold RHH, van Calster B et al (2019) Impact of predictor measurement heterogeneity across settings on performance of prediction models: a measurement error perspective. Stat Med 38(18):3444–2459. https://doi.org/10.1002/sim.8183. Epub 2019 May 31

Michiels S, Kramar A, Koscielny S (2011) Multidimensionality of microarrays: statistical challenges and (im)possible solutions. Mol Oncol 5:190–196. https://doi.org/10.1016/j.molonc.2011.01.002

Michiels S, Ternès N, Rotolo F (2016) Statistical controversies in clinical research: prognostic gene signatures are not (yet) useful in clinical practice. Ann Oncol 27:2160–2167. https://doi.org/10.1093/annonc/mdw307

Pajouheshnia R, Groenwold RHH, Peelen LM et al (2019) When and how to use data from randomised trials to develop or validate prognostic models. BMJ 365:l2154. https://doi.org/10.1136/bmj.l2154

Pauker SG, Kassirer JP (1980) The threshold approach to clinical decision making. N Engl J Med 302:1109–1117. https://doi.org/10.1056/NEJM198005153022003

Peduzzi P, Concato J, Kemper E et al (1996) A simulation study of the number of events per variable in logistic regression analysis. J Clin Epidemiol 49:1373–1379

Pepe MS, Janes H, Longton G et al (2004) Limitations of the odds ratio in gauging the performance of a diagnostic, prognostic, or screening marker. Am J Epidemiol 159:882–890

Riley RD, Ensor J, Snell KIE et al (2016) External validation of clinical prediction models using big datasets from e-health records or IPD meta-analysis: opportunities and challenges. BMJ 353:i3140. https://doi.org/10.1136/bmj.i3140

Riley RD, Snell KI, Ensor J et al (2019) Minimum sample size for developing a multivariable prediction model: PART II – binary and time-to-event outcomes. Stat Med 38:1276–1296. https://doi.org/10.1002/sim.7992

Roberts S, Nowak G (2014) Stabilizing the lasso against cross-validation variability. Comput Stat Data Anal 70:198–211. https://doi.org/10.1016/J.CSDA.2013.09.008

Royston P, Altman DG (2013) External validation of a cox prognostic model: principles and methods. BMC Med Res Methodol 13:33. https://doi.org/10.1186/1471-2288-13-33

Royston P, Parmar MKB, Sylvester R (2004) Construction and validation of a prognostic model across several studies, with an application in superficial bladder cancer. Stat Med 23:907–926. https://doi.org/10.1002/sim.1691

Royston P, Altman DG, Sauerbrei W (2006) Dichotomizing continuous predictors in multiple regression: a bad idea. Stat Med 25:127–141. https://doi.org/10.1002/sim.2331

Schemper M (2003) Predictive accuracy and explained variation. Stat Med 22:2299–2308. https://doi.org/10.1002/sim.1486

Siontis GCM, Tzoulaki I, Castaldi PJ, Ioannidis JPA (2015) External validation of new risk prediction models is infrequent and reveals worse prognostic discrimination. J Clin Epidemiol 68:25–34. https://doi.org/10.1016/j.jclinepi.2014.09.007

Sterne JAC, White IR, Carlin JB et al (2009) Multiple imputation for missing data in epidemiological and clinical research: potential and pitfalls. BMJ 338:b2393. https://doi.org/10.1136/bmj.b2393

Steyerberg EW (2008) Clinical prediction models: a practical approach to development, validation, and updating: Springer Science & Business Media

Steyerberg EW, Eijkemans MJC, Harrell FE, Habbema JDF (2001) Prognostic Modeling with logistic regression analysis. Med Decis Mak 21:45–56. https://doi.org/10.1177/0272989X0102100106

Steyerberg EW, Moons KGM, van der Windt DA et al (2013) Prognosis research strategy (PROGRESS) 3: prognostic model research. PLoS Med 10:e1001381. https://doi.org/10.1371/journal.pmed.1001381

Steyerberg EW, Uno H, Ioannidis JPA et al (2018) Poor performance of clinical prediction models: the harm of commonly applied methods. J Clin Epidemiol 98:133–143. https://doi.org/10.1016/j.jclinepi.2017.11.013

Ternès N, Rotolo F, Michiels S (2017) Robust estimation of the expected survival probabilities from high-dimensional cox models with biomarker-by-treatment interactions in randomized clinical trials. BMC Med Res Methodol 17:83. https://doi.org/10.1186/s12874-017-0354-0

Tyrer J, Duffy SW, Cuzick J (2004) A breast cancer prediction model incorporating familial and personal risk factors. Stat Med 23:1111–1130. https://doi.org/10.1002/sim.1668

Vachon CM, Pankratz VS, Scott CG et al (2015) The contributions of breast density and common genetic variation to breast cancer risk. J Natl Cancer Inst 107. https://doi.org/10.1093/jnci/dju397

Van Calster B, Nieboer D, Vergouwe Y et al (2016) A calibration hierarchy for risk models was defined: from utopia to empirical data. J Clin Epidemiol 74:167–176. https://doi.org/10.1016/j.jclinepi.2015.12.005

Van Calster B, Wynants L, Verbeek JFM et al (2018) Reporting and interpreting decision curve analysis: a guide for investigators. Eur Urol 74:796–804. https://doi.org/10.1016/j.eururo.2018.08.038

Van Klaveren D, Steyerberg EW, Serruys PW, Kent DM (2018) The proposed "concordance-statistic for benefit" provided a useful metric when modeling heterogeneous treatment effects. J Clin Epidemiol 94:59–68. https://doi.org/10.1016/j.jclinepi.2017.10.021

Van Klaveren D, Balan TA, Steyerberg EW, Kent DM (2019) Models with interactions overestimated heterogeneity of treatment effects and were prone to treatment mistargeting. J Clin Epidemiol. https://doi.org/10.1016/j.jclinepi.2019.05.029

Van Smeden M, Moons KG, de Groot JA et al (2018) Sample size for binary logistic prediction models: beyond events per variable criteria. Stat Methods Med Res:96228021878472. https://doi.org/10.1177/0962280218784726

Vergouwe Y, Royston P, Moons KGM, Altman DG (2010) Development and validation of a prediction model with missing predictor data: a practical approach. J Clin Epidemiol 63:205–214. https://doi.org/10.1016/j.jclinepi.2009.03.017

Vickers AJ, Kattan MW, Sargent DJ (2007) Method for evaluating prediction models that apply the results of randomized trials to individual patients. Trials 8:14. https://doi.org/10.1186/1745-6215-8-14

Vickers AJ, Cronin AM, Elkin EB, Gonen M (2008) Extensions to decision curve analysis, a novel method for evaluating diagnostic tests, prediction models and molecular markers. BMC Med Inform Decis Mak 8:53. https://doi.org/10.1186/1472-6947-8-53

White IR, Royston P, Wood AM (2011) Multiple imputation using chained equations: issues and guidance for practice. Stat Med 30:377–399. https://doi.org/10.1002/sim.4067

Part VIII

Publication and Related Issues

Paper Writing

102

Curtis L. Meinert

Contents

Introduction	2028
The Publication Imperative	2028
Types of Study Publications	2029
Design and Methods Publications	2029
Baseline Results Publications	2029
Treatment Results Publications	2029
"Natural" History Publications	2030
Substudy Publications	2030
Other Study Publications	2030
Ancillary Study Publications	2030
Publication Issues	2030
When to Publish?	2030
Where to Publish?	2031
Journal Supplement Versus Regular Issue?	2032
When Journals Will Not Publish?	2032
Presentation Versus Publication?	2033
Paper Writing Issues	2034
Lifting Results Blackout	2034
Database Freeze	2035
Event Adjudication	2035
Reviews, Approvals, and Sign-Offs	2035
"Insider Trading"	2036
The Design Synopsis and Study Curriculum Vitae	2036
Dos and Don'ts of Paper Writing	2037
Do	2037
Don't	2039
Key Facts	2042
Summary	2042
References	2043

C. L. Meinert (✉)
Department of Epidemiology, School of Public Health, Johns Hopkins University, Baltimore, MD, USA
e-mail: cmeiner1@jhu.edu

© Springer Nature Switzerland AG 2022
S. Piantadosi, C. L. Meinert (eds.), *Principles and Practice of Clinical Trials*,
https://doi.org/10.1007/978-3-319-52636-2_182

Keywords

Publication · Paper writing

Introduction

Publication is the sine qua non of trials. In the societal sense, there is no lasting information generated from trials, absent publication. Investigators are not finished until they have published their results and have done so regardless of the nature or direction of the results.

One might think that paper writing starts when the trial ends and is finished when the results are published but the reality is that it should start early in the course of the trial and continue long after the trial is finished.

This chapter is about the paper writing process.

The Publication Imperative

The imperative to publish is implicit in the second item of the Nüremberg Code (Shuster 1997):

> *The experiment should be such as to yield fruitful results for the good of society, unprocurable by other methods or means of study, and not random and unnecessary in nature.*

Operationally, the imperative requires that:

1. The experiment be soundly designed and properly conducted.
2. The experiment has adequate precision (power) to provide a reasonable chance of producing "fruitful results for the good of society."
3. Results of the experiment be properly analyzed.
4. Results be published.

Investigators, using promises of advancing the collective knowledge of society as inducements to enrollment of persons into the trial, assume moral obligations to publish. Failure to publish renders those promises empty. One can argue, as has Iain Chalmers, that failure to publish is a violation of ethical obligations to persons enrolled for study (Chalmers 1990).

The imperative to publish comes into play with enrollment of the first person into a trial. The obligation is an outgrowth of the public trust underlying the privilege of being able to research on human beings.

Strictly speaking, investigators who start a trial but abandon it because of inability to find suitable participants or because of inadequate funding are still obliged to publish and post results. However, even if they were to write up the results of their effort, the likelihood of getting published is small, and the value of such accounts is questionable.

Beyond question, trials producing the most "fruitful results for the good of society" are those that proceed to their appointed end or that are stopped because of results indicative of benefit or harm.

The principles below apply to such results.

Principle 1: Investigators are obligated to post results and publish finished results regardless of the nature or direction of the results and to publish in peer-reviewed, indexed, medical journals.

Principle 2: Investigators are obligated to publish results of early stops as soon as practical and to do so regardless of whether the stop was because of evidence of benefit or harm.

Principle 3: The duty to analyze, summarize, write-up, and publish results rests exclusively with study investigators. The duty is not assignable and not to be infringed upon, mitigated, interdicted, directed, or controlled by study sponsors, institutional officials, or any other authority or party.

Principle 4: Study investigators should be first to analyze, write-up, and conclude regarding their results. This means they should not be obliged to data share until they have published their primary results.

Principle 5: The responsibility to data share takes priority over publication if investigators fail to publish in a timely fashion or in the absence of efforts to publish.

Types of Study Publications

Design and Methods Publications

Papers describing the design, methods, and protocol of the trial (e.g., University Group Diabetes Program 1970a); typically produced prior to or in conjunction with the initial treatment results publication. The advantage of having stand-alone papers detailing design and methods is the ability to short circuit those descriptions in results papers by simply referencing those papers.

Baseline Results Publications

Papers describing the baseline characteristics of the study population; may be part of a design and methods paper or a stand-alone paper.

Treatment Results Publications

Papers detailing treatment results by randomized assignment for one or more outcomes of the trial; may result in more than one paper in trials involving multiple treatment groups and stops at different times over the course of the trial for the different treatments represented in the trial; e.g., as in the University Group Diabetes Program (UGDP) for stops of tolbutamide (University Group Diabetes Program 1970b) and phenformin (University Group Diabetes Program 1971, 1975).

"Natural" History Publications

Publications describing results over the course of follow-up in the control-assigned group when placebo-assigned or observation only; primarily in long-term prevention trials when people enrolled are assumed to be similar to those in the general population with condition of interest., e.g., Cornary Drug Project Research Group 1982.

Substudy Publications

Papers summarizing results of studies done on selected persons enrolled in the parent trial; performed at selected study sites or select subset of persons in the trial; e.g., limited to investigators having interest or means to do an indicated substudy.

Other Study Publications

Papers describing special reading or analysis procedures used in the trial; papers responding to criticisms of the trial.

Ancillary Study Publications

An ancillary study is a supplementary study done in association with the parent trial. Ancillary studies are the result of the varying interests and pursuits of investigators in the parent trial. Most multicenter trials have procedures for reviewing and approving proposals for ancillary studies. Studies calling for the collection of additional data or the conduct of additional procedures on persons enrolled in the parent trial are not likely to be approved if seen as interfering with the parent trial or if seen as increasing the risk of dropout or missing data in the parent trial. Studies calling for use of treatment-related data are not approved or are approved with the proviso that such data will not be available until the parent trial is completed.

Publication Issues

When to Publish?

Design, Methods, and Baseline Results?
Ideally, before or in conjunction with first report of treatment results; may not be possible in the case of early stops.

Investigators in some trials have elected to summarize the design, methods, and baseline results of a trial in a "stand-alone" paper. Ideally, such papers should be published before results papers, e.g., as in the Coronary Artery Surgery Study (CASS; Coronary Artery Surgery Study Research Group 1981), or in conjunction with the first results publication, as in the University Group Diabetes Program (UGDP; University Group Diabetes Program 1970b). However, in some instances, such papers may not appear until results have been published, e.g., as in the Coronary Drug Project (CDP; Coronary Drug Project Research Group 1973).

Treatment Results?
When the trial is completed or in relation to early stops because of harm or benefit associated with a study treatment.

Investigators should forego the temptation of publishing interim treatment results not related to early stops or completion of the trial. Such publications have the potential of compromising the trial, especially in cases where the results can affect subsequent recruitment or treatment patterns in the trial. In addition, they can open the trial to criticism if seen as vehicles for promoting the trial.

Pressures on investigators to publish can arise from publications by others. Investigators in CASS faced those pressures because of publications coming from a sister study (European Coronary Surgery Study Group) (European Coronary Surgery Study Group 1982a, b, 1980, 1979). Ultimately, CASS investigators elected to forego producing an interim results publication, but not without considerable debate.

Investigators for the Rosiglitazone Evaluated for Cardiac Outcomes and Regulation of Glycaemia in Diabetes (RECORD) trial opted to publish interim results because:

A recent meta-analysis raised concern regarding an increased risk of myocardial infarction and death from cardiovascular causes associated with rosiglitazone treatment of type 2 diabetes. (Home et al. 2007)

The triggering meta-analysis was one by Nissen and Wolski entitled *Effect of rosiglitazone on the risk of myocardial infarction and death from cardiovascular causes* published in 2007 (Nissen and Wolski 2007).

Where to Publish?

Indexed medical journals. Largely, results published elsewhere are "lost" because of lack of adequate indexing to facilitate location.

Monographs, chapters in books, proceedings of meetings, and the like, are, at best, distant seconds to indexed journals.

Results with general implications should be directed to wide circulation journals. Specialty journals should be considered if the results are of primary interest to a medical subspecialty. Both kinds of journals may be used in some cases, e.g., with the phenformin results in the UGDP. The initial report appeared in JAMA in 1971.

A more extensive report appeared in *Diabetes* in 1975 (University Group Diabetes Program Research Group 1971, 1975).

There is a pecking order for choice of medical journals. The tendency is for investigators to aim as high up the pecking order as possible. Investigators will submit to journals like JAMA, NEJM, BMJ, or Lancet, if there is a chance of being published there. If they are rejected, they move down to specialty journals.

Rejections are never easy to take. The more a group receives, the more likely they are simply to "toss in the towel." In the long run, the fact that a paper appears in an indexed journal is more important than the journal in which it appears, especially in this electronic age.

Journal Supplement Versus Regular Issue?

Investigators have to decide how papers are packaged. Paper by paper or as a collection published together as a supplement to a journal.

Any writing effort involving production of a compendium of papers requires resolve and perseverance on the part of those spearheading such efforts (to say nothing about money needed to pay for publication; most journals charge for special issues). That being so, there is always the chance of those efforts faltering and, hence, it is not wise to have that approach as the only plan for publication. The better strategy is to use that approach in addition to the "individual paper approach."

Investigators in the National Emphysema Treatment Trial (NETT) used both approaches. They published their primary results in 2003 (National Emphysema Treatment Trial Research Group 2003). They produced a special issue of the Proceedings of the American Thoracic Society in May of 2008 containing a compendium of 34 papers (Criner 2008).

The virtue of a collection of manuscripts in a single journal issue rests in its completeness. It is easier for readers to grasp the significance of a study if all pertinent design details and results are contained in one journal issue than when scattered across time in the same or different journals. The downside is in the time it takes to produce a collection of papers and the fact that the collection may delay publication of the results because of delays in preparing the package of manuscripts.

When Journals Will Not Publish?

Not every results paper is publishable. A trial can be so poorly designed, done, or analyzed so as to make publication difficult if not impossible. But, even assuming the trial is well designed, conducted, and analyzed, its results may be rejected. Indeed, rejections are what researchers learn to live with.

So how many rejections should investigators take before throwing in the towel? Certainly more than one or two. Five? If the rejection rate is 50% and if acceptance is a lottery then the probability of success drops below 5% after five rejections.

The "five rule" means that the funding agency has to support the infrastructure of the trial to allow investigators to play out the sting. That typically means support for at least 2–3 years after completion of data collection.

Acceptance rates vary by journal. They are less than 10% for high circulation journals like NEJM, JAMA, and Lancet and higher for lower circulation more specialized journals.

Also, unfortunately, better acceptance rates vary depending on the nature of the result being published. Editors prefer definitive results. Hence, if there is no difference between the treatment groups, even if the trial is adequately powered, designed, and conducted, authors are likely to have a harder time publishing than if results are positive or negative.

In this electronic age and Google searches, the focus should be more on publication than where a paper is published. Each submission drains energy and resolve from the research group. Realistically, there are only so many rejections a group can absorb until it gives up. The group needs to decide how many of its rejections are spent pursuing impossible dreams with high profile journals.

Presentation Versus Publication?

A "presentation" is a paper read or a poster presented at a scientific society meeting.

Researchers are reared to value presentations as stepping stones to recognition and success. They aspire to presenting as means of advancing their careers and for making people aware of their work. They view presentations as preludes to publications, arguing that presentations will produce better publications, even speed production of a supporting publication.

But, when it comes to results of a trial, the rule should be "publish first, present later."

The rule means there are no interim reports of results during the trial. It does not preclude publications of baseline results or of design and methods of the trial, or even results over time for the control assigned group, but it does preclude presentations of results by treatment group until results have been published.

Why the rule?
Because:

1. Presentation of results may preclude publication (some journals will not take results that have been presented).
2. The presentation may reduce resolve of investigators to publish by deluding them into believing the imperative to publish has been met with a presentation of results.
3. Presentations are not substitutes for publications. The audience reached is only the people in the meeting halls, only a fraction of the audience reached with publication.
4. Media attention generated from the presentation may negatively imprint the medical community causing it to largely ignore results when published.

To be sure, there are occasions when results are so compelling to render it imprudent to wait for publication but they are few. The mechanism used by NIH for NIH-funded trials in those cases is issue of clinical alerts (since inception, 1991, 34 alerts through 27 February 2018). https://www.nlm.nih.gov/databases/alerts/clinical_alerts.html

Even when investigators agree to "no presentation of results until published," groups may look for "workarounds" when there are results to report.

The UGDP was a multicenter randomized trial designed to assess the efficacy of several different treatments for blood sugar control against a placebo treatment in people with type 2 diabetes. One of the treatments was Orinase® (tolbutamide), the most widely used oral agent at the time for type 2 diabetics and widely regarded as safe and effective.

Midway through the trial investigators stopped use of tolbutamide because of increased mortality compared to the placebo-assigned group (University Group Diabetes Program Research Group 1970b).

The investigators had long before agreed to "publish first, present later" when it came to study results, but the rule fell by the wayside when they decided to present results at the American Diabetes Association meeting (June 1970) in anticipation of the results having been published by then.

They misjudged. The publication came months after the presentation because of delays in dealing with editors' comments concerning the manuscript. In the interim, diabetologists were deluged by calls following the presentation from worried patients concerning the drug they were on. The fact that they had to answer their questions without benefit of a supporting publication rendered them hostile to the study. By the time the publication appeared, they were convinced that any study that caused them so much trouble was "no good."

Paper Writing Issues

Lifting Results Blackout

A results blackouts in conduct of trials is a state in which investigators are shielded from seeing interim results by treatment group. The state is imposed to preserve the state of equipoise in the trials. Blackouts are common in trials independent of whether or not treatments are masked. An issue in the critical path of paper writing in trials is when and how to lift the blackout.

That investigators have to be informed of results by treatment group is obvious, even if not directly involved in the writing effort, because their input is important to the writing effort and because they will have to sign off on the paper when it is submitted for publication.

The reveal may be in a face-to-face meeting of the investigator group or via a conference call of the investigator group.

Database Freeze

Databases are never final. That means investigators have to specify cutoff dates beyond which additions or changes to the database are not accepted. Data freezes are necessary so that analyses and counts across tables in a manuscript agree.

That cutoff date in normal endings of trials is when data from all persons have been harvested into the study dataset. Usually days or weeks after the last person was seen and data have been edited and cleaned.

The date in early stops is arbitrarily set by study investigators. For example, in the case of the first early stop in the UGDP because of ill-effects associated with tolbutamide, the approach was to continue follow-up through the next scheduled follow-up visit after the decision to stop. Since visits were 3 months apart, that meant the cutoff for data collection was about 3 months after the decision to stop the tolbutamide treatment.

Event Adjudication

The time for event adjudication, if there is to be any, is in real time as events occur, but that is logistically difficult if the adjudication requires readings by multiple persons and conferences to come to consensuses. Generally in those settings, it is more efficient to wait until the end of the trial to do adjudications all at once. That approach is reasonable for normal endings to trials because people can organize the activity in advance. It is a different story with early stops. In those cases, investigators have to decide if they are going to hold writing the paper until readings have been made or proceed to publication with raw unadjudicated counts of events.

Reviews, Approvals, and Sign-Offs

Issues that have to be decided are who has rights of reviews and who has approval authority over manuscripts prior to submission.

Reviews are courtesies and suggestions made; nonbinding.

Approval authority means the manuscript may not be submitted until approvals are obtained.

Suggestions made in relation to approvals are binding.

It is common, reasonable, and prudent to offer penultimate versions of manuscripts to various parties for comments with investigators left to decide how to deal with comments. Parties offered reviews typically includes sponsors and companies providing drugs or products being tested. The right of review may be extended to members of the data monitoring committee.

Investigators should limit the right of approval to study investigators. If it is extended beyond the investigatorship, the publication should indicate that fact and the names of persons or agencies having that right should be disclosed in the publication.

The sign-offs necessary for submission of a manuscript to a journal depends on authorship format. For conventional authorship, it is persons named in the masthead of the paper. Depending on the journal, it may extend to all named investigators if the format is one listing the entire research group.

"Insider Trading"

Trials involving results from proprietary products pose risks for insider trading once results are known to study investigators before dissemination to the public.

There is no way of avoiding the risk. The best that can be done is to inform investigator groups as to what constitutes insider trading and punishments for such trading.

The Design Synopsis and Study Curriculum Vitae

A design synopsis for a trial is an outline of the key design and operating features of the trial.

Samples may be found in Appendix 1 (pp. 499–516; Meinert 2013).

The synopsis should be developed when the trial is started and updated over the course of the trial. Its primary value is as a reference document when preparing talks and writing papers concerning the trial.

A study CV is akin to that for persons. It gives the history of the trial, its key design features, sample size requirements, primary and secondary outcome measures, funding sources, study centers, study personnel, and presentations and publications made on behalf of the trial.

The list below is section headings in the CV for the NETT (https://jhuccs1.us/clm/PDFs/NETTCV-2013.pdf):

1. Background and rationale
2. Design summary
3. Summary of pulmonary rehabilitation program
4. Consent, data collection, and telephone contact schedule
5. Substudies
6. Landmark events
7. Participating centers, groups, and committees
8. Publications
9. Presentations
10. Meetings
11. Site visits
12. Meetings/conference calls and site visits by year of study
13. Support statement

14. Contract numbers, funding period, and ClinicalTrials.gov number
15. Repositories
16. Items on file at the National Technical Information Service
17. NETT website
18. Accessing the NETT limited access dataset

Dos and Don'ts of Paper Writing

Do

Organization
Follow formal processes for commissioning study publications.

> *Comment*: Typically commissioning in multicenter trials done by the study chair and ratified by the study steering committee.

Limit size of writing committee to five or fewer.

> *Comment*: Generally, less is more when it comes to writing committees.

Require the writing committee to have a "kick off" organizing meeting before starting.

> *Comment*: Meeting may be phone or face-to-face.

Indicate freeze date for dataset used in the paper.
Expect the committee to meet periodically over the course of writing. Require progress reports from the chair of the writing committee.

> *Comment*: Typically reporting is to the steering committee; essential to ensuring progress.

Designate someone in the investigator structure to maintain the study CV.

> *Comment*: Typically someone in the coordinating center in multicenter trials.

Operations
Use CONSORT as a guide.
Designate someone on the writing team to keep electronic copies of all circulated drafts of the manuscript.
Separate paragraphs with extra hard returns. Indent to indicate paragraphing.
Keep copies of all iterations of the manuscript distributed to the writing team. Number and date drafts.

Comment: Important when trying to trace the history of additions or deletions to drafts or when trying to determine if the draft is the latest draft.

Number pages (upper right hand corner).

Comment: Even if drafts are distributed electronically, they will be printed. If pages get messed up, good luck getting them back in order without page numbers!

Save space by editing out "ly" words.

Comment: Most "ly" words are unnecessary adding only to word counts.

Use headers to avoid "blind entries."

Comment: Headers are necessary because manuscripts are read as reference documents. That being so, readers need headers on each page to know where they are in the manuscript.

Tables that do not fit on a page should have column headers on continuing pages.

Comment: It is frustrating to have to flip back to determine headers for columns of table on continuation pages.

Ensure that drafts have footers (lower left or right corner) on each page that provides name of the document, location of the file, and date created.

Comment: If footer is also constructed to include "print date," make certain that date is labeled as "print date" so as not to be confused with the date document was saved.

Get rid of the second space after periods.

Comment: Even if you are a "two space after periods" person, journal editors are not.

Make certain the manuscript is printer robust.

Comment: Remember. Things that look good on a computer screen may not be legible when the document is printed.

Spell check drafts before distribution! Proof read from hard copy.

Comment: Reading on computer screens is not reliable.

Proof read drafts before distributing to members of the writing committee.

Have at least two people proof read finished drafts before submission to journals; read aloud mouthing words and running one's finger over words as read.

Comment: The "mouthing" and "fingering" reduces "brain fill-ins."

Check the accuracy of counts and analyses by having them done by at least persons working independently.

Check the accuracy of references listed in the manuscript.

Comment: Checking should be done against original sources.

Provide a full credit listing that includes names and locations of participating centers and key personnel at centers and names of key leadership committees and membership.

Check the accuracy of the listings.

Comment: Nobody likes to see their name incorrectly spelled or their institutional affiliation wrong.

Maintain glossary of abbreviations.

Comment: Useful, especially when writing subsequent manuscripts.

Sign-Off, Submission, Reviews

Make sure investigators have signed-off on paper before submission.

Designate a person from the writing team to make the submission and deal with queries from editors.

Be clear as to how investigators are to deal with press queries after publication.

Don't

Organization

Commission writing committees prior to establishment of an authorship policy.

Start writing efforts prior to agreement on sign-off processes for finished manuscripts. Create writing teams having more than five members.

Pay to have the paper written.

Comment: Ghost writers are no-nos when it comes to publications.

Allow people, not part of the investigator group, to work on or write study manuscripts.

Operations
Weasel.

Comment: You might just as well talk to the hand when asking researchers not to weasel. It is in their DNA. The person in charge of drafts should delete words like perhaps, possibly, presumably, and theoretically to reduce weaseling.

Cross positive and negative terms.

Comment: "Driver carries no cash." How does the driver do that? Brewster Higley's familiar refrain *where seldom is heard a discouraging word and the skies are not cloudy all day* (Home on the Range 1904) involves crossing positive with negative terms. The line is confusing because of the use of *not* and *all*. As a result, we remain uncertain as to whether Higley is telling us that the skies are clear all day or just part of the day. Higley could have avoided the confusion with the refrain *where words are encouraging and the skies are clear all day* (assuming that is what is meant), but it certainly does not have the same ring as his original words.

Use double negatives.

Comment: Confusing.

Block paragraph.

Comment: The reason is because when the last line on a page is filled and ends with a period, readers are uncertain as to whether the first line on the next page is a continuation of the paragraph on the previous page or the start of a new one.

Use colors as the sole means of identification of graphic information.

Comment: Colors disappear when the document is printed black and white.

Use shading for emphasis.

Comment: Shading reduces contrast and legibility.

Distribute drafts as two-sided print documents.

Comment: Two-sided print is fine for finished documents but not for works in progress. Use the extra paper and print one-sided!

Intermix page orientations.

Comment: The default orientation for manuscripts is portrait. Intermixing portrait and landscape orientations requires "turns" by the reader and can cause printing problems; irritating. The "need" for turns comes with tables that have too many columns to fit when portrait orientated. Generally, turns are just because the creator did not want to take the time to make the table fit portrait orientation.

Insert frivolous comments in the text of drafts.

Comment: To be avoided because text, once inserted, may survive into the submitted manuscript.

Use different words or phrases to mean the same thing.

Comment: Standardize vocabulary. Sports announcers vary their lingo to reduce monotony like telling us that *the Yankees trounced the Red Sox, the Athletics pummeled the Angels, the Indians squeaked by the Tigers, and the Orioles were triumphant over the Twins*, but scientific writing is different. The paper writer who refers to baseline examination in one sentence and elsewhere to the same exam as an entrance exam will confuse readers.

Rely on secondary references.

Comment: Go to the original source and cite it.

Use "et al." in place of names in reference listings.

Comment: The list in drafts should be the full citation with all names listed.

Convert to journal format before submission.

Comment: Journals generally require stripped down documents devoid of headers and footers. The format is not user-friendly for readers of drafts. Strip when submitting but remember you may need what you stripped if the manuscript is rejected and is resurrected for a new submission.

Proof read from the screen.

Comment: It will give you a headache and is not a reliable mode of proofing.

Sign-Off, Submission, and Reviews

Give the funding agency rights of approval over what is written.

Comment: OK to review and offer suggestions but investigators should be free to reject suggestions without consequence.

Give drug companies or other proprietary sponsors rights of approval over what is written.

Comment: OK to review and offer suggestions but investigators should be free to reject suggestions without consequence.

Key Facts

Whereas being able to research on human beings is a privilege, granted only by an accepting society, and
Whereas research is done to advance knowledge, and
Whereas there is no advance of knowledge in the societal sense without publication.
Therefore, as a trialist, I am obliged to:
Ensure the trial I participate in is registered and that the registration is updated as the trial proceeds including the posting of results to the website when finished,
Ensure existence of a statement fashioned and approved by study investigators committing them to publication when the trial is finished or stopped,
Make a concerted effort to publish results of the trial when finished or stopped without regard to the nature or direction of results,
Ensure that study investigators, alone, are responsible for analysis and conclusions stated without interdiction by study sponsors or others,
Be satisfied that persons or agencies funding the trial will fund analyses and paper writing when the trial is finished or stopped until results are published or through multiple rejections of the results manuscript,
Publish in peer-reviewed, indexed, medical journals,

Summary

Trials are undertaken to expand the world's collective knowledge basis regarding treatments for conditions afflicting humankind. There is no viable knowledge base for results of trials in the absence of medical liberties and databases for repose of such results.

Indeed, it can be argued that trials should not be undertaken in the absence of resolve by investigators to make the world aware of their efforts and to publish when the trial is completed, regardless of the nature or direction of the results.

But there are lots of trials started and never finished and never written up. Even if finished and written up, editors may reject because the trial is seen as so poorly done so as to not justify publication, or because they do not trust or like the results. All investigators committed to publishing can do then is to keep trying with other editors. They may or may not succeed.

Alas, the world is not perfect and editors are not robots. They have their own beliefs and biases. That will not change, but a step forward in expanding the world's knowledge base of trials is by requirements of trials being registered when undertaken and for updating registrations over the course of conduct. Now, even if not published, there is a record of trials having been done. Registration is not a substitute for publication, but it is better than nothing in terms of what is done in perfecting and improving treatments for our collective aliments.

References

Chalmers I (1990) Underreporting research is scientific misconduct. JAMA 263:1405–1408

Coronary Artery Surgery Study Research Group (edited by Killip T, Fisher LD, Mock MB) (1981) National Heart, Lung, and Blood Institute Coronary Artery Surgery Study: a multicenter comparison of the effects of randomized medical and surgical treatment of mildly symptomatic patients with coronary artery disease, and a registry of consecutive patients undergoing coronary angiography. Circulation 63(Suppl I):I-1–I-81

Coronary Drug Project Research Group (1973) The Coronary Drug Project: design, methods, and baseline results. Circulation 47(Suppl I):I-1–I-50

Coronary Drug Project Research Group (by Schlant RC, Forman S, Stamler J, Canner PL) (1982) The natural history of coronary heart disease: prognostic factors after recovery from myocardial infarction in 2789 men. Circulation 66(2):401–414

Criner GJ (ed) (2008) National emphysema treatment trial (compendium of 34 parts). Proc Am Thorac Soc 5:379–574

European Coronary Surgery Study Group (1979) Coronary-artery bypass surgery in stable angina pectoris: survival at two years. Lancet 1:889–893

European Coronary Surgery Study Group (1980) Prospective randomized study of coronary artery bypass surgery in stable angina pectoris: second interim report. Lancet 2:491–495

European Coronary Surgery Study Group (1982a) Prospective randomized study of coronary artery bypass surgery in stable angina pectoris: a progress report on survival. Circulation 65(Suppl II): II-67–II-71

European Coronary Surgery Study Group (1982b) Long-term results of prospective randomized study of coronary artery bypass surgery in stable angina pectoris. Lancet 2:1173–1180

Home PD, Pocock SJ, Beck-Nielsen H, Gomis R, Hanefeld M, Jones NP, Komajda M, JJV MM, The RECORD Study Group (2007) Rosiglitazone evaluated for cardiovascular outcomes – an interim analysis. N Engl J Med 357:28–38

Meinert CL (2013) Clinical trials handbook: design and conduct. Wiley, Hoboken

National Emphysema Treatment Trial Research Group (2003) A randomized trial comparing lung-volume-reduction surgery with medical therapy for severe emphysema. N Engl J Med 348:2059–2073

Nissen SE, Wolski K (2007) Effect of rosiglitazone on the risk of myocardial infarction and death from cardiovascular causes. N Engl J Med 356:2457–2471

Shuster E (1997) Fifty years later: the significance of the Nuremberg Code. N Engl J Med 337:1436–1440

University Group Diabetes Program Research Group (1970a) A study of the effects of hypoglycemic agents on vascular complications in patients with adult-onset diabetes: I. Design, methods, and baseline characteristics. Diabetes 19(Suppl 2):747–783

University Group Diabetes Program Research Group (1970b) A study of the effects of hypoglycemic agents on vascular complications in patients with adult-onset diabetes: II. Mortality results. Diabetes 19(Suppl 2):789–830

University Group Diabetes Program Research Group (1971) Effects of hypoglycemic agents on vascular complications in patients with adult-onset diabetes: IV. A preliminary report on phenformin results. JAMA 217:777–784

University Group Diabetes Program Research Group (1975) A Study of the effects of hypoglycemic agents on vascular complications in patients with adult-onset diabetes: V. Evaluation of Phenformin therapy. Diabetes 24(Suppl 1):65–184

Reporting Biases

103

S. Swaroop Vedula, Asbjørn Hróbjartsson, and Matthew J. Page

Contents

Introduction	2046
Types of Reporting Biases	2047
Not Reporting Clinical Trials	2048
Reporting Clinical Trials in Part	2050
Reporting Clinical Trials Such That They Are Hard for Others to Access	2053
Other Issues in Clinical Trial Reporting	2055
Who Contributes to Biased Reporting of Clinical Trials?	2057
Consequences of Reporting Biases in Clinical Trials	2061
Does Biased Reporting of Clinical Trials Constitute Fraud?	2063
Addressing Reporting Biases Through Trial Registration and Access to Protocols	2063
Addressing Reporting Biases in Research Syntheses	2065
Summary and Conclusion	2066
Key Facts	2066
Cross-References	2066
References	2066

Abstract

Clinical trials are experiments in human beings. Findings from these experiments, either by themselves or within research syntheses, are often meant to evidence-based clinical decision-making. These decisions can be misled when clinical trials

---

S. S. Vedula (✉)
Malone Center for Engineering in Healthcare, Whiting School of Engineering, The Johns Hopkins University, Baltimore, MD, USA
e-mail: swaroop@jhu.edu; vedula@jhu.edu

A. Hróbjartsson
Cochrane Denmark and Centre for Evidence-Based Medicine Odense, University of Southern Denmark, Odense, Denmark
e-mail: asbjorn.hrobjartsson@rsyd.dk

M. J. Page
School of Public Health and Preventive Medicine, Monash University, Melbourne, VIC, Australia
e-mail: matthew.page@monash.edu

© Springer Nature Switzerland AG 2022
S. Piantadosi, C. L. Meinert (eds.), *Principles and Practice of Clinical Trials*,
https://doi.org/10.1007/978-3-319-52636-2_183

are reported in a biased manner. For clinical trials to inform healthcare decisions without bias, their reporting should be complete, timely, transparent, and accessible. Reporting of clinical trials is biased when it is influenced by the nature and direction of its results. Reporting biases in clinical trials may manifest in different ways, including results not being reported at all, reported in part, with delay, or in sources of scientific literature that are harder to access. Biased reporting of clinical trials in turn can introduce bias into research syntheses, with the eventual consequence being misinformed healthcare decisions. Clinical trial registration, access to protocols and statistical analysis plans, and guidelines for transparent and complete reporting are critical to prevent reporting biases.

Keywords

Reporting biases · Publication bias · Outcome reporting bias · Time lag bias · Location bias · Language bias · Duplicate reporting · Spin · Citation bias

Introduction

Clinical trials are scientific experiments in humans. Typically, clinical trials in healthcare and public health are performed to inform healthcare and policy decisions. Clinical trials can inform healthcare decisions only when they are reported such that others can access them in full and in a timely manner. Clinical trials, as with any scientific research, can be reported in many ways such as theses/dissertations, reports or presentations shared with colleagues, or publications in scientific archives or peer-reviewed journals. Regardless of where and how they are reported, clinical trials should be promptly and completely disseminated. This chapter discusses evidence on selective reporting of clinical trials in various forms, its consequences, and ways to address it.

Selective reporting of findings from scientific research is a long-known phenomenon, for example, the James Lind Library (https://www.jameslindlibrary.org/research-topics/biases/reporting-bias/. Accessed 22 June 2021) dates the earliest known reference to the seventeenth century. The James Lind Library Initiative provides an exhaustive collection of historical references to selective reporting of scientific research and its consequences (https://www.jameslindlibrary.org/research-topics/biases/reporting-bias/). A systematic study of selective dissemination of scientific research began in the 1950s in education and psychology (Sterling 1959). Selective reporting of healthcare research was identified in early studies in the 1980s, but it was not recognized as a serious concern in healthcare until the next decade (Dickersin and Chalmers 2011).

Selective reporting of healthcare research gained importance with the rapid development of methods for research synthesis. Research syntheses are based upon surveys of the literature to identify all eligible studies on a given question. Because synthesis of an incomplete and selective subset of studies can bias estimates of the overall effect, it became apparent that all studies on a given research question should be identifiable and accessible. This need for complete access to information about methods and results of studies addressing a given question was a strong motivation to study selective reporting of healthcare research.

In the case of clinical trials, selective reporting of findings can lead to incorrect conclusions on safety and effectiveness of healthcare interventions. As an example, reboxetine was approved for use in patients with depression in Europe in 1997 and in the USA in 1999. Its approval in the USA was revoked in 2001 following additional clinical trials showing no evidence of efficacy that were reported to the regulatory agency (Eyding et al. 2010). However, a systematic review showed that according to the published literature, reboxetine was two times more effective than placebo when compared with evidence from the unpublished clinical trials (Eyding et al. 2010; Ferguson et al. 2002). In addition, the unpublished clinical trials showed a significantly greater risk of adverse effects than the published reports alone. In other words, selective reporting of clinical trials significantly altered the conclusions that could be drawn for decision-making regarding the potential harm and effectiveness of reboxetine.

As with any scientific research, findings from clinical trials contribute to evidence-based decision-making only when they are reported and made available to others. Humans may participate in a clinical trial with an implicit or explicit expectation that it will benefit others contributing to the evidence base and advancing scientific discovery. This understanding is breached when clinical trials are not transparently reported. Finally, clinical trials typically require substantial investment of healthcare and research resources. These resources are wasted when the clinical trials and their findings are not promptly, accurately, and transparently reported in full for others to access. In fact, selective reporting detracts from serious scientific inquiry. For instance, several clinical trials of reboxetine for treatment of depression were not published when the findings did not favor the intervention. As a result, reboxetine was prescribed more often than it would have been if it were not selectively reported. Not only did patient care suffer but also the community lost the opportunity to inquire as to why reboxetine did not have a meaningful effect in humans even though it showed evidence of a substantial effect in animals (Malberg et al. 2000).

Types of Reporting Biases

Research on selective reporting of clinical trials has led not only to understanding reporting biases in clinical trials generally but also to different types of biases, terminologies, and contributing mechanisms. Reporting of clinical trials is biased when it is influenced by the nature or the direction of their findings (Dickersin and Chalmers 2011; Song et al. 2010). Nature and direction of findings refer to the statistical significance of findings, magnitude of the observed effect, and whether the findings support a particular hypothesis, e.g., favor a particular intervention. Biased reporting of clinical trials manifests in several ways, some of which have been studied more than others. To broadly categorize reporting biases, they include not reporting the clinical trial at all, reporting only part of the trial, reporting in a manner that is difficult for others to access, and reporting without transparency (e.g., reporting in duplicate, emphasizing or undermining certain findings). Specifically, Box 1 lists different types of reporting biases and their definitions. The rest of this chapter discusses the various types of reporting biases, mechanisms causing biased reporting, and methods to address reporting biases.

> **Box 1 Terminologies (Adapted from Boutron et al. 2019)**
> Reporting bias: Occurs when decisions about whether, when, where, or how to disseminate results of research are influenced by the nature or direction of the results (Boutron et al. 2019).
> Publication bias: Occurs when the decision to publish a study report is influenced by the nature or direction of the results (Boutron et al. 2019).
> Selective reporting bias: Occurs when the decision to report results for some outcomes or analyses is influenced by the nature or direction of the results (Boutron et al. 2019).
> Time lag bias: Occurs when the speed with which research findings are published is influenced by the nature or direction of the results (Boutron et al. 2019).
> Location bias: Occurs when the location or venue where research findings are disseminated is influenced by the nature or direction of the results (Boutron et al. 2019).
> Language bias: Occurs when the language in which research findings are disseminated is influenced by the nature or direction of the results (Boutron et al. 2019).
> Duplicate publication bias: Occurs when the decision to disseminate research findings in one or multiple venues is influenced by the nature or direction of the results (Boutron et al. 2019).
> Spin: Occurs when research findings are reported in a way that distorts their interpretation, e.g., interpreting findings in a less or more favorable light than that supported by the findings (Chiu et al. 2017).
> Citation bias: Occurs when the decision to cite a given report of research findings is influenced by the nature or direction of the results (Boutron et al. 2019).
> Funder bias: The tendency of a scientific study to support the interests of the study's financial funder (Lundh et al. 2017).

Not Reporting Clinical Trials

"Publication bias" arises when clinical trials are not at all reported because of the nature or direction of findings. The term was likely first mentioned in a scientific journal manuscript by Mary Lee Smith in a study comparing meta-analytic effect estimates from studies published in journals with those from unpublished studies, i.e., theses/dissertations (Smith 1980). Foundational research by several scientists, including Kay Dickersin, John Simes, Thomas Chalmers, Colin Begg, Jesse Berlin, Phillippa Easterbrook, Jesse Berlin, Jini Hetherington, and Iain Chalmers, among others, have shed light on publication bias in the healthcare literature, and pioneered the field of reporting biases in healthcare research (Dickersin and Chalmers 2011).

In the context of publication bias, clinical trials are often described as "positive," "negative," or "null," based upon their results or findings. While this terminology (i.e., referring to the studies and not the findings) is not correct from many perspectives (e.g., the terminology is pejorative and simplistic in that only one outcome is considered) and are therefore discouraged, the terms are explained here to facilitate placing prior research in context. Positive results or studies refer to findings of effect usually favoring one outcome, the new or experimental intervention, which are statistically significant regardless of the magnitude of effect or the outcomes examined. Null results refer to findings of no difference in effect and thus no statistical significance between the experimental and control interventions. Finally, negative results broadly refer to findings of effect favoring the control intervention or to findings that lack statistical significance.

The existence of publication bias in healthcare research was suggested by studies on the fraction of published studies reporting findings with and without statistical significance, as well as those that were in favor and against the new or experimental intervention. Subsequent research, starting in 1985, was directed toward differences between effect estimates in published and unpublished studies on the same research question (Begg 1985). This study by Begg also described a method to estimate the magnitude by which treatment effect was inflated by reliance upon published reports. The difference in estimates between published and unpublished clinical trials was initially considered to be publication bias. But its definition has since evolved to emphasize the tendency of investigators to selectively report or fail to report, and that of reviewers and editors to selectively accept for publication, reports of clinical trials based on the nature and direction of their findings (Dickersin and Chalmers 2011).

To ascertain the existence of publication bias, it is necessary to identify the full census of studies that addressed a given question. A few different methods may be employed for this purpose. Early studies relied upon retrospective registries of trials, inception cohorts (e.g., approvals by institutional review boards or IRBs), extensive search for unpublished literature, and survey of members of professional societies (Hopewell et al. 2009). More recently, inception cohorts, i.e., prospective registration or documentation of clinical trials at their inception, have enabled the study of publication bias. For example, clinical trial protocols submitted for institutional ethics review serve as documentation of the studies at their inception. Submissions to regulatory agencies constitute another source for information on extant clinical trials conducted by entities seeking to market the evaluated interventions. Submissions to regulatory agencies by themselves do not necessarily provide a complete census of existing clinical trials although they enable access to information that may not otherwise be easily obtained.

Early studies to demonstrate the existence and frequency of publication bias relied upon surveys of authors to retrospectively identify unpublished clinical trials (Dickersin 1990; Easterbrook et al. 1991; Hetherington et al. 1989). This involved clinical trial registries maintained by one or a few investigators and surveys of authors of published clinical trials for information on unpublished ones. These studies and surveys unequivocally established the existence of publication bias and reasons for nonpublication.

A systematic review synthesized data from 17 inception cohorts of studies approved by research ethics committees and 22 inception cohorts of studies included in trial registries, of which 9 included only randomized controlled trials (RCTs). In all cohort studies, investigators completely followed up all included studies and some determined whether the study was published through communication with investigators (Schmucker et al. 2014). Publication, however, was defined in different ways across the cohorts. Studies that included only RCTs found a pooled proportion of published studies of 45% (95% confidence interval [CI] 31–59%, based on two cohorts following RCTs after ethics approval) and 60% (95% CI 45–74%, based on seven cohorts following RCTs after trial registration). Furthermore, studies with statistically significant results were almost three times as likely to be published as studies with statistically nonsignificant results (pooled odds ratio 2.8; 95% CI 2.2–3.5) based on four cohort studies following studies after ethics approval.

Reporting Clinical Trials in Part

Results of clinical trials may be reported only in part because of the nature and direction of their findings, i.e., selective reporting within published clinical trials. Reporting of outcomes and analysis populations have been well studied; the former is termed outcome reporting bias.

Selective reporting within clinical trials and resulting bias have been characterized through research by An-Wen Chan, Douglas Altman, Asbjørn Hróbjartsson, Peter Gøtzsche, Karmela Krleža-Jerić, Jane Hutton, Seokyung Hahn, Paula Williamson, and Swaroop Vedula among others. In 2002, Hahn and colleagues reported evaluating 37 studies that were reviewed and approved by a single local research ethics committee in the UK (Hahn et al. 2002). Only two of these studies were RCTs. In 15/37 studies that were completed and published, only six had explicitly specified a primary outcome in the protocol. In four of these six studies, the publication consistently reported the protocol-specified primary outcome. A new primary outcome was introduced in the publication of one study, and a protocol-specified primary outcome was not reported in the publication from the sixth study.

Selective reporting of outcomes in RCTs was definitively characterized by Chan and colleagues in two subsequent cohort studies – 102 published RCTs approved by the Scientific-Ethical Committees for Copenhagen and Frederiksberg, Denmark between 1994 and 1995, and 48 published RCTs approved for funding by the Canadian Institutes of Health Research between 1990 and 1998. In addition, Chan and Altman conducted a survey of authors for 519 RCTs that had been published in

December 2000 and listed in PubMed by August 2002. These studies, along with others, revealed a few fundamental insights on selective reporting of outcomes in clinical trials listed below (Chan et al. 2004a, b; Dwan et al. 2013).

Selective outcome reporting manifests in different forms when reporting of the outcomes is influenced by the nature and direction of findings, for example:

1. Prespecified outcomes (primary, secondary, or safety) may not be reported at all in published reports
2. Prespecified primary outcomes may be reported as secondary outcomes
3. Prespecified secondary outcomes may be reported as primary outcomes
4. Prespecified outcomes may be reported such that they are differentially accessible, e.g., reporting certain outcomes in hard-to-access literature or incompletely reporting numerical findings
5. Outcomes that are not prespecified may be introduced; they may be designated as either primary or secondary, or reported as undesignated outcomes. These may be entirely new outcomes or alterations of prespecified outcomes in one or more domains described below.

Outcomes in clinical trials are described to include four domains: the specific measurement variable (e.g., systolic blood pressure), analysis metric (e.g., time to event, value at the end of follow-up), method of aggregation (e.g., average, median), and time-point of measurement (e.g., 12 months). All four domains of outcomes should be prespecified in the clinical trial protocol and the statistical analysis plan, and they should be transparently and accurately reported in the final trial report. Altering any aspect of an outcome definition results in a different outcome and it can potentially alter the conclusion of the clinical trial. More importantly, completeness in reporting outcomes can be influenced by the nature and direction of findings.

Broadly, studies to identify selective reporting within clinical trials used three methodologies – comparing prespecified trial documentation with published reports, surveys of authors, and simulations. Of these, comparing protocols that are registered before clinical trials start with publications, which are called inception cohort studies, can provide reliable estimates of association between reporting and direction or nature of findings. Inception cohorts to study selective reporting within clinical trials typically used protocols registered with institutional ethics review committees or funding agencies. More recently, clinical trial registries have begun to serve as a source of information specified in trial protocols. But such prevalence archives of clinical trials are more susceptible to selection bias than inception cohorts that can be magnified when trials were not registered before start of participant enrollment.

A systematic review of five inception cohorts by Dwan, et al., showed the association between selective reporting of outcomes, for both efficacy and harm, and statistical significance of findings (Dwan et al. 2013). Four of these cohorts estimated that efficacy outcomes had 2.2–2.7 times greater odds of being completely reported when they were statistically significant. Harm outcomes within studies in one inception cohort were 4.7 times more likely to be completely reported when they were statistically significant (95% CI 1.8–12). A comparison of primary outcomes showed that 47–74% of protocol-specified outcomes were reported with no changes, 13–31% of protocol-specified outcomes were omitted from the published report, and 10–18% of published reports introduced a primary outcome not specified in the protocol. In two out of five inception cohorts included in the systematic review, incomplete reporting (defined as not reporting the numerical results in sufficient detail to allow inclusion in a meta-analysis) was observed for a median of 31% and 59% of efficacy outcomes, and 59% and 65% of harm outcomes. Similarly, another systematic review by Jones et al., including 27 inception cohorts, showed that a median of 31% of trials had a discrepancy between the registered and published primary outcome (Jones et al. 2015). A median of 13% of published reports introduced a primary outcome not specified in the registry entry, while a median of 9% omitted a prespecified primary outcome.

Beyond outcomes, reporting clinical trials in part may involve analysis populations, i.e., the set of participants analyzed for efficacy and harm outcomes (Vedula et al. 2013). This is distinct from conducting and reporting subgroup analyses, i.e., analyses of baseline characteristics that modify effect of interventions (Chan et al. 2008). Unlike subgroups, analysis populations serve to assess sensitivity of the estimated effect to critical aspects of study design or to estimate alternative effects of interest. For example, the intent to treat population, in which all randomized participants are analyzed in the groups they were assigned, is known to assure comparability of the groups when all randomized participants are analyzed. A per protocol analysis includes participants who comply with the protocol. The effect estimated in the per protocol population indicates sensitivity of findings to deviations from the randomization assignment and the treatment protocol. Other examples of analysis populations include participants who partly comply with protocol-specified intervention or follow-up. Unlike subgroups, analysis populations differ in subtle ways that lead to considerable changes in estimated intervention effects.

Evidence of the association between reporting analysis populations and the nature and direction of findings is anecdotal and meta-epidemiological in nature (Vedula et al. 2013; Melander et al. 2003; Abraha et al. 2015). Studies on inception cohorts of clinical trials have demonstrated discrepancies between protocol/analysis plans and published reports in sample size calculations, methods to address protocol deviations and missing data, statistical methods, and subgroup and interim analyses. To determine whether these discrepancies are associated with the nature and direction of findings, published reports should be compared with results from protocol-specified analyses. Such comparisons are possible when individual patient data or other documentation of findings from the clinical trials are available. One study of a convenience sample of clinical trials in off-label uses of gabapentin showed discrepancies between protocols, research reports/clinical study reports, and published reports in description of analysis populations (Vedula et al. 2013). But there is no evidence comparing estimates from actual and published descriptions of analysis populations.

A variety of factors in design and analysis of clinical trials can influence the analysis population, including participant eligibility criteria, methods to address protocol deviations and missing data, analytical techniques, specifically adjustment for variables, and interim analyses and their impact on statistical power of the trial. To avoid selective reporting, it is essential to prespecify in the protocol/analysis plan details that can influence which set of participants are analyzed for each outcome. In addition, the prespecified analyses must be accurately reported in publications of the clinical trial regardless of the nature and direction of findings (Chan et al. 2013).

Reporting Clinical Trials Such That They Are Hard for Others to Access

It may be hard to access clinical trials because of where they are reported (grey literature bias), when they are reported (time lag bias), and the language in which they are reported (language bias). Reporting of clinical trials is a continuum that can take several forms including internal reports to study investigators and funders, abstracts of oral or poster presentations at conferences, reports to regulatory agencies, reports to participants, and, ideally, a full peer-reviewed publication.

Peer-reviewed scientific journals in major indexed bibliographic databases such as MEDLINE or Embase ensure a reliable way to identify reports on research findings. Reporting clinical trials in full in such scientific journals assures that others can retrieve them. Access to clinical trial reports is not assured when they are disseminated in certain venues such as the grey literature (e.g., conference proceedings, theses, and dissertations) or in venues that are difficult for others to access (e.g., journals that are not indexed in bibliographic databases), when reporting is delayed, or when they are reported in non-English languages.

Grey literature bias arises when the nature and direction of findings influence whether they are published in peer-reviewed scientific journals or in the harder-to-access grey literature. A 2017 systematic review identified seven studies that compared meta-analytic effect estimates using the published and grey literature (Schmucker et al. 2017). An additional study was reported after the systematic review was published (Dechartres et al. 2018). Three of the eight studies showed that the pooled treatment effect was larger and in favor of the intervention in published versus grey literature. In the remaining studies, pooled estimates of treatment effect were not significantly altered by the inclusion of studies in the grey literature. There was limited evidence on whether the difference in effect estimates can be explained by study methodological quality.

In addition, clinical trials may be reported at scientific conferences, often in part in the form of an abstract, but not fully in a journal publication. Although reporting clinical trials at scientific conferences facilitates widespread dissemination of their findings, these reports are often difficult to find because they are typically not indexed in bibliographic databases. Furthermore, they are incomplete and insufficient for decision-making purposes. A systematic review of 425 studies, which included 307,028 abstracts of biomedical research studies, discovered that only 37.3% (95% CI 35.3–39.3%) were subsequently published in full (Scherer et al. 2018). Studies that only analyzed abstracts of RCTs showed that 59.8% (95% CI 52.1–67%) were subsequently published. This fraction was 47.6% (95% CI

28.4–67.5%) for abstracts of both randomized and controlled trials. The preceding findings show that a substantial proportion of clinical trials reported as conference abstracts are not subsequently reported in a full publication. Abstracts of studies with "positive" results were associated with a 17% (95% CI 7–28%) greater probability of subsequent full publication, wherein "positive" refers to statistical significance favoring the experimental intervention. Notably, other factors were also associated with full publication include large sample size, oral presentation vs. poster presentation, acceptance of abstract, RCTs, multicenter studies, studies with funding, perceived study impact, and study quality.

Time lag bias arises when the nature and direction of findings in clinical trials determine when they are reported, i.e., the speed with which the findings are published. Time lag bias was suggested in the literature in education and psychology, and it has been studied within cohorts of trials in multiple clinical domains beginning in late 1980s. These cohorts included either clinical trials at inception or published ones. The definition for time to publication was heterogeneous, reflecting the complexity of the clinical trial process. In particular, the starting time was defined as either time from approval from institutional ethics committees, time from enrollment of the first participant, or time from start of funding. Although most studies used the date of a peer-reviewed journal publication as the end time, heterogeneity in time to publication has precluded a quantitative synthesis of studies on time to publication (Hopewell et al. 2007).

Stern and Simes observed in an inception cohort of clinical trials that the median time to publication was about 5 years and 8 years for clinical trials with positive and negative results, respectively (Stern and Simes 1997); the hazard ratio (HR) was 3.13 (95% CI 1.76–5.58). A few more studies provide additional empirical evidence of time lag bias in cohorts of both clinical trials and studies of other designs. However, Cronin and Sheldon's analysis of a cohort of studies funded by the National Health Service in the UK did not find a statistically significant association between time from study completion to publication and whether an effect was found in the study (HR 0.53; 95% CI 0.25–1.1) (Cronin and Sheldon 2004). Other studies reported findings similar to those in Cronin and Sheldon (Hall et al. 2007; Liebeskind et al. 2006).

Clinical trials are conducted all over the world. It follows that investigators may publish their findings in journals of English or non-English languages. Because the latter may not be widely accessible to decision-makers in general, publishing clinical trials in non-English languages based on the nature and direction of findings can result in bias. Studies on language bias relied upon cohorts of investigators who published clinical trials in both English and non-English languages within the same time. Analyses of pairs of RCTs in two studies showed that clinical trials with statistically significant findings were more likely to be published in English language journals (Egger et al. 1997; Heres et al. 2004). Some studies on language bias have compared pooled treatment effects of otherwise comparable trials written in English versus written in a language other than English. The latest and largest of such studies, examining 147 meta-analyses, found that treatment effects were 14% larger for trials published in a language other than English than in English (ratio of odds ratio 0.86, 95% CI 0.78–0.95) (Dechartres et al. 2018). However, studies comparing pooled treatment effects in meta-analysis of results from trials reported only in English and trials reported in any language have generally found no major differences (Morrison et al. 2012; Hartling et al. 2017).

Other factors that influence accessibility of clinical trials include impact factor and country of origin of journals in which they are published. Although the terms place of publication bias and country bias have been applied to refer to these two concepts, there is limited evidence for these types of bias. In 1986, Simes found that clinical trials with statistically significant findings favoring the experimental intervention appeared to be published in journals with high circulation whereas those with statistically nonsignificant findings were published in journals that are less widely circulated (Simes 1986). Even when clinical trials are reported in English language journals, it is conceivable that they may be published in different geographic locales based upon their findings. Ottenbacher and DiFabio found that in trials on spinal joint manipulation for low back pain, the observed intervention was smaller in reports in English language journals based in the USA compared with that in reports in journals based outside the USA (Ottenbacher and DiFabio 1985). Despite other studies in this regard (Song et al. 2010), there is no evidence from inception cohorts that the geographic location in which clinical trials are reported is influenced by the nature and direction of their findings.

Other Issues in Clinical Trial Reporting

Thus far, we have described the empirical evidence for various types of bias due to nonreporting of studies or results. In this section, we describe other issues with clinical trial reporting, including duplicate reporting and spin. Duplicate reporting, i.e., replicating reports of clinical trials, is not necessarily biased. For instance, it is common practice to report clinical trial findings in scientific conferences along with a full report in a peer-reviewed scientific journal. In this context, standard scientific practice is to acknowledge the common source of data and to transparently report the findings. However, disseminating multiple reports of clinical trials constitutes bias when the nature and direction of findings determine whether they are reported in duplicate. Such duplicate reporting is particularly problematic when systematic reviewers are unable to determine whether multiple reports are describing the same trial, which can lead to multiple counting of participants in meta-analyses. The existence of duplicate reporting of scientific research including clinical trials is well known (Easterbrook et al. 1991; Gøtzsche 1987; Vandekerckhove et al. 1993; von Elm et al. 2004). But there is limited evidence that it is driven by the nature or direction of findings. Easterbrook, et al., studied an inception cohort of studies approved by an institutional ethics review committee, and found that duplicate reporting was more likely in studies with statistically significant findings (Easterbrook et al. 1991). In summary, evidence suggests that duplicate reporting bias exists but its magnitude and factors contributing to it have yet to be elucidated.

Spin is another type of bias in reporting clinical trials. Spin within clinical trials has been subject to limited research, although it is well studied in the context of communication. Spin in scientific literature has been defined in several ways, which reflects different ways in which it can manifest (Chiu et al. 2017; Boutron and Ravaud 2018). However, most definitions include failure to faithfully communicate observations from the data and manipulating the narrative to distort science. Spin in clinical trials has been studied in the context of how outcomes of efficacy and harm were reported. For example, Boutron, et al., analyzed reports of RCTs published in December 2006 and indexed in MEDLINE (Boutron et al. 2010). They found spin while reporting primary outcomes that were not statistically significant in 18% (95% CI 10–29%) and 38% (95% CI 26–50%) in the title and results/conclusions sections of the abstract, respectively, and in 29% (95% CI 19–41%), 43% (95% CI 31–55%), and 50% (95% CI 38–62%) in the results, discussion, and conclusion section of the main text of the manuscripts, respectively. Spin is not limited to efficacy outcomes. A study of RCTs of interventions for breast cancer published between 1995 and 2011 showed that statistical significance of the primary outcome doubled the odds that safety outcomes would be spun (95% CI 1.02–3.94) (Vera Badillo et al. 2012).

Several strategies may be used to introduce spin into reports of clinical trials (Chiu et al. 2017; Boutron and Ravaud 2018). Broadly, these include misreporting, misrepresentation, and misinterpretation. Selective reporting, e.g., outcome reporting bias may be considered a misreporting strategy to introduce spin in a clinical trial report. Another example of misreporting is failure to report a protocol deviation. Misrepresentation is often focused upon presenting figures in a way that undermine unfavorable findings. Misrepresentation of findings may also take many forms, which can lead to an interpretation that is inconsistent with the observed results. For example, opinions that favor the target hypothesis may be given undue importance while interpreting findings that do not support the hypothesis. Another example is to misinterpret lack of statistical significance as evidence of no effect. Emphasizing hypotheses postulated after the results are known is another strategy to spin findings in clinical trials. In addition, rhetoric is an often-used strategy to introduce spin in reports of clinical trials. For example, rhetoric may be used to overemphasize findings that favor a target hypothesis or to undermine findings that do not, i.e., to explain away unfavorable findings (Vedula et al. 2012).

Spin may be intentional or unintentional, and it has a measurable effect on readers' perception of findings from clinical trials. Boutron, et al., randomized clinicians in cancer with experience in clinical research to read abstracts of clinical trials that were written with and without spin (Boutron et al. 2014). Using a Likert scale of 0–10, clinicians who read abstracts with spin assigned higher ratings that the experimental treatment was beneficial (mean difference 0.71; 95% CI 0.07–1.35), as well as lower ratings for methodological quality of the trial (MD -0.59; 95% CI -1.3 to -0.05), and for importance of the study (MD -0.38; 95% CI -0.95 to 0.19).

Despite evidence that spin effectively persuades clinicians' perceptions of clinical trial findings, much remains to be studied about it. While consensus on the definition and strategies for spin seems to be emerging, it has yet to be characterized as a bias.

In other words, factors driving spin are not well recognized. Specifically, its association with the nature and direction of results has not been established. This association may not be particularly relevant for spin because it may be used to overemphasize favorable findings. While the impact of spin in abstracts of clinical trial reports is understood from one study, its findings have yet to be replicated. Similarly, the impact of spin in the main text of the clinical trial report on the readers' interpretation of findings is also unknown. Furthermore, the sources of spin, i.e., the extent to which authors, reviewers, and editors contribute to spin in clinical trial reports, remain to be ascertained.

Who Contributes to Biased Reporting of Clinical Trials?

Factors driving reporting biases are better understood for publication bias than for other types. In 1959, Sterling observed that failure to publish was associated with statistical nonsignificance of findings (Sterling 1959). He also hypothesized that a "publication policy" leading to a high frequency of studies with statistically significant findings in psychology journals is driven by selection by authors instead of editorial decisions. Subsequent studies lend substantial evidence in favor of this hypothesis. Dickersin, et al., conducted a survey of 318 authors in 1981 and found that failure to submit trial results for publication was the primary reason for unpublished clinical trials, particularly when the findings were not statistically significant (Dickersin et al. 1987). These findings were replicated in another survey of investigators of clinical trials approved by the institutional review boards by the Johns Hopkins Health Institutions in or before 1980. Of 124 unpublished studies, 118 were never submitted for publication by investigators and 6 were rejected by journals (Dickersin et al. 1992). Similar findings were observed for clinical trials sponsored by the US National Institutes of Health in 1979 (Dickersin and Min 1993). A study of 487 studies approved by the Central Oxford Research Ethics Committee between 1984 and 1987 reported similar findings (Easterbrook et al. 1991). Yet another study of clinical trials presented at the Society for Pediatric Research between 1992 and 1995 also found that 8 out of 47 unpublished trials were submitted for publication (Hartling et al. 2004). Furthermore, a systematic review of 27 studies on reasons for nonpublication of biomedical research studies found that authors reported "lack of time" as the most common and most important reason for failure to publish (Scherer et al. 2015). When compared with "lack of time," investigators' expectation that journals would not accept the manuscript was a less important reason for nonpublication.

Reasons for authors' selective outcome reporting partly mirrors those for publication bias, e.g., a perception that positive results are favored by editors. Smyth, et al., conducted qualitative interviews of authors of clinical trial reports that were recognized to have selectively reported outcomes (Smyth et al. 2011). A quarter of the authors they interviewed reported that the direction of the main findings influenced their decision to not analyze other prespecified outcomes. More generally, the survey identified lack of awareness of the seriousness of underreporting clinical trial results, and a lack of clarity about the importance and feasibility of data collection for the outcomes chosen at the time of protocol development.

Evidence shows that editorial decisions are not associated with failure to publish clinical trials and biomedical research. In one of the early studies assessing the association between editorial decision-making and whether study results were positive, a sample of 745 manuscripts submitted to the *Journal of the American Medical Association* (*JAMA*) were analyzed (Olson et al. 2002). Of 745 manuscripts, 133 were accepted for publication in the journal. Adjusted analyses suggested that positive results were more likely to be published but the association was not statistically significant (OR 1.30; 95% CI 0.87–1.96). A more recent study analyzed publication status of 15,972 manuscripts submitted to one general medical and seven specialty medical journals between 2010 and 2012 (van Lent et al. 2014). In a multivariate analysis, the study found no evidence of an association between positive study findings and editorial decision to accept the manuscript (OR 1.00; 95% CI 0.61–1.66). Similar findings were observed in an analysis of manuscripts submitted to the *British Medical Journal*, the *Lancet*, and the *Annals of Internal Medicine* between January and April 2003 and between November 2003 and January 2004 (Lee et al. 2006). The odds ratio of acceptance for statistical significance of findings was 0.83 (95% CI 0.34–1.96) in a multivariate analysis. In addition, a qualitative analysis of editorial discussions on manuscripts submitted to the *JAMA* indicates that the scientific rigor of studies is of most concern in decisions about accepting the manuscripts (Olson et al. 2002). A meta-analysis of studies on editorial decisions showed that the direction or strength of findings in biomedical research studies did not have a significant association with their acceptance (OR 1.06; 95% CI 0.80–1.39) (Song et al. 2010).

However, existing research on whether and how editorial decisions contribute to publication bias only analyzed studies that were submitted for consideration by a journal. These studies included only journals with high impact factors. Authors who responded to surveys in studies that ascertained existence of publication bias have reported the perceived chance of being accepted by journals as a reason for failure to publish (Song et al. 2014). A common perception among authors is that studies with statistically nonsignificant findings have a lower chance of being accepted. Separately, surveys have found that journal editors weighed importance of the research more than other factors including the nature and direction of findings (Song et al. 2010). The recent advent of pay-to-publish and open access models may have altered how editorial decisions influence whether clinical trials are published, but it is not well studied.

Peer reviewers may influence editorial decisions through recommendations on whether to accept reports of clinical trials for publication. There is no evidence whether recommendations by peer reviewers are associated with the nature and direction of findings in manuscripts. Other biases in reviewers affect their recommendations, however. For example, reviewers were less likely to recommend acceptance of studies with findings that were inconsistent with their own perspectives – this is termed confirmatory bias (Mahoney 1977). Geographic location of the reviewer and language of publication are other factors influencing recommendation of acceptance of clinical trial reports, but the evidence is limited and inconsistent.

Sponsors of clinical trials, commercial sponsors in particular, can determine whether and how they are disseminated, either directly as decision-makers or indirectly through their influence on investigators (Bero 2017; Wang et al. 2010), sometimes referred to as sponsorship bias. Support from any sponsor was shown to be associated with acceptance for publication by journals. In studies funded by the UK National Health Service, the amount of funding was associated with publication of findings (Cronin and Sheldon 2004). A few studies reported that support from industry funding is associated with nonpublication or delayed publication. There is some evidence that outcomes in clinical trials sponsored by for-profit entities, such as pharmaceutical companies, favor the experimental intervention (i.e., the sponsor-supported therapy) (Lundh et al. 2017). Two systematic reviews estimated odds ratios of 3.60 (95% CI 2.63–4.91) and 4.05 (95% CI 2.98–5.51) for the association between industry funding of clinical trials and findings that favor the experimental intervention (Lundh et al. 2017; Bekelman et al. 2003; Lexchin et al. 2003). This observation may be explained by a few factors, including publication bias, but qualitative research studies illustrate several other strategies (Lexchin et al. 2003). These strategies include selection of inactive or less active interventions as the control group, outcome specification to facilitate rejection of the null hypothesis or minimize detection of adverse events, selective reporting of outcomes and analyses, multiple publication, reporting studies not as stand-alone publications but within narrative reviews, and reporting trials with spin (Bekelman et al. 2003; Lexchin et al. 2003; Østengaard et al. 2020; Melander et al. 2003; Sismondo 2008a, b; de Vries et al. 2019).

Studies of within-trial reports provide evidence of the different strategies that contribute to the high likelihood that industry-sponsored clinical trials favor the sponsor-supported intervention (Jefferson et al. 2018). The source of within-trial reports included submissions to regulatory agencies, clinical study reports (CSRs), clinical trial registry records, and others such as press releases. Numerous comparisons have been reported in the literature (McGauran et al. 2010), and a few examples are described here. One of the influential studies was enabled by the litigation involving Merck & Co. Analysis of the internal company data from two clinical trials on rofecoxib for Alzheimer's disease or cognitive impairment showed a nearly threefold increased risk of death with rofecoxib (hazard ratio 2.99; 95% CI 1.55–5.77) (Psaty and Kronmal 2008). Published reports of the two trials failed to report these findings and instead concluded that rofecoxib was well tolerated. Published reports from other studies on rofecoxib for additional indications did not include data, which were evident in data available to the US Food and Drug Administration (FDA), on significantly elevated risk of serious cardiovascular thrombotic events (Mukherjee et al. 2001; McCormack and Rangno 2002; Bombardier et al. 2000).

Another study used data available through litigation against Glaxo Smith Kline on pediatric antidepressants. A systematic review including data that were not published by the company found a different risk-benefit profile, compared with that using published data alone, for some antidepressants. Two further studies comparing regulatory submissions to the US FDA on antidepressants for adults revealed similar findings, i.e., different risk-benefit profiles with data from published reports versus regulatory submissions (Turner et al. 2008; Kirsch et al. 2008). A second notable instance involves gabapentin, a medication that was approved for a narrow indication but was extensively used for several off-label indications. Studies of documents made public through litigation revealed publication bias, outcome reporting bias, and inconsistent assessment and reporting of outcomes on harm (Vedula et al. 2009, 2012). In effect, data from CSRs and other internal sources had information that could alter the perceived risk-benefit profile for some uses of gabapentin (Mayo-Wilson et al. 2019).

Furthermore, there is a prevalent notion that clinical trials may be conducted for purposes other than to publish them, i.e., clinical trials serve a nonscientific purpose. This perspective is not new. Investigators surveyed in one of the earliest studies on publication bias in clinical trials reported "Publication not aim of study" as a reason for failure to publish (Easterbrook et al. 1991). More recently, there is a notion that clinical trials, particularly when they are sponsored by for-profit entities, are marketing tools. In other words, clinical trials serve marketing purposes instead of addressing a scientific hypothesis for healthcare decision-making (Vedula et al. 2012; Barbour et al. 2016; Matheson 2017). In fact, a study of internal company documents in one instance revealed that a clinical trial of 2785 patients enrolled by 600 investigators was a "seeding" trial (Hill et al. 2008). That is, the trial was performed solely for the purpose of enabling many physicians to be familiar with the medication a few months before its launch in the market. In the absence of documentation that a clinical trial is being performed for marketing purposes, it is unclear how its published report can be differentiated from a report of a trial conducted to address a legitimate scientific hypothesis. This distinction is relevant because studies show that reporting of clinical trials for marketing purposes is driven by systematic publication planning and strategy. Effectively, it represents management of scientific communication of clinical trials and their findings to optimize marketing goals, which is sometimes referred to as "ghost management" (Sismondo 2007). However, there is limited evidence to ascertain whether reporting biases are more often observed for clinical trials performed for marketing versus scientific purposes.

Other mechanisms in dissemination of clinical trial findings serve to amplify biased reporting. For instance, citation bias refers to a practice in which reports of trial results that favor a targeted hypothesis are cited more often than reports of opposing trial results. This phenomenon was identified in the 1980s among clinical trials evaluating nonsteroidal anti-inflammatory agents for rheumatoid arthritis and called reference bias. Citation bias has been subsequently illustrated for clinical trials (Song et al. 2010; Kjaergard and Gluud 2002), studies of diagnostic accuracy (Frank et al. 2019), and more widely across different domains of biomedical research (Duyx et al. 2017).

Consequences of Reporting Biases in Clinical Trials

Clinical trials are scientific exercises that should be performed with informed consent from its participants. Findings from clinical trials inform healthcare decisions, by patients, providers, payers, and/or policymakers. Biased reporting of clinical trials can lead to incorrect healthcare decisions that they are meant to inform. Regardless of whether individual clinical trials or a systematic review of clinical trials support healthcare decisions, biased reporting can mislead. The impact of the erroneous decisions on patients depends upon the direction and extent of bias as well as the nature of information subject to bias. For example, statistically significant risk of serious adverse events that are not reported can harm patients. A classic instance is an RCT on an anti-arrhythmic drug, lorcainide, to prevent abnormal heart rhythms in patients who have a myocardial infarction. The trial was completed in 1980 but was not published until 1993. In this trial, 9 patients among 48 assigned to lorcainide had died compared with 1 among 47 in the placebo group (Cowley et al. 1993). A separate trial of drugs in the same class as lorcainide published in 1989 found more than threefold increase in risk of death from cardiac causes (risk ratio 3.6; 95% CI 1.7–8.5) (Cardiac Arrhythmia Suppression Trial (CAST) Investigators 1989). Prior to 1989, the company had stopped developing lorcainide for commercial reasons (Cowley et al. 1993).

While the lorcainide story illustrates a potential for significant consequences of biased reporting of a single trial, reporting biases result in misleading overall evidence. When statistically nonsignificant efficacy outcomes are not reported, then the summary effect from a meta-analysis of published reports is likely to be an overestimate. A study of simulated trials suggests that when statistically significant findings are four times more likely to be reported than nonsignificant findings, depending upon statistical heterogeneity and number of clinical trials, a meta-analysis of the simulated trials nearly always inaccurately estimated a nonzero effect when none existed (Kicinski 2014). There is also empirical evidence of discrepancy in findings between meta-analyses using published and unpublished data and biased reporting (Jüni et al. 2002; Hart et al. 2012). Thus, reporting biases can make the summary evidence inaccurate.

The spurious evidence of efficacy from biased reports can obfuscate subsequent meta-analyses that in turn support healthcare decisions. For instance, Mayo-Wilson, et al., analyzed data from multiple sources for trials of gabapentin and quetiapine including published reports, documents from submissions to the FDA, CSRs, and individual patient data (Mayo-Wilson et al. 2017). This analysis showed that cherry-picking among 68 trials with 98 meta-analyzable results, the overall standardized mean difference (SMD) for pain intensity with gabapentin could vary from effective (SMD −0.45; 95% CI −0.63 to −0.27) to ineffective (SMD −0.06; 95% CI −0.24 to 0.12). For depression, the magnitude of effect with quetiapine could vary from moderate (SMD −0.55; 95% CI −0.85 to −0.25) to small (SMD −0.26; 95% CI −0.41 to −0.1). Similar consequences of cherry-picking among multiple possible estimates for outcomes have been demonstrated through meta-analyses using Monte Carlo simulations and bootstrap techniques, which showed large variation between the smallest and largest values of SMD for the treatment effect (Li et al. 2018; Tendal et al. 2011).

Outcome reporting bias can have an impact on validity of findings from systematic reviews. An empirical study investigating the potential impact of outcome reporting bias in RCTs on 42 meta-analyses, each with a statistically significant result, found that after adjusting for selective reporting (using the maximum bias bound approach), the meta-analytic effect estimate became nonsignificant in 8 (19%) meta-analyses, and 11 (26%) meta-analyses would have overestimated the treatment effect by 20% or more (Kirkham et al. 2010). In another study, the addition of unreported results from both published and unpublished drug trials to 41 meta-analyses caused 46% of the meta-analytic effect estimates to show lower efficacy of the drug, 7% to show identical efficacy, and 46% to show greater efficacy. These findings suggest that the impact of selective reporting of results can be unpredictable (Hart et al. 2012).

Delayed reporting of clinical trials can affect evidence to support healthcare decisions. For example, it can manifest as a reduction in the overall estimate in cumulative meta-analyses. In this phenomenon, called "fading of reported effectiveness" by Gehr et al. (2006), clinical trials with smaller and statistically nonsignificant treatment effects that are published with a delay result in a temporal trend in cumulative meta-analyses. A few other studies analyzed temporal trends in meta-analytic effect estimates (Gehr et al. 2006; Jennions and Møller 2002). However, factors confounding temporal trends in meta-analytic effect estimates have yet to be studied.

Despite research on the quantitative and qualitative impact of reporting biases on estimates of treatment effects in clinical trials, much needs to be studied regarding their consequences for healthcare decisions. While there is ample research that reporting biases can falsify evidence and show the potential for misled healthcare decisions, the incidence of erroneous or "near miss" healthcare decisions due to biased reports of clinical trials has not been well characterized.

In summary, biased reporting of clinical trials distorts facts while assuming scientific credibility associated with the study design. Biased reporting of clinical trials can make them inaccessible, uninformative, and wasteful (Chan et al. 2014; Glasziou et al. 2014). Unreported studies can lead to repetitive research to test the same hypothesis and put patients at unreasonable risk as illustrated by clinical trials evaluating anti-arrhythmic drugs. Unnecessary repetitive research is also wasteful. Reporting biases lead to wasteful research because clinical trials fail to serve their purpose, i.e., their findings are not available in a complete and accurate form to healthcare decision-makers. Wasteful research diverts scientific resources from other productive endeavors.

From an ethical perspective, clinical trial participants volunteer for research with the understanding that the study findings will benefit either themselves, others, or both (Brassington 2017). Thus, there is an implicit contract between clinical trial investigators and participants that the study findings will be disseminated in a manner that contributes to scientific progress. Biased reporting violates this contract. It is unclear, from empirical research, whether potential clinical trial participants would consent to the study if they were informed that its findings would either never be reported at all, reported with substantial delay, reported in part or untruthfully, or reported only to serve the sponsor's marketing interests.

Does Biased Reporting of Clinical Trials Constitute Fraud?

There is insufficient understanding about whether and when biased reporting meets a legal standard for fraud. From an academic perspective, biased reporting is considered scientific misconduct particularly when it is driven by a desire to perpetuate or suppress a certain view about study interventions (Wallach and Krumholz 2019). In one perspective, clinical trials are considered tools to market healthcare interventions. This is particularly the case when clinical trials are conducted or sponsored by the for-profit industry with a goal to market the intervention if it is found to be effective (Boutron et al. 2014). In other words, clinical trials are a marketing tool. In fact, commercial entities that sponsor clinical trials are bound by a fiducial duty to its shareholders to generate revenue and profit through its products. This dual role for commercial sponsoring entities leads to tension between scientific and ethical responsibility, particularly when clinical trials reveal no evidence of effectiveness of the study intervention. Willfully suppressing or misrepresenting data, e.g., product sale, for commercial purposes or to regulatory authorities attracts legal penalties. Whether biased reporting of clinical trials by itself constitutes fraud, with commensurate penalties, is uncertain.

Addressing Reporting Biases Through Trial Registration and Access to Protocols

Beginning with the earliest studies, it was evident that publication bias with clinical trials is best addressed by registering them at their inception. At the minimum, clinical trial registries ensure that the existence of trials is transparently reported. Such registries, typically maintained by government and public agencies, enabled research that established the existence of publication bias (Dickersin and Chalmers 2011). Systematic research to characterize the nature and extent of reporting biases, and their potential consequences has eventually led to legislation and policy mandating registration of clinical trials. Several seminal events that shaped the current landscape of clinical trial registration are mentioned below, without attempting to exhaustively catalog them.

In 1997, the US Congress passed the Food and Drug Administration Modernization Act (FDAMA), which mandated registration of clinical trials of drugs evaluated for serious or life-threatening conditions. In response, the National Institutes of Health created and maintained a clinical trial registry, ClinicalTrials.gov. In 2005, the International Committee of Medical Journal Editors (ICMJE) issued a policy that required prospective registration of clinical trials as a prerequisite for publication of the clinical trial. In 2006, the World Health Organization (WHO) coordinated a global initiative to establish the International Clinical Trials Registry Platform (ICTRP). This initiative called for registration of all clinical trials in humans. The ICTRP links clinical trial registers from across the world to enable a single point of access. The WHO subsequently stipulated international standards for clinical trial registries. In 2007, the US Congress passed legislation, the FDA Amendments Act (FDAAA), that broadened the scope of clinical trials that must be registered in ClinicalTrials.gov. Per this legislation, all clinical trials other than Phase 1 trials evaluating drugs, biologics, or devices that are subject to regulation by the FDA must be registered at their inception in ClinicalTrials.gov. In addition, results from these clinical trials were required to be reported to the public through ClinicalTrials.gov within 12 months of trial completion and/or 30 days of FDA approval of the drug, biologic, or device. Additional initiatives support transparency in reporting of clinical trials. These include guidelines for reporting clinical trials and minimum content of clinical trial protocols.

In the European Union, the European Medicines Agency (EMA) chose a more open policy than the FDA. All trials performed in the EU must be registered in the European Union Clinical Trial Register (EUCTR) affiliated with the EMA. Since 2011, data on the recorded trials have been publicly available, and since 2012, all trials have been required to publish their results within 12 months of the end of the trial.

A census of clinical trials at inception, through trial registration, alone is not sufficient to mitigate reporting biases. Access to clinical trial protocols (including statistical analysis plans and all amendments) is necessary for all clinical trials. Public access to protocols is essential for preserving the societal value of clinical trials (Chan and Hróbjartsson 2018). They provide information that complements what is available in clinical trial registries and results databases. While some trial registries such as ClinicalTrials.gov allow deposition of the full clinical trial protocol, there are limited universally accessible venues for protocols to be easily made publicly accessible. While access is important, standardization of clinical trial protocols enhances their transparency and utility. To this end, the Standard Protocol Items: Recommendations for Interventional Trials (SPIRIT) statement provides a checklist of items and guidance on standardized content for clinical trial protocols (Chan et al. 2013).

Public access to CSRs for commercially sponsored trials conducted for regulatory approval or marketing purposes is critical to identify reporting biases and to avoid reaching incorrect conclusions from clinical trial findings. Typically, CSRs are available from regulatory agencies such as the FDA and EMA. However, CSRs for all clinical trials may not be available. For example, the FDA is not required to disclose reviews of clinical trials for which it denies approval. If these clinical trials are also not reported in the scientific literature, then their findings do not benefit healthcare decisions and can potentially harm patients. Finally, clinical trials supported by noncommercial sponsors are typically not required to prepare CSRs or to report about the conduct and findings in as much detail as that in CSRs.

Addressing Reporting Biases in Research Syntheses

In the context of evidence synthesis, reporting biases lead to bias in syntheses either because the available results have been cherry-picked from among multiple outcome measurements or analyses, or because of missing results. Several approaches are available to assess the risk of reporting biases in reports of clinical trials, which represents a risk of bias due to missing evidence (Page et al. 2018). A tool to assess the risk of bias due to missing evidence (ROB-ME) has recently been developed. The tool is designed for users to assess risk of bias in syntheses of quantitative data about the effects of interventions, regardless of the type of synthesis (e.g., meta-analysis of effect estimates, or calculation of the median effect estimate across studies). The framework underpinning the tool is described in detail in the second edition of the *Cochrane Handbook for Systematic Reviews of Interventions* (Page et al. 2019).

The ROB-ME tool consists of four steps. In Step 1, researchers ascertain which syntheses to assess for risk of bias and consider which types of results are eligible for inclusion in each synthesis. This may include a determination of whether to include only inception cohorts in the synthesis. In Step 2, researchers evaluate whether results known or presumed to have been generated during the clinical trial are unavailable. Some approaches for this evaluation include searching beyond journal articles, retrieving and comparing published reports against clinical trial registry records, and protocols and analysis plans available within CSRs or other regulatory agency reports. In Step 3 of the ROB-ME tool, researchers consider qualitative signals that imply some eligible clinical trials may not have been identified.

Finally, in Step 4 of the ROB-ME tool, researchers use signaling questions that draw upon observations from the first three steps. These questions aim to elicit information relevant to an assessment of risk of bias. Users consider how many studies are missing from the synthesis because no result was available consequent to the nature or direction of findings (based on information gathered in Step 2), and whether qualitative signals suggest the synthesis is likely to be missing results that were systematically different to those observed (based on information gathered in Step 3) (Page et al. 2018). In addition, users consider evidence from graphical and statistical methods, including funnel plots and tests of their symmetry. Funnel plots are scatter plots of effect size vs. precision of effect size. They are often simplistically presented and interpreted as adequate tests for publication bias, but it is important to realize their considerable limitation. Asymmetrical funnel plots can be caused by other factors than publication bias, such as more pronounced bias in small trials or heterogeneity. It is therefore more appropriate to consider funnel plots as tests for "small study effects" (caused by several factors, of which publication bias is one) (Vevea et al. 2019). Other statistical methods have been proposed to evaluate sensitivity of findings from meta-analyses to assumptions about the nature and extent of missing evidence. These methods for sensitivity analyses include trim-and-fill, selection models, and regression-based adjustment methods, and emphasize either selective reporting of clinical trials or selective nonreporting of outcomes but not both. Readers are referred to other sources for statistical details of these methods (Vevea et al. 2019; Marks-Anglin and Chen 2020).

Summary and Conclusion

Reporting of clinical trials, whose core purpose in healthcare and public health is to support healthcare decisions, is biased when it is influenced by the nature or direction of their findings. Reporting biases manifest in several ways. Reporting biases have been consistently observed across clinical disciplines and over time. Empirical research shows existence of several types of reporting biases and resulting impact on estimates of effect of different healthcare interventions. Despite availability of statistical methods to address certain types of reporting biases, registration of clinical trials at their inception and transparently reporting them are critical to prevent reporting biases.

Key Facts

- Reporting of clinical trials is biased when it is influenced by the nature and direction of their findings.
- Reporting biases can take many forms, depending on whether clinical trials are published, and when they are published, whether they are fully published in a manner accessible to others.
- Reporting biases typically result in spurious exaggeration of beneficial effects and suppression of harmful effects of interventions.
- Clinical trial registration, access to protocols and statistical analysis plans, and guidelines for transparent and complete reporting are critical to prevent reporting biases.

Cross-References

- ▶ ClinicalTrials.gov
- ▶ Clinical Trials on Trial: Lawsuits Stemming from Clinical Research
- ▶ Fraud in Clinical Trials
- ▶ Introduction to Meta-Analysis
- ▶ Introduction to Systematic Reviews
- ▶ Paper Writing
- ▶ Reading and Interpreting the Literature on Randomized Controlled Trials
- ▶ Study Name, Authorship, Titling, and Credits

References

Abraha I, Cherubini A, Cozzolino F, De Florio R, Luchetta ML, Rimland JM, Folletti I, Marchesi M, Germani A, Orso M, Eusebi P, Montedori A (2015) Deviation from intention to treat analysis in randomised trials and treatment effect estimates: meta-epidemiological study. BMJ 350:h2445

Barbour V, Burch D, Godlee F, Heneghan C, Lehman R, Perera R et al (2016) Characterisation of trials where marketing purposes have been influential in study design: a descriptive study. Trials 17:31

Begg CB (1985) A measure to aid in the interpretation of published clinical trials. Stat Med 4(1):1–9

Bekelman JE, Li Y, Gross CP (2003) Scope and impact of financial conflicts of interest in biomedical research: a systematic review. JAMA 289(4):454–465

Bero L (2017) Addressing bias and conflict of interest among biomedical researchers. JAMA 317 (17):1723–1724

Bombardier C, Laine L, Reicin A, Shapiro D, Burgos-Vargas R, Davis B et al (2000) Comparison of upper gastrointestinal toxicity of Rofecoxib and Naproxen in patients with rheumatoid arthritis. N Engl J Med 343(21):1520–1528

Boutron I, Ravaud P (2018) Misrepresentation and distortion of research in biomedical literature. Proc Natl Acad Sci 115(11):2613–2619

Boutron I, Dutton S, Ravaud P, Altman DG (2010) Reporting and interpretation of randomized controlled trials with statistically nonsignificant results for primary outcomes. JAMA 303(20): 2058–2064

Boutron I, Altman DG, Hopewell S, Vera-Badillo F, Tannock I, Ravaud P (2014) Impact of spin in the abstracts of articles reporting results of randomized controlled trials in the field of cancer: the SPIIN randomized controlled trial. J Clin Oncol 32(36):4120–4126

Boutron I, Page MJ, Higgins JPT, Altman DG, Lundh A, Hróbjartsson A (2019) Chapter 7: considering bias and conflicts of interest among the included studies. In: Higgins JPT, Thomas J, Chandler J, Cumpston M, Li T, Page MJ, Welch VA (eds) Cochrane handbook for systematic reviews of interventions. Version 6.0 (updated July 2019). Available from www. training.cochrane.org/handbook. Cochrane

Brassington I (2017) The ethics of reporting all the results of clinical trials. Br Med Bull 121(1): 19–29

Cardiac Arrhythmia Suppression Trial (CAST) Investigators (1989) Preliminary report: effect of encainide and flecainide on mortality in a randomized trial of arrhythmia suppression after myocardial infarction. N Engl J Med 321(6):406–412

Chan AW, Hróbjartsson A (2018) Promoting public access to clinical trial protocols: challenges and recommendations. Trials 19(1):116

Chan AW, Hróbjartsson A, Haahr MT, Gøtzsche PC, Altman DG (2004a) Empirical evidence for selective reporting of outcomes in randomized trials: comparison of protocols to published articles. JAMA 291(20):2457–2465

Chan AW, Krleza-Jerić K, Schmid I, Altman DG (2004b) Outcome reporting bias in randomized trials funded by the Canadian Institutes of Health Research. CMAJ 171(7):735–740

Chan AW, Hróbjartsson A, Jørgensen KJ, Gøtzsche PC, Altman DG (2008) Discrepancies in sample size calculations and data analyses reported in randomised trials: comparison of publications with protocols. BMJ 337:a2299

Chan A-W, Tetzlaff JM, Altman DG, Laupacis A, Gøtzsche PC, Krleža-Jerić K et al (2013) SPIRIT 2013 statement: defining standard protocol items for clinical trials. Ann Intern Med 158(3):200–207

Chan A-W, Song F, Vickers A, Jefferson T, Dickersin K, Gøtzsche PC et al (2014) Increasing value and reducing waste: addressing inaccessible research. Lancet 383(9913):257–266

Chiu K, Grundy Q, Bero L (2017) 'Spin' in published biomedical literature: a methodological systematic review. PLoS Biol 15(9):e2002173

Cowley AJ, Skene A, Stainer K, Hampton JR (1993) The effect of lorcainide on arrhythmias and survival in patients with acute myocardial infarction: an example of publication bias. Int J Cardiol 40(2):161–166

Cronin E, Sheldon T (2004) Factors influencing the publication of health research. Int J Technol Assess Health Care 20(3):351–355

de Vries YA, Roest AM, Turner EH, de Jonge P (2019) Hiding negative trials by pooling them: a secondary analysis of pooled-trials publication bias in FDA-registered antidepressant trials. Psychol Med 49(12):2020–2026

Dechartres A, Atal I, Riveros C, Meerpohl J, Ravaud P (2018) Association between publication characteristics and treatment effect estimates: a meta-epidemiologic study. Ann Intern Med 169: 385–393

Dickersin K (1990) The existence of publication bias and risk factors for its occurrence. JAMA 263 (10):1385–1389

Dickersin K, Chalmers I (2011) Recognizing, investigating and dealing with incomplete and biased reporting of clinical research: from Francis Bacon to the WHO. J R Soc Med 104(12):532–538

Dickersin K, Min YI (1993) NIH clinical trials and publication bias. Online J Curr Clin Trials Doc No 50

Dickersin K, Chan S, Chalmers TC, Sacks HS, Smith H (1987) Publication bias and clinical trials. Control Clin Trials 8(4):343–353

Dickersin K, Min Y-I, Meinert CL (1992) Factors influencing publication of research results: follow-up of applications submitted to two Institutional Review Boards. JAMA 267(3):374–378

Duyx B, Urlings MJE, Swaen GMH, Bouter LM, Zeegers MP (2017) Scientific citations favor positive results: a systematic review and meta-analysis. J Clin Epidemiol 88:92–101

Dwan K, Gamble C, Williamson PR, Kirkham JJ (2013) Systematic review of the empirical evidence of study publication bias and outcome reporting bias – an updated review. PLoS One 8(7):1–37

Easterbrook PJ, Gopalan R, Berlin JA, Matthews DR (1991) Publication bias in clinical research. Lancet 337(8746):867–872

Egger M, Smith GD, Schneider M, Minder C (1997) Bias in meta-analysis detected by a simple, graphical test. BMJ 315(7109):629–634

Eyding D, Lelgemann M, Grouven U, Härter M, Kromp M, Kaiser T et al (2010) Reboxetine for acute treatment of major depression: systematic review and meta-analysis of published and unpublished placebo and selective serotonin reuptake inhibitor controlled trials. BMJ 341:c4737

Ferguson JM, Mendels J, Schwartz GE (2002) Effects of reboxetine on Hamilton depression rating scale factors from randomized, placebo-controlled trials in major depression. Int Clin Psychopharmacol 17(2):45–51

Frank RA, Sharifabadi AD, Salameh J-P, McGrath TA, Kraaijpoel N, Dang W et al (2019) Citation bias in imaging research: are studies with higher diagnostic accuracy estimates cited more often? Eur Radiol 29(4):1657–1664

Gehr BT, Weiss C, Porzsolt F (2006) The fading of reported effectiveness. A meta-analysis of randomised controlled trials. BMC Med Res Methodol 6(1):25

Glasziou P, Altman DG, Bossuyt P, Boutron I, Clarke M, Julious S et al (2014) Reducing waste from incomplete or unusable reports of biomedical research. Lancet 383(9913):267–276

Gøtzsche PC (1987) Reference bias in reports of drug trials. Br Med J Clin Res Ed 295(6599): 654–656

Hahn S, Williamson PR, Hutton JL (2002) Investigation of within-study selective reporting in clinical research: follow-up of applications submitted to a local research ethics committee. J Eval Clin Pract 8(3):353–359

Hall R, de Antueno C, Webber A (2007) Publication bias in the medical literature: a review by a Canadian research ethics board. Can J Anesth 54(5):380–388

Hart B, Lundh A, Bero L (2012) Effect of reporting bias on meta-analyses of drug trials: reanalysis of meta-analyses. BMJ 344:d7202

Hartling L, Craig WR, Russell K, Stevens K, Klassen TP (2004) Factors influencing the publication of randomized controlled trials in child health research. Arch Pediatr Adolesc Med 158(10): 983–987

Hartling L, Featherstone R, Nuspl M, Shave K, Dryden D, Vandermeer B (2017) Grey literature in systematic reviews: a cross-sectional study of the contribution of non-English reports, unpublished studies and dissertations to the results of meta-analyses in child-relevant reviews. Syst Rev 17:64

Heres S, Wagenpfeil S, Hamann J, Kissling W, Leucht S (2004) Language bias in neuroscience – is the Tower of Babel located in Germany? Eur Psychiatry 19(4):230–232

Hetherington J, Dickersin K, Chalmers I, Meinert CL (1989) Retrospective and prospective identification of unpublished controlled trials: lessons from a survey of obstetricians and pediatricians. Pediatrics 84(2):374–380

Hill KP, Ross JS, Egilman DS, Krumholz HM (2008) The ADVANTAGE seeding trial: a review of internal documents. Ann Intern Med 149(4):251

Hopewell S, Clarke M, Stewart L, Tierney J (2007) Time to publication for results of clinical trials. Cochrane Database Syst Rev 2007(2):MR000011

Hopewell S, Loudon K, Clarke MJ, Oxman AD, Dickersin K (2009) Publication bias in clinical trials due to statistical significance or direction of trial results. Cochrane Database Syst Rev 1: MR000006

Jefferson T, Doshi P, Boutron I, Golder S, Heneghan C, Hodkinson A et al (2018) When to include clinical study reports and regulatory documents in systematic reviews. BMJ Evid-Based Med 23 (6):210–217

Jennions MD, Møller AP (2002) Relationships fade with time: a meta-analysis of temporal trends in publication in ecology and evolution. Proc R Soc Lond B Biol Sci 269(1486):43–48

Jones CW, Keil LG, Holland WC, Caughey MC, Platts-Mills TF (2015) Comparison of registered and published outcomes in randomized controlled trials: a systematic review. BMC Med 13:282

Jüni P, Holenstein F, Sterne J, Bartlett C, Egger M (2002) Direction and impact of language bias in meta-analyses of controlled trials: empirical study. Int J Epidemiol 31(1):115–123

Kicinski M (2014) How does under-reporting of negative and inconclusive results affect the false-positive rate in meta-analysis? A simulation study. BMJ Open 4(8):e004831

Kirkham JJ, Dwan KM, Altman DG, Gamble C, Dodd S, Smyth R, Williamson PR (2010) The impact of outcome reporting bias in randomised controlled trials on a cohort of systematic reviews. BMJ 340:c365

Kirsch I, Deacon BJ, Huedo-Medina TB, Scoboria A, Moore TJ, Johnson BT (2008) Initial severity and antidepressant benefits: a meta-analysis of data submitted to the Food and Drug Administration. PLoS Med 5(2):e45

Kjaergard LL, Gluud C (2002) Citation bias of hepato-biliary randomized clinical trials. J Clin Epidemiol 55(4):407–410

Lee KP, Boyd EA, Holroyd-Leduc JM, Bacchetti P, Bero LA (2006) Predictors of publication: characteristics of submitted manuscripts associated with acceptance at major biomedical journals. Med J Aust 184(12):621–626

Lexchin J, Bero LA, Djulbegovic B, Clark O (2003) Pharmaceutical industry sponsorship and research outcome and quality: systematic review. BMJ 326(7400):1167–1170

Li T, Mayo-Wilson E, Fusco N, Hong H, Dickersin K (2018) Caveat emptor: the combined effects of multiplicity and selective reporting. Trials 19(1):497

Liebeskind DS, Kidwell CS, Sayre JW, Saver JL (2006) Evidence of publication bias in reporting acute stroke clinical trials. Neurology 67(6):973–979

Lundh A, Lexchin J, Mintzes B, Schroll JB, Bero L (2017) Industry sponsorship and research outcome. Cochrane Database Syst Rev 2(2):MR000033

Mahoney MJ (1977) Publication prejudices: an experimental study of confirmatory bias in the peer review system. Cogn Ther Res 1(2):161–175

Malberg JE, Eisch AJ, Nestler EJ, Duman RS (2000) Chronic antidepressant treatment increases neurogenesis in adult rat hippocampus. J Neurosci 20(24):9104–9110

Marks-Anglin A, Chen Y (2020) A historical review of publication bias. Res Synth Methods 11(6): 725–742

Matheson A (2017) Marketing trials, marketing tricks – how to spot them and how to stop them. Trials 18:105

Mayo-Wilson E, Li T, Fusco N, Bertizzolo L, Canner JK, Cowley T et al (2017) Cherry-picking by trialists and meta-analysts can drive conclusions about intervention efficacy. J Clin Epidemiol 91(Suppl C):95–110

Mayo-Wilson E, Fusco N, Li T, Hong H, Canner JK, Dickersin K et al (2019) Harms are assessed inconsistently and reported inadequately Part 2: nonsystematic adverse events. J Clin Epidemiol 113:11–19

McCormack JP, Rangno R (2002) Digging for data from the COX-2 trials. CMAJ 166(13):1649–1650

McGauran N, Wieseler B, Kreis J, Schüler Y-B, Kölsch H, Kaiser T (2010) Reporting bias in medical research – a narrative review. Trials 11:37

Melander H, Ahlqvist-Rastad J, Meijer G, Beermann B (2003) Evidence b(i)ased medicine – selective reporting from studies sponsored by pharmaceutical industry: review of studies in new drug applications. BMJ 326(7400):1171–1173

Morrison A, Polisena J, Husereau D, Moulton K, Clark M, Fiander M, Mierzwinski-Urban M, Clifford T, Hutton B, Rabb D (2012) The effect of English-language restriction on systematic review-based meta-analyses: a systematic review of empirical studies. Int J Technol Assess Health Care 28:138–144

Mukherjee D, Nissen SE, Topol EJ (2001) Risk of cardiovascular events associated with selective COX-2 inhibitors. JAMA 286(8):954–959

Olson CM, Rennie D, Cook D, Dickersin K, Flanagin A, Hogan JW et al (2002) Publication bias in editorial decision making. JAMA 287(21):2825–2828

Østengaard L, Lundh A, Tjørnhøj-Thomsen T, Abdi S, Gelle MHA, Stewart LA, Boutron I, Hróbjartsson A (2020) Influence and management of conflicts of interest in randomised clinical trials: qualitative interview study. BMJ 371:m3764

Ottenbacher K, DiFabio RP (1985) Efficacy of spinal manipulation/mobilization therapy. A meta-analysis. Spine 10(9):833–837

Page MJ, McKenzie JE, Higgins JPT (2018) Tools for assessing risk of reporting biases in studies and syntheses of studies: a systematic review. BMJ Open 8(3):e019703

Page MJ, Higgins JPT, Sterne JAC (2019) Chapter 13: assessing risk of bias due to missing results in a synthesis. In: Higgins JPT, Thomas J, Chandler J, Cumpston M, Li T, Page MJ, Welch VA (eds) Cochrane handbook for systematic reviews of interventions. Version 6.0 (updated July 2019). Available from www.training.cochrane.org/handbook. Cochrane

Psaty BM, Kronmal RA (2008) Reporting mortality findings in trials of Rofecoxib for Alzheimer disease or cognitive impairment: a case study based on documents from Rofecoxib litigation. JAMA 299(15):1813–1817

Scherer RW, Ugarte-Gil C, Schmucker C, Meerpohl JJ (2015) Authors report lack of time as main reason for unpublished research presented at biomedical conferences: a systematic review. J Clin Epidemiol 68(7):803–810

Scherer RW, Meerpohl JJ, Pfeifer N, Schmucker C, Schwarzer G, von Elm E (2018) Full publication of results initially presented in abstracts. Cochrane Database Syst Rev 11(11):MR000005

Schmucker C, Schell LK, Portalupi S, Oeller P, Cabrera L, Bassler D, Schwarzer G, Scherer RW, Antes G, von Elm E, Meerpohl JJ (2014) Extent of non-publication in cohorts of studies approved by research ethics committees or included in trial registries. PLoS One 9:e114023

Schmucker CM, Blumle A, Schell LK, Schwarzer G, Oeller P, Cabrera L, von Elm E, Briel M, Meerpohl JJ (2017) Systematic review finds that study data not published in full text articles have unclear impact on meta-analyses results in medical research. PLoS One 12:e0176210

Simes RJ (1986) Publication bias: the case for an international registry of clinical trials. J Clin Oncol 4(10):1529–1541

Sismondo S (2007) Ghost management: how much of the medical literature is shaped behind the scenes by the pharmaceutical industry? PLoS Med 4(9):e286

Sismondo S (2008a) Pharmaceutical company funding and its consequences: a qualitative systematic review. Contemp Clin Trials 29(2):109–113

Sismondo S (2008b) How pharmaceutical industry funding affects trial outcomes: causal structures and responses. Soc Sci Med 66(9):1909–1914

Smith ML (1980) Publication bias and meta-analysis. Eval Educ 4:22–24

Smyth RM, Kirkham JJ, Jacoby A, Altman DG, Gamble C, Williamson PR (2011) Frequency and reasons for outcome reporting bias in clinical trials: interviews with trialists. BMJ 342:c7153

Song F, Parekh S, Hooper L, Loke YK, Ryder J, Sutton AJ, Hing C, Kwok CS, Pang C, Harvey I (2010) Dissemination and publication of research findings: an updated review of related biases. Health Technol Assess 14(8):iii, ix–xi, 1–193

Song F, Loke Y, Hooper L (2014) Why are medical and health-related studies not being published? A systematic review of reasons given by investigators. PLoS One 9(10):e110418

Sterling TD (1959) Publication decisions and their possible effects on inferences drawn from tests of significance – or vice versa. J Am Stat Assoc 54(285):30–34

Stern JM, Simes RJ (1997) Publication bias: evidence of delayed publication in a cohort study of clinical research projects. BMJ 315(7109):640–645

Tendal B, Nüesch E, Higgins JPT, Jüni P, Gøtzsche PC (2011) Multiplicity of data in trial reports and the reliability of meta-analyses: empirical study. BMJ 343:d4829

Turner EH, Matthews AM, Linardatos E, Tell RA, Rosenthal R (2008) Selective publication of antidepressant trials and its influence on apparent efficacy. N Engl J Med 358(3):252–260

van Lent M, Overbeke J, Out HJ (2014) Role of editorial and peer review processes in publication bias: analysis of drug trials submitted to eight medical journals. PLoS One 9(8): e104846

Vandekerckhove P, O'Donovan PA, Lilford RJ, Harada TW (1993) Infertility treatment: from cookery to science. The epidemiology of randomised controlled trials. BJOG Int J Obstet Gynaecol 100(11):1005–1036

Vedula SS, Bero L, Scherer RW, Dickersin K (2009) Outcome reporting in industry-sponsored trials of gabapentin for off-label use. N Engl J Med 361(20):1963–1971

Vedula SS, Goldman PS, Rona IJ, Greene TM, Dickersin K (2012) Implementation of a publication strategy in the context of reporting biases. A case study based on new documents from Neurontin litigation. Trials 13:136

Vedula SS, Li T, Dickersin K (2013) Differences in reporting of analyses in internal company documents versus published trial reports: comparisons in industry-sponsored trials in off-label uses of gabapentin. PLoS Med 10(1):e1001378

Vera Badillo FE, Shapiro R, Ocana A, Amir E, Tannock I (2012) Bias in reporting of endpoints of efficacy and toxicity in randomized clinical trials (RCTs) for women with breast cancer (BC). J Clin Oncol 30(Suppl 15):6043–6043

Vevea JL, Coburn K, Sutton A (2019) Publication bias. In: Cooper H, Hedges LV, Valentine JC (eds) The handbook of research synthesis and meta-analysis. Russell Sage Foundation, pp 383–430, New York, USA

von Elm E, Poglia G, Walder B, Tramèr MR (2004) Different patterns of duplicate publication: an analysis of articles used in systematic reviews. JAMA 291(8):974–980

Wallach JD, Krumholz HM (2019) Not reporting results of a clinical trial is academic misconduct. Ann Intern Med 171(4):293

Wang AT, McCoy CP, Murad MH, Montori VM (2010) Association between industry affiliation and position on cardiovascular risk with rosiglitazone: cross sectional systematic review. BMJ 340: c1344

CONSORT and Its Extensions for Reporting Clinical Trials

104

Sally Hopewell, Isabelle Boutron, and David Moher

Chapter dedicated to Professor Doug Altman

Contents

What Is CONSORT and Why Is It Important	2074
History of CONSORT and How It Was Developed	2074
CONSORT 2010 Statement	2075
CONSORT Flow Diagram	2075
Extensions of CONSORT	2079
CONSORT for Abstracts	2080
Impact of CONSORT	2081
Development and Evaluation of Tools to Increase Adherence	2083
Future Plans	2084
Cross-References	2084
References	2085

Keywords

CONSORT · Randomized controlled trial · Reporting guideline · Bias

---

S. Hopewell (✉)
Centre for Statistics in Medicine, Nuffield Department of Orthopaedics, Rheumatology and Musculoskeletal Sciences, University of Oxford, Oxford, UK
e-mail: sally.hopewell@csm.ox.ac.uk

I. Boutron
Epidemiology and Biostatistics Research Center (CRESS), Inserm UMR1153, Université de Paris, Paris, France
e-mail: isabelle.boutron@aphp.fr

D. Moher
Centre for Journaology, Clinical Epidemiology Program, Ottawa Hospital Research Institute, Canadian EQUATOR centre, Ottawa, ON, Canada
e-mail: dmoher@ohri.ca

© Springer Nature Switzerland AG 2022
S. Piantadosi, C. L. Meinert (eds.), *Principles and Practice of Clinical Trials*,
https://doi.org/10.1007/978-3-319-52636-2_188

What Is CONSORT and Why Is It Important

Well-designed and properly executed randomized controlled trials provide the most reliable evidence on the efficacy of healthcare interventions. However, there is overwhelming evidence that the quality of reporting of randomized trials is not always optimal. Without transparent reporting, readers cannot judge the reliability and validity of trial findings nor extract information for systematic reviews. Trials with inadequate methods are also associated with bias, especially exaggerated treatment effects (Savovic et al. 2012; Wood et al. 2008). Critical appraisal of the quality of clinical trials is only possible if the design, conduct, and analysis of randomized trials are thoroughly and accurately reported. The CONSORT (CONsolidated Standards of Reporting Trials) statement is comprised of a checklist of essential items that should be included in reports of randomized controlled trials and a diagram documenting the flow of participants through a trial. The objective of CONSORT is to provide guidance to authors about how to improve the reporting of their trials and ensure trial reports are clear, complete, and transparent (Moher et al. 2010a; Schulz et al. 2010a). Readers, peer reviewers, and editors can also use CONSORT to help them interpret the reports of randomized trials. CONSORT is not meant to be used as a quality assessment instrument, rather, the content of CONSORT relates to the internal and external validity of trials. Many items not explicitly mentioned in CONSORT may also be included in a report, such as information about approval by an ethics committee, informed consent from participants, and, where relevant, existence of a data and safety monitoring committee. The CONSORT statement thus addresses the minimum trial reporting criteria and should not deter authors from including other information they consider important (Moher et al. 2010a).

History of CONSORT and How It Was Developed

Efforts to improve the reporting of randomized trials gathered impetus in the mid-1990s. Two groups of journal editors, trialists, and methodologists independently published recommendations on the reporting of randomized trials: the Standards of Reporting Trials (The Standards of Reporting Trials Group 1994) and Asilomar (Working Group on Recommendations for Reporting of Clinical Trials in the Biomedical Literature 1994), both of which were published in 1994. In a subsequent editorial, Drummond Rennie, deputy editor of JAMA, urged the two groups to meet and develop a common set of recommendations (Rennie 1995). The outcome was the development of the CONSORT statement which was first published in 1996 (Begg et al. 1996). Further methodological research and empirical evidence underpinning the CONSORT initiative led to a revision of the CONSORT statement which was published in 2001 (Moher et al. 2001).

CONSORT is an ongoing initiative and the CONSORT statement is revised periodically. A meeting of 31 members of the CONSORT Group was convened in January 2007, in Canada, to revise the 2001 CONSORT statement (Moher et al.

2001) and its accompanying explanation and elaboration document (Altman et al. 2001). Prior to the meeting, some participants were given responsibility for aggregating and synthesizing relevant evidence on a particular checklist item. Based on the evidence, the group deliberated the value of each item and, as in prior CONSORT versions, only items deemed fundamental to reporting a randomized trial were included. After the meeting, the CONSORT Executive convened regular teleconferences and face-to-face meetings to revise the checklist. After a number of major iterations, a revised checklist was distributed to the larger CONSORT Group for feedback. Based on the feedback received, the Executive met on two subsequent occasions to consider comments and produce a penultimate version of the updated CONSORT statement which was published in 2010.

CONSORT 2010 Statement

CONSORT 2010 was published simultaneously in nine journals (Schulz et al. 2010a, b, c, d, e, f, g, h) and is comprised of a 25-item checklist (Table 1) and a flow diagram (Fig. 1). The CONSORT checklist items focus on reporting how a randomized trial was designed, executed, analyzed, and interpreted. When authors use CONSORT, it's recommended that they abide by the journal style they are submitting to, editorial directions, and research area studied. CONSORT is not intended to standardize the structure of reporting but that authors should simply address checklist items somewhere within the article and with sufficient detail and clarity (Schulz and Altman 2014). Along with the CONSORT 2010 statement, an updated Explanation and Elaboration article was also published in two journals (Moher et al. 2010a, b). The aim of the Explanation and Elaboration article is to explain the meaning, rationale, and importance of each CONSORT checklist item and provide published examples of good reporting. It is strongly recommended that the CONSORT checklist is used in conjunction with the accompanying Explanation and Elaboration document. The current version of all CONSORT publications, including the CONSORT checklist, can be downloaded from the CONSORT website (www.consort-statement.org).

CONSORT Flow Diagram

The design and conduct of some randomized trials is relatively straight forward and the flow of study participants, particularly when there are no losses to follow-up or exclusions, through each phase of the study can be relatively easy to describe. However, in more complex trials it may be difficult for readers to discern whether and why some participants did not receive treatment as allocated, were lost to follow-up, or were excluded from the analysis. This information is crucial to assessing both the internal and external validity of the trial (Moher et al. 2010a). A diagram showing the flow of participants through a trial is strongly recommended by CONSORT; the suggested template is shown in Fig. 1 and can be downloaded

Table 1 CONSORT 2010 checklist of information to include when reporting a randomized trial

Section/topic	Item no.	Checklist item	Reported on page no.
Title and abstract			
	1a	Identification as a randomized trial in the title	
	1b	Structured summary of trial design, methods, results, and conclusions (for specific guidance see CONSORT for abstracts)	
Introduction			
Background and objectives	2a	Scientific background and explanation of rationale	
	2b	Specific objectives or hypotheses	
Methods			
Trial design	3a	Description of trial design (such as parallel, factorial) including allocation ratio	
	3b	Important changes to methods after trial commencement (such as eligibility criteria), with reasons	
Participants	4a	Eligibility criteria for participants	
	4b	Settings and locations where the data were collected	
Interventions	5	The interventions for each group with sufficient details to allow replication, including how and when they were actually administered	
Outcomes	6a	Completely defined prespecified primary and secondary outcome measures, including how and when they were assessed	
	6b	Any changes to trial outcomes after the trial commenced, with reasons	
Sample size	7a	How sample size was determined	
	7b	When applicable, explanation of any interim analyses and stopping guidelines	
Randomization:			
Sequence generation	8a	Method used to generate the random allocation sequence	
	8b	Types of randomization; details of any restriction (such as blocking and block size)	
Allocation concealment mechanism	9	Mechanism used to implement the random allocation sequence (such as sequentially numbered containers), describing any steps taken to conceal the sequence until interventions were assigned	
Implementation	10	Who generated the random allocation sequence, who enrolled participants, and who assigned participants to interventions	

(continued)

Table 1 (continued)

Section/topic	Item no.	Checklist item	Reported on page no.
Blinding	11a	If done, who was blinded after assignment to interventions (for example, participants, care providers, those assessing outcomes) and how	
	11b	If relevant, description of the similarity of interventions	
Statistical methods	12a	Statistical methods used to compare groups for primary and secondary outcomes	
	12b	Methods for additional analyses, such as subgroup analyses and adjusted analyses	
Results			
Participant flow (a diagram is strongly recommended)	13a	For each group, the number of participants who were randomly assigned received intended treatment and were analyzed for the primary outcome	
	13b	For each group, losses and exclusions after randomization, together with reasons	
Recruitment	14a	Dates defining the periods of recruitment and follow-up	
	14b	Why the trial ended or was stopped	
Baseline data	15	A table showing baseline demographic and clinical characteristics for each group	
Numbers analyzed	16	For each group, number of participants (denominator) included in each analysis and whether the analysis was by original assigned groups	
Outcomes and estimation	17a	For each primary and secondary outcome, results for each group, and the estimated effect size and its precision (such as 95% confidence interval)	
	17b	For binary outcomes, presentation of both absolute and relative effect sizes is recommended	
Ancillary analyses	18	Results of any other analyses performed, including subgroup analyses and adjusted analyses, distinguishing prespecified from exploratory	
Harms	19	All important harms or unintended effects in each group (for specific guidance see CONSORT for harms)	
Discussion			
Limitations	20	Trial limitations, addressing sources of potential bias, imprecision, and, if relevant, multiplicity of analyses	
Generalizability	21	Generalizability (external validity, applicability) of the trial findings	

(continued)

Table 1 (continued)

Section/topic	Item no.	Checklist item	Reported on page no.
Interpretation	22	Interpretation consistent with results, balancing benefits and harms, and considering other relevant evidence	
Other information			
Registration	23	Registration number and name of trial registry	
Protocol	24	Where the full trial protocol can be accessed, if available	
Funding	25	Sources of funding and other support (such as supply of drugs), role of funders	

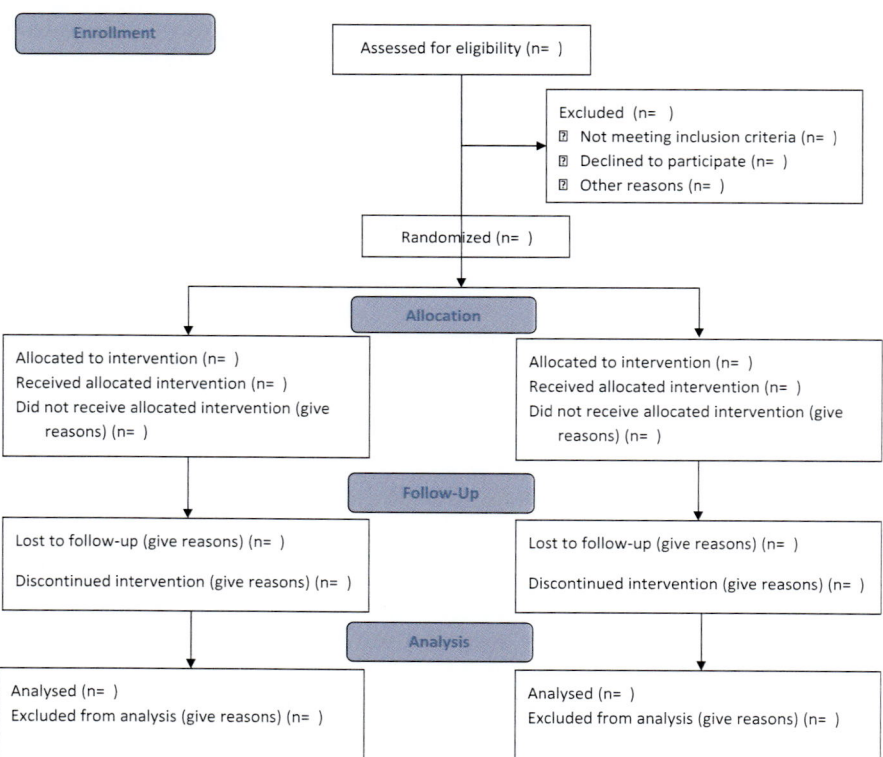

Fig. 1 Flow diagram of the progress through the phases of a parallel randomized trial of two groups (that is, enrolment, intervention allocation, follow-up, and data analysis)

from the CONSORT website (www.consort-statement.org). The exact form and content of the flow diagram may vary according to specific features of a trial. A study evaluating the reporting of flow diagrams in published reports of randomized trials found that journals endorsing CONSORT are more likely to include a flow diagram (Hopewell et al. 2011). However, not all information was adequately reported; the number of people in each arm who actually received the intervention as allocated were lost to follow-up or discontinued the intervention and were included in the main analysis that was often lacking.

Extensions of CONSORT

The CONSORT statement is primarily aimed at primary reports (i.e., reporting the main findings) of randomized trials with two group parallel designs. Extensions to CONSORT have been developed to tackle the methodological issues associated with reporting different types of trial designs, data, and reporting different types of interventions (Fig. 2). Examples of different types of trial design extension include the CONSORT extensions for cluster randomized trials (Campbell et al. 2012), cross-over trials (Dwan et al. 2019), non-inferiority and equivalence trials (Piaggio et al. 2012), pragmatic trials (Zwarenstein et al. 2008), multiarm trials (Juszczak et al. 2019), N of 1 trials (Vohra et al. 2016), pilot and feasibility trials (Eldridge et al. 2016a, b), and within person trials (Pandis et al. 2017). Different types of intervention extension include the CONSORT extensions for non-pharmacologic treatments (Boutron et al. 2017), social and psychological interventions (Montgomery et al. 2018), herbal interventions (Gagnier et al. 2006), acupuncture (MacPherson et al. 2010), and Chinese herbal medicine (Cheng et al. 2017). Extensions for reporting different types of data include patient-reported outcomes (Calvert et al. 2013), harms (Ioannidis et al. 2004), abstracts (Hopewell et al. 2008a, b), and health equity (Welch

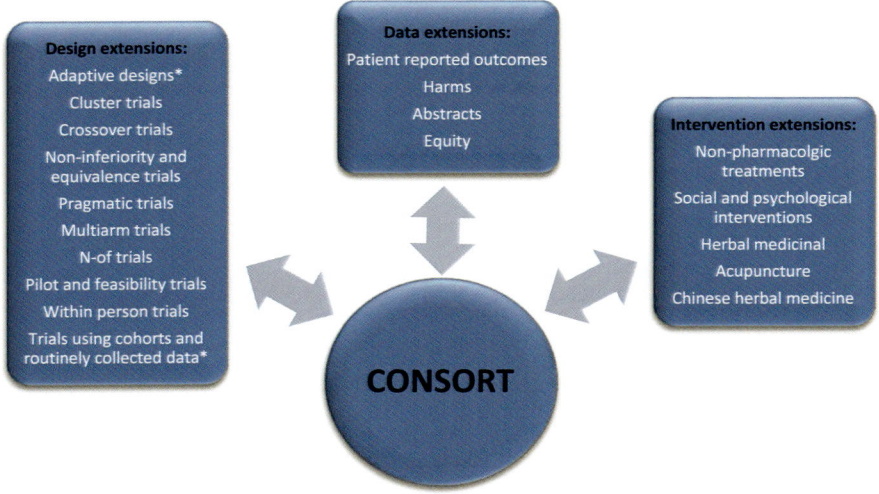

*CONSORT extension in development

Fig. 2 Extensions of the CONSORT statement

et al. 2017). Several CONSORT extensions are also in development, including reporting trials using adaptive designs (Dimairo et al. 2018) and trials using cohorts and routinely collected health data (Kwakkenbos et al. 2018). Each of these extensions includes the original CONSORT checklist items followed by the modified/ extended items, with explanations and examples of good reporting.

A number of authors have developed reporting guidelines based on CONSORT but have done so without the knowledge or participation of anyone from the CONSORT Group. These are unofficial CONSORT extensions and so have not been included here.

A randomized trial may require more than one CONSORT extension, for example, in a pragmatic trial evaluating a non-pharmacological treatment with cluster randomization, the main CONSORT checklist should be combined with three extensions: pragmatic trial, cluster trial, and non-pharmacological extensions. This can be cumbersome and difficult to apply in practice. Initiatives are underway to develop tools to simplifying this process (see "Development and Evaluation of Tools to Increase Adherence"). A recent study evaluating the impact of a web-based tool called WebCONSORT, which allows authors to obtain a customized CONSORT checklist and flow diagram specific to their trial design and type of intervention showed that the most common CONSORT extensions selected were non-pharmacologic (n = 93/197 manuscripts), pragmatic (n = 36/197), and cluster randomized trials (19/197). Over two-thirds of manuscripts were registered as requiring one or more CONSORT extension (Hopewell et al. 2016).

CONSORT for Abstracts

The CONSORT group has also published specific guidance for reporting abstracts of randomized trials (Hopewell et al. 2008a, b). The CONSORT for abstracts checklist provides a list of essential items (Table 2) that authors should include when reporting the main results of a randomized trial in a journal or conference abstract. This checklist has also been extended to provide specific guidance for reporting abstracts of trials using a cluster design (Campbell et al. 2012), non-inferiority and equivalence trials (Piaggio et al. 2012), multiarm trials (Juszczak et al. 2019), N of 1 trials (Vohra et al. 2016), pilot and feasibility trials (Eldridge et al. 2016a, b), within person trials (Pandis et al. 2017), and trials of non-pharmacologic treatments (Boutron et al. 2017). Clear, transparent, and sufficiently detailed abstracts of randomized trials are important because readers often base their assessment of a trial base on such information. A properly constructed and well-written abstract helps individuals to quickly assess the relevance of the findings and should accurately reflect what is included in the full journal article. Studies comparing the accuracy of information reported in journal abstracts have found claims that are inconsistent with, or missing from, the body of the full article which could seriously mislead someone's interpretation of the trial findings (Hopewell et al. 2008a).

Table 2 Items to include when reporting a randomized trial in a journal abstract or conference abstract[a]

Item	Description	Reported on line number
Title	Identification of the study as randomized	
Authors[a]	Contact details for the corresponding author	
Trial design	Description of the trial design (e.g., parallel, cluster, non-inferiority)	
Methods		
Participants	Eligibility criteria for participants and the settings where the data were collected	
Interventions	Interventions intended for each group	
Objective	Specific objective or hypothesis	
Outcome	Clearly defined primary outcome for this report	
Randomization	How participants were allocated to interventions	
Blinding (masking)	Whether or not participants, care givers, and those assessing the outcomes were blinded to group assignment	
Results		
Numbers randomized	Number of participants randomized to each group	
Recruitment	Trial status	
Numbers analyzed	Number of participants analyzed in each group	
Outcome	For the primary outcome, a result for each group and the estimated effect size and its precision	
Harms	Important adverse events or side effects	
Conclusions	General interpretation of the results	
Trial registration	Registration number and name of trial register	
Funding	Source of funding	

[a]This item is specific to conference abstracts

Impact of CONSORT

The CONSORT is the most well-known reporting guideline on which many reporting guidelines have been based (Schulz and Altman 2014). It has been listed among the top health research milestones of the twentieth century according to the Patient-Centered Outcomes Research Institute (Gabriel and Normand 2012). CONSORT 2010 is among the top 1% of article-level metrics (views, downloads, citations, social media shares) tracked by PLoS Medicine. Since its original publication in 1996, the main CONSORT publications have been cumulatively cited over

8000 times. In addition, the CONSORT website (www.consort.statement.org), on which all CONSORT publications and information about CONSORT and related initiatives are available, averages around 30,000 hits per months. CONSORT 2010 has also been translated into 13 different languages including Chinese, French, German, Greek, Italian, Japanese, Persian, Portuguese, Russian, Spanish, Turkish, and Vietnamese, which can be downloaded from the CONSORT website.

Perhaps the most telling indicator of CONSORT's impact is its uptake by journals and subsequent impact on the completeness of reporting of trials. It is currently known to be endorsed by over 600 biomedical journals and endorsed by several prominent editorial organizations, including the International Committee of Medical Journal Editors, the World Association of Medical Editors, and the Council of Science Editors. Journal endorsement of CONSORT and other reporting guidelines typically occurs in the form of a supportive statement in a journal's Instructions to authors. A Cochrane review assessed the effect of journal endorsement of CONSORT on the reporting of trials they publish (Turner et al. 2012). In 50 included studies evaluating the reporting of 16,604 trials, 25 of 27 CONSORT-related items measured were more completely reported in trials published in endorsing journals than those in non-endorsing journals; five items were significantly better reported. The results of this review suggest that journal endorsement of CONSORT may benefit the completeness of reporting of randomized trials they publish. Several studies have also reported some improvement in reporting over time. One such study examined the reporting characteristics and methodological details of randomized trials indexed in PubMed in 2000 and 2006 and assessed whether the quality of reporting had improved after publication of the CONSORT Statement in 2001. While reporting of several important aspects of trial methods has improved, the quality of reporting remains well below an acceptable level (Hopewell et al. 2010).

Journal endorsement of CONSORT does not imply any active attempt to ensure adherence to the guideline. Journals need to take further action regarding their endorsement and implementation of CONSORT to facilitate accurate, transparent, and complete reporting of trials. In a study examining the online "Instruction to Authors" of 168 high-impact factor journals published in 2014, 68% mentioned CONSORT in their "Instructions to Authors" and 42% explicitly stated that authors "must" use CONSORT to prepare their trial manuscript (Shamseer et al. 2016). However, only 38% required an accompanying completed CONSORT checklist as a condition of submission and 39% explicitly requested the inclusion of a flow diagram with the submission. Only 22 of the 168 included journals (13%) mentioned any of the nine CONSORT extensions published at the time of searching (Shamseer et al. 2016).

Submission of a CONSORT checklist by authors alongside their submitted manuscript, by itself, does not necessarily lead to improvement in the completeness of reporting. A recent study found that there are often a number of inconsistencies between what authors claimed on the submitted checklist and what was actually reported in the published article (Blanco et al. 2018). Journals should take further action to help ensure that these checklists reflect what is reported in the manuscript. A study which investigated the effect of the different editorial policies used by five leading general medical journals to implement the CONSORT for abstracts checklist found that journals with an active policy to enforce the checklist showed an immediate increase in the level of mean number of items reported after publication of the guideline. The change in level or trend did not increase in journals without policy to enforce the checklist, showing that active implementation of the CONSORT guidelines by journals can lead to improvements in the reporting (Hopewell et al. 2012).

Development and Evaluation of Tools to Increase Adherence

One of the biggest challenges for the CONSORT Group is now to better facilitate endorsement and implementation, including adherence, of CONSORT and its related extensions. Several initiatives are underway to develop and evaluate tools that make it easier for authors, journal editors, and editorial staff to facilitate the uptake of CONSORT. The first of these initiatives are aimed at the authors of randomized trials. WebCONSORT is a simple web-based tool which incorporates a number of different CONSORT extensions (Hopewell et al. 2016). The tool allows authors to obtain a customized CONSORT checklist and flow diagram specific to their trial design and type of intervention. The hypothesis being that the tool would allow optimal use of the CONSORT Statement and its extensions, thus leading to an improvement in the transparency of articles related to randomized trials. The tool was evaluated by authors of randomized trials who were asked to use the tool at the manuscript revision stage; authors registering to use the tool were randomized to receive either WebCONSORT or control. The customized tool failed to show benefit in terms of improvement in reporting. However, in a quarter of manuscripts, authors either wrongly selected an extension or failed to select the right extension when using the WebCONSORT tool. This suggests that better education is needed, earlier in the publication process, on when and how to implement CONSORT and, in particular, CONSORT-related extensions.

CobWEB (CONSORT-based WEB tool) is an example of an online writing aid tool, aimed at early career researchers. The CobWEB tool aims to increase adherence to CONSORT much earlier in the publication process and at the writing stage of a manuscript. The writing tool combines different CONSORT extensions and provides examples of adequate reporting. The tool was evaluated using a "split-manuscript" randomized trial whereby participants were asked to write the methods section of a manuscript. The methods section was divided into six different domains: trial design, randomization, blinding, participants, interventions, and outcomes. Participants had to draft all six domains with access to the CobWEB tool for a random three of the six domains. Completeness of reporting was significantly higher with the CobWEB tool for all domains except for blinding and outcomes (Barnes et al. 2015).

The second main group of initiatives aimed at facilitating the endorsement and implementation of CONSORT and its related extensions are aimed at journals and peer reviewers. Most peer reviewers are not formally trained. Without training, it is more difficult to detect problems in reporting and despite their good intentions, peer reviewers often fail to detect important deficiencies in the reporting of methods and results of randomized trials (Hopewell et al. 2014). Stat Reviewer is an automated software tool which scans manuscripts to assess the completeness of reporting against CONSORT checklist items (www.statreviewer.com). It then produces a detailed report on CONSORT compliance, highlighting any gaps in reporting. Stat Reviewer is now integrated within Editorial Manager, a commonly used journal manuscript submission and peer review tracking system, and can provide a quick assessment of reporting of randomized trials submitted for publication. In principle, journals can then use this report to identify manuscripts which fall below a certain level of compliance and be sent back to author's to revise before sending out to peer review.

A number of tasks are expected from peer reviewers when assessing reports of randomized trials, in addition to assessing completeness of reporting (Chauvin et al. 2015), and it may be unrealistic to expect a peer reviewer to adequately complete all of these tasks. A current study is assessing the use of a simple online peer review tool (CobPeer) and training module, aimed at early career peer reviewers, which has been developed according to the same principles used for the CobWeb tool (Barnes et al. 2015). The online peer review tool is being evaluated to compare the performance of early career peer reviewers who use the peer reviewer tool with usual journal peer reviewers in identifying inadequate reporting and switching of outcomes in completed reports of randomized trials (Chauvin et al. 2017). If found to be successful, use of the online tool by early career peer reviewers could help to improve the efficiency of the peer review system and the quality of trial reporting.

Future Plans

Clear, transparent, and complete reporting of research is essential in order to be able to assess the reliability of the results of randomized trials. Twenty years since its first publication, poor adherence to CONSORT recommendations remains common in published reports of randomized trials. In order to maximize the impact of CONSORT and its related extensions it's essential to better understand and met the needs of its different users including authors, journal editors, and peer reviewers. There is a clear need for better education much earlier in the publication process for authors and journal editorial staff on when and how to implement CONSORT and, in particular, CONSORT-related extensions. Authors need to have CONSORT in mind when they start to write the manuscript of their trial and not just at the manuscript submission stage to a journal as this may be too late. The development of tools for authors to increase adherence when writing the results of a randomized trial and for journals and peer reviewers when submitting a manuscript to journal could also help facilitate better reporting.

Cross-References

▶ Controlling for Multiplicity, Eligibility, and Exclusions
▶ Implementing the Trial Protocol
▶ Issues for Masked Data Monitoring

- Masking of Trial Investigators
- Masking Study Participants
- Paper Writing
- Power and Sample Size
- Principles of Clinical Trials: Bias and Precision Control
- Reporting Biases
- Variance Control Procedures

References

Altman DG, Schulz KF, Moher D, Egger M, Davidoff F, Elbourne D et al (2001) The revised CONSORT statement for reporting randomized trials: explanation and elaboration. Ann Intern Med 134(8):663–694

Barnes C, Boutron I, Giraudeau B, Porcher R, Altman DG, Ravaud P (2015) Impact of an online writing aid tool for writing a randomized trial report: the COBWEB (Consort-based WEB tool) randomized controlled trial. BMC Med 13:221

Begg C, Cho M, Eastwood S, Horton R, Moher D, Olkin I et al (1996) Improving the quality of reporting of randomized controlled trials. The CONSORT statement. JAMA 276(8):637–639

Blanco D, Biggane AM, Cobo E (2018) Are CONSORT checklists submitted by authors adequately reflecting what information is actually reported in published papers? Trials 19(1):80

Boutron I, Altman DG, Moher D, Schulz KF, Ravaud P (2017) CONSORT statement for randomized trials of nonpharmacologic treatments: a 2017 update and a CONSORT extension for nonpharmacologic trial abstracts. Ann Intern Med 167(1):40–47

Calvert M, Blazeby J, Altman DG, Revicki DA, Moher D, Brundage MD (2013) Reporting of patient-reported outcomes in randomized trials: the CONSORT PRO extension. JAMA 309(8):814–822

Campbell MK, Piaggio G, Elbourne DR, Altman DG (2012) Consort 2010 statement: extension to cluster randomised trials. BMJ (Clin Res Ed) 345:e5661

Chauvin A, Ravaud P, Baron G, Barnes C, Boutron I (2015) The most important tasks for peer reviewers evaluating a randomized controlled trial are not congruent with the tasks most often requested by journal editors. BMC Med 13:158

Chauvin A, Moher D, Altman D, Schriger DL, Alam S, Hopewell S et al (2017) A protocol of a cross-sectional study evaluating an online tool for early career peer reviewers assessing reports of randomised controlled trials. BMJ Open 7(9):e017462

Cheng CW, Wu TX, Shang HC, Li YP, Altman DG, Moher D et al (2017) CONSORT extension for Chinese herbal medicine formulas 2017: recommendations, explanation, and elaboration. Ann Intern Med 167(2):112–121

Dimairo M, Coates E, Pallmann P, Todd S, Julious SA, Jaki T et al (2018) Development process of a consensus-driven CONSORT extension for randomised trials using an adaptive design. BMC Med 16(1):210

Dwan K, Li T, Altman DG, Elbourne D (2019) CONSORT 2010 statement: extension to randomised crossover trials. BMJ (Clin Res ed) 366:l4378

Eldridge SM, Chan CL, Campbell MJ, Bond CM, Hopewell S, Thabane L et al (2016a) CONSORT 2010 statement: extension to randomised pilot and feasibility trials. BMJ (Clin Res Ed) 355:i5239

Eldridge SM, Chan CL, Campbell MJ, Bond CM, Hopewell S, Thabane L et al (2016b) CONSORT 2010 statement: extension to randomised pilot and feasibility trials. Pilot Feasibility Stud 2:64

Gabriel SE, Normand SL (2012) Getting the methods right – the foundation of patient-centered outcomes research. N Engl J Med 367(9):787–790

Gagnier JJ, Boon H, Rochon P, Moher D, Barnes J, Bombardier C (2006) Reporting randomized, controlled trials of herbal interventions: an elaborated CONSORT statement. Ann Intern Med 144(5):364–367

Hopewell S, Clarke M, Moher D, Wager E, Middleton P, Altman DG et al (2008a) CONSORT for reporting randomized controlled trials in journal and conference abstracts: explanation and elaboration. PLoS Med 5(1):e20

Hopewell S, Clarke M, Moher D, Wager E, Middleton P, Altman DG et al (2008b) CONSORT for reporting randomised trials in journal and conference abstracts. Lancet (London) 371(9609):281–283

Hopewell S, Dutton S, Yu LM, Chan AW, Altman DG (2010) The quality of reports of randomised trials in 2000 and 2006: comparative study of articles indexed in PubMed. BMJ (Clin Res Ed) 340:c723

Hopewell S, Hirst A, Collins GS, Mallett S, Yu LM, Altman DG (2011) Reporting of participant flow diagrams in published reports of randomized trials. Trials 12:253

Hopewell S, Ravaud P, Baron G, Boutron I (2012) Effect of editors' implementation of CONSORT guidelines on the reporting of abstracts in high impact medical journals: interrupted time series analysis. BMJ (Clin Res Ed) 344:e4178

Hopewell S, Collins GS, Boutron I, Yu LM, Cook J, Shanyinde M et al (2014) Impact of peer review on reports of randomised trials published in open peer review journals: retrospective before and after study. BMJ (Clin Res Ed) 349:g4145

Hopewell S, Boutron I, Altman DG, Barbour G, Moher D, Montori V et al (2016) Impact of a web-based tool (WebCONSORT) to improve the reporting of randomised trials: results of a randomised controlled trial. BMC Med 14(1):199

Ioannidis JP, Evans SJ, Gotzsche PC, O'Neill RT, Altman DG, Schulz K et al (2004) Better reporting of harms in randomized trials: an extension of the CONSORT statement. Ann Intern Med 141(10):781–788

Juszczak EA, Altman DG, Hopewell S, Schulz K (2019) Reporting of multi-arm parallel group randomized trials: extension of the CONSORT 2010 statement. JAMA 321(16):1610–1620

Kwakkenbos L, Juszczak E, Hemkens LG, Sampson M, Frobert O, Relton C et al (2018) Protocol for the development of a CONSORT extension for RCTs using cohorts and routinely collected health data. Res Integr Peer Rev 3:9

MacPherson H, Altman DG, Hammerschlag R, Youping L, Taixiang W, White A et al (2010) Revised Standards for reporting interventions in clinical trials of acupuncture (STRICTA): extending the CONSORT statement. PLoS Med 7(6):e1000261

Moher D, Schulz KF, Altman D (2001) The CONSORT statement: revised recommendations for improving the quality of reports of parallel-group randomized trials. JAMA 285(15):1987–1991

Moher D, Hopewell S, Schulz KF, Montori V, Gotzsche PC, Devereaux PJ et al (2010a) CONSORT 2010 explanation and elaboration: updated guidelines for reporting parallel group randomised trials. BMJ (Clin Res Ed) 340:c869

Moher D, Hopewell S, Schulz KF, Montori V, Gotzsche PC, Devereaux PJ et al (2010b) CONSORT 2010 explanation and elaboration: updated guidelines for reporting parallel group randomised trials. J Clin Epidemiol 63(8):e1–e37

Montgomery P, Grant S, Mayo-Wilson E, Macdonald G, Michie S, Hopewell S et al (2018) Reporting randomised trials of social and psychological interventions: the CONSORT-SPI 2018 extension. Trials 19(1):407

Pandis N, Chung B, Scherer RW, Elbourne D, Altman DG (2017) CONSORT 2010 statement: extension checklist for reporting within person randomised trials. BMJ (Clin Res Ed) 357:j2835

Piaggio G, Elbourne DR, Pocock SJ, Evans SJ, Altman DG (2012) Reporting of noninferiority and equivalence randomized trials: extension of the CONSORT 2010 statement. JAMA 308(24):2594–2604

Rennie D (1995) Reporting randomized controlled trials. An experiment and a call for responses from readers. JAMA 273(13):1054–1055

Savovic J, Jones HE, Altman DG, Harris RJ, Juni P, Pildal J et al (2012) Influence of reported study design characteristics on intervention effect estimates from randomized, controlled trials. Ann Intern Med 157(6):429–438

Schulz KM, Altman DG (2014) CONSORT [Chapter 7] published in guidelines for reporting health research: a users guide. Wiley Blackwell, Chichester

Schulz KF, Altman DG, Moher D (2010a) CONSORT 2010 statement: updated guidelines for reporting parallel group randomized trials. Ann Intern Med 152(11):726–732

Schulz KF, Altman DG, Moher D (2010b) CONSORT 2010 statement: updated guidelines for reporting parallel group randomized trials. Open Med 4(1):e60–e68

Schulz KF, Altman DG, Moher D (2010c) CONSORT 2010 statement: updated guidelines for reporting parallel group randomized trials. Obstet Gynecol 115(5):1063–1070

Schulz KF, Altman DG, Moher D (2010d) CONSORT 2010 statement: updated guidelines for reporting parallel group randomised trials. PLoS Med 7(3):e1000251

Schulz KF, Altman DG, Moher D (2010e) CONSORT 2010 statement: updated guidelines for reporting parallel group randomised trials. J Clin Epidemiol 63(8):834–840

Schulz KF, Altman DG, Moher D (2010f) CONSORT 2010 statement: updated guidelines for reporting parallel group randomised trials. BMC Med 8:18

Schulz KF, Altman DG, Moher D (2010g) CONSORT 2010 statement: updated guidelines for reporting parallel group randomised trials. Trials 11:32

Schulz KF, Altman DG, Moher D (2010h) CONSORT 2010 statement: updated guidelines for reporting parallel group randomised trials. BMJ (Clin Res Ed) 340:c332

Shamseer L, Hopewell S, Altman DG, Moher D, Schulz KF (2016) Update on the endorsement of CONSORT by high impact factor journals: a survey of journal "Instructions to authors" in 2014. Trials 17(1):301

The Standards of Reporting Trials Group (1994) A proposal for structured reporting of randomized controlled trials. JAMA 272(24):1926–1931

Turner L, Shamseer L, Altman DG, Schulz KF, Moher D (2012) Does use of the CONSORT statement impact the completeness of reporting of randomised controlled trials published in medical journals? A Cochrane review. Syst Rev 1:60

Vohra S et al (2016) CONSORT extension for reporting N-of-1 trials (CENT) 2015 statement. BMJ (Clin Res Ed) 355:i5381

Welch VA, Norheim OF, Jull J, Cookson R, Sommerfelt H, Tugwell P (2017) CONSORT-equity 2017 extension and elaboration for better reporting of health equity in randomised trials. BMJ (Clin Res Ed) 359:j5085

Wood L, Egger M, Gluud LL, Schulz KF, Juni P, Altman DG et al (2008) Empirical evidence of bias in treatment effect estimates in controlled trials with different interventions and outcomes: meta-epidemiological study. BMJ (Clin Res Ed) 336(7644):601–605

Working Group on Recommendations for Reporting of Clinical Trials in the Biomedical Literature (1994) Call for comments on a proposal to improve reporting of clinical trials in the biomedical literature. Ann Intern Med 121(11):894–895

Zwarenstein M, Treweek S, Gagnier JJ, Altman DG, Tunis S, Haynes B et al (2008) Improving the reporting of pragmatic trials: an extension of the CONSORT statement. BMJ (Clin Res Ed) 337:a2390

Publications from Clinical Trials 105

Barbara S. Hawkins

Contents

Introduction	2090
Publications of Comparisons of Trial Arms Regarding Primary Outcomes	2091
Analysis Database	2091
Authors and Writing Teams	2092
Manuscript Development Process	2093
Selection of Journal for Publication and Interactions with Editors	2093
Dissemination of Findings to Trial Investigators Before Publication	2094
Dissemination of Findings to Trial Participants Before Publication	2095
Public Dissemination of Trial Findings	2095
Publications of Comparisons of Trial Arms Regarding Secondary Outcomes	2095
Publications of Trial Design and Methods	2096
Other Publications	2097
Coordination and Management of Publications	2098
Publication Policy Issues	2098
Authorship Models	2098
Public Presentation of Outcomes Before Publication	2099
Prospective Publication Plans	2099
Summary and Conclusion	2099
Key Facts	2100
Cross-References	2100
References	2100

Abstract

Publication of findings in a scientific journal, in an electronic or print format, is an obligation of those who conduct clinical trials, whether as investigators or sponsors. The process of preparing manuscripts for publication in the multicenter, multidisciplinary setting typically is subject to the trial's publication policy that

---

B. S. Hawkins (✉)
Johns Hopkins School of Medicine and Bloomberg School of Public Health, The Johns Hopkins University, Baltimore, MD, USA
e-mail: bhawkins@jhmi.edu

© Springer Nature Switzerland AG 2022
S. Piantadosi, C. L. Meinert (eds.), *Principles and Practice of Clinical Trials*,
https://doi.org/10.1007/978-3-319-52636-2_184

may specify authorship models, internal review, and approval, creation and expectations of writing teams, and dissemination of findings before journal publication. Publication in a peer-reviewed, indexed journal validates the design, methods, and findings of the study for dissemination to the healthcare community. The focus of this chapter is on practices commonly followed in publicly funded multicenter randomized clinical trials and may not address issues and policies commonly found in trials with industry sponsorship.

Keywords

Analysis database · Authorship model · CONSORT · Credit roster · Internal review · Peer review · Presentation · Primary outcome · Secondary outcome · Writing team

Introduction

A major goal and responsibility of clinical trial investigators is to disseminate findings from their trials in a timely fashion and in an appropriate manner. Publication of a well-crafted article in a respected journal is the ideal method of initial dissemination because of the discipline required to organize and report findings accurately in a transparent manner and because revisions in response to comments from peer reviewers may result in a better manuscript. Although the target readers of many publications may be colleagues interested in the medical specialty of the trial, other readers may include personnel from agencies that fund research, policy-makers, methodologists, and others. Because articles in medical and other scientific journals are not designed to convey information to patients, whether trial participants or others, other methods typically are more useful to inform them of trial findings.

Publication of comparisons of trial intervention arms with respect to primary outcome data usually is the first trial report that comes to mind when planning and designing a trial. However, publications of comparisons based on secondary outcomes and other findings from all or a subgroup of participants and description and evaluation of methods used in a trial also have proven to be important. Thus, multiple types of manuscripts from an individual trial suitable for journal publication are discussed in this chapter. Although many publications of studies ancillary to a clinical trial may result, those are not addressed.

Publications from publicly-funded multicenter, multidisciplinary randomized clinical trials are the focus of the descriptions and discussions in this chapter. The principles and many of the issues apply equally to single-center trials but they may be easier to apply and to resolve in that setting. The process and practices described herein may differ in various ways from those of trials sponsored by industry (Foote 2003; Royer 1986; Tauber and Paul 2017).

In a large multidisciplinary group of trial investigators, coordination and tracking of progress with manuscript preparation and monitoring of adherence to the publication policy can be challenging. The policy may establish authorship guidelines, approval process for topics to be addressed in individual manuscripts, the method of assigning the group of investigators to be responsible for drafting each manuscript (writing team), process for review and approval by trial leadership groups and sponsor, selection of the target journal, expectations regarding timelines, and other issues.

Publications of Comparisons of Trial Arms Regarding Primary Outcomes

Despite the primacy of publications to report comparison of primary outcome findings between the intervention arms of the trial, preparation of these manuscripts usually does not begin until fairly late during the course of a trial, typically either as a result of a recommendation from a data monitoring committee to halt enrollment and randomization and to publish interim results to date (BHAT Research Group 1981a; MPS Group 1984) or after participant accrual and follow-up of trial participants have been completed. Occasionally, publication of one or more reports of interim findings may be incorporated into the trial design (COMS Group 1998, 2001).

Analysis Database

Regardless of the reason for publication, trial resources must be devoted to assuring that accumulated data on which a manuscript is based are reported accurately and completely. Many of the data analyses to be presented in the manuscript may have been reported to the data monitoring committee and discussed at one or more meetings. Those may require only minor additions or changes in format or may require updating when a more recent version of the trial database is to be the basis of the manuscript. To assure consistency of the data reported within a manuscript, the same version of the trial database, the analysis database, is used for all data displays and analyses (McBride and Singer 1995); any information included in the manuscript that was acquired after the date of the analysis database should be labeled with the later date.

A copy of the analysis database, software programs used to create the data displays, and any ancillary information are retained so as to be able to respond to requests and queries from the journal editor and peer reviewers. Preferably, the copy of the analysis database and programs eventually is stored in a repository that provides long-term curation, beyond the period of funding for trial activities. Because of the complexity of the typical master database, especially for a large, long trial, the analysis database may be the most useful for eventual sharing with others who wish to access trial data.

For some outcomes, for example, death or other major events related to benefit or harm of interventions, special effort may be required to assure that ascertainment is complete. For trials conducted in the United States (U.S.) he National Death Index

(National Center for Health Statistics, U.S. Department of Health and Human Services, Rockville, Md). may be accessed to search for trial participants lost to clinical follow-up who may have died in the interval since last contact (COMS Group 1998, 2001). Special on-site or remote reviews of clinical events may be conducted to identify types or severity of events. The perceived importance of these activities, the time they will require, and the time remaining for trial completion may influence whether they are judged essential before publication or may be postponed and outcome data updated in a later manuscript.

Authors and Writing Teams

Although policies regarding authorship of manuscripts to report trial findings and methods should be developed by the trial leadership as part of trial design and accepted by investigators who participate in the trial (Archer et al. 2016; Long et al. 2000; Pielen et al. 2014; Rosenberg et al. 2015), it may be necessary to remind investigators of policies when preparation of important manuscripts, such as reports of primary trial outcomes, are initiated (Long et al. 2000). As with all manuscripts, reports of treatment comparisons of primary outcomes from trials sponsored by public funds typically are drafted by one or a small number of trial investigators appointed by the trial leader(s) on the basis of expertise, contributions to the trial, or other criteria (Archer et al. 2016; Whellan et al. 2015).

Members of the writing team may volunteer or be appointed to draft sections of the manuscript pertinent to their special expertise or role within the trial. The trial statistician is a key member of the writing team (Archer et al. 2016) and typically is assigned responsibility for drafting the descriptions of sample size estimation and key statistical analysis methods in less detail than in a statistical analysis plan provided in the trial protocol. The trial statistician also may suggest key data displays (tables and figures) to be included in the manuscript and their format. Clinical members of the writing team advise the statistician regarding likely accessibility of proposed statistical analysis methods to readers of clinical journals (Emerson and Colditz 1983; Marsh and Hawkins 1994). Less familiar statistical methods and their application may be described in an appendix or supplement to the manuscript.

Various authorship models have been used in multicenter clinical trials and are discussed later in this chapter. It usually is not desirable or acceptable to editors to list all investigators as authors of publications from multicenter trials in which many centers and many types of personnel participate (Kassirer and Angell 1991; Rennie et al. 1997). In order to assure that all participating investigators and personnel receive credit for their contributions to the trial, a credit roster (acknowledgement of all contributing trial investigators and personnel) often is published as part of the report of primary outcome data (Meinert 1993). Study policy may specify whether all past and current investigators are listed or only a subgroup based on contributions to the trial, such as term of participation or number of participants enrolled and treated. Credit rosters usually appear at the end of published articles, but there have been exceptions (CDP Reearch Group 1973).

Manuscript Development Process

The timeline for drafting the manuscript, completing internal review and approval, and submitting the final version of the manuscript for publication are negotiated by the trial leaders with the writing team leader. Once the decision to prepare a manuscript for publication has been made, the goal is to develop the manuscript for publication expeditiously but in a manner that assures that the methods are reported transparently and the findings are reported accurately.

Ideally, an outline of the manuscript content is prepared promptly by the writing team leader and reviewed by other team members. The writing team leader may wish to consult the CONSORT checklist and guidance (Moher et al. 2010; Schulz et al. 2010; http://www.consort-statement.org/) while preparing the outline. When a manuscript that describes the design of the trial has been published before primary outcome data are available for publication, it may be possible to cite the design publication and to present some of the trial methods in summary form in the report of primary outcome data. The writing team may elect to post the trial protocol document (or manual of trial procedures) online, either independently or as a supplement to the website of the journal in which the manuscript is to be published.

All members of the writing team must review and approve the complete draft prepared or assembled by the writing team leader (ICMJE 1997). As promptly as possible, a draft is distributed to the study leaders, a representative of the sponsor, and often the chair of the data monitoring committee for rapid review and comment. After comments and suggestions have been addressed, the final version of the manuscript is prepared for approval by the study leaders and submission to the selected journal for publication. The CONSORT checklist is completed by a member of the writing team before the final version of the manuscript is submitted for publication, regardless of the journal policy regarding inclusion of the CONSORT checklist with the manuscript.

The writing team leader may decide that responding to all comments and suggestions from internal and external reviewers would result in an unjustified delay of manuscript submission or in an unacceptably long manuscript. In such cases and with the approval of the trial leaders, some topics may be set aside to be the focus or part of another manuscript.

Selection of Journal for Publication and Interactions with Editors

Selection of the journal to which a manuscript from a trial is submitted for publication may depend on several factors, including the reputation of the journal, policy regarding open access, and the targeted readership, that is, practitioners of a medical specialty or subspecialty or a broader group of medical practitioners. Preference should be given to journals indexed in large bibliographic databases. Editors of such journals typically welcome manuscripts from well-designed and -conducted clinical trials. Some journals provide "in review" services; under this model, a document identifier (DOI) is assigned as soon as a manuscript is submitted, and the content is publicly available. The peer review comments and revisions are tracked and open to public scrutiny. Although this model expedites dissemination of trial outcome data, it may not appeal to all trial sponsors and writing teams.

Although the trial findings may not be widely disseminated until publication or acceptance of the manuscript, the lead trial investigator may find it helpful to advise the editor-in-chief of the preferred journal that primary outcome findings are being prepared for publication and to seek assurance of prompt peer review, feedback, and publication of the final manuscript before the manuscript is submitted. Leaders of high-profile trials may find that editors-in-chief of multiple journals solicit reports of trial outcomes even before such findings are available for publication.

In advance of receipt of the manuscript, the editor-in-chief of the selected journal may contact potential peer reviewers to alert them to the expected date of receipt of the manuscript and to solicit their commitment to an expeditious review. In the case of a trial with many participating centers and investigators, the editor may have difficulty identifying peer reviewers with sufficient expertise who are not engaged in conduct or monitoring of the trial or who do not have other actual or potential conflicts of interest (Frohlich and Pepine 2004). The editor-in-chief also may reserve space for the manuscript in a future journal issue consistent with the timeline discussed with the lead investigator.

When multiple related trials are completed at about the same time, whether conducted by the same group or different groups of investigators, and manuscripts to report primary outcome findings are to be submitted to the same journal, the editor-in-chief may wish to coordinate publication of findings from all trials in the same issue of the journal. Alternatively, when findings are to be reported in multiple journals, the editors may wish to coordinate time of publication. Such situations require close collaboration of writing teams with journal editors. Regardless of the goal of rapid review and publication, clinical trial writing teams must respond thoughtfully and promptly to comments and requests from editors and peer reviewers.

Dissemination of Findings to Trial Investigators Before Publication

In trials in which knowledge of interim outcome comparisons by intervention has been restricted to members of the trial's data monitoring committee, a key issue is when to share findings with the other trial investigators. The trial statistician, and possibly the lead investigator, may have been present at one or more meetings of the data-monitoring committee and thus be familiar with the data displays and with comments and recommendations of the committee members. However, other trial investigators, including those who may be invited to join the writing team, likely will require a thorough presentation and discussion of the relevant data. They may provide useful suggestions for improving data displays and insightful explanations or caveats regarding data interpretation. Depending upon the authorship model adopted and trial policy, all investigators may be required to approve the manuscript before submission for publication. All trial investigators should receive a copy of the final version of the manuscript submitted for publication.

Dissemination of Findings to Trial Participants Before Publication

An equally important issue is timing and method of notification of trial participants of primary outcome findings from the trial that are about to be published and how those findings relate to their treatment, future care, and participation in the trial. Such notifications should precede publication or other public announcements (MPS 1984). Whenever participant follow-up will continue in order to assess other outcomes, trial investigators ascertain that participants understand that the trial has not ended and that their continued participation will be necessary to achieve all goals of the trial. Participants may or may not be informed of their randomly assigned treatment, depending upon the importance of maintaining participant (and investigator) masking. In some situations, it may be necessary or desirable to renew consent for continued treatment and data collection.

Public Dissemination of Trial Findings

Sponsors of clinical trials sometimes wish to make public announcements regarding trial findings, particularly primary outcome comparisons of interventions from large, high-profile trials. Ideally, the timing of such announcements is coordinated with notification of participants and publication.

Dissemination of findings outside the group of trial investigators before publication may be subject to an embargo by the journal or by trial policy. Trial leaders, writing team members, other trial investigators, and sponsors must honor the embargo.

In summary, publication of primary trial outcome findings requires thorough analysis of pertinent data, checks of the accuracy and completeness of the analysis database, clear presentation of methods and data, and diligent coordination of related activities to avoid premature dissemination of inaccurate, incomplete, or contradictory information. Consequently, the published article that results will be of high quality and a source of pride for all contributors to the trial.

Publications of Comparisons of Trial Arms Regarding Secondary Outcomes

Most investigators who design clinical trials intend to assess one or more outcomes in addition to the primary outcome or set of outcomes. For example, recent trials of various interventions for medical conditions have been designed to assess "quality of life" and other patient-reported outcomes in addition to clinical outcomes. Findings regarding secondary outcomes may be published in conjunction with primary outcomes or may be analyzed and reported in one or more additional manuscripts (SST Research Group 2005a, b). The timing of publication of secondary outcome findings may depend on how closely secondary outcomes are linked to primary outcomes.

Writing teams for manuscripts to disseminate secondary outcomes, as for manuscripts to present primary outcomes, typically are appointed by the trial leaders; often investigators with a special interest in such outcomes volunteer to lead or to join the writing team. The writing team includes a trial statistician or epidemiologist and at least one clinical investigator.

In general, manuscripts to present secondary outcome data should follow the CONSORT recommendations. However, when the trial methods have been reported in sufficient detail in one or more publications, reference may be made to those publications so that the focus of the methods section of the manuscript under development is on the secondary outcomes presented. In other respects, such as internal review of the manuscript, trial policy regarding publication of secondary outcome findings typically follows the same course as publication of primary outcome findings.

Trial leaders or writing team members may elect to submit manuscripts that report secondary outcome findings to the same journal that was selected for publication of primary outcome data or may target a different journal. Manuscripts may be submitted for publication as completed and approved or may be grouped for publication in a single journal issue or supplement (Fishman et al. 2008).

Publications of Trial Design and Methods

Many groups of trial investigators, especially those participating in multicenter trials or trials with complex designs, have found it useful to publish early in the course of the trial a description of the trial design, organization, and methods (COMS Group 1993; Babiker et al. 2013; BHAT Research Group 1981b; SOCA Research Group 1992). When published before accrual of the target number of participants has been achieved, these publications call attention to the trial and may encourage referral of candidates. Investigators in some trials have elected to complete accrual to the trial and to publish not only design and methodologic information but also information about the baseline characteristics of trial participants (BHAT Research Group 1981b; CDP Research Group 1973; Gravenstein et al. 2016; Kiel et al. 2010; SOCA Research Group 1992). Design publications typically provide considerably more detailed information about design and methods than may be acceptable to editors of journals to whom manuscripts are submitted to present findings for primary and secondary outcomes from a trial. Design publications often can be cited in manuscripts that present trial data to shorten descriptions of some trial methods or design features.

Investigators of high-profile trials may encounter no problem with acceptance of design and methods manuscripts for publication in the journals they select, particularly when those journals also have been selected for publication of primary outcome findings. Investigators participating in other trials may not find ready acceptance of such manuscripts in clinical journals, but other journals, such as Clinical Trials (https://journals.sagepub.com/home/ctj), Contemporary Clinical Trials (https://www.journals.elsevier.com/contemporary-clinical-trials/), and Trials (https://trialsjournal.biomedcentral.com/) welcome such manuscripts. Although publication of the full trial protocol or selected portions of it in a methodology journal may not generate the same interest in the trial within the medical community as publication in a clinical journal, nevertheless the information is available for citation in other publications from the trial. In addition, the information is available to peer reviewers of manuscripts from the trial and to other researchers, including designers of future trials and systematic reviewers. Some trial investigators elect to publish the complete trial protocol on a dedicated trial website, on a journal website, or on another site accessible through the Internet (Paul et al. 2005). A reporting standard for the content of trial protocols is provided at https://www.spirit-statement.org/.

There is no standard format for publications that summarize the design and methods of clinical trials. Many of the sections of the CONSORT recommendations apply to trial design and methods and should be consulted. Individual journal policy may provide guidance (Goodman 2004).

Other Publications

Not all publications from clinical trials are of the three types described. Examination of the chronology of publications from any large trial reveals a variety of types of publications, including topics such as the rationale for selection of a particular design feature (Earle et al. 1987), details of a treatment procedure (MPS Group 1991), or procedures followed in one of the trial resource centers (Toth et al. 2015). These publications assure that the rationale for design decisions, methods used in the trial, issues that arose in the trial, and ancillary findings from the trial have been thoughtfully considered and documented. They also provide many opportunities for trial investigators to serve on writing teams other than those for reports of primary and secondary outcomes (Whellan et al. 2015).

Leaders of some large multicenter, multidisciplinary trials have found it useful to create "working groups" to propose and analyze data relevant to selected issues and topics that may result in publications from the trial. Investigators may volunteer for working groups of special interest to them or may be invited to participate because of their expertise. In addition to the clinicians and other volunteers, it is useful to have as a member of each working group a trial statistician or epidemiologist who is thoroughly familiar with the trial protocol and data collected. The statistician or epidemiologist commonly prepares and presents to the other working group members data summaries and analyses for their review. Each working group may develop an analysis plan that results in a single manuscript or multiple manuscripts for publication. One member of the working group is assigned responsibility for reporting progress to the trial leadership group.

Trial policies for authorship or recognition of the writing teams for this diverse group of manuscripts may differ from those for manuscripts that report comparisons of interventions regarding primary or secondary outcomes from the trial. The trial policies regarding internal review and approval of manuscripts, presentation of unpublished data, and other issues usually apply also to manuscripts that emanate from working groups.

Coordination and Management of Publications

In a large multicenter trial, the preparation of manuscripts usually accelerates once outcome data are available to investigators. Thus, reports from writing teams and working groups become important tools for tracking progress. Typically, the task of monitoring progress has been assigned either to someone at the resource center headed by the trial chair (principal or lead investigator) or to a member of the (data) coordinating center team.

A database to monitor progress with manuscripts and to maintain a record of publications is helpful and may be essential in a trial with a large number of investigators and working groups. In addition to the working title of each manuscript in preparation, the database may contain the members of the writing team and the projected timeline and current status (Bialy et al. 2013; Cook et al. 2010; Snow et al. 2011; Weiner et al. 2010; Williams et al. 2006). Assignment of an identifying number or code to each manuscript when first drafted (or even earlier) facilitates coordination and management.

In addition to monitoring and tracking, the publication coordinator/monitor may be assigned responsibility for maintaining an online record of publications on the trial website or elsewhere. This person also may be responsible for notifying trial personnel when publications appear in electronic or print format and the information needed to access them. The publication coordinator/monitor also may be responsible for maintaining a record of all personnel who have participated in the trial at each of the clinical centers and resource centers in order to assure that credit rosters in individual manuscripts are correct before submission for publication. Whenever a Publication Committee is part of the trial organization, the publication coordinator/monitor is an important member.

Publication Policy Issues

Authorship Models

Meinert defined four authorship models (Meinert 1993): *traditional, modified traditional, corporate,* and *modified corporate.* In the *traditional model* (or conventional model), the names of the writing team members are listed in the authorship byline; the contributions of other trial personnel may be recognized in an acknowledgement or a credit roster. In the *modified traditional model*, the writing team members are listed along with an acknowledgement such as "for the XYZ Trial investigators" or "on behalf of the XYZ Trial investigators." When the *corporate model* is used, only the name of the trial group appears in the authorship byline. When the *modified corporate model* is selected, the name of the trial group appears in the authorship byline but the members of the writing team are listed in a footnote, acknowledgment, or appendix. Examples of all models can be found among the publications from multicenter clinical trials. Meinert also has summarized advantages and disadvantages of traditional and corporate models (Meinert and Tonascia 1986).

Trial policy regarding authorship models may specify one model for all publications from a trial or may specify different models for different types of publications to assure that credit is distributed equably among trial investigators and other personnel. No single model is likely to satisfy all trial investigators. One group of researchers found that it was difficult to identify all publications from a trial in bibliographic databases when all or some had been published using the corporate model for authorship (Dickersin et al. 2002). Improvements in indexing terms, search tools, and methods have evolved in the interval since they conducted their investigation and may have ameliorated the problem they identified.

Public Presentation of Outcomes Before Publication

Because trial investigators wish to disseminate trial findings promptly so that they can be applied in clinical practice, many may believe that it is important that the first announcement be made in a platform or poster presentation at a large national or international meeting of their colleagues. Several researchers have investigated the effect of presentation first on the time to publication of trial findings (Hopewell and McDonald 2003; Hopewell et al. 2006; Unalp et al. 2007; Scherer et al. 2018). They found that presentation first had delayed (or precluded) publication of findings from many trials. Also, findings reported in abstracts for presentations, including number of trial participants, often differed from those in subsequent publications.

Prospective Publication Plans

At least one group of trial leaders has reported experience with a publication and authorship plan implemented at the beginning of a multicenter clinical trial before any data were available (Whellan et al. 2015). The strategy they adopted resulted in 50 publications with 504 "authorship slots" filled by 137 trial investigators. They concluded that the strategy was highly successful when they compared their experience to publications from trials of similar size that dealt with related topics. Other researchers also have advocated early publication planning (Archer et al. 2016).

Summary and Conclusion

Publication of findings and methods from a clinical trial may require negotiating a complex process that mandates adherence to trial policy and extensive review by and advice from many trial colleagues. However, regardless of the superiority (or inferiority) of an intervention evaluated and the quality of the resulting article, publication of findings may not result in their wide dissemination. Implementation by clinical practitioners may require other activities to achieve broad dissemination to healthcare providers (Bartholomew et al. 2009).

Key Facts

- Publications from clinical trials may be of several types and are not limited to comparisons of outcomes between arms although those have priority.
- Trial leaders should establish publication and dissemination policies well in advance of preparation of the first manuscript from the trial and assure that all investigators are aware of and agree to adhere to the policies.
- The publication process entails attention to more issues and activities than describing trial findings, as documented in trial publication policies.

Cross-References

▶ Data Sharing and Reuse

References

Archer SW, Carlo WA, Truog WE, Stevenson DK, Van Meurs KP, Sanchez PJ, Das A, Devaskar U, Nelin LD, Huitema CMP, Crawford MM, Higgins RD (2016) Improving publication rates in a collaborative clinical trials network. Semin Perinatol 40:410–417

Babiker AG, Emery S, Fatkenheuer G, Gordin FM, Grund B, Lundgren JD, Neaton JD, Pett SL, Phillips A, Touloumi G, Vjecha MJ, for the INSIGHT START Study Group (2013) Considerations in the rationale, design and methods of the Strategic Timing of AntiRetroviral Treatment (START) study. Clin Trials 10(Suppl):S5–S36

Bartholomew LK, Cushman WE, Cutler JA, Davis BR, Dawson G, Einhorn PT, Graumlich JF, Piller LB, Pressel SL, Roccella EJ, Simpson L, Whelton PK, Willard A, ALLHAT Collaborative Research Group (2009) Getting clinical trial results into practice: design, implementation, and process evaluation of the ALLHAT Dissemination Project. Clin Trials 6(4):329–343

ß-Blocker Heart Attack [BHAT] Study Group (1981a) The ß-blocker heart attack trial. JAMA 246(18):2073–2074

Beta Blocker Heart Attack Trial [BHAT] Research Group (1981b) Beta blocker heart attack trial: design features. Control Clin Trials 2:275–285

Bialy S, Blessing JA, Stehman FB, Reardon AM, Blaser KM (2013) Gynecologic [O]ncology [G]roup (GOG) strategies to improve timeliness of publication. Clin Trials 10:617–623

Collaborative Ocular Melanoma Study [COMS] Group (1993) Design and methods of a clinical trial for a rare condition: the Collaborative Ocular Melanoma Study. COMS report no. 3. Control Clin Trials 14:362–391

Collaborative Ocular Melanoma Study [COMS] Group (1998) The COMS randomized trial of pre-enucleation radiation of large choroidal melanoma. II. Initial mortality findings. COMS report no. 10. Am J Ophthalmol 125:779–796

Collaborative Ocular Melanoma Study [COMS] Group (2001) The COMS randomized trial of iodine 125 brachytherapy for choroidal melanoma. III: initial mortality findings. COMS report no. 18. Arch Ophthalmol 119:969–982

Cook DR, Stowe C, Griffin J (2010) Monitoring publications and presentations submissions for a multi-center clinical trial. Clin Trials 7:455

Coronary Drug Project [CDP] Research Group (1973) The Coronary Drug Project. Design, methods, and baseline results. Circulation 47(3 Suppl 1):I-1–I-50

Dickersin K, Scherer R, Suci EST et al (2002) Problems with indexing and citation of articles with group authorship. JAMA 287(21):2772–2774

Earle J, Kline RW, Robertson DM (1987) Selection of iodine 125 for the Collaborative Ocular Melanoma Study. Arch Ophthalmol 125:763–764

Emerson JD, Colditz GA (1983) Use of statistical analysis in *The New England Journal of Medicine*. N Engl J Med 309(12):709–713

Fishman AP, Criner GJ, Sternberg AL et al (2008) National Emphysema Treatment Trial. Proc Am Thorac Soc 5(4):379–574

Foote MA (2003) Review of current authorship guidelines and the controversy regarding publication of clinical trial data. Biotechnol Annu Rev 9:303–313

Frohlich ED, Pepine CJ (2004) Subliminal editorial conundra confounding publication of multicenter trials. Am J Cardiol 94:1268–1269

Goodman SN (2004) Update on position and design papers. Clin Trials 1:415–416

Gravenstein S, Dahal R, Gozalo PL, Davidson HE, Han LF, Taljaard M, Mor V (2016) A cluster randomized controlled trial comparing relative effectiveness of two licensed influenza vaccines in US nursing homes: design and rationale. Clin Trials 13(3):264–274

Hopewell S, McDonald S (2003) Full publication of trials initially reported as abstracts in the *Australian and New Zealand Journal of Medicine* 1980–2000. Intern Med J 33(4):192–194

Hopewell S, Clarke M, Askie L (2006) Reporting of trials presented in conference abstracts needs to be improved. J Clin Epidemiol 53:681–684

International Committee of Medical Journal Editors [ICMJE] (1997) Uniform requirements for manuscripts submitted to biomedical journals. N Engl J Med 336(4):309–316

Kassirer JP, Angell M (1991) On authorship and acknowledgments. N Engl J Med 325(21):1510–1512

Kiel DP, Hannan MT, Barton BA, Bouxsein ML, Lang TF, Brown KM, Shane E, Magaziner J, Zimmerman S, Rubin CT (2010) Insights from the conduct of a device trial in older persons: low magnitude mechanical stimulation for musculoskeletal health. Clin Trials 7:354–367

Long E, Dunn D, Gordon M, Ocular Hypertension Treatment Study (OHTS) Group (2000) A publications and presentation policy for a multicenter clinical trial. Control Clin Trials 21(2 Suppl):77

Macular Photocoagulation Study [MPS] Group (1984) Changing the protocol: a case report from the Macular Photocoagulation Study. Control Clin Trials 5:203–216

Macular Photocoagulation Study [MPS] Group (1991) Subfoveal neovascular lesions in age-related macular degneration. Guidelines for evaluation and treatment in the Macular Photocoagulation Study. Arch Ophthalmol 109(9):1242–1257

Marsh MJ, Hawkins BS (1994) Publications from multicentre clinical trials: statistical techniques and accessibility to the reader. Stat Med 13:2303–2406

McBride R, Singer SW (1995) Interim reports, participant closeout, and study archives. Control Clin Trials 16(2 Suppl):137–167

Meinert CL (1993) In defense of the corporate author for multicenter trials. Control Clin Trials 14:255–260

Meinert CL, Tonascia S (1986) Clinical trials: design, conduct, and analysis. Oxford University Press, New York, p 259

Moher D, Hopewell S, Schulz KF, Montori V, Gøtzsche PC, Devereaux PJ, Elbourne D, Egger M, Altman DG (2010) CONSORT 2010 explanation and elaboration: updated guidelines for reporting parallel group randomised trials. J Clin Epidemiol 63:e1–e37

Paul J, Seib R, Prescott T (2005) The internet and clinical trials: background, online resources, examples and issues. J Med Internet Res 7(1):e5. https://doi.org/10.2196/jmir.7.1.e5

Pielen A, Wilhelm B, Holz F, fur die Arbeitsgruppe Klinische Studienzentren der DOG (2014) Empfehlungen der DOG zu publikationsregelungen in multizenterstudien. [DOG guidelines for publications in multicenter studies]. Ophthalmologe 111:498–499

Rennie D, Yank V, Emanuel L (1997) When authorship fails: a proposal to make contributors accountable. JAMA 278:579–585

Rosenberg J, Burcharth J, Pommergaard HC, Vinther S (2015) Authorship issues in multi-centre clinical trials: the importance of making an authorship contract. Dan Med J 62(2):A5009

Royer MG (1986) Preparing manuscripts for publication: a team approach. Drug Inf J 20:97–102

Scherer RW, Meerpohl JJ, Pfeifer N, Schmucker C, Schwarzer G, von Elm E (2018) Full publication of results initially presented in abstracts. Cochrane Database Syst Rev (11): Art. No. MR000005. https://doi.org/10.1002/14651858.MR000005.pub4

Schulz KF, Altman DG, Moher D, for the CONSORT Group (2010) CONSORT 2010 statement: updated guidelines for reporting parallel group randomized trials. Open Med 4(1):e60

Snow KK, Stoddard AM, Curto TM, Bell MC (2011) An organizational structure to manage analyses and manuscript development in the Hepatitis C Antiviral Long-Term Treatment Against Cirrhosis (HALT-C) Trial. Clin Trials 8:471–472

Studies of Ocular Complications of AIDS (SOCA) Research Group in collaboration with the AIDS Clinical Trials Group (ACTG) (1992) Studies of Ocular Complications of AIDS Foscarnet-Ganciclovir Cytomegalovirus Retinitis Trial: 1. Rationale, design, and methods. Control Clin Trials 13(1):22–39

Submacular Surgery Trials Research Group (2005a) Surgery for subfoveal choroidal neovascularization in age-related macular degeneration: I. Ophthalmic findings: SST report no.11. Ophthalmology 111:1967–1980

Submacular Surgery Trials Research Group (2005b) Surgery for subfoveal choroidal neovascularization in age-related macular degeneration: II. Quality-of-life findings: SST report no. 12. Ophthalmology 111:1981–1992

Tauber M, Paul C (2017) Authorship selection in industry-sponsored publications of dermatology clinical trials. Br J Dermatol 176(6):1669–1671

Toth CA, Decroos FC, Ying GS, Stinnett SS, Heydary CS, Burns R, Maguire M, Martin D, Jaffe GJ (2015) Identification of fluid on optical coherence tomography by treating ophthalmologists versus a reading center in the Comparison of Age-Related Macular Degeneration Treatments Trial. Retina 35(7):1303–1314

Unalp A, Tonascia S, Meinert CL (2007) Presentation in relation to publication of results from clinical trials. Contemp Clin Trials 28(4):358–369

Weiner S, for the Eunice Kennedy Shriver NICHD, MFMU Network (2010) Publications management in a multicenter clinical trials network. Clin Trials 7:473

Whellan DJ, Kraus WE, Kitzman DW, Rooney B, Keteyian SJ, Pifia IL, Ellis SJ, Ghali JK, Lee KL, Cooper LS, O'Connor CM (2015) Authorship in a multicenter clinical trial: the heart failure – a controlled trial investigating outcomes of exercise training (HF-ACTION) authorship and publication (HAP) scoring system results. Am Heart J 169:457–463

Williams C, Speas C, Espeland M, Hodges M, Knowler W, Ryan D, for the LOOK-AHEAD Research Group (2006) Design and implementation of an automated publications tracking system in a clinical trial. Clin Trials 3:196

Study Name, Authorship, Titling, and Credits

106

Curtis L. Meinert

Contents

Umbrella Names	2104
Study Names and Acronyms	2105
Titling Publications	2107
Headline Type	2108
Descriptive Type	2108
Authorship Models	2109
International Committee of Medical Journal Editors Authorship Requirements	2110
Authors per Publication	2111
Credits, Disclosures, and Acknowledgments	2111
References	2112

Abstract

This chapter deals with names and acronyms for trials, whose name goes in mastheads of publications from the trial, how papers are titled, and credit listings in manuscripts.

The issue of whose names goes on publications is reasonably straight forward when only a few people are involved in a work but becomes progressively more complicated as the size of the investigator group increases.

Should attribution be to the entire research group without any persons listed in the publication masthead, or should it be to named persons? If the format is to list names, then who should be listed and in what order?

How should results papers from the trial be titled? Titling is important because title is what is used to attract readers. What should it be? Should it be headline style announcing results of the trial, or should it be descriptive indicating the nature of the trial producing the results?

C. L. Meinert (✉)
Department of Epidemiology, School of Public Health, Johns Hopkins University, Baltimore, MD, USA
e-mail: cmeiner1@jhu.edu

© Springer Nature Switzerland AG 2022
S. Piantadosi, C. L. Meinert (eds.), *Principles and Practice of Clinical Trials*,
https://doi.org/10.1007/978-3-319-52636-2_187

Credits serve to inform readers who were involved and provide insights into how the trial was done. What goes in the credits sections of papers and in what format?

Keywords

Publication · Authorship · Credits · Study name

Umbrella Names

An umbrella name is a name intended to encompass a number of studies. For example, Studies of Ocular Complications of AIDS to encompass trials and studies done under that banner.

A fair number of trials emerge from structures originally created for a trial, for example, as with the Macular Photocoagulation Study (MPS). The MPS came into being as a result of investigator initiative to evaluate laser-induced photocoagulation of neovascularization associated with age-related macular degeneration. Ultimately, the MPS Research Group carried out several trials under the MPS structure (Macular Photocoagulation Study Group 1983a, b, 1982). One surmises, with the perspective of hindsight, that investigators would have preferred to have had an umbrella name for the collection of trials performed. As it was, they used the name for the first trial as the umbrella name.

Often the name of a group comes to serve the function of an umbrella name, for example, as with the Eastern Cooperative Oncology Group (ECOG). Originally the name referred to a group of collaborating oncologists from the eastern region of the USA but now to a network of researchers from across the country, hence rendering "eastern" meaningless.

Originally the Adult AIDS Clinical Trials Group (AACTG) was the surname for a group doing AIDS trials in adult populations but now serves as the name for a much broader set of activities.

Names, once established, are difficult to change – a fact to keep in mind when establishing one.

Reminders and recommendations

- Choose in favor of brevity, crispness, and succinctness
- Avoid restrictive terms likely to render a name obsolete later.
- Choose a neutral, descriptive, nonpromotional name.
- Avoid redundancies or contradictory terms.
- Keep other likely uses in mind, as in funding applications, presentations, and manuscripts.
- Avoid choosing to create a desired or "cute" acronym.
- Avoid names likely to produce undesirable names from letters of the name; remember a meaningless sequence of letters in one language can have an undesirable meaning in another.

Study Names and Acronyms

Shakespeare, in Romeo and Juliet, asserts that "a rose, by any other name would smell as sweet." By analogy, a trial by any other name is still a trial. Indeed. But the name by which it goes may cause it to be overlooked and, hence, never smelled.

If you are planning a trial, you will not have a choice regarding umbrella name if it is part of an umbrella structure, but you do have choices for the name of the trial. The name should:

1. Have "trial" as the base term (avoid less informative terms such as "study," "interventional study," "project," "program," or "investigation").
2. Have no more than eight words.
3. Be free of unnecessary or redundant terms (e.g., as with "controlled" in "randomized controlled").
4. Convey information as to the nature of the treatments being tested and the condition or disease being treated.
5. Be spelled out in consent documents, study protocols, study forms, author masthead listings, and study manuscripts.

The acronym should:

1. Be formed from the first letter of key words in the name (proper acronym)
2. Not be contrived to produce a pronounceable name
3. Be specified when the name is chosen
4. Be of eight or fewer printable characters
5. Not be used in place of name in study documents or masthead listings

Examples
Good: "Trial" as base term; name produces proper acronym
    Alzheimer's Disease Anti-inflammatory Prevention Trial (2009)   ADAPT
    National Emphysema Treatment Trial (1999)   NETT
    Long-term Oxygen Treatment Trial (2016)   LOTT
    Multiple Risk Factor Intervention Trial (1979)   MRFIT
Fair: Does not include "trial" as base term but produces proper acronym
    Coronary Drug Project (1973)   CDP
    Childhood Asthma Management Program (1999)   CAMP
    University Group Diabetes Project (1970a).   UGDP
Bad: Does not include "trial" and does not produce proper acronym
    Study **T**o **U**nderstand Fall **R**eduction and Vitamin **D** in **Y**ou (Michos et al. 2018).
    STURDY Investigation of Serial Studies to Predict Your Therapeutic Response through Imaging and
        Molecular Analysis 2 (Park et al. 2016).   I-SPY 2

The preferred base term is *trial* because it is the most accurate descriptor of what is being done. Other terms like *study* (e.g., Coronary Artery Surgery Study), *project* (e.g., Coronary Drug Project), or *program* (e.g., University Group Diabetes Program) are less informative than *trial*.

The name may include modifiers, such as *randomized* and *masked* or *blind* to characterize the nature of the trial. The name may also include terms to characterize the phase of the trial and terms to convey information about the treatment structure (e.g., parallel, crossover, or factorial).

The name should contain terms intended to indicate the type of treatments being tested (e.g., drugs, vaccines, diets, etc.) and the condition or disease treated (e.g., hypertension, diabetes, prostate cancer). Also the name may contain demographic terms to indicate the population enrolled (e.g., women, men, children, elderly).

Ideally, the name should remain accurate in the presence of changes to the study design during conduct. Everyday life is rich in names that have been sapped of their original meaning; Big Ten, Motel 6, Dime Savings, and Dollar Car Rental to name a few.

The need for accuracy argues for staying clear of descriptors related to selection criteria because they may change over the course of enrollment.

Names indicative of area are useful only so long as the trial remains confined to that area.

The term *National* or *International* to indicate spread is questionable. Both terms are subject to being rendered inaccurate with expansion of "National" to "International" or contraction from "International" to "National" with the addition or loss of sites during the trial.

Repeating a term, e.g., as with *Study* in *African American Study of Kidney Disease and Hypertension Pilot Study* (Wright et al. 1996), should be avoided if the reference is to a single study.

Most study names are shortened for everyday use. Hence, the National Cooperative Gallstone Study is also the NCGS, the Coronary Drug Project is also the CDP, and the University Group Diabetes Program is also the UGDP. Shorthand names are acceptable provided documents in which they appear contain the full name to establish equivalence.

Sometimes groups choose study names to produce a pronounceable name from letters of the names, for example, as with STRUDY from **S**tudy **T**o Understand Fall **R**eduction and Vitamin **D** in **Y**ou. The practice is questionable to the extent that it leads to contrived study names. As noted above, the practice should be to select an appropriate name and then the shortened name, not the reverse.

Reminders in choosing study names:

- Chose in favor of brevity; the fewer words and characters the better.
- Choose being mindful of the use of the name in publications and study documents.
- Choose in favor of a neutral, nonpromotional, name.
- Keep likely uses in mind, as in funding applications, publications, presentations, and other study documents.
- Keep likely contractions of name and acronyms in mind when choosing.
- Avoid choosing to create a desired or "cute" acronym.
- Avoid unnecessary words.

Characteristics of good study names:

- Succinct
- Neutral; not favoring one treatment in the trial over another
- Robust; does not become obsolete or inaccurate with changes to the trial
- Indicates nature of treatment and population being studied
- Includes the term **trial** and other currency terms like **randomized**
- Does not contain unprintable graphic characters
- Does not contain abbreviations

Shortened names (acronyms):

- Useful.
- Avoid creating study names to produce pronounceable acronyms.
- Focus on name first, then on producing a shortened name; avoid the reverse starting with an acronym and then fashioning a name to match the acronym.
- Stress test before adopting (e.g., by use in different settings and by screening for different meanings in other settings or languages).

Numbering-related trials:

- Avoid if trial is a descendent of one done by another group.
- Questionable if follow-on trial involves different study population or treatment regimens different from predecessor trial.
- Numbering (e.g., the **XYZ Trial 2**) acceptable when the trial is a repeat of a previous.
- Number reminds readers of related trials; connection may not be advantageous if the precursor trial was a "bust"; numbering usually indicates previous success; Rocky II; Queen Elizabeth 2 (QE2), but no Titanic 2.

Numbering publications:

- Useful in reminding readers of other publications from the same trial (e.g., as with publications from the University Group Diabetes Program 1970a, b).
- Do not implement unless certain of multiple publications.
- Can be confusing if only some publications are numbered.
- Can be confusing if numbering is not in order of publication.

Titling Publications

The title is the most important part of a manuscript. It is the first thing read and may be the only thing read to the extent that readers use titles to screen for articles of interest.

A good title will be devoid of "ly" words, superfluous words, and redundant words or terms. It should be succinct, should contain the word "trial," and should convey information about the mode of treatment and disease or condition being treated.

Broadly, titles are of two types.

Headline Type

Naproxen and celecoxib do not prevent AD in early results from a randomized controlled trial
 (Alzheimer's Disease Anti-inflammatory Prevention Trial Research Group 2007)

Descriptive Type

Cognitive Function Over Time in the Alzheimer's Disease Anti-inflammatory Prevention Trial (ADAPT): Results of a Randomized, Controlled Trial of Naproxen and Celecoxib (Alzheimer's Disease Anti-inflammatory Prevention Trial Research Group 2008)

The predominant "standard" in medical journals is descriptive titles.

The mean number of words in the titles of the 263 publications appearing in the *BMJ, JAMA, Lancet,* and *NEJM,* published in 2014 and indexed in PubMed to the publication types [randomized controlled trial] AND [multicenter study], was 16, range 5–37 words.

	No. publications	Mean no. words in title	Range	"Trial" in title
BMJ	13	18	12–24	13
JAMA	58	18	9–27	55
Lancet	75	23	12–33	67
NEJM	117	9	5–13	23
Total	**263**	**16**	**5–37**	**158**

The longest title was in *Lancet*:

A bioresorbable everolimus-eluting scaffold versus a metallic everolimus-eluting stent for ischaemic heart disease caused by de-novo native coronary artery lesions (ABSORB II): an interim 1-year analysis of clinical and procedural secondary outcomes

Detailed maybe but hardly succinct.

The shortest title was in *NEJM*:

Sodium zirconium cyclosilicate in hyperkalemia

Short but not informative.

It is obvious that journals have different titling preferences. Most of the publications in the BMJ, JAMA, and Lancet had "trial" in the title compared to just 20% of the publications in NEJM.

Authors are not shrinking violets. They have a say in how papers are titled. If their title included the term "trial" but deleted by journal editors, they should argue for it. Titling is a two-way street. Editors can be argued with.

Design words like *randomized* and *masked* or *blind* are useful title words. Fifty-four of the *JAMA* titles included the word "random" or forms of it. Only nine of the titles in the other three journals included the term.

Laudatory terms in characterizing one's own work like "novel," "unique," "original," "innovative," "ground breaking," or "definitive" should be avoided. Let readers decide if such terms apply.

Authorship Models

A key issue in any research effort has to do with who authors the work. Doing trials may involve the efforts of hundreds of people, and yet only a few will have the opportunity to "author." Who will they be? Experienced investigators will address the issue long before there are papers to write.

Experience with proposals for authorship in investigator groups is that the first time it is presented it is greeted with silence, almost as if members of the team cannot be concerned with such mundane matters. The second time the proposal is greeted with a few polite comments. The third time produces real debate and discussion.

Authorship forms, as represented in mastheads of publications of trials, are:

Conventional
Only persons named in the masthead of the publication (e.g., *Pernelda V Applebee, Richard L Harris, Roger W McFarland, and Franklin B Casper*)

Modified Conventional
Conventional form of attribution plus attribution to the research group (e.g., *Pernelda V Applebee, Richard L Harris, Roger W McFarland, and Franklin B Casper **and**/or **for** the POS Trial Research Group*)

Corporate
Only the corporate name of the research group in the masthead of the publication (e.g., *The POS Trial Research Group*; no writing committee listed)

Modified Corporate
Corporate form of attribution plus designation of the writing committee for the paper; writing committee designated in a footnote to the masthead page or listed in the credits section of the manuscript (e.g., *The POS Trial Research Group* in the masthead; footnote to the masthead or in credits section of the paper: Writing committee for the POS Trial Research Group: *Pernelda V Applebee, Richard L Harris, Roger W McFarland, and Franklin B Casper*)

Groups producing multiple publications over the life of the trial may use all four authorship formats, for example, as seen in publications from the National Emphysema Treatment Trial (NETT) (http://jhuccs1.us/clm/PDFs/NETTCV-2013.pdf).

The advantage of corporate modes of attribution is that it eliminates the "listing problem" involved in choosing whose names are listed in the masthead and "jockeying" for a place in the listing. The other advantage is that it forces people to use the name of the trial rather names of authors in references to the work, e.g., as in the "POS research group" as opposed to the work of "Applebee and coworkers."

The downside for editors (Kassirer and Angell 1991) under the uniform requirements for manuscripts is that they have no one to attest to the veracity of the paper in the absence of named writing committee. The Canadian Critical Care Trials Group solved that problem by indicating (on the front page of the article) that:

The steering committee of the Canadian Critical Care Trials Group assumes responsibility for the overall content and integrity of the article. (Canadian Critical Care Trials Group 2006)

The downside for investigators under the straight corporate format is absence of recognition in the published paper. The issue of recognition is especially important for people in academic institutions where promotions depend, in large measure, on authorship. Promotions committee may have difficulty evaluating the merits of candidates with curricula vitae filled with papers with corporate authorship attributions. The usual "fix" is for letters attesting to the candidate's involvement in the work to the promotion committee.

The advantage to people looking for publications from groups using corporate authorship formats lies in the ability to find publications from those groups identified by corporate authorship formats. The National Library of Medicine (NLM) introduced corporate name [CN] as a searchable tag in 2000.

Entry of "Canadian Critical Care Trials Groups"[CN] in the search box in PubMed produces citation of the primary results of the trial (2006) and other publications from the group.

International Committee of Medical Journal Editors Authorship Requirements

Standards for authorship of medical publications date back to 1978, when a small group of medical editors met in Vancouver, Canada, to establish guidelines for papers submitted to their respective journals; known as the International Committee of Medical Journal Editors (ICMJE) (Vancouver Protocol; https://research.ntu.edu.sg/rieo/Documents/Foundational Documents/Vancouver Protocol.pdf).

The ICMJE requirements for authorship are:

1. Conception and design or analysis and interpretation of data
2. Drafting the article or revising it critically for important intellectual content
3. Final approval of the version to be published

Conditions 1, 2, and 3 must all be met.

Table 1 Authors represented in 2016 BMJ, JAMA, Lancet, and NEJM publications indexed to randomized controlled trial in PubMed (24 March 2017)

	Number publications	Median number authors per publication	Range
BMJ	11	9	3–18
JAMA	67	14	4–65
Lancet	91	19	5–47
NEJM	138	19	6–58
Total	308	17	3–65

Authors per Publication

How many people does it take to write a paper?

Not many. Most of the writing is done by two or three people. That reality stands in marked contrast with the table below giving median number of authors represented in year 2016 publications for papers indexed in PubMed to the publication type [randomized controlled trial] and published in the BMJ, JAMA, Lancet, and NEJM. The median number of authors for the 308 publications is 17 (range 3–65) (Table 1).

One of the reasons for the large numbers of authors is because issues of authorship are not usually addressed until there is a paper to write. Then it is too late for any rational system of authorship, so the default is to list "everybody"; basically use of authorship listing as a form of credit listing.

Credits, Disclosures, and Acknowledgments

A credit is a recognition by name of a person, group, agency, or business firm having performed specific duties or functions in relation to the trial in question. People like to see their names in print (except on the crime page or in mastheads of publications withdrawn because of fraud!).

Years ago, I was dragged to "Who Framed Roger Rabbit?" by my three daughters. The film, for me, was a bore. The most interesting part was the credits. The film had the longest running list of credits of any film I had seen up to then. The credits revealed that the film was a technological masterpiece (even if boring).

In publications, credits are important to persons claiming credit for work on a trial. The listing may be the only way persons seeking academic promotions have of documenting work in a trial if only the study name is listed in the masthead of the publication.

But credits are also important to readers because they provide information about where the trial was done and who did it, akin to the credits in "Who Framed Roger Rabbit?".

For multicenter trials, the credits should include a listing of participating centers, their locations and associated personnel. They should also include membership listings of key committees. Lists of names without any indication of where the persons are located or functions performed is the operational equivalent of movie producers running a list of people involved in producing a film without any indication of role or function.

As a rule, credit rosters are not improved by journals. It is difficult to believe that the Digitalis Investigation Group submitted the list as published in the *NEJM* (Digitalis Investigation Group 1997) – an unsorted list of 459 names in 6 point font, not even alphabetized. Journals are space conscious leading editors to conserve space by using smaller fonts for credit rosters and to delete spacing in copy provided to make rosters unreadable, but editors are people too. They will listen if authors raise a fuss. Fortunately, the space issue becomes less important as journals move inexorable to electronic forms of publication.

"Disclosures" in the vernacular of publications relate to sources of funding and activities or relationships that have the potential of being viewed as conflicts of interest by the public. They are disclosed to editors in submissions and are listed in publications.

Acknowledgments are expressions of appreciation or thanks, typically appearing at the end of a manuscript, offered to persons, groups, or agencies for help provided in relation to the trial in question. Such expressions should not be included without knowledge of the persons or parties acknowledged.

References

Alzheimer's Disease Anti-inflammatory Prevention Trial Research Group (2007) Naproxen and celecoxib do not prevent AD in early results from a randomized controlled trial. Neurology 68:1800–1808

Alzheimer's Disease Anti-inflammatory Prevention Trial Research Group (2008) Cognitive function over time in the Alzheimer's disease anti-inflammatory prevention trial (ADAPT): results of a randomized, controlled trial of Naproxen and Celecoxib. Arch Neurol 65(7):896–903

Alzheimer's Disease Anti-inflammatory Prevention Trial Research Group (2009) Alzheimer's disease anti-inflammatory prevention trial: design, methods, and baseline results. Alzheimers Dement 5:93–104

Canadian Critical Care Trials Group (2006) A randomized trial of diagnostic techniques for ventilator- associated pneumonia. N Engl J Med 355:2619–2630

Childhood Asthma Management Program Research Group (1999) The Childhood Asthma Management Program (CAMP): design, rationale, and methods. Control Clin Trials 20:91–120

Coronary Drug Project Research Group (1973) The coronary drug project: design, methods, and baseline results. Circulation 47(Suppl I):I-1–I-50

Digitalis Investigation Group (1997) The effect of digoxin on mortality and morbidity in patients with heart failure. N Engl J Med 336:525–533

Kassirer JP, Angell M (1991) On authorship and acknowledgments. N Engl J Med 325:1510–1512

Long-Term Oxygen Treatment Trial Research Group (2016) A randomized trial of long-term oxygen for COPD with moderate desaturation. N Engl J Med 375:1,617–1,627

Macular Photocoagulation Study Group (1982) Argon laser photocoagulation for senile macular degeneration: results of a randomized clinical trial. Arch Ophthalmol 100:912–918

Macular Photocoagulation Study Group (1983a) Argon laser photocoagulation for ocular histoplasmosis: results of a randomized clinical trial. Arch Ophthalmol 101:1,347–1,357

Macular Photocoagulation Study Group (1983b) Argon laser photocoagulation for idiopathic neovascularization. Results of a randomized clinical trial. Arch Ophthalmol 101:1,358–1,361

Michos ED, Mitchell CM, Miller ER 3rd, Sternberg AL, Juraschek SP, Schrack JA, Szanton SL, Walston JD, Kalyani RR, Plante TB, Christenson RH, Shade D, Tonascia J, Roth DL, Appel LJ, STURDY Collaborative Research Group (2018) Rationale and design of the study to understand fall reduction and vitamin D in You (STURDY): a randomized clinical trial of vitamin D supplement doses for the prevention of falls in older adults. Contemp Clin Trials 73:111–122

Multiple Risk Factor Intervention Trial Group (1979) The MRFIT behavior pattern study – I: study design, procedures, and reproducibility of behavior pattern judgments. J Chronic Dis 32:293–305

National Emphysema Treatment Trial Research Group (1999) Rationale and design of the National Emphysema Treatment Trial (NETT): a prospective randomized trial of lung volume reduction surgery. Chest 116:1,750–1,761

Park JW, Liu MC, Yee D, Yau C, van't Veer LJ, Symmans WF, Paoloni M, Perlmutter J, Hylton NM, Hogarth M, De Michele A, Buxton MB, Chien AJ, Wallace AM, Boughey JC, Haddad TC, Chui SY, Kemmer KA, Kaplan HG, Isaacs C, Nanda R, Tripathy D, Albain KS, Edmiston KK, Elias AD, Northfelt DW, Pusztai L, Moulder SL, Lang JE, Viscusi RK, Euhus DM, Haley BB, Khan QJ, Wood WC, Melisko M, Schwab R, Helsten T, Lyandres J, Davis SE, Hirst GL, Sanil A, Esserman LJ, Berry DA, I-SPY 2 Investigators (2016) Adaptive randomization of neratinib in early breast cancer. N Engl J Med 375(1):11–22

University Group Diabetes Program Research Group (1970a) A study of the effects of hypoglycemic agents on vascular complications in patients with adult-onset diabetes: I. Design, methods, and baseline characteristics. Diabetes 19(suppl 2):747–783

University Group Diabetes Program Research Group (1970b) A study of the effects of hypoglycemic agents on vascular complications in patients with adult-onset diabetes: II. Mortality results. Diabetes 19(suppl 2):785–830

Wright JT Jr, Kusek JW, Toto RD, Lee JY, Agodoa LY, Kirk KA, Randall OS, Glassock R, The AASK Pilot Study Investigators (1996) Design and baseline characteristics of participants in the African American Study of Kidney Disease and Hypertension (AASK) pilot study. Control Clin Trials 16:3S–16S

# De-identifying Clinical Trial Data

107

Jimmy Le

Contents

Introduction	2116
Ethical Considerations	2117
Defining "De-identified" Clinical Trial Data	2118
Identifiers in Clinical Trial Data	2119
Protected Health Information	2120
Options for Implementing Clinical Trial Data De-identification and Other Considerations	2123
"Safe Harbor" De-identification	2125
Expert Determination	2127
Examples of Approaches to De-identifying Clinical Trial Data and Additional Considerations	2129
Where to Begin and Future Directions	2131
Summary and Conclusion	2133
Key Facts	2134
Cross-References	2134
References	2134

Abstract

Conducting clinical trials involves collecting detailed health information about participants. Privacy of individual participants is important and must be protected especially when individual participant data are shared broadly. De-identification refers to the process of removing or obscuring identifiable

---

The content of this chapter is solely the responsibility of the author and should not be interpreted as representing the viewpoint of the U.S. Department of Health and Human Services, the National Institutes of Health, or the National Eye Institute.

J. Le (✉)
National Eye Institute, Bethesda, MD, USA
e-mail: jimmy.le@nih.gov

© This is a U.S. Government work and not under copyright protection in the U.S.; foreign copyright protection may apply 2022
S. Piantadosi, C. L. Meinert (eds.), *Principles and Practice of Clinical Trials*,
https://doi.org/10.1007/978-3-319-52636-2_191

information in data. The resulting "de-identified" clinical trial dataset minimizes the risk of unintended disclosure of the identity of participants and information about them. This chapter presents different types of identifiers that may be present in clinical trial data and outlines two commonly used approaches to de-identifying data that are provided in the Privacy Rule of the United States Health Insurance Portability and Accountability Act as examples.

Keywords

Data de-identification · Good clinical practice · Metadata · Individual Participant Data · Data sharing · HIPAA · Data use agreements · Clinical trials

Introduction

Conducting clinical trials involves collecting vast amounts of data, including detailed health information about individual study participants (Institute of Medicine 2015). There are many compelling reasons to share clinical trial data – such as to promote transparency and increase accountability in research – and many examples of how secondary analyses and meta-analyses of shared individual-level participant data have advanced scientific discovery and informed health-care decision-making (Chan et al. 2014; Committee on Strategies for Responsible Sharing of Clinical Trial Data; Board on Health Sciences Policy; Institute of Medicine 2015; Lo 2015; Sim 2020). Sharing clinical trial data, however, cannot proceed without assurance that data will be shared in a way that protects individual study participants (Committee on Strategies for Responsible Sharing of Clinical Trial Data; Board on Health Sciences Policy; Institute of Medicine 2015; Lo 2015). It is important to safeguard the rights and privacy of individuals who participate in clinical trials at all times and eliminate reasonable risk that they may be identified based on the information made available.

De-identification refers to the collection of approaches to removing personal information from an organized collection of individual participant data (or "dataset") to decrease the probability of discovering (or "re-identifying") an individual's identity (Garfinkel 2015). Procedures for de-identifying data should maximize opportunities for re-use and minimize potential loss of privacy or breaches of confidentiality. A dataset that does not contain personal information is less likely to violate privacy of individuals when it is shared.

The focus of this chapter is on de-identifying structured, clinical trial individual participant data in a dataset, which often contains more-detailed information than data typically included in a clinical study report or publication. The ethical context is introduced, followed by an introduction to definitions and guiding principles. Common approaches to de-identifying clinical trial data are described along with examples and considerations for future steps.

Ethical Considerations

Researchers who conduct clinical trials have a responsibility to collect and ensure that the use of data is in accordance with ethical principles. There has been an increasing recognition that these principles need to extend beyond conducting the trial to including a proactive duty to seek out opportunities to archive and share data, including participant-level data (Brakewood and Poldrack 2013; Tom et al. 2020). Conducting research under an ethical framework means balancing priorities of different stakeholder groups: investigators of the clinical trial want recognition for their achievements and fair opportunity to analyze and publish results; other researchers want timely access to data not available elsewhere; study sponsors want to maximize scientific yield and to ensure that there are appropriate measures for preserving intellectual property; and participants want their contributions in research to be meaningful while staying informed on how their data are being used (Institute of Medicine 2015). Thus, there is an ethical responsibility for researchers conducting clinical trials and sharing clinical trial data to protect the identity of participants while preserving integrity of that data (EU General Data Protection Regulation (GDPR) 2016).

In the United States, most research involving human participants operate under the Common Rule (45 CFR Part 46) and/or the United States Food and Drug Administration's human subject protection regulations (21 CFR Parts 50 and 56) (U.-S. Department of Health and Human Services 2003). These regulations include protections (e.g., via ethic review committees, informed consent procedures, management of identifiable private information, etc.) to help ensure the privacy of participants and confidentiality. The United States Health Insurance Portability and Accountability Act (HIPAA), which includes a Privacy Rule that is described later in this chapter, builds upon these protections (U.S. Department of Health and Human Services 2003).

In general, researchers may use and disclose health information about individual research participants for research purposes if they are authorized to do so by the participant (see ▶ Chap. 23, "Long-Term Management of Data and Secondary Use" for a discussion on "The Role of Consent" in data sharing; ▶ Chap. 21, "Consent Forms and Procedures" for information on "Consent forms and Procedures") using procedures approved by their Institutional Review Boards (IRBs) (▶ Chaps. 23, "Long-Term Management of Data and Secondary Use" and ▶ 21, "Consent Forms and Procedures"). Note that authorization may be combined with or in addition to informed consent (U.S. Department of Health and Human Services 2003). In the United States, for example, the latter is a requirement under federal research regulations for the protection of human research participants (and should explicitly discuss future research use and broad data sharing, even if the data are to be de-identified), whereas the former is a legal requirement for the protection of patients' privacy (and may involve signing detailed documents that specify a number of elements including descriptions of information to be used or disclosed, the person authorized to make the use or disclosure and to whom, an expiration date, and, in some cases, the purpose for which the information may be used or disclosed)

(US Department of Health and Human Services 2015; 45 CFR Part 160). When data have been de-identified, some regulations and requirements may no longer be applicable, assuming risks to participants have been adequately minimized (National Institutes of Health 2007). Thus, de-identifying clinical trials data and sharing of the resulting datasets should be undertaken with care and in a way that is consistent with information conveyed to participants during the informed consent process.

Defining "De-identified" Clinical Trial Data

De-identified data are defined as data stripped of certain elements that are associated with individual people (Meinert 2012). De-identified *clinical trial data* reduce risks to privacy and confidentiality loss when they are shared or disseminated because it is assumed that information in a de-identified clinical trial dataset cannot be linked back to individual participants of the clinical trial. The process which produces de-identified data is referred to as de-identification; in contrast, the process that reestablishes links between de-identified data and individuals' identities is known as re-identification (Garfinkel 2015; Meinert 2012; Rothstein 2010).

De-identifying clinical trial data involves making trade-offs. The National Academy of Medicine (formerly known as the Institute of Medicine) describes these trades-offs in data de-identification on a two-dimensional space (Lo 2015). A curve is plotted on a graph where one axis represents data quality – ranging from no utility to maximum utility – and the other, privacy – ranging from no protections to maximum protection (Institute of Medicine 2015). It is impossible to have both absolute utility and absolute privacy. Removing names and addresses may be sufficient in making information *less* specific (or *more* anonymous); yet, the data could still contain other personal information such as birthdate or health status that can be used to re-identify individuals. Conversely, guaranteeing complete anonymity requires removing or replacing all values from the data, making the data useless for subsequent secondary analyses. Investigators and data managers responsible for de-identification must therefore determine the optimal intersection on the curve that represents an acceptable balance of data utility and privacy risks.

De-identifying clinical trial data also involves calculating how likely an individual may be re-identified. For example, it has been estimated that over half of people residing in the United States could be uniquely described using a combination of their birthdate, sex/gender, and five-digit ZIP code (US Department of Health and Human Services 2015; Golle 2006). Calculating this risk in a clinical trial data context requires considering the potential that an adversary (i.e., an individual/entity who attempts to re-identify one or more individuals in a dataset) knows the individual whose data are in a dataset and the types of "attacks" that adversaries may undertake to expose the identity of the individuals (El Emam and Dankar 2008). Specific examples of attacks are reported in in the National Academy of Medicine 2015 Report and elsewhere in the literature (Institute of Medicine 2015). The main point is that de-identification is most conservative when one assumes that an adversary either knows or can find out whether information about an individual is in a given dataset, that is, to assume that a potential adversary is aware that an individual of interest is a participant of a clinical trial and thus aware that the individual's information is available somewhere in the clinical trial dataset that is shared.

Finally, de-identifying clinical trial data involves understanding the "release model" or context of how clinical trial data will be made available and re-used (Institute of Medicine 2015; Garfinkel 2015). For example, sharing a dataset to a trusted researcher with strong mitigating controls (e.g., established security and privacy practices, protected cloud environments, etc.; see Sim (2020) and ▶ Chap. 23, "Long-Term Management of Data and Secondary Use") and signed confidentiality agreements may require less protections, while distributing data via a public website may require further scrutiny and de-identification to the fullest extent (Sim 2020; ▶ Chap. 23, "Long-Term Management of Data and Secondary Use"). Additionally, if data are to be shared internationally, there may be additional requirements and regulatory obligations to consider, and they may differ between countries and jurisdictions (EU General Data Protection Regulation (GDPR) 2016).

Identifiers in Clinical Trial Data

Conducting clinical trials involves collecting and storing information about individual participants. While some of this information, regardless of clinical relevance, is not useful for determining participants' identities, other information can be used to identify, contact, or locate an individual who participated in a study. Personally identifiable information or personal "identifiers" are terms often used to describe the latter (Meinert 2012). Examples of identifiers include names, marital status, place of birth, and credit card numbers, which can all be used to distinguish or trace an individual's identity either alone or in combination with other identifiers (Keerie et al. 2018; Hrynaszkiewicz et al. 2010).

Whether a piece of information is considered an identifier depends on its meeting certain characteristics. The United States Department of Health and Human Services, for example, describes "principles used by experts in the determination of the identifiability" of information in terms of (1) replicability, (2) distinguishability, and (3) data source availability (US Department of Health and Human Services 2015; Malin et al. 2010). Other agencies and organizations (e.g., the National Institute of Standards and Technology) adopt similar definitions and criteria (Garfinkel 2015; McCallister et al. 2010). Information is *replicable* if it remains sufficiently stable over time so that the values will occur consistently in relation to that individual. For example, the social security number of a person with glaucoma is unlikely to change between annual clinic visits, whereas their intraocular pressure may fluctuate over time. Information is *distinguishable* if there is sufficient variability among individuals in a dataset to differentiate between individuals. For example, in a dataset of people who all have diabetic retinopathy, a diagnosis code for diabetes would be indistinguishable because everyone with diabetic retinopathy, by definition, also has diabetes; however, each patient has a unique, distinguishing medical record number. Information is *available* if it can be known. For example, people's

Table 1 Examples of direct and indirect identifiers

Direct identifiers	Indirect identifiers
Names and initials	Sex/gender
Email addresses and telephone numbers	Race/ethnicity
Vehicle identifiers	Place of birth
Names of relatives	Socioeconomic data such as income and education
Biometric data (e.g., fingerprints)	Anthropometric measures

name, contact, and demographics information are often available in public data sources (e.g., vital records, birth, death, and marriage registries), whereas the results of a laboratory report are not often disclosed beyond the healthcare environment (US Department of Health and Human Services 2015). Therefore, a piece of information that is replicable, distinguishable, and available and can be used to identify an individual meets the definition of an identifier (Committee on Strategies for Responsible Sharing of Clinical Trial Data; Board on Health Sciences Policy; Institute of Medicine 2015; McCallister et al. 2010).

Identifiers can be classified as direct or indirect (Table 1) (Committee on Strategies for Responsible Sharing of Clinical Trial Data; Board on Health Sciences Policy; Institute of Medicine 2015; Hrynaszkiewicz et al. 2010). Direct identifiers are information such as names and telephone numbers that uniquely identify an individual, either by themselves or in combination with other readily available information but are often not useful for data analysis purposes. Indirect or quasi-identifiers are variables such as sex/gender or age that are analytically useful but not necessarily unique to an individual (Meinert 2012). The distinction between direct and indirect identifiers in clinical trial data is notable because it is easier to remove direct identifiers or they can be made more anonymous through a process known as data masking, which the National Academy of Medicine defines as a technique to remove or replace direct identifiers with random values and pseudonyms (Institute of Medicine 2015). And although indirect identifiers are not necessarily unique and not always removed or replaced, risk of re-identification increases if they can be combined with other information to identify specific individuals.

Protected Health Information

In most jurisdictions, privacy regulations are bimodal (Rothstein 2010): identifiable information is subjected to all applicable rules and protections, while data that are not identifiable (e.g., de-identified clinical trial data) may be exempted from those conditions. For example, Exemption 4 of the Common Rule exempts research from certain Common Rule requirements as long as the research involves "information recorded by the investigator in such a manner that the identity of the human subjects cannot readily be ascertained directly or through identifiers linked to the subjects, the investigator does not contact the subjects, and the investigator will not re-identify subjects" (45 CFR Part 46). Similarly, the HIPAA Privacy Rule applies only to health data that contain a specific subset of identifiers referred to as protected health information (PHI) (Fig. 1) (45 CFR Part 160).

Clinical Trials Data

Conducting clinical trials involves collecting data about individual study participants.

Data collected in a clinical trial includes information about participants and their health status, such as laboratory results, medical services, and diagnoses.

Personal Identifiers

Clinical trial data include personally identifiable information (identifiers) about individual study participants.

*Research involving data with personally identifiable information is human subjects research and may require IRB approval and/or be subject to regulations and protections including those in the **Health Insurance Portability and Accountability Act** (HIPAA).*

Protected Health Information

Some personal identifiers known as Protected Health Information or "PHI" are regulated under *HIPAA*.

*The **HIPAA Privacy Rule** defines PHI as information about the health status, provision of health care, or payment for health care that can be linked to a specific individual.*

De-identification

*The HIPAA Privacy Rule describes two approaches to de-identifying data: **Expert Determination** & **Safe Harbor**.*

De-identified Data

Clinical trial data with PHI removed are considered as de-identified and no longer regulated by *HIPAA*.

HIPAA permits use and disclosure of data that have been de-identified without obtaining authorization of each data subject (study participant) and without further restrictions on use or disclosure because de-identified data are not PHI and, therefore, are not subject to the Privacy Rule.*

---

* *In certain instances, it may not be possible to de-identify data. A **limited data set** may be disclosed without individual participants' prior authorizations if certain conditions are met. Because a limited data set contains PHI, it is still regulated by HIPAA. Recipients must enter into a **data-use agreement** with the data provider, which establishes the permitted uses and disclosures of the limited data set; identifies who may use or receive the information; prohibits recipients from using or further disclosing information except as permitted by the agreement (or by the law); requires recipients to use appropriate safeguards to prevent a use or disclosure that is not permitted by the agreement; requires recipients to report any unauthorized use or disclosure; requires recipients ensure that any agents (e.g., subcontractors) to whom it provides data will agree to the restrictions provided; and prohibits recipients from identifying or contacting individuals. In contrast, sharing of a de-identified dataset does not necessarily require a data-use agreement.*

Fig. 1 Overview of data de-identification. Personal identifiers refer to information about an individual that can be used to distinguish or trace an individual's identity (e.g., name, social security number, date and place of birth, or mother's maiden name). It includes information that is linked or linkable to an individual, such as medical, educational, and financial information. Protected Health Information or "PHI" refers to a subset of identifiers that are regulated under the United States law. PHI is any information about the health status, provision of health care, or payment for health care that is created or collected by a "covered entity" that can be linked to a specific individual. The United States Health Insurance Portability and Accountability Act (HIPAA) Privacy Rule provides federal protections for data containing PHI, as well as standards for de-identification of PHI, by which identifiers are removed from the health information to mitigate privacy risks

The HIPAA Privacy Rule regulates how health information are used and disclosed in the United States. "Covered entities" (i.e., health plans, health care clearinghouses, and those health care providers and professionals who transmit health information electronically) may only use or disclose data containing PHI if either (1) the HIPAA Privacy Rule specifically permits or requires it or (2) the individual who is the subject of the information provides written authorization that that grants covered entities permission to use PHI for specified purposes (▶ Chap. 23, "Long-Term Management of Data and Secondary Use"; 45 CFR Part 46). Covered entities can be institutions, organizations, or persons. Although the HIPAA only applies to covered entities, it may affect other types of entities that are not directly regulated if they rely on covered entities to provide health data with PHI. Clinical trials also often include researchers who meet the definition of a "covered entity" because they furnish health care services to individuals, including research participants, and transmit information containing PHI in electronic forms. Additionally, it is important to note that HIPAA is often implemented at the organizational or institutional level, consistent with local policies and procedures.

PHI is health- or medical-related information about an individual that can be used to identify them (Committee on Strategies for Responsible Sharing of Clinical Trial Data; Board on Health Sciences Policy; Institute of Medicine 2015). Specifically, HIPAA defines PHI as any information that "relates to an individual's past, present or future physical or mental health; provision of health care to the individual; or the past, present or future payment for the provision of health care to the individual" for which there is a reasonable basis to believe the individual can be identified (45 CFR Part 160; Meinert 2012). For example, information created or used to provide medical services for an individual such as their hospital bill or laboratory results would be considered PHI because these documents contain their name and/or other information associated with the health data content. In contrast, health or medical information presented in aggregate form that was compiled by combining data across large groups of patients in a hospital system and does not identify (or cannot be used to identify) individual patients of that hospital system is not necessarily PHI.

Under current regulations, sharing of a clinical trial dataset that contains PHI may violate the privacy of participants or require authorization from each participant prior to disclosure of the data. A clinical trial dataset that does not contain PHI, however, would be considered as "de-identified" under HIPAA and thus no longer regulated by HIPAA (▶ Chap. 23, "Long-Term Management of Data and Secondary Use"; 45 CFR Part 160). The HIPAA Privacy Rule offers widely accepted standards and methods for which information such as data from a clinical trial can be de-identified in the United States (e.g., in section 164.514(a)) (45 CFR Part 160). In the absence of their own standards for de-identification, many organizations in the United States look to standards described in the HIPAA Privacy Rule as guidance.

Outside of the United States, various regulations associated with data de-identification and protection also exist. Investigators conducting international trials should be aware of applicable rules and policies. For instance, the European Union General Data Protection Regulation (GDPR) and United Kingdom GDPR

Table 2 Comparison of de-identification, anonymization, and pseudonymization

De-identification, in the health care context, refers to the removal or obscuring of identifiers, such as protected health information, in a dataset to mitigate privacy risks to individuals by minimizing the risk of unintended disclosure of the identity of individuals and information about them
Anonymization refers to a de-identification process whereby direct and indirect identifiers in a dataset have been eliminated permanently and safeguards implemented to the extent that data can never be re-identified
Pseudonymization refers to de-identification process whereby identifiers in a dataset have been replaced by nonidentifying references (pseudonyms) so that anyone working with the data will not be able identify individuals. For example, names might be coded with an identification number. The key linking back to participants' names is kept separately but can be used to restore pseudonymized data back to their original state

regulate processing of personal information such as health and medical data collected from people located in the European Union or United Kingdom, respectively. Similar to HIPAA, there are exceptions (e.g., GDPR Recital 26) that states how "principles of data protection should therefore not apply to anonymous information, namely information which does not relate to an identified or identifiable natural person or to personal data rendered anonymous in such a manner that the data subject is not or no longer identifiable" (EU General Data Protection Regulation (GDPR) 2016). Unlike the HIPAA, GDPR does not describe specific methods to "de-identify" data. It provides, however, that data may be "anonymized" or "pseudonymized" (Table 2). Therefore, data considered "de-identified" under HIPAA (and thus not regulated under HIPAA) are not necessarily considered "anonymized" or "pseudonymized" under GDPR (and thus may still be regulated under GDPR, if applicable).

Options for Implementing Clinical Trial Data De-identification and Other Considerations

Approaches to de-identifying clinical trial data each have unique pros and cons as well as different resource demands. Investigators and data managers sharing clinical trial data must consider administrative and operational burdens associated with making the data available and conforming to relevant data protection and regulations (Sim 2020; ▶ Chap. 23, "Long-Term Management of Data and Secondary Use"). There are several options available: adopt homegrown (or "in-house") approaches, engage with external experts, or explore commercially available tools and software in combination with the above (▶ Chap. 23, "Long-Term Management of Data and Secondary Use"; Privacy Analytics (IQVIA) 2019).

In-house solutions are often based on existing standards such as HIPAA and involve simple, definitive methods that do not require much judgment to adequately de-identify data (Privacy Analytics (IQVIA) 2019). Typically a member of the research team (e.g., the data manager or statistician) has already developed preset routines or programs to remove and redact sensitive data elements (e.g., participant names, contact information, and dates). Some institutions and organizations may also have technology or privacy offices that offer in-house solutions for their faculty and staff members. As a downside, there may be less emphasis on retaining analytic value of the dataset given the "cook-book" or checklist nature of this approach and reliance on existing protocols that allow for little flexibilities.

Engaging with experts is a more customizable approach because the expert tackles de-identification on a case-by-case basis. The expert may be an outside consultant or a collaborator already on the team. The difference between this approach and in-house solutions is that de-identification procedures and considerations will be developed specifically for the project at hand. Rules and regulations such as HIPAA permit sharing of information provided that an expert certifies that the risk of reidentification via residual information in a de-identified dataset is low (Institute of Medicine 2015). There is, however, a notable lack of consensus on what qualifies someone as an expert and finding the appropriate expertise may be challenging or require extending beyond the organization or institution. Furthermore, approaches involving experts are not one size fits all: expert consultation does not scale well for larger studies that may contain millions of observations or variables as the process may become unmanageable (Privacy Analytics (IQVIA) 2019).

Commercial software and automated tools may address some of the complexities and challenges involved in de-identifying clinical data. By automating some aspects of de-identification, software and tools, when used in combination with the other two approaches, may provide a more systematic, cost-effective strategy to de-identify data while retaining analytic value (Kayaalp 2017; Privacy Analytics (IQVIA) 2019).

Additionally, the choice of de-identification approach may depend on how data are organized in a dataset. Data can be structured, unstructured, or a combination of both (Garfinkel 2015). Structured data are highly organized, often stored in a predefined format, and easily searchable; unstructured data are conglomerations of various formats (e.g., audio, video, images, and maps). Most approaches to de-identifying data were developed with structured data in mind. For example, it is easier to aggregate age and dates into categorical variables, and more difficult to mask images showing people's faces. Some methods are directly applicable to unstructured data (e.g., the GPS information identifying a participant's home address that is embedded in an image file can be removed). Other times, the data may be impossible to effectively de-identify (e.g., biometric identifiers such as a fingerprint and photographs that cannot be altered or redacted), thus warranting sharing through a different modality (e.g., limited data set) that may involve more-restrictive data-use agreements and vetting (see ▶ Chap. 23, "Long-Term Management of Data and Secondary Use") or require additional authorizations from participants (see ▶ Chaps. 23, "Long-Term Management of Data and Secondary Use" and ▶ 21, "Consent Forms and Procedures"). In these instances, it is especially important to consult with IRBs, study sponsors, and other parties responsible for monitoring participant safety and data integrity (see Sim 2020).

In the next two sections, we expand on two approaches to de-identifying data in the HIPAA Privacy Rule for illustrative purposes; the United States Department of Health and Human Services website or equivalent (e.g., GDPR, if applicable) should be consulted for full, up-to-date, details and requirements (US Department of Health and Human Services 2015). Additionally, some sponsors and funders of clinical trials (e.g., specific institutes of the National Institutes of Health) and the investigators own institutions or organizations may have additional requirements and considerations (National Institutes of Health 2007).

"Safe Harbor" De-identification

"Safe Harbor" refers to a highly prescriptive approach to de-identifying data that is described in HIPAA. No special software, statistical modeling, or advance analyses are required. Instead, this approach relies on the removal of 18 HIPAA-defined identifiers of an individual who is the subject of the information and of their relatives, employers, or household members. Health information, without the 18 identifiers, is not considered to be PHI if that information can no longer be used alone or in combination with other information to identify an individual who is a subject of the information and that there is no "actual knowledge" that the remaining information could be used to re-identify an individual (45 CFR Part 160). Accordingly, a clinical trial dataset can be identified under "Safe Harbor" by removing all 18 identifiers in the Box 1.

Sixteen out of the 18 "Safe Harbor" identifiers (i.e., Box 1, items 1 and 4–18) must be completely eliminated. The other two (Box 1, items 2 and 3), in most cases, can be generalized: all dates must be reported as years and the smallest allowable geographic subdivision is the first three digits of a postal ZIP code. Elimination means that no parts or derivatives or combinations of any of the listed identifiers may be disclosed. Therefore, a data set that contains participants' initials or the last four digits of their telephone number, for example, would not meet the "Safe Harbor" requirements because this information is derived from HIPAA identifiers, that is, names (Box 1, item 1) and telephone numbers (Box 1, item 4). Care must also be taken when interpreting "other unique identifying number, characteristic or code" (Box 1, item 17) because this category of identifiers corresponds to any unique feature not explicitly enumerated above. For example, a unique characteristic of a participant could be their occupation if it was listed in the dataset as "current Chancellor of 'XYZ' University" or the barcode corresponding to their records in an electronic health record database. Additionally, although age of participants may be maintained, participants over age 89 years must be aggregated into a single category (e.g., "age 90 or older") (Box 1, item 2).

Note that some images may qualify as PHI under HIPAA. During development of the Privacy Rule, patient photography was weighed carefully and proposed drafts originally considered all photographic images direct patient identifiers that could not be de-identified (Nettrour et al. 2019). In contrast, final versions of the HIPAA Privacy Rule allow for photographs as long as they are not full-face (Box 1, item 15) or contain biometric identifiers (Box 1, item 13) and unique characteristics (Box 1, item 17). Yet, neither HIPAA nor the Privacy Rule specifies exactly what characteristics should be removed or redacted when deidentifying photographs. Thus, care must be taken when photos collected as part of clinical trial data contain potentially identifying elements that are intrinsic to the participant (e.g., anatomic anomalies, birthmarks, and scars), on the participant (e.g., unique clothing, piercings and tattoos), and around the participant (e.g., unique setting or location) to determine whether those elements constitute PHI (Nettrour et al. 2019). It is also possible that there is PHI in the metafile and file names that accompany an image or that PHI is printed on the image itself (e.g., a date or name apart of the figure legend/caption or in the headers and annotations). PHI on, in, or associated with an image collected in a clinical trial must either be removed completely or replaced/redacted during de-identification; if not, then its inclusion in an otherwise de-identified dataset likely requires authorization from individual participants.

Genetic data also pose unique privacy challenges for de-identification (El Emam 2011). Although not mentioned specifically under the HIPAA Privacy Rule, some genetic sequences are highly individualistic and genetic information is routinely collected and deposited in databanks (Garfinkel 2015; Martinez and Jonker 2020; McGuire and Gibbs 2006). If sharing a clinical trial dataset that contains genetic data, it is important to ensure that genetic data are in no way associated with any of the above 18 identifier elements. Further, as more genetic datasets are produced and shared, risk of re-identification grows and this risk often implicates not only the individual but their family members and future generations (McGuire and Gibbs 2006). Thus, when managing clinical trial data containing genetics information, it may be more appropriate to consider alternative methods of de-identification (e.g., expert determination) or adopt different modalities of data sharing (e.g., limited data set) (Martinez and Jonker 2020; McGuire and Gibbs 2006).

"Safe Harbor" is a rule-based approach, and the same methods (i.e., removal of 18 identifiers) are applied regardless of context. Successful implementation of "Safe Harbor" requires assuming that investigators and data managers employing "Safe Harbor" to de-identify data must have no knowledge that data de-identified through this approach could be used to re-identify participants. Additionally, at the time of its development, "Safe Harbor" was not conceived with longitudinal data (i.e., data collected over a period of time) in mind (El Emam 2011). In practice, this means removal of critical temporal and geospatial information. For example, it would be impossible to include exact dates of when recurring adverse events occur for an individual within the same year of follow-up in a clinical trial dataset that was de-identified via the "Safe Harbor" method.

The list of identifiers enumerated under "Safe Harbor" is also not exhaustive (Keerie et al. 2018). Therefore, as mentioned earlier, the "Safe Harbor" approach on its own does not necessarily meet the de-identification standards of other jurisdictions outside of the United States. Additionally, it is important to recognize that the "Safe Harbor" approach is sometimes used alongside another HIPAA Privacy Rule provision known as "Limited Data Set" (US Department of Health and Human Services 2015; Meinert 2012). Under this provision, a limited data set of information may be disclosed to an outside party without a patient's prior authorization (permission) if certain conditions are met, namely: (1) the purpose of this disclosure may only be for research, public health, or health care operations; and (2) the party receiving the *limited data set* must sign a data-use agreement that specifies the terms under which the data can be used and includes stipulations that the recipient will use appropriate safeguards to prevent disclosure of the information except as provided for in the agreement (45 CFR Part 160; 45 CFR Part 46). Many identifiers listed under "Safe Harbor" will still be removed in a *limited data set*; however, "minimum necessary" information such as dates of hospital admission or discharge, date of birth or death, exact ZIP codes, genetics information, and certain photographs or images may remain in the disclosed information (US Department of Health and Human Services 2015). Because a *limited data set* still contains PHI, however, it remains regulated under HIPAA and is not considered de-identified (Lo 2015).

Expert Determination

Expert Determination refers to the second approach in HIPAA, and it applies current best practices from research to determine the likelihood that an individual could be identified from information in a dataset. This method requires an investigator, data manager, or team "with appropriate knowledge of and experience with generally accepted statistical and scientific principles and methods for rendering information not individually identifiable" to apply such principles and methods to a dataset; determine the risk is "very small" that the information could be used by an anticipated recipient, either alone or in combination with other reasonably available information, to identify an individual who is subject of the information (US Department of Health and Human Services 2015); and document the methods and results of the analysis informing such determination (National Institutes of Health 2007).

Implementation of Expert Determination, as the name implies, varies depending on the expert. HIPAA does not require this individual (or team of individuals) to hold a specific professional degree or certification, and relevant expertise may be gained through a combination of education, academic, and professional experience (Institute of Medicine 2015; US Department of Health and Human Services 2015). From an enforcement perspective, the United States Office for Civil Rights, which enforces HIPAA, "would review the relevant professional experience and academic or other training of the expert used by the covered entity, as well as actual experience of the expert using health information de-identification methodologies" (US Department of Health and Human Services 2015). Although there is no one-size-fits-all model for executing expert determination, United States Department of Health and Human Services does provide a general workflow for the process which is applicable to de-identifying clinical trial data (US Department of Health and Human Services 2015). To summarize:

(1) **First,** the expert determines the extent to which the data can or cannot be identified by the anticipated recipients (National Heart, Lung, and Blood Institute (NHLBI) 2020). This involves working with the covered entity to identify potential adversaries who may attempt to re-identify individuals from the data

and assessing safeguards that are in place. For example, will the data be disseminated through a publicly accessible website (e.g., "open-access") or will they be shared using a controlled-access model? Are there images or pictures with biometric identifiers in the dataset that can be used to re-identify participants? Are there security controls and contractual obligations to support data protection? Will there be data-use agreements and routine audits to ensure adequate privacy and security practices are maintained?

(2) **Then,** the expert provides guidance on which scientific methods could be applied to the data and applies (or work with the team to apply) those methods as deemed acceptable by the covered entity (Fig. 2). This involves performing detailed assessments of risks under various scenarios and quantifying the potential to re-identify an individual participant from the data. These may also involve transforming variables or data elements in the clinical trial data set, such as:

- **Removal (or suppression)**, the expert could eliminate some identifiers (or content) completely from the dataset. These are often direct identifiers such as email addresses or social security numbers that have no analytic value but may include more unique indirect identifiers such as information on serious adverse events.
- **Masking (or pseudonymization)**, the expert could replace some identifiers with coded pseudonyms (e.g., Patient A, Patient B, ... Patient Z). Note that the purpose of this technique is to retain structure and functional usability of the data, and data that have been pseudonymized can be readily reversed if the expert who performed the pseudonymization retains a table (code key) linking original identities to pseudonyms, or if the masking is performed using an algorithm for which the parameters are either known or can be discovered. Photographs could be redacted or made less specific (e.g., cropped) to prevent participant identification.

Name	~~Phone number~~	Email address	ZIP Code	Sex	Age category	Treatment group	Hospital discharge status	Length of stay (days)
Participant 1	-	NA	209XX	Male	40 – 49 years	Placebo	Yes	30
Participant 2	-	EMAIL_ADDRESS	209XX	Male	60 – 69 years	Intervention	Yes	7
Participant 3	-	EMAIL_ADDRESS	212XX	Female	50 – 59 years	Placebo	No	NA
Participant 4	-	NA	212XX	Female	60 – 69 years	Placebo	Yes	60
Participant 5	-	NA	212XX	Male	40 – 49 years	Intervention	Yes	3
Participant 6	-	EMAIL_ADDRESS	209XX	Male	30 – 39 years	Intervention	Yes	1
. . .								
Participant 999	-	EMAIL_ADDRESS	217XX	Female	30 – 39 years	Placebo	No	NA
Participant 1000	-	EMAIL_ADDRESS	212XX	Female	40 – 49 years	Intervention	Yes	7

Fig. 2 Example of application of broad classes of methods to protect data. Overarching goal of methods to protect data is to balance risk of disclosure against utility. In the table above, participant names have been *pseudonymized*, that is, coded as Participant 1, Participant 2, ... Participant 1000. Phone number and email addresses, determined to have no analytic value, were *removed* and *encoded*, respectively. ZIP codes were *generalized* to the first three digits; age, into categories (e.g., 40–49 years in lieu of a specific number); and exact date of hospital discharge, into length of stay (e.g., 21 days in lieu of an actual date). Sex, treatment groups, and hospital discharge status, in this case, were determined not to be uniquely identifying features among the 1000 participants and thus left intact

- **Encoding (or character masking),** the expert could replace some identifiers with category names (e.g., name elements can be replaced with generic phrases such as "FIRST NAME" or "LAST NAME"), information type (e.g., "EMAIL_ADDRESS"), symbols (e.g., "XXXXX"), or random, meaningless values (e.g., "Z$Y%#").
- **Aggregation (or generalization/bucketing),** the expert could combine data elements so that there are fewer groups for a given variable, for example, date of birth could be aggregated to the month and year of birth (e.g., January 1990) or further aggregated so that only the year of birth is provided (e.g., 1990) or range of years (1990–1999); continuous variables (e.g., age in years) could be converted into categorical data elements (e.g., "younger than 18 years" vs "18 years and older").
- **Perturbation,** the expert makes small changes (e.g., add random noise) to the data to prevent identification. For example, specific values for certain data elements could be swapped or changed so that the distribution of data is preserved but the actual values have been altered to introduce uncertainty; however, this technique is likely only acceptable if accurate data are not required.

(3) **Finally,** the expert assesses risk of re-identification. If the risk that individual participants are still identifiable is very small when disclosed to anticipated recipient, then de-identification is complete and the expert provides their certification; otherwise, the expert returns to the first step and repeats. It is critical that, throughout the entire process, the expert documents their methods and the results of any (statistical) analyses to justify that de-identification has been achieved because the risk (or probability) of reidentification is small and unlikely to occur.

It should be clear that expert determination is a statistical, risk-based approach. Based on the level of risk, identifiers in a dataset can be removed or modified so that the de-identified dataset retains greatest value for research while still protecting individual participants. No standard definition of what risk is acceptable exists because the amount of de-identification applied through this method varies based on assessment of the risks related to the use or disclosure of a particular dataset (Rothstein 2010). There is also an overarching responsibility to ensure compliance through IRBs and with other regulatory or institutional policies. For example, the investigator conducting the trial may need to keep any certification made by the expert, in written or electronic format, for at least 6 years from the date of its creation (National Institutes of Health 2007).

Examples of Approaches to De-identifying Clinical Trial Data and Additional Considerations

There are many examples and step-by-step guidance in the literature that report on de-identification in practice, many often applying the HIPAA-defined approaches described previously. Investigators sharing clinical trial data may want to consult with their institutions and sponsors (National Institutes of Health 2007). The examples and resources named below and throughout this chapter do not constitute endorsements or formal recommendation; rather, they are presented here to highlight the complexities involved in removing PHI from a clinical trial data set and to demonstrate that data de-identification is an evolving field. Examples include:

- The **El Emam and Malin methodology** presented as part of "Concepts and Methods for De-identifying Clinical Trial Data" in the National Academy of Medicine 2015 Report and "**k-anonymization**" introduced in ▶ Chap. 23, "Long-Term Management of Data and Secondary Use" are examples of Expert Determination (Institute of Medicine 2015; ▶ Chap. 23, "Long-Term Management of Data and Secondary Use"). An expert consultant pools individual study participants' data into a larger group comprising "k" number of people, meanwhile generalizing (aggregating) some identifying attributes and removing others entirely. In the end, information in the group could correspond to any single member rather than a particular individual, and there is no reasonable basis to believe that the containing information can be used to identify one specific individual (45 CFR Part 160).
- The United States **Department of Health and Human Services** hosted a workshop in 2010 that produced an extensive guidance on methods and approaches to achieve de-identification in accordance with the HIPAA Privacy Rule (US Department of Health and Human Services 2015).
- **Garfinkel et al.**, via a National Institute of Standards and Technology report, summarize an 11-step process for de-identifying data based on expert classification of identifiers (Garfinkel 2015). This report also introduces recommendations for de-identifying unstructured data, namely medical text, photographs and video, medical imagery, genetic information and biological materials, and geographic and map data.
- **Keerie et al.** outline a rules-based approach to anonymizing a clinical trial dataset (Keerie et al. 2018), which involves deleting or modifying 28 types of indirect and direct identifiers identified previously by **Hrynaszkiewicz et al.** (2010). They introduce two checkpoints ("Is it accurate?" and "Is it anonymous?") to evaluate prior to sharing a dataset.
- **Tucker et al.** offer recommendations to utilize a de-identification approach in line with "Safe Harbor" but with further generalization and masking of some indirect identifiers (Tucker et al. 2016).
- **Wilkinson et al.** describe and then challenge the "**cell size less than five**" approach, a rules-based practice of releasing aggregate data about individuals only if the number of individuals counted for each cell of a table is greater than or equal to five (Wilkinson et al. 2020). Authors propose an alternative risk-based expert approach in an applied public health setting.
- **Kayaalp et al.** outline different modes of de-identification involving automatic de-identification systems (e.g., on-demand, scientist-involved, patient-involved, and physician-involved) (Kayaalp 2017; Kayaalp et al. 2014).
- The **National Heart, Lung, and Blood Institute** (NHLBI) provides guidelines for Guidelines for Preparing Clinical Study Data Sets for Submission to the

NHLBI Data Repository, which includes six steps taken to protect participant privacy that must be documented and approved by the NHLBI prior to implementation (NHLBI 2020).
- The **NIH Genomic Data Sharing Policy** includes recommendations for steps to de-identifying human genomic data that are submitted to NIH-designated data repositories (National Institutes of Health 2020a).
- The **Immunology Database and Analysis Portal**, supported by a contract from the National Institute of Allergy and Infectious Diseases, describes procedures to sever connection to "subject identifiers in the source data" by following "Safe Harbor" principles (ImmPort 2020).
- **The Cancer Imaging Archive**, which is a National Cancer Institute-supported service that de-identifies and hosts a large archive of medical images of cancer accessible for public download, lays out a process that "ensures that the HIPAA de-identification standard is met by following the Safe Harbor Method" for clinical radiology and pathology images (The Cancer Imaging Archive 2020).

Tools and software also exist to assist in de-identification of data collected in clinical trials. For example, **NLM-Scrubber** (https://scrubber.nlm.nih.gov/) is a clinical text de-identification tool that uses natural language processing to automatically redact direct identifiers that are typically found in medical records (e.g., names, dates, and alphanumeric identifiers) (Kayaalp et al. 2014); and **DicomCleaner™** provides users with control over removing and replacing information that is stored in the "DICOM header" of image files collected following Digital Imaging and Communications in Medicine standards (PixelMed DicomCleaner 2016). The header of many medical images may contain demographic information about individuals, acquisition parameters, image dimensions, etc. The **National Institute of Standards and Technology** also maintains a catalog of additional tools and user-contributed examples (National Institute of Standards and Technology 2020): https://www.nist.gov/itl/applied-cybersecurity/privacy-engineering/collaboration-space/focus-areas/de-id

Where to Begin and Future Directions

Clinical trialists who intend to share data should think carefully about the study design, informed consent procedures, and structure of the resulting dataset before initiating their study (National Institutes of Health 2020b). De-identification requires collaboration among all parties involved in collecting, handling, storing, and transmitting health information. The responsibility of protecting rights and privacy of clinical trial participants lies ultimately with the researchers involved in the conduct and management of the trial and with their institutions and IRBs. Although de-identification happens after data have been collected, researchers must also ensure a priori that the informed consent procedures anticipate data uses and sharing so that individuals have an opportunity to make an informed decision whether to participate in a research study or not. The information provided in this chapter serves as a starting point for discussion with institutional staff and technical experts (e.g., statisticians, IRBs and ethics/privacy coordinators, and legal counsel). It is equally important to consider guidance for data sharing (Sim 2020), which includes topics such as seeking participant consent, establishing data-use agreements, and obtaining IRB approval.

Anyone beginning the de-identification process must also consult federal and local regulations and policies. In the United States, this includes the HIPAA Privacy Rule. Funding agencies may also have additional guidelines (e.g., NHLBI, https://www.nhlbi.nih.gov/grants-and-training/policies-and-guidelines/guidelines-for-preparing-clinical-study-data-sets-for-submission-to-the-nhlbi-data-repository; NIH, https://grants.nih.gov/grants/policy/data_sharing/data_sharing_guidance.htm) (National Institutes of Health 2007; National Heart, Lung, and Blood Institute (NHLBI) 2020; National Institutes of Health 2020b), and researchers may also want to consult and coordinate with the channels, platforms, or repositories by which they plan to share de-identified data. The National Library of Medicine, for example, maintains a list of National Institutes of Health (NIH)-supported data repositories and their requirements (https://www.nlm.nih.gov/NIHbmic/nih_data_sharing_repositories.html) (National Library of Medicine 2020).

Literature is currently sparse on the exact resource needs for de-identification (Institute of Medicine 2015). Future studies could examine the exact person hours involved in de-identifying a dataset and the infrastructure, software, and equipment required. In the interim, funding agencies such as the NIH have encouraged researchers to "request funds for data sharing and archiving in their grant application" because those who incorporate "data sharing in the initial design of the study may more readily and economically establish adequate procedures for protecting the identities of participants and share a useful dataset with appropriate documentation" (National Institutes of Health 2020b). There may also be resource needs in order to perform regular audits and monitoring to minimize any potential threat of re-identification.

Equally important, it must be recognized that like de-identification, data re-identification is a growing field. Even under approaches such as those described in HIPAA, de-identified clinical trial data may still contain private information and therefore pose some risk of re-identification (Rothstein 2010). New datasets become available at an exponential rate and, when combined with previously shared data, may provide means of re-establishing links to individual people. Similarly, advancements in statistical programming and computing allow for extracting information from large volumes of data that existed previously in disparate spaces, thus changing the risk profile of a de-identified dataset if it were to be used on its own. Future studies could examine how risk of re-identification grows as more data are de-identified, shared, and then meta-analyzed. Downstream use and re-use of de-identified data may also dramatically change a risk assessment or decisions made at time of initial de-identification; however, it is unclear how prospective risk of re-identification could be measured or quantified as this risk depends on availability and disclosure of data in the future (Institute of Medicine 2015; Garfinkel 2015; Privacy Analytics (IQVIA) 2019; McGuire and Gibbs 2006).

Finally, some data remain impossible to de-identify and cannot be shared as de-identified data without complete distortion. In these instances, perhaps risks are better managed or mitigated by releasing highly redacted datasets for general use and restricting access to more sensitive data (e.g., images and photographs) to controlled sites (i.e., "data enclaves") with stricter controls and signed data-use agreements (Institute of Medicine 2015; Garfinkel 2015; Rothstein 2010). Otherwise, use and disclosure of this information may require permission from individual participants in the form of an authorization. Our discussion thus advances onwards into the realms of data management (▶ Chap. 23, "Long-Term Management of Data and Secondary Use") and data sharing (Sim 2020).

> **Box 1 18 identifiers that are considered personally identifiable information under the Privacy Rule of the United States Health Insurance Portability and Accountability Act (HIPAA)**
>
> (1) Names
> (2) All geographic subdivisions smaller than a state (except for the initial three digits of the ZIP code) including street address, city, county, precinct, zip code, and their equivalent.
> (3) All elements of dates (except year) for dates that are directly related to an individual, and all ages over 89 and all elements of dates (including year) indicative of such age, except that such ages and elements may be aggregated into a single category of age 90 or older.
> (4) Telephone numbers
> (5) Vehicle identifiers and serial numbers
> (6) Fax numbers
> (7) Device identifiers and serial numbers
> (8) Email addresses
> (9) Web Universal Resource Locators (URLs)
> (10) Social security numbers
> (11) Internet Protocol (IP) addresses
> (12) Medical record numbers
> (13) Biometric identifiers, including finger and voice prints
> (14) Health plan beneficiary numbers
> (15) Full-face photographs and any comparable images
> (16) Account numbers
> (17) Any other unique identifying number, characteristic, or code
> (18) Certificate/license numbers

Summary and Conclusion

Data de-identification is intended to protect privacy and confidentiality of individuals while enabling important secondary use of that data. A de-identified clinical trial dataset in the United States, for example, would not contain PHI and would thus no longer be subjected to the provisions of regulations such as the HIPAA Privacy Rule. Risks to privacy and confidentiality when sharing de-identified data are reduced because information in a de-identified clinical trial dataset cannot be linked back to individual participants. Implementing de-identification requires balancing data utility and privacy concerns. Common approaches to de-identification are often rules-based or require expert determination. When de-identifying data, it is important to consider institutional and IRB policies, informed consent procedures that address anticipated data uses and sharing, requirements from sponsors, and local and federal regulations as what is considered "de-identified" may vary depending on the context or change with time.

Key Facts

- De-identified clinical trial data are data stripped of certain data elements that are associated with individual people.
- De-identifying clinical trial data requires making trade-offs: higher privacy means very little to no useful data and higher utility means less privacy.
- Personal identifiers refer to information that is uniquely attributable to specific individuals.
- Protected Health Information (PHI) is a subset of identifiers that refer to information about health status, provision of health care, or payment for health care.
- In the United States, the Health Insurance Portability and Accountability Act (HIPAA) outlines 18 PHI identifiers that must be treated with special care.
- The HIPAA Privacy Rule provides for two common approaches to de-identifying data that contains PHI: "Safe Harbor" and Expert Determination.
- The regulations governing data sharing, re-use, and de-identification will vary depending on legal jurisdiction, institutional/funding policies, and time.
- Protecting the privacy of clinical trial participants is paramount.

Cross-References

▶ Consent Forms and Procedures
▶ Data Sharing and Reuse
▶ Long-Term Management of Data and Secondary Use

References

45 CFR Part 160. https://www.ecfr.gov/current/title-45/subtitle-A/subchapter-C/part-160
45 CFR Part 46. https://www.ecfr.gov/current/title-45/subtitle-A/subchapter-A/part-46?toc=1
Brakewood B, Poldrack RA (2013) The ethics of secondary data analysis: considering the application of Belmont principles to the sharing of neuroimaging data. NeuroImage 82:671–676
Chan AW, Song F, Vickers A et al (2014) Increasing value and reducing waste: addressing inaccessible research. Lancet 383(9913):257–266

Committee on Strategies for Responsible Sharing of Clinical Trial Data; Board on Health Sciences Policy; Institute of Medicine (2015) Appendix B. Concepts and methods for de-identifying clinical trial data. In: Sharing clinical trial data: maximizing benefits, minimizing risk. Committee on Strategies for Responsible Sharing of Clinical Trial Data; Board on Health Sciences Policy; Institute of Medicine, Washington, DC

El Emam K (2011) Methods for the de-identification of electronic health records for genomic research. Genome Med 3(4):25

El Emam K, Dankar FK (2008) Protecting privacy using k-anonymity. J Am Med Inform Assoc 15 (5):627–637

EU General Data Protection Regulation (GDPR) (2016) Regulation (EU) 2016/679 of the European Parliament and of the Council of 27 April 2016 on the protection of natural persons with regard to the processing of personal data and on the free movement of such data, and repealing Directive 95/46/EC (General Data Protection Regulation), OJ 2016 L 119/1

Garfinkel S (2015) De-identification of personal information. National Institute of Standards and Technology, Gaithersburg

Golle P (2006) Revisiting the uniqueness of simple demographics in the US population. In: Proceedings of the 5th ACM workshop on privacy in electronic society, Alexandria

Hrynaszkiewicz I, Norton ML, Vickers AJ, Altman DG (2010) Preparing raw clinical data for publication: guidance for journal editors, authors, and peer reviewers. BMJ 340:c181

ImmPort (2020) ImmPort de-identification process. https://www.immport.org/docs/BISC-Subject-De-identification.pdf. Accessed 1 June 2021

Institute of Medicine (2015) Sharing clinical trial data: maximizing benefits, minimizing risk. The National Academies Press, Washington, DC

Kayaalp M (2017) Modes of de-identification. AMIA Annu Symp Proc 2017:1044–1050

Kayaalp M, Browne AC, Dodd ZA, Sagan P, McDonald CJ (2014) De-identification of address, date, and alphanumeric identifiers in narrative clinical reports. AMIA Annu Symp Proc 2014: 767–776

Keerie C, Tuck C, Milne G, Eldridge S, Wright N, Lewis SC (2018) Data sharing in clinical trials – practical guidance on anonymising trial datasets. Trials 19(1):25

Lo B (2015) Sharing clinical trial data: maximizing benefits, minimizing risk. JAMA 313(8): 793–794

Malin B, Karp D, Scheuermann RH (2010) Technical and policy approaches to balancing patient privacy and data sharing in clinical and translational research. J Investig Med 58(1):11–18

Martinez C, Jonker E (2020) A practical path toward genetic privacy in the United States. Privacy analytics. Available at https://fpf.org/wp-content/uploads/2020/04/APracticalPathTowardGeneticPrivacy_April2020.pdf. Accessed 1 July 2021

McCallister E, Grance T, Scarfone K (2010) SP 800-122. Guide to protecting the confidentiality of personally identifiable information (PII). National Institute of Standards and Technology, Gaithersburg

McGuire AL, Gibbs RA (2006) No longer de-identified. Science 312(5772):370–371

Meinert CL (2012) Clinical trials dictionary: terminology and usage recommendations. Wiley, Hoboken

National Heart, Lung, and Blood Institute (NHLBI) (2020) Guidelines for preparing clinical study data sets for submission to the NHLBI data repository. https://www.nhlbi.nih.gov/grants-and-training/policies-and-guidelines/guidelines-for-preparing-clinical-study-data-sets-for-submission-to-the-nhlbi-data-repository. Accessed 1 June 2021

National Institute of Standards and Technology (2020) De-identification. https://www.nist.gov/itl/applied-cybersecurity/privacy-engineering/collaboration-space/focus-areas/de-id. Accessed 1 June 2021

National Institutes of Health (2007) How can covered entities use and disclose protected health information for research and comply with the privacy rule?. https://privacyruleandresearch.nih.gov/pr_08.asp. Accessed 1 June 2021

National Institutes of Health (2020a) NIH genomic data sharing policies. https://osp.od.nih.gov/scientific-sharing/policies/. Accessed 1 June 2021

National Institutes of Health (2020b) NIH data sharing policy and implementation guidance. https://grants.nih.gov/grants/policy/data_sharing/data_sharing_guidance.htm. Accessed 1 June 2021

National Library of Medicine (2020) Data sharing resources. https://www.nlm.nih.gov/NIHbmic/nih_data_sharing_repositories.html. Accessed 1 June 2021

Nettrour JF, Burch MB, Bal BS (2019) Patients, pictures, and privacy: managing clinical photographs in the smartphone era. Arthroplast Today 5(1):57–60

National Heart, Lung, and Blood Institute (2020) Guidelines for preparing clinical study data sets for submission to the NHLBI data repository. https://www.nhlbi.nih.gov/grants-and-training/policies-and-guidelines/guidelines-for-preparing-clinical-study-data-sets-for-submission-to-the-nhlbi-data-repository. Accessed 1 June 2021

PixelMed DicomCleaner (2016) What is DicomCleaner™?. http://www.dclunie.com/pixelmed/software/webstart/DicomCleanerUsage.html. Accessed 1 June 2021

Privacy Analytics (IQVIA) (2019) De-identification 101: how to protect private health information

Rothstein MA (2010) Is deidentification sufficient to protect health privacy in research? Am J Bioeth 10(9):3–11

Sim I (2020) Data sharing and reuse. In: Piantadosi S, Meinert CL (eds) Principles and practice of clinical trials. Springer, Cham, pp 1–22

The Cancer Imaging Archive (2020) The Cancer Imaging Archive – submission and de-identification overview. https://wiki.cancerimagingarchive.net/display/Public/Submission+and+De-identification+Overview. Accessed 1 June 2021

Tom E, Keane PA, Blazes M et al (2020) Protecting data privacy in the age of AI-enabled ophthalmology. Transl Vis Sci Technol 9(2):36

Tucker K, Branson J, Dilleen M et al (2016) Protecting patient privacy when sharing patient-level data from clinical trials. BMC Med Res Methodol 16(Suppl 1):77

U.S. Department of Health and Human Services (2003) Research. Health information privacy. https://www.hhs.gov/hipaa/for-professionals/privacy/guidance/research/index.html. Accessed 1 July 2021

U.S. Department of Health and Human Services (2015) Guidance regarding methods for de-identification of protected health information in accordance with the Health Insurance Portability and Accountability Act (HIPAA) Privacy Rule. https://www.hhs.gov/hipaa/for-professionals/privacy/special-topics/de-identification/index.html#rationale. Accessed 1 June 2021

Wilkinson K, Green C, Nowicki D, Von Schindler C (2020) Less than five is less than ideal: replacing the "less than 5 cell size" rule with a risk-based data disclosure protocol in a public health setting. Can J Public Health 111(5):761–765

Data Sharing and Reuse

108

Ida Sim

Contents

Introduction	2138
Policy Context	2139
FAIR Data Sharing Principles	2140
Landscape: Current Data Platforms	2141
Findability	2144
Accessibility	2147
Interoperability	2148
Syntactic Interoperability	2149
Semantic Interoperability	2149
Reusability	2150
Culture of Data Sharing	2151
Costs and Sustainability	2153
Future Issues	2153
Summary and Conclusions	2154
Key Facts	2155
Cross-References	2156
References	2156

Abstract

Traditionally, clinical trials influence science through publications of their results. Increasingly, however, summary-level and individual participant-level results data are being shared with the scientific community and are influencing science through data reuse. Journal and funder mandates are compelling the sharing of summary-level as well as individual participant-level data (IPD) by industry and academic trialists. Patients, too, are becoming more vocal in demanding that their data contributions to clinical trials be re-used to accelerate findings.

I. Sim (✉)
Division of General Internal Medicine, University of California San Francisco, San Francisco, CA, USA
e-mail: Ida.sim@ucsf.edu

© Springer Nature Switzerland AG 2022
S. Piantadosi, C. L. Meinert (eds.), *Principles and Practice of Clinical Trials*,
https://doi.org/10.1007/978-3-319-52636-2_190

The move toward clinical trial data sharing is part of a wider movement toward open science in general. Four principles underlie scientific data sharing: Findability, Accessibility, Interoperability, and Reusability (FAIR). To handle the global volume of clinical trials, automated implementation of these principles is needed to complement more manual methods. Close to 100 clinical trial data sharing platforms currently exist worldwide, each meeting the FAIR data sharing principles to varying degrees of automation.

This chapter reviews the history, motivations, and current landscape of clinical trial data sharing and reuse. A culture of data sharing is now the norm in the pharmaceutical industry and is starting to take hold in academia, where new mechanisms for crediting and rewarding data sharing are needed. The benefits of data sharing go beyond new publishable findings to include improvements in future study designs informed by analyses of prior IPD. Clinical trial data sharing honors participant contributions to research, enhances public trust in clinical trials, and promises to accelerate scientific findings by maximizing the value of clinical trials data.

Keywords

Data sharing · Data reuse · Individual Participant-level Data · IPD · FAIR data sharing principles · Data repositories · Data sharing platforms · Interoperability

"A scholar's positive contribution is measured by the sum of the original data that he contributes. Hypotheses come and go but data remain. Theories desert us, while data defend us. They are our true resources, our real estate, and our best pedigree." (Santiago Ramón y Cajal, 1897)

Introduction

Traditionally, clinical trials influence science through publications of their results. Increasingly, however, summary-level and individual participant-level results data are being shared with the scientific community and are influencing science through data reuse. Summary-level results data are not only reported through publications but are also expected to be posted on ClinicalTrials.gov 12 months after study completion. The sharing of individual participant-level data (IPD) is more challenging due to concerns about privacy, "rogue analyses," and the sheer logistics of sharing IPD and associated study documents.

As clinical trial results data acquire a life of their own after completion of the original trial, methodological, technical, and policy issues arise on how to manage the sharing and reuse of these data. Who owns these data? What restrictions, if any, should be placed on access and reuse? How can data from disparate sources be found and aggregated? What are the most scientifically productive uses and reuses of results data? A key tenet of data sharing is that sharing by itself does not generate scientific value; shared data must be reused either to reproduce the original analysis or for new analyses. The more value that is generated from reuse, the greater will be the interest and willingness of clinical trialists to share. The more data that are shared, the greater will be the value of data sharing. This virtuous cycle is on the cusp of occurring. This chapter reviews the history, motivations, and current landscape of clinical trial data sharing and reuse, focusing primarily on the sharing of IPD.

Policy Context

The long road to clinical trial data sharing begins with the storied history behind trial transparency. A seminal paper by Dickersin in 1990 (Dickersin 1990) called out publication bias in the medical literature, wherein studies with positive results are more likely to be published than those with negative results. This systematic skewing toward favorable results for tested interventions has a corrosive effect on science and on health policy. Subsequent scandals involving the suppression of negative and unfavorable study results of marketed drugs (Melander et al. 2003; Turner et al. 2008) heightened the need for transparent identification of all existing trials so that complete results can be tracked down regardless of their direction of benefit. Increased transparency and accountability were also needed to restore public trust in clinical trials. Thus, decades after the initial call for international trial registration (Simes 1986), trial registration became global policy in 2006 under the leadership of the World Health Organization's International Clinical Trials Registry Platform (ICTRP) (Sim et al. 2006). ICTRP launched a network of approved trial registers across the world, with the pre-existing United States' ClinicalTrials.gov register being the largest. To date, trial registration is still not complete (Zarin et al. 2017), but the expectations are clear.

While trial registration ensures transparency of the existence of a trial, bias in results reporting is reduced only if all results from all registered trials are made available to the scientific community. The first step toward this vision was the US Food and Drug Administration Amendments Act (FDAAA) of 2007, which mandated the reporting of summary-level results in ClinicalTrials.gov "for those clinical trials that form the primary basis of an efficacy claim or are conducted after the drug involved is approved or after the device involved is cleared or approved" (2007). The US National Institutes of Health (NIH) adopted these requirements for summary-level reporting, but adherence has been less than complete due to the absence of strong sanctions for non-adherence. Nevertheless, just as incomplete achievement of trial registration moved the needle on trial transparency, incomplete achievement of summary-level results reporting has moved the needle on clinical trial data sharing.

The scientific value of having summary-level results available for all trials is to guard against results reporting bias and to enable meta-analysis. Substantially greater scientific value arises from sharing IPD, which allows for more complex and flexible analyses than is possible with only summary-level results. For example, with IPD, an analyst can standardize or redefine outcomes across studies, check analysis assumptions (e.g., normality), model heterogeneity within and between studies, explore covariates and treatment-covariate interactions, conduct new subgroup analyses, or model prognostic or diagnostic data (Debray et al. 2015). IPD are particularly valuable for reusing and meta-analyzing studies with time-to-event outcomes such as survival.

Movement toward requiring IPD sharing started in Europe with the European Medicines Agency's (EMA) Policy 0070 (2014, p. 70). The initial version of Policy 0070 mandated the automatic release of IPD for all studies supporting any drug approved by the EMA. The pushback from industry and other quarters was strong and sustained such that the policy was suspended. Regardless, the culture of data sharing had shifted: in 2015, an influential National Academy of Medicine report stated "The issue is no longer whether to share clinical trial data, but what specific data to share, at what time, and under what conditions" (The National Academies Press 2015). In 2018, the International Committee of Medical Journal Editors (ICMJE) began requiring that all clinical trial manuscripts provide a statement detailing how the IPD will be shared, to whom, and under what conditions, and all trials started after January 1, 2019, must include an IPD sharing plan in their trial registration (Taichman et al. 2017). Because ICMJE includes some of the leading medical journals (e.g., *New England Journal of Medicine*, *JAMA*, *Annals of Internal Medicine*, *Lancet*), ICMJE policies are highly influential in medical publishing and in academic research communities. Additional drivers toward IPD sharing include over 50 funders worldwide – predominantly in Europe and the UK – who require IPD sharing (Nature 2018). The NIH is in the midst of proposing that IPD sharing be required for all NIH-funded trials and that evidence of actual data sharing be factored into future funding decisions (National Institutes of Health 2018). The policy momentum toward routine IPD sharing in industry and academia is indisputable.

The push for clinical trial data sharing is part of a wider open science movement touching fields as disparate as economics, climate science, and education (Vicente-Saez and Martinez-Fuentes 2018). In clinical research, the voices of trial participants – questioning why clinical trial data are not being shared more widely to accelerate findings – are insistent and provide additional moral pressure behind results data sharing (Mello et al. 2018). Motivated initially by the need for transparency and accountability that led to trial registration, results data sharing has now evolved into sharing for science's sake with increasing recognition that effective data reuse is the means by which data sharing will generate scientific and social value.

FAIR Data Sharing Principles

With the open science movement, the sharing and reuse of scholarly data are of interest across many scientific fields. Notwithstanding unique privacy concerns when sharing human clinical data, the foundations for scholarly data sharing are similar across clinical and non-clinical data. In 2016, a diverse group of stakeholders representing academia, industry, funding agencies, and scholarly publishers defined and endorsed "a concise and measurable set of principles" for "scientific data management and stewardship" (Wilkinson et al. 2016). These FAIR Data Principles center around four foundational principles: Findability, Accessibility,

> **Box 2 | The FAIR Guiding Principles**
>
> **To be Findable:**
> F1. (meta)data are assigned a globally unique and persistent identifier
> F2. data are described with rich metadata (defined by R1 below)
> F3. metadata clearly and explicitly include the identifier of the data it describes
> F4. (meta)data are registered or indexed in a searchable resource
>
> **To be Accessible:**
> A1. (meta)data are retrievable by their identifier using a standardized communications protocol
> A1.1 the protocol is open, free, and universally implementable
> A1.2 the protocol allows for an authentication and authorization procedure, where necessary
> A2. metadata are accessible, even when the data are no longer available
>
> **To be Interoperable:**
> I1. (meta)data use a formal, accessible, shared, and broadly applicable language for knowledge representation.
> I2. (meta)data use vocabularies that follow FAIR principles
> I3. (meta)data include qualified references to other (meta)data
>
> **To be Reusable:**
> R1. meta(data) are richly described with a plurality of accurate and relevant attributes
> R1.1. (meta)data are released with a clear and accessible data usage license
> R1.2. (meta)data are associated with detailed provenance
> R1.3. (meta)data meet domain-relevant community standards

Fig. 1 **FAIR data sharing principles**. From Scientific Data, 3:160018 | https://doi.org/10.1038/sdata.2016.18. (Copyright permission from Nature under Creative Commons Attribution 4.0 International License.)

Interoperability, and Reusability. These principles underpin the goal of *machine-actionable* data sharing (Fig. 1). The importance of machine actionability cannot be overstated. Every year, ClinicalTrials.gov adds over 30,000 trials, and PubMed adds almost 40,000 new trial publications. Manual approaches to finding, accessing, or re-using clinical trial data are insufficient for the volume and complexity of clinical trials. For clinical trial data sharing to be scientifically valuable, the data sharing infrastructure must be machine-actionable to assist humans in finding, accessing, and re-using data.

Of the four FAIR principles, Reusability is the crowning one. Data can be said to be shared if they are Findable and Accessible, but without Reusability, little new scientific value will be generated. Since its publication, the FAIR principles have been adopted by NIH and many other funding agencies and research groups worldwide. These principles will be the organizing framework for the rest of this chapter.

Landscape: Current Data Platforms

Clinical trial data platforms can be categorized as data archiving platforms that primarily support Findability and Accessibility, and data sharing platforms that support some aspects of Reusability in addition to Findability and Accessibility. This section introduces the landscape of existing platforms. Greater detail is presented in the following discussion of how these platforms do or do not meet the FAIR principles.

General purpose data repositories. Data platforms that primarily support data archiving retain data in long-term storage (aka repositories) to meet regulatory compliance and other needs. Data in these repositories must be Findable and Accessible to regulators and other users. Typically, such repositories will assign a Digital Object Identifier (DOI) to each dataset to serve as a persistent unique identifier and as a mechanism for dataset search, reference, and citation. To ensure that each DOI is unique and that it always points to the digital object referenced, DOIs are issued by centralized DOI registration agencies. Two widely used registration agencies are DataCite and CrossRef. The DOIs from each registration agency include a common set of high-level metadata (data about data) that describe the digital object. For example, a DataCite DOI for a dataset will include information about the dataset's creator, title, publication year, version, and description. By providing a persistent unique identifier with standard metadata, DOIs ensure that data objects are not only Findable but also uniquely identifiable. Unique Findability is critical for machine-actionable data archiving, sharing, scholarly data reuse, and citation and attribution.

Dryad and Figshare are examples of independent general-purpose data repositories. Some universities and institutions also maintain repositories to archive their own research products (e.g., University of California's DASH). These repositories accept datasets from any discipline in a wide range of data types and formats, and generally do not impose any metadata description requirements beyond those needed for DOIs. These datasets are therefore Findable, but usually only by high-level descriptors such as title, author, or keyword. Furthermore, these repositories generally permit anyone to download any dataset without restriction, an Accessibility approach that is reasonable for many scholarly datasets but not for clinical trial data, where participant privacy is a concern. Because general-purpose data repositories impose little standardization on format or content and provide no technical support for data integration or analysis, they do not directly support Interoperability or Reusability and cannot be said to be FAIR data repositories.

In contrast, Sage Bionetworks exemplifies a general-purpose approach that is highly tuned to the needs of clinical trial data sharing. Sage is a non-profit organization that promotes and supports open science approaches for advancing human health. They partnered with Apple Inc. to support clinical research using ResearchKit, a user-friendly trial recruitment and data collection platform for iPhones. As a condition of running a ResearchKit study with Sage's technical infrastructure, researchers must agree to ask participants for broad data sharing consent and to make all study data available via Sage's Synapse data sharing and analysis platform under Sage's data request and review processes. The initial set of Sage-supported ResearchKit studies involved tens of thousands of participants in observational studies of heart, asthma, Parkinson's, and other conditions, with some enrolling over 10,000 participants each. For example, the mPower Parkinson's study enrolled 12,201 participants of whom 78% opted to share broadly (Bot et al. 2016), yielding a dataset that has to date been accessed by over 183 separate Sage-approved projects.

Likewise, the Yale University Open Data Access (YODA) Project is tuned for clinical trial data sharing. The YODA Project requires that data partners give the YODA Project team full jurisdiction to make decisions regarding data access. Initial YODA Project data partners include Medtronic, Inc. and Johnson & Johnson.

Vivli is a general clinical research data sharing platform launched in 2018 that explicitly aims to implement the FAIR principles (Sim et al. under review). Datasets on Vivli are uniquely identifiable via a Datacite DOI and are made "Findable" based on curated rich metadata. IPD are made "Accessible" via harmonized data request and review policies, and through either direct download or in secure research environments. Interoperability is partially addressed by recommendations on data formatting. Reusability is supported by rich metadata, availability of associated study documents, clear usage licenses, and user support to ensure a user-friendly experience for both data contributors and data requesters. Unique among IPD sharing platforms, Vivli partners provide data request review and secure data access services to other IPD sharing platforms. This bridging serves to break down data silos and expand the scope and scale of IPD sharing globally.

Institutional data sharing platforms. Many academic medical institutions maintain their own secure data platforms that are provisioned with common analytic tools (e.g., STATA, MATLAB). These platforms support data sharing but typically require that all data users be from that institution. For example, faculty can store their trial data in such a platform and other investigators from the same institution can access that data, but collaborators from outside that institution either cannot access that data or must complete onerous forms to do so. Such barriers limit data sharing and preclude data aggregation as investigators cannot aggregate data from different institutions. Thus, institutional platforms tend to provide too little Accessibility to clinical trial data, whereas general-purpose repositories like Dryad and Figshare provide too much Accessibility. One final challenge to using institutional platforms for data sharing is that these platforms are not meant to serve as long-term storage, and investigators often lack the funds to continue storing data in these platforms beyond the funding period of the trial.

Study-specific and disease-specific platforms. Some large studies maintain their own data sharing platforms. The Framingham Heart Study has shared data for decades under a model that requires data requesters to collaborate with the original investigators. The Alzheimer's Disease Neuroimaging Initiative (ADNI) has been sharing imaging and clinical data via direct download from observational studies of dementia since 2004. ADNI has resulted in over 1700 publications. Study-specific data sharing platforms are thus one way to share data but require substantial technical and administrative resources that are beyond the capacity of most studies. Disease-specific platforms that bring a disease community together to share IPD from multiple trials include the Worldwide Antimalarial Resistance Network (WWARN), the TB-Platform for Aggregation of Clinical TB Studies (TB-PACTS), and Project Datasphere that shares data from cancer trials. Disease-specific platforms require a level of community organization that is the exception rather than the rule for most research communities around specific diseases. Neither study-specific nor disease-specific platforms thus are likely to meet broader clinical trial data sharing needs.

Industry platforms: In 2013, the pharmaceutical trade group PhRMA and the European Federation of Pharmaceutical Industries and Associations issued a statement committing their members to sharing participant-level data from clinical trials underlying approved medicines and indications in the United States and the European Union (PhRMA and EFPIA 2013). This commitment accelerated the development of several IPD sharing platforms. The largest one is ClinicalStudyDataRequest (CSDR), which started as a consortium of 13 pharmaceutical companies that coalesced around a common web portal, a single process for data requests and review, and the ability to combine datasets from multiple sponsors in a secure SAS environment. CSDR has now expanded to include several non-profit funders such as The Bill and Melinda Gates Foundation and the Wellcome Trust. An example of sponsor-specific platform is Supporting Open Access for Researchers (SOAR), which is managed by the Duke Clinical Research Institute for sharing trials from Bristol-Myers Squibb.

Funder platforms: The NIH maintains 82 data sharing repositories spanning organisms (e.g., xenopus), diseases (e.g., influenza), and NIH institutes (U.S. National Library of Medicine). One of the largest is BioLINCC from the National Heart, Lung, and Blood Institute (NHLBI). BioLINCC was started in 2000 and has since generated over 270 articles from the sharing of 47 trials (Coady et al. 2017).

The landscape for clinical trial data sharing is therefore best described as a patchwork, with varying levels of FAIR data sharing as described below. Such a patchwork is inefficient for data sharing and reuse, with duplicated processes, differing access and security policies, and siloed data access. Moreover, a substantial portion of clinical trials are not served by any of the funder-, disease-, or study-specific platforms described above. The newest platform, Vivli, aims to provide global capacity for sharing clinical trials from any country, funder, sponsor, investigator, or disease area, and uniquely seeks to bridge existing platforms through partnerships that bring data from multiple platforms together. No doubt the landscape for data sharing platforms will evolve as new data sharing mandates from funders and journals come into force over the coming years.

Findability

Findability is a prerequisite for any data archiving, sharing, or reuse. A clinical trial must be uniquely findable – if you are looking for Trial X, you should not be pointed to multiple variations of Trial X that may or may not be valid. To be uniquely findable, a trial must have a globally unique and persistent identifier like a DOI as described above. Data subsets for the same trial should have DOIs that are related to each other in a well-documented way. For example, the datasets underlying specific publications and derivative datasets must be reliably identified with the trial's main dataset.

The accuracy of findability depends on the detail, accuracy, and standardization of the metadata that describes the trial. Metadata can be as high level as the study title or as granular as standardized codes describing the 25th secondary outcome. Indeed, the quality of metadata underlies Findability, Interoperability, and Reusability because for all these actions, one must know enough about the data to properly find, combine, or re-use them. Many data sharing platforms provide a fixed set of terms that can be used to filter a search. For example, the YODA Project lists all the generic intervention names (e.g., acetaminophen), therapeutic areas (e.g., Neurosciences), and conditions studied (e.g., AIDS) for all trials available on that platform. Users can then scroll through the lists to select their studies of interest. While this approach nominally supports Findability, it does not meet the FAIR principles because the trials are not described by rich metadata "with a plurality of accurate and relevant attributes" (Wilkinson et al. 2016) for scholarly data reuse.

To fully satisfy the Findability principle, a data sharing platform should be able to accurately respond to queries such as: find studies that test glucagon-like peptide-1 receptor agonists against placebo only for patients with HgbA1c levels over 8.0% who are already on metformin, for a primary composite outcome of major cardiovascular events (cardiovascular mortality, non-fatal myocardial infarction, and non-fatal stroke) measured at least 6 months after randomization. Automated execution of queries like this requires that all studies in the repository be described in a common clinical trial model using standardized terms from a controlled vocabulary. Vivli uses a clinical trial model based on the Ontology of Clinical Research (OCRe) (Sim et al. 2014) with terms from the Cochrane vocabulary, which is based on the SNOMED, MEDRA, and WHO-ATC standard medical terminologies (Dodd et al. 2018). Both OCRe and the Cochrane vocabulary are specially built to support machine-actionability on clinical research studies. However, accurately curating trial descriptions using standardized trial models and vocabularies is difficult. Various groups are working on machine learning approaches to augment manual curation of study descriptions from study protocols, article abstracts, or full-text articles (Thomas et al. 2017). Clinical trial data findability would be improved if a common clinical trial model and controlled vocabulary were adopted across trial registries and IPD sharing platforms.

Once studies are described using rich metadata, researchers must be able to express queries against that metadata. The Vivli platform offers a novel query interface based on the PICO (Population, Intervention, Comparison, Outcome) framework that allows researchers to pose more scientifically precise queries (Fig. 2).

For example, the Vivli interface allows the researcher to query for GLP-1 studies that include stroke only as an outcome and not as an eligibility criterion. The user can also navigate to broader or narrower terms in the Cochrane vocabulary tree (e.g., for diabetes mellitus in Fig. 2) to calibrate the specificity of their desired search. Another benefit of coding studies against a controlled vocabulary is that visualization techniques can be applied to make large retrieval sets more understandable than simply listing hundreds of returned studies (Fig. 3).

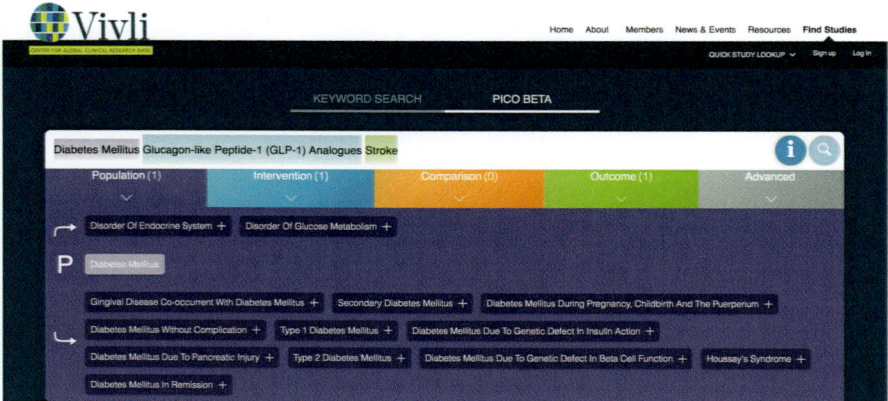

Fig. 2 Example of a search interface. This example from the Vivli data sharing platform illustrates the Participant Intervention Comparison Outcome (PICO) formulation for specifying queries for finding clinical trials. Users can assign search terms to one of the PICO categories and can select broader or narrower terms based on the Cochrane vocabulary. (Copyright permission from Vivli, Inc.)

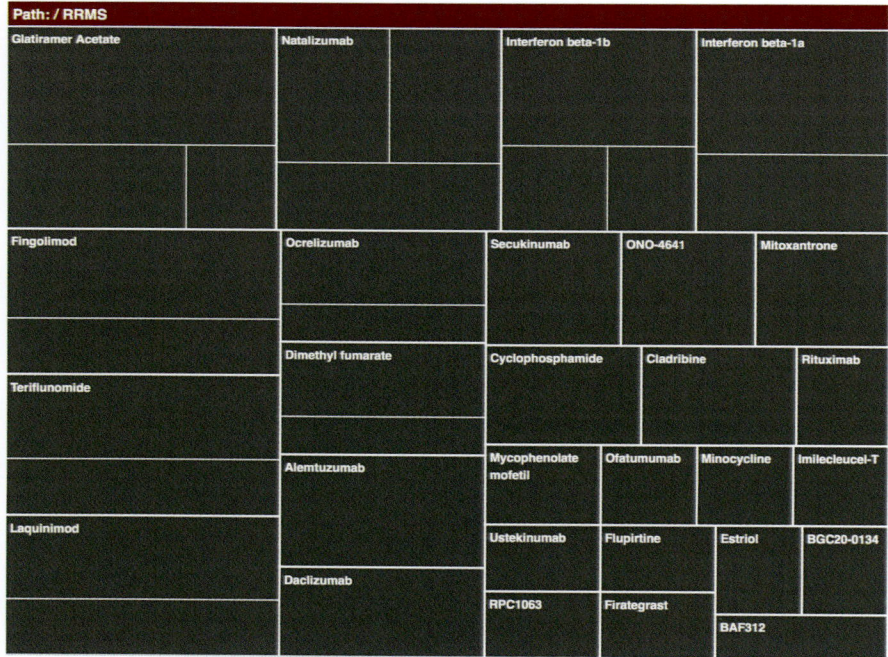

Fig. 3 Treemap of multiple sclerosis trials. This treemap is a visual representation of 108 trials on relapsing remitting multiple sclerosis (RRMS). Each box represents the proportionate number of trials testing a particular intervention (e.g., glatiramer acetate). Subdivisions within the larger boxes show the proportion of studies in Phase II, III, and IV. Treemaps are an example of interactive graphics that allow users to easily see patterns in and browse large retrieval sets. (Copyright permission from Multiple Sclerosis Discovery Forum, CC BY 3.0.)

Accessibility

Once a dataset is found, it needs to be accessed. Access control encompasses authorization, authentication, and physical access. Authorization is whether you have the right or are allowed to access the data. Authentication is whether you are who you say you are, usually addressed by requiring at least a login account. Physical access may be temporary or permanent and may involve restrictions on how and where the data are accessed.

Authorization to access clinical trial IPD ranges from fully open to highly restricted. An example of fully open authorization is the National Institute for Allergy and Infectious Disease's ImmPORT site, where anyone can download IPD immediately without further request or review. Platforms like ImmPORT that offer fully open and downloadable datasets require neither authorization nor authentication.

Most other clinical trial data sharing platforms impose some degree of authorization restriction that is often implemented through a data request process with or without request review. The main motivation for requiring researchers to submit a data request for review is a fear of "rogue analyses," i.e., analyses that are inappropriate, incorrect, or intentionally misleading. Data sharing platforms that require submission of a formal data request include CSDR, Vivli, the YODA Project, and BioLINCC. Data request forms typically ask for a description of the planned hypotheses and analyses, team composition and qualifications, funding source, and potential conflicts of interest. Data requests are then reviewed internally (e.g., BioLINCC) or by an independent review panel (IRP) with levels of review ranging from minimal to very involved. For example, Vivli uses an IRP managed by the Wellcome Trust to review requests for their scientific rationale and relevance, the ability of the proposed research plan to meet the scientific objectives, real or potential conflicts of interest that may impact the planning, conduct or interpretation of the research, and proposals to manage these conflicts of interest. The objective of data request review is to determine if the data request reflects legitimate scientific interest rather than a biased agenda (Christakis and Zimmerman 2013). Some data contributors wish to screen requests for potential competition with their own publication plans. Other data contributors waive their right to screen requests. Published reports of data request experience indicate that the vast majority of data requests are approved (ClinicalStudyDataRequest.com; Coady et al. 2017; Ross et al. 2018). Common reasons for refusal include requests for data that are not in the requested dataset, and for some sponsors, requests are refused if they compete with the sponsor's own publication plans. To date, there have been no clear cases of rogue analyses from data sharing.

Once access is authorized and the requester is authenticated, physical access is granted. Physical access can be restricted or unrestricted. Allowing requesters to download IPD to their own machine equates to permanent, unrestricted physical access because once that data are on a personal machine, they can be copied and distributed ad libitum. Such freedom to redistribute data defeats the purpose of restricted authorization, so IPD that requires data request and review is almost never freely downloadable. Instead, physical access is granted under policy and technical restrictions. BioLINCC, for example, allows requesters to download IPD to a personal machine but only if they attest to certain security features on their machine and to a commitment not to share the IPD. This approach, which relies solely on policy to restrict physical access, is weaker than approaches that impose technical constraints on physical access. For example, CSDR and Vivli can make all approved IPD for a particular project available together within a single secure environment (e.g., a virtual machine) that is pre-populated with analytic tools such as statistical packages and from which no data can be removed. This approach is called "bringing data to the compute" because data from multiple sources are brought to one machine (the Microsoft Azure cloud in the case of Vivli) where the computation occurs. A technically more sophisticated approach is to "bring compute to the data." In this approach, IPD datasets reside in multiple distributed secure environments, and computations (e.g., logistic regression) are "federated" or sent to each of the data environments. The data requester never sees or directly touches the IPD. This approach requires that the federated datasets be pre-aligned so that analytic commands can be executed reproducibly across all the data (Guinney and Saez-Rodriguez 2018). Such pre-alignment can occur in a consortium where the number and nature of datasets are known and fixed (e.g., FDA Sentinel network), but pre-alignment is not a feasible approach for data sharing platforms that aim to support ad hoc and novel analyses across ever growing numbers of new datasets.

Access control – authorization, authentication, physical access control – is especially important for lowering the risk of re-identification of individual participants in a clinical trial, which can, for example, have adverse consequences for participants with stigmatized diseases. The new Common Rule allows for sharing of "de-identified" data without requiring explicit consent of the trial participant. De-identification involves removing Protected Health Information (PHI) (e.g., birth dates) that are identifiers. Caution must be taken that a nominally de-identified dataset can, when combined with another dataset, result in re-identification of individuals who are in both datasets. A famous example is the re-identification of a Massachusetts governor's health data by linking de-identified hospital data with voter rolls that resulted in only one record for a male with the governor's birthdate residing at his zip code (2017). However, de-identification may remove so much information that the dataset is rendered useless for scientific purposes. De-identification is thus always a tradeoff between privacy and utility of the data, and the risk of re-identification varies depending on which other datasets it is combined with. In any case, the risk of re-identification is never zero, which raises the importance of access control as a complement to de-identification to make it more difficult for nefarious actors to re-identify participants.

Interoperability

In the context of data sharing, interoperability refers to the ability to combine and make sense of multiple datasets. Interoperability is required for any pooled analysis such as IPD meta-analysis, pooled subgroup analyses, or identifying better estimates of effect size. Testing for reproducibility of a single trial does not require interoperability, but experience with data sharing shows that only a small minority of data requests is for reproducibility (Coady et al. 2017). Thus, interoperability is extremely critical for unlocking the full value of data sharing. Interoperability is of two types. Syntactic interoperation is the ability to combine the format of the data, e.g., the structure of the data tables. Semantic interoperation is the ability to combine the meanings of individual variables, e.g., whether the definition of heart failure in one dataset is the same as in another data set.

Syntactic Interoperability

Clinical trials conducted to support regulatory approval by the FDA or the EMA are required to be submitted in CDISC Study Data Tabulation Module (SDTIM) format (CDISC 2019a). SDTM stipulates how clinical trial IPD datasets are to be prepared, with a standard format for the tables and data dictionary. Another CDISC standard, the Analysis Data Model (ADaM), stipulates the data format for the analyses that were conducted by the company (CDISC 2019a). While having IPD in ADaM would facilitate reproducibility checks, having IPD in SDTM would be more useful for facilitating unrestricted pooled analyses. However, non-industry trials are rarely in SDTM or any standard format, although there is nascent interest in academia to adopt SDTM. There are paid services available to convert datasets into SDTM.

Syntactic interoperability is also an issue for specialized data types. Almost all imaging data is available in DICOM format (DICOM 2019). Variant Call Format (VCF) is the standard format for genomic variant data. Newer formats that do not yet have extensive uptake include the Open mHealth standard format for mobile health and sensor data.

Semantic Interoperability

How does one know whether two variables capture the same phenomenon in the real world? If two datasets label an outcome variable as "heart failure" but one defines heart failure as systolic dysfunction and the other as heart failure with preserved ejection fraction (HFpEF), those variables are not "about" the same thing despite the identical label. Certainly, one can laboriously read the data dictionaries to manually align the meaning of variables across datasets, but the ideal would be automated alignment to allow interrogation of datasets on the fly. There are two major current approaches to semantic interoperability.

The first approach is for studies to use Common Data Elements (CDEs) up front in their study design so that variables will have the same definition across studies. CDEs can be standardized within subfields, e.g., "heart failure" for cardiology trials. Because this idea is so attractive in the abstract, there is no shortage of CDE efforts. The National Library of Medicine's CDE Repository currently lists over 26,000 CDEs (National Library of Medicine 2019). For industry, CDISC offers CDEs in

31 Therapeutic Areas including Breast Cancer, Diabetes, and Traumatic Brain Injury (CDISC 2019c). The International Consortium for Health Outcomes Measurement (ICHOM) defines CDEs across 28 areas including Breast Cancer, Diabetes, and Overactive Bladder (ICHOM – International Consortium for Health Outcomes Measurement 2019). There is, however, low uptake of any CDEs in any disease domain. Reasons include little harmonization across the profusion of "common" data elements, the lack of any requirements for using CDEs, and no obvious benefit to trialists to use CDEs. However, as data sharing becomes more widespread and data alignment becomes a pain point for more researchers, CDE uptake may finally occur to enable automated alignment of at least major demographic and disease variables across trials.

A second approach to semantic interoperability is realistically the only approach currently available: post hoc manual alignment of variables. This is a challenging and time-consuming task that severely limits the usability of shared datasets. There is at present no way to share or reuse alignment mappings. Automated approaches to post hoc alignment are also challenging and not ready for prime time. Automation first requires that each variable be "annotated" or labelled with a term from a controlled vocabulary such as MeSH or SNOMED to describe what the variable is about. If this annotation process is accurate and reproducible for all variables across all datasets, then it will be easy to align variables across datasets. Moreover, one can exploit the tree structure of a controlled vocabulary to adjust the alignment: if two variables are both called "heart failure" but are labelled accurately as systolic heart failure and as HFpEF, then depending on the research question, a researcher can choose not to align them or can "go up the tree" to find a common parent term "heart failure" to justify the alignment. Unfortunately, the state-of-the-art in annotation accuracy is not yet good enough for fully automated alignment. The most pragmatic approach to semantic interoperability would be to use CDEs up front for demographic and major disease variables with machine-assisted manual alignment of all other variables post hoc. Semantic interoperability will likely remain the most difficult FAIR principle to implement for many years to come.

Reusability

The last principle of FAIR data sharing is Reusability that data can be reused by researchers other than the original trialists. Reuse may be for reproducibility, meta-analysis, informing new studies, generating new hypotheses, or other purposes as described above. Regardless of the purpose, proper interpretation and reuse of IPD require that the final study protocol, the data dictionary, and the statistical analysis plan be available for reference. While data contributors may redact commercially sensitive and other confidential information, there is no current consensus on the limits of redaction. Additional study materials such as case report forms or the original analytic code could also be helpful. However, past experience with data sharing and IPD meta-analysis suggests that there is no substitute for communication between the original trialist and data re-users to ensure proper reuse of clinical trial data.

The availability of different types of data impacts on reusability. The authoritative National Academy of Medicine report on clinical trial data sharing encouraged the sharing of entire final cleaned datasets (The National Academies Press 2015), but there is variation on what IPD are actually shared. GlaxoSmithKline, for example, routinely shares its entire final cleaned datasets while other companies elect to share only the data needed for specific approved data requests. Project Datasphere initially shared only the control arms of trials from participating partners, but more and more of their datasets now include active arms as well. Datasets shared to satisfy journal requirements for IPD sharing (e.g., PLoS or BMJ) may only include the data underlying that publication. Certain analyses may require access to the raw data from before cleaning and imputation, but raw data are rarely shared. The availability of the original analytic code permits checking of reproducibility but requires that clear documentation of the code be available.

Practical aspects of reusability include the user-friendliness of finding, requesting, accessing, and computing across IPD datasets. Platforms that support richer, more precise search queries and that provide harmonized data request forms and data use and data contributor agreements are closer to satisfying the Reusability principle. As discussed under Accessibility above, privacy concerns often require that IPD be made available only within secure computing environments such as virtual machines that are inherently less flexible and user-friendly than unrestricted compute environments.

Finally, reusability is recursive. Aggregated datasets that have been cleaned and aligned could themselves be reused. To support recursive reuse, derivative data sets should also be uniquely identified with DOIs to permit tracking and credit sharing for the original datasets.

Culture of Data Sharing

The National Academy of Medicine's seminal 2015 report on sharing clinical trial data directly addressed the culture of data sharing: "Stakeholders in clinical trials should foster a culture in which data sharing is the expected norm, and should commit to responsible strategies aimed at maximizing the benefits, minimizing the risks, and overcoming the challenges of sharing clinical trial data for all parties" (The National Academies Press 2015). In the pharmaceutical industry, data sharing is indeed the expected norm, propelled by policies such as EMA Policy 0070 and codified in an industry-wide principles statement (PhRMA 2013). On the other hand, the culture of academia and other sectors of the life sciences industry such as biotechnology are only just starting to shift, propelled by journal mandates and funders that are increasingly factoring in past data sharing as a condition of future funding.

While journal and funder edicts may change behavior, communities will fully embrace data sharing as a cultural norm only if there are tangible benefits to data contributors themselves and to the scientific enterprise as a whole. For academic data contributors, pertinent benefits include the potential for co-authorship with data requesters, new collaborations, and more citations of their original work. Early evidence suggests that making study data available in a public repository increases paper citations by 9% to 70% (Piwowar et al. 2007; Piwowar and Vision 2013). Additional benefits can accrue if datasets can themselves be cited and rewarded as research products in their own right separate from publications. Assigning DOIs to datasets, as platforms like Figshare and Vivli do, facilitates development of dataset citation and credit mechanisms. Ultimately, the academic promotions process will need to holistically assign and reward fair credit for data sharing.

For the scientific enterprise as a whole, tangible benefits of data sharing need to be visible and commensurate to the effort of sharing. One obvious metric of benefit is the number of publications arising from data sharing. Table 1 shows the number of requests received and the number of publications from the BioLINCC, CSDR, and the YODA Project platforms.

It is difficult to directly compare publication output in Table 1 because the platforms vary in the number of studies available and in the scientific importance of the studies available. Also, some of the studies have only recently been available so publications would not yet be expected. Nevertheless, these data raise the question of whether this output is a reasonable return on effort. Answering this question requires asking another question: are publications the only metric of the value of data sharing? Tierney et al. discuss multiple ways that pooled IPD analysis can inform the design of future trials, including definition of study populations, choice of comparators and outcomes, definitions and collection of outcome data, and better estimates of effect size (Tierney et al. 2015). These analysis results may lead to more efficient studies that ask better questions and generate better answers – in other

Table 1 Number of data requests and publications from selected data sharing platforms

Platform	# Trials Available (as of)	# of Requests received	# of Publications	# of Manuscripts under review	Time frame
BioLINCC[a]	194 (April 2019)	370	270	–	2000–2017
CSDR[b]	3682 (April 2019)	487	42	28	2013–April 2019
The YODA project[c]	270 (August 2018)	104	12	7	2013–2018
Vivli[d]	4788 (January 2020)	91	2	–	July 2018–January 2020

[a]Coady et al. (2017)
[b]ClinicalStudyDataRequest.com
[c]Ross et al. (2018)
[d]Vivli.org

words, better science. Yet these results will often not be substantial enough on their own to be publishable. As data sharing proceeds, it will be vital to fully and accurately define the benefits of data sharing and not rely only on narrow metrics such as publication count.

One intriguing aspect of the culture of data sharing is how data contributors and data requesters should interact. Ideally, data requesters should be able to ask questions of the original investigators, and data contributors should have the option to collaborate in secondary uses of their data. However, investigators may be overwhelmed by having to respond to numerous data requesters, or it may be infeasible to conduct a secondary analysis with a large number of original investigators. What responsibilities do investigators have to re-users of their data? Are citations of publications and datasets sufficient acknowledgement of the original study? Should data contributors be allowed to embargo their data, for how long and for what reasons? Should data contributors be allowed to review or even veto manuscripts arising from reuse of their data? These and other questions will have to be resolved as the culture of data sharing evolves.

Costs and Sustainability

The costs of data sharing are not insubstantial. Definable costs include storage, de-identification, data request review and management, and computational environment costs. Less definable costs include the time spent preparing datasets for sharing, documenting sharing plans, finding and requesting datasets, aligning datasets, and time responding to data requester or data contributor queries. Potential benefits accrue to data contributors in the form of co-authorship and citations and to data requesters in the form of better future study designs or new publishable findings. Because both sides benefit, both sides should share the costs. Funding for existing data sharing platforms is coming from a mix of industry contributions, membership models, foundation grants, and revenue from services. As data sharing infrastructures mature, the costs and benefits will become more apparent, and more robust sustainability models will be developed.

Future Issues

Routine sharing and re-use of participant-level clinical trial data can potentially transform the science of clinical trials through changes in how trials are designed, selected for funding, executed, and reported. Several consequences may flow from mandating IPD sharing. First, knowing that their study protocol and participant-level data will be open to community scrutiny may cause investigators to improve data quality and accuracy. Clinical trial management systems may become more standardized and streamlined to efficiently provide clean data and metadata for machine-actionable FAIR data sharing. If shared IPD is also interoperable and re-usable, funders may expect investigators to routinely justify their study designs based on analysis of prior data, resulting in better, more efficient, and more reproducible science. These transformations, if they occur, will take many years but may ultimately be the most enduring benefits of clinical trial data sharing.

Much work remains to be done on the informatics of sharing scientific data. Advances in curation, metadata management, data alignment, and search and visualization are needed. Machine-assisted approaches will no doubt play an increasingly large role over time. However, human capital needs remain paramount. A new generation of data curators and data wranglers will need to be trained and rewarded with viable career paths, while new technical and policy foundations need to be built for new incentive and reward structures (Blasimme et al. 2018).

The rise of real-world evidence (RWE) poses some challenges to the current model of clinical trial data sharing. RWE is evidence on interventions derived from analysis of data routinely collected during the course of daily life or health care from data sources such as electronic health records, claims, disease registries, and patient-generated health data from mobile apps and sensors (FDA 2019). Traditional RCTs are conducted on selected populations in ideal controlled circumstances that do not reflect the diversity and complexity of real-world decision-making. RWE studies – such as pragmatic clinical trials based on real-world data – aim to provide a more complete understanding of treatment usage, effectiveness, and value to inform "care, research, safety surveillance, and public health" (The National Academies Press 2017). This broad remit challenges data sharing platforms to serve data re-users beyond researchers. How can the principles, processes, and infrastructure described in this chapter support data sharing for studies that are continually generating RWE for frontline clinical decision-making? What new types of metadata are needed to ensure that the rich context of real-world studies is adequately described for appropriate re-use? As clinical research methods change, data sharing platforms will be at the forefront of driving changes in the technology, policies, and culture of data sharing.

Summary and Conclusions

The present state of clinical trial data sharing is the culmination of a decades-long process of increasing trial transparency and accountability. Triggered initially by several scandals in the early 2000s of selective reporting of results, mandatory trial registration became global policy. This was followed in 2016 by legislation in the US mandating summary-level results reporting. Since then, increasing numbers of funders and journals have moved toward requiring the sharing of individual-participant-level data (IPD), a movement that is part of a wider movement toward open data for open science. In fact, a consensus has arisen around four principles for effective scientific data sharing: Findability, Accessibility, Interoperability, and Reusability (FAIR). Existing clinical trial data sharing platforms meet the FAIR principles to varying degrees.

Findability requires that each dataset be uniquely identifiable and be sufficiently well-described with metadata to support accurate search and retrieval. **Accessibility**

has three components: authorization, authentication, and physical access. The process for authorizing researchers to access IPD often involves requiring researchers to complete a data request form detailing their planned analyses followed by scientific review of the request by an independent review panel. Approved IPD access can occur via direct download or via secure locked-down computing environments. Most platforms require that IPD be de-identified before being placed there, with privacy concerns managed by a combination of technical (de-identification, secure computing environments) and policy approaches (e.g., data use agreements). **Interoperability** of IPD – the ability to combine and make sense of multiple datasets – is critical for data sharing to generate scientific value. Interoperability is facilitated by common data formats (such as CDISC SDTM) and by common data elements (CDEs). There is a profusion of CDEs in many disease domains but low adoption in both industry and academia. Until CDEs are more commonly used, interoperability will be a challenge requiring manual alignment of variables across datasets. Finally, **Reusability** requires that data sharing be user-friendly with sufficient reference material and access to data contributors for questions. Achieving machine-actionable Findability, Interoperability, and Reusability will be facilitated if data sharing platforms shared a common clinical trial data model along with detailed metadata. Machine-learning approaches are being used to augment humans in the challenging task of metadata curation.

A culture of data sharing is now the norm in industry and is starting to take hold in academia. To shift the culture in academia, data sharing must be rewarded in the promotions process. While papers have higher citation rates if the underlying data are available for sharing, publication and citation of the datasets themselves should also be metrics for promotion. Another critical driver is if grant funding is contingent on data sharing plans and past data sharing behavior.

Broader shifts in the culture of data sharing will occur when there is a greater track record of the benefits. These benefits will include but are not limited to the number of publications generated. For example, improvements in study design due to analyses of prior data can be of substantial scientific and societal value even if those analyses are never published. In the same vein, routine IPD sharing may result in improved data quality because researchers know their data will be scrutinized by others, and in improved research integrity through increased data transparency and accountability. Finally, clinical trial data sharing honors participant contributions to research, enhances public trust in clinical trials, and promises to accelerate scientific findings by maximizing the value of clinical trials data.

Key Facts

- Clinical trial data sharing involves sharing summary-level and individual participant-level results.
- Over 50 funders globally require sharing of participant-level data as a condition of clinical trial funding.

- The International Committee of Medical Journal Editors requires that all clinical trial manuscripts include a statement describing plans for sharing participant-level data.
- There exist close to 100 clinical trial data sharing platforms worldwide, with a range of policies, constituents, and scopes.
- Four foundational principles for scientific data sharing are Findability, Accessibility, Interoperability, and Reusability.
- Most data requests are approved.
- Only a minority of data requests are for reproducibility.

Cross-References

▶ Archiving Records and Materials
▶ De-identifying Clinical Trial Data

References

Blasimme A, Fadda M, Schneider M, Vayena E (2018) Data sharing for precision medicine: policy lessons and future directions. Health Aff (Millwood) 37:702–709. https://doi.org/10.1377/hlthaff.2017.1558

Bot BM, Suver C, Neto EC et al (2016) The mPower study, Parkinson disease mobile data collected using ResearchKit. Sci Data 3:160011. https://doi.org/10.1038/sdata.2016.11

CDISC (2019a) Study data tabulation model (SDTM). In: Study Data Tabul. Model SDTM. https://www.cdisc.org/standards/foundational/sdtm. Accessed 28 Jun 2018

CDISC (2019b) Analysis data model (ADaM). In: Anal. Data Model ADaM. https://www.cdisc.org/standards/foundational/adam. Accessed 13 Apr 2019

CDISC (2019c) CDISC therapeutic areas. In: Publ. User Guid. https://www.cdisc.org/standards/therapeutic-areas. Accessed 13 Apr 2019

Christakis DA, Zimmerman FJ (2013) Rethinking reanalysis. JAMA 310:2499–2500. https://doi.org/10.1001/jama.2013.281337

ClinicalStudyDataRequest.com Metrics. In: Metrics. https://clinicalstudydatarequest.com/Metrics.aspx. Accessed 13 Apr 2019

Coady SA, Mensah GA, Wagner EL et al (2017) Use of the National Heart, Lung, and Blood Institute data repository. N Engl J Med 376:1849–1858. https://doi.org/10.1056/NEJMsa1603542

Debray TPA, Moons KGM, van Valkenhoef G et al (2015) Get real in individual participant data (IPD) meta-analysis: a review of the methodology. Res Synth Methods 6:293–309. https://doi.org/10.1002/jrsm.1160

Dickersin K (1990) The existence of publication bias and risk factors for its occurrence. JAMA 263:1385–1389

DICOM (2019) DICOM standard. In: DICOM Stand. https://www.dicomstandard.org/. Accessed 13 Apr 2019

Dodd S, Clarke M, Becker L et al (2018) A taxonomy has been developed for outcomes in medical research to help improve knowledge discovery. J Clin Epidemiol 96:84–92. https://doi.org/10.1016/j.jclinepi.2017.12.020

FDA (2019) Real world evidence. In: Real World Evid. https://www.fda.gov/ScienceResearch/SpecialTopics/RealWorldEvidence/default.htm. Accessed 13 Apr 2019

Guinney J, Saez-Rodriguez J (2018) Alternative models for sharing confidential biomedical data. Nat Biotechnol 36:391–392. https://doi.org/10.1038/nbt.4128

ICHOM – International Consortium for Health Outcomes Measurement (2019) ICHOM Standard Sets. In: ICHOM – Int. Consort. Health Outcomes Meas. https://www.ichom.org/standard-sets/. Accessed 9 Dec 2018

Melander H, Ahlqvist-Rastad J, Meijer G, Beermann B (2003) Evidence b(i)ased medicine – selective reporting from studies sponsored by pharmaceutical industry: review of studies in new drug applications. BMJ 326:1171–1173. https://doi.org/10.1136/bmj.326.7400.1171

Mello MM, Lieou V, Goodman SN (2018) Clinical trial participants' views of the risks and benefits of data sharing. N Engl J Med 378:2202–2211. https://doi.org/10.1056/NEJMsa1713258

National Institutes of Health (2018) Proposed provisions for a draft NIH data management and sharing policy. National Institutes of Health, Bethesda

National Library of Medicine (2019) NIH common data elements (CDE) repository. In: NIH Common Data Elem. CDE Repos. https://cde.nlm.nih.gov/. Accessed 9 Apr 2019

Nature RD at S (2018) Accelerating data sharing. In: Res. Data Springer Nat. https://researchdata.springernature.com/users/8075-grace-baynes/posts/40275-how-can-we-accelerate-data-sharing. Accessed 6 Nov 2018

PhRMA, EFPIA (2013) Principles for responsible clinical trial data sharing. Principles for responsible clinical trial data sharing. http://phrma-docs.phrma.org/sites/default/files/pdf/PhRMAPrinciplesForResponsibleClinicalTrialDataSharing.pdf. Accessed 4 May 2020

Piwowar HA, Vision TJ (2013) Data reuse and the open data citation advantage. PeerJ 1. https://doi.org/10.7717/peerj.175

Piwowar HA, Day RS, Fridsma DB (2007) Sharing detailed research data is associated with increased citation rate. PLoS One 2:e308. https://doi.org/10.1371/journal.pone.0000308

Ross JS, Waldstreicher J, Bamford S et al (2018) Overview and experience of the YODA project with clinical trial data sharing after 5 years. Sci Data 5:180268. https://doi.org/10.1038/sdata.2018.268

Sim I, Chan A-W, Gülmezoglu AM et al (2006) Clinical trial registration: transparency is the watchword. Lancet 367:1631–1633. https://doi.org/10.1016/S0140-6736(06)68708-4

Sim I, Tu SW, Carini S et al (2014) The ontology of clinical research (OCRe): an informatics foundation for the science of clinical research. J Biomed Inform 52:78–91. https://doi.org/10.1016/j.jbi.2013.11.002

Sim I, Wood J, Baskaran A et al (under review) Vivli: a practical implementation of FAIR clinical trial data sharing. Trials

Simes RJ (1986) Publication bias: the case for an international registry of clinical trials. J Clin Oncol Off J Am Soc Clin Oncol 4:1529–1541. https://doi.org/10.1200/JCO.1986.4.10.1529

Taichman DB, Sahni P, Pinborg A et al (2017) Data sharing statements for clinical trials – a requirement of the International Committee of Medical Journal Editors. N Engl J Med 376:2277–2279. https://doi.org/10.1056/NEJMe1705439

The National Academies Press (2015) Sharing clinical trial data: maximizing benefits, minimizing risk. The National Academies Press, Washington, DC

The National Academies Press (2017) Real-world evidence generation and evaluation of therapeutics: proceedings of a workshop. In: Real-World Evid. Gener. Eval. Ther. Proc. Workshop. http://www.nationalacademies.org/hmd/Reports/2017/real-world-evidence-generation-and-evaluation-of-therapeutics-proceedings.aspx. Accessed 13 Apr 2019

Thomas J, Noel-Storr A, Marshall I et al (2017) Living systematic reviews: 2. Combining human and machine effort. J Clin Epidemiol 91:31–37. https://doi.org/10.1016/j.jclinepi.2017.08.011

Tierney JF, Pignon J-P, Gueffyier F et al (2015) How individual participant data meta-analyses have influenced trial design, conduct, and analysis. J Clin Epidemiol 68:1325–1335. https://doi.org/10.1016/j.jclinepi.2015.05.024

Turner EH, Matthews AM, Linardatos E et al (2008) Selective publication of antidepressant trials and its influence on apparent efficacy. N Engl J Med 358:252–260. https://doi.org/10.1056/NEJMsa065779

U.S. National Library of Medicine NIH Data Sharing Repositories. https://www.nlm.nih.gov/NIHbmic/nih_data_sharing_repositories.html. Accessed 8 Apr 2019

Vicente-Saez R, Martinez-Fuentes C (2018) Open Science now: a systematic literature review for an integrated definition. J Bus Res 88:428–436. https://doi.org/10.1016/j.jbusres.2017.12.043

Wilkinson MD, Dumontier M, Aalbersberg IjJ, et al (2016) The FAIR guiding principles for scientific data management and stewardship. In: Sci Data https://www.nature.com/articles/sdata201618. Accessed 28 Jun 2018

Zarin DA, Tse T, Williams RJ, Rajakannan T (2017) The status of trial registration eleven years after the ICMJE policy. N Engl J Med 376:383–391. https://doi.org/10.1056/NEJMsr1601330

(2007) Food and Drug Administration Amendments Act

(2014) European Medicines Agency policy on publication of clinical data for medicinal products for human use

(2017) Re-identification of "anonymized" data. In: Georget Law Technol Rev. https://georgetownlawtechreview.org/re-identification-of-anonymized-data/GLTR-04-2017/. Accessed 13 Apr 2019

Introduction to Systematic Reviews

109

Tianjing Li, Ian J. Saldanha, and Karen A. Robinson

Contents

Introduction: What Is a Systematic Review? 2160
Why Do a Systematic Review? 2161
Steps in Completing a Systematic Review 2163
    Step 1. Framing the research question (PICO) and determining which study designs to
    include.. 2163
    Step 2. Searching for and selecting studies. 2164
    Step 3. Extracting data and assessing risk of bias 2165
    Step 4. Conducting a qualitative synthesis 2167
    Step 5. Conducting a quantitative synthesis 2167
    Step 6. Grading the certainty of the evidence and drawing conclusions 2167
    Step 7. Writing the systematic review report 2168
How Can Systematic Reviews be Found? 2169
How Is the Methodological Rigor of Systematic Reviews Assessed? 2169
Common Challenges of Systematic Reviews from the Viewpoint of Trialists 2171
    Systematic Reviewers Rely on Clinical Trial Data 2171
    Garbage In Garbage Out 2172
    Time, Effort, and Funding 2172
    Systematic Reviews Can Go Out of Date Quickly 2173
Technology and Innovations 2173
Summary and Conclusions 2174
Key Facts 2174
Cross-References 2174
References 2174

T. Li (✉)
Department of Ophthalmology, University of Colorado Anschutz Medical Campus, Aurora, CO, USA
e-mail: tianjing.li@cuanschutz.edu

I. J. Saldanha
Department of Health Services, Policy, and Practice and Department of Epidemiology, Brown University School of Public Health, Providence, RI, USA

K. A. Robinson
Department of Medicine, Johns Hopkins University, Baltimore, MD, USA

© Springer Nature Switzerland AG 2022
S. Piantadosi, C. L. Meinert (eds.), *Principles and Practice of Clinical Trials*,
https://doi.org/10.1007/978-3-319-52636-2_194

Abstract

A systematic review identifies and synthesizes all relevant studies that fit pre-specified criteria to answer a research question. Systematic review methods can be used to answer many types of research questions. The type of question most relevant to trialists is the effects of treatments and is thus the focus of this chapter. We discuss the motivation for and importance of performing systematic reviews and their relevance to trialists. We introduce the key steps in completing a systematic review, including framing the question, searching for and selecting studies, collecting data, assessing risk of bias in included studies, conducting a qualitative synthesis and a quantitative synthesis (i.e., meta-analysis), grading the certainty of evidence, and writing the systematic review report. We also describe how to identify systematic reviews and how to assess their methodological rigor. We discuss the challenges and criticisms of systematic reviews, and how technology and innovations, combined with a closer partnership between trialists and systematic reviewers, can help identify effective and safe evidence-based practices more quickly.

Keywords

Systematic review · Meta-analysis · Research synthesis · Evidence-based · Risk of bias

Introduction: What Is a Systematic Review?

A systematic review identifies and synthesizes all relevant studies that fit pre-specified criteria to answer a research question (Lasserson et al. 2019; IOM 2011). What sets a systematic review apart from a narrative review is that it follows consistent, rigorous, and transparent methods established in a protocol in order to minimize bias and errors. Systematic review methods can be used to answer many types of research questions, such as questions about the effectiveness and safety of a preventive or therapeutic intervention (while interventions are often treatments, we have used the broader term intervention in this chapter), etiology and/or prognosis of a disease, and accuracy of a screening or diagnostic test. The type of question most relevant to trialists – the majority readers of this book – is likely the effects of interventions and is thus the focus of this chapter.

Systematic review uses a highly structured and, at least theoretically, reproducible methodology that includes several key steps (Fig. 1; IOM 2011). The first step is to specify the research question in terms of its population, intervention(s), comparator intervention(s), and outcomes. The scope of the review determines which studies are eligible for inclusion. Then, every effort is made to identify all potentially relevant studies, including searching multiple electronic bibliographic databases and other resources that may be more difficult to access. The next step is to collect data from and assess the risk of bias in included studies. When appropriate, a systematic review

PREPARE TOPIC	SEARCH FOR STUDIES	SCREEN STUDIES	ABSTRACT DATA	ANALYZE AND SYNTHESIZE DATA	REPORT FINDINGS
• Formulate research question(s) • Develop analytic framework	• Define eligibility criteria • Search for relevant studies	• Screen studies for inclusion	• Abstract data from included studies • Assess risk of bias • Construct evidence tables	• Conduct qualitative synthesis • Conduct quantitative synthesis (ie, meta-analysis) if appropriate • Assess the strength of evidence	

Fig. 1 Steps in completing a systematic review

may include a meta-analysis (i.e., a statistical combination of the results from multiple independent studies), which may improve the precision of the estimate of effect and can quantify the amount of heterogeneity among studies. Finally, after analyzing information both qualitatively and, if appropriate, quantitatively, conclusions are formed with an indication of certainty of the evidence. Reporting of a systematic review should follow pertinent reporting guidelines (Equator Network). Section 2 elaborates on each of these steps.

Why Do a Systematic Review?

> The hundreds of hours spent conducting a scientific study ultimately contribute only a piece of an enormous puzzle. The value of any single study is derived from how it fits with and expands previous work, as well as from the study's intrinsic properties. Through systematic review the puzzle's intricacies may be disentangled.
> – Cynthia D. Mulrow, M.D., M.Sc., Senior Deputy Editor, *Annals of Internal Medicine* 1994

Systematic reviews were developed out of a need to ensure that health and healthcare decisions can be informed by the totality of research evidence. One well-known and classic example that illustrates the need for keeping track of evidence in an ongoing fashion is the use of intravenous streptokinase as thrombolytic therapy for acute myocardial infarction (Lau et al. 1992). Between 1959 and 1988, 33 trials evaluating this therapy were conducted. A consistent, statistically significant reduction in total mortality (odds ratio, 0.74; 95% confidence interval, 0.59–0.92) was achieved by 1973, after findings from only eight trials involving 2432 participants had been published. However, this pooled odds ratio was not calculated in 1973; instead, another 25 trials enrolled an additional 34,542 patients through 1988, and the results of these trials had little or no effect on the odds ratio establishing efficacy. Two very large trials, the Gruppo Italiano per lo Studio della Streptochinasi nell'Infarto Miocardico trial published in 1986 (11,712 patients) and the Second International Study of Infarct Survival trial published in

1988 (17,187 patients), did not modify the odds ratio substantively. This example and many others (Chalmers et al. 2014) clearly demonstrate that, had researchers kept track of the evidence systematically while it was accumulating, some beneficial and harmful effects of interventions could have been identified earlier than they were, and clinical practice guidelines and medical textbooks could have recommended the most effective treatments sooner (Lau et al. 1992; Rouse et al. 2016).

In the example of streptokinase for acute myocardial infarction, there was a considerable delay in the identification and widespread use of effective interventions. A perhaps more compelling question for trialists is why were thousands of patients randomized to placebo after the benefit of the treatment should have already been known? Today, it is expected that decisions about health are informed by evidence (evidence-based medicine, evidence-based healthcare, and evidence-based public health). "Evidence-based research" is also needed to ensure that trials (and other types of research) are scientific, ethically justified, and not wasteful. Evidence-based research is the use of prior research in a systematic and transparent way to inform a new study so that it answers the questions that matter in a valid, efficient, and accessible manner (Lund et al. 2016; Robinson 2009). For trials to be evidence-based, they should be informed by systematic reviews of existing evidence *before* the trial. A comprehensive and systematic assessment of existing literature will avoid unnecessary duplication and provide the most scientific and ethical justification for a new trial. In addition, pitfalls of previous work and important design considerations (e.g., expected treatment effect, response rate in the control group, outcomes to measure) can be identified to inform the design of the new trial. In addition, the trial should be followed by a systematic review (or an update to the previous one) to set the new results within the context of what was already known.

While it has been advocated for more than 20 years that clinical trials should begin and end with systematic reviews of relevant evidence (Clarke and Chalmers 1998), much work is still needed to see this become standard practice (Cooper et al. 2005; Djulbegovic et al. 2011; Robinson and Goodman 2011). The National Institute of Health Research, a major public funder of clinical trials in the United Kingdom (UK), explicitly requires justification for new research both in terms of time and relevance, and emphasizes that it "will only fund primary research where the proposed research is informed by a review of the existing evidence" (NIHR 2020). However, few ethics review boards or funding agencies require explicit consideration of existing research. The Evidence-Based Research Network (ebrnetwork.org) and EVBRES (EVidence-Based RESearch) (evbres.eu), a COST-Action project with participation of all European countries, are working to encourage and support the use of systematic reviews in research. The European Cooperation in Science and Technology (COST) is a funding organization for the creation of research networks, called COST-Actions. These networks offer an open space for collaboration among scientists across Europe and beyond and thereby give impetus to research advancements and innovation (cost.eu).

Steps in Completing a Systematic Review

Well-conducted systematic reviews, like any other type of well-conducted research, follow a set of rigorous steps. These steps are usually detailed a priori in a protocol. It is strongly encouraged that protocols of systematic reviews be registered in a registry, such as the International Prospective Register of Systematic Reviews (PROSPERO; available at https://www.crd.york.ac.uk/prospero/).

Before starting a systematic review, it is crucial to gather the appropriate team. This involves incorporating and balancing the relevant expertise, perspectives, and experience to ensure that the systematic review addresses the most relevant question(s) (including specifying the appropriate outcomes of interest), follows the most appropriate methodology, and interprets the findings accurately for the context at hand. To these ends, systematic review teams should, at the minimum, include clinicians with expertise in the topic area of the review, methodologists (e.g., statisticians, epidemiologists) with expertise in methodology for systematic review and meta-analysis, and information specialists or librarians.

We describe below the steps in completing a systematic review once the appropriate team has been gathered (Fig. 1).

Step 1. Framing the research question (PICO) and determining which study designs to include.

Research questions in systematic reviews are typically framed using a framework comprising four main elements: Population, Interventions, Comparators, and Outcomes (PICO) (AHRQ 2015; IOM 2011; Thomas et al. 2019). Within each of these four elements, systematic reviewers specify details about study characteristics that would determine whether a given study is eligible.

A few addenda and caveats to the PICO framework are worth noting. *First*, some systematic reviewers add elements to this framework, such as timing (T) and setting (S). While that approach is reasonable, a simpler use of the framework (that we describe) incorporates aspects of timing in the interventions/comparators (e.g., duration of intervention/comparator) and/or outcomes (e.g., time-points of outcome measurement) (elements I and O, respectively), and aspects of setting in the population (e.g., patients admitted to an intensive care unit) and/or interventions/comparators (e.g., treatment at home). *Second*, while outcomes are a critical element in the PICO framework, systematic reviews of interventions do not usually exclude a given study (either during screening or subsequent steps) solely because it does not report any outcomes of interest, provided all other eligibility criteria are satisfied. Excluding abstracts based on the lack of relevant outcomes runs the risk of excluding studies that report relevant outcomes in the full-text publication but not in the abstract. *Third*, in the context of a systematic review that focuses on non-interventional exposures (e.g., air pollution), the interventions (I) element is replaced by exposures (E).

In addition to defining the elements of the PICO framework, it is important to specify the types of study designs that would be eligible for the systematic review, such as randomized trials, cohort studies, and case-control studies.

Step 2. Searching for and selecting studies.

After specifying the details of each element of the PICO framework, systematic reviewers design a search strategy with the objective of identifying all relevant studies that address the research question(s).

Key Principles during Searching
- *Comprehensiveness* – What sets apart a systematic review from other types of reviews, such as narrative reviews, is that its objective is to summarize *all* existing relevant studies that address the research question(s).
- *Specificity* – To make the screening process manageable within the constraints of time, financial and human resources available to the team, systematic reviewers try to design searches that are as specific as possible. However, specificity and comprehensiveness can be at odds with each other; systematic review teams must balance these to ensure that the review is both comprehensive and manageable.
- *Transparency* – It is important that the search strategy that is used for the systematic review (databases, search dates, search terms, and syntax) is documented clearly and completely so that it can be replicated, verified, and reused (such as during updates of the systematic review).

To help abide by these principles and design the most rigorous search strategy, it is imperative that systematic review teams involve or consult with an information specialist with expertise in designing searches for systematic reviews.

Design and Execution of the Search Search terms include both free-text words that might appear in a title, abstract, or keywords of a record in a database as well as controlled vocabulary terms that denote how the record has been indexed in that database.

Typically, systematic reviewers designing searches for health-related topics begin with a MEDLINE search. However, no single electronic database is considered to be comprehensive enough to merit being the only database that is searched in a systematic review. Systematic reviews generally search multiple electronic databases, including topic area-specific databases, if available. Once search terms and syntax are developed for one database, the next step is to translate them into search terms and syntax that can be used in each of the other databases (e.g., Embase).

In addition to searching electronic databases, systematic reviewers implement a set of strategies to identify studies that were either not in the chosen databases or not identified by the search. First, systematic reviewers search for ongoing studies using study registries, such as ClinicalTrials.gov. This allows systematic reviewers to identify ongoing studies even though their results might not yet be publicly available. In addition, examining the ClinicalTrials.gov record enables systematic reviewers to identify outcomes that may have been prespecified but were not reported in any of the publications associated with a given study. Second, systematic reviews conduct a search of other literature that is outside of traditional peer-reviewed journals. Examples of such types of literature include conference abstracts, websites, materials from the regulatory bodies (e.g., the U.S. Food and Drug Administration), clinical study reports, and others. Third, systematic reviews read the bibliographies of studies included in the systematic review and of other systematic reviews to find other studies that might have been missed by the electronic searches. This process is called "handsearching."

Selecting Studies Once the searches have been run, the records obtained from each of the searches need to be downloaded and de-duplicated. The next step is to conduct title and abstract screening, typically independently by two screeners (preferably one topic area expert and one methodological expert). Discrepancies should be resolved through discussion or by a third screener.

Citation screening is usually conducted using systematic review platforms, such as AbstrackR, DistillerSR®, Rayyan, and Covidence®. The advantage of many systematic review platforms, such as AbstrackR, is that they employ advanced machine-learning algorithms that learn from the screening behavior of screeners and, after a threshold of number of abstracts has been reached, predict the likelihood of relevance of the remaining abstracts.

Citations that are accepted during title and abstract screening are then advanced to the stage of full-text screening. In this stage, which is also typically conducted independently and in duplicate, screeners apply the same study eligibility criteria to the full-text articles to confirm whether the studies described in them truly are eligible for the systematic review. The reasons for excluding the full-text articles are usually documented and reported.

Step 3. Extracting data and assessing risk of bias

Once the set of studies to be included in the systematic review has been identified, the next step is to extract all relevant data and assess the risk of bias from each study. Data that are relevant for extraction for each study relate to the following aspects (at a minimum):

- Study citation information, e.g., year, authors.
- Study characteristics, e.g., number of participants, country, study design.
- Participant characteristics at baseline, e.g., age, gender, comorbidities, and health characteristics that are relevant to the research question.
- Intervention and comparator characteristics, e.g., dose, frequency, duration, components (for complex interventions), setting.

- Outcomes (for each relevant categorical or continuous outcome), e.g., results data for each domain, specific measurements, methods of aggregation, and time-points of interest for the systematic review.
- Methodological aspects that are related to risk of bias.

A risk of bias assessment is conducted for each study included in the systematic review. Various tools for assessing risk of bias have been developed for various study designs, such as the revised Cochrane Risk of Bias tool for randomized trials (RoB 2) (Sterne et al. 2019), the Risk of Bias in Nonrandomized Studies of Interventions (ROBINS-I) (Sterne et al. 2016), and the Newcastle-Ottawa Scale (for observational studies of exposure-outcome associations) (available at http://www.ohri.ca/programs/clinical_epidemiology/oxford.asp). Because this is a book for trialists, we briefly summarize below the Cochrane Risk of Bias tool for randomized trials (RoB 2).

RoB 2 has been developed for individually randomized parallel group trials, cluster-randomized parallel group trials, and individually randomized crossover trials. For each trial, the tool requires systematic reviewers to (1) select a single numerical result for which the risk of bias will be assessed, and (2) decide whether the aim is to assess the effect of assignment to the intervention (intention-to-treat effect) or the effect of adhering to the intervention (per-protocol effect). Next, the tool requires systematic reviewers to assess the trial under the following five main domains:

1. Risk of bias arising from the randomization process.
2. Risk of bias due to deviations from the intended interventions.
3. Risk of bias due to missing outcome data.
4. Risk of bias in measurement of the outcome.
5. Risk of bias in selection of the reported result.

For each of the five domains, the RoB 2 tool incorporates a set of signaling questions and an algorithm to guide systematic reviewers to arrive at a judgment regarding the risk of bias (low risk of bias, some concerns, and high risk of bias). Each of the signaling questions has been carefully designed to address specific aspects of the trial and minimize subjectivity, while still allowing room for uncertainty in responses (e.g., the tool allows "Yes" and "Probably Yes" as responses, although both lead to similar judgments regarding risk of bias). Finally, the tool guides systematic reviewers in summarizing the five domain-specific judgments of risk bias into an overall risk of bias judgment for the chosen result for the trial.

Even with helpful tools, such as RoB 2, part of the challenge with assessing risk of bias in included studies remains the often-poor quality of reporting in studies. Most, if not all, items in RoB 2 can be readily assessed if trials appropriately adhered to existing reporting guidelines, such as the CONSORT Statement.

Tools and software to facilitate data extraction and risk of bias assessment vary from word processing software, such as Microsoft Word® and Google Documents®, to spreadsheet software, such as Microsoft Excel® and Google Sheets®, to relational database software, such as Microsoft Access®, to online, cloud-based relational database platforms. It is generally recommended that systematic reviewers use online cloud-based relational database platforms, such as the Systematic Review Data Repository (SRDR), DistillerSR®, Covidence®, and EPPiReviewer. These platforms offer advantages in terms of specific development for systematic reviews, flexibility, online collaborative ability, in-built risk of bias assessment tools, and, in the case of SRDR, a public, free, open-access platform for sharing data.

Step 4. Conducting a qualitative synthesis

Before exploring the potential for conducting a quantitative synthesis, that is, meta-analysis, of the included studies, systematic reviewers summarize the existing evidence narratively in what is known as a "qualitative synthesis." It should be clarified that this is a distinct concept from "qualitative research." According to the Institute of Medicine, a qualitative synthesis is an "assessment of the body of evidence that goes beyond factual descriptions or tables that, for example, simply detail how many studies were assessed, the reasons for excluding other studies, the range of study sizes and treatments compared, or quality scores of each study as measured by a risk of bias tool" (IOM 2011). The purpose of the qualitative synthesis is "to develop and convey a deeper understanding of the diversity of questions addressed, designs, strength of evidence, methods used in the underlying literature and the combinability of the studies" (IOM 2011).

Step 5. Conducting a quantitative synthesis

Meta-analysis is the statistical combination of the results obtained for an outcome from two or more studies in a systematic review. Given that individual trials can be underpowered to determine the relative effects between two interventions, meta-analyses are advantageous because they may generate effect estimates with increased precision. Meta-analysis can also be used to explore different or even contradicting findings among individual studies. To perform a meta-analysis, a relative effect measure (e.g., risk ratio, odds ratio, mean difference, hazard ratio) and its associated uncertainty (e.g., standard error, variance, confidence interval) are needed from each study. A separate chapter introduces the methods for meta-analysis.

Step 6. Grading the certainty of the evidence and drawing conclusions

An important aspect of the systematic review process is to grade the certainty of the evidence and draw conclusions accordingly. The certainty of the evidence is usually graded separately for the body of evidence addressing each comparison and outcome in the systematic review. Various frameworks have been developed for assessing certainty. Examples include those from the GRADE Working Group (Guyatt et al. 2011), the United States Preventive Services Task Force (USPSTF) (USPSTF 2017), and the AHRQ Program (Berkman et al. 2015). We briefly summarize here the key domains or concepts that underlie these frameworks. Each domain is assessed separately for each comparison and outcome:

- *Risk of bias* – To what extent did the relevant studies minimize the risk of bias?
- *Directness* – To what extent is the evidence presented in the relevant studies directly applicable to this particular comparison in the systematic review?
- *Consistency* – To what extent were the relevant studies consistent in their results?
- *Precision* – How narrow is the range of uncertainty associated with the results in the relevant studies?
- *Publication bias* – Is it likely that some relevant studies were not published and therefore missing from the evidence identified? Is this missingness likely to have impacted the results of the synthesis?

Most of the frameworks for assessing certainty require systematic reviewers to assess the body of evidence addressing each comparison in the review using these domains. Generally, the procedure for assessing the certainty of the evidence involves downgrading the certainty each time a domain is identified as having a challenge. After the assessment of all the domains for a given body of evidence, systematic reviewers arrive at a certainty of evidence rating of "high," "moderate," "low," or "very low." The certainty of evidence is usually presented in tables that are called "evidence profiles."

Step 7. Writing the systematic review report

An important component of the work conducted in a systematic review is communicating the methods and findings of the review in a clear, accurate, and comprehensive report. This involves a description of the various methods used in the systematic review (including any changes to the methods from those detailed in the protocol), characteristics of the included studies, results of individual included studies, risk of bias in individual included studies, the qualitative synthesis, any quantitative syntheses, and the evidence profiles reflecting the certainty of the evidence. These should be followed by a discussion that interprets the review findings in the context of what was previously known and current clinical practice, mentions the limitations of the studies and of the systematic review methods, and provides conclusions.

The Preferred Reporting Items for Systematic Reviews and Meta-Analyses (PRISMA) is a recommended reporting guideline for systematic review reports (Moher et al. 2009; Liberati et al. 2009); a specific version of PRISMA is tailored to reporting systematic review protocols (PRISMA-P) (Moher et al. 2015). Extensions of PRISMA to systematic reviews of other types are available from the Enhancing the Quality and Transparency Of health Research (EQUATOR) Network (Equator Network).

How Can Systematic Reviews be Found?

Conducting a systematic review takes time, resources, and a team with diverse expertise. Before embarking on a new systematic review, one should first assess whether a relevant systematic review already exists or is underway. There are two aspects that are relevant to the issue of finding systematic reviews, and both present challenges.

First, there is no singular accepted search tool or filter that is specific enough to only identify reviews that are truly "systematic." Several filters have been developed. For instance, one can simply add "AND systematic[sb]" to PubMed/MEDLINE searches. However, not all articles that are tagged as systematic reviews truly are systematic reviews.

Second (and related to the first aspect described above), not all systematic reviews are of good methodologic quality. Typically, systematic reviews considered to be of good quality will report: (1) a research question, (2) the sources that were searched, with a reproducible search strategy, (3) the inclusion and exclusion criteria, (4) the methods used to select studies, (5) critical appraisals of the risk of bias or quality of the included studies, and (6) information about data analysis and synthesis that allows the results to be reproduced (Krnic Martinic et al. 2019). Additional ways to identify systematic reviews of generally good methodological quality include searching online resources and databases of systematic reviews (see Box 1).

How Is the Methodological Rigor of Systematic Reviews Assessed?

Although the importance of systematic reviews is increasingly recognized and the number of reviews published over time is growing rapidly, the conduct and reporting of systematic reviews are variable and often poor (Page et al. 2016). When Page and colleagues examined all systematic reviews indexed in MEDLINE in 1 month (February 2014), they found a threefold increase in the number of reviews published in that month (682 reviews) compared with a month from a decade earlier (2004). In many cases, important methodology was either not used or not reported: unpublished data were rarely sought, risk of bias assessment was not performed or rarely incorporated into analysis, and at least a third of the reviews used statistical methods discouraged by leading organizations (Page et al. 2016). This suggests that readers should not accept the findings of systematic reviews uncritically.

Importantly, systematic reviewers should follow widely adopted methodological standards in performing and reporting reviews. For example, Cochrane has formally adopted the Methodological Expectations of Cochrane Intervention Reviews (MECIR) (Higgins et al. 2019a, b); the Institute of Medicine in the USA has recommended standards for conducting high-quality systematic reviews (IOM 2011); and the Agency for Healthcare Research (AHRQ) in the USA has developed and maintained a methods guide for effectiveness and comparative effectiveness reviews (AHRQ 2015).

For users of systematic reviews, several instruments have been developed for undertaking critical appraisal of the methodological rigor of systematic reviews.

Box 1 Searchable databases for identifying systematic reviews of generally good methodological quality

Resource/Database	URL	Type of systematic review
Agency for Healthcare Research and Quality effective healthcare program	https://www.ahrq.gov/research/findings/evidence-based-reports/search.html	Health interventions, diagnostic tests, etiologic associations
Cochrane library	https://www.cochranelibrary.com/	Health interventions and diagnostic tests
Campbell collaboration library	https://campbellcollaboration.org/library.html	Crime and justice, education, international development, knowledge translation and implementation, nutrition, and social welfare
Epistemonikos	https://www.epistemonikos.org/	Health interventions, diagnostic tests, etiologic associations
Joanna Briggs institute EBP database	http://know.lww.com/JBI-resources.html	Health-related systematic reviews, specifically targeted for allied healthcare professionals
PROSPERO	https://www.crd.york.ac.uk/prospero/	Systematic review protocols in health, social care, welfare, public health, education, crime, justice, and international development
Open Science framework	https://osf.io/	No restriction by discipline
SYRCLE	https://www.radboudumc.nl/en/research/departments/health-evidence/systematic-review-center-for-laboratory-animal-experimentation	Animal research

---

Box 2. AMSTAR 2 critical items
- Protocol registered before commencement of the review (item 2)
- Adequacy of the literature search (item 4)
- Justification for excluding individual studies (item 7)
- Risk of bias from individual studies being included in the review (item 9)
- Appropriateness of meta-analytical methods (item 11)
- Consideration of risk of bias when interpreting the results of the review (item 13)
- Assessment of presence and likely impact of publication bias (item 15)

Box 2 AMSTAR 2 critical items

Although none have been universally adopted, A MeaSurement Tool to Assess systematic Reviews (AMSTAR), published in 2007 (Shea et al. 2007) and subsequently revised in 2017 to AMSTAR 2 (Shea et al. 2017), is among the most popular tools. AMSTAR 2 includes 16 items, of which seven are regarded as critically important and can affect the validity of a review and its conclusions (Shea et al. 2017) (Box 2).

	Phase 2				Phase 3
	1. Study eligibility criteria	2. Identification and selection of studies	3. Data collection and study appraisal	4. Synthesis and findings	Risk of bias in the review
Signaling questions	1.1 Did the review adhere to predefined objectives and eligibility criteria?	2.1 Did the search include an appropriate range of databases/ electronic sources for published and unpublished reports?	3.1. Were efforts made to minimize error in data collection?	4.1. Did the synthesis include all studies that it should?	A. Did the interpretation of findings address all of the concerns identified in domains 1 to 4?
	1.2 Were the eligibility criteria appropriate for the review question?	2.2 Were methods additional to database searching used to identify relevant reports?	3.2. Were sufficient study characteristics available for both review authors and readers to be able to interpret the results?	4.2. Were all predefined analyses reported or departures explained?	B. Was the relevance of identified studies to the review's research question appropriately considered?
	1.3 Were eligibility criteria unambiguous?	2.3 Were the terms and structure of the search strategy likely to retrieve as many eligible studies as possible?	3.3. Were all relevant study results collected for use in the synthesis?	4.3. Was the synthesis appropriate given the nature and similarity in the research questions, study designs, and outcomes across included studies?	C. Did the reviewers avoid emphasizing results on the basis of their statistical significance?
	1.4 Were all restrictions in eligibility criteria based on study characteristics appropriate?	2.4 Were restrictions based on date, publication format, or language appropriate?	3.4. Was risk of bias (or methodologic quality) formally assessed using appropriate criteria?	4.4. Was between-study variation minimal or addressed in the synthesis?	
	1.5 Were any restrictions in eligibility criteria based on sources of information appropriate?	2.5 Were efforts made to minimize error in selection of studies?	3.5. Were efforts made to minimize error in risk of bias assessment?	4.5. Were the findings robust, for example, as demonstrated through funnel plot or sensitivity analyses?	
				4.6. Were biases in primary studies minimal or addressed in the synthesis?	
Judgment	Concerns regarding specification of study eligibility criteria	Concerns regarding methods used to identify and/or select studies	Concerns regarding methods used to collect data and appraise studies	Concerns regarding the synthesis	Risk of bias in the review

Box 3 Summary of phase 2 ROBIS domains, phase 3, and signaling questions

Another tool is the Risk Of Bias In Systematic reviews (ROBIS) tool (Whiting et al. 2016). ROBIS is completed in three phases: (1) assess relevance (optional), (2) identify concerns with the review process, and (3) judge risk of bias. Phase 2 covers four domains through which bias may be introduced into a systematic review: study eligibility criteria, identification and selection of studies, data collection and study appraisal, and synthesis and findings. Signaling questions are included to help assess specific concerns about potential biases with the review. The ratings from these signaling questions help assessors to judge overall risk of bias (Box 3) (Whiting et al. 2016).

Common Challenges of Systematic Reviews from the Viewpoint of Trialists

Systematic Reviewers Rely on Clinical Trial Data

In the evidence-based healthcare paradigm, clinical trials impact practice by virtue of their results being incorporated into systematic reviews that inform practice guidelines. This model of flow of information from clinical trials to practice is sometimes short-circuited, especially in the context of emergencies and/or the release of findings of a large, definitive trial. For this paradigm to work effectively, systematic reviews rely on the existence, rigorous conduct, and complete and unbiased reporting of data from clinical trials (and other primary studies). However, even if a trial's results are published in a peer-reviewed journal, assessing completeness of trial reporting is not straightforward. A recently developed tool provides a framework to facilitate such assessment (Page et al. 2019).

Moreover, not all trials included in a systematic review may have reported data for outcomes that are chosen for the review (Saldanha et al. 2017), or data may not have been reported for all relevant subgroups. In these situations, conducting analyses for such outcomes and subgroups in the review is not possible in the absence of individual participant data (IPD) from the trials. IPD are sometimes requested years after the trial is done. The trialists may not have the resources to deidentify data for release or to reanalyze the data for the purpose of the review, leading to suboptimal use of a trial's results in a systematic review. To minimize the burden on trialists of responding to multiple data requests from systematic reviewers, to facilitate such analyses and, more broadly, to support the concept of transparency and open science, the authors of this chapter support the concept of clinical trial data sharing and reuse, as mandated by many funders and journals (see ▶ Chap. 108, "Data Sharing and Reuse"). Patients, too, are becoming more vocal in demanding that their data contributions to clinical trials be reused to accelerate evidence-based practice. We believe that the recently proposed Findable, Accessible, Interoperable, and Reusable (FAIR) metadata standards, if widely adopted, can greatly aid this process.

Garbage In Garbage Out

The quality of information synthesized and reported in systematic reviews is only as good as the information that feeds into the review. The old adage "garbage in, garbage out" is frequently used to describe the challenge in this context especially when meta-analyses are performed. While a meta-analysis can increase the power and precision of the estimated treatment effect, it cannot "fix" problems that might exist in the underlying data. For example, a meta-analysis of studies that are individually at high risk of bias will render a summary estimate that is also at high risk of bias. Worse still, it generates a precisely biased result. Therefore, when individual studies are at high risk of bias, conducting a meta-analysis may not be appropriate. It is more important to critically appraise the within-study bias and, if a meta-analysis includes a sizeable proportion of studies at high risk of bias, the certainty of evidence should be downgraded when interpreting the results and drawing conclusions.

Time, Effort, and Funding

As the scientific literature continues to grow, an immense amount of time and effort is needed to generate high-quality, comprehensive systematic reviews. While the time needed to produce a review can be quite variable, estimates range from 6 months when an investigator devotes 10–20 h per week (Whitaker 2015) to, on average, 16 months involving five coauthors (Borah et al. 2017). Cochrane reviews currently take a median of 29 months from review registration to publication (Andersen et al. 2020). One study estimated that each systematic review costs appropriately $141,195 (Michelson and Reuter 2019). These calculations of time and effort did not account for the time and effort needed to assemble the team, frame and refine the research question, and obtain funding (if the review is funded). The true time to publication and resources required may therefore be much more substantial than these estimates. Interestingly, funded reviews took significantly longer to complete and publish (mean = 42 vs. 26 weeks) and involved more authors and team members (mean = 6.8 vs. 4.8 individuals) than reviews that did not report funding (Borah et al. 2017). One possible reason, speculated by authors of this chapter, is that funded reviews may generally be broader in scope and more likely to adhere to contemporary methodological guidance and expectations.

Systematic Reviews Can Go Out of Date Quickly

Results reported in systematic reviews represent a snapshot of knowledge gained from studies identified at the time of the latest search. Systematic reviews can go out of date quickly, especially in fast-evolving fields with primary studies emerging at an unprecedented speed. The relevance of review findings can be threatened if new studies have not been included in a timely fashion. Signals indicating the need to update systematic reviews may occur frequently and within relatively short timelines (Shojania et al. 2007), but the decisions about whether and when to update a review need to take into account whether the review addresses a current question, uses valid methods, and is well conducted; and whether there are new review methods, new studies, or new information on existing included studies (Garner et al. 2016).

Technology and Innovations

Emerging technological advances, such as increased use of artificial intelligence, for the systematic review tasks of informational retrieval, screening, data extraction, and risk of bias assessment can revolutionize the efficiency of systematic review production and updating (Lau 2019). Recent years have seen the development and advancement of methodology and tools for "living systematic reviews" (Elliott et al. 2017). These types of reviews incorporate findings from clinical trials (and other types of studies) soon after they become available. Technologic tools to automate some systematic review steps already exist and are in early use. For example, a machine learning-based routine has been developed to automatically distinguish between randomized trials, quasi-randomized trials, and non-randomized studies (the "RCT classifier"; Marshall et al. 2018). Other tools have been developed to automatically extract PICO information (e.g., number of participants, their age, sex, country, recruiting centers, intervention groups, outcomes, and time points), study design and results (e.g., objectives, study duration, participant flow), and risk of bias information (Jonnalagadda et al. 2015). While these advances have somewhat minimized the demands on human time and effort, many strides remain to be made for automation for systematic reviews to become the norm.

Summary and Conclusions

As providers of key data for input into systematic reviews, clinical trialists can help make the production of systematic reviews more efficient and impactful. As discussed, the authors of this chapter support the FAIR metadata standards to facilitate widespread data sharing. We recognize that this vision requires clinical trial and systematic review communities to work together more than ever before. After all, both communities share the common goal of efficiently identifying the most evidence-based interventions for humanity.

Key Facts

1. By synthesizing the results of individual studies, systematic reviews present a summary of all the avilable evidence to answer a question, and in doing so can uncover important gaps for future research.

Cross-References

- ▶ CONSORT and Its Extensions for Reporting Clinical Trials
- ▶ Data Sharing and Reuse
- ▶ Introduction to Meta-Analysis

References

AHRQ (2015) Methods guide for effectiveness and comparative effectiveness reviews. Available from https://effectivehealthcare.ahrq.gov/products/cer-methods-guide/overview. Accessed on 27 Oct 2019

Andersen MZ, Gülen S, Fonnes S, Andresen K, Rosenberg J (2020) Half of Cochrane reviews were published more than two years after the protocol. J Clin Epidemiol 124:85–93. https://doi.org/10.1016/j.jclinepi.2020.05.011

Berkman ND, Lohr KN, Ansari MT, Balk EM, Kane R, McDonagh M, Morton SC, Viswanathan M, Bass EB, Butler M, Gartlehner G, Hartling L, McPheeters M, Morgan LC, Reston J, Sista P, Whitlock E, Chang S (2015) Grading the strength of a body of evidence when assessing health care interventions: an EPC update. J Clin Epidemiol 68(11):1312–1324

Borah R, Brown AW, Capers PL, Kaiser KA (2017) Analysis of the time and workers needed to conduct systematic reviews of medical interventions using data from the PROSPERO registry. BMJ Open 7(2):e012545. https://doi.org/10.1136/bmjopen-2016-012545

Chalmers I, Bracken MB, Djulbegovic B, Garattini S, Grant J, Gülmezoglu AM, Howells DW, Ioannidis JP, Oliver S (2014) How to increase value and reduce waste when research priorities are set. Lancet 383(9912):156–165. https://doi.org/10.1016/S0140-6736(13)62229-1

Clarke M, Chalmers I (1998) Discussion sections in reports of controlled trials published in general medical journals: islands in search of continents? JAMA 280(3):280–282

Cooper NJ, Jones DR, Sutton AJ (2005) The use of systematic reviews when designing studies. Clin Trials 2(3):260–264

Djulbegovic B, Kumar A, Magazin A, Schroen AT, Soares H, Hozo I, Clarke M, Sargent D, Schell MJ (2011) Optimism bias leads to inconclusive results-an empirical study. J Clin Epidemiol 64(6):583–593. https://doi.org/10.1016/j.jclinepi.2010.09.007

Elliott JH, Synnot A, Turner T, Simmonds M, Akl EA, McDonald S, Salanti G, Meerpohl J, MacLehose H, Hilton J, Tovey D, Shemilt I, Thomas J (2017) Living systematic review network. Living systematic review: 1. Introduction-the why, what, when, and how. J Clin Epidemiol 91:23–30

Equator Network. Reporting guidelines for systematic reviews. Available from https://www.equator-network.org/?post_type=eq_guidelines&eq_guidelines_study_design=systematic-reviews-and-meta-analyses&eq_guidelines_clinical_specialty=0&eq_guidelines_report_section=0&s=+. Accessed 9 Mar 2020

Garner P, Hopewell S, Chandler J, MacLehose H, Schünemann HJ, Akl EA, Beyene J, Chang S, Churchill R, Dearness K, Guyatt G, Lefebvre C, Liles B, Marshall R, Martínez García L, Mavergames C, Nasser M, Qaseem A, Sampson M, Soares-Weiser K, Takwoingi Y, Thabane L, Trivella M, Tugwell P, Welsh E, Wilson EC, Schünemann HJ (2016) Panel for updating guidance for systematic reviews (PUGs). When and how to update systematic reviews: consensus and checklist. BMJ 354:i3507. https://doi.org/10.1136/bmj.i3507. Erratum in: BMJ 2016 Sep 06 354:i4853

Guyatt G, Oxman AD, Akl EA, Kunz R, Vist G, Brozek J, Norris S, Falck-Ytter Y, Glasziou P, DeBeer H, Jaeschke R, Rind D, Meerpohl J, Dahm P, Schünemann HJ (2011) GRADE guidelines: 1. Introduction-GRADE evidence profiles and summary of findings tables. J Clin Epidemiol 64(4):383–394

Higgins JPT, Thomas J, Chandler J, Cumpston M, Li T, Page MJ, Welch VA (eds) (2019a) Cochrane handbook for systematic reviews of interventions, 2nd edn. Wiley, Chichester

Higgins JPT, Lasserson T, Chandler J, Tovey D, Thomas J, Flemyng E, Churchill R (2019b) Standards for the conduct of new Cochrane intervention reviews. In: JPT H, Lasserson T, Chandler J, Tovey D, Thomas J, Flemyng E, Churchill R (eds) Methodological expectations of Cochrane intervention reviews. Cochrane, London

IOM (2011) Committee on standards for systematic reviews of comparative effectiveness research, board on health care services. In: Eden J, Levit L, Berg A, Morton S (eds) Finding what works in health care: standards for systematic reviews. National Academies Press, Washington, DC

Jonnalagadda SR, Goyal P, Huffman MD (2015) Automating data extraction in systematic reviews: a systematic review. Syst Rev 4:78

Krnic Martinic M, Pieper D, Glatt A, Puljak L (2019) Definition of a systematic review used in overviews of systematic reviews, meta-epidemiological studies and textbooks. BMC Med Res Methodol 19(1):203. Published 4 Nov 2019. https://doi.org/10.1186/s12874-019-0855-0

Lasserson TJ, Thomas J, Higgins JPT (2019) Chapter 1: Starting a review. In: Higgins JPT, Thomas J, Chandler J, Cumpston M, Li T, Page MJ, Welch VA (eds) Cochrane handbook for systematic reviews of interventions version 6.0 (updated July 2019). Cochrane. Available from www.training.cochrane.org/handbook

Lau J, Antman EM, Jimenez-Silva J, Kupelnick B, Mosteller F, Chalmers TC (1992) Cumulative meta-analysis of therapeutic trials for myocardial infarction. N Engl J Med 327(4):248–254

Lau J (2019) Editorial: systematic review automation thematic series. Syst Rev 8(1):70. Published 11 Mar 2019. https://doi.org/10.1186/s13643-019-0974-z

Liberati A, Altman DG, Tetzlaff J, Mulrow C, Gøtzsche PC, Ioannidis JP, Clarke M, Devereaux PJ, Kleijnen J, Moher D (2009) The PRISMA statement for reporting systematic reviews and meta-analyses of studies that evaluate health care interventions: explanation and elaboration. PLoS Med 6(7):e1000100. https://doi.org/10.1371/journal.pmed.1000100

Lund H, Brunnhuber K, Juhl C, Robinson K, Leenaars M, Dorch BF, Jamtvedt G, Nortvedt MW, Christensen R, Chalmers I (2016) Towards evidence based research. BMJ 355:i5440. https://doi.org/10.1136/bmj.i5440

Marshall IJ, Noel-Storr A, Kuiper J, Thomas J, Wallace BC (2018) Machine learning for identifying randomized controlled trials: an evaluation and practitioner's guide. Res Synth Methods 9(4):602–614. https://doi.org/10.1002/jrsm.1287

Michelson M, Reuter K (2019) The significant cost of systematic reviews and meta-analyses: a call for greater involvement of machine learning to assess the promise of clinical trials. Contemp Clin Trials Commun 16:100443. https://doi.org/10.1016/j.conctc.2019.100443. Erratum in: Contemp Clin Trials Commun 2019 16:100450

Moher D, Liberati A, Tetzlaff J (2009) Altman DG; PRISMA group. Preferred reporting items for systematic reviews and meta-analyses: the PRISMA statement. Ann Intern Med 151(4):264–269. W64

Moher D, Shamseer L, Clarke M, Ghersi D, Liberati A, Petticrew M, Shekelle P, Stewart LA, PRISMA-P Group (2015) Preferred reporting items for systematic review and meta-analysis protocols (PRISMA-P) 2015 statement. Syst Rev 4(1):1. https://doi.org/10.1186/2046-4053-4-1

NIHR HTA Stage 1 guidance notes. Available from https://www.nihr.ac.uk/documents/hta-stage-1-guidance-notes/11743; Accessed 10 Mar 2020

Page MJ, Shamseer L, Altman DG, Tetzlaff J, Sampson M, Tricco AC, Catalá-López F, Li L, Reid EK, Sarkis-Onofre R, Moher D (2016) Epidemiology and reporting characteristics of systematic reviews of biomedical research: a cross-sectional study. PLoS Med 13(5):e1002028. https://doi.org/10.1371/journal.pmed.1002028

Page MJ, Higgins JPT, Sterne JAC (2019) Chapter 13: assessing risk of bias due to missing results in a synthesis. In: Higgins JPT, Thomas J, Chandler J, Cumpston M, Li T, Page MJ et al (eds) Cochrane handbook for systematic reviews of interventions, 2nd edn. Wiley, Chichester, pp 349–374

Robinson KA (2009) Use of prior research in the justification and interpretation of clinical trials. Johns Hopkins University

Robinson KA, Goodman SN (2011) A systematic examination of the citation of prior research in reports of randomized, controlled trials. Ann Intern Med 154(1):50–55. https://doi.org/10.7326/0003-4819-154-1-201101040-00007

Rouse B, Cipriani A, Shi Q, Coleman AL, Dickersin K, Li T (2016) Network meta-analysis for clinical practice guidelines – a case study on first-line medical therapies for primary open-angle glaucoma. Ann Intern Med 164(10):674–682. https://doi.org/10.7326/M15-2367

Saldanha IJ, Lindsley K, Do DV et al (2017) Comparison of clinical trial and systematic review outcomes for the 4 most prevalent eye diseases. JAMA Ophthalmol 135(9):933–940. https://doi.org/10.1001/jamaophthalmol.2017.2583

Shea BJ, Grimshaw JM, Wells GA, Boers M, Andersson N, Hamel C, Porter AC, Tugwell P, Moher D, Bouter LM (2007) Development of AMSTAR: a measurement tool to assess the methodological quality of systematic reviews. BMC Med Res Methodol 7:10

Shea BJ, Reeves BC, Wells G, Thuku M, Hamel C, Moran J, Moher D, Tugwell P, Welch V, Kristjansson E, Henry DA (2017) AMSTAR 2: a critical appraisal tool for systematic reviews that include randomised or non-randomised studies of healthcare interventions, or both. BMJ 358:j4008. https://doi.org/10.1136/bmj.j4008

Shojania KG, Sampson M, Ansari MT, Ji J, Doucette S, Moher D (2007) How quickly do systematic reviews go out of date? A survival analysis. Ann Intern Med 147(4):224–233

Sterne JA, Hernán MA, Reeves BC, Savović J, Berkman ND, Viswanathan M, Henry D, Altman DG, Ansari MT, Boutron I, Carpenter JR, Chan AW, Churchill R, Deeks JJ, Hróbjartsson A, Kirkham J, Jüni P, Loke YK, Pigott TD, Ramsay CR, Regidor D, Rothstein HR, Sandhu L, Santaguida PL, Schünemann HJ, Shea B, Shrier I, Tugwell P, Turner L, Valentine JC, Waddington H, Waters E, Wells GA, Whiting PF, Higgins JP (2016) ROBINS-I: a tool for assessing risk of bias in non-randomised studies of interventions. BMJ 355:i4919. https://doi.org/10.1136/bmj.i4919

Sterne JAC, Savović J, Page MJ, Elbers RG, Blencowe NS, Boutron I, Cates CJ, Cheng HY, Corbett MS, Eldridge SM, Emberson JR, Hernán MA, Hopewell S, Hróbjartsson A, Junqueira DR, Jüni P, Kirkham JJ, Lasserson T, Li T, McAleenan A, Reeves BC, Shepperd S, Shrier I, Stewart LA, Tilling K, White IR, Whiting PF, Higgins JPT (2019) RoB 2: a revised tool for assessing risk of bias in randomised trials. BMJ 366:l4898. https://doi.org/10.1136/bmj.l4898

Thomas J, Kneale D, McKenzie JE, Brennan SE, Bhaumik S (2019) Chapter 2: determining the scope of the review and the questions it will address. In: Higgins JPT, Thomas J, Chandler J, Cumpston M, Li T, Page MJ, Welch VA (eds) Cochrane handbook for systematic reviews of interventions version 6.0 (updated July 2019). Cochrane. Available from www.training.cochrane.org/handbook

USPSTF U.S. Preventive Services Task Force Procedure Manual (2017). Available from: https://www.uspreventiveservicestaskforce.org/uspstf/sites/default/files/inline-files/procedure-manual2017_update.pdf. Accessed 21 May 2020

Whitaker (2015) UCSF guides: systematic review: when will i be finished? https://guides.ucsf.edu/c.php?g=375744&p=3041343, Accessed 13 May 2020

Whiting P, Savović J, Higgins JP, Caldwell DM, Reeves BC, Shea B, Davies P, Kleijnen J (2016) Churchill R; ROBIS group. ROBIS: a new tool to assess risk of bias in systematic reviews was developed. J Clin Epidemiol 69:225–234. https://doi.org/10.1016/j.jclinepi.2015.06.005

Introduction to Meta-Analysis

110

Theodoros Evrenoglou, Silvia Metelli, and Anna Chaimani

Contents

Introduction	2180
Working Example	2181
Data Required for a Meta-Analysis	2181
Data Synthesis	2182
Common Effect Meta-Analysis	2182
What Is Heterogeneity	2183
Random-Effects Meta-Analysis	2183
Identifying Heterogeneity	2184
Interpreting Results	2186
Exploring Heterogeneity	2187
Subgroup Analysis	2187
Meta-Regression	2188
Within-Trial Bias	2190
Small-Study Effects and Publication Bias	2190
Meta-Analysis of Individual Participant Data	2192
Network Meta-Analysis	2192
Summary and Conclusion	2193
Key Facts	2193

T. Evrenoglou
Université de Paris, Research Center of Epidemiology and Statistics (CRESS-U1153), INSERM, Paris, France

S. Metelli
Université de Paris, Research Center of Epidemiology and Statistics (CRESS-U1153), INSERM, Paris, France

Assistance Publique - Hôpitaux de Paris (APHP), Paris, France
e-mail: silvia.metelli@parisdescartes.fr

A. Chaimani (✉)
Université de Paris, Research Center of Epidemiology and Statistics (CRESS-U1153), INSERM, Paris, France

Cochrane France, Paris, France
e-mail: anna.chaimani@inserm.fr

© Springer Nature Switzerland AG 2022
S. Piantadosi, C. L. Meinert (eds.), *Principles and Practice of Clinical Trials*,
https://doi.org/10.1007/978-3-319-52636-2_287

Cross-References 2194
References 2194

Abstract

Studies within a systematic review are often combined statistically in a meta-analysis, which quantitatively synthesizes all available evidence about the relative effects of two healthcare interventions for the same clinical outcome. A key issue in every meta-analysis is whether the identified randomized control trials (RCTs) are similar enough to be combined together since important differences in trial- or patient-level characteristics may affect the treatment effects. Such differences, called *heterogeneity*, need to be properly investigated and accounted for in the analysis. In this chapter, we introduce the basic concepts of meta-analyses of RCTs and we describe the two main meta-analytical models, namely, the common effect and the random effects models. Then, we present several ways to identify and assess heterogeneity. We discuss the interpretation of results from a meta-analysis using two exemplar datasets. The chapter closes with a brief introduction to more sophisticated meta-analytical techniques such as the use of individual participant data and network meta-analysis.

Keywords

Evidence synthesis · Heterogeneity · Random effects · Publication bias

Introduction

Systematic reviews are essential for summarizing all available evidence in a reliable way using predefined methods and criteria. Meta-analysis is the quantitative component of a systematic review that combines estimates obtained from two or more RCTs for the same outcome. Meta-analysis of RCTs, when properly conducted, is usually ranked above individual RCTs in hierarchies of evidence for health-care decisions (Higgins et al. 2019). Findings from meta-analyses can change clinical practice. One well-known example is streptokinase administration on the risk of death from acute myocardial infarction (Lau et al. 1992). Although 33 RCTs had been published until then, only six of them clearly showed favorable results for streptokinase. The contradictory findings from RCTs had made investigators being skeptical about the benefit of the drug. However, the meta-analysis of all RCTs showed a highly significant effect of streptokinase (RR: 0.79, 95% CI: [0.72, 0.87]) and since then, streptokinase has been more widely recommended and used.

Given that RCTs are sometimes underpowered to determine the relative effects between interventions, meta-analyses, by combining several studies together, can often increase the precision. While individual RCTs are often targeted to a specific type of participants and interventions, summary of evidence from a collection of RCTs allows for investigating the consistency of effect across different, yet similar populations. Despite the aforementioned advantages of meta-analyses, investigators should always consider whether a meta-analysis is appropriate. Even in well-conducted systematic reviews, results from meta-analysis can be misleading if the required synthesis assumptions are not fulfilled or when results are interpreted in isolation from trial characteristics.

This chapter aims to introduce the basic concepts of meta-analysis including the underlying assumptions of the two commonly used statistical models, the notion of heterogeneity and its impact on the interpretation of the findings, and the role of potential sources of bias in the overall conclusions. Throughout we provide examples from a previously published meta-analysis in the field of mental health.

Working Example

To illustrate the methods presented in the chapter, we use data from a published meta-analysis investigating the relative efficacy and acceptability of repetitive transcranial magnetic stimulation (rTMS) for major depressive disorder (Brunoni et al. 2017). The full review includes 81 RCTs comparing nine different rTMS interventions. Here, we use a subset of 15 RCTs that compare high frequency rTMS (HF-rTMS) versus sham (i.e., the control intervention). The outcome of interest is response to the intervention after 10 sessions, where response is defined as 50% or greater improvement from baseline on a depression scale.

Data Required for a Meta-Analysis

Meta-analysis can combine any type of outcome data such as binary data (e.g., death, no death), continuous data (e.g., blood pressure, weight loss), and time-to-event data (e.g., time from virus infection until death). Meta-analysis of other types of data, for example, ordinal data, is also possible but not discussed in this chapter due to its greater complexity.

Typically, RCTs estimate the difference between two interventions in the form of summary results; hence by reporting a measure of effect and a measure of precision (i.e., standard error, variance, or confidence interval [CI]). Such type of data are *aggregate data*. For binary data, the most common effect measures are risk ratio (RR), odds ratio (OR), and risk difference. For continuous data, the most frequent choices are mean difference and the standardized mean difference. Standardized mean difference is used when a continuous outcome of interest is measured in different scales across studies and thus the values are not directly comparable (e.g., all studies measure anxiety but they use different psychometric scales). It is defined as the difference of the mean values between the two groups divided by the common standard deviation of the two groups. Time-to-event data are usually expressed through hazard ratios.

Obtaining a measure of effect (e.g., mean difference for a continuous outcome) and its precision (e.g., variance) from every RCT is the first step to perform a meta-analysis. Precision is necessary for assigning each RCT a *weight* in the synthesis reflecting the uncertainty of the trial results. In this way, larger RCTs, which are usually more precise, would have a greater impact on the combined results. Very often the necessary data for meta-analyses are not reported from all RCTs. For example, p-values or hypothesis testing statistics may be given instead of standard errors or variances. In such situations data transformations or approximations may be used but reviewers should be aware that some of these approaches are based on assumptions that need to be carefully checked (Deeks et al. 2019). An additional issue that may arise during data extraction is that different RCTs may provide different effect measures (e.g., RR in some RCTs and OR in others). In such situations, review authors could extract arm-level data (e.g., number of events and number of participants per arm) and re-calculate the effect of intervention using a common effect measure for the purpose of meta-analysis. In the absence of arm-level data, transformations between effect sizes are possible under certain conditions (Deeks et al. 2019).

Data Synthesis

The two main meta-analytical methods for data synthesis are the *common effect* model and the *random effects* model. The two models differ primarily in their underlying assumptions. A choice between the two models should always be made through careful consideration of which assumption is more plausible given the research question and the characteristics of RCTs expected to be included in the meta-analysis.

Common Effect Meta-Analysis

The *summary effect* of the meta-analysis is a weighted average of the relative effect estimates obtained from the individual RCTs. All RCTs within a meta-analysis are weighted according to their precision, which is defined as the inverse of their variance. The mathematical expression of this *inverse variance* meta-analysis is:

$$\widehat{\theta} = \frac{\sum_i w_i y_i}{\sum_i w_i}, w_i = \frac{1}{var(y_i)}$$

where y_i and $var(y_i)$ are the observed relative effect and its variance respectively in RCT i, w_i is the weight of RCT i, and $\widehat{\theta}$ is the summary estimate of the common relative effect comparing the two interventions of interest. This is called a *fixed effect* or *common effect* meta-analysis. The underlying assumption being made here is that all RCTs in the meta-analysis are estimating a common "true" relative effect and the only source of variation across their results is random error (Borenstein et al. 2010). However, this assumption is unrealistic in most situations as it is unlikely that all included RCTs would share a common type of population in an identical clinical setting, and utilize a uniform design (Deeks et al. 2019). The inverse variance weights presented here can be used for any type of data. For binary data, other commonly used weighting schemes for the RCTs are the Mantel-Haenszel (Mantel and Haenszel 1959) and Peto (Yusuf et al. 1985) methods, which might be more appropriate when events are not frequent.

What Is Heterogeneity

Heterogeneity refers to important differences in the characteristics of the RCTs. There are three types of heterogeneity: clinical, methodological, and statistical. Clinical heterogeneity may arise due to variation in the population (e.g., inclusion criteria, geographical location), the interventions (e.g., dose, nature of control interventions), and the outcomes (e.g., follow-up duration, cut-off points). For example, when different doses of a drug are administered across RCTs and the effect of the drug varies by dose, a common effect meta-analysis that ignores differences in dose is inappropriate. Methodological heterogeneity occurs when there is variability in the design of the RCTs, the quality of conduct, and approach to analysis. For example, meta-epidemiological studies have suggested that when the sequence of assigning participants to treatment groups is not concealed, RCTs tend to estimate larger treatment effects (Pildal et al. 2007; Savović et al. 2012). When clinical and/or methodological heterogeneity are present, we expect that they would be reflected in the form of statistical heterogeneity, which is the discrepancy in the effects of the interventions across RCTs. Statistical heterogeneity occurs when the 'true' treatment effects are more different than one would expect due to chance alone. This may include contradictory findings (benefit vs. harm) or differences in the degree of benefit (or harm) found across RCTs. Statistical heterogeneity might not be always observed despite the presence of clinical and/or methodological heterogeneity, and thus, lack of statistical heterogeneity should not be interpreted as evidence for the lack of heterogeneity.

Random-Effects Meta-Analysis

Because common effect meta-analysis assumes no heterogeneity, such an analysis is inappropriate in the presence of important differences among RCTs. To allow for heterogeneity when synthesizing RCTs, we employ an approach in which we assume that the 'true' effects of the RCTs are similar (i.e., coming from a common – usually normal – distribution) but not identical. This is the assumption of the *random effects meta-analysis*, which implies that apart from within-trial random error there is a second source of variation across RCTs; that is heterogeneity (usually denoted with τ^2) (Nikolakopoulou et al. 2014). A graphical representation of the common and random effects model assumptions is shown in Fig. 1. In practice, random-effects meta-analysis incorporates heterogeneity in the weights of the RCTs and then the summary effect is obtained as before:

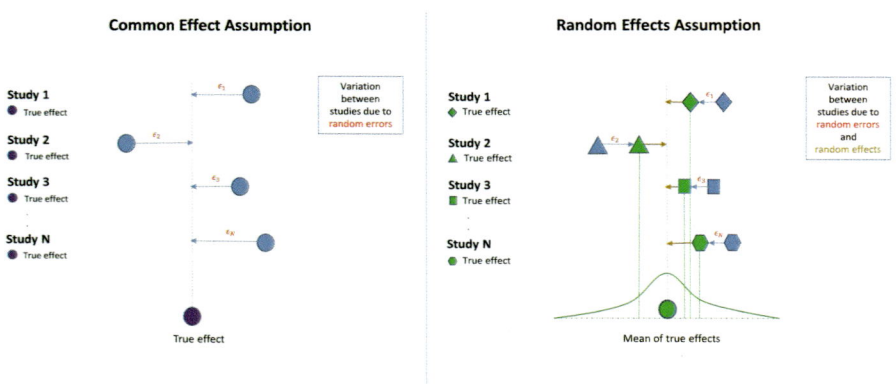

Fig. 1 Graphical representation of the common and the random effects model assumptions

$$\widehat{\theta}^* = \frac{\sum_i w_i^* y_i}{\sum_i w_i^*}, w_i^* = \frac{1}{var(y_i) + \tau^2}$$

where τ^2 is the between-trial variance (i.e., heterogeneity), w_i^*s are the weights under random effects and $\widehat{\theta}^*$ is the summary estimate from the meta-analysis. It is important to note that the summary effect ($\widehat{\theta}^*$) of the random effects model represents the mean of the assumed distribution for the trial-specific underlying effects. The only difference between the two formulae for common and random effects models is the incorporation of the heterogeneity parameter in the RCT weights. However, this additional source of uncertainty added to the model may impact the results as it usually leads to wider confidence intervals. Clearly, in the case of $\tau^2 = 0$, the two models give identical results.

Multiple estimators have been proposed for τ^2 such as the Der Simonian and Laird (Der Simonian and Laird 1986) (DL), the restricted maximum likelihood and maximum likelihood (ML), the Paul-Mantel (Paule and Mandel 1982) (PM). Although DL is the most commonly used estimator of heterogeneity, a lot of criticism has been made to that choice. Results from simulations suggest that PM estimator under certain conditions provides a less biased choice (Sidik and Jonkman 2007) while ML estimator performs better when heterogeneity is small (Petropoulou and Mavridis 2017). For binary data, estimation of the heterogeneity parameter can be challenging when the events are infrequent (Efthimiou 2018). In those cases, τ^2 can sometimes be estimated to be zero due to lack of power; hence results coincide to those obtained from the common effect model. An extended discussion on the properties of the different estimators can be found elsewhere (Petropoulou and Mavridis 2017; Veroniki et al. 2016).

Identifying Heterogeneity

Typically, meta-analyses are presented in *forest plots*, where both trial-specific and summary results are depicted along with their CIs. Visual inspection of the forest plot is always the first step in the identification of heterogeneity. Large variation among the results of the RCTs and lack of overlap of their CIs suggest that heterogeneity might be present. Figure 2 shows the forest plot of the 15 RCTs that compared rTMS to sham intervention. The size of the squares is proportional to the weights of the RCTs according to the random-effects model. The plot suggests that there is some variation between the effects estimated in different RCTs but the amount of variation seems to be reasonable for combining these RRs. The summary results appear at the bottom of the graph. Both common (fixed) and random effects meta-analyses suggest that the chances of response are higher in the HF-rTMS group. However, the two models give somewhat different results in terms of magnitude of summary RR; the random effects model also gives a wider CI.

Q-test (a chi-square test) for homogeneity and the I-square statistic may be used to assess statistically heterogeneity but caution is needed to avoid mis- and over-interpretations. A non-significant result of the Q-test suggests the absence of heterogeneity but the test usually has low power to detect heterogeneity when there are few RCTs while it has excessive power to detect clinically unimportant heterogeneity in the presence of many RCTs. For this reason, a p-value of 0.1 (rather than 0.05) is recommended as a threshold for statistical significance of the Q-test. Since clinical and methodological differences across a set of RCTs inevitably exist, the Q-test is often seen as investigating an irrelevant question and so the emphasis should rather be placed on measures that aim to quantitatively describe the amount of heterogeneity (Higgins and Thompson 2002).

Study	Randomized HF-rTMS	Randomized Sham		Weights Fixed (%)	Weights Random (%)	RR [95% CI]
Anderson, 2007	13	16		1.55 %	2.31 %	7.38 [1.01, 53.83]
Avery, 2006	35	33		2.99 %	4.19 %	5.19 [1.24, 21.66]
Bakim, 2012	11	12		3.53 %	4.83 %	4.36 [1.17, 16.27]
Blumberger, 2012	24	22		1.13 %	1.71 %	0.46 [0.04, 4.71]
Blumberger, 2016	40	41		2.58 %	3.67 %	3.08 [0.66, 14.34]
Boutros, 2002	12	9		1.97 %	2.89 %	0.75 [0.13, 4.36]
Garcia-Toro-JAD, 2001	20	29		1.43 %	2.14 %	7.25 [0.91, 57.46]
Garcia-Toro-JNNP, 2001	11	11		3.96 %	5.32 %	1.33 [0.39, 4.62]
George, 2010	92	98		6.35 %	7.77 %	2.98 [1.12, 7.95]
Hernandez-Ribas, 2013	10	11		5.57 %	7.02 %	2.57 [0.90, 7.31]
Herwig, 2007	62	65		22.35 %	17.05 %	1.00 [0.59, 1.68]
Huang, 2012	30	30		14.42 %	13.52 %	1.30 [0.68, 2.49]
Kreuzer, 2015	15	15		2.98 %	4.18 %	1.00 [0.24, 4.18]
Loo, 2007	19	21		3.98 %	5.34 %	2.21 [0.64, 7.63]
O"Reardon, 2007	155	146		25.23 %	18.03 %	1.79 [1.09, 2.93]
Q=18.33, df=14, p=0.19, I²=23.2%, τ²=0.08			Random effects	---	100.00 %	1.82 [1.33, 2.49]
			Common effects	100.00 %	---	1.69 [1.32, 2.16]
			Prediction interval	---	---	--- [0.96, 3.43]

Fig. 2 Forest plot of 15 RCTs comparing the response of high-frequency (HF) rTMS vs Sham for major depressive episodes. Squares represent the risk ratios (RR) estimated from the RCTs with size proportional to their weight and the diamonds are the summary estimates from random (blue) and common (red) effects meta-analysis. The blue horizontal line at the bottom represents the prediction interval

The I-square statistic expresses the proportion of the total variation that is due to heterogeneity. Although, the I-square is more informative than the Q-test, it should always be considered along with τ^2 – the estimate of between-trial variance (Borenstein et al. 2017). A common mistake in the interpretation of I-square is to treat it as an absolute measure, although, in fact, it does not provide any information about the amount of heterogeneity among RCTs. Large values of I-square indicate that a large percentage of the total variation is due to heterogeneity, but this does not necessarily mean that there is a lot of heterogeneity across the RCTs and vice versa.

In Fig. 2, although the Q-test gives a nonsignificant p-value and the I-square is rather small (23.2%), the magnitude of the between-trial variance (τ^2) is estimated to be 0.08. A decision upon the importance of this observed heterogeneity should be made considering the clinical question and the outcome under investigation. Such decisions may be assisted by comparing the estimated between-trial variance with the empirical distributions that have been provided in the literature (Turner et al. 2012; Rhodes et al. 2015). Here, we see that the estimated $\tau^2 = 0.08$ is smaller than the median of the empirical distribution given by Turner et al. (2012) (i.e., 0.12) but it is larger than the first quantile of the distribution (i.e., 0.02); hence overall we may say that heterogeneity is low to moderate.

Finally, *prediction intervals* (Higgins and Thompson 2002; Borenstein et al. 2017) provide the range within which we expect the true effect in a future RCT to fall in. Prediction intervals offer a more intuitive way to assess the level of heterogeneity as they show how it will impact the effects in future RCTs. However, prediction intervals strongly rely on the assumption of normal distribution, which can be implausible when the total number of the available RCTs is small (Borenstein et al. 2017). The use of prediction intervals is strongly encouraged when there are at least 10 RCTs available. In the absence of statistical heterogeneity ($\tau^2 = 0$), the prediction interval would coincide with the CI. In the rTMS example we see that the prediction interval marginally crosses the line of no effect but overall it doesn't seem to challenge the superiority of HF-rTMS over sham.

It is important to note that the decision between common effect and random effects meta-analysis should be made a priori in the protocol of a systematic review and not based on the above statistics or the summary results. Meta-analysts should consider whether the RCTs they expect to identify are likely to be homogenous enough or not, based on their experience, their understanding of the clinical field, and the research question (Deeks et al. 2019).

Interpreting Results

The diamond in a forest plot gives important information about the magnitude, direction, and the uncertainty of the summary effect. The corresponding diamonds for both common and random effects models in the rTMS example suggest an increase to the probability of response of 82% and 69% respectively, in favor of the HF-rTMS group. Moreover, for both models the confidence intervals do not cross the no-effect line, thus indicating that both summary estimates are statistically significant.

The interpretation of results from meta-analyses should not only focus on the summary estimate (i.e., the diamond). Forest plot inspection, assessment of the plausibility of the model assumptions, and the biases arising from the design and conduct of RCTs are crucial for interpreting the numerical results. For instance, if some RCTs are at high risk of bias, the result of a meta-analysis, although more precise, can be biased. Results obtained from random-effects models are usually easier to be generalized in wider populations, as they take into account heterogeneity across RCTs, but interpretation of the summary effect becomes more challenging. This is because the summary effect of a random effects meta-analysis represents a distribution of effects and not a common average effect. Also, in the presence of heterogeneity, review authors should further explore possible sources of this between-trial variation using explorative analyses. Of course, when the amount of heterogeneity across RCTs is substantial, it may be preferable not to perform a meta-analysis.

Exploring Heterogeneity

The presence of excessive heterogeneity across RCTs renders the summary effect meaningless. In such a case, combing results from multiple RCTs in a meta-analysis may not be the best approach. Review authors would need to explore what makes RCTs being different, and with scientific rationale, they may restrict the meta-analysis to a more homogenous set of RCTs. When a considerable amount of heterogeneity is observed, investigation of its sources should be carried out through *subgroup analysis* and *meta-regression*. These types of analyses allow to explore the impact of trial-level characteristics, considered potential effect modifiers (e.g., average age of participants, publication year of RCTs, dose of the intervention) on the relative effects. Subgroup analysis can be used only for exploring discrete characteristics, while meta-regression is both for discrete and continuous characteristics.

Subgroup Analysis

Subgroup analysis splits RCTs into different subsets and performs a meta-analysis in each subset separately to explore their potential differences. Differences between subgroups should be examined using formal statistical tests (Borenstein and Higgins 2013). The test for subgroup differences is a chi-square test for testing the presence of heterogeneity across subgroups. A nonsignificant test implies that results from different subgroups are in statistical agreement; in such a case, review authors may decide to present primarily the results from the overall analysis. When only two subgroups are present, the confidence intervals of the summary estimates can be informative about potential subgroup differences as an overlap between the confidence intervals would indicate non-significant differences between the two

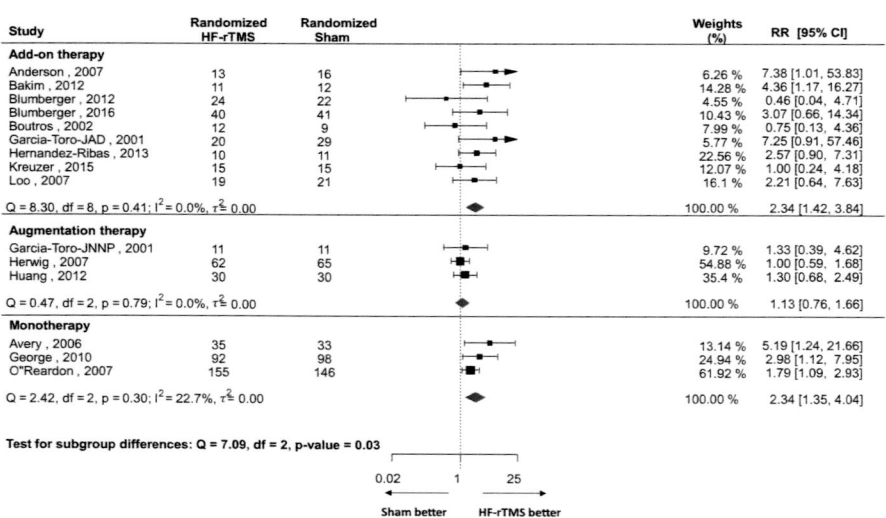

Fig. 3 Subgroup analysis of the rTMS example according to the type of intervention (add-on therapy, augmentation therapy, monotherapy)

subgroups. Figure 3 shows the results of a subgroup analysis in which RCTs were grouped by how HF-rTMS was used (add-on therapy, augmentation therapy, or monotherapy). According to the graph, the benefit from receiving HF-rTMS is higher when it is given as add-on therapy or monotherapy, whereas results are not so favorable for HF-rTMS as an augmentation therapy. These findings are supported by the test for subgroup differences that suggest important discrepancies across the three subgroups (p-value = 0.03). However, it is important to consider that there are only 3 RCTs that evaluated HF-rTMS as augmentation therapy and it might worth to perform further RCTs to explore the effectiveness of this approach. The fact that the within-subgroup τ^2s are 0 suggests that this intervention-specific characteristic may explain some of the overall heterogeneity.

Meta-Regression

Meta-regression is a meta-analysis model that includes covariates. Conceptually, a meta-regression model resembles a weighted regression model in which the outcome variable is the effect estimate and the covariates are the characteristics of the RCTs judged to be potentially influential on the intervention effect. Mathematically, a random effects meta-regression model can be expressed through the following equations:

$$y_i = \theta + x_1\beta_1 + \cdots + x_k\beta_\kappa + u_i + \varepsilon_i,$$

$$u_i \sim N(0, \tau^2),$$

$$\varepsilon_i \sim N(0, var(y_i)),$$

where $x_1, \ldots, x_k$ are the covariates (i.e., potential effect moderators), $\beta_1, \ldots, \beta_k$ are the coefficients of the covariates, u_i the random effects, ε_i the random errors. As before, y_i and $var(y_i)$ are respectively the observed effect and its variance for RCT i. The coefficients are the key parameters of the model as they show how the outcome changes when the respective covariates change. The characteristics to be investigated in meta-regression should always be pre-specified at the protocol stage and chosen according to scientific rationale. In practice, only a small number of characteristics should be chosen to mitigate the risk for false positive findings (identification of statistically significant associations when there is no real association).

Results of meta-regression are typically presented through a *bubble plot* when the model includes only one covariate. This is a scatter plot showing the treatment effect on the y-axis and the covariate of interest on the x-axis. In this plot, RCTs are represented by circles with size proportional to the weight of each RCT in the meta-analytical model. Figure 4 shows the results of meta-regression in the rTMS example where the number of sessions undertaken in each RCT was used as covariate. The slope of the line indicates that as the number of sessions increases the RR of response for HF-rTMS vs sham also increases. Specifically, with one more session the log-RR of response increases by 0.04. This means that the RR increases on average by 4% ($\exp(0.04) = 1.04$) for each additional session. The intercept of the model represents

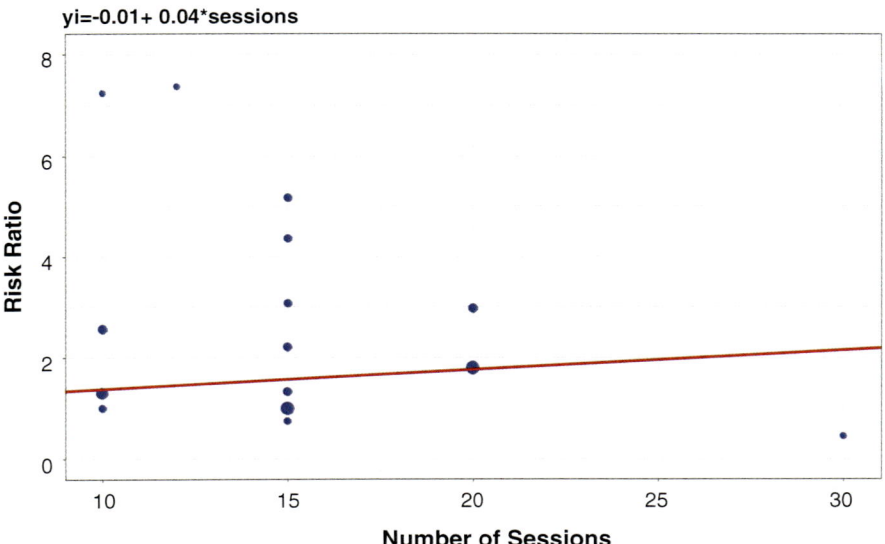

Fig. 4 Bubble plot showing the results of meta-regression with number of sessions as explanatory variable. The red line represents the meta-regression line and the blue circles are the RCTs. The size of the circles is proportional to the weight of each RCT

the RR when number of sessions is equal to 0. To obtain more meaningful interpretation of the intercept, it is preferable to use transformations of the explanatory variable (number of session). For example, we may center the number of sessions at the mean value; this would give an intercept representing the log-RR of response at the mean number of sessions.

A rough threshold of at least 10 RCTs is generally needed for each covariate explored in a meta-regression because with fewer studies the model would have limited power to detect any association even when it is present. Review authors should also consider the size of the included RCTs. For subgroup analysis both common and random effects models are valid, while for meta-regression the common effect model has been proved not suitable, as it likely leads to high false-positive rates (Deeks et al. 2019).

Within-Trial Bias

Findings of meta-analyses should always be interpreted in light of the credibility of the data. If the majority of the included RCTs have important limitations, hence high risk of bias, this would threaten the validity of the results. Often to assess the impact of 'suspicious' RCTs, we run *sensitivity analyses* by excluding them and monitor changes in the summary effect. The incorporation of a sensitivity analysis is strongly encouraged as it represents an important tool for assessing the robustness of the results. When conducting a systematic review and a meta-analysis, many decisions – such as eligibility criteria, modeling choice, or choice of covariates – are not always straightforward. Sensitivity analysis allows the investigators to assess whether findings are robust against those decisions, making it possible to draw conclusions with a higher degree of certainty.

Small-Study Effects and Publication Bias

Although random-effects meta-analysis is generally considered more reasonable than common effect meta-analysis, it gives more weight to smaller RCTs and can yield misleading or biased results when smaller RCTs are systematically different from larger RCTs. This phenomenon is known as *small-study effects* and can be due to several reasons. Small RCTs might be of lower methodological quality, include restricted populations, have different eligibility criteria, include populations of higher baseline risk, etc. Another explanation of small-study effects is *publication bias*: the systematic selection of RCTs for publication depending on their results. Small RCTs are known to be more prone to selective publication than larger RCTs and this might explain why they provide different conclusions. Moreover, empirical evidence has shown that small studies tend to favor active or new treatments more than large studies do (Turner et al. 2013).

The presence of small-study effects can be assessed graphically (Mavridis and Salanti 2014) when enough RCTs (e.g., ten) are available. This is done using a *funnel plot* which is a scatter plot of the measure of effect against its precision (e.g., the standard error). By inverting the vertical axis, large RCTs lie at the top of the graph and small RCTs at the bottom. In the absence of small-study effects, we expect that points will be distributed symmetrically around the summary effect of the meta-analysis. It should be noted that an asymmetrical funnel plot suggests the presence of small-study effects, but not necessarily the presence of publication bias. Funnel plot asymmetry can also be due to the presence of substantial heterogeneity across RCTs.

Statistical tests may be used to assess the significance of funnel plot asymmetry, such as the Egger's test (Egger et al. 1997). However, results from statistical tests of funnel plot asymmetry are underpowered in the case of less than 10 RCTs; thus, conclusions about funnel plot asymmetry should not rely on statistical test significance only (Mavridis and Salanti 2014). The funnel plot of the 15 RCTs from the exemplar meta-analysis is shown in Fig. 5. The graph is somewhat asymmetrical as most of the small RCTs (except two) tend to show larger effects in comparison to the larger RCTs. Several statistical methods aiming to adjust the results for small-study effects or publication bias are also available (Egger et al. 1997; Duval 2005; Moreno et al. 2009a, b; 2011; Peters et al. 2006). Probably the best way, though, to mitigate the risk of publication bias is to follow a comprehensive search strategy, identifying and including unpublished RCTs. On the other hand, including unpublished literature sometimes can raise several concerns because of the absence of a proper peer-review process, thus making it difficult to judge the study quality.

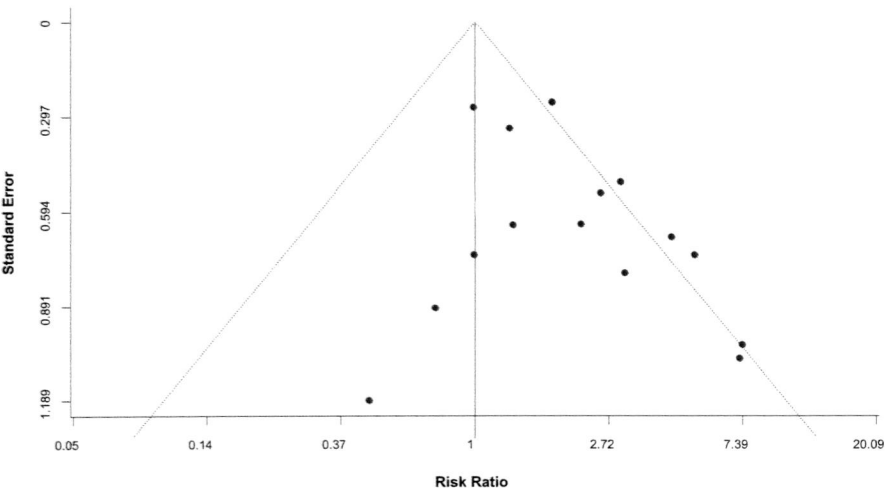

Fig. 5 Funnel plot of the rTMS example

Meta-Analysis of Individual Participant Data

To date, most meta-analyses use aggregate data meaning that only a relative effect and a measure of its uncertainty (e.g., the standard error) are extracted from each RCT for analysis. Such data do not provide information about potential associations between participants' characteristics and their outcomes. Therefore, when possible, review authors are seeking the *individual participant data* (IPD) (i.e., the raw data) from the RCTs. The use of IPD in meta-analyses has several advantages (Debray et al. 2015; Thomas et al. 2014). It allows better assessment and investigation of heterogeneity across RCTs as patient-level covariates are available. It allows recalculation of outcomes and mitigates problems of poor reporting. It also enables different approaches to handling missing data (e.g., with multiple imputation techniques (Mavridis et al. 2014)), and it allows more accurate inference about subgroups of the population and free of aggregation bias that arises when the associations observed across RCTs do not exist within RCTs or vice versa.

Despite all the aforementioned advantages, obtaining IPD is a time-consuming and costly procedure as it usually involves multiple repeated requests and long-lasting discussions with trialists to get the raw data for a proportion of the eligible RCTs. It is very rare to have available IPD for all the RCTs within a meta-analysis. Further, even after obtaining the desired data, meta-analyses of IPD are more complex statistically than those using aggregate data only. As a result, when planning a meta-analysis, it is necessary to estimate whether the benefit of using IPD would overweigh the additional efforts required.

Network Meta-Analysis

So far, we have only discussed meta-analysis of a pair of interventions. For most clinical conditions multiple interventions are available and thus comparing only two interventions at a time cannot answer the most interesting question: *among all possible options, which interventions work best?* Such questions can be addressed through *network meta-analysis* (NMA), an extension of standard pair-wise meta-analysis. NMA can synthesize simultaneously RCTs comparing different interventions. In this way, NMA exploits all available evidence and provides relative effect estimates usually with improved precision compared to pair-wise meta-analysis. NMA generates relative effect estimates for comparisons that have never been evaluated against each other in an RCT, and it ranks the competing interventions according to the outcomes of interest (Caldwell et al. 2005; Mavridis et al. 2015). To decide what kind of RCTs, populations, and interventions can feed into the same NMA, review authors should be aware of the fundamental assumption of NMA, called *transitivity*. Transitivity suggests that the anchor treatments (e.g., A) are "transitive" to allow validly comparing indirectly any interventions B and C when RCTs comparing directly A with B and A with C exist. Transitivity requires several conditions to be met, such as similar distributions of effect modifiers across direct comparisons, similar definitions of the anchor treatments in different trials, etc. More

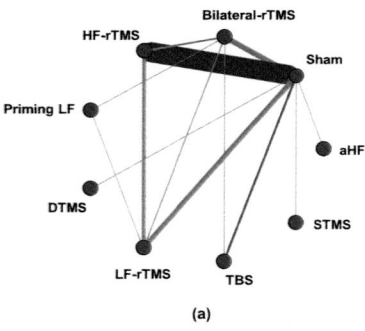
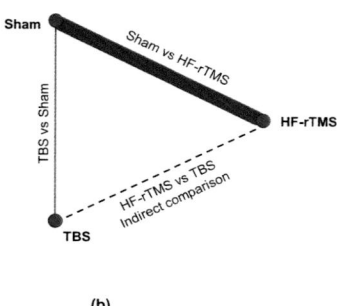

Fig. 6 Full network diagram of the rTMS example comparing 9 interventions major depressive episodes (**a**) with a focus on a loop of three interventions (**b**). The thickness of the lines corresponds to the number of RCTs comparing each pair of interventions. [aTMS = accelerated TMS; dTMS = "deep" (H-coil) TMS; HF = high frequency; LF = low frequency; pTMS = priming TMS; sTMS = synchronized TMS; TBS = θ-burst stimulation]

details on the concept of NMA and its assumptions can be found elsewhere (Salanti 2012; Chaimani et al. 2019). Figure 6a depicts as an example the full network of the 9 rTMS interventions. Panel (b) shows how an indirect comparison for HF-rTMS vs. Sham can be obtained through θ-burst stimulation (TBS) but also through any other connected route in the network.

Summary and Conclusion

Meta-analysis can combine any number of RCTs that compare two interventions for the same condition and usually results in more precise estimates of the treatment effects than individual RCTs. Discrepancies across RCTs can be taken into account in the analysis by the random effects model that allows for the presence of heterogeneity. Interpretation of results should consider, along with the summary treatment effect, the amount of heterogeneity, the risk of bias of the RCTs, and the risk for across study bias such as publication bias. Subgroup analysis and meta-regression or sensitivity analysis can be used to investigate the impact of different characteristics on the treatment effects and the robustness of the results. Comparisons of more than two interventions can be made through network meta-analysis.

Key Facts

- Meta-analysis is the quantitative component of a systematic review.
- The summary effect of the meta-analysis is a weighted average of the study results with weights the inverse of their variance.
- Clinical and methodological heterogeneity across RCTs may be reflected as discrepancies in their treatment effects.

- The choice between fixed and random effects should be made a priori in the protocol.
- Forest plot inspection should take place before interpreting the results of the meta-analysis.
- The risk for within- and across-trial biases as well as potential sources of heterogeneity should be investigated thoroughly before drawing conclusions.

Cross-References

▶ Introduction to Systematic Reviews

References

Borenstein M, Higgins JP (2013) Meta-analysis and subgroups. Prev Sci 14(2):134–143

Borenstein M, Hedges LV, Higgins JP, Rothstein HR (2010) A basic introduction to fixed-effect and random-effects models for meta-analysis. Res Synth Methods 1(2):97–111

Borenstein M, Higgins JP, Hedges LV, Rothstein HR (2017) Basics of meta-analysis: I2 is not an absolute measure of heterogeneity. Res Synth Methods 8(1):5–18

Brunoni AR, Chaimani A, Moffa AH et al (2017) Repetitive transcranial magnetic stimulation for the acute treatment of major depressive episodes: a systematic review with network meta-analysis. JAMA Psychiat 74(2):143–152

Caldwell DM, Ades AE, Higgins JPT (2005) Simultaneous comparison of multiple treatments: combining direct and indirect evidence. BMJ 331(7521):897–900

Chaimani A, Caldwell DM, Li T, Higgins JP, Salanti G (2019) Undertaking network meta-analyses. In: Cochrane handbook for systematic reviews of interventions. Wiley, pp 285–320. https://doi.org/10.1002/9781119536604.ch11

Debray TP, Moons KG, van Valkenhoef G et al (2015) Get real in individual participant data (IPD) meta-analysis: a review of the methodology. Res Synth Methods 6(4):293–309

Deeks JJ, Higgins JP, Altman DG, Group CSM (2019) Analysing data and undertaking meta-analyses. In: Cochrane handbook systematic reviews of interventions. John Wiley & Sons, Ltd; Published online 2019, pp 241–284. https://doi.org/10.1002/9781119536604.ch10

DerSimonian R, Laird N (1986) Meta-analysis in clinical trials. Control Clin Trials 7(3):177–188

Duval S (2005) The trim and fill method. In: Publication bias in meta-analysis prevention assessment and adjustments. John Wiley & Sons, Ltd; Published online, pp 127–144. https://doi.org/10.1002/0470870168.ch8

Efthimiou O (2018) Practical guide to the meta-analysis of rare events. Evid Based Ment Health 21(2):72. https://doi.org/10.1136/eb-2018-102911

Egger M, Smith GD, Schneider M, Minder C (1997) Bias in meta-analysis detected by a simple, graphical test. BMJ 315(7109):629–634

Higgins JP, Thompson SG (2002) Quantifying heterogeneity in a meta-analysis. Stat Med 21(11):1539–1558

Higgins JP, Thomas J, Chandler J et al (2019) Cochrane handbook for systematic reviews of interventions. Wiley, Chichester

Lau J, Antman EM, Jimenez-Silva J, Kupelnick B, Mosteller F, Chalmers TC (1992) Cumulative meta-analysis of therapeutic trials for myocardial infarction. N Engl J Med 327(4):248–254. https://doi.org/10.1056/NEJM199207233270406

Mantel N, Haenszel W (1959) Statistical aspects of the analysis of data from retrospective studies of disease. J Natl Cancer Inst 22(4):719–748

Mavridis D, Salanti G (2014) Exploring and accounting for publication bias in mental health: a brief overview of methods. Evid Based Ment Health 17(1):11. https://doi.org/10.1136/eb-2013-101700

Mavridis D, Chaimani A, Efthimiou O, Leucht S, Salanti G (2014) Addressing missing outcome data in meta-analysis. Evid Based Ment Health 17(3):85–89

Mavridis D, Giannatsi M, Cipriani A, Salanti G (2015) A primer on network meta-analysis with emphasis on mental health. Evid Based Ment Health 18(2):40–46

Moreno SG, Sutton AJ, Turner EH et al (2009a) Novel methods to deal with publication biases: secondary analysis of antidepressant trials in the FDA trial registry database and related journal publications. BMJ b2981:339

Moreno SG, Sutton AJ, Ades AE et al (2009b) Assessment of regression-based methods to adjust for publication bias through a comprehensive simulation study. BMC Med Res Methodol 9(1):2

Moreno SG, Sutton AJ, Ades AE, Cooper NJ, Abrams KR (2011) Adjusting for publication biases across similar interventions performed well when compared with gold standard data. J Clin Epidemiol 64(11):1230–1241

Nikolakopoulou A, Mavridis D, Salanti G (2014) Demystifying fixed and random effects meta-analysis. Evid Based Ment Health 17(2):53. https://doi.org/10.1136/eb-2014-101795

Paule RC, Mandel J (1982) Consensus values and weighting factors. J Res Natl Bur Stand 87(5):377–385

Peters JL, Sutton AJ, Jones DR, Abrams KR, Rushton L (2006) Comparison of two methods to detect publication bias in meta-analysis. JAMA 295(6):676–680

Petropoulou M, Mavridis D (2017) A comparison of 20 heterogeneity variance estimators in statistical synthesis of results from studies: a simulation study. Stat Med 36(27):4266–4280

Pildal J, Hrobjartsson A, Jørgensen KJ, Hilden J, Altman DG, Gøtzsche PC (2007) Impact of allocation concealment on conclusions drawn from meta-analyses of randomized trials. Int J Epidemiol 36(4):847–857

Rhodes KM, Turner RM, Higgins JPT (2015) Predictive distributions were developed for the extent of heterogeneity in meta-analyses of continuous outcome data. J Clin Epidemiol 68(1):52–60. https://doi.org/10.1016/j.jclinepi.2014.08.012

Salanti G (2012) Indirect and mixed-treatment comparison, network, or multiple-treatments meta-analysis: many names, many benefits, many concerns for the next generation evidence synthesis tool. Res Synth Methods 3(2):80–97

Savović J, Jones HE, Altman DG et al (2012) Influence of reported study design characteristics on intervention effect estimates from randomised controlled trials: combined analysis of meta-epidemiological studies. Health Technol Assess 16(35):1–82

Sidik K, Jonkman JN (2007) A comparison of heterogeneity variance estimators in combining results of studies. Stat Med 26(9):1964–1981

Thomas D, Radji S, Benedetti A (2014) Systematic review of methods for individual patient data meta-analysis with binary outcomes. BMC Med Res Methodol 14(1):79

Turner RM, Davey J, Clarke MJ, Thompson SG, Higgins JP (2012) Predicting the extent of heterogeneity in meta-analysis, using empirical data from the Cochrane Database of Systematic Reviews. Int J Epidemiol 41(3):818–827. https://doi.org/10.1093/ije/dys041

Turner RM, Bird SM, Higgins JP (2013) The impact of study size on meta-analyses: examination of underpowered studies in Cochrane reviews. PLoS One 8(3):e59202

Veroniki AA, Jackson D, Viechtbauer W et al (2016) Methods to estimate the between-study variance and its uncertainty in meta-analysis. Res Synth Methods 7(1):55–79. https://doi.org/10.1002/jrsm.1164

Yusuf S, Peto R, Lewis J, Collins R, Sleight P (1985) Beta blockade during and after myocardial infarction: an overview of the randomized trials. Prog Cardiovasc Dis 27(5):335–371

Reading and Interpreting the Literature on Randomized Controlled Trials

111

Janet Wittes

Contents

Introduction	2198
Who Is the Reader?	2199
The Population	2200
Hypothesis	2201
Study Design	2202
Observations	2203
Operations	2203
Adherence and Follow-Up	2203
Outcomes and Multiplicity	2204
Subgroups	2205
The Accompanying Editorial and Other Related Opinions	2205
Some Caveats for Those Who Use Data from a Report to Design Their Own Trials	2206
Summary and Conclusion	2206
Cross-References	2207
References	2208

Abstract

Readers of papers describing the design, methods, or results of randomized controlled trials should exercise critical caution in interpreting what the authors have written. Readers should pay particular attention to important aspects of the design, including the scientific rationale of the study, the choice of control group, the selection of the primary and secondary outcomes, and the planned length of follow-up. In reviewing a paper describing the results of a trial, the reader should ensure that the paper describes the degree of fidelity to the protocol, the amount of missing data along with the methods used to deal with any missing data, the

---

J. Wittes (✉)
Statistics Collaborative, Inc, Washington, DC, USA
e-mail: janet.wittes@statcollab.com

methods of statistical analysis used, and the approaches taken to validate the measurements, the data, and the statistical methods.

Keywords

Bias · Control group · Study design · Study population · Missing data · Statistical methods

Introduction

Confronted with a smorgasbord of medical journals that collectively publish roughly a half million papers per year, how can the potential reader select what articles to tackle and, once having read a paper, how can the reader know that the content is likely to be scientifically valid? The careful reader will realize that the premise of this question is not relevant, because that "half million" includes all published papers in these journals; the more relevant number for this chapter would be the number of research papers that describe aspects of randomized controlled trials. Even that number would be too large; the reader-specific number should be the number of papers in the reader's fields of interest. The first rule of reading the literature is to understand why one has chosen to read a specific paper along with the underlying premise of the paper.

A second rule for reading the literature is to judge whether the conclusions are true (a very important rule that is hard to follow!). Both the scientific and lay press contain warnings concerning papers that proffer conclusions that are false. Indeed, many papers do in fact report results that are not true; sometimes the falsity stems from deliberate misrepresentation of the experiment or the data. More often, the problems arise from poor design or imperfect execution of the study or from the authors' unself-recognized bias. Metrics that purport to identify reliable papers are themselves flawed; for example, many indices measure the frequency that a given paper is cited by others, not the scientific validity of the conclusions. Ostensibly, frequent citation is one indication of the value of a paper; however, papers that present falsified data are often extremely frequently cited both because the results are so surprising – and therefore cited – and then again when the error becomes known. Wakefield's (1999) notorious paper published in the Lancet, claiming that the measles, mumps, and rubella vaccine caused autism was highly influential, leading to a drop-off in vaccinations among children (and a consequent increase in disease). Even though the editor of the Lancet had stated publically that the paper was "utterly false" and that the journal had been "deceived" (Boseley 2010), many internet sites still cite the original Wakefield paper and urge parents not to vaccinate their children (see, for example, the website Age of Autism). Note that the Wakefield paper did not describe a clinical trial or any actual experiment; instead it presented observational data.

Wakefield was not the first, nor the last, medical "researcher" who has published fraudulent results. The year 2018 saw two egregious examples of fraudulent medical research published by professors from leading institutions. Journals retracted 15 papers by Wansik (Resnick and Belluz 2018) of Cornell University and 31 by Anversa of Harvard (Kolata 2018). Both sets of papers had been widely cited before problems with them had been identified. Wansik's "research" dealt with how to present food to decrease caloric intake; Anversa's studies purported to describe stem cell treatment for damaged hearts. Their papers, like Wakefield's, had been published in leading journals; their manuscripts had passed presumably rigorous peer review. Unlike Wakefield's, these papers had described experiments.

These examples are unusual; the errors in most papers with invalid results stem not from fraud but from faulty design, execution, or analysis or from biased interpretation. This chapter provides the reader with tips on how to assess the likely validity of report of a randomized controlled trial. Colton (1974) presents an excellent summary of how to evaluate a medical research paper. The remainder of the chapter refers specifically to randomized controlled trials; the reader addressing a paper that summarizes observational data should use the caveats included here along with even more skepticism regarding possible bias.

Who Is the Reader?

Different readers have different reasons for looking at a paper. Consider five types of readers of clinical journals. Some clinicians read the literature in their eagerness to learn the best treatment for their patients. This class of reader is probably most interested in papers that address an issue relevant to their own patient population. Related to this type of reader is a second type – the public health professional, or the payer, or the hospital pharmacist who is looking to see what medicines to use, to pay for, or to keep in stock. A third type of reader is the patient or a family member who wants to be reasonably certain that their or their family member's clinical care is up-to-date. These readers look to papers on the specific disease of interest to them or the specific drug being prescribed. A fourth type is the researcher wanting to ferret out data from published papers in order to inform the design of a proposed clinical trial. Finally, some people are just curious – they may not have specific need for information but they are generally interested in the state of medical knowledge. Each of these types of reader will attack the literature in a different way, choosing the papers to read and the critical stance taken in a manner consistent with their own purposes.

Several general principles are applicable to all readers. While as described above, some deeply flawed papers are published in excellent journals, and some important papers are found in journals of generally lower rank, a reasonable strategy is to limit one's reading to journals that aim to publish papers only if the journals themselves are of high quality. The journals one should choose to read are those that have a rigorous peer-review system and that are generally recognized as being careful in their selection of articles. A useful rule of thumb is that serving as an arm of a professional society usually indicates seriousness. Always avoid papers that appear in so-called "predatory" journals; these are journals that charge publication fees to authors but provide neither the editorial nor publishing services typical of legitimate journals. Readers thinking of looking at a paper published in one of these journals should resist the temptation. See, for example, the websites http://www.library.stonybrook.edu/scholarly-communication/know-journal-legitimate/ and https://thinkchecksubmit.org for guidance on how to judge whether a journal is legitimate.

Having determined that the journal is respectable, the next step is to decide whether to read the paper and then, once having read it, whether its results are probably reliable. The title and keywords should describe the content of the paper. The abstract, especially if it is a structured abstract, should give a helpful indication of the contents and quality of the paper. The conclusion section should indicate whether the paper is likely to be useful to the reader. Stopping here will be sufficient in many cases – if the reader wants only a general view of what the paper purports to say, these sections – title, keywords, abstract, and conclusion (and maybe the discussion) should suffice. The reader who wants to know how the authors came to their conclusions should read the entire paper, with particular care to understand the population studied, the methods – medical, scientific, and statistical – used, and the limitations of the paper. For the latter, most papers will have a paragraph that starts, "This paper has some limitations." Of course it does – no paper is comprehensive enough to be perfect. The reader should be wary, however, that the described limitations rarely comprise the entire list; other problems may be subtly embedded in the text. It is these problems that the reader must weigh: what are they and whether they are important enough to render the conclusions invalid or inapplicable to the population of interest.

The next sections describe some important parts of reports pertaining to randomized controlled trials. Some of these reports will be papers describing the study design; some will be summaries of the results; and some will describe particular special aspects of the trials.

The Population

The protocol for a randomized controlled trial typically defines the study population through a set of inclusion and exclusion criteria, collectively called the entry criteria. These criteria specify the population to be studied (the inclusion criteria) excluding those who, for one reason or another, should not enter the trial. Sometimes the protocol-defined entry criteria do not accurately characterize the actual study population. This type of issue frequently arises in trials where the upper age range is very high, say a trial of heart failure where the age range is 21 through 85 or even "21 and above." If the actual age range is only 42–78, or the proportion of participants above 75 is low, applying the results to patients above, say 85, is extrapolating beyond the data. Such extrapolation may be valid; the reader should recognize, however, that the exercise is, in fact, extrapolation (Cowan and Wittes 1994).

Now consider the classes of readers mentioned above. The treating physician should look at the entry criteria as well as the actual baseline distribution of the participants in the trials. The population in the trial is relevant to physicians treating patients that fit the entry criteria. On the other hand, suppose the physician's patients come primarily from a frail elderly population and the actual study had very few such participants. Further, because of a host of exclusion criteria, the elderly participants actually in the trial may have been composed of a relatively healthy cohort compared to the average elderly person. In such a situation, the results of the study may not be applicable to the physician's patient cohort. Similar considerations apply to the patient, the public health professional, and the payers. The hospital pharmacist may not care about the details of the entry criteria because stocking the drug may make sense. As for curiosity seekers, as long as they understand the population actually studied, the discordance between the entry criteria and the actual population may not matter.

Hypothesis

Papers describing the design of the trial and those that report the trial's results need to state the primary and important secondary hypotheses clearly; moreover, these hypotheses should be the ones actually described in the protocol. All too often, the protocol-defined hypotheses do not match the hypotheses reported in the paper. Unfortunately, the reader is rarely privy to the protocol so is often unable to know whether what the paper claimed were the initial hypotheses were in fact the prespecified ones. Several journals now require that the authors of a paper reporting the results of a clinical trial supply the protocol and perhaps the statistical analysis plan to the editors so that the reviewers can make sure that the paper's hypotheses are the ones the protocol specified. Websites that register trials often list the primary hypothesis the study was designed to address. Thus, in some situations the interested reader has the ability to check whether what the paper reports comports with the actual design of the study. If it does, the reader can be reassured that the authors did not dredge the data to find hypotheses that matched the findings. On the other hand, the reader should be wary of bias if the prespecified primary hypothesis does not match precisely the hypothesis stated in the paper. (Now this assumes that the reader will have the time and energy to check. Once more, the need for such checking depends on the reason for selecting this particular paper to read.)

Secondary hypotheses are often more difficult to interpret than is the primary hypothesis. Many protocols list a host of secondary hypotheses but the published report of the trial describes only a subset of them, often the subset that show nominally significant p-values. Even when the paper says something like, "These secondary outcomes were prespecified," the skeptical reader may suspect that these were not the only prespecified ones. All too often, the reader is at the mercy of the rigor of the referees and the editors. Fortunately, in the current era, many relevant documents are available as supplementary material on the website associated with the article, which gives the interested reader the tools for matching the plan with the report of the trial.

Study Design

A design paper and a report of a trial should clearly describe the study design. Elements should include such features as the type of randomization, the stratification used, the extent and nature of the blinding, the treatment and control groups, the visit schedule, and the length of follow-up. For studies that are not double blind, this part of the paper should describe whether the assessment of the outcome was performed in a blinded manner. If the design is simple (e.g., a two arm parallel group study), this section can be succinct.

On the other hand, papers reporting on trials with a complicated design need to include enough details so that the reader can understand what actually happened. All too often, perhaps in an attempt to address journal-imposed word limits, papers fail to describe crucial aspects of the design. For example, some studies have built-in strategies for recalculating sample size or they may have other adaptive features. These methods affect the way to estimate the primary outcome and to calculate the final test statistic. Some papers describing the results of many such trials fail to describe this central aspect of the design. The reader who does not read the protocol often has no clue that what appears to be a simple parallel group trial actually had a much more complicated design.

The reader should pay special attention to the control group. Consider two types of controls: placebo and active control. In a two-arm placebo-controlled trial, the typical design specifies that all participants receive the standard of care. Some participants are randomly allocated to placebo and other to the experimental arm. Thus, the question such a trial asks is, "For patients on standard of care, is the experimental treatment superior to placebo?" Some trials mandate the specific standard of care; others leave the decision concerning background therapy to the investigators. In some situations, a small number of standard regimens are in frequent use. Suppose, for example, two common standards are available. Then the design might stratify by type of standard of care. When placebo is the control intervention, interpretation of the results is clear: the estimate and the statistical test will refer to the effect of the experimental intervention relative to placebo. Physicians who use a very different standard of care, however, may question whether the results are relevant to their patients.

A more challenging inferential problem arises in open-label trials where randomization is between the experimental treatment and standard of care. Here the experimental treatment is compared to a heterogeneous control group. In the situation where no standard of care is effective (e.g., in disease characterized by inexorable decline) and the outcome is unambiguous (e.g., mortality), such a design can lead to interpretable results. This design, however, does not allow clear results when a several effective treatments are available.

Active control trials, even when they are double blind, are often more difficult than placebo-controlled trials to interpret, especially if the active control is not the typically used therapy for the condition. Consider, for example, age-related macular degeneration (AMD). In that condition, a recommended regimen for ranibizumab is 0.5 mg administered by intravitreal injection once a month (Lucentis prescribing information 2018). Trials of AMD often use noninferiority designs with the control group defined by an FDA-labeled indication. If such a trial shows noninferiority of the new drug to ranibizumab, the conclusion would be that the new treatment is not unacceptably worse than the labeled regimen of ranibizumab. In practice, however, only a small proportion of patients actually receive monthly injections (Holz et al. 2015). More typical is injection when needed. Readers, in applying the results of such a paper to their patients or themselves, need to interpret the data in terms of a control group that is relevant to them.

Observations

Over the course of a trial, the protocol may specify that the participants make a number of visits to the clinic and that the investigators make many measurements. The paper should describe those measurements clearly. The reader needs to know, for example, what diagnostic criteria were used and how measurements were made.

Operations

Results from a well-run trial are more useful than results from a trial that is operationally weak. The reader should try to glean from the paper information on how faithfully executed the trial was; often such information is hard to learn from the report of a trial.

An important clue into the rigor of the trial is an unambiguous reporting of the number of randomized participants who stopped study intervention during the course of the trial and the number who failed to complete the study. If a large proportion (say more than 10%) of participants did not complete the study, or stopped intervention early, the reader needs to pay careful attention to how the analysis accounted for these participants.

Adherence and Follow-Up

Many well-designed randomized controlled trials suffer an important failure – adherence to the protocol is often less stringent than desirable and many participants fail to complete the trial. These two features, lack of adherence and failure to complete, differ in their inferential implications.

If lack of adherence reflects a true characteristic of the use of the product, and if those who fail to adhere to their assigned regimen are followed for the outcome of interest in the trial, the intent-to-treat analysis may in fact reflect the effect that would be observed in a population not involved in a trial. Some pairings – lack of adherence but full follow-up – are common in trials of interventions for prevention of clinical outcomes. In cardiovascular clinical trials where the outcome is death or myocardial infarction, many people fail to adhere to their therapy but the investigators follow them through the course of the trial. Three examples are trials of hormone therapy (Writing Group for the Women's Health Initiative Investigators 2002), lipid-altering drugs (Ridker et al. 2008), and drugs for patients at high risk for vascular events (ONTARGET Investigators 2008). Similarly, in trials of drugs for prevention of fracture in people with osteopenia or osteoporosis, many people stop taking their assigned medication but the investigators capture their frequency of fracture even after participants have ceased adhering to their regimen. Some of these trials have led to the development of long acting, or slow-release, versions of the intervention on the theory that better adherence would be likely to lead to higher efficacy.

Failure to have complete follow-up is a more serious problem than failure to complete the study regimen because in the absence of data on the study outcome, the investigators are forced to make assumptions, either implicit or explicit, about what the missing observations would have been. When the results are strongly favorable, or strongly unfavorable, and fewer than 10% of the observations in any treatment group are missing, the lack of follow-up data does not pose a serious threat to inference; however, a larger percentage of missing data renders the estimated effect size and the statistical test questionable. In interpreting the results of a trial, the reader should carefully consider how much data are missing and what methods the authors have used to deal with those unmeasured would-be observations. Some analyses commonly reported are anticonservative; that is, they inflate the estimate and decrease the p-value by simply reporting the observed data. One informal rule-of-thumb says that the method used for missing data should not give a larger effect size than seen in the observed data themselves; that is, investigators should not be rewarded for missing data. Another rule of thumb is to devise a strategy for missing values that will discourage investigators from failing to follow participants (Proschan et al. 2001).

Outcomes and Multiplicity

The typical trial has a single primary outcome, one or more secondary outcomes, and a host of exploratory outcomes. Some protocols lump all the nonprimary outcomes into a single category called "secondary." The report of the trial describes results pertinent to the primary outcome and then summarizes the secondaries. If the report fails to give a clue about which of these secondaries were allocated Type I error rate, the reader is at a loss to deduce what results the data rigorously support and what data-dredging has caught. Hiding behind a statement that calls many secondaries "prespecified" is not sufficient – having many hypotheses with no error control is close to not specifying any hypothesis.

If the report describes the results of a clinical trial that has led to drug approval, the label of the drug will distinguish between those secondary hypotheses that the data strongly support from others. The former will constitute claims in the label; the others may be in the clinical trial section of the label. Remember, even careful reviewers are at the mercy of documents; the FDA has access to the actual data. Thus, the label of a drug represents the summary of results written by the two groups that have access to actual data: the sponsor of the trial and the regulators at the FDA. In journals, only the authors and their team member see the actual raw data.

Subgroups

In a rigorous report of a randomized controlled trial, the authors will describe the results of the intention-to-treat analysis, which will generally include all randomized participants, and then often present a summary of the results in subgroups of the population. The paper will often say something like, "Although the effects in subgroups appear to show differences in effect size, the reader should consider these data cautiously." (Such papers fail to tell the reader how to interpret "cautiously.") The sophisticated reader will understand that variability in results by subgroup may reflect true differences in effect, but more often simply reflect the natural variability spawned by small sample sizes.

Sometimes, investigators will write a paper that analyzes only a subgroup and report those results without telling the reader than the overall results of the trial did not show statistically significant evidence of benefit on the entire study population. Readers should be wary of reports of clinical trials that appear to present only a slice of the data from the study as a whole. Sometimes, a paper will present the main results of the trial, but subsequent papers will address individual subgroups or specific prespecified or post hoc analyses. The reader on finding such a paper should be sure to read the main paper as well in order to help interpret the findings of the subsequent paper.

In a few instances, the primary paper will fail to describe certain very important aspects of the trial because they were not prespecified and the journal has a policy not to publish post hoc analyses. In these cases, a subsequent paper may be more useful in interpreting the data than is the primary report of the trial. See, for example, the original report of the TOPCAT trial (Pitt et al. 2014) and an important secondary analysis that put the data in clearer context (Pfeffer et al. 2014).

The Accompanying Editorial and Other Related Opinions

If the paper describes the results of a randomized controlled trial that the editors judge important, perhaps because the intervention is novel or the treatment studied is likely to change practice, the journal may publish an accompanying editorial. Such an opinion piece is often very useful to the reader especially if it reflects the reasoned judgment of an expert in the field who has no conflict of interest. Similarly, press reports (as distinguished from press releases by the authors or the Sponsor of the trial), review papers, discussion at FDA Advisory Committees, reports of treatment guideline committees, and other publications that critically assess the paper, together with the paper itself, provide the interested reader with a range of views. Taken together, the body of discussion related to the paper can help the reader put the results in context.

Some Caveats for Those Who Use Data from a Report to Design Their Own Trials

In describing various types of readers, this chapter mentioned the type of researcher who uses a paper not for its results, but to learn about statistics relevant for planning another trial. In designing a trial, the investigators must make assumptions about such parameters as the effect predicted to be seen in the control group, the likely magnitude of the effect in the treated group, and the expected variability in each. Reports of trials studying the same condition to be investigated in the planned trial will include tables with summary data relevant to some of those assumptions. The reader should be wary of simply plucking out the numbers from tables without first reading the methods part of the paper very carefully to make sure that the parameters in the paper were estimated in an unbiased way. Often the standard deviations reported in papers are smaller than those observed in a future trial because the population studied was more homogeneous than the cohort to be recruited. In some cases, the authors deleted outliers from the data but failed to report their removal. The effect of such deletion may have only a small effect on the mean and, especially, the median; in fact, the measure of central tendency thus produced may be more accurate than the statistic would have been had the outliers been included. On the other hand, such trimming of outliers may unrealistically deflate the true variance. Unwary readers who use the reported variance from a paper as a predictor of the variance in the trial being planned may be in for a rude shock when the actual variance may turn out to be much larger than anticipated. A useful strategy in projecting the variance of the planned primary endpoint is to collect data from several papers, written by different teams of authors, and then to construct one's assumptions conservatively.

Summary and Conclusion

Few papers describing a trial revolutionize treatment; research tends to be incremental. Even the results of major randomized controlled trials often do not tell either the complete story to date or the final story that will emerge. Every paper describing the results of a trial probably was preceded by papers describing the chemistry and biology of the drug, experiments with animals, as well as randomized, or non-randomized, Phase 1 and Phase 2 trials of the product. There may have been reports of other trials with the same drug, perhaps at different doses or different regimens or different populations or that used different outcome measures. There might have been similar trials of a drug in the same class. Thoughtful readers (if they are not too busy) will consider all of these related papers, past and future, in coming to an interpretation of the report of the trial they are currently reading.

After the paper reporting the trial is published, a host of other related papers will appear. Some will be reanalyses of the current paper or analyses of data collected in the trial but not reported in the paper. Some will be extensions of the current paper (can we modify the regimen and still find benefit? Can we add another intervention to yield even more benefit?). Perhaps a study team will try to replicate the result in somewhat different population. Papers may emerge with data from long-term follow-up either of the study group of the primary paper or from observational data in populations using the drug. Relevant information about long-term safety of the drug and rare adverse experiences may emerge. All of these will modify the interpretation of this first paper.

Thus far, the chapter has had a rather negative cast. It has warned readers to be suspicious of what they see in papers because often results are overstated, details are missing, and analyses are not ideal. But that negativity flies in the face of the global changes that have occurred in medicine and public health. Human health has improved over the centuries and even over recent decades. Some of that improvement has been due to better treatments of disease and some to better strategies for prevention (Caldwell et al. 2019). The data from randomized controlled trials have led to a portion of those improvements. So how should one square the negativity of the chapter with the overall improvement?

First, many of the errors, omissions, and misstatements in papers do not overturn the overall results. Consider the classic case of Mendel's peas. Scientists generally concur with the Fisher's (1936) opinion that the monk must have fabricated his data because the data fit his theory too perfectly to be true. Nonetheless, science accepts Mendelian genetics. So as one critically reads a paper, one needs to remember that when one plays "gotcha" with details, one should not necessarily disbelieve the results. The reader should keep in mind that the protocol was probably over 50,000 words long; the statistical analysis plan another 20,000; the complete report may have included hundreds of tables and figures (but many of these were probably unnecessary). The paper distilled that huge amount of information into under 5000 words along with a handful of tables and figures. Authors, in selecting what to include in the paper, are forced to decide what to emphasize and what to ignore. Thus, it is hardly surprising that a hypercritical reader can almost always find something with which to quibble.

The critical reader should be just that; "critical" not in the sense of quick to find fault, but rather in the more positive sense of exercising careful, detailed judgment.

Cross-References

▶ Estimation and Hypothesis Testing
▶ Fraud in Clinical Trials
▶ Intention to Treat and Alternative Approaches
▶ Missing Data
▶ Paper Writing
▶ Principles of Clinical Trials: Bias and Precision Control
▶ Reporting Biases
▶ Trials Can Inform or Misinform: "The Story of Vitamin A Deficiency and Childhood Mortality"

References

Age of Autism: daily web newspaper of the autism epidemic. https://www.ageofautism.com/. Accessed 20 Jan 2019

Boseley S (2010) Lancet retracts 'utterly false' MMR paper. The Guardian. https://www.theguardian.com/society/2010/feb/02/lancet-retracts-mmr-paper. Accessed 20 Jan 2019

Caldwell M, Martinez M, Foster JC et al (2019) Prospects for the primary prevention of myocardial infarction and stroke. J Cardiovasc Pharmacol Ther 24:207–214

Colton T (1974) Statistics in medicine. Little Brown and Company, Boston

Cowan C, Wittes J (1994) Intercept studies, clinical trials, and cluster experiments: to whom can we extrapolate? Control Clin Trials 15:24–29

Fisher RA (1936) Annals Sci.1.115. Reprinted in: Stern C, Sherwood ER (eds) (1966) The origin of genetics; a Mendel source book. W.H. Freeman, San Francisco/London

Genentech (2018) Lucentis prescribing information. https://www.gene.com/download/pdf/lucentis_prescribing.pdf. Accessed 26 Jan 2019

Holz FG, Tadayoni R, Beatty S et al (2015) Multi-country real-life experience of anti-vascular endothelial growth factor therapy for wet age-related macular degeneration. Br J Opthalmol 99:220–226

Kolata G (2018) Harvard calls for retraction of dozens of studies by noted cardiac researcher. New York Times. https://www.nytimes.com/2018/10/15/health/piero-anversa-fraud-retractions.html. Accessed 20 Jan 2019

ONTARGET Investigators (2008) Telmisartan, ramipril, or both in patients at high risk for vascular events. N Engl J Med 358:1547–1559

Pfeffer MA, Clagget B, Assman SF et al (2014) Regional variation in patients and outcomes in the treatment of preserved cardiac function heart failure with an aldosterone antagonist (TOPCAT) Trial. Circulation 131:34–42

Pitt B, Pfeffer MA, Assman SF et al (2014) Spironolactone for heart failure with preserved ejection fraction. N Engl J Med 370:1383–1392

Proschan M, McMahon R, Shih J et al (2001) Sensitivity analysis using an imputation method for missing binary data in clinical trials. J Stat Plan Inference 96:155–165

Resnick B, Belluz J (2018) A top Cornell food researcher has had 15 studies retracted. Vox. That's a lot. https://www.vox.com/science-and-health/2018/9/19/17879102/brian-wansink-cornell-food-brand-lab-retractions-jama. Accessed 20 Jan 2019

Ridker PM, Danielson E, Fonseca FAH et al for the JUPITER Study Group (2008) Rosuvastatin to prevent vascular events in men and women with elevated C-reactive protein. N Engl J Med 359:2195–2207

Stony Brook University. http://www.library.stonybrook.edu/scholarly-communication/know-journal-legitimate/. Accessed 31 Jan 2019

Think. Check submit. https://thinkchecksubmit.org. Accessed 26 Jan 2019

Wakefield AJ (1999) MMR vaccination and autism. Lancet 354:949–950

Writing Group for the Women's Health Initiative Investigators (2002) Risks and benefits of estrogen plus progestin in healthy postmenopausal women. JAMA 288:321–333

Trials Can Inform or Misinform: "The Story of Vitamin A Deficiency and Childhood Mortality"

112

Alfred Sommer

Contents

Introduction	2210
Setting the Stage	2211
Origins of the Issue: An Unexpected Epidemiologic Observation	2211
The First Randomized Community Clinical Trial Testing the Impact of Improving Vitamin A Status on Subsequent Childhood Mortality	2211
Confirming RCT	2212
Hospital-Based RCT of Measles Mortality in Tanzania	2213
Other Investigators Join the Hunt (Ignoring Truly Miserable Attempts!)	2213
An Initial Foray, in the Sudan, Suffered from Deficient Design and Compromised Execution	2213
Replication RCT that was Under-Resourced, Overly Complicated, Under-Supervised, and (Initially) Misinterpreted But Looked Perfectly Respectable When Published	2214
Replication RCT, Madurai, India: Confusing Clinical with Statistical Significance	2214
"The Million Child Trial" DEVTA Study	2217
Expanding the New Paradigm to Solve Adjacent Public Health Problems – Excess Maternal Mortality in Low-Income Populations: Perfect Symmetry – Misunderstood	2219
Dosing Newborns: Controversy and Context Continue to Confound	2221
Conclusion	2221
Key Facts	2221
Cross-References	2222
References	2222

Abstract

This "case study" documents the ways in which a variety of epidemiologic studies and the data they generated (which challenged existing beliefs and public

A. Sommer (✉)
Johns Hopkins Bloomberg School of Public Health, Baltimore, MD, USA
e-mail: asommer@jhu.edu

health constructs) were greeted by established "experts" in relevant fields. Just as Virchow described over a century ago, results of an initial observational study, which raised the issues, were entirely ignored. Prominent publication of a randomized clinical trial, which both supported the observational study's associations and proved that they were causal, was greeted with intense hostility, disbelief, and rejection. Only the subsequent accrual of additional, similar RCTs slowly changed scientific opinion, especially when replications were eventually conducted by others than the original investigators. A halt was brought to this slowly changing scientific climate by the timely gathering of those involved in a week-long meeting that evaluated the quality and interpretation of all available data and discussed their relevance and validity. That many investigators had not understood the importance of the context in which their own studies had been conducted was startling, particularly regarding the two variables of greatest relevance: the study population's baseline risk of vitamin A deficiency and mortality. Investigators of some of the best conducted studies misinterpreted their own data. The resulting 10-year effort eventually changed global health policy, but some "deniers," without a shred of evidence to back their claims, still refuse to accept this outcome.

Keywords

Observational studies · Randomized clinical trials · Controversies · Contradictory evidence · Context · Interpretation · Scientific acceptance · Persistent disagreement · Public health policy

Introduction

The ultimate purpose of most randomized clinical trials (RCTs), whether explicitly stated or not, is to investigate whether a new therapeutic or preventive intervention is superior to the prevailing form of treatment or existing health policies. Whether or not a positive trial actually changes clinical practice or public policy depends upon numerous factors, sometimes simply the inflexibility of established "wisdom." Virchow recognized this over a century ago, when he advised that new knowledge is often greeted in the same way as "bad news": at first it is ignored; when subsequently supported by additional data, the whole premise is attacked; when the data become irrefutable, these same "experts" claim it is nothing new – "we've known this all along" (Sommer 1997).

This is a case study of how epidemiologic data and RCTs in one area of nutrition were repeatedly ignored and misinterpreted; how poorly conducted trials appeared peerless in published form; how perfectly good trial data were misinterpreted, by both the authors and the journal's editors; the importance of "context," which was often ignored in the interpretation of study data; and a striking instance in which "clever" trial design trumped quality and interpretation.

I've been blessed with a long and productive career in clinical and population epidemiologic research (McCarthy 2005). While my investigations have covered a wide variety of health issues (proving that I'm motivated more by curiosity than by design), I'm most closely associated with the question and policy implications of the relationship between vitamin A status and childhood mortality (Sommer 1997). The latter arose from a wholly unanticipated observation.

Setting the Stage

Origins of the Issue: An Unexpected Epidemiologic Observation

A series of three inter-related studies were conducted in Indonesia between 1976 and 1979, primarily to document clinically important aspects of the ocular disease, *xerophthalmia* (literally, "dry eye"), which was thought to be responsible for large numbers of children going blind in the developing world (Sommer 1982). Medical experts long knew that xerophthalmia was caused by vitamin A deficiency. The clinical manifestations of deficiency were universally associated with this ocular disease. The mildest manifestation was thought to be "nightblindness," whereby "mildly deficient" children could not see at dusk or early dawn, followed, with more severe deficiency, by foamy accretions of keratinized material on the surface of the eye ("Bitot's spots"). These were known to be entirely reversible with vitamin A treatment. The most serious manifestation, associated with severe vitamin A deficiency, was corneal ulceration, which inevitably left corneal scarring if treated quickly and blindness if not.

One of those 3 inter-related Indonesian studies followed 3500 children, 6 months to 5 years of age, in 6 villages, who were examined at baseline and again every 3 months for 18 months (seven examinations). Each examination included an assessment of the families' economic status (inevitably poor or poorer) and a dietary and clinical history, pediatric and ophthalmic examination, and the biochemical (vitamin A) status of the child. The original purpose was to identify factors that distinguished those children who would go on to develop mild xerophthalmia from their village peers.

Analysis revealed a wholly unexpected finding: "mild" xerophthalmia was associated with increased mortality over the succeeding 3 months and the more advanced the degree of xerophthalmia, the higher the subsequent mortality (by factors of three- to eightfold) (Sommer et al. 1983). Tellingly, this publication did not elicit a single letter to the editor, nor any interest, by others, to further investigate the reproducibility of this apparent association, its potential causality, or its possible clinical and policy implications.

The First Randomized Community Clinical Trial Testing the Impact of Improving Vitamin A Status on Subsequent Childhood Mortality

The opportunity existed to test whether the apparent association between vitamin A status and early childhood mortality was real, and, if so, causal, at relatively low cost. The Indonesian government had already decided to begin twice-annual vitamin A supplementation (200,000 IU) of children 1–5 years of age in an area of Sumatra identified as the most seriously vitamin A deficient. While the government would not countenance the use of a placebo in testing the benefits of this approach, they did allow us to randomize the order in which the villages were enrolled in the program. Specially trained teams, unrelated to the government program, mapped and enumerated all households in the 400 study villages. Half the villages had been randomly assigned to enter the program over the course of that year, and half the following year 1 month before government teams distributed vitamin A supplements. The two groups of villages contained 25,000 children who were between 1 and 5 years of age. Within 1 month of each of the two distribution cycles, by government workers, the specially trained and supervised, independent study teams determined that over 80% of all children in the villages assigned to the dosing program had actually received at least one large dose. The study teams returned to each village 1 year later to ascertain the status of the children enumerated at the start of the study. The conservative estimate of the impact of the distribution program (all deaths of children identified at baseline, whether or not they had actually received a supplement) was a 34% reduction in mortality over the 12 months since baseline enumeration (Sommer et al. 1986). Adjusting for those who did not receive the vitamin A supplement, the reduction in mortality exceeded 70% (Tarwotjo et al. 1987; Sommer and Zeger 1991).

Despite (or because of) a supportive accompanying editorial (Lancet 1986), this publication elicited an outpouring of letters to the editor (Martinez et al. 1986); none of which were supportive. No group attempted to prove or disprove these findings, presumably because they fell outside the range of beliefs about the origin(s) of excessive childhood morbidity and mortality in deprived populations of low-income countries.

Confirming RCT

As it was estimated that vitamin A deficiency might well be responsible for half a million children being blinded every year (Sommer et al. 1981), and now, possibly, even many more dying unnecessarily, we carried out a second RCT in Nepal. In this instance, village wards were randomized for their pre-school children to receive either 200,000 IU vitamin A or identical-looking placebos every 4 months. The study had to be discontinued after four rounds because of a highly statistically significant (SS) reduction of 30% mortality among children in the vitamin A recipient villages. To solidify these findings, two more distribution rounds were conducted, in which unbeknownst to the teams vitamin A supplements were substituted for the placebos, such that all recipient children actually received vitamin A. Confirming the initial results, the subsequent childhood mortality in the original placebo villages fell to the same rates as in the vitamin A villages (West et al. 1991). "Oral autopsies" of childhood deaths in this study revealed that the greatest reduction in mortality was attributable to deaths from diarrhea and measles (each reduced by roughly 50%).

The few letters to the editor were more balanced than they had been for the previous trial.

Hospital-Based RCT of Measles Mortality in Tanzania

The unanticipated observation that many of the children hospitalized with measles in Mvumi, Tanzania, were developing corneal ulcers and blindness led to the documentation that many of these complications were the result of previously unrecognized vitamin A deficiency (Foster and Sommer 1987). Given the high (roughly 15%) mortality of hospitalized measles cases, a relatively small therapeutic RCT was initiated: all children hospitalized with measles, who did not have ocular involvement (such cases were immediately treated with vitamin A), were randomized to receive either one large oral dose of vitamin A on admission and again the following day or only routine therapy. Those receiving vitamin A died at only half the rate of those who didn't (Barclay et al. 1987).

A 50% reduction in mortality, related to either treatment of acute measles or community-based vitamin A supplementation prior to developing measles, soon approached the regularity of Avogadro's number! Vitamin A supplementation does not appear to reduce the incidence of measles infection, only its clinical severity and resultant mortality.

Other Investigators Join the Hunt (Ignoring Truly Miserable Attempts!)

An Initial Foray, in the Sudan, Suffered from Deficient Design and Compromised Execution

An early RCT by another team was launched in the Sudan (Herrera et al. 1992). An unfortunate choice, given the available study population, recurrent political upheavals, and an unforeseeable flood.

Using household (rather than village) randomization, the study population differed greatly from Indonesia and Nepal and many other trials that followed. Rather than being a truly "deprived" population, half the households had indoor plumbing, and fewer than 7% of the children suffered "wasting" malnutrition. The actual conduct was, to some degree, difficult to document: the Principle Investigator was unable to obtain a visa to enter the country during the entire conduct of the trial (Herrera 1992, personal communication). Making matters worse, the study area suffered a prolonged flood, during which NGOs distributed large-dose vitamin A to children throughout the study site. Not surprisingly, there was no difference in the subsequent incidence of xerophthalmia between the two arms of the trial, nor in their risk of death, both consistent with potential contamination of the assigned supplement across the two arms of the trial and the relatively low, overall, 1–5-year mortality. The investigators were sufficiently surprised by the results that they reported that children having greater vitamin A intake from a combination of dietary sources and the study supplements (they had no documentation of which children received supplements during NGO-relief activities) suffered fewer deaths than those with less vitamin A intake from all sources (Fawzi et al. 1994).

Replication RCT that was Under-Resourced, Overly Complicated, Under-Supervised, and (Initially) Misinterpreted But Looked Perfectly Respectable When Published

This highly publicized, village-cluster RCT, conducted by the Indian Research Council's National Nutrition Research Institute, in Hyderabad, India, suffered several serious limitations (Vijayaraghavan et al. 1990). One of the most serious was vastly insufficient resources (a problem which will recur in the "Million Child Trial," discussed later); the Indian Council for Medical Research severely restricted the funds they were allowed to employ (less than $100,000 versus the several million dollars spent on both the Indonesian and Nepal trials). The Achilles heel of the quality of any community-based, large-scale RCT involving over 10,000 children in rural, remote areas is the ability to ensure high-quality data collection; and that, in turn, depends upon careful, repeated training, testing, validating, and supervising the work of hundreds of field workers, something difficulty if not impossible to ensure on so limited a budget. Exacerbating the situation, "trained" field and medical workers visited each family on a frequent basis, advising all those whose children appeared ill to seek medical attention – thereby inducing a serious Hawthorne effect (studying a problem inevitably alters its outcome), a problem identified in an accompanying editorial (Lancet 1990) and several letters to the editor (Sommer and West 1991).

The published results showed only a modest (6%), non-SS reduction in mortality among the (allegedly) supplemented children.

Despite all these shortcomings, this RCT is regularly included in most major meta-analyses of the impact of vitamin A supplementation on childhood survival.

Replication RCT, Madurai, India: Confusing Clinical with Statistical Significance

This well-designed and conducted trial in Madurai, India, employed a different dosing schedule – one not suited to policy implications but likely yielding maximum potential benefits of supplementation. Rather than supplement 1–5-year-olds with one large dose twice a year, they supplemented every child in the vitamin A arm with a weekly dose – weekly. This would maximize the potential benefit of improving vitamin A status: re-visiting children weekly dramatically reduces the number of children in the active arm likely to miss their vitamin A supplementation, since they have many more chances to be home and receive at least some supplement than they would with dosing once every 4 or 6 months; weekly dosing with relatively small doses of vitamin A also maximizes retention, thereby better improving vitamin A status and liver stores. Less than half the large, twice-yearly dose is retained and stored in the liver for later use; serum retinol levels rise rapidly following a single, large, twice-yearly dose, but retinol levels return to baseline values within 2–3 months. Giving smaller, weekly doses causes a slow, gradual, but steady increase in liver stores and serum retinol levels and is therefore likely to have a more profound impact (though it is impractical as a population-based intervention). Indeed, this particular RCT, with its weekly dosing, yielded the greatest impact: those assigned to vitamin A died at less than half the rate of those assigned the placebo.

Now the confusion begins. The quality of the study, and size of its impact, earned it a lead in the *New England Journal of Medicine* (Rahmathullah et al. 1990). The study's results agreed with virtually every finding in the Indonesian and Nepalese RCTs, and the hospital treatment trial in Tanzania (which they apparently did not understand, calling it a "case-control" study), save one: they did not, they concluded, find any impact of vitamin A supplementation on measles mortality. They offered several potential explanations for why their results might have differed so dramatically from ours: perhaps, they posited, measles was very different in India than it was in sub-Saharan Africa or Nepal; the protein-energy nutritional status of the populations might have differed; or the large, twice-yearly "mega-doses" we had employed acted differently than the small, weekly doses they used (which should have increased their impact!).

This important article was accompanied by a very supportive editorial (Keusch 1990), one in which the author explains that he has changed his views, and now accepts the importance of vitamin A status, and the impact of vitamin A supplementation on childhood mortality in deficient populations. But he, too, highlights the unexpected absence of any impact on measles mortality and how that differs from the previously referenced trials. He offers the same list of explanations for this seemingly important discrepancy. Who knows how many readers, policy makers, and other investigators decided, on this evidence, to dismiss the potential impact of vitamin A status on the clinical severity and mortality of measles?

Fortunately for science – though not for those who failed to study the article or editorial closely – the actual numbers of deaths, by cause (ascertained from "verbal autopsies"), were provided (Table 1). As can be readily seen, 12 children died of measles in the control arm; and 7 in the vitamin A arm. One could hardly have come closer to a 50% reduction! Had the authors (and editorialist) understood simple statistics, they would have worded their conclusions quite differently: "our results are compatible with previous reports that vitamin A supplementation of deficient children can dramatically reduce subsequent measles mortality, but the numbers were small and not statistically significant."

By 1992, essentially all the well-funded, well-designed, and well-executed RCTs, including an excellent population-based study in Ghana (Ghana VAST Study Team 1993), where malaria was prevalent, and impacted, by vitamin A supplementation, had been published. Their findings were further bolstered by a large number of hospital- and field-based clinical and immunologic studies. The "never-ending"

Table 1 Symptom- and disease-specific mortality, according to treatment group

Symptoms or disease	Control group No. of children	Treated group	Relative risk[a]
Measles	12	7	0.58 (0.17, 1.92)
Diarrhea	33	16	0.48 (0.24, 0.96)[b]
Respiratory	3	2	–
Malnutrition	1	1	–
Convulsions	12	3	0.25 (0.07, 0.85)[b]
Other	19	6	0.31 (0.12, 0.78)[b]
Total deaths	80	37	

Originally published in Rahmathullah et al. (1990)
[a]Relative risk for the treated group, as compared with the control group. Values in parentheses are 95% confidence limits
[b]$P = 0.05$

debate about the importance of vitamin A's influence on infectious morbidity and mortality was brought to a definitive conclusion (as far as major agencies and respected scientists and clinicians were concerned) at a small (23-person) workshop held at Villa Serbelloni (the Rockefeller Foundation's study retreat in Bellagio, Italy) (Bellagio 1993). The assembled experts in child survival, nutrition, statistics, and epidemiology were charged with reviewing all available data to answer four critical questions: (1) Did vitamin A deficiency increase infectious mortality among malnourished children? (2) Did twice-yearly supplementation (or any other approach that improved vitamin A status) of children 1–5 years of age significantly reduce their mortality? (3) Was vitamin A deficiency particularly important in measles mortality? (4) Should all children from potentially deficient populations receive vitamin A supplementation as a routine part of their treatment for measles? By the end of the week, the group unanimously agreed with each of these propositions, many returning home to publish these conclusions. One such report was published in the *Lancet* (Sommer 1992).

Less than a year after the Bellagio meeting, the World Health Organization and UNICEF, supported by outside donors (particularly Canada), embarked on a global program to improve the vitamin A status of 1–5-year-olds in deficient populations – in effect, almost all children in rural Asia, Africa, and Central and South America (UNICEF 2007).

A new paradigm had emerged, in which it was now understood that the earliest clinical impact of vitamin A deficiency was an impaired immune response, which increases the severity and lethality of infectious disease, and that even the mildest ocular manifestations, nightblindness and Bitot's spots, only emerge with more severe deficiency (Fig. 1) (Sommer and West 1996; Sommer 1997).

A Global Program Launched

Within 1 year of the Bellagio meeting, the Director General of the World Health Organization and the Executive Director of UNICEF launched a "global program" to curtail the ravages of vitamin A deficiency among pre-school-age children.

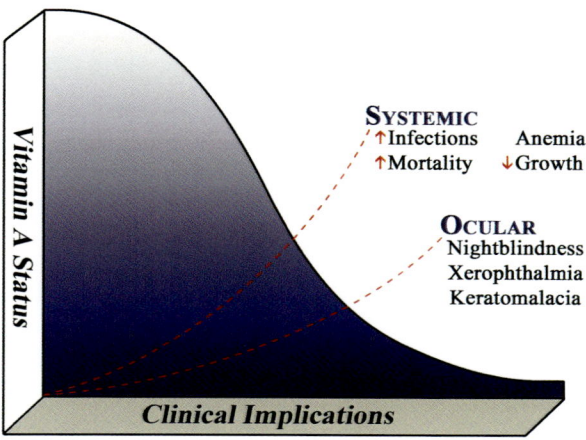

Fig. 1 Schematic representation of temporal relationship between decline in vitamin A status and onset of systemic and ocular complications. (Originally published in Sommer A (1997); with kind permission of *Nature Medicine* (Springer Nature). All rights reserved)

Over 50 low- and middle-income countries adopted twice-annual vitamin A supplementation as the most practical strategy for improving the vitamin A status of 1–5-year-old children in vitamin A-deficient populations. Some countries were able to employ alternative strategies for improving vitamin A intake, like the fortification of sugar, a staple product consumed by most of the population. This global program is now well into its third decade and is estimated, by UNICEF, to be saving the lives (and sight) of 350,000 children every year. The number would be still larger if coverage rates were higher. Both the World Bank and the Copenhagen Consensus have estimated that vitamin A supplementation is one of the most cost-effective of all health interventions. The program has made considerable progress, but still falls short of its full potential (Hamer and Keusch 2015).

"The Million Child Trial" DEVTA Study

A trial that was not a "trial" and certainly not an RCT – but whose results were reported as if it were, creating considerable controversy and confusion among health planners and policy makers.

Nearly a decade after the "global program" was launched, a senior, highly respected epidemiologist/statistician from Oxford had (what he conceived as) a brilliant idea: undertake an extremely low-cost, opportunistic, and uniquely large – on the basis of the number of potential "participants" – "trial" of the impact that vitamin A distribution with or without albendazole would have on child mortality in the desperately poor Indian state of Uttar Pradesh (Awasthi et al. 2013). Large blocks of villages in poverty-stricken Uttar Pradesh were "randomized" to be either "vitamin A blocks" (vitamin A with or without albendazole was provided to the local health centers – called Anganwadi Centers or AWCs – that were "officially" staffed by a local worker) or "control blocks" (AWCs that were not provided vitamin A).

Note that according to an official Indian evaluation, fewer than two-thirds of all such centers in Uttar Pradesh are actually staffed at any one time and fewer than 22% of the children under 6 years ever receive any intervention. The areas included in the study contained 1 million children 1–5 years of age; since an annual cohort entered and left each year, this 5-year study reports results on roughly 2 million children (and 5 million child-years of study).

However, with only $250,000 to spend on the entire enterprise (versus millions of dollars spent on each of the previous studies of roughly 20,000 children each, generally over 1–2 years), they conducted no mapping, no census, and enumerated no families or their children, the reason the publication lacks a CONSORT diagram (Awasthi et al. 2013; personal communication, University of Oxford Clinical Trials Service Unit 2008). Nor did they hire, pay, train, or supervise teams to distribute the supplements; only 18 study monitors provided ongoing supervision of the roughly 8400 local workers purportedly staffing these centers (463 workers per supervisor) or validate their supplement coverage. All capsule distribution relied on listings maintained by the local Anganwadi workers, who had received, at most, half a day's training, with no follow-up testing and little if any supervision. These workers were also responsible for alerting a "flying squad" of motorcycle riders any time that a child died in their village, in order to confirm the death. The "flying squad" had never visited any of the houses previously and had no independent census listing the children who'd previously been born or lived in the households.

At the end of 5 years, and an alleged 5 million children-years of "observation," they concluded that vitamin A supplementation had no impact on 1–5-year-old child mortality. Despite the absence of any reasonable standards of control and oversight – they spent roughly 5 cents per child-year of "observation," roughly one-2000th that of the other trials – they performed a meta-analysis, in which the enormous "sample size" (as they describe it) of their "study" overwhelmed the results of all the positive, carefully conducted RCTs that had preceded it. They generously concluded that the meta-analysis could not rule out a "modest" impact, of perhaps 11% (Confidence Interval [CI]: 5–16%). Not surprisingly, the study also failed to find any impact of deworming with albendazole, contradicting prior RCTs of that intervention.

Astonishingly, the *Lancet* was unstinting in its praise of this poorly conducted "trial," blaming any (and all) concern within the wider scientific community on "belief disconfirmation bias" (Garner et al. 2013). The *Lancet* editorial extolled the "simplicity" and "size" as "definitive," ignoring problems in the study's design and execution or even its context: one small area of India. Of the few among many letters received by the *Lancet* that were published, some highlighted the study's many failings as a purported "trial" (Sommer et al. 2013), while others noted how it did not even meet the standards expected of a valid evaluation of a programmatic effort (Habicht and Victora 2013). The real tragedy was that the study publication, and supportive *Lancet* editorial, caused considerable confusion and consternation among health planners and ministries, who began questioning the value and necessity of their vitamin A policies and programs.

Fortunately, the serious limitations of the DEVTA "study" were soon widely recognized, and its publication had only a transitory impact on the progress of the global vitamin A supplementation program. Bizarrely, there are those who still stridently claim that supplementation is not only useless, but actually harmful, despite the lack of supporting evidence from any reputably conducted trial (Delisle 2018).

The global program's biggest constraint, as expressed both by an editorial in the *Lancet* (Hamer and Keusch 2015) and by UNICEF (its lead international agency) (UNICEF 2018), is that coverage rates fall short of what is needed, in part because of the limited means by which the supplements can be efficiently distributed and administered to the target population. Nutrition researchers recognize that more efficient means of improving vitamin A status of deficient populations are needed, potentially including the use of genetically modified crops.

Why studies in low- and middle-income countries, particularly those addressing issues critical to the health of disadvantaged populations, are so often poorly designed and conducted – but still published in reputable peer-reviewed journals – remains a mystery. Fortunately, insights into the importance of improving the vitamin A status of deficient children have weathered the tribulations of naysayers and poor science; in fact, global policy changed in a relatively short time: it took barely a decade between publication of our original observational study demonstrating the apparent association between vitamin A status and mortality (1983) and the launch of the global program to correct the problem (1993).

These results encouraged us, and others, to explore the potential implications of vitamin A deficiency, and its correction, at other stages of life. Those studies have proved equally interesting (and contentious); despite what would appear to be adequate evidence for rational policies, they have yet to yield any sustainable commitment to action. The greatest obstacles are once again the failure to recognize the importance of context – the health and nutritional status of the population being addressed – and an inability to properly interpret one's own results. Two such life stages are discussed, briefly, below: the potential benefits of improving the vitamin A status of deficient, pregnant women who experience high maternal mortality; and the potential for reducing infant mortality by supplementing vitamin A-deficient newborns – the time of highest childhood mortality.

Expanding the New Paradigm to Solve Adjacent Public Health Problems – Excess Maternal Mortality in Low-Income Populations: Perfect Symmetry – Misunderstood

Poor women in nutritionally deprived populations are at increased risk of vitamin A deficiency, particularly during their third trimester of pregnancy. Might improving their vitamin A status reduce the risk of death in populations with high maternal mortality? We approached this question by conducting an RCT in the same, deprived population in Nepal in which we had carried out the earlier pre-school-aged child mortality study. Because large, "mega" doses of vitamin A can be teratogenic, and because the nutrition community insisted that improving dietary sources of vitamin A ("pro-vitamin A beta-carotene," the primary source of vitamin A available from fruits and vegetables) was a "natural" long-term solution, women of childbearing age were randomized to receive on a weekly basis a small (7000 µg) vitamin A supplement, a retinol-equivalent amount of beta-carotene, or placebo. All-cause maternal mortality during pregnancy and up to 12 weeks post-partum was reduced by a SS 40% among those randomized to receive vitamin A, and a SS 49% among those randomized to receive a retinol-equivalent amount of beta-carotene, for a SS average reduction among those receiving either form of vitamin A of 44% (West et al. 1999).

As positive as this trial appeared, no policy makers would act without a confirming RCT.

We conducted a nearly identical RCT in a nearby population in Bangladesh no more than a few hundred miles away – as the crow flies, whose (government supplied) health statistics were similar to those of the study population in Nepal (West et al. 2011).

Approximately 80% of women in the Bangladesh study consumed at least 94% of their assigned supplement (weekly vitamin A, beta-carotene, or placebo).

In contrast to the results of the Nepal study, neither vitamin A nor beta-carotene supplementation caused an appreciable reduction in pregnancy-related maternal mortality! A number of commentators concluded that this "disproved" the value of vitamin A supplementation of pregnant women. In fact, it "proved the rule"!

The government health data on rural Bangladeshi women upon which we planned the study was clearly outdated, at least as far as this population of women was concerned: the Bangladeshi women were less than a third as likely as their Nepalese counterparts to be vitamin A deficient; consumed a more nutritious diet; were half as likely to suffer wasting malnutrition; were twice as likely to be delivered by a trained birth-attendant; and experienced a maternal mortality (in the placebo group) less than one-third that of the Nepalese. Clearly, this population of women were far better off than existing Bangladesh statistics suggested and were now considerably healthier and better nourished than those we had studied only a few years earlier in nearby Nepal. Context matters! The Bangladesh study did not disprove the potential value of improving the vitamin A status of vitamin A-deficient women suffering particularly high pregnancy-related mortality; instead, it confirmed that supplementing populations with lower pregnancy-related mortality and better vitamin A status would likely make little difference! Had it dramatically reduced maternal mortality in Bangladesh, we would have been hard-pressed to explain the results!

A similar study, among Ghanaian women, who were also better nourished, suffered far lower pregnancy-related mortality, and had less vitamin A deficiency than the women in Nepal, was understandably also negative (Kirkwood et al. 2010). Taken together, these studies should have helped to sharply define those populations in which vitamin A supplementation of women of childbearing age might have reduced needless maternal mortality. Instead, the value (and limitations) of a potentially effective, life-saving, inexpensive intervention has proved contentious, and the potential benefits of thoughtful, targeted intervention have been largely ignored (WHO 2017).

Dosing Newborns: Controversy and Context Continue to Confound

There is now active discussion about the value of dosing newborn children with vitamin A to reduce infant mortality. Studies in India (Mazumder et al. 2015; Tielsch et al. 2007) and Bangladesh (Klemm et al. 2008), where newborn mortality is high and vitamin A deficiency is prevalent, have shown a roughly (SS) 12% reduction in infant mortality (a time at which mortality is highest, and therefore the absolute impact greatest). Similar studies in two African countries, where mortality is lower and vitamin A deficiency far less prevalent and severe, were negative. Yet ongoing discussions, meta-analyses, and unpublished recommendations are treating these as identical trials, despite dramatic differences in the relevant characteristics of the study populations. "Experts" continue to ignore (or simply don't understand) the importance of **context**; one would not recommend routine cataract surgery in patients who lack cataracts or bypass surgery in patients without coronary artery disease!

Conclusion

RCTs are only as good as their design and conduct. They are also only as good as their interpretation and the degree to which "policy experts" understand, interpret, and rationally apply the totality of the "information" they provide, though nothing appears to prevent senior "experts" from continuing to deny the obvious, even after it has been adopted as global policy (UNICEF 2018; Latham 2010).

Key Facts

- Observational studies can yield important, unanticipated outcomes.
- Pursuing unanticipated epidemiologic outcomes often leads to important contributions to biomedical knowledge.
- Randomized clinical trials can be a powerful means of corroborating associations found in observational studies and proving causal relationships.
- The "context" in which epidemiologic studies are conducted can powerfully influence their outcome.
- Unanticipated relationships are often initially rejected by subject experts, because they challenge established wisdom and scientific consensus.
- Persistence is critical in overcoming existing "wisdom" and best accomplished by "burying opponents in data" rather than with arguments and "debates."
- This author believes that whenever epidemiologic data suggest new or alternative prevention and treatment paradigms, the investigator is ethically bound to continue to study the matter, until they either disprove their own initial results or prove them, and change medical practice accordingly.

Cross-References

▶ Adherence Adjusted Estimates in Randomized Clinical Trials
▶ Causal Inference: Efficacy and Mechanism Evaluation
▶ Clinical Trials in Children
▶ Consent Forms and Procedures
▶ Cross-over Trials
▶ End of Trial and Close Out of Data Collection
▶ Intention to Treat and Alternative Approaches
▶ Interim Analysis in Clinical Trials
▶ International Trials
▶ Introduction to Systematic Reviews
▶ Investigator Responsibilities
▶ Issues for Masked Data Monitoring
▶ Issues in Generalizing Results from Clinical Trials
▶ Introduction to Meta-Analysis
▶ Participant Recruitment, Screening, and Enrollment
▶ Power and Sample Size
▶ Prevention Trials: Challenges in Design, Analysis, and Interpretation of Prevention Trials
▶ Publications from Clinical Trials
▶ Randomized Selection Designs
▶ Reading and Interpreting the Literature on Randomized Controlled Trials
▶ Reporting Biases
▶ Selection of Study Centers and Investigators
▶ Study Name, Authorship, Titling, and Credits

References

Awasthi S, Peto R, Read S, Clark S, Pande V (2013) Vitamin A supplementation every 6 months with retinol in 1 million pre-school children in North India: DEVTA, a cluster-randomised trial. Lancet 381(9876):1469–1477

Barclay AJG, Foster A, Sommer A (1987) Vitamin A supplements and mortality related to measles: a randomised clinical trial. Br Med J 294(6567):294–296

Bellagio Meeting on vitamin A Deficiency and Childhood Mortality (1993) Proceedings of the "Public health significance of vitamin A deficiency and its control" conference, Bellagio Study and Conference Center of the Rockefeller Foundation, Bellagio, 3–7 February 1992. https://pdfs.semanticscholar.org/6986/cf87fedd6c27dd46e469985aeceb0d660893.pdf. Accessed 17 Sept 2018

Delisle H (2018) Vitamin A in danger: should we worry? Lancet 392(10148):631

Fawzi WW, Herrera MG, Willett WC, Nestel P, el Amin A (1994) Dietary vitamin A intake and the risk of mortality among children. Am J Clin Nutr 59:401–408

Foster A, Sommer A (1987) Corneal ulceration, measles, and childhood blindness in Tanzania. Br J Ophthalmol 71(5):331–343

Garner P, Taylor-Robinson D, Sachdev HS (2013) DEVTA: results from the biggest clinical trial ever. Lancet 381(9876):1439–1441

Ghana VAST Study Team (1993) Vitamin A supplementation in northern Ghana: effects on clinic attendances, hospital admissions, and child mortality. Lancet 342(8862):7–12

Habicht JP, Victora C (2013) Vitamin A in Indian children. Lancet 382(9892):592

Hamer DH, Keusch GT (2015) Vitamin A deficiency: slow progress towards elimination. Lancet Glob Health 3(9):e502–e503. https://doi.org/10.1016/S2214-109X(15)00096-0

Herrera MG, Nestel P, el Amin A, Fawzi WW, Mohamed KA, Weld L (1992) Vitamin A supplementation. Lancet 340(8814):267–271

Keusch GT (1990) Vitamin A supplements – too good not to be true. N Engl J Med 323(14):985–987

Kirkwood BR, Hurt L, Amenga-Etego S, Tawiah C, Zandoh C et al (2010) Effect of vitamin A supplementation in women of reproductive age on maternal survival in Ghana (ObaapaVitA): a cluster-randomised, placebo-controlled trial. Lancet 375(9726):1640–1649

Klemm RD, Labrique AB, Christian P, Rashid M, Shamim AA et al (2008) Newborn vitamin A supplementation reduced infant mortality in rural Bangladesh. Pediatrics 122:e242–e250. https://doi.org/10.1542/peds.2007-3448

Lancet (ed) (1986) Fall and rise of the anti-infective vitamin (Editorial). Lancet 1(8941):1191

Lancet (ed) (1990) Vitamin A and malnutrition/infection complex in developing countries (Editorial). Lancet 336(8727):1349–1351

Latham M (2010) The great vitamin A fiasco. World Nutr 1:12–45

Martinez H, Shekar M, Latham M (1986) Vitamin A supplementation and child mortality. Lancet 2(8504):451–452

Mazumder S, Teneja S, Bhatia K, Yoshida S, Kaur J et al (2015) Efficacy of early neonatal supplementation with vitamin A to reduce mortality in infancy in Haryana, India (Neovita): a randomised, double-blind, placebo-controlled trial. Lancet 385(9975):1333–1342

McCarthy M (2005) Profile: Alfred Sommer: a life in the field and in the data. Lancet 365(9460):649

Rahmathullah L, Underwood BA, Thulasiraj RD, Milton RC, Ramaswamy K et al (1990) Reduced mortality among children in southern India receiving a small weekly dose of vitamin A. N Engl J Med 323(14):929–935

Sommer A (1982) Nutritional blindness: xerophthalmia and keratomalacia. Oxford University Press, New York

Sommer A (1992) Vitamin A deficiency and childhood mortality (conference at Bellagio). Lancet 339(8797):864

Sommer A (1997) 1997 Albert Lasker award for clinical research. Clinical research and the human condition: moving from observation to practice. Nat Med 3(10):1061–1063

Sommer A, West KP (1991) Vitamin A and childhood mortality. Lancet 337(8746):925

Sommer A, West KP (1996) Vitamin A deficiency: health, survival, and vision. Oxford University Press, New York/Oxford

Sommer A, Zeger SL (1991) On estimating efficacy from clinical trials. Stat Med 10:45–52

Sommer A, Tarwotjo I, Hussaini G (1981) Incidence, prevalence and scale of blinding malnutrition. Lancet 82(1):1407–1408

Sommer A, Tarwotjo I, Hussaini G, Susanto D (1983) Increased mortality in children with mild vitamin A deficiency. Lancet 322(8350):585–588

Sommer A, Tarwotjo I, Djunaedi E, West KP, Loedin AA et al (1986) Impact of vitamin A supplementation on childhood mortality: a randomised controlled community trial. Lancet 1(8491):1169–1173

Sommer A, West JP Jr, Martorell R (2013) Vitamin A in Indian children. Lancet 382(9892):591

Tarwotjo I, Sommer A, West KP, Djunaedi E, Mele L et al (1987) Influence of participation on mortality in a randomized trial of vitamin A prophylaxis. Am J Clin Nutr 45:1466–1471

Tielsch JM, Rahmathullah L, Thulasiraj RD, Katz J, Coles C et al (2007) Newborn vitamin A dosing reduces the case fatality but not incidence of common childhood morbidities in South India. J Nutr 137(11):2470–2474

UNICEF (2007) Vitamin A supplementation: a decade of progress. United Nations Children's Fund (UNICEF), UNICEF House, New York

UNICEF (2018) Coverage at a crossroads: new directions for vitamin A supplementation programmes. UNICEF House, New York

Vijayaraghavan K, Radhaiah G, Prakasam BS, Sarma KV, Reddy V (1990) Effect of massive dose vitamin A on morbidity and mortality in Indian children. Lancet 336(8727):1342–1345

West KP Jr, Pokhrel RP, Katz J, LeClerq SC, Khatry SK et al (1991) Efficacy of vitamin A in reducing preschool child mortality in Nepal. Lancet 338(8759):67–71

West KP Jr, Katz J, Khatry SK, LeClerq SC, Pradhan EK et al (1999) Double blind, cluster randomised trial of low dose supplementation with vitamin A or β carotene on mortality related to pregnancy in Nepal. Br Med J 318:570–575

West KP, Christian P, Labrique AB, Rashid M, Shamim AA et al (2011) Effects of vitamin A on beta carotene supplementation on pregnancy-related mortality and infant mortality in rural Bangladesh: a cluster randomized trial. JAMA 305(19):1986–1995

WHO (2017) Vitamin A supplementation during pregnancy. World Health Organization. Available via eLENA. http://www.who.int/elena/titles/vitamina_pregnancy/en/. Accessed 17 Sept 2018

Part IX
Special Topics

Issues in Generalizing Results from Clinical Trials

113

Steven Piantadosi

Contents

Introduction	2228
Example	2229
Lessons from the Laboratory	2229
Sampling as a Basis for Generalization	2231
Accounting for New Findings and Old Data	2233
Fit for Purpose Data	2234
Shared Biology	2235
Harmful Effects Double Standard	2237
Final Comments	2238
Summary	2239
Key Facts	2239
Cross-References	2239
References	2240

Abstract

Generalization is inference from the specific circumstances of a clinical trial to other settings or populations with the condition of interest. Accomplishing this is complex because trials are not population samples, methods supporting both internal and external validity must be assessed, the trial data must be fit for purpose, and relevant shared biology must be a foundation for extrapolation of results. In the context of the large-scale randomized evidence from the COVID-19 vaccine trials, this chapter discusses these issues and how generalizations might be enhanced. Laboratory experiments are a useful microcosm of the same issues and carry important lessons for this process.

S. Piantadosi (✉)
Department of Surgery, Division of Surgical Oncology, Brigham and Women's Hospital, Harvard Medical School, Boston, MA, USA
e-mail: spiantadosi@bwh.harvard.edu

© Springer Nature Switzerland AG 2022
S. Piantadosi, C. L. Meinert (eds.), *Principles and Practice of Clinical Trials*,
https://doi.org/10.1007/978-3-319-52636-2_236

Keywords

External validity · Generalizing results · Clinical trial analyses · Metadata · Data reduction · Biological similarity

Introduction

To perform a fair evaluation of therapeutics, we must compare like with like. Today this idea is familiar, but it has taken many years for scientific medicine to come to terms with all its implications. To generalize the results of the evaluation of therapeutic, we must also compare like with like. This chapter will suggest that we also know the methods and implications of how to accomplish that, but do not always do so effectively.

Generalization is inference from the specific circumstances of a clinical trial to other settings or populations with the condition of interest. I will make a distinction between objective methods that support external validity versus our willingness to generalize or apply results in broader circumstances. Thus, generalization is more subjective than assessing validity. For example, inclusion and exclusion criteria may cleanly define the disease being studied in a trial, supporting external validity. However, we might hesitate to generalize the results to a disease subgroup characterized by a factor that was not controlled by the trial.

Generalizations are especially challenging when the intent is to alter clinical practice, as will be assumed in this chapter, rather than merely supporting early steps in therapeutic development. For regulated treatments such as drugs and biologics, external validity of the relevant trial(s) is assessed as part of safety and efficacy review and a market approval. After a drug becomes available, general applications depend on the judgment of individual practitioners. Assessing the extent to which findings are applicable to people who were not in the study cohort can be complex for several reasons. First, trials are not representative population samples, removing the most familiar empirical basis of generalization. Second, all inferences including generalizations must account simultaneously for the new findings, old data or prior evidence, and trial methodology.

Third, just as with internal validity, reliable generalization depends on the data being fit for purpose. Evidence for this is in the meta data – features of how data production was designed and executed. Fourth, extrapolation requires knowledge of shared biology. Such knowledge is external to the clinical trial. Each of these complicating factors is a challenge to simplistic assessments of external validity. The goal of this chapter is not to provide a comprehensive solution to the difficulties but to explain these issues and suggest improvements in how we approach the problem.

Journal club is a common venue for discussions about generalization. There, investigators dissect studies to test their own critical judgment, the robustness of the trial, and the quality of the journal report. This process sometimes concludes that the results do not generalize because one or more of the following is true: (a) the study cohort lacks diversity, (b) trial requirements such as eligibility and randomization create an irrelevant microcosm, (c) the sociodemographic characteristics of the trial cohort is unlike "my clinic" or the population with the disease, (d) biological differences between the trial cohort and other individuals with the disease are evident. The extent to which selection enhances or restricts extrapolation of results is a topic that this chapter will address.

We will begin with a brief contemporary example for which generalization from clinical trials is critical. Then the discussion will briefly explore why (preclinical) laboratory experiments appear so efficient compared to clinical trials for extrapolations. As a microcosm for clinical trials they carry useful lessons. Then the four complexities surrounding generalizations mentioned above will be individually discussed. Finally, a double standard regarding harmful effects will be explored for its relevance to the perspectives offered in the chapter.

Example

A striking example of the consequences of generalizing results can be seen in the major vaccine trials in the COVID-19 pandemic of 2020–2021 (Baden et al. 2020; Polack et al. 2020; Sadoff et al. 2021). Three vaccines were developed independently, and each relied on their own body of basic science, clinical development, large definitive clinical trials, regulatory review, and application to a heterogeneous population. Each of the trials in question was large, diverse, included subjects at high risk of serious illness and death, and reflected strong preventive and safety results for the respective vaccines. For example, although the vaccines were each a different construct, the total enrollment on the three COVID-19 vaccine trials was over 113,000 subjects. By the fall of 2021 following extensive reviews all three vaccines had achieved FDA and CDC approval including boosters, and hundreds of millions of people had received the products worldwide. This combination of efficacy, safety, strength of evidence, and application experience exceeds what we can typically find for other therapeutics aimed at a given disease in a small subset of the population.

Vaccines for a pandemic are intended to be applied universally. Generalizing results to the world's diversity by representative participation is not achievable even in a large trial. The vaccine trials presented obvious questions of applicability based on risk due to age, comorbidities, and underlying immune function. The age question was addressed in additional trials. Beyond those issues, how were experts certain that efficacy and safety results from a nonrepresentative sample of less than one hundred thousandth of those in need could be applied to the world's diverse population? The perspectives in this chapter may help answer this question.

Lessons from the Laboratory

The only method to control random variation is replication. This law of nature causes sample sizes for clinical trials to be large because we often seek effects smaller than natural variation. Laboratory (preclinical) experiments by virtue of their small size appear to escape the law of variability. Laboratory studies use animals bred to be genetically homogeneous, small sample sizes, and artificial controlled conditions. Despite this, they generalize effectively and contribute strongly to understanding of the biology of the treatment under study (Weber 2014; Stackhouse et al. 2019; Conn 2017; Fukushima et al. 2015). This success is accomplished using three methods: reduced variation, relevant mechanistic models, and shared biology. Reduced overall variation comes from the similarity of test subjects often created by selective breeding or simple screening. Mechanistic models are constructed using methods such as selection, xenografts, genetic modifications, breeding, treatments to induce a disease or condition, and many others. Shared biology is based on evolutionary conservation of genes, metabolic pathways, and drug targets that assure that a result from the laboratory will be relevant to humans, at least as far as guiding the next experiments (Weber 2014; Stackhouse et al. 2019; Conn 2017).

All these methods are available to help clinical trials generalize in principle, but do not seem to be as highly leveraged as they are in preclinical experiments. Reduced variation is partially used in clinical trials by restricted eligibility and exclusion criteria. However, doing so is routinely criticized as working against inclusiveness and empirical (sampling-based) validity. The use of mechanistic models seems superficially to be irrelevant to human trials. However, selection criteria and certain biomarkers can assure that the cohort under study is homogeneous in key features of the disease. A good example of this is testing of targeted agents in cancer where the therapeutic mechanism pertains only to genetic or other subsets of disease selected by predictive biomarkers.

Shared biology is the most powerful but possibly least used principle for generalizations from human trials. The closeness of single species biological similarity is routinely fractured by skepticism derived from age, sex, sociodemographic, and other non-biological constructs. Such characteristics are trivial to measure and passively test but difficult to prove therapeutically consequential.

The implications of many laboratory experiments cross species boundaries easily. For example:

> It may seem as somewhat paradoxical that it is exactly these experimental disciplines of biology that limit their research to the smallest part of life's diversity that aspire to the greatest degree of universality. For the point of studying model organism is often to gain knowledge that is not only valid for one species but for many species, sometimes including humans. (Weber 2012)

Yet we often struggle to draw firm conclusions from a clinical trial within our single species. To the extent that humans are more complex or heterogeneous than other experimental subjects, interpretation of clinical trials might be more difficult than laboratory studies. Human heterogeneity can arise from biological diversity, behavior, or environment, for example. Each of these could potentially modify a treatment effect to a clinically significant degree. Hence, we need to understand these discrete sources of variation to generalize a trial result. More correctly, we need to understand *if* these sources of heterogeneity explain a large fraction of overall variation *and* do so in a way that carries therapeutic importance. Unfortunately, our trial designs often do not actively control biological diversity and rarely attempt to account for variation due to behavior or environment. Even so, analytical methods for assessing potential effect modifiers, such as subgroup comparisons, are simple and can be performed without being supported by design.

Sampling as a Basis for Generalization

This leads to the first and simplest aspect of external validity which relates to population subgroups (design), cohort subgroups (results), and the extent to which effect estimates are homogeneous. This question can be approached by subgroup analyses using familiar methods, results, and empirical extrapolations. One of the most famous subgroup analyses was in the Second International Study of Infarct Survival (ISIS-2) trial testing the effects of streptokinase and aspirin on myocardial infarction (ISIS-2 (Second International Study of Infarct Survival) Collaborative Group 1988). It showed consistent effects across subsets of the trial population, but also illustrated the danger of type 1 error inflation using such methods. Some of the subgroups examined were based on signs of the zodiac, with two of them showing trends significantly different from the overall results.

Consistent subgroup effects support the existence of a common overall effect, which is a good case for generalizability. Subgroups should be defined in advance but might become interesting based on findings in the data or new information from outside the trial. Although we are reassured by observing consistent treatment effects in subgroups, random variation must be present in the granules of a clinical trial. We cannot properly account for that variation without prior design, which is seldom done. Approaches to subgroup analyses have been much discussed and will not be reviewed here. See Wang et al. (2020) for a recent reference.

Contrary to the way many investigators think, clinical trials do not sample randomly from a population and generalize results back based on that sample. The unattainable ideal is shown in Figure 1. Filters on representative sampling are

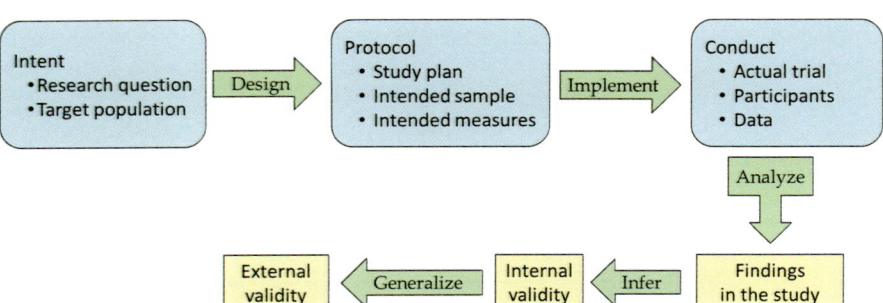

Fig. 1 Frames of reference and inferences in a clinical trial. External validity depends on design, implementation, and analysis and factors external to the experiment that support generalization

unavoidable. For example, eligibility and exclusion criteria improve safety and reduce variation in the study cohort. Self-selection and consent are essential to satisfy the ethics of human subjects research. But both filters prevent representative sampling and the type of direct inference that might otherwise come from a population survey.

The simplest approach to generalization is derived from such representative sampling. A key aspect of this is to demonstrate homogeneity of effects across subsets of the sample, which is then usually taken as support for generalizations. The subsets in question are often small, leading to underpowered comparisons and a potential error: no evidence of differences is interpreted as evidence of no differences. While this is as far as some observers get, it is not a solid, or the only, basis for generalization.

Here we should distinguish simple random variation from heterogeneity due to fixed covariates. Many statistical procedures have been developed to do just that. For example, part of the overall variation in human height might be explained by sex using an analysis of covariance, with considerable random variation remaining within both males and females. Similar thinking might apply to the study of variation in a treatment effect attributable to covariates.

We try to understand if discrete factors explain large fractions of overall variability because (1) it might yield biological insights and (2) different methods of variance control might then be necessary in our experiments. For example, it has been important in the COVID-19 pandemic to understand if the wide variability in mortality is partly attributable to specific risk factors, or simply reflects a highly variable disease process. Experiment design is the right tool for such questions but post hoc analyses of existing data are widely used to assess risk factors or covariates.

This thinking leads to one basis to support external validity – searching for, and failing to find, fixed sources of significant heterogeneity. This search can be undertaken only if the covariates of interest, subgroups, are available in the data for study. This is one element of the data being fit for purpose. Study design could assure this if the hypothesis was made prior to the trial. But the usual procedure is to examine many variables after the fact. While technically easy, the search is often done without much regard for plausibility and is error prone.

Suppose a large randomized controlled trial (RCT) were to reveal subgroup differences in the treatment effect. Assuming they are internally valid and clinically important, search for a mechanistic explanation would follow. It would be preferable to have a plausible biological mechanism in mind ahead of time and design the RCT accordingly. In either case, mechanism and data combine to improve the inference. When a covariate explains part of the variability in a treatment effect, it does not provide a secure basis for external validity until we fully understand the biology behind how the treatment effect is modulated.

If subgroup findings result from prior hypothesis, we presumably had some mechanistic basis that was strong enough to incorporate into the design of the trial. If the findings result only from data exploration, they typically would not be taken as conclusive until independently verified. A third possibility is that strong findings from the trial reinforce a prior idea that was not convincing enough to incorporate into its design. Here again, independent verification would be required for reliable generalizations. When independent verification is necessary, prior hypothesis and a plausible mechanism would be part of the research design.

Not all heterogeneity in treatment effects due to covariates is created equal. It matters whether the treatment effect is altered in magnitude (quantitatively) versus direction (qualitatively). This defines quantitative versus qualitative interaction (Poulson et al. 2012). Suppose we have an RCT testing treatment A versus B and a dichotomous covariate, X. Treatment-covariate interactions examine the AB difference as a function of levels of X. Suppose A is preferred. If the AB difference changes only in magnitude across X, the interaction is quantitative and preference for A is consistent. However, if the AB difference changes direction across X, the interaction is qualitative and A is preferred in one subset while B is preferred for the other. The distinction matters, because a qualitative interaction requires us to account for X when choosing treatment whereas a quantitative interaction does not.

This provides another tool to help our assessment of external validity. While we may be scientifically interested in large quantitative interaction attributable to some factor, qualitative interactions are important therapeutically because they affect the choice of treatment. Luckily, large interactions are uncommon, and factors that reverse therapeutic choice from A to B are even more rare – few if any examples exist. It is also useful to remember that interactions require large sample sizes to detect in addition to whatever mechanistic rationale supports them.

Accounting for New Findings and Old Data

It is possible for an experiment to be internally valid but externally invalid. This is implied in Figure 1 showing external validity as a final assessment. Suppose our randomized controlled trial (RCT) investigates the wrong disease subset or variant. This statement already implies knowledge of the disease and treatment mechanism based on prior evidence. Perhaps we were unlucky or unwise in the selection of the original study cohort. The treatment effect in this RCT may not be the same as in the disease variant of interest. Hence the RCT result could be internally valid but not externally valid.

Alternatively, the observed treatment effect could still be valid for the non-represented disease variant if the treatment works through a mechanism common to both disease types. An example where this might happen is a centrally acting analgesic like an opiate. Any type of pain might be reduced by a drug acting on a common pathway in the brain. This could be detected in in a clinical trial using subjects selected without regard to condition or source of pain. Similarly, an antiviral found effective in one strain of influenza might also be useful for a different virus if the mechanism of action is common to both.

A basis for external validity stronger than simple representation is mechanism of action, implying consistency with established knowledge. Though clinical trials are operationally very empirical, their external validity relies heavily on prior knowledge external to the experiment. The key point is the basis used to establish similarity between the trial population and the target population. Valid similarity is based on biology (like with like) whereas unreliable similarity is based on superficial characteristics. Sometimes superficial traits are correlated with biological differences, but they are usually poor surrogates for genetic, physiologic, metabolic, and similar definitive determinants. When similarity or representation is founded on a common biological mechanism, then external validity is much more straightforward. If mechanistic similarities do not exist or seem to contradict established facts, then extrapolation is unwise.

What if we do not know the mechanism of the disease or the action of our therapy? Perhaps it was found by lucky accident or by trial and error. Or we might not have detailed knowledge of the disease and therapeutic mechanisms, such as for some mental illnesses and their treatments. Trials can still provide internally valid treatment comparisons in these circumstances on a purely empirical basis. A clinical trial could demonstrate that treatment A is superior to treatment B in a defined cohort – but selection factors could severely restrict generalizations. For example, certain behavioral treatments for anxiety or depression might be effective as demonstrated by empirical evidence, only in narrow subsets of the condition, perhaps depending on causes, personality traits, or environment.

Some therapeutic mechanisms are claimed not to be natural processes at all, examples being homeopathy or intercessory prayer. We could use the structure of a clinical trial for such questions but would have little or no basis on which to assure validity. Any result might be a random error; or we might need to rethink large parts of previously established science. Without a plausible mechanism for the observed effects, we are unable to interpret either internal or external validity. In other words, data from an experiment that disregards mechanism of action might be unfit for purpose.

This requirement for a plausible mechanism makes investigators uncomfortable if they prefer to focus only on operational aspects of a trial. However, it is important to understand that when a specific tool like a clinical trial is required for a scientific answer, it may not be the sole requirement.

Fit for Purpose Data

Humans do not directly interpret data from a clinical trial, or from any scientific source for that matter. We have no innate ability to understand or interpret raw data. This is unlike images or sounds for which we have highly evolved neurological structures and pathways that allow us to instantaneously process and understand those data-rich sensations. However, to understand statistical data like those from a clinical trial, we require both metadata and data reduction.

Metadata is information about data that describes where they came from and what they were designed to do. We require several types of metadata. For example, were the data produced by an experiment, or did they arise by happenstance? If data were produced by design for a given question, are the analytic methods consistent with the

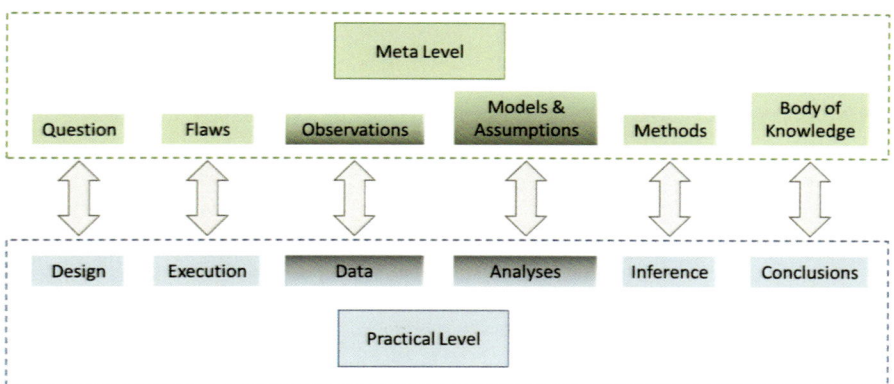

Fig. 2 Correspondence between meta level considerations and practical level methods. At each step in our practical conduct of a clinical trial we refer to considerations at the meta level for support. The methods of obtaining data and performing analyses rely on models and assumptions, for example

purpose? We also want to know what types of quality control have been applied to the data, the nature of missingness, and so on.

In addition to metadata, we require reduction or simplification of data using summaries (statistics) and models to understand them. For example, thousands of raw observations could be summarized as a mean and standard deviation which becomes easy to comprehend under the normal distribution model. Data reduction replaces large numbers of observations by a handful of numerical values that have biological interpretations. Examples of numerical quantities that have biological interpretations are proportions, time rates, risks, or relative treatment effects.

To arrive at correct conclusions for good or bad data, we need meta-level considerations to be paired with familiar procedures at the practical level as shown in Fig. 2. Also, the literal process of analysis requires that we reduce or simplify raw data using assumptions and statistical models to make inferences about the clinical effects of interest. At every step in the practical level we reference the meta level for validation, as in Fig. 2. All the processes discussed here are necessary to establish internal validity for trial findings, so it should not be surprising that additional requirements are necessary to establish external validity.

Shared Biology

Biological models are distinct from the statistical models just discussed. Commonalities among various types of models are fascinating and extensive (Rothenberg 1989; Widman et al. 1989) but cannot be discussed here. Biological models are inextricably linked to experiments just as statistical models are integral to data analysis. Models capture essentials of the object of study in a simple or convenient form. For example, preclinical experiments often use disease models based on laboratory animals. The animals have the disease of interest or something very similar by virtue of breeding, genetic alterations, or other interventions to induce it. For example, in a cancer explant model (Weber 2014), the actual human cancer is placed in the animal where it will grow and can be treated with experimental agents to assess its responsiveness. In animal models of myocardial or neurological injury for example, the vascular supply to an organ might be interrupted surgically to test rescue drugs or devices. Models of traumatic injuries have been created in anesthetized animals.

In some cases, the animal *is* the model. An important example is carcinogenicity testing of chemicals or radiation (Fukushima et al. 2015). The agent is administered to rodents (say) at doses higher than humans would encounter in the environment. Outcome frequencies are then mathematically extrapolated back to low doses to judge if environmental exposures constitute a risk for humans. This is an interesting example because it involves both an animal model and a mathematical model of effect. Scientists accept this type of modeling and associated extrapolation and we have all likely benefitted greatly from its validity. Sweeping cautions regarding risks to humans are based on these types of assessment. While these modeling methods are generally valid, they can also illustrate a double standard regarding harmful effects which will be discussed below.

Many animal models are less anatomical, more physiologically intricate, or employ species quite distant evolutionarily from humans (Conn 2017). Examples are guinea pigs, zebrafish, and drosophila (fruit flies). The evolutionary divergence of the human and drosophila genomes happened about 783 million years ago, yet eight Nobel Prizes have been awarded for elucidating fundamental genetic mechanisms via fruit flies. Model behavior is informative regarding the human condition based on biological similarity. Essential features of the disease are present in the model along with essential normal features so that observations of treatment effects are likely to apply to humans. Ultimately what is a good model depends on factors such as those listed in Table 1. Equally important are factors not usually relevant to a model, also listed in Table 1.

Absence of models is a significant shortcoming for efficient therapeutic development. One example is in neurodegenerative conditions such as Alzheimer's disease where good laboratory models do not presently exist. This limits preclinical

Table 1 Features of Biological Models

Important	Unimportant
Disease mechanisms	Similarity unrelated to the disease
Treatment mechanisms	Diet
Genes and regulation	Behavior
Cellular pathways	Age
Metabolism and organ function	Population heterogeneity
Anatomical similarities	Species
Judgment and experience	

exploration and makes it more difficult to develop new therapeutic drugs or biologicals that might prevent or alter the disease.

Human volunteers in a clinical trial are biological models for other humans who did not participate. When we are skeptical that the results of a trial are relevant to an external population, we are essentially rejecting the adequacy of the human model as a basis for extrapolation of the treatment effect. This seems to happen much more frequently than we can justify based on mechanism. We should make these assessments based on relevant biological similarities as in Table 1.

Harmful Effects Double Standard

Most investigators have a double standard when generalizing results from research studies. The double standard is that we are quick to extrapolate negative or harmful effects (environmental exposures or adverse effects of treatment, for example) but hesitant to generalize beneficial effects of treatments. A bias toward safety is one reason for this asymmetry, but it does not fully explain the phenomenon. Why should this be the case?

Harmful effects are often immediately taken to be externally valid even in the presence of considerable contrary evidence. For example, at the time of writing this chapter, there are numerous lawsuits pending over the herbicide glyphosate and its possible role as a causative agent in non-Hodgkin's lymphoma, a lymphatic cancer. Several juries in civil trials have awarded millions of dollars to plaintiffs exposed to the chemical. In many cities, there are constant fishing advertisements by law firms for additional plaintiffs. The International Agency for Research on Cancer (IARC) has classified glyphosate as a "probable carcinogen," whereas other agencies such as the U.S. Environmental Protection Agency have indicated no risk (International Agency for Research on Cancer 2017; Guyton et al. 2015; Benbrook 2019; U.-S. Environmental Protection Agency 2021; EPA 2017). Clearly this is not a question to be answered by a clinical trial. The putative risk is widely generalized and strongly sympathetic to juries.

The clearly established risks of many exposures such as cigarette smoking, ultraviolet light, lead paint, and other toxins have been generalized to populations dissimilar to the original studies with respect to sex, ethnicity, sociodemographic factors, environment – essentially universally. It is appropriate to impute risk based on mechanistic knowledge of how such exposures produce their harmful effects. These are not empirical or representation-based generalizations.

In contrast, hesitation to generalize beneficial therapeutic effects from clinical trials has reached large proportions. Presently, we are seeing this in the delay or refusal of some people to be vaccinated against coronavirus. Although this phenomenon is complex, at the core lies disbelief in efficacy coupled with belief in elevated risk of vaccination. Both are completely at odds with the considerable experimental evidence from the vaccine trials as well as the utilization data from hundreds of millions of people. Whatever else is going on in the minds of those leaving themselves at risk, the circumstance does illustrate the double standard of reluctance to generalize benefit and willingness to extrapolate risk essentially regardless of the evidence.

Recent decades have focused strongly on sex and ethnic representation in trial cohorts to support generalizations based on sampling. In addition to those mandates, we routinely try to enhance external validity by removing eligibility restrictions and using patient centric outcomes. Patient reported outcomes are discussed in another chapter in this book (▶ Chap. 51, "Patient-Reported Outcomes"). In recent years, clinical trials were explicitly defined as being outside the "real world" in mandates to the FDA (2018; Sherman et al. 2016). "Real world" is not a well-defined term but has been weaponized by some to suggest that there is a more appropriate basis than clinical trials in utilization or transactional data to establish safety and efficacy of new therapeutics. The ability to accomplish this, and its value in therapeutic comparisons, is presently undetermined. Pragmatic trials (Patsopoulos 2011; Gamerman et al. 2019) have for many years attempted to correct the artificial environment required by a typical clinical trial. Among other methods, expanded eligibility criteria and group rather than individual randomization may be used in pragmatic trials. These are intended to show if or how an intervention might perform in health care environments more broadly.

There is no analogous "real world" or pragmatic approach to harmful effects which are not and should not be discounted when they appear in a controlled environment. Typical healthcare environments are messier than clinical trials which seem more likely to increase risks associated with treatment. Weak research designs often allow inversion of the efficacy and safety mindset – unimpressive efficacy is often generalized when or if risk appears to be minimal. Examples of this low-risk low-reward phenomenon can be seen in the explosion of dietary or nutritional supplements in the "nutraceutical" industry in the last few decades.

Final Comments

Much of this chapter has been written during the COVID-19 pandemic. Literally the world was waiting for the results of several large vaccine clinical trials and the respective regulatory decisions. Although the relevant trials involved (only) tens of thousands of participants, we are extrapolating vaccine effects to billions of humans. This cannot be done empirically. Decisions on generalizing the results of the vaccine trials are weighty and ongoing, and aligned with the considerations of this chapter. Trial populations have not captured the cultural, ethnic, or genetic diversity of the world's populations. But the more important question is if they have captured the relevant immunologic commonality to support universal usage. The answer is undoubtedly yes. Humans seem to be similar enough to each other to support the infection, so why not immunity?

It is given that rare adverse effects will be seen in large experiences using the vaccines. Some members of the population, especially in the USA, are laden with an anti-vaccination fervor based partly on such events but fueled mainly by point sources of ignorance and misinformation. See the Wakefield story (Deer 2020) for one example where anti-vaccination opinion was sustained by false information. Their process for refusing a safe, effective, free, and available vaccine will not be analysis of the trial but closed mindedness. Some will pay for their ignorance with their lives. It remains to be seen if coronavirus can escape vaccine immunity by mutation. However that question evolves, generalizing the results of the vaccine trials is likely to be an important enduring example of assessing external validity.

Summary

The COVID-19 vaccine trials illustrate how important generalizing clinical trial results can be and how effectively and appropriately it can be accomplished. Although the COVID-19 vaccine trials constitute large-scale randomized evidence, smaller trials and laboratory experiments carry the same issues regarding generalization. The wisdom of employing large, broad, and diverse populations in clinical trials can be seen in the COVID-19 vaccine trials but is not the sole foundation for external validity. The full set of tools for extrapolating results must consider the mechanism of action for treatment effects, biological modifiers of those effects, as well as empirical representativeness. The strongest basis for generalizing clinical trial results comes from knowing there is shared biology between the study participants and those we intend to treat. That key information is external to the trial but must be brought into the assessment of external validity. The principle of shared biology partially explains why our concerns for harmful effects are so universal. Extrapolation of beneficial effects should be supported by similar reasoning.

Key Facts

Simple generalization regarding the results of a clinical trial is typically based on sampling or population representation. This is adequate for some purposes, but there are stronger bases for extrapolating results, especially considering that clinical trials are not random samples of any population or subgroup with a given disease. The external validity of findings relies on internal validity, previously established knowledge, having data that are fit for purpose, and shared biology. Shared biology is the critical similarity necessary between the study population and subgroups of interest. This basis for generalization is readily used in laboratory experiments and when considering harmful effects but appears to be less widely used in clinical trials. The best recent example of the role and effective use of these principles is the worldwide application of new vaccines for COVID-19.

Cross-References

▶ Patient-Reported Outcomes

References

Baden LR, El Sahly HM, Essink B et al (2020) Efficacy and safety of the mRNA-1273 SARS-CoV-2 vaccine. N Engl J Med 384(5):403–416

Benbrook CM (2019) How did the US EPA and IARC reach diametrically opposed conclusions on the genotoxicity of glyphosate-based herbicides? Environ Sci Eur 31:2. https://doi.org/10.1186/s12302-018-0184-7

Conn PM (2017) Animal models for the study of human disease, 2nd edn. Academic Press

Deer B (2020) The doctor who fooled the world : Andrew Wakefield's war on vaccines. Johns Hopkins University Press, Baltimore

EPA (2017) Revised glyphosate issue paper: evaluation of carcinogenic potential. https://cfpub.epa.gov/si/si_public_file_download.cfm?p_download_id=534487

FDA (2018) Framework for FDA's real-world evidence program. https://www.fda.gov/media/120060/download

Fukushima S et al (2015) Qualitative and quantitative approaches in the dose–response assessment of genotoxic carcinogens. Mutagenesis 31(3):341–346

Gamerman V, Cai T, Elsäßer A (2019) Pragmatic randomized clinical trials: best practices and statistical guidance. Health Serv Outcomes Res Methodol 19(1):23–35. https://doi.org/10.1007/s10742-018-0192-5

Guyton KZ et al (2015) Carcinogenicity of tetrachlorvinphos, parathion, malathion, diazinon, and glyphosate. Lancet Oncol 16(5):490–491

International Agency for Research on Cancer (2017) Some organophosphate insecticides and herbicides. IARC monographs on the evaluation of carcinogenic risks to humans, vol 112. https://publications.iarc.fr/549

ISIS-2 (Second International Study of Infarct Survival) Collaborative Group (1988) Randomised trial of intravenous streptokinase, oral aspirin, both, or neither among 17,187 cases of suspected acute myocardial infarction: ISIS-2. Lancet 2(8607):349–360

Patsopoulos NA (2011) A pragmatic view on pragmatic trials. Dial Clin Neurosci 13(2):217–224. https://doi.org/10.31887/DCNS.2011.13.2/npatsopoulos

Polack FP, Thomas SJ, Kitchin N et al (2020) Safety and efficacy of the BNT162b2 mRNA Covid-19 vaccine. N Engl J Med 383(27):2603–2615. https://doi.org/10.1056/NEJMoa2034577

Poulson RS, Gadbury GL, Allison DB (2012) Treatment heterogeneity and individual qualitative interaction. Am Statist 66(1):16–24. https://doi.org/10.1080/00031305.2012.671724

Rothenberg J (1989) The nature of modeling. RAND Corporation. https://www.rand.org/pubs/notes/N3027.html

Sadoff J, Gray G, Vandebosch A et al (2021) Safety and efficacy of single-dose Ad26.COV2.S vaccine against Covid-19. N Engl J Med 384(23):2187–2201. https://doi.org/10.1056/NEJMoa2101544

Sherman RE et al (2016) Real-world evidence – what is it and what can it tell us? N Engl J Med 375:2293–2297. https://doi.org/10.1056/NEJMsb1609216

Stackhouse CT, Gillespie GY, Willey CD (2019) Cancer explant models. In: Current topics in microbiology and immunology. Springer, Berlin, Heidelberg

U.S. Environmental Protection Agency (2021) Glyphosate. https://www.epa.gov/ingredients-used-pesticide-products/glyphosate

Wang X, Piantadosi S, Le-Rademacher J, Mandrekar S (2020) Statistical considerations for subgroup analyses. J Thor Onc 16(3):375–380. https://doi.org/10.1016/j.jtho.2020.12.008

Weber M (2012) Experiment in biology. In: Zalta EN (ed) The Stanford encyclopedia of philosophy. The Metaphysics Research Lab, Center for the Study of Language and Information, Stanford University, Stanford. http://plato.stanford.edu/entries/biology-experiment/

Weber M (2014) Experimental modeling in biology: in vivo representation and stand-ins as modeling strategies. Phil Sci 81(5):756–769. https://doi.org/10.1086/678257

Widman L, Loparo K, Nielsen N (1989) Artificial intelligence, simulation & modeling. Wiley

Leveraging "Big Data" for the Design and Execution of Clinical Trials

114

Stephen J. Greene, Marc D. Samsky, and Adrian F. Hernandez

Contents

Introduction	2242
Current Challenges to Traditional Clinical Trials	2243
Low Enrollment Rate	2244
Representativeness of the General Population	2246
High Costs	2247
Emergence of the Electronic Health Record and "Big Data"	2249
There Is No Substitute for Randomization	2250
Potential Avenues for Improving Clinical Trials Through "Big Data"	2251
Research Networks with Common Data Models	2251
Pragmatic Trials Within Individual Health Systems	2253
Connecting Multiple Health Systems as a Single Research Network	2254
Registries for Improving Clinical Trials and Curating Big Data	2254
Digital Health Devices to Decrease the Burden of Trial Participation for Patients	2255
Embedding Machine Learning Within Clinical Trials	2257
Summary and Conclusion	2260
References	2260

Abstract

Randomized clinical trials form the cornerstone of evidence-based medicine and are required to accurately determine cause-effect relationships and treatment effects of medical interventions. Nonetheless, contemporary clinical trials are becoming increasingly difficult to execute and are hampered by slow patient enrollment, burdensome and extensive data collection, and high costs. Over the past decades, there has been an infusion of digital technology and computing power within healthcare. "Big data," defined as data so large and complex that traditional mechanisms and software used to store and analyze data are

S. J. Greene · M. D. Samsky · A. F. Hernandez (✉)
Duke Clinical Research Institute, Durham, NC, USA

Division of Cardiology, Duke University School of Medicine, Durham, NC, USA
e-mail: stephen.greene@duke.edu; marc.samsky@duke.edu; Adrian.hernandez@duke.edu

© Springer Nature Switzerland AG 2022
S. Piantadosi, C. L. Meinert (eds.), *Principles and Practice of Clinical Trials*,
https://doi.org/10.1007/978-3-319-52636-2_161

insufficient, offers the potential of innovation and improvement for contemporary clinical trials. The primary focus of health technology to date has been direct patient care, but these platforms offer further potential to change the paradigm for conducting clinical trials and generating medical evidence. The digitalization of medical information allows data across multiple health systems to be integrated and centralized within readily analyzable common data models with standardized data definitions. Moreover, these technologies favor embedding clinical research within everyday clinical care, offering the benefits of generalizable study results, "re-use" of data already collected during routine patient care, and minimal burden of trial participation on patients and local study sites. "Big data" approaches and machine learning also may aid in phenotyping complex medical conditions and identifying optimal patient subsets for study in clinical trials. In this chapter, we review the current challenges facing traditional clinical trials and discuss the conceptual framework and rationale for merging clinical trials with the evolving field of health data science. We follow by outlining specific avenues through which "big data" have potential to reshape the way clinical trials are performed and by discussing respective advantages for purposes of generating high-quality, highly actionable, and patient-centered medical evidence.

Keywords

Clinical trials · Data · Pragmatic · Electronic health record

Introduction

Randomized clinical trials represent the cornerstone of evidence-based medicine and are central in shaping contemporary clinical practice guidelines and patient care. Evidence generated from such trials is directly responsible for the widespread use of numerous medical therapies central to the modern-day medical practice. These evidence-based therapies have in turn led to drastic improvements in patient outcomes across numerous major medication conditions, such as heart attack, stroke, and many forms of cancer. In many cases, these programs have fundamentally shaped the current understanding of human health and disease. As such, many have argued that the design and execution of the clinical trial, in itself, represent among the single biggest advances in the practice of medicine.

However, while the critical importance of the clinical trial is clear, the healthcare environment in which such trials are conducted is rapidly changing. Technological advances in the way people communicate and store information have fundamentally changed the human existence as compared with decades prior. These innovations have led to entirely new industries and a wide array of digital tools, and with them an evolving societal expectation for increased speed, convenience, and efficiency of communication, while simultaneously maintaining accuracy and security. These expectations have infiltrated medicine and the standard to which healthcare providers use existing patient data and evidence to guide ongoing patient care and

Table 1 Key terms and definitions

Big data	Data so large and complex that traditional mechanisms and software used to store and analyze data are insufficient
Electronic health record	Digital longitudinal repository of electronic health information for an individual patient that provides medical staff with the information necessary for delivering clinical care
Health data science	Field of study centered on generating data-driven observations, solutions, and actionable knowledge regarding real-world health problems by applying advanced analytics to big data
Machine learning	Statistical programs that harness substantial computing power to execute algorithms that learn from raw data without human interaction
Prospective registry	Observational studies used by study sponsors to collect standardized data from patients seen in a variety of settings. Data can be used for a variety of purposes, including to describe practice patterns and trends, identify outliers, detect safety signals, or assess comparative effectiveness
"Traditional" randomized clinical trial	Generally characterized as randomized, double-blind (i.e., investigator and participant both unaware of treatment assignment), double-dummy (when appearance of study medication cannot be made identical), placebo-controlled, and with narrow inclusion and extensive exclusion criteria. Patient data are collected specifically for purposes of the trial, and participants attend scheduled follow-up visits for additional study-related testing and data collection. Trial endpoints are adjudicated centrally by blinded reviewers using standardized definitions

medical decision-making. In this era of digitalization, more patient data are collected than ever before and, if properly harnessed, offer the potential to revolutionize the way clinical trials are performed and the way medical evidence is generated. Nonetheless, despite this tremendous promise, the current state of incorporating "big data" within clinical trials of medical interventions remains at an early stage and has generally lagged behind more rapid uptake within other industries. In this chapter, we will review the current challenges facing traditional clinical trials and will discuss the conceptual framework and rationale for merging clinical trials with the evolving field of health data science (Table 1). We follow by outlining specific avenues through which "big data" have the potential to reshape the way clinical trials are performed and by discussing the respective advantages for purposes of generating high-quality, highly actionable, and patient-centered medical research.

Current Challenges to Traditional Clinical Trials

To thoroughly understand the potential advantages of incorporating "big data" approaches into clinical trials, it is critical to review the current challenges facing traditional clinical trials. Although wide variation does exist, traditional clinical trials may be generally characterized as randomized, double-blind (i.e., both investigator and participant unaware of treatment assignment), double-dummy (when appearance of study medication cannot be made identical), placebo-controlled, and with narrow inclusion and extensive exclusion criteria (Fanaroff et al. 2018a). Patient data are collected by research staff specifically for purposes of the clinical trial, and participants attend scheduled study follow-up visits (independent of follow-up visits for their usual medical care) for additional study-related testing and data collection (Fanaroff et al. 2018a). Trial endpoints, such as all-cause death, cause-specific death (e.g., cardiovascular death), and hospitalization, are adjudicated centrally by blinded reviewers using standardized definitions. While the prior success of this paradigm in advancing medicine cannot be understated, the evolving landscape of clinical and site-based research has made the effective use of this approach increasingly challenging for a variety of reasons.

Low Enrollment Rate

Among the most significant problems facing contemporary clinical trials is a low enrollment rate. For example, recent trials among patients with cardiovascular disease often enroll <1 patient/site/month, and this rate has decreased over time (Fig. 1). This is particularly the case in the United States where representation in global mega-trials generally lags behind other parts of the world. Data from a leading academic clinical trial coordinating center suggest only approximately 5% of acute care hospitals in the United States consistently participate in trials and approximately 1% account for the vast majority of participant accrual (Califf and Harrington 2011).

There are multiple reasons underlying the patient enrollment problem for conventional clinical trials. One notable contributor is generally extensive inclusion and exclusion criteria, resulting in only a small subset of the general population with the disease of interest being eligible for the trial. However, independent of the trial selection criteria, there are additional obstacles, and it is reasonable to consider these barriers separately from the patient and study site perspective.

Patient Perspective: Typical clinical trials often involve extensive data collection, laboratory tests, and extra in-person visits. Some may even require invasive procedures. The majority of these elements represent testing patients would otherwise not receive as part of their standard care. Often many patients with the disease of interest inherently have a degree of associated disability and/or comorbidities that make enduring extra procedures or in-person healthcare visits unappealing or unfeasible. Even among patients without significant functional limitation, missing work or traveling to a particular site for additional testing may be impractical. In addition, the informed consent process for patients is often complex, intimidating, and time-consuming and may be particularly unattractive to patients already coping with the added stress of a medical condition.

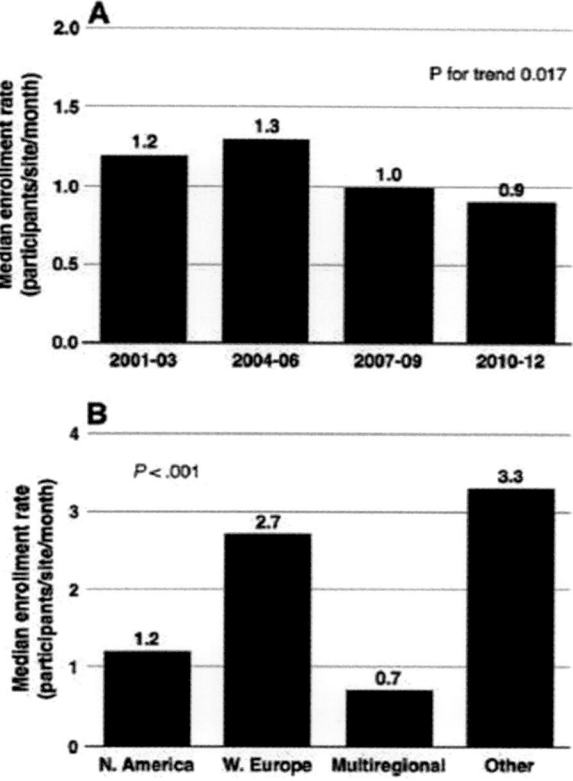

Fig. 1 (a) Between 2001–2003 and 2009–2012, enrollment rates (expressed as participants/site per month) in cardiovascular clinical trials have overall decreased significantly (P for trend = 0.017). (b) The highest enrollment rates were observed in trials done exclusively in countries outside North America or Western Europe, whereas multiregional trials had the lowest enrollment rates. (Reproduced with permission from Butler et al. (2015))

Site Investigator/Site Perspective: The extensive data collection and schedule of on-site assessments common to traditional clinical trials are often onerous for site investigators and staff. This workload limits the number of study sites who wish to or are able to participate. Moreover, juxtaposed to this time and resource burden, many have argued that there are diminishing incentives for site investigators to enroll patients in clinical trials. Due to financial pressures, there has been a progressive decline in the amount of time local investigators can dedicate to trials. This is particularly the case in the United States, where investigator salaries are generally tied to generation of relative value units (RVUs) from pure clinical work, making the role of local site investigator a potential detractor from time spent doing mandatory and/or more lucrative clinical activities. For example, in a study surveying physician perceptions regarding research, 86% reported less likely to perform activities that did not count toward their clinical work target (Summer et al. 2012). In addition, site investigators frequently get minimal recognition and/or promotion within their own institution for trial participation and are inconsistently afforded authorship on trial manuscripts or any subsequent academic output.

Consequences of Low Enrollment Rates

Concurrent with trends toward declining US enrollment is a continued movement toward globalization of clinical research. Although inclusion of multiple global populations in research may align with the worldwide prevalence of disease and foster collaboration, there are concerns that globalization is driven by relative inability to conduct large trials in high-income countries where enrollment is consistently slower and the regulatory environment more bureaucratic and expensive. Especially concerning is the observation that despite comprising the majority of the study population, lower-income countries may be paradoxically more likely to find newly approved therapies prohibitively expensive and may only have routine access after years of use in wealthier countries. Ideally, for both ethical and scientific reasons, clinical trials should be conducted in populations in proportion to their potential use of the therapy should it eventually gain approval. Indeed, despite technological and scientific advances in high-income countries, there is evidence of a widening gap between their desire for high-quality evidence and the capacity to produce it.

Low enrollment rates among US centers also pose serious problems regarding the generalizability of trial results to US patients. Despite uniform selection criteria that apply to all sites in all countries, patients enrolled in global clinical trials frequently show marked variation by the geographic region of enrollment. For example, in the ASTRONAUT (Aliskiren Trial on Acute Heart Failure Outcomes) trial among patients hospitalized for heart failure, rates of all-cause death at 12-month follow-up were 7.3% in North America, 14.7% in Western Europe, and 26.7% in Asia (Greene et al. 2015). Although the pattern of heterogeneity may vary (i.e., specific regions do not always have lowest or highest event rates in every clinical trial for a given condition), notable global and regional differences in patient profiles and outcomes are frequently observed in clinical trials across multiple fields of medicine. Whether secondary to geographic differences in patient factors (e.g., disease pathophysiology/genetics, race/ethnicity, comorbidities), trial site factors (e.g., interpretation of selection criteria, accuracy of data collection, protocol adherence), healthcare practice factors (e.g., adherence to clinical practice guidelines, local standards of care), or healthcare environment factors (e.g., physician/hospital reimbursement incentives, patient access to healthcare, socioeconomics of the population, medicolegal liability climate), the exact mechanism of these differences in each particular example is often unclear. Nonetheless, the modest North American enrollment of many trials amplifies the ramifications of this geographic variation in the United States. Specifically, global heterogeneity in the types of patients included in a trial presents challenges for regulators, guideline writers, third-party payers, and practicing clinicians who must determine whether results from an international trial are relevant to their respective patients.

Representativeness of the General Population

By virtue of multiple inclusion and exclusion criteria and need for rigorous longitudinal data collection and in-person visits, patients enrolled in a clinical trial may differ substantially from patients with the same medical condition in the general population. For example, comorbidities are frequently responsible for many patients failing to qualify for a clinical trial (e.g., a clinical trial for patients with heart disease will exclude patients with concurrent kidney disease). However, in routine practice, clinicians see patients with multiple simultaneous health conditions, and overlap between medical problems is common (e.g., obesity, diabetes, kidney disease, heart disease, stroke). Even when landmark clinical trial results are available and widely publicized, due to these comorbid conditions and other trial selection criteria, clinicians may be unsure if the available evidence reflects individuals akin to the patient sitting across from them in the exam room.

Trial representativeness may be particularly problematic for particular patient subsets. Although minorities represent nearly one fourth of the US population, they remain significantly underrepresented in clinical trials. Similarly, clinical trials across many health conditions continually struggle to enroll high numbers of women and patients of older age. This persistent enrollment bias toward white men has persisted despite government and regulatory efforts to enhance inclusion of women and minorities in clinical trials (FDA U 2017). Given that most health conditions span a wide range of demographic groups, representation of these groups in clinical trial populations should ideally match the proportion of patients with clinical need in routine practice. Moreover, given biologic differences by age, sex, and race/ethnicity, the risk and benefits of tested therapies may differ across subsets. Extrapolation from homogenous trial populations to underrepresented groups increases uncertainty regarding effectiveness and may increase the potential for unexpected efficacy or harm.

To date, reasons underlying the underrepresentation of women and minorities across many clinical trials remain uncertain. From the patient perspective, it is plausible that differential attitudes toward research or the consent process between white men, women, and minorities contribute to differences in clinical trial participation. Such patient perceptions among underrepresented groups may, in part, relate to similar underrepresentation among enrolling clinicians and site investigators. It is also possible that differential social or economic barriers exist for women and racial/ethnic minorities that make compliance with a study protocol particularly difficult (e.g., travel to and from study site, home or family responsibilities). Likewise, it is unclear if healthcare providers and clinical trial personnel demonstrate selection bias for trial participation based on gender or race (independent of trial selection criteria) or if study sites serving higher proportions of underrepresented minorities are less likely to participate in clinical trials.

High Costs

Financial Cost
The costs of clinical trials and bringing new drugs or devices to market are of high concern to all study sponsors. For perspective, a recent analysis including seven major pharmaceutical companies and 726 clinical trials conducted across several

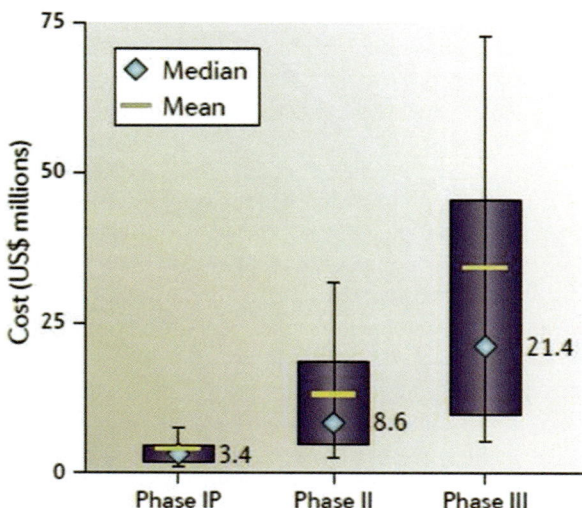

Fig. 2 Data from 726 studies conducted by seven major companies (all of which are in the top 20 biopharma companies ranked by revenue in 2016) from 2010 to 2015. Medians and means are indicated with diamonds and lines. Boxes indicate the 25th to 75th percentiles, and whiskers indicate the 10th and 90th percentiles. Phase IP = phase I study involving patients. (Reproduced with permission from Martin et al. (2017a))

medical conditions from 2010 to 2015 found that median costs from conducting a study from protocol approval to final report were as follows: US$3.4 million for phase I, US$8.6 million for phase II, and US$21.4 million for phase III trials (Fig. 2) (Martin et al. 2017a). Multiple study design elements were associated with increased cost, including number of patients enrolled, number of regions and countries included, and the number of site visits in the protocol. In addition, other factors related to operational performance (i.e., how well a sponsor executes a trial according to their chosen design) also explained variability in trial costs. Overall, these high costs present a relative barrier to evidence generation and therapeutic discovery. Sponsors are increasingly needing to consider the likelihood of return of investment in considering the high upfront costs of executing a clinical trial. Conceivably, these budgetary constraints may challenge innovation or favor overly conservative behavior whereby companies with modest resources or expertise abandon "high-risk/high-reward" pursuits.

Opportunity Cost

From time of program inception to final completion, clinical trials (particularly phase III trials with clinical event endpoints) typically take several years to complete. These timelines are further lengthened for sponsors seeking approval of new drugs or devices, where the development process is generally prolonged through a series of phase I/II/III trials. For example, the time from drug target identification to first drug approval in a major market has been estimated at 13.8 years (Martin et al. 2017b). The combination of long cycle times with the large size of many clinical trials requires substantial sustained resource allocation from sponsors, possibly limiting investigation in alternate areas and limiting the number of scientific questions that can be simultaneously explored.

However, irrespective of sponsor perspective, patients and clinicians share the burden of the opportunity cost associated with clinical trials. The slow pace of evidence generation delays availability of therapies that will eventually be shown efficacious while in other cases prolongs patient exposure to interventions ultimately shown ineffective or harmful. These long timelines for clinical trial completion are often compounded by further delays in clinical adoption of new medical evidence. For instance, a landmark study from the Institute of Medicine reported that it takes an average of 17 years for new medical knowledge generated by randomized clinical trials to be reasonably incorporated into clinical practice (Institute of Medicine 2017).

Emergence of the Electronic Health Record and "Big Data"

The healthcare industry has always generated incredible amounts of data. Historically however, data was recorded using pen and paper. An early example of generating digital data via a computer occurred at Duke University in the Cardiac Care Unit. Dr. Eugene Stead, Chair of Medicine from 1947 to 1967, arranged for a computer to be at the bedside of patients following myocardial infarction. The computer's purpose was to serve as a resource for information storage and retrieval. Dr. Stead intended to prognosticate mortality by recording serial observations in every patient following myocardial infarction. Nurses were instructed to enter prespecified characteristics of patients over time while in the intensive care unit and in the catheterization lab. The generated database was called "The Duke Databank for Cardiovascular Disease" and was one of the earliest examples of a digital-based registry used to record clinical observations and conduct research rather than rely on experiences limited to case series of patients.

Subsequent "big data" approaches to clinical research have paralleled the integration of technology into the healthcare system and other facets of care delivery. Over the past 20–30 years, computers, the Internet, automation, and numerous other major technological advances have changed the landscape of "everyday" life in the United States and countries throughout the world. However, despite this infusion of digitalization and innovation into the private sector, the uptake of technology within healthcare has been slow by comparison. For example, as recently as 2–3 years ago, multiple major academic medical centers in the United States had components of the patient medical record that were handwritten and/or not accessible remotely. Although widespread adoption was sluggish, the vast majority of today's US hospitals and clinics utilize an electronic health record (EHR). An EHR can be defined as a digital longitudinal repository of electronic health information for an individual patient that provides medical staff with the information necessary for delivering clinical care (Raman et al. 2018; Hayrinen et al. 2008). Since the institution of the Health Information Technology for Economic and Clinical Health Act in 2009, 90% of office-based clinicians and 100% of hospital-based clinicians are using an EHR in some capacity.

The digitalized modern healthcare system produces exponentially increasing quantities of data on an annual basis. Indeed, projections suggest that the US healthcare system alone will produce zettabytes (10^{21} gigabytes) and yodabytes (10^{24} gigabytes) of data in the coming years. "Big data" is defined as data so large and complex that traditional mechanisms and software used to store and analyze data are insufficient (Hilbert and Lopez 2011). Today's generated data are also heterogenous, and when combined with the increasing rate of generation, the vastness of data is overwhelming. Practically, "big data" in healthcare refers not only to data generated but also to methods of generation, processing to render it useful, and computational methods used to analyze data and generate evidence that guides clinical practice. Moreover, with the emergence of EHRs and advanced analytics, data elements now have the potential to serve a dual purpose and contribute to both direct patient care and clinical research or trials. While continually evolving its structure and functionality, EHRs and "big data" technology offer the potential to streamline and increase the speed of clinical research. Never before has health information for so many people spread among various locations been readily accessible and captured in centralized platforms.

There Is No Substitute for Randomization

To date, "big data" and the digitalization of healthcare information and delivery have allowed for numerous analyses addressing the current state and changes in medical practice, including (but not limited to) uptake of evidence-based practices, patterns and disparities of care, characterization of risk factors for various outcomes, and detection of potential treatment-related safety signals. However, while these observational studies can be critically important, perhaps the most impactful role of "big data" in medical research involves potential use in randomized controlled trials.

When assessing the effect of a medical therapy or intervention, randomization is required to prove causality. Assignment of treatment is mandatory to eliminate selection bias and confounding that inevitably occurs when patients or physicians are allowed to choose the therapy received (Fonarow 2016). Nonetheless, there has been increasing interest in using observational data for comparing outcomes and safety with different therapies. In efforts to account for selection bias related to receiving a therapy, multiple sophisticated statistical approaches have been developed, including multivariable risk modeling, propensity score risk adjustment (e.g., inverse probability weighting), propensity matching, and instrumental variable analysis (Fonarow 2016). While some have suggested these methods can simulate results from a randomized trial, it is increasingly recognized that even these approaches are subject to hidden bias and unmeasured and residual confounding. Perhaps most striking, multiple examples have highlighted that these approaches may not only fail to align with available results from randomized trials but that the specific type of statistical approach used may dictate the conclusions from observational data. For example, an observational cohort of patients with recent coronary artery stenting as treatment for heart attack evaluated the association between treatment with two different anti-platelet medications and subsequent cardiovascular outcomes (Federspiel et al. 2016). They evaluated these associations using two frequently utilized state-of-the-art statistical methods, inverse probability weighting and instrumental variable analysis, and produced different results with each. Moreover, there were concerning findings with falsification endpoints (i.e., endpoints with no biologic means of being influenced by exposure to the therapy and thus used to evaluate the rigor of the statistical methods).

Despite the need for randomized trials to prove cause-effect relationships, randomized trials are not logistically possible for all scientific questions, and patients with a given condition in trials may differ substantially from patients with the condition in general practice. Aside from other advantages for clinical trial conduct, "big data" approaches offer a chance to navigate these dilemmas by potentially facilitating randomization within routine clinical care. In the following sections, we discuss the possible avenues by which "big data" may improve randomized clinical trial execution and the subsequent impact of trial results.

Potential Avenues for Improving Clinical Trials Through "Big Data"

Research Networks with Common Data Models

In their present state, randomized clinical trials require significant infrastructure in order to enroll patients, conduct data collection/analysis, and ensure regulatory compliance. Programs to execute these trials are usually tailored to a specific project and separate from clinical practice. These infrastructures are highly inefficient; they are expensive, require extensive planning prior to execution, and cannot be recycled to answer future questions.

The Patient-Centered Outcomes Research Institute (PCORI) and resulting National Patient-Centered Clinical Research Network (PCORnet) were established to address inefficiencies of current clinical research. The institute and research network constitute a "network of networks" and are comprised of 13 Clinical Data Research Networks (CDRN) and 21 Patient-Powered Research Networks (PPRN). Each CDRN is a collection of local healthcare systems including academic health centers, community hospitals, health plans, and outpatient health centers. PPRNs are organizations of patients, families, and advocates that have coalesced and tackle issues relevant to a specific condition, usually in collaboration with clinical investigators and an associated academic health center (PCORnet). PCORnet is represented in all 50 US states and collects data from >40 million people at >100 healthcare entities. When patients receive care at participating PCORnet sites, healthcare data and insurance claims are standardized into a template, transferred to a centralized warehouse, and stored in an analysis-ready format called a Common Data Model (CDM). The key advantage of CDMs is the use of standardized data definitions. Standardization allows for rapid and efficient transmission of data generated from clinical practice into a format that is immediately analyzable.

ADAPTABLE: The Aspirin Study. A Case Example of a Pragmatic Trial Leveraging Research Networks and Common Data Models

PCORnet's ongoing "Aspirin Dosing: A Patient-Centric Trial Assessing Benefits and Long-Term Effectiveness" (ADAPTABLE) trial exemplifies the power and potential of a research network utilizing a common data model (Fig. 3) (Jones et al. 2016). ADAPTABLE aims to determine the optimal dosing of aspirin for the secondary prevention of atherosclerotic cardiovascular disease while simultaneously testing the ability to conduct a highly efficient randomized comparative effectiveness trial embedded in usual clinical practice (Johnston et al. 2016). The central premise of ADAPTABLE is to leverage EHR data at every phase of a trial while not disrupting routine clinical care. Specifically, trial recruitment and enrollment involve

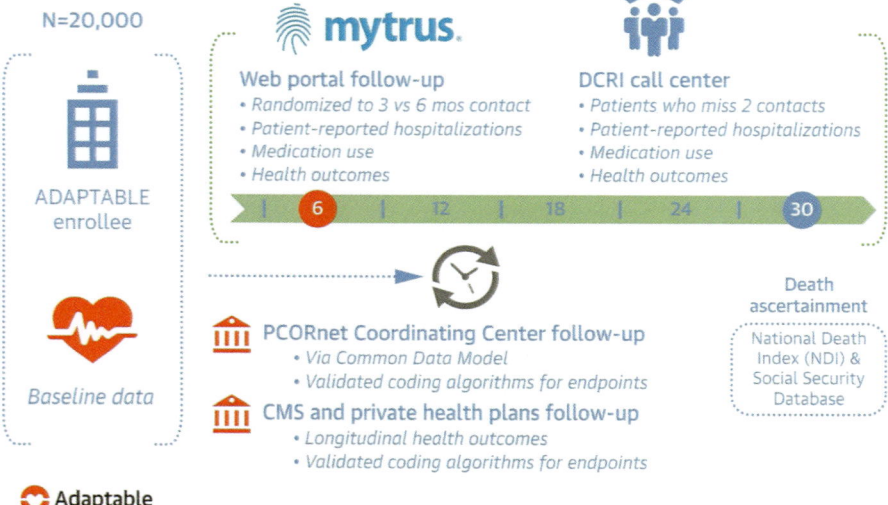

Fig. 3 ADAPTABLE data flow and follow-up. The figure depicts the ADAPTABLE trial as an example of how patients will be engaged throughout a pragmatic patient-centered clinical trial. Patients will directly log into the patient Internet portal or be contacted by the Duke Clinical Research Institute (DCRI) call center at intervals of 3 or 6 months. During these encounters, patients will be asked about prior hospitalizations, health status, and concomitant medication use (including dosage of study medication). Ascertainment of cause-specific hospitalizations with International Classification of Diseases, 10th Revision codes for nonfatal endpoints, such as MI, stroke, and major bleeding, will be performed via queries of administrative and clinical data (i.e., the common data element) within each CDRN and linked administrative claims data from Medicare and private health plans. Death status will be ascertained by routine queries of the Social Security Administration and National Death Index. CDRN = clinical data research network; CMS = Centers for Medicare & Medicaid Services; PCORnet = Patient-Centered Outcomes Research Institute's National Patient-Centered Clinical Research Network. (Reproduced with permission from Jones et al. (2016))

applying algorithms to data warehouses at participating sites to identify eligible patients, followed by email invitations. Patients can consent electronically via computer, mobile device (including smartphones), or in clinic. Patients are randomized electronically and notified of treatment assignment via a secure electronic portal (traditional enrollment/consent will also occur when desired by patients). Finally, data on clinical course and trial endpoints will be longitudinally collected electronically via data harvests from the PCORnet CDM.

Aside from the benefits of reducing burden on patient and site investigators, the design of ADAPTABLE and PCORnet facilitates a randomized trial that is efficient and inexpensive. Projected costs appear to be approximately $1,000 per patient, significantly less than the historical figure of approximately $25,000 per trial participant. Reduced costs stem largely from fewer research staff required to screen, consent/enroll, and collect data and the "re-use" of data already generated from routine care.

Pragmatic Trials Within Individual Health Systems

As exemplified from ADAPTABLE, pragmatic trials seek to establish effects of a therapy under "real-world" conditions by embedding themselves into routine clinical care. Infrastructures used to conduct pragmatic trials require upfront investment but may be recyclable. While ADAPTABLE leverages the PCORnet infrastructure and CDM to quickly amass computable data from routine clinical care, there are other ways pragmatic trials can integrate within health systems to efficiently conduct research.

The real-world Salford Lung Study was an open-label phase III pragmatic randomized trial evaluating a novel inhaled medication for patients with lung disease in and around the city of Salford, United Kingdom (New et al. 2014). Several characteristics of Salford made it a favorable location for a pragmatic trial, including a relative static population served by a single hospital and an integrated EHR between the hospital and surrounding primary care practices and pharmacies. Through this single electronic database, all study-related medications were easily provided, and events could be easily ascertained. General practitioners in Salford served as the primary investigators and were responsible for recruitment/enrollment, follow-up visits, and adjudication of safety events/study outcomes. As a similar example, the integrated Vanderbilt University health system EHR was recently leveraged to simultaneously and rapidly conduct 2 large-scale pragmatic trials enrolling >28,000 combined patients over a 2-year period. The SMART (Isotonic Solutions and Major Adverse Renal Events Trial) and SALT-ED (Saline against Lactated Ringer's or Plasma-Lyte in the Emergency Department) compared two different isotonic intravenous fluids frequently administered to hospitalized patients (Semler et al. 2018; Self et al. 2018). Both trials were conducted without interruption to ongoing clinical care across multiple settings including the emergency department, general inpatient wards, and intensive care units. For both studies, data were extracted entirely from the EHR. The US National Institutes of Health (NIH) Common Fund has also recently sponsored multiple ongoing and completed examples of embedded pragmatic clinical trials (Huang et al. 2019; Mor et al. 2017).

The Salford Lung Study, SMART, and SALT-ED trials highlight the power of an integrated individual healthcare system to conduct pragmatic and efficient research. These trials all demonstrate that minimal inclusion/exclusion criteria combined with streamlined digitized data collection and extraction lower the barriers to conduct efficient, large-scale clinical research. National initiatives such as the NIH Collaboratory aim to engage healthcare delivery systems as research partners in order to conduct efficient, large-scale, pragmatic research studies. Data, tools, and resources produced by the collaboratory are made available to the greater research community to promote partnerships with healthcare systems and propel a transformation in how clinical research is conducted.

Connecting Multiple Health Systems as a Single Research Network

By virtue of utilizing a single health system (e.g., SLS, SMART, and SALT-ED) or a pre-existing research network (e.g., ADAPTABLE and PCORNet), the abovementioned pragmatic trials all share the common theme of using an integrated research database to extract curated, computable data ready to be analyzed. On the other hand, when involving multiple healthcare systems with different EHR platforms, extracted data requires further processing and standardization before it can be compiled and analyzed. This necessity stands as a major obstacle hindering current abilities to pool data across healthcare systems. In efforts to improve this process, Fast Healthcare Interoperability Resources (FHIR; pronounced "fire") is in development as a technology designed to export and share data from a specific EHR. However, although FHIR provides an interface for compiling large real-world datasets across multiple EHRs, it remains limited in that its final product is raw, unanalyzable data that must still undergo processing and standardization.

As an example of how a service such as FHIR may be extended, Flatiron Health is a data network designed to both acquire and analyze big data to help cure cancer. Flatiron's OncologyCloud platform provides services and technology that include a full-fledged EHR with included claims and billing services that can be utilized by community oncologists. Through this platform and its partnership with the National Comprehensive Cancer Network, Flatiron may integrate with academic medical centers and hospital-based EHRs to curate and export local data. Together, information from over 265 community clinics and academic institutions is combined and curated into a clinico-genomic database with cancer genetics linked to patient demographics, previous/ongoing therapies, and outcomes. These data can then be analyzed to generate real-world evidence.

Registries for Improving Clinical Trials and Curating Big Data

Prospective registries can generally be described as observational studies used by professional societies, government agencies, private corporations, and independent researchers to collect standardized data from patients seen in a variety of settings.

Data can be used for a variety of purposes, including description of practice patterns and trends, identification of outliers, detection of safety signals, or assessment of comparative effectiveness.

More recently, the concept of "registry-based randomized trials" has been introduced. Such programs use existing registry infrastructure and data capture to streamline the process of establishing trial sites, enrolling patients, and maintaining follow-up. The trial then randomizes patients who would otherwise be in the registry to a given intervention and thus remains able to determine causality similar to a traditional randomized trial. Two prominent examples of this registry-based randomized trial approach have been recently completed in the interventional cardiology space. The SAFE-PCI for Women trial was able to use an existing registry to execute a trial of radial versus femoral vascular access for coronary stent placement (Rao et al. 2014). Much of the basic patient data for the trial, including demographics, medical history, medications, and index hospitalization clinical outcomes, were electronically harvested from the registry database of consenting patients and auto-populated into the trial's electronic case report form. Study leadership estimated that this feature decreased study coordinator workload by 65%. Similarly, the TASTE (Thrombus Aspiration in ST-Elevation Myocardial Infarction in Scandinavia) trial comparing thrombus aspiration plus coronary stenting to coronary stenting alone was conducted within a large national Swedish registry.(Frobert et al. 2013). Using this registry platform, the trial randomized >7200 patients, >6 times more than a previous landmark trial of the same intervention (Svilaas et al. 2008). In summary, both SAFE-PCI and TASTE illustrate the possibility of inserting randomization into established registries.

Digital Health Devices to Decrease the Burden of Trial Participation for Patients

Combining big data approaches with digital health technologies has the significant potential to reduce the burden of clinical trials on patients and make trial participation more attractive. Although still relatively uncommon, the use of digital technologies within clinical trials has been increasing over time (Fig. 4).

Patient Recruitment and Consent

Aside from the above-noted ADAPTABLE trial, a small but increasing number of cohort studies have shown the feasibility of using a web-based or app-based platform for patient recruitment. For example, the MyHeart Counts Cardiovascular Health Study recruited and consented 48,968 patients over a 10-month period in 2015 using the Apple Research Kit (McConnell et al. 2017; Sharma et al. 2018). Likewise, the Health eHeart Study, a PPRN within PCORnet, enrolled and consented >140,000 patients using digital technology (Sharma et al. 2018). Many of the patients from this broad cardiology-focused e-cohort have then been secondarily recruited to disease-specific ancillary studies.

As a key factor related to recruitment, digital health has the potential to make the consent process less onerous and confusing for patients. Innovative strategies to

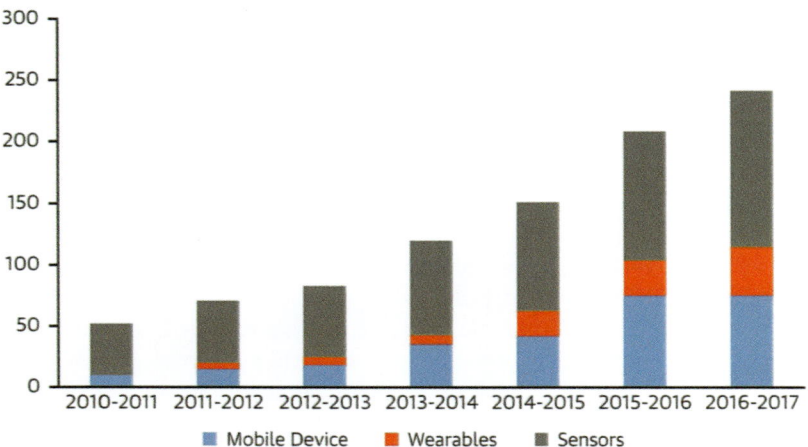

Fig. 4 Use of digital health technologies within clinical trials. Data reflect the number of initially registered trials on clinicaltrials.gov per year (accessed March 20, 2017). Posted entries are defined based on investigator description of proposed devices used. (Reproduced with permission from Sharma et al. (2018))

improve the consent experience include electronic informed consent, mobile-app based consent, and video consent. These platforms offer benefits of allowing patients to learn and proceed at their own pace and on their own schedule while potentially using patient-centered language and less medicolegal jargon. Recently, the Provider Assessment of Lipid Management (PALM) registry published findings related to a novel tablet-based video informed consent tool (Fanaroff et al. 2018b). Of 153 sites participating in the registry, 44% obtained IRB approval for video consent, while remaining sites used a conventional consent process (Fanaroff et al. 2018b). Although sites in PALM using video and traditional consent enrolled similar numbers of overall patients, the video consent process was associated with shorter time from site approach to first patient enrolled and increased enrollment of traditionally underrepresented patient groups, including older patients ≥75 years and nonwhite patients (Fanaroff et al. 2018b). Although PALM was a non-interventional registry program, these data generate the hypothesis that similar processes could be practically applied and be useful in the consent for randomized trials.

Study Endpoints

Contrary to the traditional model of study-specific in-person visits, digital health offers the potential for convenient and remote collection of patient data. Web-based portal, mobile apps, and other devices may allow data to be transmitted directly from patient's homes or during usual activities, thus better blending clinical research participation with everyday life. Moreover, by making data collection more convenient, studies may be able to collect a greater amount of information while still reducing in-person visits and the burden of participation compared to the conventional randomized trial. For example, the NEAT-HFpEF (Nitrate's Effect on Activity Tolerance in Heart Failure

With Preserved Ejection Fraction) trial randomized patients with heart failure with preserved ejection fraction (HFpEF) to isosorbide mononitrate or placebo and evaluated the primary endpoint of daily activity level, defined by patient wearable activity monitors containing high-sensitivity accelerometers (Redfield et al. 2015). Although activity level has been a frequent endpoint in HF trials, most have evaluated activity level at discrete time points during in-person study visits using the 6-minute walk test (i.e., measuring the maximal distance patients can walk in 6 min). However, like most traditional study follow-up assessments, the 6-minute walk test reflects only a brief snapshot in time and may not be fully representative of patient health status during everyday life. The NEAT-HFpEF study demonstrated that compared with placebo, isosorbide dinitrate caused notable worsening of patient activity level as measured by the activity monitor, but no difference in 6-minute walk test (Redfield et al. 2015). This discrepancy between endpoints intended to measure the same thing (i.e., activity level) illustrates the potential advantages and added sensitivity of continuous data for detecting treatment effects. In this context, digital health technologies may help facilitate more complete or continuous data capture for study endpoints without increasing demands on patients. These approaches to centralize data collection for study endpoints and follow-up may also decrease study costs and the demands on local study personnel and infrastructure.

Embedding Machine Learning Within Clinical Trials

Machine learning can be defined as statistical programming that harnesses substantial computational power to execute algorithms that learn from raw data without human interaction (Darcy et al. 2016). The term "machine learning" is often used interchangeably with artificial intelligence, but more precisely, machine learning represents the set of techniques that enable artificial intelligence (Johnson et al. 2018). These advanced analytic approaches are able to use objective and data-driven processes to examine large datasets for purposes of identifying relationships and making predictions (Fig. 5).

Phenotyping Complex Diseases

Despite significant research, many common medical conditions remain relatively poorly understood. Given the high numbers of patients afflicted by these diseases and the associated healthcare resource utilization, these select conditions represent areas where advancement in therapy and care delivery could pay the largest dividends. One such example is HFpEF. HFpEF comprises roughly half of the ~38 million people worldwide with HF and is projected to be the most common form of heart failure (HF) in the coming years. Despite this increasing burden of disease and a long-term prognosis comparable to many forms of cancer, the etiology and pathophysiology of HFpEF remain unclear. Despite numerous clinical trials, uncertainty in the definition and mechanism of disease has directly contributed to the current lack of available treatments proven to improve patient outcomes. Specifically, the heterogeneity of the HFpEF syndrome and patient profile has been a key challenge to studying the

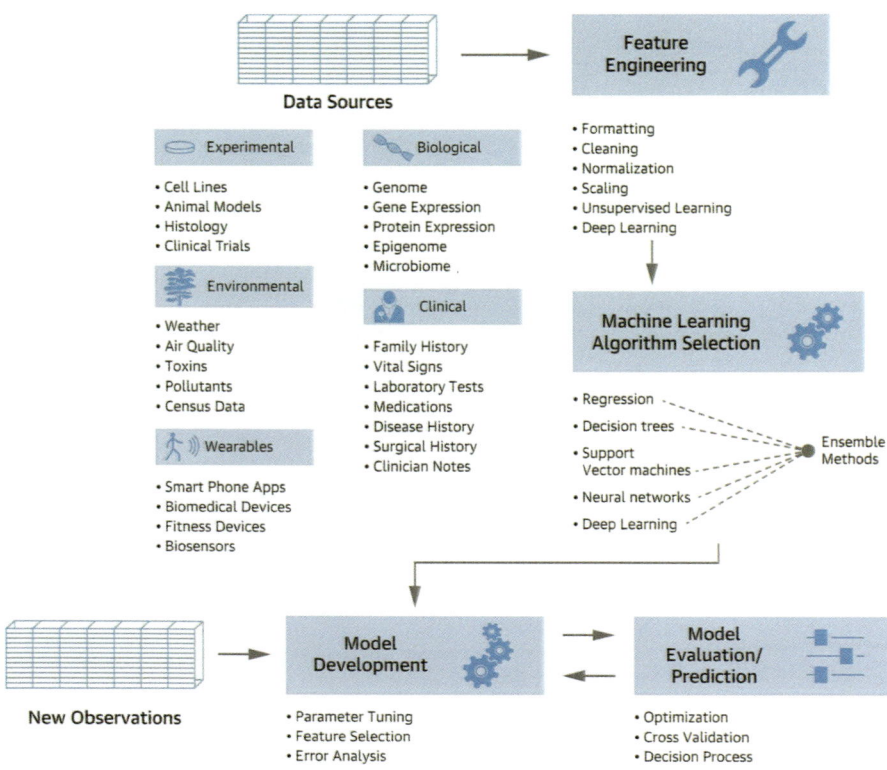

Fig. 5 Overview of the machine learning workflow. The central promise of machine learning is to incorporate data from a variety of sources (clinical measurements and observations, biological omics, experimental results, environmental information, wearable devices) into sensible models for describing and predicting human disease. The typical machine learning workflow begins with data acquisition, proceeds to feature engineering and then to algorithm selection and model development, and finally results in model evaluation and application. (Reproduced from Johnson et al. (2018))

condition and therapeutic advancement. While traditional clinical trial subgroup analyses by baseline patient characteristics have generally been unrevealing, many experts have argued that HFpEF patient phenotypes are complex and that future clinical trials must match investigational therapies with the phenotype most likely to benefit. Given the uncertainty and relative subjectivity regarding ideal definitions for specific phenotype, Shah et al. used an innovative "big data" machine learning approach to phenomap a detailed HFpEF database (Shah et al. 2015). An objective unbiased machine learning algorithm used data from 67 continuous variables to define three mutually exclusive HFpEF clusters (Shah et al. 2015). Each group differed markedly in clinical characteristics and risk for clinical events, and the classification scheme was prospectively validated in a second cohort. While the utility of this classification scheme in subsequent HFpEF trials remains to be seen, this example illustrates the power of "big data" to classify complex medication conditions into clinically relevant subsets when simple clinical criteria or clinician judgement may be inadequate. Aside from enriching clinical trial populations with a specific subset of patients, these sophisticated "big data" phenotypes may also be important in the emerging era of "precision medicine" where tailoring interventions and treatment strategies to particular patients is increasingly emphasized.

Risk Prediction

As an alternative to characterization of patients by phenotype, machine learning may also be used within clinical trials to characterize patients by level of risk. Statistical power calculations are based on expected accrual of clinical events, with higher event rates inversely proportional to sample size required. Thus, for feasibility purposes, traditional clinical trials frequently utilize "enrichment criteria" within eligibility criteria to select for higher-risk patients. Nonetheless, despite these efforts, trials frequently encounter lower than expected event rates and jeopardize study power. In this context, machine learning algorithms have the potential to predict downstream risk better than simple clinical variables or even multivariable risk models. For example, a sophisticated machine learning analysis including >44,000 HF patients demonstrated excellent calibration and discrimination for 1-year survival, while ejection fraction (a simple and commonly referenced variable used in trial selection criteria) did not (Ahmad et al. 2018). Although applying a machine learning calculation to identify patients could appear more complicated than using traditional clinical variables, this concern may be alleviated by embedding such automated tools within the EHR. One could imagine the scenario where patient data would be pulled in real time from the EHR and the final output continually calculated and presented back to the practicing clinician within the EHR. Such a platform would take advantage of robust statistical analytics and improved predictive power while presenting data in a simplified and easily actionable form to the clinician or study coordinator.

Patient Recruitment and Engagement

Aside from the trial protocol and intervention itself, prior studies have suggested that objective patient factors such as age, race, sex, and socioeconomic status influence likelihood of participation, as well as subjective factors such as patient attitudes toward research. Nonetheless, despite general awareness of these specific challenges to recruitment among researchers, these barriers to enrollment persist. In this context, machine learning may offer the ability to use automated algorithms to provide granular detail on patient subsets by likelihood of trial participation and predict the chances of patient participation should they be approached. A novel study by Ni et al. explored this hypothesis (Ni et al. 2016). Investigators collected 3,345 patient responses to trial invitations from 18 trials ongoing at a pediatric hospital emergency department at single center over a 3-year period (Ni et al. 2016). They then leveraged machine learning to construct automated algorithms based on available patient-level data and found the model to perform well for predicting patient response. If confirmed across other care settings and disease states, this innovative application of machine learning has the potential to reshape current approaches to patient recruitment. Specifically, these methods could be used to (1) more specifically identify challenging patient subsets and improve their representation or (2) identify patients who are likely to participate, thus increasing recruitment efficiency and optimizing allocation of resources at enrolling study sites.

Summary and Conclusion

Randomized clinical trials are necessary to definitively determine treatment effects of medical interventions and are instrumental in informing patient care and clinical decisions. Nonetheless, contemporary clinical trials are becoming increasingly difficult to execute and are hampered by slow patient enrollment, burdensome data collection beyond that required for standard care, and high costs. The current infusion of digital technology and computing power within healthcare has given birth to the new field of health data science and possibility of using "big data" approaches to innovate and improve upon traditional clinical trials. The primary focus of health technology to date has been direct patient care, but these platforms offer further potential to change the paradigm for conducting clinical research and generating medical evidence. The digitalization of medical information allows data across multiple health systems to be pooled and centralized within readily analyzable common data models with standardized data definitions. Moreover, these technologies favor embedding clinical research within everyday clinical care, offering the benefits of generalizable study results, "re-use" of data already collected during routine patient care, more rapid patient accrual, and minimizing the burden of trial participation on patients and local study sites. "Big data" approaches and machine learning also may aid in phenotyping complex medical conditions and identifying patient subsets for study in clinical trials. Moving forward, the rise of "big data" within healthcare signals the realization of a new emerging clinical research paradigm. Harnessing the capabilities of "big data" and integrating these elements within clinical trials offer a vision of an efficient, cost-effective, and patient-centered system for generating actionable medical evidence and improving human health.

Disclosures Dr. Greene has received a Heart Failure Society of America/Emergency Medicine Foundation Acute Heart Failure Young Investigator Award funded by Novartis, receives research support from the American Heart Association, Amgen, AstraZeneca, Bristol-Myers Squibb, Merck, and Novartis; serves on advisory boards for Amgen and Cytokinetics; and serves as a consultant for Amgen and Merck.

References

Ahmad T, Lund LH, Rao P, Ghosh R, Warier P, Vaccaro B, Dahlstrom U, O'Connor CM, Felker GM, Desai NR (2018) Machine learning methods improve prognostication, identify clinically distinct phenotypes, and detect heterogeneity in response to therapy in a large cohort of heart failure patients. J Am Heart Assoc 77(8):e008081. https://doi.org/10.1161/JAHA.117.008081

Butler J, Tahhan AS, Georgiopoulou VV, Kelkar A, Lee M, Khan B, Peterson E, Fonarow GC, Kalogeropoulos AP, Gheorghiade M (2015) Trends in characteristics of cardiovascular clinical trials 2001–2012. Am Heart J 170:263–272

Califf RM, Harrington RA (2011) American industry and the U.S. Cardiovascular Clinical Research Enterprise an appropriate analogy? J Am Coll Cardiol 58:677–680

Darcy AM, Louie AK, Roberts LW (2016) Machine learning and the profession of medicine. JAMA 315:551–552

Fanaroff AC, Steffel J, Alexander JH, Lip GYH, Califf RM, Lopes RD (2018a) Stroke prevention in atrial fibrillation: re-defining 'real-world data' within the broader data universe. Eur Heart J 39(32):2932–2941

Fanaroff AC, Li S, Webb LE, Miller V, Navar AM, Peterson ED, Wang TY (2018b) An observational study of the Association of video- versus text-based informed consent with multicenter trial enrollment: lessons from the PALM study (Patient and Provider Assessment of Lipid Management). Circ Cardiovasc Qual Outcomes 11:e004675

FDA U. http://www.fda.gov/ucm/groups/fdagov-public/@fdagov-afda-gen/documents/document/ucm126396.pdf. Accessed 20 Jan 2017

Federspiel JJ, Anstrom KJ, Xian Y, McCoy LA, Effron MB, Faries DE, Zettler M, Mauri L, Yeh RW, Peterson ED, Wang TY (2016) Treatment with adenosine diphosphate receptor inhibitors-longitudinal assessment of treatment P and events after acute coronary syndrome I. Comparing inverse probability of treatment weighting and instrumental variable methods for the evaluation of adenosine diphosphate receptor inhibitors after percutaneous coronary intervention. JAMA Cardiol 1:655–665

Fonarow GC (2016) Randomization-there is no substitute. JAMA Cardiol 1:633–635

Frobert O, Lagerqvist B, Olivecrona GK, Omerovic E, Gudnason T, Maeng M, Aasa M, Angeras O, Calais F, Danielewicz M, Erlinge D, Hellsten L, Jensen U, Johansson AC, Karegren A, Nilsson J, Robertson L, Sandhall L, Sjogren I, Ostlund O, Harnek J, James SK, Trial T (2013) Thrombus aspiration during ST-segment elevation myocardial infarction. N Engl J Med 369:1587–1597

Greene SJ, Fonarow GC, Solomon SD, Subacius H, Maggioni AP, Bohm M, Lewis EF, Zannad F, Gheorghiade M, Investigators A (2015) Coordinators. Global variation in clinical profile, management, and post-discharge outcomes among patients hospitalized for worsening chronic heart failure: findings from the ASTRONAUT trial. Eur J Heart Fail 17:591–600

Hayrinen K, Saranto K, Nykanen P (2008) Definition, structure, content, use and impacts of electronic health records: a review of the research literature. Int J Med Inform 77:291–304

Hilbert M, Lopez P (2011) The world's technological capacity to store, communicate, and compute information. Science (New York, NY) 332:60–65

Huang SS, Septimus E, Kleinman K, Moody J, Hickok J, Heim L, Gombosev A, Avery TR, Haffenreffer K, Shimelman L, Hayden MK, Weinstein RA, Spencer-Smith C, Kaganov RE, Murphy MV, Forehand T, Lankiewicz J, Coady MH, Portillo L, Sarup-Patel J, Jernigan JA, Perlin JB, Platt R, team AIt (2019) Chlorhexidine versus routine bathing to prevent multidrug-resistant organisms and all-cause bloodstream infections in general medical and surgical units (ABATE infection trial): a cluster-randomised trial. Lancet 393:1205–1215

Institute of Medicine (2017) Crossing the quality chasm: a new health system for the 21st century. The National Academies of Sciences, Engineering, and Medicine. National Academy Press (Washington DC)

Johnson KW, Torres Soto J, Glicksberg BS, Shameer K, Miotto R, Ali M, Ashley E, Dudley JT (2018) Artificial Intelligence in Cardiology. J Am Coll Cardiol 71:2668–2679

Johnston A, Jones WS, Hernandez AF (2016) The ADAPTABLE trial and aspirin dosing in secondary prevention for patients with coronary artery disease. Curr Cardiol Rep 18:81

Jones WS, Roe MT, Antman EM, Pletcher MJ, Harrington RA, Rothman RL, Oetgen WJ, Rao SV, Krucoff MW, Curtis LH, Hernandez AF, Masoudi FA (2016) The changing landscape of randomized clinical trials in cardiovascular disease. J Am Coll Cardiol 68:1898–1907

Martin L, Hutchens M, Hawkins C, Radnov A (2017a) How much do clinical trials cost? Nat Rev Drug Discov 16:381–382

Martin L, Hutchens M, Hawkins C (2017b) Trial watch: clinical trial cycle times continue to increase despite industry efforts. Nat Rev Drug Discov 16(3):157. https://doi.org/10.1038/nrd.2017.21

McConnell MV, Shcherbina A, Pavlovic A, Homburger JR, Goldfeder RL, Waggot D, Cho MK, Rosenberger ME, Haskell WL, Myers J, Champagne MA, Mignot E, Landray M, Tarassenko L, Harrington RA, Yeung AC, Ashley EA (2017) Feasibility of obtaining measures of lifestyle from a smartphone app: the MyHeart counts cardiovascular health study. JAMA Cardiol 2:67–76

Mor V, Volandes AE, Gutman R, Gatsonis C, Mitchell SL (2017) PRagmatic trial of video education in nursing homes: the design and rationale for a pragmatic cluster randomized trial in the nursing home setting. Clin Trials 14:140–151

New JP, Bakerly ND, Leather D, Woodcock A (2014) Obtaining real-world evidence: the Salford Lung Study. Thorax 69:1152–1154

Ni Y, Beck AF, Taylor R, Dyas J, Solti I, Grupp-Phelan J, Dexheimer JW (2016) Will they participate? Predicting patients' response to clinical trial invitations in a pediatric emergency department. J Am Med Inform Assoc 23:671–680

PCORnet: The National Patient Centered Clinical Research Network. https://www.pcori.org/research-results/pcornet-national-patient-centered-clinical-research-network. Accessed 10 May 2018

Raman SR, Curtis LH, Temple R, Andersson T, Ezekowitz J, Ford I, James S, Marsolo K, Mirhaji P, Rocca M, Rothman RL, Sethuraman B, Stockbridge NL, Terry S, Wasserman S, Peterson ED, Hernandez AF (2018) Leveraging electronic health records for clinical research. Am Heart J 202:13–19. https://doi.org/10.1016/j.ahj.2018.04.015

Rao SV, Hess CN, Barham B, Aberle LH, Anstrom KJ, Patel TB, Jorgensen JP, Mazzaferri EL Jr, Jolly SS, Jacobs A, Newby LK, Gibson CM, Kong DF, Mehran R, Waksman R, Gilchrist IC, McCourt BJ, Messenger JC, Peterson ED, Harrington RA, Krucoff MW (2014) A registry-based randomized trial comparing radial and femoral approaches in women undergoing percutaneous coronary intervention: the SAFE-PCI for women (Study of Access Site for Enhancement of PCI for women) trial. JACC Cardiovasc Interv 7:857–867

Redfield MM, Anstrom KJ, Levine JA, Koepp GA, Borlaug BA, Chen HH, LeWinter MM, Joseph SM, Shah SJ, Semigran MJ, Felker GM, Cole RT, Reeves GR, Tedford RJ, Tang WH, McNulty SE, Velazquez EJ, Shah MR, Braunwald E, Network NHFCR (2015) Isosorbide mononitrate in heart failure with preserved ejection fraction. N Engl J Med 373:2314–2324

Self WH, Semler MW, Wanderer JP, Wang L, Byrne DW, Collins SP, Slovis CM, Lindsell CJ, Ehrenfeld JM, Siew ED, Shaw AD, Bernard GR, Rice TW, Investigators S-E (2018) Balanced crystalloids versus saline in noncritically ill adults. N Engl J Med 378:819–828

Semler MW, Self WH, Wanderer JP, Ehrenfeld JM, Wang L, Byrne DW, Stollings JL, Kumar AB, Hughes CG, Hernandez A, Guillamondegui OD, May AK, Weavind L, Casey JD, Siew ED, Shaw AD, Bernard GR, Rice TW, Investigators S, the Pragmatic Critical Care Research G (2018) Balanced crystalloids versus saline in critically ill adults. N Engl J Med 378:829–839

Shah SJ, Katz DH, Selvaraj S, Burke MA, Yancy CW, Gheorghiade M, Bonow RO, Huang CC, Deo RC (2015) Phenomapping for novel classification of heart failure with preserved ejection fraction. Circulation 131:269–279

Sharma A, Harrington RA, McClellan MB, Turakhia MP, Eapen ZJ, Steinhubl S, Mault JR, Majmudar MD, Roessig L, Chandross KJ, Green EM, Patel B, Hamer A, Olgin J, Rumsfeld JS, Roe MT, Peterson ED (2018) Using digital health technology to better generate evidence and deliver evidence-based care. J Am Coll Cardiol 71:2680–2690

Summer R, Wiener RS, Carroll D, Sager A (2012) Physician perception of the impact of productivity measures on academic practice. Arch Intern Med 172:967–969

Svilaas T, Vlaar PJ, van der Horst IC, Diercks GF, de Smet BJ, van den Heuvel AF, Anthonio RL, Jessurun GA, Tan ES, Suurmeijer AJ, Zijlstra F (2008) Thrombus aspiration during primary percutaneous coronary intervention. N Engl J Med 358:557–567

Trials in Complementary and Integrative Health Interventions

115

Catherine M. Meyers and Qilu Yu

Contents

Introduction	2264
Trials of Natural Products	2266
Defining the Intervention and Appropriate Controls	2266
Randomization and Masking	2267
Assessing Intervention Quality	2268
Compliance and Contamination	2269
Alternative Trial Designs	2269
Trials of Mind and Body Approaches	2270
Defining the Intervention and Appropriate Controls	2270
Randomization and the Trial Design	2271
Masking	2274
Assessing Intervention Quality	2275
Fidelity of Intervention Delivery	2275
Adherence to the Intervention	2276
Contamination	2277
Missing Data	2277
Other Considerations for Trials of Complementary and Integrative Health Approaches	2278
Participant Recruitment and Retention	2278
Efficacy Outcomes Assessment	2279
Safety Outcomes Assessment	2280
Reporting Research Results	2280
Conclusion	2283
Key Facts	2284
Cross-References	2284
References	2285

C. M. Meyers (✉) · Q. Yu
Office of Clinical and Regulatory Affairs, National Institutes of Health, National Center for Complementary and Integrative Health, Bethesda, MD, USA
e-mail: cm420i@nih.gov; meyersc@mail.nih.gov; yuq6@nih.gov; qilu.yu@nih.gov

© This is a U.S. Government work and not under copyright protection in the U.S.;
foreign copyright protection may apply 2022
S. Piantadosi, C. L. Meinert (eds.), *Principles and Practice of Clinical Trials*,
https://doi.org/10.1007/978-3-319-52636-2_162

Abstract

Trials of complementary and integrative health approaches study a variety of health interventions, such as natural products and mind and body practices, in diverse clinical settings. The nature and level of pre-existing information on these interventions have a large impact on trial planning, as lack of a standardized intervention and potential intervention complexity pose unique challenges for trial planning and analysis. Natural products, including dietary supplement trials, are in many ways similar to conventional drug trials but typically require considerable early-phase data prior to actually launching efficacy studies. Some botanical or herbal natural products are mixtures of compounds that are challenging for reliable product characterization. By contrast, mind and body approaches encompass a number of practices that are delivered in either individual or group sessions, and trials by design are not fully masked. Standardizing intervention delivery remains a critical factor for many of these interventions; and those delivered in a group setting bring greater complexity to trial designs and analyses. With widespread use by the public of these interventions, there is expanding interest in performing appropriately designed clinical trials to generate an evidence base for both safety and efficacy of complementary and integrative health approaches.

Keywords

Natural product · Dietary supplement · Herbal · Probiotic · Mind and body · Yoga · Meditation · Acupuncture · Chiropractic

Introduction

Complementary and integrative health approaches include a variety of interventions that are not typically part of conventional medical care and that may have origins outside of traditional Western medical practice. Complementary refers to the use of these interventions together with conventional medical care, whereas integrative health refers to a more coordinated approach that uses both complementary and conventional medical care. The National Health Interview Survey (NHIS) data on trends in use of complementary and integrative health approaches suggests that less than 5% of US adults use such approaches as alternatives to conventional medical care but rather use them in addition to conventional care (Clarke et al. 2015). These interventions are broadly divided into two distinct categories, natural products and mind and body practices. Natural products include dietary supplements, herbal or botanical products, and probiotics, which are widely marketed in the USA. Mind and body approaches, however, comprise a number of different interventions, practices, and practitioner disciplines such as acupuncture, yoga, meditation, tai chi, massage, and chiropractic and osteopathic manipulation.

There is considerable use of complementary and integrative health approaches in the USA. The NHIS data suggest that perhaps 40% of the general population use one or more complementary health practices on a regular basis (Clarke et al. 2015). Table 1 relates the trend in these observations since 2002, which indicates sustained widespread use of natural products and a marked increase in yoga exposure over time. The five most common natural product supplements reported in the 2012 NHIS data (Table 2) are fish oil, glucosamine or chondroitin, probiotics or prebiotics, melatonin, and coenzyme Q, although trends of use from 2007 to 2012 suggest some changes in supplements taken by US adults. A further increase in the use of yoga and meditation are noted in the recent NHIS data report from 2017. NHIS data reports reveal that women and non-Hispanic whites are more likely to use these approaches, with some geographic variability around the USA. Similar use trends are also reported for US children (aged 4–17 years). With such widespread use, there is substantial interest in conducting clinical trials of interventions commonly used by

Table 1 Use trends for selected complementary health approaches by adults in the USA (2002–2012). Age-adjusted percentages

Approach	2002	2007	2012
Natural products – dietary supplements, herbal products, and probiotics	18.9	17.7	17.7
Yoga, tai chi, and qi gong	5.8	6.7	10.1
Manipulation (chiropractic and osteopathic)	7.5	8.6	8.4
Meditation	7.6	9.4	8.0
Massage	5.0	8.3	6.9
Acupuncture	1.1	1.4	1.5

Adapted from Clarke et al. (2015)

Table 2 Use trends for selected natural products by adults in the USA (2007–2012). Age-adjusted percentages

Dietary supplement	2007	2012
Fish oil*	4.8	7.8
Glucosamine or chondroitin*	3.2	2.6
Probiotics or prebiotics*	0.4	1.6
Melatonin*	0.6	1.3
Coenzyme Q-10	1.2	1.3
Echinacea*	2.2	0.9
Cranberry (pills or capsules)	0.7	0.8
Garlic supplements*	1.4	0.8
Ginseng*	1.5	0.7
Ginkgo biloba*	1.3	0.7
Green tea pills or EGCG pills	0.7	0.6
Combination herb pill*	1.5	0.6
MSM (methylsulfonylmethane)*	0.6	0.4
Milk thistle (silymarin)	0.4	0.4
Saw palmetto*	0.7	0.4
Valerian	0.4	0.3

Adapted from Clarke et al. (2015)
*$p < 0.05$ for change from 2007 to 2012

the public. Moreover, there is a critical public health need to generate an evidence base for most complementary approaches, which can assess not only their potential efficacy for clinical symptoms or conditions but also, perhaps more importantly, can assess their safety profile for routine use.

Several design considerations have unique issues for trials of natural products and for trials of mind and body approaches. These considerations include defining the intervention and appropriate controls, randomization, masking, assessing intervention quality, participant compliance, and contamination. As trials of the two broad categories of complementary and integrative health approaches have distinct investigative challenges, the categories will be discussed separately.

Trials of Natural Products

The strength of pre-existing evidence on a specific natural product largely dictates the appropriate preclinical investigative pathway toward testing in clinical trials. This evidence base includes preliminary information on product characterization and chemistry, to dosing and potential human toxicity. Understanding the putative mechanism of action of a given product is also an important aspect of the knowledge base, as it strengthens the plausibility of the intervention and, most importantly, facilitates identification of biomarkers to document in vivo effect of the natural product. If a biomarker is identified that can be used to document exposure or activity of a product, it permits a rational approach to dosing, makes it possible to determine which patients might be responding to the intervention, and can inform choice of outcome measure (s) that are maximally sensitive (Hawke et al. 2010; Hersch et al. 2006). In addition, identifying the optimum target population and outcome marker (s) are critical milestones in the pathway to large-scale clinical trials (Hersch et al. 2006). The absence of this evidence base on a given product frequently limits expansion of clinical studies beyond early-phase testing of natural products.

Defining the Intervention and Appropriate Controls

Unlike conventional drugs, natural products, including dietary supplements, can be sold in the USA without a specific indication and without the need for clinical use data. The US Food and Drug Administration (FDA) regulates most natural products differently from conventional drugs, under the Dietary Supplement Health and Education Act for 1994, which considers dietary supplements as a special category of foods. As such, dietary supplements are typically labeled with information on how they might impact structure or function of the body (FDA/CDER 2016). Conventional drugs, by contrast, are products marketed to diagnose, cure, mitigate, treat, or prevent disease. All products meeting this drug definition are required to conduct extensive early-phase preclinical and clinical testing, which are performed during product development, prior to launching extensive clinical trials. Such early-phase testing is conducted with oversight from the FDA, typically via an Investigational New Drug (IND) application. These kinds of early-phase testing data, however, are not usually available for most natural product supplements and must therefore be generated on a specific natural product prior to planning an efficacy trial in a specific disease setting (FDA/CDER 2016). FDA generally requires that such trials also be conducted under an IND, with standard preclinical and clinical data reporting requirements (FDA/CDER 2016).

A clinical trial testing a previously uncharacterized natural product will therefore require a substantial amount of information to document safety, stability, and reproducibility of that product. This information also includes detailed knowledge about steps in the product chain of custody from harvest to patient administration. FDA released an updated Botanical Drug Development Guidance in 2016, which is a comprehensive resource on quality control procedures for trials of herbal products (FDA/CDER 2016). Investigators intending to conduct clinical studies generally contact FDA to determine if an IND application is required and for specific guidance regarding type of information required and level of detail for product characterization and preclinical testing.

In addition to product characterization and preclinical testing of natural products, early-phase testing also is facilitated by developing a bioassay for assessing product levels and performing pharmacokinetic studies. Such analyses are critical for testing study product across dose ranges, for identifying doses and dose frequencies to test in early clinical trials. Although natural products used by the public are sold with recommended daily use levels, these use levels are not typically derived from formal dose testing in a specific disease condition.

Like conventional drug studies, natural product trials must also include developing an acceptable inert placebo product for all phases of clinical testing. Some products possess physical properties that may make placebo generation challenging, or resource intensive, but an acceptable placebo in terms of appearance, size, and tablet number is an obvious critical component for conducting randomized trials that are appropriately masked (Barry et al. 2011). Also, like conventional drugs it is not anticipated that most natural products will have major clinical effects for most diseases or conditions. For clinical trials assessing the efficacy of natural product in settings where the primary outcome measure is a patient reported outcome (PRO), a mild to modest clinical effect size can be diluted by non-specific effects noted in placebo-treated groups. This has largely been observed in the setting of pain management trials, where placebo treatment can be associated with a higher than anticipated response rate, such that it is comparable to improvement in the product-treated group (Clegg et al. 2006).

Randomization and Masking

As the modern standard for safety and efficacy testing of natural products remains the inert placebo-controlled randomized clinical trials (RCT), physical characteristics of some supplements may be problematic for product masking. Strong odor, taste, or color of supplements, such as fish or peppermint oil or turmeric, require special attention in generating a masked placebo. Manufacturing strategies for such placebos, with capsules or coatings may be necessary. Some natural products may also induce characteristic clinical symptoms, such as dyspepsia or gastrointestinal upset, or induce predictable changes in clinical chemistries. These notable alterations have been described for products such as fish oil or creatine and can jeopardize study product masking during a trial (Hersch et al. 2017). These clinical side effects of the active product may also precipitate differential dropout across treatment groups in a trial. Formally assessing study masking during a natural product supplement trial is frequently undertaken (Hersch et al. 2017). In early-phase trials of supplements for which there is no pre-existing safety data, dose comparisons for supplements are frequently conducted sequentially, with dose escalation over time, rather than in a parallel group design. Such a strategy provides essential safety data on a given dose prior to subsequent product exposure at a higher dose (Barry et al. 2011). If the design includes randomization across parallel groups of differing doses, product requires matching not only physical characteristics but the number or quantity of product assigned to participants (Fried et al. 2012).

Assessing Intervention Quality

A particular challenge for natural product research is that many products are complex, a mixture of compounds, and their composition can be quite variable. This issue makes developing a standardized regimen for clinical testing difficult for many supplements. Some single-component supplements, such as resveratrol, can be accurately characterized and readily reproduced, but most plant extracts are considerably more complex. For herbal or botanical products, there is a high level of complexity and natural variability, based on climate, soil conditions, and time of harvest, which prevent investigators from completely characterizing or reproducing a particular extract (DeKosky et al. 2006; FDA/CDER 2016; Reddy et al. 2012). Moreover, some individual plant species can produce thousands of metabolites at varying concentrations. Additional variables for these products include the observation that the same species grown in different places, or even different years in the same place, will generate the different metabolic profiles. A certain amount of product variability for some supplements may be expected, but parameters must be defined in early-phase studies. An additional complexity for botanical products is that they may undergo a variety of chemical extraction methods during the manufacturing process. Manufacturers frequently use different methods for the formulations they market, and choice of method can significantly alter chemical components of an extract.

Despite these challenges, researchers must still implement a thorough analysis of products for clinical testing. Extensive characterization of a natural product supplement is a critical first step, so that subsequent study results can be appropriately interpreted and reliably reproduced. Furthermore, as has been widely documented, there can be considerable inconsistency in batch-to-batch, bottle-to-bottle, and brand-to-brand content of "off-the-shelf" dietary supplements. Degradation of supplements over time has also been well-described for many botanical extracts and must be addressed in a standardized manner prior to, and during, clinical trials (FDA/CDER 2016). Study product integrity for natural product supplement trials must be addressed in early-phase testing. Conventional drugs typically have extensive product characterization and standardized formulation, and these data must be collected prior to efficacy trials of natural product supplements.

Compliance and Contamination

As clinical trials need to ensure adequate product exposure in distinct treatment groups, planning efforts typically address issues of participant compliance and potential contamination across groups. Some supplement trials rely solely on pill counts for assessing participant compliance with the intervention, if a specific assay for detecting circulating product levels is unavailable (Hawke et al. 2010; Hersch et al. 2006). If an assay is available, monitoring product levels can be incorporated into study procedures, either at specific time points pre- or post-dose administration. Assessing study product levels can be cost-prohibitive during a trial, however, and some trials have adopted strategies of performing levels for all active treatment participants with only random sampling of placebo treatment participants (Hawke et al. 2010; Hersch et al. 2006). In view of widespread availability of dietary supplements, randomly assessing control group participants can be most useful. Although participants are usually requested to avoid taking the same or related supplements while participating in the trial, contamination with such product "drop-in" can occur (Hersch et al. 2017).

Alternative Trial Designs

Recent trends in clinical trial design have attempted to facilitate methods for improving trial strategies for medical product development. In clinical studies of new potential therapies, investigators and regulatory agencies have considered adaptive designs in both early-phase trials and large-scale confirmatory efficacy trials (FDA/CDER/CBER 2018). To facilitate optimizing final trial design, adaptations in interventional studies may include changes made to the trial procedure such as enrollment criteria (target subject population), product dose and study endpoints, and/or statistical procedure such as samples size, randomization, interim analysis, and analytic methods (FDA/CDER/CBER 2018). As previously discussed, the knowledge base for many products is lacking in several critical aspects, including target subject population, dose, and appropriate endpoints. Although adaptive design methods provide a mechanism for informed changes to study design after study initiation, appropriate analytic methods must be implemented in the planning of studies such that the scientific validity and integrity of the study is maintained (FDA/CDER/CBER 2018).

As natural products are frequently tested in settings of chronic conditions, individualized medication effectiveness tests (n of 1 trials) have been considered a potential strategy for specific products (Nikles et al. 2005). Unlike the typical RCT design, the n of 1 trial is individualized within-patient randomized and placebo-controlled and includes multiple crossover comparisons of product versus placebo or versus another active treatment (Nikles et al. 2005). Also, unlike the RCT, the n of 1 trial provides a mechanism for assessing intervention effects in individual patients who might not otherwise be included in a targeted RCT subject population (Nikles et al. 2005). These less commonly employed designs can provide a means for adequate data collection, markedly enhancing a product's knowledge base, such that more definitive clinical trials can be optimally designed and implemented.

Trials of Mind and Body Approaches

Defining the Intervention and Appropriate Controls

Similar to trials of natural products, trials of mind and body interventions must also address standardizing or characterizing the intervention delivered to participants, as well as the setting in which the intervention takes place. Development of treatment manuals or practitioner guidelines must be performed prior to a trial, to outline parameters for intervention delivery during the study (Ali et al. 2012). Manuals facilitate delivering more uniform interventions across study groups and provide a mechanism for assessing quality control during study implementation. Some mind and body interventions, such as chiropractic, massage, and acupuncture, are typically delivered via individual practitioner–patient interactions. Most other mind and body interventions, such as meditation, yoga, and tai chi, are delivered by an instructor in a group or class setting. Delineating group size (minimum and maximum number of participants), composition (research participants only or mixture of research and non-research participants), and the frequency of group sessions are essential aspects of trial planning.

In addition to the intervention that is delivered during treatment sessions, most trials of mind and body approaches are also supplemented with individual home practice sessions during the intervention phase of the study. Moreover, in the digital age, mobile apps have been developed that allow intervention delivery remotely and in a variety of settings. These variable aspects of mind and body interventions provide additional complexity and require specific attention in trial planning.

The choice of the experimental control in trials of mind and body approaches depends on the primary research question for the study. Many efficacy trials include active controls, to address factors such as time and attention, to mimic patient experience. For group interventions, the control could include a group intervention, such as an education control, which provides the social interaction with other participants and the practitioner. For individual interventions like acupuncture or chiropractic therapy, active controls could include sham or simulated interventions. The sham intervention in this setting mimics contextual effects of the primary intervention and controls for the practitioner–participant interactions(Briggs and Shurtleff 2017). It should be noted that trials of mind and body interventions, like many behavioral intervention trials, typically observe clinical benefit from active control interventions. The apparent non-specific effects of mind and body interventions, particularly in the setting of pain management, remind investigators of the importance of better understanding the context of care delivery to design trials that can improve symptom management (Briggs and Shurtleff 2017).

A waitlist is a common control arm choice for mind and body intervention trials. It includes a contemporaneous group that is not exposed to the intervention but undergoes all the required assessments, with the promise of receiving the active intervention either after study completion or during a later follow-up period of the study (Avis et al. 2016). The waitlist control strategy is useful for assessing more immediate treatment effects during the initial intervention phase of a trial, but is not an optimal choice for assessing more delayed or sustained treatment effects for mind and body approaches.

Mind and body intervention trials that focus on treatment effectiveness outcomes typically include a control group that receives usual care or other commonly available interventions (Cherkin et al. 2016). Since usual care frequently changes over time, it is important that studies track how it changes during the trial and document interventions delivered to participants. Understanding the variation in usual care over time is critical for interpreting trial findings. One design strategy to address the potential drift in usual care is to include a two-group comparison of usual care versus usual care with the add-on active intervention.

Prior to launching large-scale trials of mind and body interventions, it is important to assess the feasibility and acceptability of a specific control group in the target population. As participants in trials of these interventions will not be masked to group assignment, studies may experience greater than expected study dropout rates due to participant disappointment at group assignment. Participants may have expectations for benefit with a specific intervention and may be less likely to remain in a trial with an active control intervention (education control for meditation interventions or walking control for tai chi trials) (Eisendrath et al. 2016; Wang et al. 2010). Including a waitlist control may address this dropout issue, by ultimately offering the intervention to all participants, but it will not provide information on the potential time and attention aspects of the intervention.

Randomization and the Trial Design

As outlined in Table 3, trials of mind and body interventions implement a variety of randomization strategies, based on how the intervention is typically administered. Individual-randomized mind and body trials, such as acupuncture, massage, or chiropractic therapy, can be conducted at a single site or multiple sites (Eisendrath et al. 2016; Goertz et al. 2013; Perlman et al. 2019). Single site trials are more commonly conducted in early-phase studies, whereas multisite studies are larger-scale trials with greater power to test study hypotheses and obtain more generalizable

Table 3 Design and randomization strategies for trials of mind and body interventions

Design	Unit of randomization	Intervention
Individual-randomized trial	Individual	Individual level
Individually randomized group treatment trial	Individual	Group level
Partially nested randomized trial	Individual	Group level for one intervention arm; individual level for the other intervention arm
Group-randomized trial	Group	Group level
Stepped-wedge group-randomized trial	Group	Group level

findings. To ensure balance across intervention arms, stratified randomization is frequently performed on patient characteristics related to outcomes within site. For mind and body intervention trials, these characteristics typically focus on gender, age, previous exposure, to the intervention and chronicity of the underlying condition or symptom assessed (Eisendrath et al. 2016; Goertz et al. 2013; Perlman et al. 2019). With complex interventions, training and retention of study teams at each site may become challenging during such trials, due to issues in remote training and monitoring, quality assurance, and competing demands of staff's responsibilities.

Another common design for mind and body interventions is individually randomized group treatment (IRGT) trials, in which the unit of randomization is the individual, but interventions are delivered in a group setting. Examples include studies of meditation, tai chi, or yoga in which participants receive the intervention in small groups or classes (Eisendrath et al. 2016; Wang et al. 2010). Cohorts are typically randomized across treatment groups, once a sufficient number of participants are identified. Participants in these groups can have the same interventionist or instructor and/or have various level of interactions with other participants in the same group. The timing of randomization for trials of group interventions can be challenging, however. Depending upon the group size, the waiting period between randomization and initiation of the group intervention can be quite long due to a number of logistical factors. Loss of participants in this phase between randomization and intervention delivery significantly impacts trial success and interpretation of trial results.

Study design and analysis becomes even more complex with partially nested randomized trials, where unbalanced design is precipitated by clustering in only one study arm. For example, participants in one arm may receive a group meditation intervention, while those in the other arm receive individualized usual care. Clustering introduced by group treatment in either one or both study arms must be accounted for in the sample size calculations and statistical analysis.

Compared to individual-randomized or IRGT trials, group or cluster randomized trials (GRT) are randomized controlled trials in which the unit of randomization is a group or cluster and measurement of outcomes is obtained among members of the groups or clusters (Turner et al. 2017). This trial design has been useful for interventions that assess effectiveness of mind and body interventions, administered either at a clinician, clinic, or health system level (DeBar et al. 2018). Group randomization is often adopted when the intervention is operated naturally at a group level or when individual randomization is not feasible or could lead to treatment group contamination. For example, in a trial studying a single or combination of mind and body interventions in patients with chronic low back pain, randomization at the patient level could be associated with substantial risk of contamination across study arms due to shared knowledge of the treatments in the same clinic and/or overlap in clinic personnel. Randomization is therefore carried out at the clinic or health plan level.

The randomization in GRTs in the setting of mind and body studies needs to balance baseline characteristics across intervention arms, including balancing of baseline covariates as well as group sample size. Methods for balancing covariates include stratification, pair matching, and constrained randomization (Wright et al. 2015). Variability in group size can also be adjusted for in sample size calculations on the basis of the mean and variance of the group size or on the basis of relative efficiency (Carter 2010). In GRTs, since interventions are carried out at group level, outcomes for participants of the same group are likely to be more similar to each other than to outcomes for members from other groups. Such clustering needs to be accounted for in the design and in the data analysis. Power and sample size calculations for GRTs can be implemented in currently available software systems (Turner et al. 2017).

Decisions regarding randomization and study design are typically made based on criteria including nature of the interventions, participation of study sites, potential control group contamination, as well as power considerations (Torgerson 2001). If interventions are conducted at the individual level and group contamination is not likely, individual-randomized multi-site study with randomization stratified within sites can be more efficient than a GRT. For interventions with group settings, deciding between GRTs and IRGTs of mind and body interventions is typically made based on practical considerations such as feasibility of recruitment and retention, timing of the grouping (i.e., before or after randomization), nature of the grouping (i.e., in all intervention arms or partial), and baseline data collection. As in other trials, the use of the baseline data collection period is important for balancing among intervention arms, especially for GRTs with small numbers of groups.

There are many alternative designs to the traditional GRT. In situations where it is important for all study sites to eventually receive intervention due to practical or ethical considerations, the stepped-wedge GRT design could be implemented. The stepped-wedge GRT (Hemming et al. 2015) is a one-directional crossover GRT that involves random and sequential crossover of groups/clusters from control to intervention so that eventually all groups are exposed to intervention. The stepped-wedge design allows investigators to conduct group- or site-level intervention that involves multiple health-care providers and guarantees that every site will benefit from participation by receipt of the intervention. In a stepped-wedge design, more groups are exposed to the intervention toward the end of the study than in its early stages. Thus, the effect of intervention might be confounded with any underlying temporal trend. This could be observed, for example, in secular trends toward more exposure to practices such as meditation and yoga in participants of an efficacy trial. Sample size calculations and statistical analysis need to adjust for both the clustered nature of the design and the confounding effect of time.

Masking

The randomized, double-masked, placebo-controlled study remains a modern standard for clinical trials. The purpose of masking is to minimize bias in many aspects of trial implementation, including participants and the research team involved in intervention delivery, participant management, outcome assessment, and data management and analysis. Therefore, trial planning requires careful review of how these different aspects will be protected from potential bias. This is particularly important for trials of most mind and body interventions, which cannot be conducted with a full double-masked design. As previously described, some trials of individual interventions (such as acupuncture) may select a sham or simulated treatment as a control group to address participant masking, but a full double-masked design is not feasible. Table 4 provides an overview of the differences in distinct elements of study masking between the "ideal" double-masked and typical single-masked RCTs for mind and body interventions, all of which require specific attention in trial planning.

In single-masked RCTs of mind and body interventions, it is critical that all study personnel involved in screening and enrollment remain masked to upcoming randomization assignment. While study personnel delivering the interventions cannot be masked to the assignment, they should remain masked to trial outcome measures. Trial outcome assessors are therefore independent of intervention delivery and trained in ensuring unbiased data collection. Additionally, outcome assessors generally remain masked to study assignment until database lock.

Table 4 Comparison of different aspects of trial masking in double-masked trials vs single-masked trials of mind and body approaches

Target of masking	Ideal double-masked RCT		Typical single-masked mind and body trial	
	Intervention assignment	Outcome measures	Intervention assignment	Outcome measures
Participants	Yes	No	No	No
Practitioners	NA	NA	No	Yes
Outcome assessors	Yes	No	Yes	No
Investigators	Yes	Yes	Yes	Yes
Statisticians (masked)	Yes	No	Yes	No
Statisticians (unmasked)	No	No	Yes	No

Yes masked, *No* not masked, *NA* not applicable as practitioners cannot be masked for mind and body interventions

During the study and following completion of study enrollment and data collection, study statisticians are not masked to outcome measures. Therefore, it is best to mask them to the intervention group assignment (Table 4). Intervention group allocation and/or data management is typically carried out by a designated unmasked statistician, who is not involved in final analysis of the trial data. During interim analyses and adverse event monitoring, it is still possible to mask statisticians to group assignment since the interest is to see if any group is benefiting more or has a higher than expected adverse event rate. However, sometimes there are different outcome measures collected for different intervention groups, and the statistician can figure out randomization during data analyses. In such situations it is crucial to plan statistical analyses and tests a priori and make sure that no excessive additional analyses are carried out to look for results in favor of the *intervention of interest*.

Assessing Intervention Quality

The quality of the mind and body intervention delivery is typically assessed by factors related to both practitioners and participants. Practitioner factors include verifying adequate training and the adequate number of practitioners for a trial, as well as monitoring practitioner fidelity to the study regimen. Even for small early-phase trials, it is important that practitioners are appropriately credentialed and of sufficient number so the study can reliably be performed, and results are reproducible. Participant factors focus primarily on adherence to study session attendance and home practice assignments that may be part of the study intervention(s).

Fidelity of Intervention Delivery

Fidelity of intervention delivery refers to the extent to which the trial practitioners comply with the study protocol when delivering interventions. Along with participants' adherence to the invention, fidelity of intervention delivery may act as a moderator of the intervention's effect on outcome measures. Appropriate evaluation of intervention fidelity needs to be implemented so that a potential moderating effect can be assessed. Moreover, fidelity of intervention delivery will also need to be quantified. This is particularly important given the greater potential for inconsistencies in intervention delivery in some mind and body interventions that are delivered in a group setting. Regular checks can be scheduled for outcome accessors as well as interventionists. For example, a convenience sample of in-person cognitive behavioral therapy (CBT) sessions were audiotaped and reviewed for content and quality related to specific characteristics of the intervention by an experienced clinician in an efficacy study of interactive voice response-based CBT for chronic back pain (Heapy et al. 2017). By evaluating study team's fidelity to intervention, the internal and external validity of the intervention can be established to assess how well it is conducted within a study and how well it can be generalized to other clinical settings.

Adherence to the Intervention

Adherence refers to the extent to which participants comply with the study intervention. For mind and body approaches, this includes both session attendance, level of session participation, and performance of home practice assignments. Aspects of adherence measures include both level and direction of adherence. They need to be defined to provide information on dose-response relationships and the consequences of nonadherence. If no dose-response is involved, the adherence definition can be straightforward. However, the pragmatic nature of mind and body interventions often complicates such definition. For example, in a study of early physical therapy versus usual care in patients with recent onset low back pain, the early physical therapy consisted of education and four sessions of therapy, while usual care involved only education and no intervention sessions (Fritz et al. 2015). Percent adherence may not be very meaningful given the different denominators for intervention sessions. Adherence was assessed by the number of participants that attended two, three, and four sessions of intervention in the early physical therapy group and number of participants that deviated from the protocol in the usual care group. Participants may also exhibit nonadherence at directions of either underexposure or overexposure to the intervention. One strategy to quantitatively assess level of adherence is to categorize adherence into three groups: non-adherent, partially adherent, and fully adherent. However, such categorization fails to take into account the heterogeneity among the partially adherent participants. In this scenario, intervention adherence and the association of adherence and outcome measures are best assessed within intervention arms, but not across arms.

Adherence monitoring is typically implemented in real-time during mind and body intervention trials, so that feedback can be provided to investigators and barriers addressed for improving adherence. Frequency and routine for assessing and collecting adherence information is preestablished prior to initiating a trial. As these trials typically involve weekly individual or group treatment sessions that span 8–12 weeks, adherence monitoring is critical for preventing implementation failure. For some trials, adherence information such as number of treatment sessions attended may be collected via the electronic health record. Depending on the frequency of health record data checks, real-time monitoring for these assessments may be challenging.

Monitoring adherence and maximizing it during a mind and body intervention trial has been made easier, as some interventions such as meditation and yoga increasingly incorporate technologies like audiovisual aids, email, internet, and smartphone apps. This allows for more standard interventions and adherence tracking. In addition, intervention delivered via videos or smartphone apps can help maintain masking of those conducting outcome assessments, thus further minimize trial bias.

While remediation plans can be established when barriers to participant adherence are identified, thresholds for failure of intervention adherence are also determined based on measures such as delivery of key intervention contents and level of attendance of intervention sessions. For multi-center trials of mind and boy interventions, overall study site levels of participant adherence are also tracked during the trial. An analytical approach most frequently applied to adjust for suboptimal adherence mind and body intervention trials is the per-protocol analysis. Compared to intention-to-treat analysis where all randomly allocated patients are included in the analysis and analyzed in the groups to which they are assigned, per-protocol analysis does not include data from individuals who fail to achieve a minimal level of adherence. Other statistical methods used less frequently for these trials include the marginal structural model with inverse-probability weighting (Rochon et al. 2016) and an instrumental variables strategy (Dunn et al. 2005).

Contamination

Cross contamination in mind and body intervention trials is a consideration at both practitioner and participant levels. The typical lack of full masking can increase the possibility of cross contamination by practitioners, if they are delivering an intervention across treatment arms. A practical solution adopted by many such trials is assigning practitioners to just one treatment arm, rather than multiple arms, and each arm served by multiple practitioners.

As most mind and body interventions are widely available to the general public in the USA, there may be considerable "drop-in" use of the experimental intervention in a given trial. Participants may also use other treatment regimens during the conduct of the study. Some studies have implemented strategies to address this issue by carefully communicating elements of the protocol to participants and collecting concomitant use of other products and treatment modalities during a study. It is important to note that if there is disproportionate use of concomitant interventions between treatment groups, the study results may be confounded by potential non-comparable treatment groups. Other design strategies could be considered to address this cross contamination, including using a control that is less likely to foster use of other concomitant therapies. Depending upon the goal of the study, it may also be possible to target an alternative study endpoint.

For example, in many studies of chronic back pain, it is difficult to discern significant improvement in pain between treatment groups, which may result from a lack of efficacy of an intervention or from dilution of its apparent benefit by use of widely available of analgesics or other methods of pain relief by research participants (Cherkin et al. 2016). Careful data collection and analysis of concomitant use of other interventions might provide greater insight into observed findings from such studies.

Missing Data

Missing data is a common data challenge in mind and body intervention trials and can lead to a loss of statistical power and potential bias in the comparison of intervention groups. Missingness in outcome and covariate data can arise for a variety of reasons. Mind and body intervention trials frequently incorporate many PROs measures as study outcomes, which include a variety of validated instruments such as those for pain, physical function, and quality of life. For such PROs, missing data can be missing items or missing questionnaires. Loss to follow-up is also a typical source of missingness in trials with complex study design and/or outcomes measured repeated over time. In addition, intermittent missing data can be due to the inability or unwillingness of participants to meet appointments for evaluation. Studies need to be designed and conducted carefully to limit the amount and impact of missing data. For example, sample size is often inflated to accommodate an expected percent of dropouts to ensure the power of a study. It is also critical to assess the extent and nature of missing data to help with data interpretation and selections of missing data approaches in data analyses. Missing data mechanisms and different statistical approaches under different mechanism assumptions have been discussed intensively in literature (Little et al. 2012; Rubin 2002). Statistical analysis needs to be performed to make full use of information on all randomized participants and be based on careful attention to the assumptions about the nature of the missing data underlying estimates of intervention effects. In the presence of missing data, it is imperative to perform sensitivity analyses to examine the robustness of results to assumptions made for the missing data mechanism.

Other Considerations for Trials of Complementary and Integrative Health Approaches

Participant Recruitment and Retention

Trials of complementary and integrative health interventions experience similar recruitment and retention challenges to those noted in conventional medical treatment trials (Sherman et al. 2009). Extensive interest and public use of natural products and mind and body interventions can significantly impact participant willingness to be randomized to a control intervention and adhere to a study regimen. This is particularly evident in mind and body intervention trials, whereby participants are aware of the treatment arm assignment at randomization. If randomized to a control intervention, participants may choose to dropout of the trial or choose to remain in the study but participate in the active intervention outside of the trial. Differential dropout may result in unbalanced study arms and reduce internal validity. The impact of differential dropout is typically addressed and adjusted for in the statistical analyses when planning for missing data. Such analyses may start with an assumption of missing at random, with careful examination and documentation of the missingness mechanism(s), and include sensitivity analyses if missing not at random data are suspected.

Another potential obstacle to enrollment results from widespread use of complementary and integrative health approaches by the public. There is frequently considerable pre-existing use or intervention exposure in the targeted patient population for a given trial. Most efficacy trials of natural product and mind and body interventions target patients who are either naïve to the active intervention or who have not used the active intervention for at least a year. If there is high level of use of the intervention in the target population, identifying an eligible cohort for the trial is particularly challenging.

For clinical trials of complementary interventions that focus on PRO measures, many small trials have observed significant improvement in outcomes when assessed immediately following the intervention phase of the trial. These short-term benefits frequently extinguish over time, and trials therefore typically require more extensive follow-up to determine whether there is a lingering impact of the intervention. This is particularly relevant for trials of symptom management in a chronic disease setting, where disease activity varies over time. As a result, most trials attempt to address outcomes at 9 or 12 months post intervention; and retaining subjects to obtain outcome data for extended follow-up can be challenging for trial implementation.

Efficacy Outcomes Assessment

Efficacy outcome measures of natural product trials share many similarities with those of conventional drug trials, if testing in the setting of a medical disease or condition. Such primary efficacy outcomes typically focus on clinical measures, including clinical laboratory or radiologic markers of disease activity over time, as well as assess the need for other conventional drugs to manage disease activity (Barry et al. 2011; Clegg et al. 2006; Fried et al. 2012; Hersch et al. 2017). Natural product efficacy trials also frequently collect secondary measures tracking a variety of PRO measures that can inform outcomes on symptom management (fatigue, sleep quality, anxiety, quality of life, and pain). With the growing popularity of wearable devices (actigraphy, wristwatch, or phone technology with mobile applications), trials can also collect a number of secondary measures that readily track participant activity and symptoms.

Efficacy outcome measures of mind and body intervention trials do not typically focus on primary measures of disease activity. By contrast, such trials target the potential role of these interventions in managing troubling symptoms. Most commonly, these trials address the potential utility of incorporating interventions into the usual care that participants otherwise receive for a given condition and then focus on primary PRO measures. There are many validated PRO instruments that have been developed to evaluate pain, fatigue, physical function, sleep quality, and quality of life (Avis et al. 2016; Cherkin et al. 2016; Eisendrath et al. 2016; Fritz et al. 2015). Clinical trials of these approaches have a variety of primary and secondary measures from which to choose for specific investigative strategies.

Multiplicity issues are not uncommon in either natural product or mind and body intervention trials. Multiple testing occurs when there are multiple outcome measures, comparisons across multiple treatment arms, multiple subgroup comparisons, or analyses of the same outcome at multiple time points. As a result, the potential inflation of the type I error may be introduced. The probability of making a false-positive finding in multiple testing, i.e., family-wise error rate, needs to be controlled. Specific strategies for dealing with multiplicity are typically incorporated into the analytic plan, to ensure reliability of statistical inferences and maximize the probability of success in a trial at its design, analysis, and interpretation stages. For example, in trials of acupuncture or chiropractic therapy assessing multiple outcomes such as pain, disability, and quality of life, several solutions can be applied. One option for the study design phase is to identify one single outcome as primary and the remaining as secondary outcomes. In this case, findings for the secondary outcomes would be exploratory. Another option could include composite outcomes, for example, a combined outcome of pain and physical function measures for trials assessing the impact of mind and body approaches for pain management. Relevant statistical methods that can be used to adjust for multiplicity and control family-wise error rate in sample size calculations and data analyses, include the Bonferroni correction, Holm procedure, Hochberg procedure, and control of the false discovery rate (Dmitrienko and D'Agostino Sr 2013).

Safety Outcomes Assessment

Despite widespread and longstanding use of natural products and mind and body interventions, there is surprisingly little published safety data on their chronic use. Many consider that these interventions are of low risk to participants, but there have been episodic reports of serious adverse events. Some natural products can be toxic to humans, and hepatotoxicity has been observed for some concentrated herbal extracts. Natural products may also interfere with drug metabolism for individuals who are taking other medications, and toxicity resulting from these interactions have also been described. Clinical trials of natural products have provided a mechanism for collecting patient safety data in a standardized manner, to objectively assess level of risk to the public (Barry et al. 2011; Clegg et al. 2006; DeKosky et al. 2008; Fried et al. 2012; Hersch et al. 2017). Similarly, mind and body interventions have not been studied extensively in a standardized manner. Clinical trials of these interventions provide an opportunity to collect evidence on safety in targeted populations that chronically practice them (Avis et al. 2016; Cherkin et al. 2016; Eisendrath et al. 2016; Fritz et al. 2015). Safety profiles for the interventions may vary considerably for specific populations with a chronic medical condition (s) versus healthy users.

Reporting Research Results

In view of the many unique considerations described for RCT of complementary and integrative approaches, investigators must address a number of issues when reporting research results in peer-reviewed journals. In view of existing Consolidated Standards of Reporting Trials (CONSORT) recommendations followed by most journals, special elements of the CONSORT items have been expanded for trials of herbal interventions, nonpharmacologic treatments, and acupuncture (Boutron et al. 2017; Gagnier et al. 2006; MacPherson et al. 2010). These elaborations or extensions of the CONSORT items provide recommendations for better characterizing or standardizing several elements of a trial manuscript (Table 5).

Table 5 CONSORT extensions for manuscripts reporting clinical trials of natural products and mind and body interventions

Section/topic	Herbal medicine interventions	Nonpharmacologic treatments	Acupuncture
Title and abstract	State the herbal medicinal product's Latin binomial, the part of the plant used, and the type of preparation	When applicable, report eligibility criteria for centers where the intervention is performed and for care providers; report any important changes to the intervention delivered from what was planned	In the abstract, description of the experimental treatment, comparator, care providers, centers and masking status
Introduction			
Background	Including a brief statement of reasons for the trial with reference to the specific herbal medicinal product being tested and, if applicable, whether new or traditional indications are being investigated		
Methods			
Participants	If a traditional indication is being tested, a description of how the traditional theories and concepts were maintained		When applicable eligibility criteria for centers and for care providers
Interventions	Herbal medicinal product name; characteristics of the herbal product; dosage regimen and quantitative description; qualitative testing; placebo/control group; practitioner	Precise details of both the experimental treatment and comparator; description of the different components of the interventions and, when applicable, description of the procedure for tailoring the interventions to individual participants; details of whether and how the interventions were standardized; details of whether and how adherence of care providers to the protocol was assessed or enhanced; details of	Precise details of both the experimental treatment and comparator

(continued)

Table 5 (continued)

Section/topic	Herbal medicine interventions	Nonpharmacologic treatments	Acupuncture
		whether and how adherence of participant to interventions was assessed or enhanced	
Objectives			
Outcomes	Outcome measures should reflect the intervention and indications tested considering, where applicable, underlying theories and concepts		
Sample size		When applicable, details of whether and how the clustering by care providers or centers was addressed	When applicable, details of whether and how the clustering by care providers or centers was addressed
Randomization – sequence generation			When applicable, how care providers were allocated to each trial group
Masking (blinding)		If done, who was masked after assignment to interventions (e.g., participants, care providers, those administering co-interventions, those assessing outcomes) and how; if masking was not possible, descriptions of any attempts to limit bias	Whether or not those administering co-interventions were masked to group assignment. If masked, method of masking and description of the similarity of interventions
Statistical methods		When applicable, details of whether and how the clustering by care providers or centers was addressed	When applicable, details of whether and how the clustering by care providers or centers was addressed
Results			
Participant flow		The number of care providers or centers performing the intervention in each group and the number of patients treated by each care provider or in	The number of care providers or centers performing the intervention in each group and the number of patients treated by

(continued)

Table 5 (continued)

Section/topic	Herbal medicine interventions	Nonpharmacologic treatments	Acupuncture
		each center; for each group, the delay between randomization and the initiation of the intervention; details of the experimental treatment and comparator as they were implemented	each care provider or in each center
Baseline data	Including concomitant medication, herbal, and complementary medicine use	When applicable, a description of care providers (case volume, qualification, expertise, etc.) and centers (volume) in each group	When applicable, a description of care providers (case volume, qualification, expertise, etc.) and centers (volume) in each group
Discussion			
Limitations/ interpretation	Interpretation of the results in light of the product and dosage regimen used	In addition, take into account the choice of the comparator, lack of or partial masking, and unequal expertise of care provider or centers in each group	In addition, take into account the choice of the comparator, lack of or partial masking, unequal expertise of care providers or centers in each group
Generalizability	Where possible, discuss how the herbal product and dosage regimen used relate to what is used in self-care and/or practice	Generalizability (external validity) of the trial findings according to the intervention, comparators, patients, and care providers and centers involved in the trial	Generalizability (external validity) of the trial findings according to the intervention, comparators, patients and care providers, and centers involved in the trial
Overall evidence	Discussion of the trial results in relation to trials of other available products		

Adapted from Boutron et al. (2017), Gagnier et al. (2006), and MacPherson et al. (2010)

Implementation of these standards enhances the quality of reports such that research findings can be interpreted in the appropriate context.

Conclusion

Extensive public use of complementary and integrative health approaches has prompted a need for more trials assessing both safety and efficacy of these health approaches. Historically, natural products derived from botanicals have been a rich source for many conventional drugs and remain an important reservoir for new products. Nearly half of the new pharmaceuticals developed over the last 20 years, which were approved by FDA, were natural products or a synthetic derivative from a natural product (Newman and Cragg 2016). Despite the investigative challenges outlined here, however, there remains strong interest in natural product supplements. With growing interest in probiotics, many trials are being conducted to assess safety and efficacy of these products. Similarly, many mind and body approaches have a long history of clinical use, derived from a variety of practitioner disciplines. Emerging evidence on such approaches in the setting of chronic pain, in particular, suggests a need for more expanded testing in light of the current opioid crisis and obvious need for enhanced and targeted nonpharmacologic treatment strategies (DeBar et al. 2018). NHIS data suggest most complementary and integrative health approaches are used by the public to maintain health and well-being. Generating a larger, more rigorous evidence base on the safety and impact of these approaches with chronic use remains an important public health goal.

Key Facts

- There is widespread use of complementary and integrative health approaches in the USA, which include both natural product and mind and body practices.
- Natural products typically require considerable early-phase testing prior to launching a clinical trial.
- Natural products can be complex and variable mixtures many different compounds, and extensive testing is required to ensure product integrity.
- Many efficacy trials of natural products require oversight from the FDA, if conducted in an affected population.
- Trials of mind and body approaches test interventions that are delivered in a variety of settings and are not fully masked.
- Assessing intervention quality in a mind and body intervention trial is complex and requires tracking both practitioner fidelity and participant adherence to the intervention.
- Recruitment and retention can be challenging in all trials of complementary and integrative health approaches due to the widespread availability of the interventions and hence the ability of participants to continue or initiate the intervention independently of a clinical trial.
- Widespread use of complementary and integrative health approaches by the public, in the absence of evidence for both safety and efficacy, remains a primary motivation for further clinical trials of these interventions.

Cross-References

▶ Administration of Study Treatments and Participant Follow-Up
▶ Cluster Randomized Trials
▶ CONSORT and Its Extensions for Reporting Clinical Trials

- ▶ Controlling for Multiplicity, Eligibility, and Exclusions
- ▶ Dose-Finding and Dose-Ranging Studies
- ▶ Intention to Treat and Alternative Approaches
- ▶ Issues for Masked Data Monitoring
- ▶ Issues in Generalizing Results from Clinical Trials
- ▶ Masking of Trial Investigators
- ▶ Masking Study Participants
- ▶ Missing Data
- ▶ N-of-1 Randomized Trials
- ▶ Participant Recruitment, Screening, and Enrollment
- ▶ Patient-Reported Outcomes
- ▶ Principles of Clinical Trials: Bias and Precision Control
- ▶ Publications from Clinical Trials
- ▶ Qualifications of the Research Staff
- ▶ Safety and Risk Benefit Analyses

References

Ali A, Kahn J, Rosenberger L, Perlman AI (2012) Development of a manualized protocol of massage therapy for clinical trials in osteoarthritis. Trials 13(1):185. https://doi.org/10.1186/1745-6215-13-185

Avis NE, Coeytaux RR, Isom S, Prevette K, Morgan T (2016) Acupuncture in Menopause (AIM) study: a pragmatic, randomized controlled trial. Menopause 23(6):626–637. https://doi.org/10.1097/GME.0000000000000597

Barry MJ, Meleth S, Lee JY, Kreder KJ, Avins AL, Nickel JC, Roehrborn CG, Crawford ED, Foster HE Jr, Kaplan SA, McCullough A, Andriole GL, Naslund MJ, Williams OD, Kusek JW, Meyers CM, Betz JM, Cantor A, McVary KT (2011) Effect of increasing doses of saw palmetto extract on lower urinary tract symptoms: a randomized trial. JAMA 306(12):1344–1351. https://doi.org/10.1001/jama.2011.1364

Boutron I, Altman DG, Moher D, Schulz KF, Ravaud P, Group CN (2017) CONSORT statement for randomized trials of nonpharmacologic treatments: a 2017 update and a CONSORT extension for nonpharmacologic trial abstracts. Ann Intern Med 167(1):40–47. https://doi.org/10.7326/M17-0046

Briggs JP, Shurtleff D (2017) Acupuncture and the complex connections between the mind and the body. JAMA 317(24):2489–2490. https://doi.org/10.1001/jama.2017.7214

Carter B (2010) Cluster size variability and imbalance in cluster randomized controlled trials. Stat Med 29(29):2984–2993. https://doi.org/10.1002/sim.4050

Cherkin DC, Sherman KJ, Balderson BH, Cook AJ, Anderson ML, Hawkes RJ, Hansen KE, Turner JA (2016) Effect of mindfulness-based stress reduction vs cognitive behavioral therapy or usual care on Back pain and functional limitations in adults with chronic low Back pain: a randomized clinical trial. JAMA 315(12):1240–1249. https://doi.org/10.1001/jama.2016.2323

Clarke TC, Black LI, Stussman BJ, Barnes PM, Nahin RL (2015) Trends in the use of complementary health approaches among adults: United States, 2002–2012. Natl Health Stat Rep 79:1–16

Clegg DO, Reda DJ, Harris CL, Klein MA, O'Dell JR, Hooper MM, Bradley JD, Bingham CO 3rd, Weisman MH, Jackson CG, Lane NE, Cush JJ, Moreland LW, Schumacher HR Jr, Oddis CV, Wolfe F, Molitor JA, Yocum DE, Schnitzer TJ, Furst DE, Sawitzke AD, Shi H, Brandt KD, Moskowitz RW, Williams HJ (2006) Glucosamine, chondroitin sulfate, and the two in combination for painful knee osteoarthritis. N Engl J Med 354(8):795–808. https://doi.org/10.1056/NEJMoa052771

DeBar L, Benes L, Bonifay A, Deyo RA, Elder CR, Keefe FJ, Leo MC, McMullen C, Mayhew M, Owen-Smith A, Smith DH, Trinacty CM, Vollmer WM (2018) Interdisciplinary team-based care for patients with chronic pain on long-term opioid treatment in primary care (PPACT) – protocol for a pragmatic cluster randomized trial. Contemp Clin Trials 67:91–99. https://doi.org/10.1016/j.cct.2018.02.015

DeKosky ST, Fitzpatrick A, Ives DG, Saxton J, Williamson J, Lopez OL, Burke G, Fried L, Kuller LH, Robbins J, Tracy R, Woolard N, Dunn L, Kronmal R, Nahin R, Furberg C, Investigators G (2006) The Ginkgo Evaluation of Memory (GEM) study: design and baseline data of a randomized trial of Ginkgo biloba extract in prevention of dementia. Contemp Clin Trials 27(3):238–253. https://doi.org/10.1016/j.cct.2006.02.007

DeKosky ST, Williamson JD, Fitzpatrick AL, Kronmal RA, Ives DG, Saxton JA, Lopez OL, Burke G, Carlson MC, Fried LP, Kuller LH, Robbins JA, Tracy RP, Woolard NF, Dunn L, Snitz BE, Nahin RL, Furberg CD (2008) Ginkgo biloba for prevention of dementia: a randomized controlled trial. JAMA 300(19):2253–2262. https://doi.org/10.1001/jama.2008.683

Dmitrienko A, D'Agostino R Sr (2013) Traditional multiplicity adjustment methods in clinical trials. Stat Med 32(29):5172–5218. https://doi.org/10.1002/sim.5990

Dunn G, Maracy M, Tomenson B (2005) Estimating treatment effects from randomized clinical trials with noncompliance and loss to follow-up: the role of instrumental variable methods. Stat Methods Med Res 14(4):369–395. https://doi.org/10.1191/0962280205sm403oa

Eisendrath SJ, Gillung E, Delucchi KL, Segal ZV, Nelson JC, McInnes LA, Mathalon DH, Feldman MD (2016) A randomized controlled trial of mindfulness-based cognitive therapy for treatment-resistant depression. Psychother Psychosom 85(2):99–110. https://doi.org/10.1159/000442260

FDA/CDER (2016) Botanical drug development guidance for industry. The Center for Drug Evaluation and Research, the US Food and Drug Administration. Retrieved from https://www.fda.gov/downloads/Drugs/Guidances/UCM458484.pdf

FDA/CDER/CBER (2018) Adaptive designs for clinical trials of drugs and biologics guidance for industry. The Center for Drug Evaluation and Research and the Center for Biologics Evaluation and Research, the US Food and Drug Administration. Retrieved from https://www.fda.gov/downloads/drugs/guidances/ucm201790.pdf

Fried MW, Navarro VJ, Afdhal N, Belle SH, Wahed AS, Hawke RL, Doo E, Meyers CM, Reddy KR (2012) Effect of silymarin (milk thistle) on liver disease in patients with chronic hepatitis C unsuccessfully treated with interferon therapy: a randomized controlled trial. JAMA 308(3):274–282. https://doi.org/10.1001/jama.2012.8265

Fritz JM, Magel JS, McFadden M, Asche C, Thackeray A, Meier W, Brennan G (2015) Early physical therapy vs usual care in patients with recent-onset low back pain: a randomized clinical trial. JAMA 314(14):1459–1467. https://doi.org/10.1001/jama.2015.11648

Gagnier JJ, Boon H, Rochon P, Moher D, Barnes J, Bombardier C (2006) Reporting randomized, controlled trials of herbal interventions: an elaborated CONSORT statement. Ann Intern Med 144(5):364–367

Goertz CM, Long CR, Hondras MA, Petri R, Delgado R, Lawrence DJ, Owens EF, Meeker WC (2013) Adding chiropractic manipulative therapy to standard medical care for patients with acute low back pain: results of a pragmatic randomized comparative effectiveness study. Spine (Phila Pa 1976) 38(8):627–634. https://doi.org/10.1097/BRS.0b013e31827733e7

Hawke RL, Schrieber SJ, Soule TA, Wen Z, Smith PC, Reddy KR, Wahed AS, Belle SH, Afdhal NH, Navarro VJ, Berman J, Liu Q-Y, Doo E, Fried MW (2010) Silymarin ascending multiple oral dosing phase I study in noncirrhotic patients with chronic hepatitis C. J Clin Pharmacol 50(4):434–449. https://doi.org/10.1177/0091270009347475

Heapy AA, Higgins DM, Goulet JL, LaChappelle KM, Driscoll MA, Czlapinski RA, Buta E, Piette JD, Krein SL, Kerns RD (2017) Interactive voice response-based self-management for chronic back pain: the COPES noninferiority randomized trial. JAMA Intern Med 177(6):765–773. https://doi.org/10.1001/jamainternmed.2017.0223

Hemming K, Haines TP, Chilton PJ, Girling AJ, Lilford RJ (2015) The stepped wedge cluster randomised trial: rationale, design, analysis, and reporting. BMJ 350:h391. https://doi.org/10.1136/bmj.h391

Hersch SM, Gevorkian S, Marder K, Moskowitz C, Feigin A, Cox M, Como P, Zimmerman C, Lin M, Zhang L, Ulug AM, Beal MF, Matson W, Bogdanov M, Ebbel E, Zaleta A, Kaneko Y, Jenkins B, Hevelone N, Zhang H, Yu H, Schoenfeld D, Ferrante R, Rosas HD (2006) Creatine in Huntington disease is safe, tolerable, bioavailable in brain and reduces serum 8OH2'dG. Neurology 66(2):250–252. https://doi.org/10.1212/01.wnl.0000194318.74946.b6

Hersch SM, Schifitto G, Oakes D, Bredlau AL, Meyers CM, Nahin R, Rosas HD (2017) The CREST-E study of creatine for Huntington disease: a randomized controlled trial. Neurology 89(6):594–601. https://doi.org/10.1212/wnl.0000000000004209

Little RJ, D'Agostino R, Cohen ML, Dickersin K, Emerson SS, Farrar JT, Frangakis C, Hogan JW, Molenberghs G, Murphy SA, Neaton JD, Rotnitzky A, Scharfstein D, Shih WJ, Siegel JP, Stern H (2012) The prevention and treatment of missing data in clinical trials. N Engl J Med 367(14):1355–1360. https://doi.org/10.1056/NEJMsr1203730

MacPherson H, Altman DG, Hammerschlag R, Youping L, Taixiang W, White A, Moher D, Group SR. (2010) Revised STandards for Reporting Interventions in Clinical Trials of Acupuncture (STRICTA): extending the CONSORT statement. PLoS Med 7(6):e1000261. https://doi.org/10.1371/journal.pmed.1000261

Newman DJ, Cragg GM (2016) Natural products as sources of new drugs from 1981 to 2014. J Nat Prod 79(3):629–661. https://doi.org/10.1021/acs.jnatprod.5b01055

Nikles CJ, Clavarino AM, Del Mar CB (2005) Using n-of-1 trials as a clinical tool to improve prescribing. Br J Gen Pract 55(512):175–180

Perlman A, Fogerite SG, Glass O, Bechard E, Ali A, Njike VY, Pieper C, Dmitrieva NO, Luciano A, Rosenberger L, Keever T, Milak C, Finkelstein EA, Mahon G, Campanile G, Cotter A, Katz DL (2019) Efficacy and safety of massage for osteoarthritis of the knee: a randomized clinical trial. J Gen Intern Med 34(3):379–386. https://doi.org/10.1007/s11606-018-4763-5

Reddy KR, Belle SH, Fried MW, Afdhal N, Navarro VJ, Hawke RL, Wahed AS, Doo E, Meyers CM (2012) Rationale, challenges, and participants in a phase II trial of a botanical product for chronic hepatitis C. Clin Trials 9(1):102–112. https://doi.org/10.1177/1740774511427064

Rochon J, Bhapkar M, Pieper CF, Kraus WE (2016) Application of the marginal structural model to account for suboptimal adherence in a randomized controlled trial. Contemp Clin Trials Commun 4:222–228. https://doi.org/10.1016/j.conctc.2016.10.005

Rubin DBLR (2002) Statistical analysis with missing data. Wiley, Hoboken

Sherman KJ, Hawkes RJ, Ichikawa L, Cherkin DC, Deyo RA, Avins AL, Khalsa PS (2009) Comparing recruitment strategies in a study of acupuncture for chronic back pain. BMC Med Res Methodol 9:69. https://doi.org/10.1186/1471-2288-9-69

Torgerson DJ (2001) Contamination in trials: is cluster randomisation the answer? BMJ 322(7282):355–357

Turner EL, Li F, Gallis JA, Prague M, Murray DM (2017) Review of recent methodological developments in group-randomized trials: part 1-design. Am J Public Health 107(6):907–915. https://doi.org/10.2105/ajph.2017.303706

Wang C, Schmid CH, Rones R, Kalish R, Yinh J, Goldenberg DL, Lee Y, McAlindon T (2010) A randomized trial of tai chi for fibromyalgia. N Engl J Med 363(8):743–754. https://doi.org/10.1056/NEJMoa0912611

Wright N, Ivers N, Eldridge S, Taljaard M, Bremner S (2015) A review of the use of covariates in cluster randomized trials uncovers marked discrepancies between guidance and practice. J Clin Epidemiol 68(6):603–609. https://doi.org/10.1016/j.jclinepi.2014.12.006

Orphan Drugs and Rare Diseases

116

James E. Valentine and Frank J. Sasinowski

Contents

Introduction	2290
Orphan Drug Designation	2292
Requesting Orphan Drug Designation	2292
Identification of the Disease or Condition	2292
Scientific Rationale for Use of the Drug	2293
Population Estimate to Establish Rarity of the Disease or Condition	2294
Amendments to Orphan Drug Designation	2294
Incentives of Orphan Drug Designation	2294
Orphan Drug Exclusivity	2295
Priority Review Voucher	2296
Tax Credits	2298
Orphan Drug Grants	2298
Written Protocol Assistance	2299
User Fee Exemption	2299
Other Considerations Related to Orphan Drug Development	2299
Challenges with Clinical Trial Design for Rare Diseases	2300
Evidence Required for Orphan Drug Approval	2300
The Patient Voice in Orphan Drug Development	2302
Natural History Studies to Support Orphan Drug Development	2303
New Horizons: Targeted Therapies for Rare Disease	2304
Summary and Conclusion	2305
Key Facts	2305
Cross-References	2305
References	2306

J. E. Valentine
University of Maryland Carey School of Law, Baltimore, MD, USA
e-mail: JValentine@HPM.com

F. J. Sasinowski (✉)
University of Rochester School of Medicine, Department of Neurology, Rochester, NY, USA
e-mail: FSasinowski@HPM.com

© Springer Nature Switzerland AG 2022
S. Piantadosi, C. L. Meinert (eds.), *Principles and Practice of Clinical Trials*,
https://doi.org/10.1007/978-3-319-52636-2_253

Abstract

There are approximately 8,000 recognized rare diseases affecting close to 30 million people in the United States. Sponsors choosing to engage in research and development of drugs for rare diseases, known as orphan drugs, face challenges and opportunities that are unique to orphan drug development. Small population size, disease heterogeneity, and unknown natural histories, among other factors, must be considered when designing clinical trials for orphan drugs. Additionally, sponsors need to consider the quality and quantity of clinical trial information needed to support the approval of an orphan drug. To further understand these unique challenges, sponsors should partner with patient groups who can provide disease-specific perspectives and experiences, as well as conduct natural history studies, to better inform the design and evaluation of results from clinical trials. Novel technologies are changing the clinical trial landscape which provide sponsors a unique opportunity to employ novel, lifesaving technologies that can truly "cure" rare diseases. Incentives provided by the Orphan Drug Act and other FDA policies, such as market exclusivity, priority review vouchers, and tax credits, recognize the unique status of orphan drugs and serve to stimulate the development of these products.

Keywords

Food and Drug Administration · Rare disease · Orphan drugs · Orphan Drug Act · Incentives · Challenges · Flexibility · Patient-focused drug development · Natural history studies · Targeted therapies

Introduction

The Food and Drug Administration (FDA) defines a "rare disease" as a disease or condition that affects less than 200,000 persons in the United States (Federal Food, Drug, and Cosmetic Act (FDCA) § 526(a)(2)). There are approximately 8,000 recognized rare diseases in the United States (National Institutes of Health, National Center for Advancing Translational Sciences n.d.). While individually, each rare disease affects a small number of people, when taken in aggregate, rare diseases affect close to 30 million Americans. Rare diseases became known as "orphan diseases" because sponsors were not developing therapies that had limited markets. Despite the challenges related to developing treatments for orphan diseases, or orphan drugs, orphan drug development has become a key area of growth in the pharmaceutical industry. To date, over 600 orphan drug indications have been approved from over 450 distinct drug products (see Table 1). This chapter explores the incentives and other regulatory programs put in place to facilitate clinical development of orphan drugs, as well as challenges and strategies for conducting clinical trials in rare diseases.

Prior to 1983, only ten drugs for rare diseases had been approved by FDA (Mikami 2017). To facilitate the development of drugs for rare diseases, the

Table 1 Examples of recently approved orphan drugs

Drug name	Orphan designation	Approved indication	Designation date (approval date)
Spinraza (nusinersen)	Treatment of spinal muscular atrophy	Treatment of spinal muscular atrophy in pediatric and adult patients	4/8/2011 (12/23/2016)
Luxturna (voretigene neparvovec-rzyl)	Treatment of inherited retinal dystrophy due to biallelic RPE65 gene mutations	Treatment of patients with confirmed biallelic RPE65 mutation-associated retinal dystrophy	3/18/2015 (12/19/2017)
Galafold (migalastat hydrochloride)	Treatment of Fabry disease	Treatment of adults with a confirmed diagnosis of Fabry disease and an amenable galactosidase alpha gene (GLA) variant based on in vitro assay data	2/25/2004 (8/10/2018)

Orphan Drug Act of 1983 was signed into law (Pub. L. No. 97-414, 96 Stat. 2049 (1983)). The Orphan Drug Act amended the FDCA to provide incentives for manufacturers to develop and market products for rare diseases. The Orphan Drug Act also created FDA's Office of Orphan Products Development (OOPD) which evaluates scientific and clinical data submissions to identify and authorize orphan drug designations for products that demonstrate promise for the diagnosis and/or treatment of rare diseases. OOPD also administers incentives provided by the Orphan Drug Act, including orphan products grants, and works with medical and research communities, professional organizations, academia, governmental agencies, industry, and rare disease patient groups to address various issues related to rare disease product development.

Sponsors choosing to engage in research and development of drugs for rare diseases face unique challenges and opportunities when designing clinical trials. Small population size, disease heterogeneity, and unknown natural histories, among other factors, must be considered when designing clinical trials for orphan drugs (Food and Drug Administration 2018c; Food and Drug Administration 2019a). Additionally, sponsors need to consider the quality and quantity of clinical trial information needed to support the approval of an orphan drug. Sponsors should not underestimate the power of the patient voice in designing and evaluating clinical trials since they are uniquely positioned to inform the understanding of the therapeutic context for trial design. Lastly, novel technologies are changing the clinical trial landscape which provide sponsors a unique opportunity to employ novel, lifesaving technologies for rare disease patients who have often been overlooked. Incentives provided by the Orphan Drug Act and other FDA policies recognize the unique status of orphan drugs and serve to stimulate the development of these products. This chapter begins with a discussion of these incentives in order to establish the current environment in which orphan drug development exists, which then drives the needs to design and conduct clinical trials to support marketing approval.

Orphan Drug Designation

The Orphan Drug Act provides for granting special status to a drug or biological product ("drug") to treat a rare disease or condition upon request of a sponsor. A "rare disease or condition" is one that "affects fewer than 200,000 persons in the United States" or "affects more than 200,000 persons in the United States and for which there is no reasonable expectation that the cost of developing and making available in the United States a drug for such disease or condition will be recovered from sales in the United States of such drug" (FDCA § 526(a)(2)). For a drug to qualify for orphan drug designation, both the drug and the disease must meet certain criteria specified in the Orphan Drug Act and FDA's implementing regulations (Pub. L. No. 97-414, 96 Stat. 2049 (1983); 21 C.F.R § 316).

Requesting Orphan Drug Designation

In order to obtain orphan drug designation, a sponsor must submit a formal request to OOPD that includes a scientific rationale for the use of the drug and the prevalence of the disease. These requests are commonly known as orphan drug designation requests (ODDRs). ODDRs can be submitted early in the development process since FDA does not require that an investigational new drug (IND) application be in effect at the time of the ODDR submission. Therefore, a sponsor may submit a request for orphan drug designation at any time prior to submitting a marketing application. FDA generally responds to an ODDR within 90 days of submission. The content and format of an ODDR is described in 21 C.F.R § 316.20.

The key elements addressed in an ODDR are (1) identification of the disease or condition; (2) a description of the scientific rationale for the use of the drug for the disease or condition of interest; and (3) a determination of the population estimate to support that the disease or condition is rare. If a drug has already been approved for the same disease indication, the ODDR must demonstrate that the drug that is the subject of the request is clinically superior to the already approved drug (21 C.F.R. § 316.20(b)).

Identification of the Disease or Condition

First and foremost, a sponsor must identify the disease or condition for which the drug is being or will be investigated. Unlike marketing applications, orphan drug designation is only given to a drug for a particular disease or condition, not an indication. The way a sponsor defines the disease or condition could directly affect whether the disease or condition is considered rare (i.e., affects fewer than 200,000 persons in the United States). The practice of sponsors narrowly tailoring a disease or condition definition to only include a specified subgroup is known as "subsetting."

Table 2 Examples of orphan subsets

Drug	Common disease	Orphan subset
Gilotrif (afatinib)	Non-small cell lung cancer	Non-small cell lung cancer with EGFR mutation
Viread (tenofovir)	HIV	Treatment of pediatric HIV infection
Yervoy (ipilimumab)	Melanoma	Treatment of high-risk stage II, stage III, and stage IV melanoma

FDA has anticipated the creative ways a sponsor could subset a "common disease" with a population over 200,000 in order to fulfill the prevalence requirement and has implemented regulations to minimize inappropriate subsetting. These regulations state that an "[o]rphan subset of a non-rare disease or condition ('orphan subset') means that use of the drug in a subset of persons with a non-rare disease or condition may be appropriate but use of the drug outside of that subset (in the remaining persons with the non-rare disease or condition) would be inappropriate owing to some property(ies) of the drug, for example, drug toxicity, mechanism of action, or previous clinical experience with the drug" (21 C.F.R. § 316.3(b)(13)). An example of a proper orphan subset would be a subset of patients who are refractory to, or intolerant of, less toxic drugs as appropriate candidates for treatment with a highly toxic drug for purposes of orphan drug designation for that drug (see Table 2). It is important to note that if a disease is common (i.e., the prevalence of the disease is 200,000 persons or greater), but the prevalence of the pediatric population affected by the disease is less than 200,000, the drug may be eligible for orphan designation for the pediatric population as an orphan subset, but there is no stand-alone pediatric subpopulation designation (Food and Drug Administration 2018a). In addition, FDA does not allow sponsors to create arbitrary criteria when defining an orphan subset. If a sponsor requests orphan drug designation for a drug for only a subset of persons with a particular disease or condition, the sponsor must explain why the drug is expected to treat that subset and not the entire disease population.

When considering orphan drug designation of a drug for a particular disease or condition, the FDA considers factors such as the mechanism of action of the drug, pathophysiology, etiology, treatment options, and prognosis. More than one sponsor may receive orphan drug designation of the same drug for the same rare disease or condition if separate ODDRs are received from each sponsor.

Scientific Rationale for Use of the Drug

The second major component of an ODDR is the sponsor's discussion of the scientific rationale to "establish a medically plausible basis for the use of the drug for the rare disease or condition." This includes providing OODP with all relevant data from in vitro laboratory studies, preclinical studies in animal models, and any clinical experience with the drug (21 C.F.R. § 316.20(b)(4)). Importantly, sponsors must provide scientific data, not merely theories, that demonstrates a promise of the drug's ability to treat, diagnose, or prevent the disease or condition in the intended population, whether defined as the general disease population or an orphan subset.

Population Estimate to Establish Rarity of the Disease or Condition

Lastly, a sponsor must demonstrate that the disease or condition meets the statutory definition of a rare disease or condition. In determining whether the disease or condition for which the drug is to be developed affects less than 200,000 persons, prevalence, not incidence, is the deciding factor for FDA (21 C.F.R. § 316.21). Prevalence is defined as the number of persons in the United States who have been diagnosed as having the disease or condition at a particular time. Conversely, incidence is the number of new cases of a disease or condition in the United States in a given time period. Only if the disease is an acute illness lasting less than 1 year will FDA consider incidence to estimate the prevalence of a disease or condition that is the subject of an orphan drug designation request. If a drug that is the subject of an orphan drug designation request will have an indication for prevention of a rare disease or condition, rather than treatment, the relevant population that FDA will consider is the population at risk for the disease. FDA recognizes that prevalence data may be difficult to obtain but expects sponsors to "make every effort to survey the literature and obtain all information available on the prevalence of the indicated disease" counting only "diagnosed symptomatic patients" (Orphan Drug Regulations, 57 Fed. Reg. 62,076, 62,081 (Dec. 29, 1992)).

Amendments to Orphan Drug Designation

FDA permits sponsors to amend its orphan drug designation at any time prior to marketing approval of the designated drug. An amendment request to the designated use of the drug must be due to new and unexpected findings during research on the drug, information arising from FDA recommendations, or unforeseen developments in treatment or diagnosis of the disease or condition. An approval of an amendment is conditioned upon a finding that the original ODDR was submitted in good faith and the amendment does not make the drug ineligible for designation (21 C.F.R. § 316.26).

Incentives of Orphan Drug Designation

The Orphan Drug Act, in combination with other FDA policies, offers a combination of incentives to sponsors that receive an orphan drug designation for a product. Major incentives to encourage sponsors to develop orphan drugs include 7 years of marketing exclusivity and priority review vouchers. Other incentives are intended to lower research and other development-related costs through research tax credits, orphan drug grants, consultation with staff on acceptable research designs, and exemption from user fees.

Orphan Drug Exclusivity

The Orphan Drug Act provides a 7-year period of marketing exclusivity to the first sponsor who obtains marketing approval for a designated orphan drug. Orphan drug exclusivity is broader than other types of exclusivity. During the period of exclusivity, FDA cannot approve a marketing application from a different sponsor for the same orphan drug for the same indication, regardless of any independent clinical data of safety or efficacy (FDCA § 527(a)). Orphan drug exclusivity is highly valued by sponsors because it acts as an additional layer of protection, on top of 20 years of patent protection, to delay the approval of generic drugs. Therefore, orphan drug exclusivity provides incentives for companies to invest in drugs for orphan conditions despite the limited market size.

Upon approval of a designated drug, FDA cannot approve another sponsor's product for 7 years from the date of approval if it is the same drug for the same disease. However, FDA may approve a subsequent drug under certain circumstances. In the first instance, FDA may approve a subsequent drug if the sponsor who has the original orphan drug approval agrees to the additional approval. Secondly, FDA may approve a subsequent drug if the sponsor of the original orphan drug approval is found to be unable to supply sufficient quantities of the product to meet the needs of persons with the disease or condition. Finally, FDA may approve a subsequent orphan drug if the drug is different from the approved orphan drug (FDCA § 527(b)). Importantly, FDA will not recognize an orphan drug's exclusivity if the sponsor fails to demonstrate upon approval that the drug is clinically superior to the previously approved drug (21 C.F.R. § 316.34.).

One way a sponsor can demonstrate that its drug is different from the approved orphan drug is by showing that its drug is either chemically or structurally distinct and therefore not the "same drug." The degree of chemical or structural similarity that allows FDA to determine whether two drugs are the same depends on whether the drugs are small molecules or macromolecules. In the case of small molecules, drugs are considered the same if they have identical chemical structure. For macromolecules, a subsequent drug is considered the same as the approved drug if it "contains the same principal molecular structural features (but not necessarily all of the same structural features) and is intended for the same use . . . ." Posttranslational events, infidelity in the translation or transcription processes, or minor differences in amino acid sequence would not warrant a finding by FDA that two macromolecules were different (21 C.F.R. § 316.3(b)(14)).

In addition to showing that its drug is not the same drug, a subsequent sponsor can show clinical superiority (see Table 3). A clinically superior drug is one that is "shown to provide a significant therapeutic advantage over and above that provided by an approved drug (that is otherwise the same drug)" in at least one of three ways (21 C.F.R. § 316.3(b)(3)).

Table 3 Examples of "clinically superior drugs"

Type	Approved drug(s) (Clinically superior drug)	Rationale
Greater effectiveness	Avonex (Interferon beta-1a)	Clinical data demonstrated a meaningful improvement in the frequency of multiple sclerosis exacerbations
	Rebif (Interferon beta-1a)	
Greater safety	Remodulin (Treprostinil) (injection)	Greater safety with inhaled product compared to injection in relation to widespread and severe nature of pain associated with administration
	Tyvaso (Treprostinil) (inhalation)	
Major contribution to patient care	Dantrium IV (Dantrolene sodium for injection)	Decreased time for anesthesiologist to reconstitute and administer Ryanodex allowed for more time for supportive care and treatment of patients with malignant hyperthermia
	Ryanodex (Dantrolene sodium)	

First, the subsequent drug has greater effectiveness as assessed by effect on a clinically meaningful endpoint in adequate and well-controlled trials. A showing of greater effectiveness generally requires the same kind of evidence as is required to support a comparative effectiveness claim for two different drugs. FDA regulations also provide that, in most cases, direct comparative clinical trials would be necessary to demonstrate greater effectiveness.

Second, the subsequent drug has greater safety in a substantial portion of the target population. A demonstration of greater safety usually requires that the subsequent product provides greater safety in a "substantial portion of the target populations, for example, by the elimination of an ingredient or contaminant that is associated with relatively frequent adverse effects" (21 C.F.R. § 316.3(b)(3)(ii)). FDA acknowledges that in some cases, the sponsor may have to perform direct comparative clinical trials.

Lastly, in unusual cases, the sponsor demonstrates that the drug makes a major contribution to patient care (21 C.F.R. § 316.3(b)(3)). One such example would be the development of an oral dosage form where the originally approved orphan drug was available only by parenteral administration. FDA has indicated that the cost of treatment and the hardships of complying with treatment cannot be used to demonstrate a major contribution to patient care.

Priority Review Voucher

As a means to further incentivize the development of therapies for rare diseases, FDA has the power to grant priority review vouchers (PRV) to sponsors who obtain approval for qualifying tropical disease and rare pediatric disease products (FDCA §§ 524, 529). A PRV is a voucher issued to the sponsor of a tropical or rare pediatric disease product application that entitles the holder of such a voucher to priority review of a single new drug application (NDA) or biologics license application (BLA) after the date of approval of the tropical or rare pediatric disease product application. Priority review is a very powerful tool for sponsors because it gives them the opportunity to expedite FDA review of a future application of any product, not just orphan drugs. A PRV requires FDA to review a sponsor's NDA or BLA not later than 6 months upon receipt of the application, compared to the standard review time of 10 months. An additional incentive of the PRV program is that a sponsor that receives a PRV can either use the voucher to expedite the review of its own therapies or sell the voucher to another sponsor that wishes for a faster review of its products. PRVs have sold between $67.5 million and $350 million, proving that the program can help offset the cost of orphan drug development by expediting a sponsor's future drug to market or by offsetting the cost of research and development if the voucher is sold.

While the tropical and rare pediatric disease PRV programs are similar with regard to the benefits the program provides to sponsors, the two programs have several key differences worth noting. In order for a tropical disease product application to qualify for a PRV, the product must meet four requirements: (1) it must address a listed tropical disease; (2) it must be submitted under FDCA § 505(b)(1) or Public Health Service Act (PHSA) § 351; (3) the drug that is the subject of the application must not contain a previously approved active moiety; and (4) the application must qualify for priority review (FDCA § 524(a)(4); Food and Drug Administration 2016). Tropical diseases that qualify for priority review include "infectious disease[s] for which there is no significant market in developed nations and that disproportionately [affect] poor and marginalized populations" which are listed under the FDCA or designated by FDA through an order (FDCA § 524(a)(3)).

A rare pediatric disease product application qualifies for priority review if it meets the following five criteria: (1) it must prevent or treat a rare pediatric disease; (2) it must be submitted under FDCA § 505(b)(1) or PHSA § 351; (3) the drug that is the subject of the application must not contain a previously approved active moiety; (4) the application must qualify for priority review; and (5) the application must rely on clinical data derived from studies examining a pediatric population and dosages of the drug intended for that population (FDCA § 529(a)(4); Food and Drug Administration 2019c). FDA defines a "rare pediatric disease" as a "serious or life-threatening disease in which the serious or life-threatening manifestations primarily affect individuals aged from birth to 18 years" and that meets the criteria for orphan drug designation (FDCA § 529(a)(3)). A sponsor must notify FDA of its intent to use a PRV within 90 days of submitting an NDA or BLA and pay an additional fee to use the voucher. This fee is determined by FDA every fiscal year but has generally been between $2 million and $4 million. It is important to note that there is no limit on the number of times a voucher can be transferred (FDCA § 529(b)). These PRV programs provide incentives to spur the development of new treatments for diseases that would otherwise not attract development interest from companies due to the cost of development and the lack of market opportunities. While the tropical diseases PRV program does not sunset, the rare pediatric disease PRV program is set to expire in October 2022 unless extended by Congress.

Tax Credits

One of the Orphan Drug Act's key provisions is the Orphan Drug Tax Credit (ODTC) which is administered under the Internal Revenue Code. The ODTC allows sponsors to receive a tax credit for 50% of their "qualified clinical testing expenses" for orphan drug development. If a sponsor pays taxes in the United States, it may use its ODTC against its federal income tax liability. To qualify for the credit, clinical testing must (1) be conducted under an IND; (2) relate to a drug and an indication that has received an orphan drug designation from the FDA; (3) occur after FDA designation as an orphan drug and before FDA approval; and (4) be conducted by or on behalf of the taxpayer to whom the orphan drug designation applies. In order for sponsors to qualify for the ODTC, clinical testing must have been performed in the United States unless there was an insufficient testing population (26 U.S.C. § 45C). A testing population is considered insufficient if there are not enough subjects available in the United States "to produce reliable data from the clinical investigation" (26 C.F.R. § 1.28-1(d)(3)(ii)(B)). Eligible expenses include both in-house research expenses, such as wages and non-depreciable supplies, and contract research expenses.

Similar to other incentives in the Orphan Drug Act, the ODTC aids sponsors before orphan drugs have received market approval which helps to alleviate some of the risk sponsors face when making large investments in treatments for rare diseases where the ability to recover costs from the small patient population may be uncertain. Since the ODTC is a non-refundable tax credit, sponsors cannot use their ODTC immediately. However, sponsors can apply their ODTC forward to future tax years and accumulate unused tax credits for up to 20 years.

Orphan Drug Grants

The Orphan Drug Act also empowers FDA to award grants and contracts to sponsors to defray the costs of developing orphan drugs (Orphan Drug Act § 5(a)). One such grant is the Orphan Products Clinical Trials Grant which fosters and encourages the development of new safe and effective medical products for rare diseases and conditions and ensures that product development occurs in a timely manner with a modest investment. This grant program has facilitated the marketing approval of more than 60 products since the passage of the Orphan Drug Act in 1983. A second type of grant is the Orphan Products Natural History Grant which helps fund sponsors engaging in natural history studies of a rare disease or condition. A natural history study describes the course of a disease or condition over time, identifying demographic, genetic, environmental, and other variables that correlate with its development and outcomes. This grant program was launched in 2016 and in fiscal year 2017, and FDA funded six natural history studies in an effort to understand how rare diseases progress over time. In fiscal year 2019, of its approximately $15.5 million budget, OOPD intends to fund approximately $2,000,000 in support of orphan drug natural history research and makes up to five awards.

A third type of grant is the Pediatric Device Consortia Grant, which provides funding to events that bring together individuals and institutions that support pediatric medical device progression. This grant furthers the clinical need for pediatric devices through business planning, regulatory advising, intellectual property protections, and scientific, engineering, preclinical, and clinical services and capabilities.

Written Protocol Assistance

An additional incentive under the Orphan Drug Act is a written guidance by FDA, upon request by a sponsor, on the nonclinical and clinical studies needed to obtain marketing approval of its orphan drug (FDCA § 525). This type of development support is not as highly valued by sponsors, compared to other incentives of the orphan drug program, since FDA generally provides informal advice to any sponsor, regardless of whether it is developing an orphan drug or not.

User Fee Exemption

Under the FDCA, a human drug application for a product that has an orphan drug designation is not subject to an application fee unless the application includes an additional indication that is not for a rare disease or condition (FDCA § 736(a)(1)(F)). Additionally, a product with an orphan drug designation is exempt from the program fee if the sponsor can demonstrate that it has less than $50 million in gross worldwide revenue during the year preceding the request for exemption and the designated drug meets the public health requirements contained in the FDCA as such requirements are applied to requests for waivers of the program fee (FDCA § 736(k)).

Other Considerations Related to Orphan Drug Development

While the Orphan Drug Act provides several powerful incentives for sponsors to engage in orphan drug development, sponsors should be aware of potential disadvantages to developing and marketing an orphan drug. First, and the most obvious, is that there is no guarantee of cost recovery in the orphan drug market. In fact, the Orphan Drug Act requires sponsors, for drugs intended to treat a disease or condition with a population of 200,000 or greater in the United States, to show evidence of "no reasonable expectation that costs of research and development of the drug for the indication can be recovered by sales of the drug in the United States" (21 C.F.R. § 316.20(b)(8)(ii)). This must be made through a showing of all costs that the sponsor has incurred and expects to incur during development and an estimate of revenues for the first 7 years of marketing.

Second, a sponsor should consider whether they will need to demonstrate clinical superiority to obtain orphan drug designation. As discussed previously, clinical superiority can result from greater effectiveness, greater safety, or a major contribution to patient care. In order to adequately demonstrate clinical superiority when it is based on efficacy, a sponsor will likely have to perform a comparative study which further adds to the cost of development of the orphan product.

Third, FDA publicly announces all orphan designations in its *Approved Drug Products with Therapeutic Equivalence Evaluations* (the "Orange Book") and on the OOPD website. Therefore, once a drug obtains orphan drug designation, a sponsor's plan to develop a drug for the declared rare disease or condition becomes public knowledge. This provides notification to a sponsor's competitors of its development plans, which may not have previously been disclosed through publications, presentations at scientific meetings, or other public disclosures.

Fourth, the sponsor of any approved orphan drug must give notice at least 1 year before discontinuing production of its orphan drug. This requirement may complicate corporate decision-making since the decision to cease marketing must be made so far in advance.

Challenges with Clinical Trial Design for Rare Diseases

Once a promising compound that may prevent or treat a rare disease or condition has been identified, sponsors proceed with preclinical and clinical developments which are necessary steps in bringing a product to market. However, sponsors who develop therapies for rare diseases encounter several unique challenges that are not present when designing clinical trials for common ones (Food and Drug Administration 2018c; Food and Drug Administration 2019a). First, the small population size provides limited study opportunities relating to enrollment, adequately powering the study, and replication of results. Second, rare diseases display high heterogeneity across patients with the same disease and across similar diseases. Third, rare diseases are poorly understood due to incomplete natural histories. This tends to make diagnosis difficult, with years between the first presentation of symptoms and actual diagnosis of the rare disease or condition. On average, diagnosis of a rare disease or condition takes 7 years. Additionally, only a small number of doctors and medical facilities have experience diagnosing and treating rare diseases and conditions. Fourth, most rare diseases and conditions are serious or life-threatening, with most patients having unmet medical needs due to a lack of drugs developed. Fifth, since rare diseases and conditions are poorly understood, clinical endpoints are difficult to identify, and outcome assessment tools often lack sensitivity. Lastly, many rare diseases and conditions affect pediatric patients which poses additional ethical considerations and constraints when designing clinical trials (Food and Drug Administration 2017).

Evidence Required for Orphan Drug Approval

A key underlying issue facing the development of drugs, particularly orphan drugs, is the level of evidence FDA requires for approval (e.g., the quality and quantity of clinical trial information needed). A shortfall of the Orphan Drug Act is that it did not amend or revise the statutory standards for the quantum of evidence required for establishing that an orphan drug is safe and effective for its proposed use (Sasinowski et al. 2015). Therefore, a strict interpretation of the law would warrant that the standard of approval for orphan drugs is identical to the standard required for all other drugs, namely, that "substantial evidence" demonstrates effectiveness through "adequate and well-controlled [clinical] investigations." An adequate and well-controlled trial is one that has been designed well enough so as to be able "to distinguish the effect of a drug from other influences, such as spontaneous change... , placebo effect, or biased observation" (21 C.F.R. § 314.126). FDA has interpreted this standard to mean, generally, a minimum of two such adequate and well-controlled clinical trials, and traditionally, the Agency has accepted two such trials when each meets its primary endpoint by its prespecified primary analysis and is statistically significant (a P value of ≤ 0.050). However, FDA has continuously shown flexibility in the quantum of effectiveness evidence required to meet the "substantial evidence" standard.

First, FDA has administrative discretion found in formal FDA statute, regulation, or guidance. There are two different ways that FDA flexibility can manifest: either by affecting the number of studies required (i.e., less than two adequate and well-controlled trials) or by affecting the type of effectiveness evidence required (i.e., basing evidence of effectiveness on a finding on a surrogate endpoint or intermediate clinical endpoint under the "accelerated approval" pathway). With regard to flexibility in number of studies required, between the FDCA and guidance issued by FDA, there are two distinct pathways in which a single study may provide the quantum of effectiveness evidence required for approval of a drug. One of these is described in FDA guidance: a single adequate and well-controlled study with certain characteristics including and especially "a statistically very persuasive finding" (Food and Drug Administration, *Providing Clinical Evidence of Effectiveness for Human Drug and Biological Products* (May 1998)). The other comes from Section 115 of the Food and Drug Administration Modernization Act (FDAMA): an adequate and well-controlled study plus "confirmatory evidence."

Then, with regard to flexibility in the type of evidence of effectiveness, the accelerated approval pathway was created by FDA in response to the AIDS crisis in the mid-1980s, designed for therapies for serious diseases for which there is an unmet medical need (21 C.F.R. §§ 312, 314; Food and Drug Administration 2014). Under this pathway, FDA can establish evidence of effectiveness based either on an unvalidated surrogate that is reasonably likely to predict a clinical outcome or on an outcome other than irreversible morbidity or mortality that is reasonably likely to predict irreversible morbidity and mortality. For any such approval, there is an additional postapproval requirement to conduct a study to establish the ultimate clinical outcome benefit, and if that study fails to do so, FDA may withdraw its approval on an expedited basis.

In the review of orphan drugs, there are times when FDA has had to consider a marketing application with fewer than two positive adequate and well-controlled studies, and where FDA cannot rely upon one of its administrative programs for flexibility, yet the Agency determines that there is substantial evidence of effectiveness to support approval of the drug. In fact, recent studies have shown that in approximately two-thirds of approvals for orphan drugs, FDA deviated from its traditional requirement for two or more adequate and well-controlled studies by employing administrative flexibility or case-by-case flexibility (Sasinowski 2011; Sasinowski et al. 2015). In exercising this flexibility, FDA has reinforced the notion that orphan drugs are deserving of special considerations when assessing safety and effectiveness.

The Patient Voice in Orphan Drug Development

Input from stakeholders on trial design is important for ultimate approval of an orphan drug (Clinical Trials Transformation Initiative 2015), and patients have increasingly been recognized as key partners in this process and have led to more patient-focused drug development (PFDD). Through PFDD, patient advocacy groups, healthcare providers, researchers, and industry can overcome many of the existing hurdles in orphan drug development that were discussed previously. In recent years, patients have become an increasingly important force in providing experiences, perspectives, needs, and priorities which can then be captured and meaningfully incorporated into drug development and evaluation, as well as inform FDA regulatory decision-making. Since patients are the experts on what it is like to live with a particular rare disease or condition, they are uniquely positioned to inform the understanding of the therapeutic context for trial design.

Patients became significantly more involved in FDA's review process after the passage of the Food and Drug Administration Safety and Innovation Act (FDASIA) in 2012. This legislation added patients' perspectives to the drug development process by requiring FDA to "implement strategies to solicit the views of patients ... and consider the perspectives of patients during regulatory discussions" (FDCA § 569C(a)). At this time, FDA established the PFDD initiative to more systematically obtain the patient perspective on specific diseases and available treatments by conducting a series of meetings with patients and their caregivers to solicit their experiences and perspectives on these topics. The main goal of this initiative is to better incorporate the patient voice in drug development and evaluation.

Since enactment of the twenty-first Century Cures Act in 2015 and the FDA Reauthorization Act in 2017, PFDD has been expanded to include a broader range of qualitative and quantitative methods and systematic approaches to collecting and utilizing robust and meaningful patient and caregiver input. The goals are to more consistently inform drug development and regulatory decision-making, encourage identification and use of approaches and best practices to facilitate patient enrollment and minimize the burden of patient participation in clinical trials, enhance the understanding and appropriate use of methods to capture information on patient preferences and the potential acceptability of trade-offs between treatment benefit and risk outcomes, and identify the information that is most important to patients and how to best communicate that information to support their decision-making (Food and Drug Administration 2018b). For example, patient perspectives can be invaluable early during drug development, such as in the selection of endpoints, which are often not well-established in rare diseases. To establish treatment benefit to support approval, a product must have a meaningful effect on how patients feel, function, or survive. There are key questions that must be answered when selecting and developing measures of these effects for use in clinical trials: (1) How do we know the right concept of interest to measure?; (2) What opportunities are there to measure a concept of interest in patients' daily life?; and (3) Do we know what result on a measure is considered clinically meaningful? These are the types of questions that the patient experience can help answer.

Despite efforts to select and develop fit-for-purpose endpoints, the heterogeneity so common in many rare diseases reduces their sensitivity, which, when combined with small numbers of patients, can lead to concerns of type II errors. Novel methods have been employed that bulwark against such false negatives by capturing patients' and their caregivers' perceptions of change using semi-structured video interviews that can be implemented before, during, and after a clinical trial (Contesse et al. 2019).

Other examples of PFDD initiatives include utilizing a patient representative as a Special Government Employee to be part of the internal FDA review team or on an FDA advisory committee, having patients provide testimony during the open hearing segment of Advisory Committee meetings, initiating Rare Disease Listening Sessions to meet with FDA officials, and hosting externally led PFDD meetings or conduct PFDD surveys. Through these initiatives, the patient voice has become a key factor in evaluating both the safety and efficacy of new drugs as well as establishing what is clinically meaningful to patients with rare diseases and conditions.

Natural History Studies to Support Orphan Drug Development

The natural history of a disease is traditionally defined as the course a disease takes in the absence of intervention in individuals with the disease, from disease onset until resolution of the disease or the individual's death. Knowledge of a disease's natural history is important for planning drug development which poses a challenge for orphan drug development since there is only limited information about the natural history of most rare diseases. To address this challenge, FDA has provided guidance on how sponsors can conduct and use information from natural history studies to inform orphan drug development throughout all phases of development. A natural history study is a preplanned observational study intended to track the course of disease in order to identify demographic, genetic, environmental, and other variables that correlate with a disease's progression and outcomes (Food and Drug Administration 2019b). Information obtained from a natural history study can better inform the drug development process, from drug discovery to trial design through to the post-marketing period. Specifically relating to trial design, knowledge of the natural history of a rare disease can help sponsors design and conduct adequate and well-controlled trials of adequate duration that measure clinically meaningful endpoints.

First, natural history studies may be useful in understanding the patient population with a particular rare disease and identifying which patient subgroup(s) may benefit from a particular trial design. Second, natural history studies may be useful in the identification or development of clinical outcome assessments. A clinical outcome assessment is an assessment that describes or reflects how an individual feels, functions, or survives and can be used during trials to assess the safety and efficacy of an orphan drug. Third, natural history studies can help identify or develop biomarkers that can diagnose disease, prognose the progression of disease, predict treatment response, or guide patient and dose selection. Relatedly, natural history studies provide an opportunity to collect images and specimens over a long period of time that, when validated, can serve as endpoints or surrogate endpoints in clinical trials. Fourth, natural history study data can serve as external controls if substantial evidence of effectiveness can still be demonstrated as previously discussed.

New Horizons: Targeted Therapies for Rare Disease

Approximately 80% of rare diseases are genetic in nature, creating an evolution and broader application of targeted therapies for rare diseases and conditions. One such strategy is to target disease-associated genes at the ribonucleic acid (RNA) level such that specific disease-associated proteins are degraded. This is known as oligonucleotide therapy, which utilizes antisense oligonucleotides (ASOs) and small interfering RNAs (siRNAs) to prevent the expression of proteins that cause a particular disease or condition. Each ASO must be synthesized to bind to a specific RNA target which then goes on to affect gene expression in various ways. ASOs have been used as a robust platform for gene knockdown and have demonstrated clinical efficacy for the treatment of multiple diseases such as hereditary transthyretin-mediated amyloidosis (hATTR) and spinal muscular atrophy (SMA). The mechanistic characteristics of oligonucleotide therapies result in high specificity, ability to address targets that are otherwise inaccessible with traditional therapies, and reduced toxicity owing to limited systemic exposure. This greatly expands the numbers and types of selectable targets.

A second novel strategy is to utilize viral vectors for gene therapy in order to promote or suppress the expression of genes that contribute to the manifestation of a rare disease or condition (Food and Drug Administration 2020). For example, adeno-associated viral (AAV) vectors have proved to be very useful for clinical studies since the vector is very successful in tissue-specific gene delivery. Due to AAV vectors' non-integrating nature, this type of therapy is generally considered safe from a regulatory perspective. AAV vectors have demonstrated clinical efficacy for several rare diseases including SMA- and RPE-65-mediated retinal degeneration. A second example is retroviral vectors as ex vivo gene therapy using hematopoietic stem cells to safely and effectively treat hematologic diseases. AAV vectors appear to be an excellent platform for treating rare monogenic disorders, supporting transgene expression that persists for years in nondividing cells. A key limitation is the complexity and cost of manufacturing and production, which is vastly greater than for small molecules.

With greater biological plausibility in treatment mechanism of action, coupled with expected large magnitudes of treatment effect, targeted therapies may be able to demonstrate effectiveness in as few as one clinical trial – a departure from the traditional three phases of clinical development.

Summary and Conclusion

The development of drugs for rare diseases and conditions presents both unique opportunities and challenges for sponsors. Beginning with the Orphan Drug Act, ongoing efforts to encourage the development of orphan drugs have been successful, and the number of such approvals is continuously increasing. Sponsors must continue to improve their understanding of the unique drug development challenges that are posed by rare diseases and conditions. Such an understanding can be achieved by partnering with patient groups who can provide disease-specific perspectives and experiences, as well as through conduct of natural history studies, both of which can better inform the design and evaluation of results from clinical trials. Together, patients, industry, and FDA can work collectively to bring safe and effective orphan drugs to market, including emerging targeted therapy technologies that can truly "cure" these diseases.

Key Facts

1. A rare disease is a disease that affects fewer than 200,000 persons in the United States or affects more than 200,000 persons in the United States and for which a sponsor cannot reasonably expect to make a profit in developing a product to treat the disease or condition.
2. A rare pediatric disease is a serious or life-threatening disease in which the serious or life-threatening manifestations primarily affect individuals aged from birth to 18 years.
3. A tropical disease is an infectious disease for which there is no significant market in developed nations and that disproportionately affects poor and marginalized populations.
4. There may be as many as 8,000 rare diseases.
5. The total number of Americans living with a rare disease is estimated at 30 million or 1 in 10 people.
6. FDA has approved over 600 drugs for rare diseases.
7. Approved treatments are only available for 5% of all rare diseases.
8. 80% of rare diseases are genetic in origin.

Cross-References

▶ Advocacy and Patient Involvement
▶ Clinical Trials, Ethics, and Human Protections Policies
▶ Patient-Reported Outcomes
▶ Safety and Risk Benefit Analyses
▶ Use of Historical Data in Design

References

Clinical Trials Transformation Initiative (2015) CTTI recommendations: effective engagement with patient groups around clinical trials, Oct 2015. https://www.ctti-clinicaltrials.org/sites/www.ctti-clinicaltrials.org/files/7-revised_pgct-recommendations-2019_final.pdf. Last visited 10 Mar 2020

Contesse M, Valentine J, Wall T, Leffler M (2019) The case for the use of patient and caregiver perception of change assessments in rare disease clinical trials: a methodologic overview. Adv Ther. https://doi.org/10.1007/s12325-019-00920-x

FDA (2014) Expedited programs for serious conditions – drugs and biologics, May 2014. https://www.fda.gov/media/86377/download

FDA (2016) Tropical disease priority review vouchers, Oct 2016. https://www.fda.gov/media/72569/download

FDA (2017) Pediatric rare diseases – a collaborative approach for drug development using Gaucher disease as a model, Dec 2017. https://www.fda.gov/media/109465/download

FDA (2018a) Clarification of orphan designation of drugs and biologics for pediatric subpopulations of common diseases, July 2018. https://www.fda.gov/media/109496/download

FDA (2018b) Patient-focused drug development: collecting comprehensive and representative input, June 2018. https://www.fda.gov/media/113653/download

FDA (2018c) Slowly progressive, low-prevalence rare diseases with substrate deposition that results from single enzyme defects: providing evidence of effectiveness for replacement or corrective therapies, July 2018. https://www.fda.gov/media/115408/download

FDA (2019a) Rare diseases: common issues in drug development, Jan 2019. https://www.fda.gov/media/119757/download

FDA (2019b) Rare diseases: natural history studies for drug development, Mar 2019. https://www.fda.gov/media/122425/download

FDA (2019c) Rare pediatric disease priority review vouchers, July 2019

FDA (2020) Human gene therapy for rare diseases, Jan 2020. https://www.fda.gov/media/113807/download

Mikami K (2017) Orphans in the market: the history of orphan drug policy. Soc Hist Med:1–22. https://doi.org/10.1093/shm/hkx098

National Institute of Health, National Center for Advancing Translational Sciences. (n.d.) FAQ about rare diseases. http://rarediseases.info.nih.gov/about-ordr/pages/31/frequently-asked-questions. Last visited 10 Mar 2020

Sasinowski F (2011) Quantum of effectiveness evidence in FDA's approval of orphan drugs. Ther Innov Regul Sci. https://doi.org/10.1177/0092861511435906

Sasinowski F, Panico E, Valentine J (2015) Quantum of effectiveness evidence in FDA's approval of orphan drugs: update, July 2010 to June 2014. Ther Innov Regul Sci. https://doi.org/10.1177/2168479015580383

Pragmatic Randomized Trials Using Claims or Electronic Health Record Data

117

Frank W. Rockhold and Benjamin A. Goldstein

Contents

Introduction	2308
Pragmatic Randomized Clinical Trials	2309
Differences from Explanatory Trials	2310
Identifying Eligible Patients	2311
Approaches for Ascertaining and Classifying Endpoints in Pragmatic Trials	2312
Gaps in Patient Data: "Missing" or Just Not Needed?	2313
Data Latency	2314
Data Concordance (or Lack Thereof)	2314
Clinical Trial Site Investigators Versus Practicing Physicians	2315
Conclusion/Discussion	2316
Cross-References	2316
References	2316

Abstract

Randomized clinical trials have been the accepted standard for addressing key questions in medicine for well over 60 years. The structure and process, while well documented and characterized, have been historically described in the context of "efficacy" in a targeted population as opposed to "effectiveness" objectives in the greater population. Efficacy can be defined as the performance of an intervention under ideal and controlled circumstances, whereas effectiveness refers to its performance under "real-world" conditions. Another way to think about an effectiveness trial is that it often tests a treatment strategy or "policy" of applying an intervention as opposed to the actual action of the intervention itself. Trials looking at real-world outcomes may have some aspects of greater variability in the data and therefore the precision of the question and

F. W. Rockhold (✉) · B. A. Goldstein
Department of Biostatistics and Bioinformatics, Duke Clinical Research Institute, Duke University Medical Center, Durham, NC, USA
e-mail: frank.rockhold@duke.edu; benjamin.a.goldstein@duke.edu

© Springer Nature Switzerland AG 2022
S. Piantadosi, C. L. Meinert (eds.), *Principles and Practice of Clinical Trials*,
https://doi.org/10.1007/978-3-319-52636-2_270

rigor of the hypothesis are as essential as they are in any trial. Therefore, a key component of implementing a pragmatic clinical trial (PCT) is using data that one can more easily obtain (i.e., pragmatically). In recent years, one solution to this has been to use Electronic Health Record (EHR) and/or administrative billing (claims) data. These data fall under the larger and growing rubric of "real-world data," roughly defined as data that are not primarily collected for research purposes. Instead, EHR and claims data are generated as a product of a patient's healthcare encounters. As such, from a researcher's perspective, there appears to be minimal cost with using these data for research purposes. However, the trade-off is that there is often minimal control of which data are collected and how.

In this chapter, we discuss the characteristics of these data sources, their usage within pragmatic trials, and considerations that can be challenging to practitioners' research.

Keywords

Pragmatic clinical trials · Electronic health records · Real-World data · Clinical trials

Introduction

Randomized clinical trials have been the accepted standard for addressing key questions in medicine for well over 60 years. The structure and process, while well documented and characterized, have been historically described in the context of "efficacy" in a targeted population as opposed to "effectiveness" objectives in the greater population. **Efficacy** can be defined as the performance of an intervention under ideal and controlled circumstances, whereas **effectiveness** refers to its performance under "real-world" conditions. Research on efficacy and effectiveness has also been described as explanatory versus pragmatic trials. The latter is a more outcome-based approach, whereas the former relies more on surrogate markers or measurement endpoints. In addition, looking at effectiveness usually entails outcome variables that are more relevant in the real world albeit ones that are often subject to greater measurement error. Another way to think about an effectiveness trial is that it often tests a treatment strategy or "policy" of applying an intervention as opposed to the actual action of the intervention itself. When coupled with the measurement issues highlighted below, these types of "pragmatic" trials can yield greater variability in response. So, while one still needs to apply the rigor of the scientific method, as John Tukey said, "Far better an approximate answer to the right question, which is often vague, than an exact answer to the wrong question, which can always be made precise" (Tukey 1962). Note the importance of specifying the question which underlines objective and hypothesis that while trials looking at real-world outcomes may have some aspects of greater variability in the data, the precision of the question and rigor of the hypothesis are as essential as they are in any trial. Some specifics of the characteristics of these trials are given below.

One of the primary challenges of traditional clinical trials is the cost – on both a time and monetary basis – of collecting the data that are required. Therefore, a key component of implementing a Pragmatic Clinical Trial (PCT) is using data that one can easily collect (i.e., pragmatically). In recent years, one solution to this has been to use Electronic Health Record (EHR) and/or administrative billing (claims) data. While each data source has its unique characteristics and corresponding strengths and weaknesses, for the purposes of this exposition, we will focus on the similarities. These data fall under the larger and growing rubric of *real-world data*, roughly defined as data that are not collected for research purposes (see ▶ Chap. 114, "Leveraging "Big Data" for the Design and Execution of Clinical Trials" for a discussion of EHR data). Instead, EHR and claims data are generated as a product of a patient's healthcare encounters. As such, from a researcher's perspective, there appears to be minimal cost with using these data for research purpose. However, the trade-off is that there is often minimal control as to which data are collected and how. In this chapter, we discuss the characteristics of these data sources, their usage within pragmatic trials, and considerations that might be challenging to practitioners' research.

Pragmatic Randomized Clinical Trials

The decision to implement any clinical trial involves assessment of a series of trade-offs which may hold more or less weight depending on the health question and current state of the external evidence. Pragmatic trials should not necessarily be intended to *replace* "traditional" RCTs but, rather as they answer a slightly different question with different data sources, should be used to supplement RCTs.

The concept of pragmatic clinical research dates back to the 1960s (Schwartz and Lellouch 1967). In fact, many of the "large and simple" trials conducted in the 1980s and 1990s in cardiovascular disease could be considered PCTs even though they did not employ EHR or claims data. Current pragmatic trials are primarily designed to compare *strategies* (effectiveness as described above) for the prevention, diagnosis, and treatment of diseases. They have also (rarely) been considered for the marketing authorization application of new drugs with increasing regulatory attention paid toward using real-world evidence in drug approval. GlaxoSmithKline's Salford Lung Study was the first phase 3 PCT supporting registration of a new drug (Bakerly et al. 2015; Woodcock et al. 2015). Other sponsors of pragmatic trials of medical strategies include funding agencies such as the Patient-Centered Outcomes Research Institute (PCORI). The largest PCORI funded pragmatic trial to date is the ADAPT-ABLE trial, comparing high-dose and low-dose aspirin in 15,000 patients which has been ongoing since 2016 (Johnston et al. 2016). This latest example is a trial done almost entirely within the health system. There are no "investigators" or "sites," and with the exception of patient check-ins on the patient web portal, all patient data and endpoint follow-up (death, stroke, and myocardial infarction) are done within the EHR and aligned data sources. Some of the concepts described in this chapter derive from experiences with these trials.

It should be noted that some pragmatic trials are based on "cluster" randomization where units (clusters) of participants, such as hospitals, clinics, counties, and schools, are the unit of randomization and the analysis can be done at either the "cluster" or participant-level data. The use of cluster designs can prove to be logistically easier from a participant recruitment standpoint and conversely be somewhat less efficient statistically due to the correlation among participants within a cluster. A full review of cluster designs can be found elsewhere (Turner et al. 2017). The motivation and examples upon which this chapter is based relate to trials involving individual randomization and informed consent. This is more aligned with the "RCT" approach.

Differences from Explanatory Trials

PCTs differ from a traditional "explanatory" clinical trial in important ways. As noted above, PCTs are closely associated with the concept of effectiveness rather than efficacy, or how well therapies work in a usual care setting versus an ideal setting. So, in the case of ADAPTABLE, patients are "prescribed" by randomization their aspirin dose as they would be in the real world but without defined follow-up visits or compliance checks. While this may introduce more extensive heterogeneity between treatment groups than is typically observed in more tightly controlled trials, randomized designs can help to minimize these differences and equalize the distribution of unobserved confounders. PCTs typically evaluate outcomes that are clinically observable and therefore likely to have direct relevance to diverse stakeholders and thus fit into the mold of "effectiveness" trials as noted above. Table 1 provides an overview of differences between traditional randomized clinical trials and PCTs. The extent to which one leans toward the right side of the table is a measure of the degree of pragmatism of the design. The PRECIS wheel (Loudon et al. 2015) (Fig. 1) is a more formal way of documenting this concept. In general, PCTs rely heavily on data that are already collected as part of routine clinical practice. This allows a more "real-world" approach to patient-centered research and supports generalizability of study findings to broader populations than those enrolled in traditional randomized clinical trials. However, relying on existing data necessarily introduces challenges due to the fact that these data were collected for purposes other than research as described below. Thus, some additional structure and refinements may be needed (Rockhold et al. 2020).

Of particular relevance to this chapter is the requirement that data and endpoints selected for the trial be grounded in and leverage existing healthcare workflows (see highlighted rows in Table 1). In PCTs (as considered in this chapter), this typically means using EHR or claims data for most (if not all) data analyses. However, the challenges of using EHR data for clinical research have been well described above including the fact that EHRs will not collect all data necessary for a trial. So, designers of pragmatic trials might need consider alternative data sources, including patient-reported health data (PRH). The challenge is to decide how to integrate different data sources and determine which is best for which types of data and

Table 1 Ways that randomized controlled trials (RCTs) and PCTs can differ

Classic RCT	Criterion	P"R"CT
Intentionally homogeneous to maximize treatment effect	Eligibility criteria	Heterogeneous – representative of normal treatment population
Randomization and double blind	Bias control	Randomization and rarely blinding
Clinical measures, intermediate endpoints, composite endpoints, clinical outcomes	Endpoints	Clinical outcomes as reported in the health system
Protocol defines the level and timing of testing	Routine follow-up tests	Measured according to standard practice
Fixed active control or placebo	Comparison or intervention	Standard clinical practice
Conducted only by trained and experienced investigators	Trial "investigator"	Practitioners with differing and limited experience
Visit schedule defined in the protocol	Longitudinal follow-up	Visits at the discretion of physician and patient
Compliance is monitored closely	Protocol compliance	Passive or indirect monitoring of patient compliance
Close monitoring of adherence	Adherence or treatment	Passive or indirect monitoring of practitioner adherence
Intent to treat, per protocol and completers	Estimand	All patients included ITT

what to do when there are discrepancies between an EHR and a patient-reported source. In choosing a strategy for collecting PRH data to augment the EHR, it is important to ensure that the data collected have the same meaning semantically/conceptually with what is available in the EHR. The same data may be represented in different ways across multiple health systems, and even in multiple ways within the same health system, as clinical workflows change over time.

Identifying Eligible Patients

EHR systems can be used to identify eligible patients. This identification can be done prospectively or retrospectively. Prospectively, one can create alerts that pop-up when a patient meets some enrollment criterion. This can be done in real-time as data are being entered by providers into the system. This becomes particularly useful for point-of-care trials or trials within the emergency department environment. One can also use recent retrospective EHR data to generate eligible lists. For example, if one were designing a diabetes trial, one could start by building a registry of diabetics that use the health system. Using this registry – and the knowledge of their clinical characteristics – one could then identify patients to be enrolled, thus ensuring that one recruits a study population that has the desired clinical characteristics.

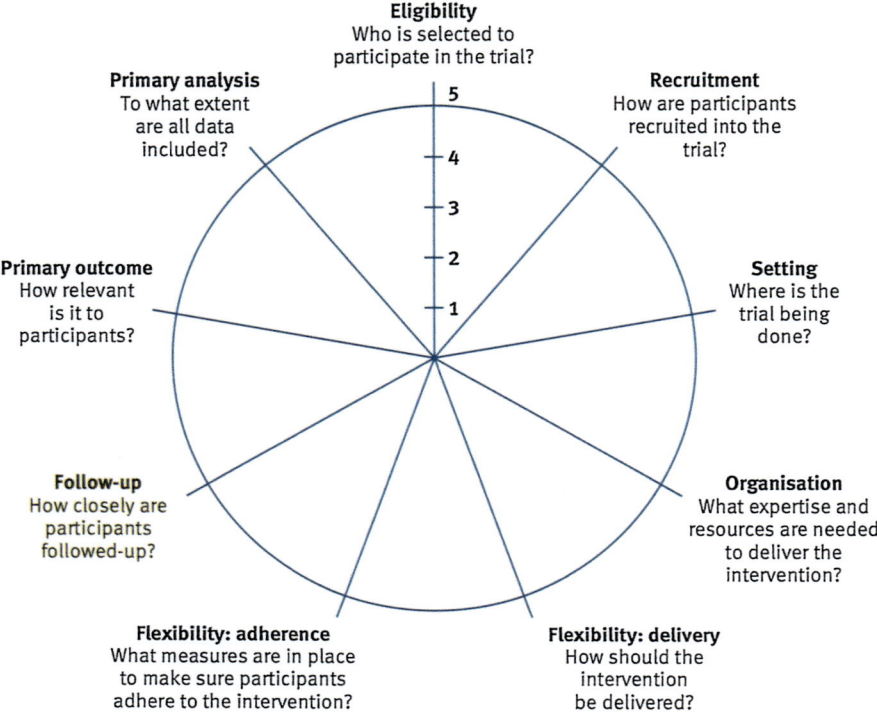

Fig. 1 PRECIS construct for the spectrum of "pragmatism" in a randomized clinical trial (Loudon et al. 2015)

Approaches for Ascertaining and Classifying Endpoints in Pragmatic Trials

There are unique features related to the ascertainment of outcomes from randomized PCTs. While some of these offer challenges over and above that of the standard randomized clinical trial, a key consideration is whether the ascertainment is in some way related to randomized treatment in an analogous manner to the concept of "missing data" as described below. This is more likely to happen if the trial is not blinded or masked, as is usually the case in pragmatic trials, and knowledge of the assigned treatment can lead to different changes in the patients' medical care or therapy. This knowledge revolving around prior beliefs of the nature of "usual care" introduces bias. Another key feature is the nature of the control, that is, (1) an "active" controlled trial where one of the therapies is known to be effective in the trial population or (2) a treatment compared to no added treatment or on top of "usual care," since it is an ethical challenge to withhold usual standard of care. While arguably in trials with "hard" endpoints (e.g., death, myocardial infarction), the effect of this "unmasking" bias should be less and the scientific hypothesis being tested is protected by the randomization scheme, there are a number clearly of potential sources of bias that make these issues far from settled (Ford and Norrie 2016).

When adjudicating endpoints from the EHR, it is important to recognize there may be no specific field that denotes the presence of event, such as a myocardial infarction or progression to diabetes. Instead one needs to use the available data – based on diagnoses, laboratory results, medications, etc. – to create a *computable phenotype*. Computable phenotypes are Boolean definitions used to indicate the presence of a condition of interest. For example, a computable phenotype for diabetes may include the presence of a diabetes diagnosis code OR a diabetes medication OR a hemoglobin A1c greater than 6.5% (Richesson et al. 2013; Spratt et al. 2017).

The exact computable phenotype will control the sensitivity and specificity of outcome ascertainment. The desired thresholds depend on the nature of the trial design. Even under ideal study design circumstances, PCTs are typically expected to have lower specificity (true negative rate) and sensitivity (true positive rate) with respect to event capture. Because secondary data sources used in pragmatic trials are not collected for research purposes, the depth and auditability will not be the same as with a standard clinical trial with a well-designed, stand-alone case report form.

For cardiovascular outcome trials of myocardial infarction and stroke such as ADAPTABLE, the lower expected sensitivity may be addressed by using other information in the EHR and by mimicking the adjudication process of a randomized controlled trial. Specificity is of course more difficult and would require supplemental resources such as claims data, National Death Index, and patient-reported information to ensure we are not missing events. Several approaches for consideration are outlined in the next section.

Gaps in Patient Data: "Missing" or Just Not Needed?

"Missingness" is a term often incorrectly applied to the PCT framework. It is carried over from traditional clinical trial terminology where a case report form contains a data element, and the concept of "missing" is clear if that data element is blank. In a pragmatic trial, the needed information may be not available for research purposes because it was not necessary for the patients' medical care; it is not clear what "missingness" implies in this context. When relying on EHR data, understanding these "gaps" becomes important, because the presence of data elements is usually informative, a process we've referred to as *informed presence* (Goldstein et al. 2019; Phelan et al. 2017). This typically manifests itself in that we have more information on sicker patients. For example, a doctor will typically only measure a certain laboratory marker if she/he is concerned about its values. This type of data collection can create feedback loops, biasing results. While these biases are inherent in real-world data, careful design consideration can mitigate these biases (Goldstein et al. 2019).

As such it is important to include information that is routinely collected in care or collect extra data to either augment or reconcile data from the EHR. A clear description is needed in the protocol about what information is reasonably expected to be routinely available in a real-world data source, like the EHR, along with how missingness or gaps will be defined for scenarios in which an *expected* value is unavailable.

As noted above, the reliability of an outcome that is tied to an administrative function like reimbursement may be different from one that is workflow-driven, like the collection of vital signs during an ambulatory visit. These differences can affect the way that an outcome could become missing or incomplete and also play a role in the strategy for PRH-based reconciliation or augmentation. Collecting information on outcomes from multiple sources, including patients, may address this incompleteness, but best practices for integrating multiple sources and reconciling differences between them have not yet been defined.

Data Latency

Because PCTs generally rely on health information that is extracted and transformed from an EHR system, they are vulnerable to incomplete information due to data latency as well as data availability. Data latency is a particular issue because, while information is uploaded quickly to billing systems from EHRs, it may be less current than information collected from other sources (such as a case report form in a traditional RCT) due to the additional step of transformation into research-ready format. This introduces special considerations for ongoing surveillance of event rates in the trial and may affect the functioning of the data monitoring committee as the lag time from event to data collection could be slower than a typical RCT. Normally a Data Monitoring Committee (DMC) gets site-based events quickly and then has to wait for adjudicated events. In the case of a PCT, those are one in the same, and the EHR version of the event could be delayed for several months due to common data model extractions from the medical center. If there is no direct contact with the patient, then the DMC could be making recommendations on data aged more than they like. Improving processes for transferring data to the coordinating center will be essential in the future for the optimal functioning of a DMC in an EHR-based PCT.

Data Concordance (or Lack Thereof)

When the EHR or claims data are augmented by PRH in a PCT, examining the level of concordance between the data reported by the patient and what was collected in the course of clinical care and entered into the EHR is important to confirm the ascertainment of events. But this is not always the case, and researchers need to identify discrepancies, research underlying causes, and make plans/protocols for what to do. For example, where the structure of the data element does not align perfectly, it may be possible to map one to the other. Consider smoking status: if a patient's smoking status is captured in the EHR as the average number of cigarettes smoked per day, and the patient is asked during the trial to report the average number of packs per week, it is relatively straightforward to translate between them or to a third representation. Though some types of data will require choosing one source or another, in other cases the sources may be combined. This issue ties back to the data or information gaps section above. For questions regarding whether the patient has ever had a given diagnosis or procedure, a combination of EHR data and the patient's memory may represent the best triangulation of ground truth.

Another consideration in deciding how to handle discordant data is the specific use case, and specifically, the relative importance of sensitivity versus specificity. If one is looking at inclusion criteria for a very rare condition, it may be best to err on the side of accepting false positives in order to cast a wide net. If one intends to perform a case-control analysis, one may want to be very certain that patients designated as cases are indeed true cases.

Owing to the numerous choices that need to be made, data models become extremely useful for organizing data collection, particularly across multiple institutions. A data model will provide rules for which data elements ought to be extracted from the underlying EHR and how similar data elements ought to be combined or how to define computable phenotypes. Since EHR systems differ across institutions, having these definitions allows for easier coordination of data across sites.

Clinical Trial Site Investigators Versus Practicing Physicians

Much of what is discussed about the usefulness of health system data in randomized PCTs is done against the backdrop of the reality that the practicing physician has in many ways replaced the role of the site investigator in a traditional RCT. These professionals while primarily responsible for patient care are not necessarily well versed in research methods, data collection standards, equipoise, trial informed consent, and other features of trials. The interaction these healthcare workers have with the patient is now the primary and only source of data for the researcher. Depending on the complexity of the trial, this can compound some of the variability and unfocused data structures present in EHR or claims databases. Thus, the "real-world" nature of these trials needs to be factored into the question being studied and the endpoints chosen for the trial. The scientific and medical question needs to come first and then a decision as to whether an EHR-based trial could address that question. Too often investigators chose the RWD data approach and then modify the question to fit. That does not serve the science and community well. Second, the trialist needs to recognize the issues noted above and determine if the data collected for medical care are extensive enough to address the research needs. If not, there is always the option of augmenting the medical record with patient-collected information or ancillary case report forms. A balance must be struck however, as the more that is added the less "pragmatic" and "real world" the trial becomes. In addition, as noted above, this could results in data concordance issues, and the trialist is well advised to have an a priori decision rule for what is "truth" and what is supportive. For recruitment, it may be that direct to patient approaches result in slow enrollment and some engagement from the patients or institution's medical staff may be needed to encourage or educate patients about the trial. This could also add cost and complexity to the trial. In summary, these EHR-based trials using data collected from healthcare practitioners collecting data to treat patients are contrasted with research trained investigators using trial-specific data collection tools and weighing the pros and cons of each should drive how and if either or both can answer the clinical question of interest. One should not let convenience and access drive the decision on how to construct the trial question.

Conclusion/Discussion

When used to address appropriate, well-defined questions, high-quality "pragmatic" clinical trials using EHR data hold great potential for informing healthcare. Our objective was to describe the characteristics and challenges involved in the use of EHR data which is primarily collected for patient care and administration of health systems. While possibly decreasing data collection and monitoring concerns, using EHR data in clinical trials may increase the burden of ensuring data integrity and methodological rigor. There are a number of differences between the "PCT" and "RCT" approaches that affect the use of the data. Nevertheless, these augmentations to traditional RCT approaches improve generalizability of trial results, thereby driving improved clinical decision-making. We identified numerous actionable steps to ensure the quality, safety, and viability of the use of the data to drive valid clinical trial endpoints. Taking these steps will help optimize the implementation and growth of high-quality, safe, and scientifically rigorous PCTs that will improve patient health.

Cross-References

▶ Leveraging "Big Data" for the Design and Execution of Clinical Trials

References

Bakerly ND et al (2015) The Salford Lung Study protocol: a pragmatic, randomised phase III real-world effectiveness trial in chronic obstructive pulmonary disease. Respir Res 16:101
Ford I, Norrie J (2016) Pragmatic trials. N Engl J Med 375(5):454–463
Goldstein BA et al (2019) How and when informative visit processes can bias inference when using electronic health records data for clinical research. J Am Med Inform Assoc 26(12):1609–1617
Johnston A, Jones WS, Hernandez AF (2016) The ADAPTABLE trial and aspirin dosing in secondary prevention for patients with coronary artery disease. Curr Cardiol Rep 18:81. https://doi.org/10.1007/s11886-016-0749-2
Loudon K et al (2015) The PRECIS-2 tool: designing trials that are fit for purpose. BMJ 350:h2147
Phelan M, Bhavsar NA, Goldstein BA (2017) Illustrating informed presence bias in electronic health records data: how patient interactions with a health system can impact inference. EGEMS (Wash DC) 5(1):22

Richesson RL et al (2013) A comparison of phenotype definitions for diabetes mellitus. J Am Med Inform Assoc 20(e2):e319–e326

Rockhold FW, Tenenbaum JD, Richesson R, Marsolo KA, O'Brien EC (2020) Design and analytic considerations for using patient-reported health data in pragmatic clinical trials: report from an NIH Collaboratory roundtable, J Am Med Inform Assoc, ocz226, https://doi.org/10.1093/jamia/ocz226

Schwartz D, Lellouch J (1967) Explanatory and pragmatic attitudes in therapeutical trials. J Chronic Dis 20(8):637–648

Spratt SE et al (2017) Assessing electronic health record phenotypes against gold-standard diagnostic criteria for diabetes mellitus. J Am Med Inform Assoc 24(e1):e121–e128

Tukey JW (1962) Future of data analysis. Ann Math Stat 33(1):1–67

Turner EL et al (2017) Review of recent methodological developments in group-randomized trials: part 1-design. Am J Public Health 107(6):907–915

Woodcock A et al (2015) The Salford Lung Study protocol: a pragmatic, randomised phase III real-world effectiveness trial in asthma. BMC Pulm Med 15:160

Fraud in Clinical Trials

118

Stephen L. George, Marc Buyse, and Steven Piantadosi

Contents

Introduction	2320
Case Studies of Fraud in Clinical Trials	2321
Roger Poisson	2321
Werner Bezwoda	2322
Robert Fiddes	2322
Harry W. Snyder, Jr. and Renee Peugeot	2322
Yoshitaka Fujii	2323
Hiroaki Matsubara	2323
Joachim Boldt	2324
Anil Potti	2324
Anne Kirkman-Campbell	2324
Piero Anversa	2325
Predisposing Factors	2325
Estimates of Prevalence	2326
Detection of Fraud	2328
Principles of Statistical Monitoring	2329

S. L. George (✉)
Department of Biostatistics and Bioinformatics, Basic Science Division,
Duke University School of Medicine, Durham, NC, USA
e-mail: stephen.george@duke.edu

M. Buyse
International Drug Development Institute (IDDI) Inc., San Francisco, CA, USA

CluePoints S.A., Louvain-la-Neuve, Belgium and I-BioStat, University of Hasselt,
Louvain-la-Neuve, Belgium

Interuniversity Institute for Biostatistics and Statistical Bioinformatics (I-BioStat), Hasselt
University, Hasselt, Belgium
e-mail: marc.buyse@iddi.com

S. Piantadosi
Department of Surgery, Division of Surgical Oncology, Brigham and Women's Hospital, Harvard
Medical School, Boston, MA, USA
e-mail: spiantadosi@bwh.harvard.edu

© Springer Nature Switzerland AG 2022
S. Piantadosi, C. L. Meinert (eds.), *Principles and Practice of Clinical Trials*,
https://doi.org/10.1007/978-3-319-52636-2_163

Implementations of Statistical Monitoring	2330
Center Scoring	2331
Summary and Conclusion	2333
Key Facts	2334
Cross-References	2334
References	2334

Abstract

Several high-profile cases of fabrication or falsification of data have occurred in clinical trials in recent years. The number of such reported cases is quite low, given the large number of clinical trials conducted worldwide. Although this suggests that the prevalence of fraud is very low, reliable evidence on prevalence is lacking. Regardless of the true prevalence, fraud is damaging to the public trust in the clinical trial process and can put patients at risk. This chapter summarizes some prominent examples of detected fraud in clinical trials, the existing evidence on prevalence, contributing predisposing factors and statistical techniques for detection of fraud.

Keywords

Fraud · Fabrication · Falsification · Prevalence of fraud · Case studies · Detection of fraud · Central statistical monitoring

Introduction

The practice of science is a human endeavor, subject to the usual human foibles, including misconduct and fraud, which bedevil any such endeavor. It should therefore not be surprising to learn that fraud has also occurred in the conduct and analysis of clinical trials, although such activity is particularly egregious in clinical trials because of the direct risk posed to patients.

In this chapter, fraud in the clinical trial setting is defined as fabrication or falsification of data in the planning, conduct, or analysis of trials. There are many definitions of general scientific misconduct, ranging from the most serious violations of scientific norms (fabrication and falsification of data) to lesser violations (selective reporting, sloppiness, use of improper statistical techniques, etc.). The US Public Health Service definition of scientific misconduct restricts attention to fabrication, falsification, or plagiarism: "Research misconduct means fabrication, falsification, or plagiarism in proposing, performing, or reviewing research, or in reporting research results" (Federal Register 2005).

In this chapter, we discuss some of the more notorious cases of discovered fraud in clinical trials, predisposing factors, and estimates of the prevalence of fraud and describe some statistical methods for the detection of suspected fraud.

Case Studies of Fraud in Clinical Trials

Recent examples of cases of fraud in different areas of science are abundant (Sovacool 2008; Stroebe et al. 2012). The US Office of Research Integrity (ORI) provides case summaries and the results of ORI investigations into cases of suspected misconduct by grant supported investigators (https://ori.hhs.gov/). Coverage of retractions of papers in the scientific literature, many of which are the result of suspected fraud, may be found at the Retraction Watch website (https://retractionwatch.com/).

In this section, ten prominent case studies are presented in which alleged fraud was committed either directly in a clinical trial or in preclinical studies that led to clinical trials. Each case is presented in a very brief summary. Several of the cases were discussed in more detail elsewhere (George and Buyse 2015; Piantadosi 2017).

Roger Poisson

One of the more highly publicized cases of fraud in clinical trials is that of Dr. Roger Poisson, a clinical investigator at St. Luc Hospital in Montreal, Canada, one of the institutions in the National Surgical Adjuvant Breast and Bowel Project (NSABP), a large clinical trials cooperative group (George 1997). In 1994 it was announced by the NSABP that Dr. Poisson had committed fraud in several clinical trials involving breast cancer patients during the period 1977 through 1990, including some important practice-changing trials. The revelation of this fraud precipitated an uproar in the media and led to congressional investigations and increased pressure on all of the cooperative groups by the National Cancer Institute. Dr. Poisson's explanation for his data manipulation was that he was doing what he felt was in the best interest of his patients by allowing them to be enrolled on NSABP trials, despite violation of certain in his opinion, unimportant eligibility criteria (Poisson 1994).

The perceived importance of the fraud was disproportionate to its actual impact on the studies involved (Peto et al. 1997). As a percentage of all patients entered on the trials in which St. Luc participated, only 0.3% were found to have any fraudulent data in the records. This alone should have been enough to temper concern that the previously published results of the trial were no longer valid. In addition, subsequent audits revealed that the falsifications were restricted primarily to selected eligibility criteria (e.g., a change in a surgical date to avoid a protocol-specified limit of the maximum number of days from surgery to registration). The tweaking of the eligibility criteria did not unduly put patients at risk. There were no fictitious patients. Once the patients were registered, the protocol was followed, and there was no alteration of any subsequent data, including outcome data. The Poisson case is a vivid example of the potential damage to trial credibility caused by fraud, beyond any rational assessment of the impact on the conclusions of the trial. The other cases in this section exhibit more serious implications.

Werner Bezwoda

In May 1999, at a plenary session at the annual meeting of the American Society of Clinical Oncology (ASCO), Dr. Werner Bezwoda, then professor and chair of the Department of Hematology and Oncology at the University of Witwatersrand in Johannesburg, South Africa, presented results from a single-institution randomized clinical trial in women with high-risk breast cancer. The experimental treatment arm involved the use of high-dose chemotherapy and stem cell rescue, a topic of intense interest in the breast cancer research community at the time. The results were strongly in favor of the high-dose treatment arm, made even more striking in comparison to the results from similar and much larger trials from two NCI-sponsored multi-institutional groups reported at the same session showing no benefit, but potential harm, from such high-dose chemotherapy.

Based on these results, the NCI decided to launch a confirmatory trial but, before proceeding, commissioned an external site visit and audit at Dr. Bezwoda's institution to verify the quality of the source data. The results of that site visit were telling (Weiss et al. 2000). There were no medical records of any kind for a majority of patients, none for control arm patients, and eligibility criteria were not available for many of those with records could be produced. Further, there was no evidence that informed consent had been obtained and no record that the trial had been reviewed by any human research oversight committee. Shortly after these results were known, Dr. Bezwoda admitted to the fraud and was removed from his position.

Robert Fiddes

In the early 1990's, Dr. Robert Fiddes, director of the Southern California Research Institute, was the lead clinical investigator on many pharmaceutical-sponsored clinical trials. Dr. Fiddes was popular as an investigator because of the high recruitment rate at his institution and the low dropout rate for the recruited patients. But after a whistleblower's notification of possible misconduct, the US Food and Drug Administration (FDA) began an extensive investigation. It was soon discovered that over many years, Dr. Fiddes had enrolled ineligible and even fictitious patients; other patients were pressured or coerced into entering trials; and clinical and laboratory data were falsified or fabricated. In 1997, Dr. Fiddes pled guilty to fraud and was sentenced to 15 months in prison. One remarkable feature of the Fiddes case is that although the fraud was conducted over many years, it was not uncovered by routine audits or other checks during that time; it was only discovered after a concerned whistleblower's report.

Harry W. Snyder, Jr. and Renee Peugeot

In 1994, a randomized clinical trial of BCX-34, a topical ointment used in the treatment of psoriasis and cutaneous T-cell lymphoma (CTCL) developed at BioCryst Pharmaceuticals, was conducted at the University of Alabama at Birmingham (UAB). In early 1995, a BioCryst press release touted highly favorable results for BCX-34 in both indications, a particularly noteworthy result in CTCL. Dr. Harry Snyder was the primary BioCryst investigator for this trial. Renee Peugeot, Dr. Snyder's wife and a registered nurse at UAB, was the study coordinator responsible for the day-to-day conduct of the trial. In June 1995, following an internal review of the trial by a newly appointed Medical Director at BioCryst, the previously issued press release was retracted with the comment that "no statistically significant drug effect" was observed. A subsequent FDA investigation of the conduct of the trial led to charges of falsification of data and alteration of the randomization assignments to favor BCX-34. Subsequently both Dr. Snyder and Ms. Peugeot received felony convictions with prison sentences of 3 years and 2.5 years, respectively, plus financial restitution and permanent FDA debarment.

Yoshitaka Fujii

A letter to the editor of *Anesthesia & Analgesia* in 2000 noted a remarkable result for 21 papers authored by Dr. Yoshitaka Fujii reporting the results of randomized clinical trials for treatment of postoperative nausea and vomiting (PONV). All 21 of the trials reported postoperative headache rates in the treatment groups that were nearly identical. The probability of such a result is so small that strong suspicions should have been raised about these studies. Unfortunately, no definitive action resulted from this initial red flag, and Dr. Fujii continued to publish at an extremely high rate, more than 200 papers by 2012, at which time a detailed analysis of 168 of his trials was published in *Anesthesia & Analgesia* (Carlisle 2012). This analysis extended the previously noted lack of expected variation to the distribution of most variables in the trials. This time, the evidence was not ignored and led to an investigation by the Japanese Society of Anesthesiologists (JSA) that concluded that of 212 papers reviewed and over 80% were fraudulent, including almost 60% that were "totally fabricated." This in turn led to the retraction of 183 papers, the current record for any author in the scientific literature. Dr. Fujii was dismissed from his University position in 2012, officially for failing to obtain prior ethical review board approval, not for fraud, and is no longer involved in research.

Hiroaki Matsubara

Dr. Hiroaki Matsubara, a cardiologist at the Kyoto Prefectural University School of Medicine (KPUM), led the Kyoto Heart Study, a 3000-patient randomized clinical trial comparing valsartan (Diovan®) with a control group. Results of this study were published in the *European Heart Journal* in August 2009 and showed a large reduction (hazard ratio = 0.55) in cardiovascular events, both fatal and nonfatal, in the valsartan treatment arm. In 2012, a short letter appeared in *The Lancet* noting an unusual statistical result in this paper: identical means and standard deviations for pre- and postsystolic and diastolic blood pressure in the two treatment groups. This led to an in-depth investigation by KPUM of this study with the conclusion that "the data were manipulated" and that, after the manipulations were corrected, there was no longer any statistically significant difference in the cardiovascular events between the two treatment groups. In 2013, the *European Heart Journal* retracted the paper and Dr. Matsubara resigned from his position.

Joachim Boldt

In December 2009, the results of a small randomized clinical trial by Dr. Joachim Boldt and colleagues were published in the journal *Anesthesia & Analgesia*. This study compared the effects of a hydroxyethyl starch (HES) priming preparation compared to an albumin-based control regimen given prospectively to patients undergoing coronary artery bypass grafting. The results indicated reduced inflammation, less endothelial damage, and other benefits for the HES regimen. But some unusual statistical anomalies in the published paper, primarily suspiciously small variability, led to investigations resulting in the retraction of the paper and a conclusion that the trial in question may not have been conducted at all. This in turn led to additional investigation of Dr. Boldt's publications. To date, 96 publications have been retracted, second only to the total number of retractions for Dr. Yoshitaka Fujii. In 2013, a large meta-analysis of the use of HES reached different conclusions regarding mortality and acute kidney injury depending on whether the retracted papers on the topic were included or not. After exclusion of the papers, there was significant evidence of increased mortality and acute kidney injury, an indication of the important influence fraud can have on overall medical evidence.

Anil Potti

From 2004 to 2010, Dr. Anil Potti was a prominent cancer researcher at Duke University, whose work focused on the use of microarray and other types of genomic data in developing predictive models that could identify appropriate therapies for patients based on their genomic profiles. In 2008, a medical student involved in this work became concerned about the integrity of the research and wrote a letter of concern to the administration. Unfortunately, nothing came of this early whistleblowing, and only after subsequent events, including the unsuccessful attempt in 2009 to reproduce independently certain previously published analyses of Dr. Potti (Baggerly and Coombes 2009), was the earlier whistleblowing revealed. An internal investigation by Duke led to a temporary suspension, reinstatement, and then final closure of three clinical trials based on Dr. Potti's work. An NCI investigation began soon after this, and as additional evidence emerged, Dr. Potti resigned his position in 2010. Two years later an Institute Of Medicine report, instigated largely by the Potti case, laid out "best practice" procedures to be followed in developing and validating predictive "omics" models and included a detailed account of the Potti case as a case study (Institute of Medicine 2012). A formal ORI misconduct finding against Dr. Potti was issued in 2015 (Office of Research Integrity 2015). To date, 11 papers of Dr. Potti have been retracted.

Anne Kirkman-Campbell

In April 2004, the FDA approved the use of Ketek® (telithromycin), an oral antibiotic, for the treatment of various respiratory infections. In a previous study of Ketek conducted in 2001–2002, one of the study sites, a small weight loss clinic in a town in Alabama, enrolled over 400 patients during a 3-month period, for which the site received $150 for each patient enrolled and $250 per patient for follow-up. This accrual was the largest number of patients enrolled at any single study site and represented a suspiciously high accrual rate. In addition, there were no patient withdrawals, no patients were lost to follow-up, and there were suspiciously similar laboratory results among patients, all additional red flags. Sponsor monitors raised concerns, but these were not reported to the FDA. A subsequent audit revealed that only 50 patients could be confirmed to exist and, even for these patients, there were serious problems including forged signatures, lack of evidence that any drug was administered, and no history of infections as required by the eligibility criteria. The principal investigator at the site, Dr. Anne Kirkman-Campbell, a single practitioner, was subsequently charged with fraud and eventually sentenced in March 2004 to 57 months in prison, along with a $557,000 fine and $925,000 restitution to the sponsor. Further fallout from this episode included a congressional investigation of the FDA handling of the case and, in February 2007, removal of license approval for two of the three original indications.

Piero Anversa

An eminent cardiologist, Dr. Piero Anversa, based at Harvard Medical School and the Brigham and Women's Hospital (BWH) from 2007 to 2015, is a pioneer in studies involving heart muscle regeneration from stem cells. In 2012, Dr. Anversa's group published a paper in Circulation that led to concern over possible data and image manipulation. In early 2013, Harvard began an internal investigation of the publications from Dr. Anversa's lab. The Circulation paper was retracted in 2014 at the request of the paper's co-authors, and Dr. Anversa left his positions at Harvard and BWH in 2015. In April 2017, BWH agreed to a $10 M restitution to the NIH for submitting fraudulent data on research grant applications. In October 2018, Harvard and BWH released a report requesting retraction of 31 of Dr. Anversa's publications because they contained fabricated or falsified data. Dr. Anversa denied any personal wrongdoing, claiming that a colleague had betrayed him. At least one clinical trial, CONCERT-HF, indirectly derived from the work of Dr. Anversa, began in 2015 but, due to the retraction requests, was suspended pending a detailed review of participant safety and scientific integrity (U.S. NHLBI 2018). Fortunately, the trial DSMB recently determined that the data already collected from the patients enrolled in the study at the time it was suspended would provide sufficient information to provide a reliable answer to the key study questions (U.S. NHLBI 2019).

Predisposing Factors

Knowledge of the predisposing factors underlying fraud is important in developing effective prevention strategies. Unfortunately, reliable empirical evidence is lacking on the motivations of those who commit fraud in science in general or in clinical trials in particular. Information from the perpetrators themselves is often lacking and, even if available, may not be dependable for obvious reasons. However, there is no shortage of speculation and opinions on the topic. One approach is to consider three broad narratives about the primary factors contributing to fraud in science: individual traits, institutional traits, and inherent problems in the practice of scientific research itself (Sovacool 2008). The latter narrative, concerning such issues as secrecy, competition, emphasis on "first to publish," and other topics, is important for science in general but less so for clinical trials. However, the individual and institutional narratives are particularly relevant for clinical trials. At the institutional level, there may be incentives to outperform competing institutions, with corresponding pressure applied to individual researchers. However the most prevalent explanation for fraud is the "bad apple" analogy. In any human endeavor, science included, some individuals will not conform to prevailing norms so as to obtain some personal gain. Examples include direct or indirect financial gain, promotion, tenure, and scientific prestige. Some of these factors might be in play in some cases of fraud in clinical trials but are unlikely to be major factors for isolated individuals participating in multi-institutional clinical trials. In more extreme cases, some individuals may have a pathological or self-destructive predilection to fraud without any obvious potential personal gain.

Other possible individual motivations don't fall neatly in the "bad apple" narrative. In clinical trials, one reason may be a perceived conflict between the needs of patients and the rules of clinical trials. For example, in the Poisson case discussed above, Dr. Poisson admitted the fraud but explained his motivation:

> I believed I understood the reasons behind the study rules, and I felt that the rules were meant to be understood as guidelines and not necessarily followed blindly. My sole concern at all times was the health of my patients. I firmly believed that a patient who was able to enter into an NSABP trial received the best therapy and follow-up treatment... Maintaining the proper balance between good clinical care and rigid research methods is not an easy task. (Poisson 1994)

Estimates of Prevalence

The notoriety of the publicized cases of alleged fraud in clinical trials raises the important issue of estimating the prevalence of fraud. Unfortunately, the cases themselves provide no reliable information concerning the prevalence of fraud. Although fraud obviously occurs occasionally, how common is it? Is fraud a regrettable but extremely rare event perpetrated by a few "bad apple" renegades? Or, rather, are the known cases merely the "tip of the iceberg," as claimed by some journalists and others (Herold 2018; Roberts 2015), or something in between? These questions are explored in this section.

To begin, there needs to be clarity about what is meant by "prevalence." There are at least three possibilities derived from the definitions of prevalence used in epidemiology:

- Point prevalence – the proportion of patients in a defined population who exhibit a given condition at a specific time
- Period prevalence – the proportion of patients who exhibit the condition at any time during a specific period
- Lifetime prevalence – the proportion of patients who have exhibited the condition at any time

In the setting considered here, the "condition" is fraudulent activity and the population refers to a class of people (e.g., primary investigators, data managers, etc.) involved in the conduct, analysis, or reporting the results of clinical trials. Since it is difficult, if not impossible, to determine in an objective fashion whether specific individuals have committed fraud or not, the most common studies of misconduct have relied on direct surveys (Martinson et al. 2005; Kalichman and Friedman 1992; Swazey et al. 1993; Titus et al. 2008) . Most of these surveys are in general scientific research settings, not restricted to clinical trials, but there has been at least one survey of biostatisticians involved in medical research, in which it was concluded that "fraud is not a negligible phenomenon in medical research, and that increased awareness of the forms in which it is expressed seems appropriate" (Ranstam et al. 2000).

There are many difficult issues in such studies (George 2016). Two of these issues are particularly problematic: selecting a representative sample from the population of interest and obtaining truthful answers to questions about whether an investigator has committed fraud. The latter ascertainment issue is a well-known problem in behavioral research in which answers are sought on activities that are illegal, violate socially acceptable norms, or are simply embarrassing. In these settings, investigators have strong incentives to be evasive. There are statistical methods that have been developed for these situations, including randomized response designs (Blair et al. 2015) and others (Yu et al. 2007; Glynn 2013), but unfortunately, their application to surveys of fraud is rare (Roberts and St. John 2014; List et al. 2001).

In a meta-analysis of the published surveys, even without an attempt to address the underestimate bias caused by evasive answers, a surprising 2% (95% CI: 0.9–4.5%) of individuals admitted to committing fabrication or falsification themselves, and 14.1% (95% CI: 9.9–19.7%) reported having observed such practices by others (Fanelli 2009). As noted above, these results are not specific for clinical trials, but if the percentages apply to those involved in clinical trials, the number of individuals who commit fraud in clinical trials may be quite large. The number of clinical trials registered at clintrials.gov in early 2019 was nearly 300,000; the total number of individuals directly involved in these trials (investigators, nurses, data coordinators, statisticians, etc.) is unknown but is obviously a large number.

Another issue not addressed directly in the attempts to estimate prevalence is the seriousness of the fraud. The wholesale falsification and fabrication of data, perhaps including fictitious patients and falsified outcome or safety data, is not the same as an isolated instance of, say, fabrication of a single missing laboratory value for a patient. Both constitute fraud, but the former is clearly more serious than the latter, both in terms of the primary conclusions from the trial and the implications for patient safety.

In summary, the evidence on the prevalence of fraud is weak. Other forms of questionable research practices, short of fraud, may be quite common and have serious implications (Garmendia et al. 2019; Seife 2015), but the available evidence on fabrication and falsification suggests that fraud is relatively rare, but not negligible (George 2016). Nevertheless, any fraud is unacceptable, and procedures for detection, discussed below, are important in any clinical trial quality control program.

Detection of Fraud

Detection of fraud is one aspect of quality control in clinical trials (Knatterud et al. 1998). As part of good clinical practice, trial sponsors are required to monitor the conduct of clinical trials. The aim of monitoring is to ensure the patients' well-being, compliance with the approved protocol and regulatory requirements, and data accuracy and completeness (International Conference on Harmonisation 2016). Baigent et al. (2008) draw a useful distinction between three types of trial monitoring: oversight by trial committees, on-site monitoring, and central statistical monitoring. These authors argue that the three types of monitoring are useful in their own right to guarantee the quality of the trial data and the validity of the trial results. Oversight by trial committees is especially useful to prevent or detect errors in the trial design and interpretation of the results. On-site monitoring is especially useful to prevent or detect procedural errors in the trial conduct at participating centers (e.g., whether informed consents have been signed by all patients or legally acceptable representatives). Statistical monitoring is especially useful to detect data errors, whether due to faulty equipment, systematic errors, sloppiness, incompetence, or fraud.

A survey of current monitoring practices reveals that the vast majority of trials are monitored primarily through on-site visits with source data verification, which consists of comparing information recorded in the trial's case report form with the corresponding source documents (Morrison et al. 2011). While there is general agreement that some on-site monitoring is necessary, the usefulness of extensive source data verification has been questioned for some time (Smith et al. 2012). Source data verification detects discrepancies due to transcription errors from source documentation to the case report form, which have no impact whatsoever on the results of a trial. In addition, source data verification does not detect errors present in the source documents (Buyse et al. 2017). Finally, an analysis conducted on data from 1168 clinical trials showed that "full" (100%) source data verification led to corrections for only 1.1% of all site-entered data on average (Sheetz et al. 2014). The current industry standard of full source data verification leads to unnecessary on-site visits that compound the overall costs of clinical trials (Eisenstein et al. 2008; Reith et al. 2013). Recent guidance documents from the US Food and Drug Administration and the European Medicines Agency strongly favor the use of "quality by design" and risk-based monitoring approaches with targeted audits guided by central statistical monitoring (European Medicines Agency 2011; U.S. Food and Drug Administration 2013).

It seems paradoxical that statistical theory, which is so central to the design and analysis of clinical trials, has not been used so far to optimize their conduct, even though the potential of statistics to uncover fraud in multicenter trials has received attention for almost two decades (Buyse et al. 1999; Evans 2001; George and Buyse 2015; Buyse and Evans 2016). Recent regulatory guidance documents (European Medicines Agency 2011; U.S. Food and Drug Administration 2013) have spurred much interest in using central statistical monitoring as a tool to detect fraud and, more generally, any abnormal pattern in the data that could help focus monitoring activities on centers where they appear to be most needed (Bakobaki et al. 2012; Buyse 2014; Timmermans et al. 2016).

Principles of Statistical Monitoring

Statistical monitoring of clinical trials uses a few basic procedures based on the nature of data collected in multicenter clinical trials. First, statistical monitoring relies on the highly structured nature of clinical trial data, since the same protocol is implemented identically in all participating centers, where data are collected using the same case report form, usually electronically. Abnormal trends and patterns in the data can be detected by comparing the distribution of some variables in each center against all other centers (Edwards et al. 2013; Kirkwood et al. 2013; Lindblad et al. 2014). Such comparisons can be performed on all variables collected in order to compute an overall "data inconsistency score" as described below (Venet et al. 2012). Such an overall score addresses the issues of multiple testing as well as small sample sizes in some sites. Similar comparisons can also be made between other units of analysis, if the structure of the trial warrants it. When the trial is randomized, the treatment group allocated by randomization provides another design feature that allows for specific statistical tests to be performed (Buyse et al. 1999). Indeed, baseline variables are not expected to differ between the randomized groups (except for the play of chance), while outcome variables are expected to differ about equally in all centers (except for the play of chance).

A second tenet of statistical monitoring is that even when simple comparisons indicate no major differences in the data of all centers, a more in-depth investigation of the complex data structure typical of clinical trials can be informative. The multivariate structure or time dependence of the variables can provide the basis for sensitive tests of data quality. Fabricated or falsified data, even if plausible univariately, are likely to exhibit abnormal multivariate patterns that are hard to mimic and therefore easy to detect statistically (Evans 2001; Buyse and Evans 2016). The frequency of "data collisions," i.e., identical values for one or several variables for different patients, is a sensitive indicator of situations where data have simply been cut and pasted from one patient to another. Similarly, variables that are repeatedly measured over time can be statistically scrutinized for "data propagation." In addition, humans are poor random number generators and are generally forgetful of natural constraints in the data. Tests on randomness can be used to detect invented data. Benford's law on the distribution of the first digits, or tests for digit preference, can raise red flags (Al-Marzouki et al. 2005; Hill 1995). Tests on dates can also be used to detect anomalies in the distribution of days (e.g., a high proportion of visits during weekends may reveal data fabrication) (Buyse and Evans 2016).

Which of the cases of fraud discussed above could have been detected by statistical methods? Although the answer to this question remains conjectural for the examples cited, the anomalies in Dr. Poisson's center were detected by the NSABP statistical office, although not as part of a routine central statistical monitoring program. The Sudbo and Fujii cases would almost surely have been detected, since the data reported by these two investigators contained gross aberrations that in retrospect appear too large to have remained unnoticed upon close scrutiny. The Fiddes case could arguably have been detected since the trials involved were multicentric. The Snyder/Peugeot and Bezwoda cases would have been far more difficult to detect statistically because these trials were carried out at single institutions.

Statistical procedures are valuable as part of data quality control/assurance, but these procedures must be valid and judiciously applied. Apparently anomalous results alone do not imply fraud. If the detection procedure is not valid, it should not be applied routinely. For example, in the editor's comments accompanying a retraction/republication of a recent paper (Estruch et al. 2018), it was indicated that 934 RCT journal reports were screened and 11 were identified with distributions of baseline variables that did not appear consistent with randomization according to a statistical method (Carlisle 2017). The method is based on an expected uniform distribution of p-values in comparisons of baseline variables. That methods paper and its accompanying editorial (Loadsman and McCulloch 2017) raised extremely serious concerns about a possibly high frequency of fraud in published RCTs. In fact, the method is sensitive to correlation among baseline variables, which yields non-uniform distributions of p-values and many more false-positives than expected. Confounding of a serious implication (fraud) with a commonplace innocent explanation (correlation) is a fatal flaw for a screening tool.

Implementations of Statistical Monitoring

Different implementations of statistical monitoring have been proposed in the literature (Venet et al. 2012; Zink 2014; Edwards et al. 2013; Kirkwood et al. 2013; Lindblad et al. 2014; Pogue et al. 2013; Van Den Bor et al. 2017; Oba 2016). The most popular approach is based on "key risk indicators," which are clinical data variables identified as important and monitored throughout the trial against pre-specified thresholds (Edwards et al. 2013). A site that exceeds the threshold for a key risk indicator is flagged for further scrutiny. For instance, protocol violations could constitute a key risk indicator. Sites could be flagged if they experienced protocol violations in more than, say, 10% of their patients. Although key risk indicators are quite useful as part of routine clinical trial monitoring, their potential for fraud detection is extremely limited. A more sophisticated approach was developed specifically to detect fraud in cardiovascular trials, with predictive models built using the database of a multicenter trial in which data from some centers were known to have been fabricated. Simple models based on systolic and diastolic pressure measurements were shown to be predictive of fraud in independent trials in the same indication (Pogue et al. 2013). Whether such models can be generally useful requires further study.

A comprehensive statistical approach to data monitoring consists of performing as many statistical tests as possible on as many clinical data variables as possible: tests for proportions, means, global variances, within-patient variances, event counts, distributions of categorical variables, proportion of week days, outliers, missing values, correlations between several variables, and so forth (Kirkwood et al. 2013; Lindblad et al. 2014; Venet et al. 2012). The central idea is to compare the data of each center to the data of all other centers, which requires no distributional assumptions and can be easily automated (Venet et al. 2012). Extensive testing of all variables in a clinical trial raises challenging issues, including control of multiplicity and avoidance of false-positive signals, as well as allowance for natural variability in the data (e.g., due to regional differences), but there are statistical ways of addressing these issues (Desmet et al. 2014). Graphical displays can help spot centers with data anomalies (Kirkwood et al. 2013; Lindblad et al. 2014; Zink 2014). The statistical tests can also generate a high-dimensional matrix of P-values, with centers as rows and tests as columns, analogous to the gene expression matrix of a microarray experiment (Venet et al. 2012).

Center Scoring

A "data inconsistency score" (DIS) can be calculated for each center on the basis of the P-values of all statistical tests performed for this center (a row in the matrix of P-values) (Trotta et al. 2019). Statisticians at the FDA have proposed two alternative ways of scoring centers, one based on a Fisher combination test and the other on a likelihood ratio test (Xu et al. 2020). Of note, center scores can be expressed as significance probabilities (P-values), or minus the log transformation of P-values, so that scores range from 0 to 10 (or in rare instances larger) and have therefore a similar interpretation to the Richter scale for the amplitude of seismic waves. Centers with a score close to 0 have data that are compatible with data from other centers, while centers with high scores (say, 3 or above, i.e., $P < 0.001$) have data that are so inconsistent overall with data from other centers that the observed differences cannot be attributed to chance alone. Centers with extreme data inconsistency scores are worthy of further investigation, with the aim of explaining the differences, retraining the site personnel if required, or – in the worst case scenario – uncovering some fraud that might otherwise have remained undetected. Note that centers can have inconsistent data if they treat different patient populations, so high data inconsistency scores do not automatically imply that a remedial action is warranted (Timmermans et al. 2016). Also note that centers can have inconsistent data if their data are of much better quality than on average (say, for instance, if they have far fewer missing data than overall). Hence high data inconsistency scores are a statistical finding with no implied value judgment. Likewise, as we illustrate in the following two examples, inconsistent data can reveal a number of issues ranging from overt fraud to accidental causes unidentified by the investigators.

An Example of Fraud

Statistical monitoring of clinical trial data is likely to pick up many cases of fraud simply because of unusual patterns in the data. As an example, Fig. 1 shows a "bubble plot" produced using central statistical monitoring of a completed randomized clinical trial involving more than 4,500 patients treated in 160 clinical centers (details omitted to preserve anonymity). In the bubble plot, each center is represented by a bubble, the size of which is proportional to the number of patients enrolled by the center. The horizontal axis of Fig. 1 represents center size, while the vertical axis represents the data inconsistency score of the center. Bubbles falling above the horizontal line labeled "FDR = 3%" correspond to centers with extreme data inconsistency scores, indicating that the data collected in these centers differ statistically from the data collected in all other centers. The false discovery rate (FDR) above the horizontal line is less than 3%, i.e., there is less than 3% chance that any of the sites above the line was identified as having inconsistent data just by the play of chance.

Fraud was known to have occurred at center X, where 97 patients had been treated. An on-site audit had revealed that in center X some patients had not been provided with quality of life questionnaires, which had instead been completed by site personnel (Venet et al. 2012). Interestingly, statistical analysis of the data suggested that the quality of life data were equally suspicious in center Y, yet on-site visits at that center had not uncovered any problem at that center. This example illustrates the

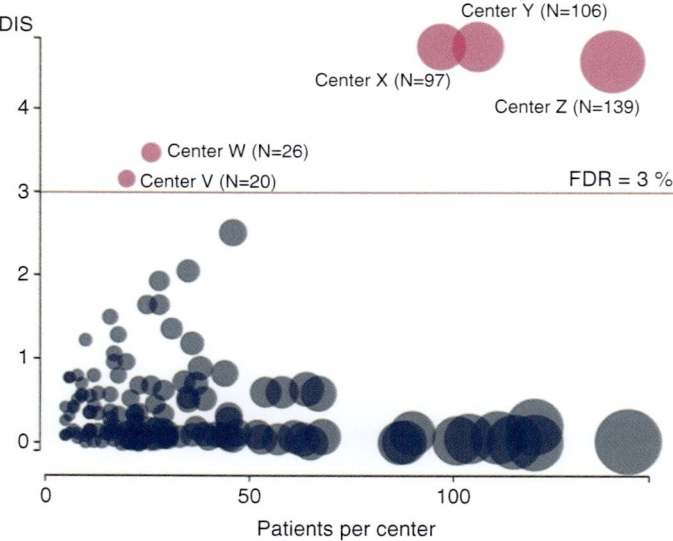

Fig. 1 Bubble plot showing the data inconsistency score as a function of the center size in a randomized clinical trial (Venet et al. 2012). The data from the centers above the horizontal line, labeled V, W, X, Y, and Z, differ statistically form the data in all other centers. Fraud was confirmed to have occurred in center X (DIS, data inconsistency score; N, number of patients per center; FDR, false discovery rate)

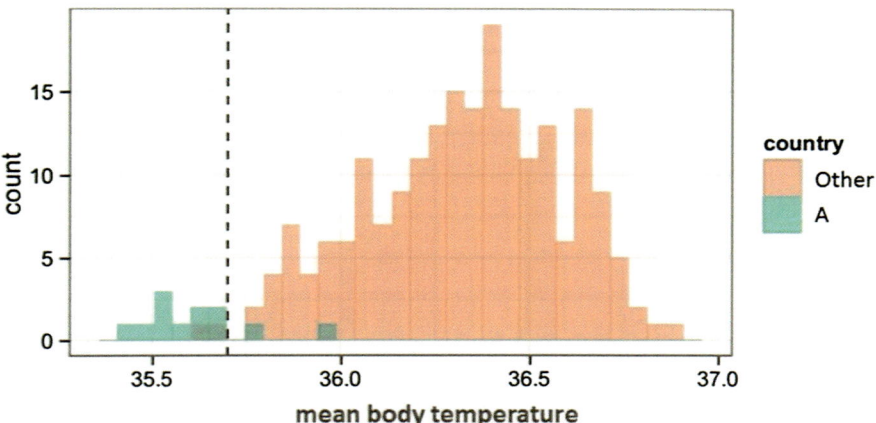

Fig. 2 Distribution of mean body temperatures (in degrees Celsius) for centers in country A and for all other centers in a randomized clinical trial. The data from 10 of the 12 centers in country A differ statistically form the data in all other centers. The difference was found to be due to a single lot of miscalibrated thermometers (Desmet et al. 2014)

effectiveness of statistical analysis to reveal fabricated data, which tend to differ in several subtle but detectable ways from actually observed data (Buyse et al. 1999).

An Example of Technical Problem

Statistical monitoring of clinical trial data may pick up *any* unusual pattern in the data, whether due to fraud, tampering, sloppiness, incompetence, misunderstanding, technical problems, or other causes. As an example, Fig. 2 shows the distribution of mean body temperatures in an on-going randomized clinical trial involving more than 16,000 patients treated in 218 clinical centers (details omitted to preserve anonymity).

The mean body temperatures in the 12 centers of country A were within the allowed range and were not flagged as suspicious by data management checks or during on-site monitoring visits. Yet when the totality of the data was submitted to statistical monitoring checks, the centers in country A were clearly identified as inconsistent with all other centers. After further investigation, it was found that a single lot of thermometers was miscalibrated in this country, causing a downward shift in the temperatures too small to be detected in a single measurement, but statistically detectable in a large number of them.

Summary and Conclusion

Although regularly occurring high-profile cases demonstrate that fraud occasionally happens in clinical trials, the existing evidence suggests that it is a rare phenomenon, although other forms of misconduct may be more common. Given human nature, it is likely to occur in the future. The damage that fraud causes, both to the clinical trial enterprise and potentially to patients on the trial itself or to future patients, is serious. Increased attention to prevention and detection is therefore warranted. Some authors have also suggested putting in place a "Fraud Recovery Plan" to mitigate the potentially devastating consequences of the discovery of a case of fraud in an otherwise well-conducted trial (Herson 2016).

Evidence about effective prevention techniques is lacking, despite efforts to increase awareness through training in research ethics adopted by many universities and other institutions. Although such efforts supposedly cannot hurt, it seems likely that attention to removing the opportunities to commit fraud and improving the detection methodology may be even more effective. Recently developed concepts of "reproducible research" in science in general are applicable to clinical trials in particular. Single-institution trials are especially vulnerable to misconduct since they often lack standardized and centralized data collection and monitoring procedures. The model of central collection of data separate from the investigator, as done in multicenter trials, may also be applied in single-institution trials and can lead to more effective monitoring of data quality.

Key Facts

- Several high-profile cases of fraud in clinical trials have raised awareness of the need for prevention and detection of any such occurrences.
- Although the prevalence of fraud is commonly thought to be quite low, reliable evidence on prevalence is lacking.
- Factors predisposing to fraud include individual characteristics, institutional policies, and structural issues.
- Central statistical monitoring can be effective in detecting fraud and other types of data errors.

Cross-References

▶ Data Capture, Data Management, and Quality Control; Single Versus Multicenter Trials
▶ Investigator Responsibilities
▶ Multicenter and Network Trials

References

Al-Marzouki S, Evans S, Marshall T, Roberts I (2005) Are these data real? Statistical methods for the detection of data fabrication in clinical trials. BMJ 331:267–270
Baggerly KA, Coombes KR (2009) Deriving chemosensitivity from cell lines: forensic bioinformatics and reproducible research in high-throughput biology. Ann Appl Stat 3:1309–1334

Baigent C, Harrell FE, Buyse M, Emberson JR, Altman DG (2008) Ensuring trial validity by data quality assurance and diversification of monitoring methods. Clin Trials 5:49–55

Bakobaki JM, Rauchenberger M, Joffe N, McCormack S, Stenning S, Meredith S (2012) The potential for central monitoring techniques to replace on-site monitoring: findings from an international multi-centre clinical trial. Clin Trials 9:257–264

Blair G, Imai K, Zhou Y-Y (2015) Design and analysis of the randomized response technique. J Am Stat Assoc 110:1304–1319

Buyse M (2014) Centralized statistical monitoring as a way to improve the quality of clinical data [Online]. http://www.appliedclinicaltrialsonline.com/centralized-statistical-monitoring-way-improve-quality-clinical-data. Accessed 5 Mar 2020

Buyse M, Evans SJW (2016) Fraud in clinical trials. Wiley StatsRef: Statistics Reference Online. Wiley, New York

Buyse M, George SL, Evans S, Geller NL, Ranstam J, Scherrer B, Lesaffre E, Murray G, Edler L, Hutton J, Colton T, Lachenbruch P, Verma BL (1999) The role of biostatistics in the prevention, detection and treatment of fraud in clinical trials. Stat Med 18:3435–3451

Buyse M, Squifflet P, Coart E, Quinaux E, Punt CJ, Saad ED (2017) The impact of data errors on the outcome of randomized clinical trials. Clin Trials 14:499–506

Carlisle JB (2012) The analysis of 168 randomised controlled trials to test data integrity. Anaesthesia 67:521–537

Carlisle JB (2017) Data fabrication and other reasons for non-random sampling in 5087 randomised, controlled trials in anaesthetic and general medical journals. Anaesthesia 72:944–952

Desmet L, Venet D, Doffagne E, Timmermans C, Burzykowski T, Legrand C, Buyse M (2014) Linear mixed-effects models for central statistical monitoring of multicenter clinical trials. Stat Med 33:5265–5279

Edwards P, Shakur H, Barnetson L, Prieto D, Evans S, Roberts I (2013) Central and statistical data monitoring in the Clinical Randomisation of an Antifibrinolytic in Significant Haemorrhage (CRASH-2) trial. Clin Trials 11:336–343

Eisenstein EL, Collins R, Cracknell BS, Podesta O, Reid ED, Sandercock P, Shakhov Y, Terrin ML, Sellers MA, Califf RM, Granger CB, Diaz R (2008) Sensible approaches for reducing clinical trial costs. Clin Trials 5:75–84

Estruch R, Ros E, Salas-Salvadó J, Covas M-I, Corella D, ArÓS F, GÓmez-Gracia E, Ruiz-GutiÉrrez V, Fiol M, Lapetra J, Lamuela-Raventos RM, Serra-Majem L, PintÓ X, Basora J, MuÑoz MA, SorlÍ JV, MartÍnez JA, FitÓ M, Gea A, HernÁN MA, MartÍnez-GonzÁlez MA (2018) Primary prevention of cardiovascular disease with a Mediterranean diet supplemented with extra-virgin olive oil or nuts. N Engl J Med 378:e34

European Medicines Agency (2011) Reflection paper on risk based quality management in clinical trials [Online]. http://www.ema.europa.eu/docs/en_GB/document_library/Scientific_guideline/2011/08/WC500110059.pdf. Accessed 5 Mar 2020

Evans S (2001) Statistical aspects of the detection of fraud. In: Lock S, Wells F, Farthing M (eds) Fraud and misconduct in medical research, 3rd edn. BMJ Publishing Group, London

Fanelli D (2009) How many scientists fabricate and falsify research? A systematic review and meta-analysis of survey data. PLoS One 4:e5738

Federal Register (2005) Public health service policies on research misconduct final rule (42 CFR part 93.103) [Online]. http://www.ecfr.gov/cgi-bin/text-idx?SID=0b07ed68cf889962cae6c2b45d89150b&node=pt42.1.93&rgn=div5. Accessed 5 Mar 2020

Garmendia CA, Nassar Gorra L, Rodriguez AL, Trepka MJ, Veledar E, Madhivanan P (2019) Evaluation of the inclusion of studies identified by the FDA as having falsified data in the results of meta-analyses: the example of the Apixaban trials. JAMA Intern Med 179:582–584

George SL (1997) Perspectives on scientific misconduct and fraud in clinical trials. Chance 10:3–5

George SL (2016) Research misconduct and data fraud in clinical trials: prevalence and causal factors. Int J Clin Oncol 21:15–21

George SL, Buyse M (2015) Data fraud in clinical trials. Clin Invest 15:161–173

Glynn AN (2013) What can we learn with statistical truth serum? Design and analysis of the list experiment. Public Opin Q 77:159–172

Herold E (2018) Researchers behaving badly: known frauds are "the Tip of the Iceberg" [Online]. https://leapsmag.com/researchers-behaving-badly-why-scientific-misconduct-may-be-on-the-rise/. Accessed 5 Mar 2020

Herson J (2016) Strategies for dealing with fraud in clinical trials. Int J Clin Oncol 21:22–27

Hill TP (1995) A statistical derivation of the significant-digit law. Stat Sci 10:354–363

Institute of Medicine (2012) Evolution of translational omics: lessons learned and the path forward. The National Academies Press, Washington, DC

International Conference on Harmonisation (2016) Integrated addendum to ICH E6(R1): Guideline for good clinical practice E6(R2) [Online]. https://database.ich.org/sites/default/files/E6_R2_Addendum.pdf. Accessed 5 March 2020

Kalichman MW, Friedman PJ (1992) A pilot study of biomedical trainees' perceptions concerning research ethics. Acad Med 67:769–775

Kirkwood AA, Cox T, Hackshaw A (2013) Application of methods for central statistical monitoring in clinical trials. Clin Trials 10:783–806

Knatterud GL, Rockhold FW, George SL, Barton FB, Davis CE, Fairweather WR, Honohan T, Mowery R, O'neill R (1998) Guidelines for quality assurance in multicenter trials: a position paper. Control Clin Trials 19:477–493

Lindblad AS, Manukyan Z, Purohit-Sheth T, Gensler G, Okwesili P, Meeker-O'connell A, Ball L, Marler JR (2014) Central site monitoring: results from a test of accuracy in identifying trials and sites failing Food and Drug Administration inspection. Clin Trials 11:205–217

List JA, Bailey CD, Euzent PJ, Martin TL (2001) Academic economists behaving badly? A survey on three areas of unethical behavior. Econ Inq 39:162–170

Loadsman JA, McCulloch TJ (2017) Widening the search for suspect data – is the flood of retractions about to become a tsunami? Anaesthesia 72:931–935

Martinson BC, Anderson MS, De Vries R (2005) Scientists behaving badly. Nature 435:737–738

Morrison BW, Cochran CJ, White JG, Harley J, Kleppinger CF, Liu A, Mitchel JT, Nickerson DF, Zacharias CR, Kramer JM (2011) Monitoring the quality of conduct of clinical trials: a survey of current practices. Clin Trials 8:342–349

Oba K (2016) Statistical challenges for central monitoring in clinical trials: a review. Int J Clin Oncol 21:28–37

Office of Research Integrity (2015) Case summary: Potti, Anil [Online]. https://ori.hhs.gov/case-summary-potti-anil. Accessed 5 Mar 2020

Peto R, Collins R, Sackett D, Darbyshire J, Babiker A, Buyse M, Stewart H, Baum M, Goldhirsch A, Bonadonna G, Valagussa P, Rutqvist L, Elbourne D, Davies C, Dalesio O, Parmar M, Hill C, Clarke M, Gray R, Doll R (1997) The trials of Dr. Bernard fisher: a European perspective on an American episode. Control Clin Trials 18:1–13

Piantadosi S (2017) Misconduct and fraud in clinical research. In: Clinical trials: a methodologic perspective, 3rd edn. Wiley, New York

Pogue JM, Devereaux PJ, Thorlund K, Yusuf S (2013) Central statistical monitoring: detecting fraud in clinical trials. Clin Trials 10:225–235

Poisson R (1994) Fraud in breast-cancer trials [letter]. N Engl J Med 330:1460

Ranstam J, Buyse M, George SL, Evans S, Geller NL, Scherrer B, Lesaffre E, Murray G, Edler L, Hutton JL, Colton T, Lachenbruch P (2000) Fraud in medical research: an international survey of biostatisticians. ISCB Subcommittee on Fraud. Control Clin Trials 21:415–427

Reith C, Landray M, Devereaux P, Bosch J, Granger CB, Baigent C, Califf RM, Collins R, Yusuf S (2013) Randomized clinical trials–removing unnecessary obstacles. N Engl J Med 369:1061–1065

Roberts I (2015) Retraction of scientific papers for fraud or bias is just the tip of the iceberg [Online]. http://theconversation.com/retraction-of-scientific-papers-for-fraud-or-bias-is-just-the-tip-of-the-iceberg-43083. Accessed 5 Mar 2020

Roberts DL, St. John FAV (2014) Estimating the prevalence of researcher misconduct: a study of UK academics within biological sciences. PeerJ 2:e562

Seife C (2015) Research misconduct identified by the US Food and Drug Administration: out of sight, out of mind, out of the peer-reviewed literature. JAMA Intern Med 175:567–577

Sheetz N, Wilson B, Benedict J, Huffman E, Lawton A, Travers M, Nadolny P, Young S, Given K, Florin L (2014) Evaluating source data verification as a quality control measure in clinical trials. Ther Innov Regul Sci 48:671–680

Smith CT, Stocken DD, Dunn J, Cox T, Ghaneh P, Cunningham D, Neoptolemos JP (2012) The value of source data verification in a cancer clinical trial. PloS One 7:e51623

Sovacool BK (2008) Exploring scientific misconduct: isolated individuals, impure institutions, or an inevitable idiom of modern science? J Bioeth Inq 5:271–282

Stroebe W, Postmes T, Spears R (2012) Scientific misconduct and the myth of self-correction in science. Perspect Psychol Sci 7:670–688

Swazey JP, Anderson MS, Lewis KS (1993) Ethical problems in academic research. Am Sci 81:542–553

Timmermans C, Venet D, Burzykowski T (2016) Data-driven risk identification in phase III clinical trials using central statistical monitoring. Int J Clin Oncol 21:38–45

Titus SL, Wells JA, Rhoades LJ (2008) Repairing research integrity. Nature 453:980–982

Trotta L, Kabeya Y, Buyse M, Doffagne E, Venet D, Desmet L, Burzykowski T, Tsuburaya A, Yoshida K, Miyashita Y, Morita S, Sakamoto J, Praveen P, Oba K (2019) Detection of atypical data in multicenter clinical trials using unsupervised statistical monitoring. Clin Trials. (in press) 16:512

U.S. Food and Drug Administration (2013) Oversight of clinical investigations – a risk-based approach to monitoring: guidance for industry [Online]. Rockville. http://www.fda.gov/down loads/Drugs/GuidanceComplianceRegulatoryInformation/Guidances/UCM269919.pdf. Accessed 5 March 2020

U.S. NHLBI (2018) Statement on NHLBI decision to pause the CONCERT-HF trial [Online]. https://www.nih.gov/news-events/news-releases/statement-nhlbi-decision-pause-concert-hf-trial. Accessed 5 Mar 2020

U.S. NHLBI (2019) CONCERT-HF study [Online]. https://www.nhlbi.nih.gov/science/concert-hf-study. Accessed 5 Mar 2020

Van Den Bor RM, Vaessen PWJ, Oosterman BJ, Zuithoff NPA, Grobbee DE, Roes KCB (2017) A computationally simple central monitoring procedure, effectively applied to empirical trial data with known fraud. J Clin Epidemiol 87:59–69

Venet D, Doffagne E, Burzykowski T, Beckers F, Tellier Y, Genevois-Marlin E, Becker U, Bee V, Wilson V, Legrand C, Buyse M (2012) A statistical approach to central monitoring of data quality in clinical trials. Clin Trials 9:705–713

Weiss RB, Rifkin RM, Stewart FM, Theriault RL, Williams LA, Herman AA, Beveridge RA (2000) High-dose chemotherapy for high-risk primary breast cancer: an on-site review of the Bezwoda study. Lancet 355:999–1003

Xu JL, Huang Z, Yao Z, Xu J, Zalkikar R, Tiwari (2020). Statistical methods for clinical study site selection. Therapeutic Innovation ≈ Regulatory Science 54:211–219

Yu J-W, Tian G-L, Tang M-L (2007) Two new models for survey sampling with sensitive characteristic: design and analysis. Metrika 67:251–263

Zink RZ (2014) Risk-based monitoring and fraud detection in clinical trials using JMP® and SAS®. SAS Institute Inc, Cary

Clinical Trials on Trial: Lawsuits Stemming from Clinical Research

119

John J. DeBoy and Annie X. Wang

Contents

Introduction	2340
Personal Injury Lawsuits	2340
Theories of Liability	2341
Legal Duties of Clinical Trial Participants	2344
Causation	2357
Damages	2358
Other Lawsuits	2358
Contractual Disputes	2358
Intellectual Property Disputes	2359
Securities Litigation	2360
Employment Lawsuits	2361
Criminal Cases and Other Government Lawsuits	2362
Lawsuits Demanding Medicines or Other Treatment	2362
Pharmaceutical and Medical Device Mass Tort Litigation	2363
Summary and Conclusion	2364
Cross-References	2365
References	2365

The authors represent pharmaceutical and medical device companies in various litigation matters. Any opinions expressed are those of the authors and do not necessarily reflect the views of their firm. This book chapter is for general information purposes and is not intended to be, nor should it be taken as, legal advice.

J. J. DeBoy (✉) · A. X. Wang
Covington & Burling LLP, Washington, DC, USA
e-mail: jdeboy@cov.com; awang@cov.com

© Springer Nature Switzerland AG 2022
S. Piantadosi, C. L. Meinert (eds.), *Principles and Practice of Clinical Trials*,
https://doi.org/10.1007/978-3-319-52636-2_164

Abstract

Clinical trials and the law routinely intersect, and as a result, litigation occasionally arises out of clinical trial activities. Such litigation includes not only personal injury suits – claims by individuals who allege they suffered injury during a clinical trial – but also breach-of-contract lawsuits, intellectual property matters, and even criminal prosecutions. This chapter provides an overview of the types of litigation that might arise out of clinical trials. The chapter focuses on personal injury litigation and, in particular, the related duties that courts have held apply to participants in clinical trials, including sponsors, investigators, and institutional review boards. Notwithstanding this focus, the chapter also provides an overview of lawsuits grounded in other areas of the law. The ultimate goal is to provide researchers with a basic understanding of litigation-related issues, in the hopes that such knowledge might aid them in avoiding pitfalls that increase litigation risk.

Keywords

Clinical trial · Clinical research · Lawsuit · Litigation · Court · Personal injury · Negligence · Product liability · Contract · Intellectual property

Introduction

Clinical trials and the law are necessarily intertwined – both because clinical research functions in a regulated environment and because such research implicates important and delicate matters involving human health, commerce, and, in many instances, life-or-death issues. In this setting, litigation – disputes between parties overseen by courts – occasionally arises.

This chapter provides an overview of litigation involving clinical trials, with a focus on the U.S. legal environment. The discussion begins with (and focuses on) an overview of personal injury lawsuits – cases in which individuals claim they suffered injuries during their participation as study subjects in clinical research. The discussion then continues with an examination of other types of lawsuits that can also arise in the setting of clinical trials. Such lawsuits include contractual disputes, intellectual property matters, securities litigation, and even criminal prosecutions.

This chapter aims to provide an overview of clinical trial-related litigation that will benefit anyone who participates in clinical research, including investigators; representatives of hospitals, universities, and other research institutions; members of industry; and academics, among others. The goal is to provide all readers with a core understanding of litigation risk in the setting of clinical trials, with an eye toward facilitating awareness of pitfalls that can lead to legal disputes.

Personal Injury Lawsuits

When one contemplates lawsuits in the healthcare setting, the personal injury lawsuit – a case in which an individual claims to have suffered an injury due to negligent or intentional misconduct by another – is probably what first comes to mind. In the clinical trial setting, such lawsuits occasionally arise when study participants believe they have suffered injuries related to their participation in clinical research.

Notably, though, clinical trials rarely lead to personal injury litigation on a mass scale – what attorneys sometimes refer to as "mass tort" litigation or complex litigation. Unlike approved pharmaceuticals and medical devices, which reach many thousands (or millions) of patients after they come to market, therapies tested in clinical trials reach relatively small populations. As a result, the economic motivations for pursuing large-scale personal injury litigation – which often depend upon the ability of personal injury lawyers to aggregate hundreds (or even thousands) of lawsuits – do not frequently arise in the setting of clinical research. Also, because clinical trials commonly involve novel therapies for patients who have failed existing treatments (such as in the oncology setting), the willingness of study subjects to accept risk might be higher than in other healthcare settings. For these reasons and others, personal injury lawsuits involving clinical trials tend to be fairly discrete, and, as a result, the legal framework in this area is not especially well-developed. Nevertheless, despite their comparatively discrete nature, personal injury lawsuits present an area of meaningful risk for those conducting legal research (Morreim 2005, at 47-48).

Examination of personal injury lawsuits in the clinical trial setting requires discussion of several topics. These include the key issues of theories of liability, legal duties of research participants, causation, and damages.

Theories of Liability

Personal injury lawsuits fall within the legal category known as torts – claims by individuals who allege injuries suffered due to wrongdoing by others. The legal frameworks that govern whether a plaintiff is entitled to a legal remedy in a tort lawsuit alleging personal injuries include negligence and product liability, among others.

Negligence

Most personal injury lawsuits arising out of clinical trials are grounded in the legal theory of negligence. Negligence occurs when an individual suffers injury due to the unreasonable conduct of another. In general, to prevail in a negligence lawsuit, a plaintiff must prove each of the following four "elements" of her negligence claim: (1) the defendant owed a legal *duty* to the plaintiff, (2) the defendant *breached* the legal duty owed, (3) the defendant's breach of duty *caused* injury to the plaintiff, and (4) the plaintiff suffered *damages* as a result of her injury (Bal 2009). If a plaintiff cannot satisfy all four of these elements, her lawsuit will fail.

Negligence lawsuits have long been a part of the healthcare landscape, particularly in the setting of medical malpractice – claims by patients that their physicians (or other healthcare providers) failed to adhere to the applicable medical standard of care (i.e., that they were negligent) in providing treatment, leading to injury. In medical malpractice cases, the basic legal framework is generally well-established, in large part because courts have long recognized that physicians owe a duty to their patients and must exercise reasonable care in providing treatment (Bal 2009).

Lawsuits involving clinical trials, however, are a comparatively recent development, and they implicate different goals and interests. Unlike the traditional practice of medicine, in which the principal goal is to treat the patient, medical research focuses on its core goals of experimentation and discovery. While study subjects in clinical trials can – and often do – benefit from the treatments they receive in research, the reason for the research's existence is not the treatment of these patients per se, but rather the advancement of medicine and science to develop new therapies for *future* patients (Tereskerz 2012, at 7–9; Morreim 2004).

In light of these differences between traditional medical practice and medical research, commentators have opined that the legal frameworks governing the two areas should differ. In particular, regarding the issue of legal duties, commentators have explained that the legal duties of clinical trial role players – such as investigators and sponsors – should be viewed differently from those of physicians in the ordinary practice of medicine, since the purposes and goals of the two undertakings (discovery in the case of research versus treatment of the patient in the case of medicine) are not the same (Tereskerz 2012, at 7–9; Morreim 2004). Put another way, many hold the view that medical malpractice and "research malpractice" are different concepts and should have different standards, particularly on the question of legal duties owed.

Courts encountering the relatively recent emergence of clinical trial negligence lawsuits often struggle to address these questions. For instance, a common threshold question in negligence lawsuits arising from clinical trials is: What legal duties do sponsors, investigators, and institutional review boards owe to study subjects, and how do these duties differ from those imposed in more traditional healthcare settings? The challenges inherent in answering such questions have resulted in conflicting and sometimes confusing court decisions, with some courts recognizing the uniqueness of clinical research and others defaulting to more traditional negligence principles, including those developed in the malpractice setting. The law on these questions remains unclear and continues to evolve, making it difficult to predict how individual courts will rule on key questions such as legal duties owed.

Another vexing question courts must consider in negligence cases – once the legal duty question is answered – is the issue of the standard of care. While the standard of care – the care that a reasonable professional would provide in fulfilling her duty (Bal 2009) – can be straightforward (or at least fairly well-established) in many medical malpractice cases, the standard can be comparatively unclear in the area of clinical research. For instance, what practice must a reasonable investigator follow in obtaining an informed consent from a study subject? What practice must a reasonable institutional review board follow in overseeing the safety of patients in a clinical trial? How do these standards differ from those recognized in more traditional settings? Although this area is still evolving, some courts have concluded that these questions can be answered only through expert testimony by individuals with expertise in the relevant areas of clinical research. As one court has held: "In a case such as the present one, which concerns complex details regarding the adequacy of a phase III clinical study and standards of care in designing experimental drugs for the treatment of relapsing-remitting multiple sclerosis, expert testimony is essential in order for the plaintiff to sustain her burden of proof" (*Milton v. Robinson*, 27 A.3d

480, 493 (Conn. App. Ct. 2011); *see also Heinrich v. Sweet*, 308 F.3d 48, 62–71 (1st Cir. 2002)).

A core goal of this chapter is to predict – based on existing law, however unclear – how courts could rule on these issues, so that clinical trial participants can be aware of risks that might arise.

Product Liability

Product liability is another legal framework that sometimes applies in lawsuits involving clinical trials. In a product liability lawsuit, an individual claims that she suffered injury due to a defect in a product. In the United States, plaintiffs' attorneys commonly bring product liability lawsuits against manufacturers and other sellers of medicines and medical devices, in many instances by aggregating hundreds or thousands of cases. Claims of product liability are sometimes founded in negligence, but they also often rest on a concept known as "strict liability" – a legal framework under which a plaintiff can prevail solely by showing that she was injured by a defective product, without having to prove fault (breach of a duty through unreasonable conduct) by the defendant.

Regardless of the underlying foundation (strict liability versus negligence), a plaintiff in a product liability suit cannot prevail without showing that her injury was caused by a product defect. Typically, a product defect takes one of three forms: (1) a design defect (a flaw in the product's design), (2) a manufacturing defect (a deviation from the product's design during manufacture, such as contamination), or (3) a flaw in the product's warnings (a failure to warn of known or reasonably knowable risks of the product) (*Moss v. Wyeth Inc.*, 872 F. Supp. 2d 162, 166 (D. Conn. 2012)). In the setting of medicines and medical devices, most product liability lawsuits involve claims of failure to warn, although design and manufacturing cases also arise.

In cases involving alleged warning defects in prescription medicines or medical devices – frequently called "failure-to-warn" cases – courts in the United States ordinarily apply the "learned intermediary" doctrine. Under this doctrine, a prescription medicine or device manufacturer's duty is not to warn the patient directly, but rather to warn the "learned intermediary" – the trained physician or other prescriber – who in turn has a duty to conduct a risk-benefit analysis and obtain the patient's informed consent (*Murthy v. Abbott Laboratories*, 847 F. Supp. 2d 958, 967–68 (S.D. Tex. 2012)). The theory underlying the learned intermediary doctrine is that, because warnings involving prescription medicines and devices require discussion of complex medical and scientific issues, the warnings should be oriented toward the prescriber, who can understand the warning information and then use it in conducting risk-benefit analyses and advising patients. In clinical trial lawsuits involving product liability claims, courts have held that the learned intermediary doctrine applies, just as it does in cases involving approved and marketed medicines and devices (*Murthy*, 847 F. Supp. 2d at 967–68; *Kernke v. The Menninger Clinic, Inc.*, 173 F. Supp. 2d 1117, 1121 (D. Kan. 2001); *Tracy v. Merrell Dow Pharmaceuticals*, 569 N.E.2d 875, 878–80 (Ohio 1991); *Gaston v. Hunter*, 588 P.2d 326, 340 (Ariz. Ct. App. 1978)).

Of course, many clinical trials involve research concerning new medicines and medical devices, and for this reason product liability lawsuits sometimes arise in this setting. As in the case of "research malpractice" suits, the unique circumstances of clinical trials – including the experimental nature of treatments and the necessarily more limited knowledge of medicine and device manufacturers who make them – counsel in favor of different standards in clinical trial cases. While some courts have not remarked on this distinction, others have explained that, in the research setting, the adequacy of a manufacturer's warnings must be viewed through the lens of what was known (or reasonably knowable) at the time – as opposed to what later became known about the medicine or device during the research (or after its conclusion). In other words, in a failure-to-warn case involving a clinical trial, a manufacturer should not be held responsible for warning about risks of which it was reasonably unaware at the time of the research, when its knowledge was, by definition, more limited. As one court held: "We find no evidence that the drug companies in this case gave inadequate warnings in view of the facts then known about [the medicine]... Plaintiff has failed to show inadequacy of [the defendant's] warnings except, possibly, when judged in the wake of subsequent developments" (*Gaston*, 588 P.2d at 340–41).

Other Theories of Liability

Personal injury litigants who claim injuries during clinical trials also sometimes bring claims founded in other legal theories. Often, plaintiffs will bring these additional claims in tandem with negligence and/or product liability claims. Such claims include claims for battery (an intentional tort), wrongful death, fraud or misrepresentation, breach of warranty, and breach of contract, among others (*Zeman v. Williams*, 2014 WL 3058298 (D. Mass. July 7, 2014); *Darke v. Estate of Isner*, 20 Mass. L. Rptr. 419, 2005 WL 3729113 (Mass. Super. Ct. Nov. 22, 2005); *Kernke v. The Menninger Clinic, Inc.*, 173 F. Supp. 2d 1117 (D. Kan. 2001); Agati 2006, at 415-16).

Legal Duties of Clinical Trial Participants

As explained above, an essential element of many tort lawsuits (especially those founded in negligence) is the establishment of a legal duty owed by the defendant (the party sued) to the plaintiff (the party bringing suit). In other words, to succeed in a personal injury suit, a plaintiff must ordinarily establish (among other things) that the defendant owed a legal duty to the plaintiff and that the defendant engaged in conduct that breached that duty.

In the setting of clinical trials, the question of what legal duties are owed – and to whom they are owed – is complex. This complexity arises in part due to the differences between clinical research and traditional medical practice. The multitude of potential participants in a clinical trial also introduces complexity. For instance, in a clinical trial assessing the efficacy and safety of a new medicine or medical device, the potential players (and thus potential parties in personal injury litigation) will commonly include study subjects (patients), investigators (often physicians or other healthcare providers) and their associated institutions (often hospitals or universities), sponsors (often pharmaceutical or medical device companies), contract research organizations ("CROs"), institutional review boards ("IRBs"), and data and safety monitoring boards ("DSMBs"), among others. In light of the uniqueness of clinical research, and given the number and diversity of potential parties involved, the legal duties owed are not always clear in the clinical trial setting, and for this reason courts frequently struggle to address the duty question.

To determine what legal duties apply in a personal injury lawsuit, attorneys and judges will consult different sources of law, including statutes (written laws promulgated by legislatures), regulations (rules created by regulatory agencies), and case law (written decisions by judges in prior cases). Although there are federal laws and regulations that govern the conduct of clinical trials, these legal sources do not directly define the legal duties that apply for purposes of a civil lawsuit, and, in any event, the existence of a legal duty is ordinarily a question answered by the *state* law, as opposed to federal law, that governs in a particular lawsuit. (As noted, federal statutes and regulations do not *directly* define legal duties arising under state law. However, as discussed in further detail below, state court judges sometimes look to federal statutes and regulations for guidance in determining the responsibilities of different role players in clinical trials. These responsibilities under federal law will, in turn, sometimes influence a judge in determining the duties that apply under state law.) For this reason, the best source for identifying legal duties is typically case law – again, written decisions by judges in other cases. As noted, though, the cases in this area are frequently unclear and conflicting, making the ascertainment of duties a challenge.

Duties Owed by Study Sponsors

In personal injury lawsuits involving clinical trials, plaintiffs sometimes name study sponsors as defendants. Sponsors of clinical trials might be named as defendants for multiple reasons. In many instances, sponsors are manufacturers of a medicine or medical device under investigation and therefore might be sued due to their role in manufacturing a product that allegedly caused injury. In addition, many sponsors are so-called "deep-pocket" entities with substantial financial resources, meaning that they might be attractive litigation targets from an economic perspective.

Several of the cases addressing the legal duties of study sponsors have concluded that sponsors owe few – if any – tort duties to study subjects. These conclusions flow, at least in part, from the fact that study sponsors typically do not have contact with study participants and therefore do not play a direct role in overseeing their treatment. This contrasts with the role of investigators, many of whom are physicians charged with managing the treatment of patients enrolled in clinical trials.

The case of *Wholey v. Amgen, Inc.* serves as a recent example of the limitations that courts have placed on the scope of sponsor duties. In *Wholey*, a woman sued the manufacturer of a treatment for inflammatory conditions, alleging that she suffered injuries attributable to the medicine during her participation in a clinical trial and also while she continued to take the medicine after her participation in the trial ended.

During the litigation, a New York state appellate court concluded that the plaintiff could not sue the manufacturer for any injuries attributable to the plaintiff's time in the clinical trial because the manufacturer, as study sponsor, owed her no duty in that context. Specifically, the court stated: "As the sponsors of a clinical trial, defendants owed no duty to [the plaintiff], an enrollee in the trial. Thus, her claims concerning the drug ... must be limited to those that allegedly arose after she stopped participating in the trial and was prescribed the drug as a patient" (*Wholey v. Amgen, Inc.*, 165 A.D.3d 458, 458 (N.Y. App. Div. 2018)).

Other courts have, like the *Wholey* court, ruled that clinical trial sponsors owe no duties to study participants. In *Sykes v. United States*, a wrongful death case involving trials for hepatitis C treatments, the Federal Court of Appeals for the Sixth Circuit upheld a lower court's dismissal of claims against pharmaceutical defendants, reasoning that "under the FDA's regulatory scheme it is not the pharmaceutical companies that are charged with ensuring the trial participants' well-being. Rather, it is the Institutional Review Board that is meant to protect the rights and welfare of trial participants during a clinical trial" (*Sykes v. U.S.*, 507 F. App'x 455, 462 (6th Cir. 2012) (quoting *Abney v. Amgen, Inc.*, 443 F.3d 540, 551 (6th Cir. 2006))). Similarly, in *Darke v. Estate of Isner*, a case involving a clinical trial of a gene therapy treatment for coronary artery disease, a Massachusetts trial court rejected claims against the treatment's manufacturer, concluding that the company, "as sponsor, did not directly owe specific duties to [the deceased patient], the breach of which gave rise to a cause of action for negligence. Instead, such duties inhered in the responsibilities imposed upon the investigators in this case" (*Darke v. Estate of Isner*, 20 Mass. L. Rptr. 419, 2005 WL 3729113, at *15 (Mass. Super. Ct. Nov. 22, 2005)).

The sound rationale underlying these no-duty rulings is that, unlike investigators, sponsors typically do not participate in the treatment of study subjects during clinical trials and therefore should not be held responsible for ensuring subjects' well-being. As support for such conclusions, courts commonly cite federal regulations defining the roles that different participants play in clinical trials. In the *Darke* case, for instance, the court pointed to section 312.3 of Title 21 of the Code of Federal Regulations, which states that, although a sponsor "takes responsibility for and initiates a clinical investigation," the "sponsor does not actually conduct the investigation unless the sponsor is a sponsor-investigator" (21 C.F.R. § 312.3; *Darke*, 2005 WL 3729113, at *15). The *Darke* court contrasted this regulatory provision with section 312.60, which states that an *investigator* (unlike a sponsor) is responsible for conducting the investigation, obtaining informed consent from human study subjects, and "protecting the rights, safety, and welfare of subjects under the investigator's care" (*Darke*, 2005 WL 3729113, at *15 (citing 21 C.F.R. § 312.60)). Noting this division of responsibilities between sponsors and investigators, the *Darke* court reasoned that the study sponsor in that case owed no "specific duties" to the deceased study subject and that the plaintiff therefore could not "prove her negligence claim against" the sponsor (*Darke*, 2005 WL 3729113, at *15).

Notwithstanding these no-duty rulings by many courts, other courts have articulated a more expansive view of sponsor duties. In the case of *Kernke v. The*

Menninger Clinic, a federal district court in Kansas oversaw a personal injury lawsuit brought by the relatives of a man who died during his participation in a trial of a novel treatment for schizophrenia and schizoaffective disorders. In ruling on the viability of the plaintiffs' negligence claim against the sponsor (a pharmaceutical company), the *Kernke* court adhered to the reasoning outlined in other cases and concluded that, because the study sponsor owed no specific duties to the deceased patient, the plaintiffs' negligence claim was not viable (*Kernke v. The Menninger Clinic, Inc.*, 173 F. Supp. 2d 1117, 1123–24 (D. Kan. 2001) (citing 21 C. F.R. §§ 50.20, 312.3 & 312.60)). At the same time, however, in analyzing the plaintiffs' separate *product liability* claim for failure to warn of the medicine's risks, the *Kernke* court implicitly concluded that the pharmaceutical defendant *did* have a duty to warn the investigators of the risks of the treatment, so that the investigators could in turn advise study subjects of the risks and obtain their informed consent (*Kernke*, 173 F. Supp. 2d at 1121). Nevertheless, the *Kernke* court concluded that the plaintiffs' failure-to-warn claim was, like their negligence claim, nonviable because the record was clear that the sponsor in fact provided adequate warnings to the investigators (*Kernke*, 173 F. Supp. 2d at 1121–22).

The case of *Zeman v. Williams* presents another example of a court articulating a more expansive view of sponsor duties. In *Zeman*, the plaintiff was a patient with young-onset Parkinson's disease who allegedly suffered injuries during a clinical trial of an innovative gene transfer therapy for the disease. Among other parties, the plaintiff sued the sponsor of the clinical trial and manufacturer of medical equipment used to facilitate the therapy under investigation. With respect to the sponsor, the plaintiff alleged that the company "negligently drafted and approved the informed consent form used in the clinical trial" (*Zeman v. Williams*, 2014 WL 3058298, at *1 (D. Mass. July 7, 2014)). On the question of legal duties owed by the sponsor, the company argued that "the responsibility for obtaining an informed consent rests exclusively with the investigator" (*Zeman*, 2014 WL 3058298, at *3). The court, however, disagreed, reasoning that a sponsor legal duty exists because the sponsor must provide investigators with information for use in informing study subjects of the risks of a treatment:

> The sponsor argues that the responsibility for obtaining an informed consent rests exclusively with the investigator. It is certainly true that the investigator has a major, if not the major, role in obtaining a properly informed consent. But that does not foreclose the possibility that some other persons, including particularly the trial's sponsor, might also have a responsibility to help assure that the investigator actually gets a properly informed consent. . . . If the investigator fails to inform a subject about some substantial risk because the sponsor has failed adequately to inform the investigator about the risk, the sponsor may be liable in tort. (*Zeman*, 2014 WL 3058298, at *3 (citations omitted))

Based on this reasoning, the *Zeman* court concluded that the plaintiff's negligence-based informed consent claim could proceed beyond the pleading stage – i.e., that it should not be thrown out at the outset – because the plaintiff had "adequately pled" "that [the sponsor] negligently failed in a duty owed to [Plaintiff]" (*Zeman*, 2014 WL 3058298, at *4). (The "general principle espoused by *Zeman*" – that "if the sponsor does not fulfill its duty to the investigator, then, by extension, it does not fulfill its duty to the participant" – has since been endorsed by a federal court in Arizona (*Spedale v. Constellation Pharmaceuticals Inc.*, 2019 WL 3858901, at *13 (D. Ariz. Aug. 16, 2019)). The *Spedale* case involved allegations of inadequate warnings of an injury that arose during a Phase I dose escalation clinical trial of a cancer medicine, and the court followed *Zeman*'s reasoning in allowing several claims – for alleged negligent drafting of the informed consent form, lack of informed consent, and failure to warn the physician investigators – to proceed to trial against the medicine's manufacturer (*Spedale*, 2019 WL 3858901, at *13–16).)

The *Zeman* court also implied, without specifically deciding, that a sponsor could be held liable for negligence if it failed in its responsibility to prepare an appropriate clinical trial protocol, stating that "[t]he sponsor and investigator of a clinical trial both participate in the clinical treatment of the subject by designing and implementing the treatment protocol" (*Zeman*, 2014 WL 3058298, at *5). Other courts have similarly suggested that a clinical trial sponsor has a duty, in preparing a clinical trial protocol, to act reasonably to ensure the safety of study subjects participating in the clinical investigation. In the case of *Liu v. Janssen Research & Development*, for instance, an appellate court ruled that, although sponsors cannot be held responsible for unforeseeable medical malpractice by study physicians, sponsors *do* have a "general duty to ensure study participants' health and safety during the study" and that this duty extends to preparation of "clinical trial protocols" and "monitor[ing] the progress of their studies to ensure compliance with study protocols" (*Liu v. Janssen Research & Development*, 2018 WL 272219, at *6–9 (Cal. Ct. App. Jan. 3, 2018) (unpublished decision)). Thus, in at least a few cases, including *Zeman* and *Liu*, courts have essentially taken the view that sponsors have a duty to act reasonably when they engage in activities that could impact patient safety.

As the various cases demonstrate, the tort duties that study sponsors owe to study subjects are hardly clear, with some courts adopting the view that no such duties are owed and others concluding that sponsors have certain duties with respect to patient safety. Further complicating matters is the fact that, because the existence of a legal duty is a question of state law, legal duties might vary significantly from state to state. In addition, a court's conclusion will often turn on the specific facts of a given case, including facts showing the extent to which the sponsor played a role in the patient safety matters at issue. Nevertheless, despite the variability and lack of clarity in the court decisions, a few key principles can be gleaned from the cases:

- **A sponsor's tort duties are limited.** Because sponsors do not participate directly in the treatment of study subjects, courts do not ordinarily hold clinical trial sponsors liable for the direct management of individual patients, including, for example, errors committed in the provision of treatment to subjects.
- **Nevertheless, sponsors might have a duty (in tort) to act reasonably when they take action that could potentially impact the safety of study subjects.** Notwithstanding their limited role in the treatment of study subjects, clinical trial sponsors engage in activities that could potentially impact patient safety,

including the development of clinical trial protocols, the provision of safety-related information to investigators, and the monitoring of trial activities. Because at least some courts have concluded that participation in such activities gives rise to a legal duty to study participants, the possibility of civil liability exists if trial sponsors do not act with reasonable care when they engage in safety-related activities.

In light of this legal framework, clinical trial sponsors incur a certain amount of legal risk when they conduct clinical investigations. Sponsors can mitigate this risk by devoting care to patient safety matters, including when they develop clinical trial protocols, provide safety information to investigators, and monitor patient safety during the administration of trials.

Duties Owed by Investigators and Associated Institutions

In the personal injury setting, the legal duties owed by clinical trial investigators are somewhat clearer than those owed by study sponsors. This relative (but hardly pristine) clarity derives in part from the fact that investigators – unlike sponsors – participate directly in the treatment of study subjects. In light of the role of investigators in administering treatment, courts have concluded that investigators have a duty to obtain a patient's informed consent. In addition, some courts have also suggested that investigators have a broader duty to oversee the patient's safety during her participation in the clinical trial. And, of course, to the extent that they administer ordinary medical treatment in the context of a physician-patient relationship, investigators have a duty to adhere to the medical standard of care in treating their patients, separate and apart from their roles as investigators (Morreim 2004).

Previously, commentators have explained that many court decisions have focused on informed consent when discussing the tort duties of investigators (Tereskerz 2012, at 34–36, 42–43). While this is true, some cases suggest that courts might cast the duty net more widely, such that it encompasses other aspects of patient safety during a trial, including those imbedded in a clinical trial protocol. If, for instance, an investigator deviated from a trial protocol in a manner that impacted patient safety, a court might well conclude that the investigator could be held liable under a negligence theory for any resulting patient injuries.

The previously discussed case of *Darke v. Estate of Isner* illustrates the reasoning that courts sometimes follow in determining the scope of investigator duties. In *Darke*, the court referenced the role that physician-investigators necessarily play in patient treatment and concluded that, in light of this role, investigators owe "specific duties" to study subjects. Relying on federal regulations governing clinical trials, the *Darke* court explained that investigators are responsible for "ensuring that an investigation is conducted according to the signed investigator statement, the investigational plan, and applicable regulations, protecting the rights, safety, and welfare under the investigator's care, and obtaining the informed consent of each human subject to whom the drug is administered" (*Darke*, 2005 WL 3729113, at *15 (citing 21 C.F.R. § 312.60)). Based in part on these duties – as well as a physician's general duty to follow the medical standard of care in treating patients with whom she has a physician-patient relationship – the *Darke* court permitted claims for negligence to proceed against the study's principal investigator and one of the sub-investigators who treated the deceased study subject (*Darke*, 2005 WL 3729113, at *3–11). (Notably, however, the *Darke* court did *not* permit the plaintiff to pursue a claim against another sub-investigator who "proposed [the deceased patient's] candidacy for the clinical trial and was aware of his participation," but who otherwise played no role in the patient's treatment (*Darke*, 2005 WL 3729113, at *11–12). Therefore, the liability of a physician-investigator might depend, at least in part, on the establishment of an actual role in the study subject's treatment. A *principal* investigator, on the other hand, might have a more expansive scope of liability, due to her responsibility for exercising "directive authority and control over" the broader clinical trial (*Darke*, 2005 WL 3729113, at *5 & n.3).)

Similarly, in the *Zeman v. Williams* case (also discussed previously), a federal court in Massachusetts concluded, based on its review of federal regulations governing clinical trials, that an "investigator is responsible for the conduct of the trial according to the applicable protocol" and "has a major, if not the major, role in obtaining a properly informed consent" (*Zeman*, 2014 WL 3058298, at *2–3). Although the role of investigator duties was not directly before the court in *Zeman*, the court implied (in the context of addressing sponsor duties) that an investigator's clinical trial responsibilities create duties to study subjects under Massachusetts law.

Importantly, an investigator's associated institution or company could also be deemed to have legal responsibilities in a personal injury case. Under a legal principle known as "vicarious liability," an individual's employer can be held liable for negligence that its employee commits, provided that the employee was acting within the scope of her employment when she committed the wrongdoing at issue. In the *Darke* case, for instance, the court concluded that the pharmaceutical company defendant could potentially be held liable under Massachusetts law for the acts of a physician-investigator who received compensation from, "possessed a significant financial share" in, and "devoted a significant portion of his professional life to" the company (*Darke*, 2005 WL 3729113, at *13–14). Additionally, apart from the question of vicarious liability, an investigator's associated institution or company could also be deemed responsible for a study subject's injuries to the extent it played an independent role in the conduct of the clinical trial, including the administration of an IRB (*Abney*, 443 F.3d at 551). (The potential duties owed by IRBs will be discussed in further detail below.) Also, some courts have held that hospitals have an independent duty – apart from the duties of individual investigators – to obtain the informed consent of study subjects participating in clinical research, although there is disagreement among the courts on this point (*Kus v. Sherman Hospital*, 644 N. E.2d 1214, 1220–21 (Ill. App. Ct. 1995); *Connelly v. Iolab Corp.*, 1995 WL 250794, at *7–8 (Mo. Ct. App. May 2, 1995); *Friter v. Iolab Corp.*, 607 A.2d 1111, 1116 (Pa. Super. Ct. 1992); *Kershaw v. Reichert*, 445 N.W.2d 16, 17–18 (N.D. 1989)).

Thus, although applicable court decisions do not provide perfect clarity on the legal duties that investigators (and their associated institutions or companies) owe to study subjects, the following general principles emerge from the cases:

- **Investigators likely have a tort duty to obtain a patient's informed consent.** Based in part on responsibilities imposed by federal regulations, courts have held that investigators have a duty to obtain the informed consent of study subjects to whom they administer treatment.
- **Investigators might also have a broader duty to ensure patient safety.** Based on applicable court decisions, clinical trial investigators might also have a broader tort duty to act reasonably to protect patient safety, including by (1) ensuring that the study is conducted according to the trial protocol and applicable regulations and (2) adhering to the medical standard of care when providing ordinary medical treatment in the context of a physician-patient relationship.
- **Associated institutions might have independent tort duties to secure informed consent and oversee patient safety and could also be held liable for the wrongful acts of their employees.** The case law is less illuminative on the duties of investigators' associated institutions (e.g., hospitals). Nevertheless, it would be prudent for institutions to assume that courts could conclude they have duties to oversee patient safety (e.g., through administration of an IRB) and ensure that study subjects in their institutions give informed consent to participating in research. In addition, under the principle of vicarious liability, institutions and companies might be deemed liable for the wrongful conduct of their employees.

Duties Owed by IRBs, DSMBs, and CROs

As with other role players in clinical trials, the duties owed by IRBs, DSMBs, and CROs are not entirely clear. Nevertheless, certain guideposts can be gleaned from the existing case law.

Institutional Review Boards

The case law addressing the liability of IRBs and their members is relatively scant. Nevertheless, given that federal regulations task IRBs with "protect[ing] the rights and welfare of human subjects involved in [clinical] investigations" (21 C.F.R. § 56.101), some courts have concluded that IRBs have a state-law duty to ensure that study subjects give their informed consent. In addition, some cases suggest that IRBs might have a broader duty to ensure the protection of patient safety during clinical trials.

The case of *Kus v. Sherman Hospital* is illustrative on the issue of informed consent. In *Kus*, the plaintiff alleged that he suffered injuries following implantation of ocular lenses. Although the plaintiff signed an informed consent form before implantation, the form did not advise him that the lenses were experimental – i.e., that they were "under investigation for efficacy and safety." In his lawsuit, the plaintiff sued the hospital where the implantation procedures were performed, asserting claims of medical battery, negligence due to lack of informed consent, and negligence for alleged failure to respond to a product recall involving the lenses (*Kus v. Sherman Hospital*, 644 N.E.2d 1214, 1216–18 (Ill. App. Ct. 1995)). At trial, the lower court dismissed the medical battery and product recall claims, and the jury issued a verdict for the defendant on the informed consent claim. However, on appeal, the appellate court ruled that the medical battery claim should have gone to the jury and that the trial court improperly instructed the jury on the informed consent claim. Although the appellate court recognized that a hospital ordinarily does not play a direct role in obtaining a patient's informed consent, the court concluded that, because the hospital had agreed to become a participant in a clinical trial, it had a state-law duty – derived at least in part from applicable federal regulations – to ensure (through its IRB) that study subjects had given their informed consent to the implantation procedures:

> By becoming a participating institution in this particular study, [the Hospital] was charged with assuring that 'legally effective informed consent' was obtained prior to the experimental surgery and that 'procedures which are experimental' needed to be identified before such surgery occurred. While we agree that generally a hospital is not in the best position to inform a patient of risks, here it is clear that [the Hospital] undertook the responsibility to inform the plaintiff of the experimental nature of his surgery. Moreover, a participating institution in the intraocular lens study is required to conduct 'continuing review of research' under the Federal guidelines, which includes the duty to review the informed consent process. Thus, [the Hospital] also had the minimal duty here of checking to ensure that the form its IRB had promulgated was being used. We determine that the particular facts in the case before us require a determination that a hospital, as well as a physician, may be liable for claims arising from the lack of informed consent in this instance. Thus, the plaintiff's medical battery count is viable under Illinois law. (*Kus*, 644 N.E.2d at 1221 (citations omitted))

Other courts have followed reasoning similar to that of the *Kus* court in concluding that IRBs have a duty to ensure that study subjects give informed consent to experimental treatment. For instance, in *Friter v. Iolab Corp.*, another case involving experimental ocular lenses, a Pennsylvania appellate court concluded that, by virtue of its participation in a clinical trial, the defendant "hospital had assumed a duty, pursuant to FDA regulations, to ensure that any patient involved in a clinical study was made aware of the clinical nature of the procedure and the risks associated with such experimentation, and had signed a consent form acknowledging that fact" (*Friter v. Iolab Corp.*, 607 A.2d 1111, 1114 (Pa. Super. Ct. 1992)).

In addition, some courts have implied that IRBs have an even broader duty – beyond just obtaining informed consent – to protect the welfare of study subjects during a clinical trial. In the *Sykes* case (discussed above), a federal appellate court rejected claims against pharmaceutical company defendants, reasoning that "it is the Institutional Review Board" – not the study sponsor – "that is meant to protect the rights and welfare of trial participants during a clinical trial" (*Sykes v. U.S.*, 507 F. App'x 455, 462 (6th Cir. 2012) (citations and internal quotation marks omitted)). In reaching this conclusion, the *Sykes* court cited *Abney v. Amgen*, an earlier case in which the same court suggested – without specifically deciding – that an IRB could be sued for breach of a fiduciary duty in light of federal regulations that require IRBs to protect the welfare of study subjects. Specifically, the *Abney* court stated:

> Although we express no ultimate view, it appears that the plaintiffs might have considered suit against the [University]'s Institutional Review Board and the physician investigators involved in the clinical trial. . . [A]s discussed above, under the FDA's regulatory scheme it is

not the pharmaceutical companies that are charged with ensuring trial participants' well-being. Rather, it is the Institutional Review Board that is meant to 'protect the rights and welfare' of trial participants during a clinical trial. 21 C.F.R. § 56.101 (requiring university conducting clinical trials to establish institutional review boards for the purpose of 'protect[ing] the rights and welfare of human subjects involved in' clinical trials); *see also* 21 C.F.R. § 56.103 (requiring institutional review boards to approve all clinical trials before initiation and requiring continuing review of clinical trials while they are being conducted). Thus, while the plaintiffs' arguments have little merit against [the pharmaceutical company], they may have merit against the University and its Institutional Review Board. (*Abney v. Amgen, Inc.*, 443 F.3d 540, 551 (6th Cir. 2006))

A take-away from cases like *Kus*, *Friter*, *Sykes*, and *Abney* is that a court might conclude that an IRB has a duty to ensure that study subjects give informed consent and possibly a broader duty to ensure study subjects' safety – including through the IRB's role in approving clinical studies and "review[ing] clinical trials while they are being conducted" (*Abney*, 443 F.3d at 551). For these reasons, an IRB could potentially face liability for any number of problems that might arise in a clinical trial, including a failure to obtain informed consent, a safety deficiency in a clinical trial protocol, or a failure to monitor – and respond to – safety issues arising in the course of a clinical trial.

On the other hand, other courts addressing the question of IRB duties have declined to impose them. In the case of *Kershaw v. Reichert*, yet another ocular implant case, the Supreme Court of North Dakota held that a personal injury lawsuit could not proceed against the defendant hospital and its IRB because (1) regulations applicable to ocular implants did not specifically "authorize a private action against hospitals, institutional review committees, or doctors for unsuccessful intraocular implants" and (2) a hospital – unlike a physician – "generally has no duty to obtain a like informed consent from the same patient" (*Kershaw v. Reichert*, 445 N.W.2d 16, 17–18 (N.D. 1989)). Similarly, in the *Zeman* case (discussed above), a federal court in Massachusetts concluded that, although a negligence claim could proceed against the study sponsor, a similar claim against IRB members was nonviable. Specifically, the *Zeman* court reasoned that, because an IRB does not play a direct role in the treatment of study subjects, "[i]ts role is more like a regulatory body, than a treating medical professional or designer of the clinical trial protocol" (*Zeman*, 2014 WL 3058298, at *5). For this reason, the *Zeman* court held that, under Massachusetts law, the IRB members did "not have any duty to [the plaintiff] (or any other specific patient) with respect to the obtaining of informed consent" (*Zeman*, 2014 WL 3058298, at *5).

As with other clinical trial participants, a review of the conflicting state and federal cases involving IRBs makes the issue of legal duties seem as clear as mud. Unfortunately, operating under an ambiguous legal structure is a fact of life in this area. Nevertheless, recognizing that some courts have articulated fairly expansive views of IRB legal duties, institutions conducting clinical trials should assume that:

- **IRBs might have a tort duty to ensure that study subjects give informed consent to study procedures.** For this reason, IRB members should take care to

ensure that informed consent forms adequately advise patients of an experimental treatment's risks (Tereskerz 2012, at 38) and that processes exist to ensure that patients actually review risk information and give informed consent before treatment begins.
- **IRBs might have a broader tort duty to protect patient safety during the conduct of a clinical trial.** In light of this possible duty, IRB members should take care to comply with applicable state and federal regulations – and to otherwise take measures to protect patient safety – during a clinical trial. Such efforts should include careful review of clinical trial designs and protocols, as well as reviewing – and responding to potential safety issues identified during – the conduct of a clinical trial.

Data and Safety Monitoring Boards

In the personal injury setting, the duties – if any – that might be owed by members of DSMBs are far from clear. Although actions by DSMBs sometimes come up in litigation, including in securities fraud cases (*see*, for instance, *In re: Immune Response Securities Litigation*, 375 F. Supp. 2d 983 (S.D. Cal. 2005)), the authors are unaware of any court decision specifically analyzing the legal duties of DSMBs in the context of a personal injury case.

To some extent, though, and despite the distinctions between them, DSMBs are analogous to IRBs. Both play a role in overseeing matters involving patient safety in clinical trials, and both stand outside of any direct role in patient treatment. For this reason, commentators have noted that (1) personal injury litigation against members of DSMBs is probably inevitable and (2) courts might conclude, as some courts have concluded in cases involving IRBs, that federal regulations and other requirements create tort duties for DSMB members in personal injury cases (Tereskerz 2012, at 55–56; Tereskerz 2010, at 30–31). At the same time, commentators have noted that members of DSMBs might be more insulated from liability (compared to IRBs) because there are fewer regulatory requirements that specifically govern the conduct and responsibilities of DSMBs (Tereskerz 2012, at 57).

In light of the potential for liability in personal injury litigation, members of DSMBs should give special attention to adhering to requirements imposed by regulations (or otherwise) and to their roles as monitors of patient safety. Also, as commentators have noted, members of DSMBs might wish to seek protection from liability through indemnification agreements with study sponsors (Tereskerz 2012, at 62–63).

Contract Research Organizations

As with other clinical trial participants, personal injury cases addressing the duties of CROs are few and far between. Nevertheless, given that CROs assume the responsibilities of the study sponsors with whom they contract, it can be fairly assumed that their potential duties (and therefore their potential liabilities) will track those of study sponsors. In addition, there is at least some precedent for the imposition of legal duties on CROs in personal injury litigation (Valdes and McGuire 2004, at 13).

Under federal regulations, a study sponsor may transfer some or all of its clinical trial obligations to a CRO, provided that the transfer of obligations is described in writing (21 C.F.R. § 312.52(a)). When such a transfer of obligations occurs, the CRO must comply with the regulations governing the responsibilities transferred and "shall be subject to the same regulatory action as a sponsor for failure to comply with any obligation assumed under these regulations" (21 C.F.R. § 312.52(b)). The regulations also specifically state that "all references to 'sponsor' in this part apply to a contract research organization to the extent that it assumes one or more obligations of the sponsor" (21 C.F.R. § 312.52(b)). Therefore, from the perspective of federal regulations – and, possibly, from the perspective of a court that relies on such regulations in determining duties under state law – a CRO's duties align with those of a sponsor, at least with respect to the activities it has agreed to conduct.

The case of *Wawrzynek v. Statprobe, Inc.*, while not directly on point, illustrates how these principles might play out in personal injury litigation. In *Wawrzynek*, a woman alleged that she developed a back infection and serious spinal column injury as a result of her use of a conditionally approved medical device. The plaintiff sued several defendants, including a CRO that, pursuant to a contract with the device manufacturer (and clinical trial sponsor), assumed responsibility for various clinical trial activities, including clinical monitoring, data management, statistical analysis, and safety data monitoring (*Wawrzynek v. Statprobe, Inc.*, 2007 WL 3146792, at *2 (E.D. Pa. Oct. 25, 2007)). Although the plaintiff was treated after the medical device's conditional approval (and thus after the clinical trial had ended), she alleged that the CRO's activities during the trial – including alleged involvement in data manipulation – led to her injuries (*Wawrzynek*, 2007 WL 3146792, at *4).

With respect to the *Wawrzynek* plaintiff's negligence claim, the CRO argued that it could not be held liable for the plaintiff's injuries because "a CRO assisting a medical device manufacturer does not owe a duty of care to individuals who may use the researched product, as the connection between a CRO and consumers is too remote to create a legal duty" (*Wawrzynek*, 2007 WL 3146792, at *13–14). The court, however, disagreed. In its analysis, the court reasoned that, because the CRO apparently had "assumed a role in the U.S. clinical study for [the medical device] that involved much more than simple, remote 'number crunching,'" it likely had a duty (under Pennsylvania law) to protect the well-being of individuals within the "foreseeable orbit" of those who could potentially be harmed by its conduct (*Wawrzynek*, 2007 WL 3146792, at *14–15). The court also stated that, "[c]learly, the performance of research, administration of clinical trials, and compilation of statistical data implicate the well-being of third parties, such as consumers, to some extent" (*Wawrzynek*, 2007 WL 3146792, at *13). Applying this reasoning, the *Wawrzynek* court held that the plaintiff's suit against the CRO could proceed to trial.

Thus, although the *Wawrzynek* court did not address an injury that occurred during a clinical trial, it held that a CRO likely has a duty to protect those who could potentially be harmed by actions taken by a CRO during a clinical study. In *Wawrzynek*, the patient within the "foreseeable orbit" of the CRO's actions was a post-approval consumer, but the same reasoning could be just as easily – if not more easily – applied to a clinical study subject.

The key take-away from federal regulations and the *Wawrzynek* case is that courts are likely to view CRO duties as similar to those of sponsors in the personal injury setting. This means that, while some courts might view CRO duties as limited or nonexistent, other courts might conclude – as the *Wawrzynek* court concluded – that a CRO has a duty to protect patient safety in carrying out the activities it has agreed to undertake.

Summary of Tort Duties Owed

Based on the foregoing discussion, and notwithstanding the considerable lack of clarity in the case law, the tort duties that might apply to the different role players in clinical trials can be summarized as outlined in the table below. (This chapter focuses on civil litigation, and the duties that apply in that setting, particularly in tort lawsuits. Of course, outside of the tort context, participants in clinical trials have other legally imposed responsibilities under federal and state laws and regulations. These responsibilities – the violation of which can have significant consequences outside of the tort setting – are beyond the scope of this chapter.)

Clinical trial participant	Tort duties potentially owed to study subjects

Sponsors	Possible duty to act with reasonable care when engaging in activities that could impact patient safety, including:
	    Provision of safety-related information to investigators (e.g., in investigator's brochure, model informed consent form, clinical trial protocol, etc.)
	    Development and implementation of clinical trial protocol
	    Monitoring of patient safety during study

Investigators and associated institutions	*Investigators*
	    Duty to obtain valid informed consent from study subjects
	    Possible duty to protect patient safety, including by ensuring that study is conducted according to protocol and applicable regulations
	    Duty to adhere to applicable standard of care when providing ordinary medical care in context of physician-patient relationship
	Associated institutions/companies
	    Possible duty to ensure patient safety through administration of IRB
	    Possible duty to obtain valid informed consent from study subjects
	    Possible liability for wrongful conduct of employees participating in clinical research

IRBs, DSMBs, and CROs	*IRBs*
	    Possible duty to obtain valid informed consent from study subjects
	    Possible broader duty to protect patient safety during conduct of clinical trial, including through:
	        Review of clinical trial designs and protocols
	        Review of – and response to – safety issues identified during trial
	DSMBs
	    Possible duty to protect patient safety during conduct of clinical trial, including through review of – and response to – safety issues identified during trial
	CROs
	    Likely assumption of sponsor duties (*see* above) for any activities transferred from sponsor to CRO

Causation

The legal concept of causation is another core element of a personal injury claim. Regardless of the underlying legal theory – negligence versus product liability, for instance – a plaintiff cannot prevail on a claim for personal injury unless she can prove that the defendant's conduct or defective product caused her injury. Therefore, even if a defendant acted negligently, or even if a medicine or device's warnings were inadequate, the plaintiff will not succeed unless her injuries were causally connected to the misconduct proven.

Many jurisdictions divide the causation concept into two distinct sub-concepts. The first is *actual* causation: whether the misconduct in fact caused the injury. The second is *proximate* or *legal* causation: whether the plaintiff's injuries were the foreseeable or direct consequence of the misconduct. A claim will fail unless both sub-elements are satisfied (*Brown v. Philadelphia College of Osteopathic Medicine*, 760 A.2d 863, 868–69 (Pa. Super. Ct. 2000); Tereskerz 2012, at 59).

Individual cases illustrate the concept of causation in action. In the *Liu* case (discussed above), the appellate court overturned a substantial jury verdict for the plaintiffs because it concluded that they had failed to prove causation. Specifically, the court held that the plaintiffs had introduced nothing more than speculative expert testimony supporting their claim that a test dose of an antipsychotic medication had caused their son's death due to cardiomyopathy. For this reason, "there was insufficient evidence that administration of the single, one-milligram dose of the study drug was a substantial factor in causing [the decedent's] death" (*Liu*, 2018 WL 272219, at *9–12).

A similar result occurred in the case of *Looney v. Moore*. In *Looney*, the parents of premature infant participants in a clinical trial of oxygen saturation levels sued various defendants, claiming that the infants suffered injuries (including neurological damage) during the trial. The lower court dismissed the plaintiffs' claims at the summary judgment stage, and the appellate court affirmed. The basis for dismissal was the plaintiffs' failure to show that the infants' injuries were caused by their participation in the trial, as opposed to their "premature births and consequent low birth-weight," which, by themselves, "carr[y] increased risks of the kinds of neurodevelopmental and respiratory impairments claimed by Plaintiffs" (*Looney v. Moore*, 886 F.3d 1058, 1062–64 (11th Cir. 2018)).

Liu and *Looney* were negligence cases, but similar causation failures lead to dismissal of product liability claims arising out of clinical trials. In *Kernke* (also discussed above), the court concluded that the plaintiffs' failure-to-warn product liability claim failed for causation reasons (among others). In particular, the plaintiffs failed to establish a causal connection between the decedent's death and alleged deficiencies in the warnings that the study sponsor provided for the schizophrenia medicine under investigation. Put another way, the plaintiffs failed to establish that the outcome would have been avoided if the defendant study sponsor had issued different warnings (*Kernke*, 173 F. Supp. 2d at 1122–23).

These cases and others demonstrate that proving negligence, or a product defect, will not alone result in liability. A plaintiff must do more by proving a causal connection between the alleged wrong and the injuries she suffered. Many personal injury cases fail due to a plaintiff's inability to prove causation.

Damages

A personal injury plaintiff must also show that she suffered damages – a compensable injury – as a result of the alleged failure by the defendant. In personal injury lawsuits, damages may include both *economic* damages (such as lost wages or the costs of medical care needed to treat an injury) and *noneconomic* damages (such as the pain and suffering endured by the plaintiff) (Bal 2009). In clinical trial lawsuits, as in other personal injury lawsuits, damages can vary widely. Factors that might impact the extent of damages include the severity of the plaintiff's injuries, the extent of out-of-pocket costs incurred by the plaintiff, the egregiousness of the misconduct proven, the extent to which the plaintiff needed the therapy provided in the clinical trial, and the varying or idiosyncratic views of judges and juries.

Damages awards can be significant, highlighting the potential risk to clinical trial participants. In the *Liu* case, for example, a jury awarded more than $5.6 million to the parents of a man who died during a trial of a schizophrenia medication, although the judgment was reversed on appeal (*Liu*, 2018 WL 272219, at *1, *5). Similarly, in the *Friter* case, a jury awarded more than $1.75 million as compensation for eye injuries experienced during a clinical trial of intraocular lenses (*Friter*, 607 A.2d at 625). These and other cases demonstrate that, while rare, judgments in clinical trial-based personal injury suits can be substantial.

Other Lawsuits

While not exhaustive, this section addresses other types of lawsuits that might arise in the context of (or in relation to) a clinical trial: contractual disputes, intellectual property disputes, securities litigation, employment lawsuits, criminal actions, lawsuits demanding medicines or treatment, and mass torts. Each of the subsections provides a discussion of actual lawsuits and offers perspectives on possible ways to mitigate the risk of litigation.

Contractual Disputes

Numerous entities – such as sponsors, investigators, clinical trial sites, and CROs – must work in collaboration to launch and run a clinical trial. The relationships between these entities are ordinarily formalized through contracts that cover the obligations of the parties. A clinical trial agreement between a sponsor and a clinical trial site, for example, typically includes provisions covering the roles of the principal investigator, sponsor, and institution, confidentiality terms, termination rights, responsibilities for payment of medical expenses in the event of subject injury, and indemnification. When any aspect of one of these relationships breaks down, a contractual dispute might arise.

For example, in *CTI Clinical Trial Services v. Gilead Sciences*, a CRO filed a lawsuit against a pharmaceutical company alleging breach of contract after the company decided to terminate a phase III clinical study early. The CRO sought payment for services it had already performed and for those it would have performed had the study not been terminated early (*CTI Clinical Trial Services, Inc. v. Gilead Sciences, Inc.*, 2013 WL 1641348, at *6 (S.D. Ohio Apr. 16, 2013)). Applying basic principles of contract law, the court first assessed whether the relevant language in the agreement was clear and unambiguous. If so, it would interpret the contract based on the plain meaning of the language, and if not, it would look to extrinsic evidence to interpret the meaning. The court ultimately determined that the plain meaning of the contract terms did not allow the CRO to recover payment for services it would have performed, but as for the exact amount due for services already performed, the court found the contract and extrinsic evidence to be sufficiently ambiguous that it remained an issue of fact for a jury to resolve (*CTI Clinical Trial Services*, 2013 WL 1641348, at *20).

As illustrated in the *CTI* case, entities working on clinical trials that seek to avoid potential protracted contractual disputes should aim to draft a clear expression of each party's rights and obligations in their agreements and ensure that any questions regarding the roles of each entity are clarified. To the extent a court determines that the contractual language is ambiguous, retaining extrinsic evidence that helps clarify the meaning of the terms might be useful as well.

Intellectual Property Disputes

Intellectual property can be a critical issue in the administration of clinical trials. Sponsors commonly test proprietary medicines and medical devices during clinical trials, with the goal of obtaining approval by the Food and Drug Administration ("FDA") to market their products. Intellectual property disputes can arise from clinical trials in several ways, including when the product being tested allegedly infringes other patents and when other companies seek to invalidate patents protecting the product under investigation.

Generally, using patented products or processes without permission from the patent owner is an act of patent infringement. The law, however, exempts certain experimental activities during research and development that would normally be considered infringement. Specifically, the use of patented medicines and devices in the context of a clinical trial – such as using a patented product as a comparator – can be protected as long as the information being generated is "solely for uses reasonably related" to obtaining FDA approval of a product (35 U.S.C. § 271(e)(1)). Questions regarding the scope of this statutory exemption have been the subject of litigation involving allegations of patent infringement. For example, courts have held that activities such as demonstrations of a medical device during medical conferences to obtain clinical investigators and reporting clinical trial progress to investors appropriately fell under the exempted category of dissemination of data developed for FDA approval (*Telectronics Pacing Systems, Inc. v. Ventritex, Inc.*, 982 F.2d 1520, 1523–24 (Fed. Cir. 1992)). The U. S. Supreme Court has also since held that certain preclinical testing, such as the screening of potential compounds for further testing, could also fall under the protected exemption (*Merck KGaA v. Integra Lifesciences I, Ltd.*, 545 U.S. 193, 202 (2005)).

To minimize the risk of successful infringement allegations, clinical trial sponsors might benefit from formulating an early action plan for submission to the FDA, as well as properly documenting the experiments and reasons for the experiments in the event it becomes necessary to show that the experiments were reasonably related to information to be submitted to the FDA (Russo and Johnson 2015).

As for disputes regarding the validity of a sponsor's own patents, challengers have argued that such patents have become invalid through "public use" during clinical trials. A claimed invention is deemed "public" if it has been accessible to the public or on sale for at least 1 year prior to the patent application (35 U.S.C. § 102). But use for purposes of experimentation negates the public use bar. As a court has explained, "a clinical trial seeking to test a particular treatment hypothesis seems to be the quintessential experimental use" (*Sanofi v. Glenmark Pharmaceuticals Inc., USA*, 204 F. Supp. 3d 665, 698 (D. Del. 2016)). Courts consider a number of factors in making a fact-intensive assessment of whether use during a clinical trial constitutes experimental use, including the length of the test period, presence of confidentiality agreements, any records of testing, monitoring of test results, and the length of the test period in relation to testing for similar inventions (*Eli Lilly & Co. v. Zenith Goldline Pharmaceuticals, Inc.*, 471 F.3d 1369, 1381 (Fed. Cir. 2006)).

In light of these considerations, a sponsor seeking to avoid a finding that a clinical trial constitutes an invalidating public use might want to consider various precautions, such as limiting the number of subjects enrolled in the trial to the smallest number that is commensurate with obtaining necessary safety and efficacy data, imposing restrictions as to whom physicians may provide the study medicine, requiring physicians to sign confidentiality agreements regarding details of the study, and requiring patients to maintain usage logs and to return any unused doses of the study medicine (Chiacchio 2017).

Securities Litigation

Sponsors of clinical trials are often publicly traded companies that are accountable to shareholders. Information presented about clinical trials has led to securities litigation in situations where investors allege that they were misled by information presented by the company, including when the outcome of a medicine's approval process or real-world data fail to meet investor expectations.

For example, in *In re: Incyte Shareholder Litigation*, a pension plan brought a securities fraud class action on behalf of all persons who purchased the common stock of a pharmaceutical company, alleging that the company made false and misleading statements about the discontinuation rates – the rates at which patients stop using a medicine for any reason – for a treatment for bone marrow disease (*In re: Incyte Shareholder Litigation*, 2014 WL 707207, at *1 (D. Del. Feb. 21, 2014)). The pension fund contended that various statements made by the company during investor calls and health conferences suggested that the discontinuation rates for prescriptions shortly after FDA approval were consistent with the rates recorded during the clinical trials, when (according to the fund) the company knew the discontinuation rates in practice were in fact much higher than those associated with the clinical trials.

The court dismissed the action because the plaintiffs failed to point to any specific statements made by the company indicating the actual discontinuation rates for the medicine shortly after FDA approval were the same or consistent with the rates recorded during the clinical trials. Instead, the court found that the company consistently communicated to investors that it was too early to tell whether the discontinuation rates in practice would be consistent with the rates observed in the clinical trials, and it repeatedly disclosed that a more severely ill patient population that was excluded from the clinical trial was approved to use the medicine by the FDA, which would account for heightened discontinuation rates in the real world (*In re: Incyte*, 2014 WL 707207, at *8).

As demonstrated in the *Incyte* case, clinical trial sponsors might be able to successfully avert prolonged securities litigation so long as they describe available data truthfully and disclose appropriate caveats for projections where data are not conclusive.

Employment Lawsuits

The various entities involved in a clinical trial – including clinical trial sponsors, clinical trial sites, and CROs – all have employees and/or contractors that act on their behalf. Thus, the full range of conflicts that can arise from any employment relationship could occur in the context of a clinical trial as well. Such conflicts can include lawsuits alleging wrongful termination, discrimination, harassment, and retaliation, among other claims.

For instance, in *Perez v. Progenics Pharmaceuticals, Inc.*, a former employee of a pharmaceutical company alleged that he was wrongfully terminated in retaliation for writing a memorandum to management stating that he believed the company was committing fraud against shareholders based on representations made to the public that, in his view, were not consistent with the actual results of a clinical trial (*Perez v. Progenics Pharmaceuticals, Inc.*, 965 F. Supp. 2d 353, 359–60 (S.D.N.Y. 2013)). The court allowed the case to proceed to the jury because, in the court's view, the employee was able to demonstrate through documentation that a genuine issue of fact remained as to whether he reasonably believed the company was committing securities fraud and because the court concluded that the company had failed to prove by clear and convincing evidence that it would have terminated the employee even in the absence of his alleged protected whistleblower activity (*Perez*, 965 F. Supp. 2d at 369).

To successfully prosecute or defend against claims brought by employees, both parties benefit from careful documentation of the events that occur during an employment relationship. Further, employers can reduce the risk of employment lawsuits by ensuring that appropriate policies regarding discrimination, harassment, and termination are available, trained on, and carefully followed.

Criminal Cases and Other Government Lawsuits

Misconduct related to clinical trial procedures and proprietary data can lead to criminal actions and other lawsuits brought by the government. Insider trading prosecutions and civil lawsuits brought under the False Claims Act are two such examples.

One of the largest insider trading convictions in U.S. history centered on information obtained about a clinical trial. In February 2014, a jury found a former hedge fund manager guilty of making $275 million in illegal gains through secret tips about the negative results of a clinical trial involving a treatment for Alzheimer's disease (ElBoghdady 2014). Prosecutors alleged that the manager illegally made use of information he learned from a neurology professor who served as chairman of the safety monitoring committee overseeing the clinical trial 2 weeks before the results were made public. The manager was sentenced to 9 years in prison and has been unsuccessful in overturning the verdict on appeal.

Lawsuits alleging violations of the False Claims Act ("FCA") can also arise out of clinical trials. The FCA imposes liability for any person who knowingly submits a false claim to the government or knowingly makes a false statement to obtain money or to avoid paying money to the government (31 U.S.C. § 3729(a)). While the government can directly initiate a lawsuit, the FCA also allows private persons to file whistleblower *qui tam* actions for violations of the FCA on behalf of the government. In the context of a clinical trial, liability can be imposed if, for example, an entity knowingly files illegal reimbursement claims with the government (McAllister 2007, at 6).

While clinical trial sponsors cannot necessarily prevent individual bad actors from committing criminal violations or fraud, sponsors can endeavor to protect themselves from liability by ensuring that confidentiality agreements and other clinical trial agreements are properly executed, conducting proper training on clinical trial conduct policies, conducting appropriate oversight, and implementing processes for efficiently escalating and acting on matters when potential issues are discovered.

Lawsuits Demanding Medicines or Other Treatment

Under its expanded access – or "compassionate use" – program, the FDA allows companies to provide their experimental medicines to patients with serious or life-threatening illnesses outside of clinical trials in certain situations. While the FDA cannot compel pharmaceutical companies to supply medicines to a patient, when a company allegedly makes representations that it would support a patient in securing access to an experimental medicine, courts have held that the company might be required to follow through.

In *Cacchillo v. Insmed Inc.*, a study subject who experienced positive results during a clinical trial filed a lawsuit challenging the sponsor's alleged refusal to support her compassionate-use application to allow her to resume treatment with the experimental medicine after the clinical trial was suspended. Based on allegations that the sponsor's website included a number of messages indicating that those who participated in clinical trials would have the sponsor's support in securing continued access to the study medicine if it proved to be safe and effective for them, the court concluded that the study participant adequately stated claims for fraud, negligent misrepresentation, and breach of contract (although the court later granted summary judgment for the sponsor and dismissed the study participant's claims) (*Cacchillo v. Insmed Inc.*, 833 F. Supp. 2d 218, 241 (N.D.N.Y. 2011); *Cacchillo v. Insmed Inc.*, 2013 WL 622220, at *19 (N.D.N.Y. Feb. 19, 2013)).

The *Cacchillo* case outlines a very narrow area of potential liability in clinical trials, but it underscores the importance of clearly articulating the sponsor's and the clinical trial site's intentions and obligations during and following a clinical trial.

Pharmaceutical and Medical Device Mass Tort Litigation

Although clinical trials rarely lead to personal injury litigation on a mass scale, clinical trials can play an important, indirect role in mass tort litigation involving FDA-approved medicines and medical devices. For instance, mass tort plaintiffs sometimes point to clinical trial data to allege that a pharmaceutical company overlooked and failed to warn about an important safety issue. Manufacturers often similarly rely on clinical trial data to help refute failure-to-warn claims brought by plaintiffs.

In the *Lipitor* multidistrict litigation, over 3000 women sued a pharmaceutical manufacturer, claiming that they developed diabetes as a result of taking Lipitor (a medicine for treating high cholesterol) and that the manufacturer failed to adequately warn about that risk (*In re: Lipitor (Atorvastatin Calcium) Marketing, Sales Practices & Products Liability Litigation*, 892 F.3d 624, 630 (4th Cir. 2018)). The plaintiffs relied in part on an expert biostatistician who performed analyses of several clinical trials and other studies and concluded that Lipitor led to a statistically significant increased risk of diabetes among those who took the medicine. However, after carefully reviewing the expert's methodology, the court excluded the expert's testimony because his "methodology and application [were] too tainted with potential bias and error to" be reliable (*In re: Lipitor*, 892 F.3d at 633). The court reached the same conclusion as to all of the plaintiffs' other causation experts. Because the plaintiffs ultimately lacked any expert testimony to support their claims, the entire litigation was dismissed. As reflected in the *Lipitor* litigation, clinical trials – and clinical trial data – can play a front-and-center role in lawsuits that do not directly arise out of the conduct of the trials.

Clinical trial-related activities have also been used for jurisdictional purposes in mass tort lawsuits. For example, plaintiffs' attorneys have argued that clinical trial activities conducted in a certain state give courts in that state jurisdiction over (i.e., the authority to decide) product liability cases, including such cases brought by out-of-state plaintiffs against out-of-state defendants – that is, cases that would otherwise have little or nothing to do with the forum state (e.g., a lawsuit brought in a California state court by a Maine resident against a pharmaceutical company based in Indiana). By way of background, in 2017, in the *BMS* case, the U.S. Supreme Court significantly limited courts' jurisdictional reach over out-of-state defendants, holding that non-California plaintiffs could not establish jurisdiction in California courts to sue an out-of-state pharmaceutical company for product liability claims (*Bristol-Myers Squibb Co. v. Superior Court of California*, 137 S. Ct. 1773, 1781 (2017)). The *BMS* decision effectively limited the ability of plaintiffs to shop for favorable forums.

Plaintiffs have since raised novel arguments in their attempts to circumvent the Supreme Court's *BMS* ruling, including arguments that the location of a pharmaceutical company's clinical trials sufficiently establishes jurisdiction in a given state (e.g., allowing a Maine resident to sue an Indiana company in California, merely because some clinical trial activities for the medicine took place in California). Most courts have rejected this strained approach, holding that clinical trials in a given state are insufficient, without more, to create jurisdiction there (*In re: Xarelto Cases*, 2018 WL 809633, at *10–11 (Cal. Super. Ct. Feb. 6, 2018); *Dyson v. Bayer Corp.*, 2018 WL 534375, at *4–5 (E.D. Mo. Jan. 24, 2018); *BeRousse v. Janssen Research & Development, LLC*, 2017 WL 4255075, at *4 (S.D. Ill. Sept. 26, 2017)). A minority of courts, however, have accepted such arguments, relying on the alleged importance of clinical trial work in bringing the product to market. For example, a California federal court exercised jurisdiction over an out-of-state pharmaceutical manufacturer where the plaintiff alleged that "nearly every pivotal clinical trial necessary for [the drugs'] approval involved studying of the ... drugs throughout the State of California" and that without these trials, "the drugs would not have been sold[.]" (*Dubose v. Bristol-Myers Squibb Co.*, 2017 WL 2775034, at *4 (N.D. Cal. June 27, 2017)). Thus, parties facing a dispute over jurisdiction might emphasize (or de-emphasize) the relevance of clinical trials (and/or clinical trial data) to the claims at issue in the litigation.

Summary and Conclusion

Although clinical trials do not ordinarily give rise to litigation on a mass scale, the intersection between clinical trials and the law naturally results in litigation in various isolated circumstances. Such litigation includes, to be sure, personal injury litigation, but it also encompasses litigation in numerous other areas, including contracts, intellectual property, and even criminal prosecutions. By obtaining a working familiarity with the issues that sometimes result in litigation in the setting of clinical trials, sponsors, investigators, and other role players might be able to avoid pitfalls that increase litigation risk in the setting of clinical research.

Cross-References

▶ Post-approval Regulatory Requirements

References

Cases

Abney v. Amgen, Inc., 443 F.3d 540 (6th Cir. 2006)
BeRousse v. Janssen Research & Development, LLC, 2017 WL 4255075 (S.D. Ill. Sept. 26, 2017)
Bristol-Myers Squibb Co. v. Superior Court of California, 137 S. Ct. 1773 (2017)
Brown v. Philadelphia College of Osteopathic Medicine, 760 A.2d 863 (Pa. Super. Ct. 2000)
Cacchillo v. Insmed Inc., 833 F. Supp. 2d 218 (N.D.N.Y. 2011)
Cacchillo v. Insmed Inc., 2013 WL 622220 (N.D.N.Y. Feb. 19, 2013)
Connelly v. Iolab Corp., 1995 WL 250794 (Mo. Ct. App. May 2, 1995)
CTI Clinical Trial Services, Inc. v. Gilead Sciences, Inc., 2013 WL 1641348 (S.D. Ohio Apr. 16, 2013)
Darke v. Estate of Isner, 20 Mass. L. Rptr. 419, 2005 WL 3729113 (Mass. Super. Ct. Nov. 22, 2005)
Dubose v. Bristol-Myers Squibb Co., 2017 WL 2775034 (N.D. Cal. June 27, 2017)
Dyson v. Bayer Corp., 2018 WL 534375 (E.D. Mo. Jan. 24, 2018)
Eli Lilly and Co. v. Zenith Goldline Pharmaceuticals, Inc., 471 F.3d 1369 (Fed. Cir. 2006)
Friter v. Iolab Corp., 607 A.2d 1111 (Pa. Super. Ct. 1992)
Gaston v. Hunter, 588 P.2d 326 (Ariz. Ct. App. 1978)
Heinrich v. Sweet, 308 F.3d 48 (1st Cir. 2002)
In re: Immune Response Securities Litigation, 375 F. Supp. 2d 983 (S.D. Cal. 2005)
In re: Incyte Shareholder Litigation, 2014 WL 707207 (D. Del. Feb. 21, 2014)
In re: Lipitor (Atorvastatin Calcium) Marketing, Sales Practices & Products Liability Litigation, 892 F.3d 624 (4th Cir. 2018)
In re: Xarelto Cases, 2018 WL 809633 (Cal. Super. Ct. Feb. 6, 2018)
Kernke v. The Menninger Clinic, Inc., 173 F. Supp. 2d 1117 (D. Kan. 2001)
Kershaw v. Reichert, 445 N.W.2d 16 (N.D. 1989)
Kus v. Sherman Hospital, 644 N.E.2d 1214 (Ill. App. Ct. 1995)
Liu v. Janssen Research & Development, 2018 WL 272219 (Cal. Ct. App. Jan. 3, 2018)
Looney v. Moore, 886 F.3d 1058 (11th Cir. 2018)
Merck KGaA v. Integra Lifesciences I, Ltd., 545 U.S. 193 (2005)
Milton v. Robinson, 27 A.3d 480 (Conn. App. Ct. 2011)
Moss v. Wyeth Inc., 872 F. Supp. 2d 162 (D. Conn. 2012)
Murthy v. Abbott Laboratories, 847 F. Supp. 2d 958 (S.D. Tex. 2012)
Perez v. Progenics Pharmaceuticals, Inc., 965 F. Supp. 2d 353 (S.D.N.Y. 2013)
Sanofi v. Glenmark Pharmaceuticals Inc., USA, 204 F. Supp. 3d 665 (D. Del. 2016)
Spedale v. Constellation Pharmaceuticals Inc., 2019 WL 3858901 (D. Ariz. Aug. 16, 2019)
Sykes v. U.S., 507 F. App'x 455 (6th Cir. 2012)
Telectronics Pacing Systems, Inc. v. Ventritex, Inc., 982 F.2d 1520 (Fed. Cir. 1992)
Tracy v. Merrell Dow Pharmaceuticals, 569 N.E.2d 875 (Ohio 1991)
Wawrzynek v. Statprobe, Inc., 2007 WL 3146792 (E.D. Pa. Oct. 25, 2007)
Wholey v. Amgen, Inc., 165 A.D.3d 458 (N.Y. App. Div. 2018)
Zeman v. Williams, 2014 WL 3058298 (D. Mass. July 7, 2014)

Statutes and Regulations

21 C.F.R. §§ 50.20, 56.101, 56.103, 312.3, 312.52 & 312.60
31 U.S.C. § 3729(a)
35 U.S.C. § 102
35 U.S.C. § 271

Secondary Sources

Agati A (2006) Clinical research trials in the courtroom. In: Clinical research law and compliance handbook. Jones & Bartlett Publishers, Sudbury
Bal S (2009) An introduction to medical malpractice in the United States. Clin Orthop Relat Res 467:339–347
Chiacchio T (2017) Avoiding drug development clinical trials from being an invalidating public use. IPWatchdog.com, November 9, 2017. https://www.ipwatchdog.com/2017/11/09/drug-development-clinical-trials-invalidating-public-use/id=89799/
ElBoghdady D (2014) SAC's Martoma found guilty of insider trading. Washington Post, February 6, 2014
McAllister D (2007) Are clinical trial sponsors the next target for false claims act enforcement. J Clin Res Best Pract 3(10):1–10
Morreim E (2004) Litigation in clinical research: malpractice doctrines versus research realities. J Law Med Ethics 32:474–484
Morreim E (2005) Clinical trials litigation: practical realities as seen from the trenches. Account Res 12:47–67
Russo A, Johnson J (2015) Research use exemptions to patent infringement for drug discovery and development in the United States. Cold Spring Harb Perspect Med 5:1–10
Tereskerz P (2010) Data safety monitoring boards: legal and ethical considerations for research accountability. Account Res 17:30–50
Tereskerz P (2012) Clinical research and the law. Wiley-Blackwell, London
Valdes S, McGuire P (2004) Contract Research Organizations (CROs) may be the next trend in clinical trials liability. J Biolaw Bus 7:11–15

Biomarker-Driven Adaptive Phase III Clinical Trials

120

Richard Simon

Contents

Introduction	2368
Predictive Biomarkers, Prognostic Biomarkers, and Surrogate Endpoints	2368
Predictive Classifiers	2369
Enrichment Design	2370
Including Both Test Positive and Test Negative Patients in the Clinical Trial	2370
Adaptive Designs for A Candidate Binary Biomarker	2372
Adaptive Threshold Determination	2374
Adaptively Determining Predictive Classifier	2375
Summary	2377
References	2377

Abstract

Developments in cancer genomics have dramatically changed oncology drug development. The discovery of important mutations in tumors has led to the development of drugs which target these alterations. This has rendered obsolete some older paradigms of clinical trial design and analysis. Newer paradigms emphasize use of narrow eligibility enrichment designs when the molecular target and drug are well characterized and adaptive designs when they are not. The pace of progress in tumor biology has accelerated and the size of treatment effects that can be expected when treating the right population has increased. Some of the conventional wisdom about effective clinical trial design that statisticians have taught to clinical investigators needs reevaluation. Success in oncology therapeutics development will be facilitated by the use of new, information-rich designs.

Keywords

Biomarker · Adaptive trial · Enrichment · Resampling · Subset

R. Simon (✉)
R Simon Consulting, Potomac, MD, USA

Introduction

Oncology has undergone major changes in therapeutics development during the past two decades. These changes were driven by the discovery of alterations in tumor genomes which drive the invasion and progression of the disease. Many of these alterations occurred in kinase genes. Such genes act as molecular on/off switches. These kinases served to activate proliferation and survival pathways that were not activated in normal cells. Some of these changes were drugable in the sense that the effect of the mutation could be modulated by treatment. This led to the development of molecularly drugs which could only be expected to be effective for patients whose tumors carried the alterations. These developments led to new paradigms for clinical trials because it was recognized that such drugs would only be effective in the subset of patients whose tumors carried the specific mutation targeted by the drug. I will review some important aspects of these developments.

Predictive Biomarkers, Prognostic Biomarkers, and Surrogate Endpoints

A *biomarker* is any measurement made on a biological system. Biomarkers are used for very different purposes, and this often leads to confusion in discussions of biomarker development, use, and validation. Predictive biomarkers are usually pretreatment measurements used to characterize the patient's disease in order to determine whether the patient is likely to benefit from a particular therapy. The term predictive denotes predicting outcome to a specific treatment. In order to determine whether the benefit is causally related to the treatment, investigators often evaluate whether outcome for biomarker positive patients receiving the treatment is better than biomarker positive patients receiving some other control regimen. The treatment specificity of predictive biomarkers is in contrast to that of prognostic biomarkers which generally are measures of the pace of disease even if patients were untreated and are therefore correlated with outcome regardless of the treatment.

The medical literature is replete with publications on prognostic factors but very few of these are used in clinical practice. For example, Pusztai et al. (2007) identified 939 publications over a 20-year period on prognostic factors in breast cancer but only four factors (ER, PR, HER2, and Oncotype DX) are recommended for use by the American Society of Clinical Oncology. Prognostic factors are often not used unless they help with therapeutic decision-making. Most prognostic factor studies are conducted using a convenience sample of patients whose tissues are available (Simon 2012). The studies are often not focused on a specific therapeutic decision for a characterized set of patients and hence the resulting prognostic factors identified have little therapeutic relevance. Often these patients are too heterogeneous with regard to treatment, stage, and standard prognostic factors to support therapeutically relevant conclusions. Prognostic biomarkers can sometimes be therapeutically relevant if they are developed with an intended use clearly in mind and used for treatment selection (e.g., Paik et al. 2006).

Predictive biomarkers identify patients who are likely or unlikely to benefit from a specific treatment. For example, HER2 amplification is a predictive biomarker for benefit from herceptin (Slamon et al. 2001). The presence of a mutation in the kinase domain of the epidermoid growth factor receptor (EGFR) gene may be a predictive marker for response to EGFR inhibitors (Zhou et al. 2011). A predictive biomarker may be used to identify patients who are poor candidates for a particular drug; for example, colorectal cancer patients whose tumors have KRAS mutations may be poor candidates for treatment with EGFR inhibitors (Lievre et al. 2006).

Many predictive biomarkers are indicators of the presence of genomic alterations important for the invasion and progression of the tumors. The discovery of these markers led to the development of specific drugs to block biochemical pathway activations resulting from the mutations.

Predictive Classifiers

In some cases there are multiple biomarkers which together are predictive for benefit from a specific drug. These biomarkers can be used to define a function whose value indicates whether the patient is likely to benefit from the test treatment or not. This function could be based on separate functions $\mu_T(X)$ and $\mu_C(X)$ which give estimates of the expected outcome for a patient with covariate vector X receiving the test treatment T or control C. The covariate vector X should contain the candidate features which individually are thought to be predictive of response. They may be based on genomic alterations in the tumor. For example, these could be based on logistic regression modeling of the treatment and control groups of an RCT with binary outcome. Then the predictive classifier would be $f(X) = 1$ if $\mu_T(X) - \mu_C(X) \geq \varepsilon$ and $f(X) = 0$ otherwise, where ε reflects clinical significance.

For survival outcome separate prognostic proportional hazards modeling for the treatment and control group is problematic because the baseline hazard functions differ. Consequently, it is preferable to use a joint model such as

$$\log\left(\frac{h(t; X, z)}{h_0(t)}\right) = \alpha z + z\beta'X + (1-z)\eta'X$$

where z is a binary (0,1) indicator of treatment and β and η are regression coefficients for the prognostic effects of the covariate vector in the treatment and control group. With this model, the expected outcome, on the log hazard scale, for the treatment group is $\mu_T(X) = \widehat{\alpha} + \widehat{\beta}'X$ and for the control group $\mu_C(X) = \widehat{\eta}'X$. Consequently the predictive classifier is defined as 1 if $\widehat{\alpha} + \left(\widehat{\beta} - \widehat{\eta}\right)' X \leq \varepsilon$ (sign reversed to reflect log hazard for treatment less than control) and the predictive classifier is 0 otherwise. The value 1 of the predictive classifier indicates that the outcome if the patient receives the active treatment is predicted to be better than otherwise.

Enrichment Design

With an enrichment design, a diagnostic test is used to restrict eligibility for a randomized clinical trial of a regimen comparing a new drug to a control regimen. This design has been used frequently over the past two decades to evaluate drugs which have been developed to inhibit oncogenes discovered by DNA sequencing of tumors.

Simon and Maitournam (2004; Maitournam and Simon 2005) studied the efficiency of this approach relative to the standard approach of randomizing all patients without measuring the diagnostic. They found that the efficiency of the enrichment design can have a dramatic effect on the number of randomized patients needed. They showed that if an enrichment design and a standard design in which the biomarker is not even measured are to have the same statistical power and significance level, the ratio of the number of patients randomized in the two designs is approximately

$$\frac{N_{enrichment}}{N_{standard}} = \left\{ \frac{\gamma_+ TE_+ + (1-\gamma_+) TE_-}{TE_+} \right\}^2$$

This is the square of the ratio of the average treatment effect for the standard design to the treatment effect for the enrichment design. TE_+ and TE_- denote the treatment effects in the biomarker positive and negative patients, respectively, where "treatment effect" indicates the expected outcome under T relative to expected outcome under C for the same biomarker subset of patients. γ_+ denotes the prevalence of positivity for biomarker positive patients. If the drug is not effective at all for negative patients, then the expression simplifies to γ_+^2. So if the biomarker has prevalence 0.50, then the standard design will require four times as many randomized patients as the enrichment design.

The enrichment design is appropriate for contexts where there is a strong biological basis for believing that test negative patients will not benefit from the new drug and that including them would raise ethical concerns.

Including Both Test Positive and Test Negative Patients in the Clinical Trial

When test positive and test negative patients are included in the randomized clinical trial comparing the new treatment to a control, it is essential that an analysis plan be predefined in the protocol for how the predictive classifier will be used in the analysis. It is not sufficient to just stratify the randomization with regard to the classifier without specifying a complete analysis plan. The analysis plan should ensure that the sample size for marker positive patients provides sufficient power for separate analysis of them. Stratifying the randomization by the biomarker serves mainly to ensure that only patients with adequate test results will enter the trial (Simon 2014).

It is important to remember that the purpose of this design is to evaluate the new treatment in the positive and negative subsets determined by the prespecified classifier. The purpose is not to modify or optimize the classifier. If the classifier is a composite gene expression-based classifier, the purpose of the design is not to reexamine the contributions of each component. If one does reexamine contributions of components, then an additional phase III trial may be needed to evaluate treatment benefit in subsets determined by the new classifier.

When biomarker negative patients are included, the objective is usually to evaluate the treatment overall for all patients and for the subset of biomarker positive patients. Because two inferences are of interest, some control for multiple hypothesis testing will generally be required to ensure that the type I error level of the trial does not exceed the targeted 0.05. Several analysis strategies were described by Simon (2013) to control for multiple testing.

(i) In cases where a priori one does not expect the treatment to be effective in the test negative patients unless it is effective in the test positive patients, one might structure the analysis in the following manner: test treatment versus control first in test positive patients using a threshold of significance of 5%. If the treatment difference in test positive patients is not significant at that level, do not perform any other statistical significance tests. If, however, the treatment is significantly better than control in test positive patients, then compare treatment to control overall using a threshold of statistical significance of 5%.

(ii) The traditional statistical analysis strategy is to first test whether there is a significant interaction between biomarker level and treatment effect. That is, test whether the treatment effect in biomarker positive patients equals that in biomarker negative patients. The interaction test is often performed using a significance threshold of 0.10 because the test has limited statistical power. If the interaction test is not significant, then the treatment versus control comparison is evaluated overall, not within levels of the second factor. If the interaction test is significant, then one is justified in evaluating treatment separately for biomarker positive and negative patients. The value of this approach is limited by the ethics of placing sufficient biomarker negative patients on study to have sufficient power for the interaction effect when a priori we have doubts that the treatment will be effective for them.

(iii) Simon and Wang (2006) proposed a fallback analysis plan in which the new treatment group is first compared to the control group overall. If that difference is significant at a reduced significance level such as 0.03, then the new treatment is interpreted to be effective for the population overall and no further testing is done. Otherwise, the new treatment is compared to the control group just for test positive patients. The latter comparison uses a threshold of significance of 0.02, or whatever portion of the traditional 0.05 not used by the initial test. This design was intended for situations where it was expected that the new treatment would be broadly effective; the subset analysis being a fallback option.

Song and Chi (2007) have proposed a refinement of the significance levels used with this option that takes into account the correlation between the test of overall treatment effect and the treatment effect within the test positive subset.

(iv) In the MAST method of Freidlin et al. (2014) one specifies in advance a value α_1 somewhat less than the 0.05 level. If $p_+ \leq \alpha_1$ then we conclude that the test treatment is effective in the biomarker positive patients. If that is the case and also $p_- \leq 0.05$ then we conclude that the treatment is significant overall. If $p_+ \leq \alpha_1$ but $p_- > 0.05$ then we conclude that the treatment is effective only for the marker positive patients. If $p_+ > \alpha_1$ and $p_0 \leq 0.05 - \alpha_1$ then we conclude that the treatment is effective for the overall population where p_0 denotes the p value for treatment effect overall.

None of these analysis plans deal with the need to limit the number of marker negative patients if interim data indicate that the treatment effect is limited to marker positive patients. This is important because the proportion of marker positive patients is generally less than one-half.

Adaptive Designs for A Candidate Binary Biomarker

The most common type of adaptive enrichment in phase III trials involves utilizing a binary candidate biomarker to restrict eligibility. Initially the biomarker is measured, patients are characterized with regard to the biomarker and then randomized to the test treatment or control, but the biomarker is not used to restrict eligibility. At some point during the trial an interim analysis is performed and one of three decisions is made. Either (i) the entire trial is closed for futility, or (ii) the trial continues accruing without any restriction of eligibility until its originally planned sample size is reached, or (iii) accrual is continued only for biomarker positive patients. In the third case, the total target accrual may be increased to adequately power the final analysis for biomarker positive patients.

Several authors have proposed designs for the binary biomarker case described above (Jennison and Turnbull 2007; Wang et al. 2009; Mehta and Gao 2011; Magnusson and Turnbull 2013; Simon and Simon 2013). They contain multiplicity adjustments to account for the fact that inferences are being made for the treatment effect overall and for biomarker positive patients. And the intended use population may be the biomarker positive patients instead of the eligible population.

Several methods have been used for making the decision of how to proceed at the interim analysis. The method of Karuri and Simon (2012) is of interest because the decision is based on a prior for the likelihood that the biomarker is truly predictive. This enables the trial design to be tailored to the degree of confidence the trialists have in that biomarker. The method of Karuri and Simon is fully Bayesian although the threshold of posterior probabilities for decision-making are calibrated to protect the type I error in a frequentist sense.

Interim decision-making may be based on a Bayesian model even when the final analysis is frequentist (Brannath et al. 2009; Simon and Simon 2018). This alleviates the traditional argument between frequentists and Bayesians; both approaches can be useful in a trial but for different purposes. Let us assume that the trial will have one interim analysis and a final analysis. The final analysis will be frequentist and will utilize log-rank p values for testing treatment effect overall and for the biomarker positive patients. The interim analysis will also test those two hypotheses and will also decide whether to continue the trial for all patients, for no patients or just for biomarker positive patients.

For simplicity two-point priors for treatment log hazard ratios are used. The two log hazard ratios are 0 and δ^*. The prior for the biomarker positive and negative strata need not be independent. See the example in Table 1. If $\delta_+ = 0$ then there is very low prior probability that $\delta_- = \delta^*$ meaning that in this case we have good confidence a priori in the biomarker. In this case we probably also would take Pr$[\delta_- = \delta^*|\delta_+ = \delta^*]$ to also be small reflecting the view that the probability of benefit for biomarker negative patients is small. For a setting where we have very little confidence in the biomarker, we might take Pr$[\delta_- = \delta^*|\delta_+ = 0] = Pr[\delta_- = \delta^*|\delta_+ = \delta^*]$ meaning that our view of whether the test treatment will be effective in marker negative patients is not influenced by whether it is effective in biomarker positive patients. We will use Pr$[\delta_- = \delta_+ = 0]$ to calibrate (by simulation) that the type I error of the trial is less than 0.05.

Suppose that at the end of the trial we perform a log-rank test for biomarker positive patients, a log-rank test for biomarker negative patients, and a log-rank test for all randomized patients. As noted above, several methods are available for testing the null hypotheses of interest. Here we suggest using the MAST method of Freidlin et al. (2014).

Using the MAST strategy at the final analysis, the type I error is preserved at 0.05 regardless of the criteria for enrichment used at the interim analysis. The power does depend on the interim analysis criteria however. Let n_2 denote the number of patients planned to be accrued after the interim analysis. Without enrichment these would be unselected patients, but with enrichment they would all be biomarker positive patients. We can compute the predictive probability of rejecting H_0 at the final analysis if we do not enrich (PP$_0$) and the predictive probability of rejecting only H_+ at the final analysis if we do enrich (PP$_+$). From a utility function viewpoint it will be best to enrich only if

$$\gamma_+ PP_+ > PP_0$$

If this is not true, then it would be best not to enrich and either complete accrual with n_2 new unselected patients or to stop for futility, depending on the size of PP$_0$ and the futility parameter ζ employed. If PP$_+ > \zeta$ but PP$_0 < \zeta$ and the above inequality is not true, then it would make sense to continue the trial with enrichment.

Table 1 Example of prior distribution: strong belief in candidate predictive biomarker

	δ_+		
δ_-		0	δ^*
	0	0.48	0.48
	δ^*	0.01	0.01

δ_+ and δ_- are the log hazard ratios of treatment effect for the biomarker positive and negative stratum, respectively. Two-point priors for log hazard treatment ratios with values of 0 and δ^* are used for these priors

Adaptive Threshold Determination

In addition to the design issues with a single binary candidate biomarker as described above, the other very common biomarker setting involves a single quantitative or semiquantitative biomarker that is thought to be predictive of which patients are most likely to benefit. Often previous studies have not established the relationship between biomarker value and likelihood of benefit and there is no adequately determined cut point for positivity. A recent example is the PD-L1 level of expression on nonsmall cell lung tumors as a predictor of response to T cell checkpoint therapy.

Because of regulators' requirements that sponsors demonstrate "statistically significant" effectiveness of the treatment for an intended use population, most sponsors want to have the intended use population defined as the eligible population. This may require using a cut point selected based on inadequate phase II trials. This unfortunately reduces the potential value of the trial for gaining a better understanding of the relationship between biomarker level and treatment effectiveness.

There are very few cases in which investigators use an adaptive design to determine an optimal cut point based on interim data perhaps because they are unaware of the new statistical designs which may achieve this in a statistically valid manner.

Jiang et al. (2007) showed how one could test the null hypothesis of no treatment effect. Their proposed analysis is performed at the end of the trial using the full dataset. This approach is easy to implement as it does not require any changes during the trial. It is "adaptive" in that the intended use population is adaptively determined at the end of the trial.

They begin with comparing outcomes for all patients receiving the new treatment to all control patients. If this difference in outcomes is significant at a prespecified significance level α_1 then the new treatment is considered effective for the eligible population as a whole. Otherwise, a second-stage test is performed using significance threshold $\alpha_2 = 0.05 - \alpha_1$. The second-stage test involves finding the candidate cut point b for the biomarker which leads to the largest treatment versus control treatment effect when restricted to patients with predictive index above b. Jiang et al. maximized the partial log likelihood for proportional hazards models for survival data restricted by each candidate cut point level in order to find b. Let S(b) denote the partial log likelihood for the treatment effect when restricted to patients with predictive index above b. Jiang et al. evaluated the statistical significance of S(b) by randomly permuting the labels of which patients were in the new treatment group and which were controls and determining the maximized partial log likelihood for the permuted data. This is done for thousands of random permutations. If the value S(b) is beyond the $1 - \alpha_2$th percentile of this null distribution created from the random permutations, then the second-stage test is considered significant. They also describe construction of a confidence interval for the optimal cut point b using a bootstrap resampling approach. Simon and Simon (2013) described a general adaptive enrichment framework for clinical trials and illustrated how an optimal cut point can be determined at an interim analysis and used to restrict subsequent eligibility in order to improve the statistical power of the trial.

If the only candidate cut point is the median value of the biomarker, then one can use the design described in section "Adaptive Designs for A Candidate Binary Biomarker" for adaptively determining whether the treatment is effective overall or just for those with biomarker values above the median or for no patients. Instead of using the bivariate prior shown in section "Adaptive Designs for A Candidate Binary Biomarker," one can use a prior giving a 50% prior probability for no treatment effect, a 25% prior probability for an overall treatment effect, and a 25% prior probability that the treatment is effective only for patients with biomarker above the median. At the final analysis, two frequentist hypothesis tests would be performed: one of no overall treatment effect and one of no treatment effect for patients with biomarker values above the median. At the interim analysis one can compute the posterior distribution of the optimal cut point (cut point 0 is interpreted as all patients benefit, cut point 1 is interpreted as no patients benefit). One also computes the predictive probability of rejecting H_0 at the final analysis if patient accrual continues unchanged and the predictive probability of rejecting $H_{0.5}$ at the final analysis if the remaining patients to be accrued are restricted to those with biomarker values above the median. Those predictive probabilities are interpreted as described in section "Adaptive Designs for A Candidate Binary Biomarker."

Adaptively Determining Predictive Classifier

Freidlin and Simon (2005) developed a method for identifying a subset of patients who benefit from the test treatment in an RCT. Although there are numerous methods for subset analysis, the "Adaptive Signature Design" was unique in that it provided an unbiased estimate of the treatment effect in this "intent to treat" subset and a valid significance test of significance for this treatment effect. The adaptive signature design is not limited to high-dimension genomic data; in fact it is best utilized with a moderate number of candidate predictive biomarkers.

At the final analysis the patients randomized in the clinical trial are partitioned randomly into a training set and a validation set. A "predictive classifier" is developed using only training set data. A predictive classifier classifies patients into a subset who are predicted to have better outcome on the test treatment than control and the complementary subset.

There are many ways to define a predictive classifier. With the adaptive signature design, however, one is only permitted to develop a single predictive classifier, and it must be completely specified before the validation set data is used in any way. Finally, the patients in the validation set are classified as likely to benefit from the active treatment ($f(X) = 1$) or not ($f(X) = 0$). The set of covariate vectors for which $f(X) = 1$ is considered the intended use subset S. $S = \{X: f(X) = 1\}$.

Having developed a single predictive classifier using training data, the next step is to evaluate the treatment effect on patients in the validation set with covariate vectors in S. Outcomes of those who received active treatment are compared to outcomes of those who received the control. Since the validation set was not used in development of the classifier, this comparison of outcomes is unbiased and independent of the test set.

Freidlin et al. suggested that the final analysis of an RCT first compare treatment groups overall using a reduced threshold of significance α_{full}, say 0.04. If that overall analysis is not significant, then the dataset is split randomly into a training set and validation set. A predictive classifier is developed on the training set. The cases in the validation set are classified and the treatment effect in classifier positive patients in the validation set is evaluated using a threshold of significance $\alpha_1 = 0.05 - \alpha_{full}$. This preserves the overall type I error level for the trial at 0.05. Practical experience in designing a clinical trial using the adaptive signature design is described by Scher et al. (2011) and by Mi (2017).

Although the adaptive signature design provides a new paradigm for subset analysis of RCTs, its statistical power is limited because of the sample splitting. Freidlin et al. (2010) introduced an improved method called the "Cross-validated Adaptive Signature Design" with improved power for establishing the significance of the treatment effect in the adaptively determined intended use subset. The adaptive signature design is employed at the final analysis after the overall treatment effect is found nonsignificant using a reduced threshold of significance α_{full} as described above. With the cross-validated approach a predictive classifier is trained on the *full* dataset using a prespecified classifier development algorithm A. We denote the resulting predictive classifier as C(A,D) where D denotes the complete dataset.

The original adaptive signature design is based on a K-fold cross-validation using a random partition $(D_1, \ldots, D_K)$. Consider the fold in which subset D_k is withheld. A classifier is trained using algorithm A on $D_{-k} = D - D_k$.

Let C_k denote the classifier developed on D_{-k}. Use this classifier to classify the omitted cases of D_k. Let $\zeta_i = 1$ if $\{i \in D_k\} \cap \{C_k(X_i) = 1\}$, that is case i is both in D_k and is classified by C_k as having better outcome on the test treatment than the control and 0 otherwise. ζ_i is the "pre-validation" classification of patient i (Höfling and Tibshirani 2008). After completing all K-folds of the cross-validation, all of the cases have been classified once. All cases have been classified using a classifier that was developed using a training set that they were not part of.

Let IU = $\{i: \zeta_i = 1\}$ the "intended use" subset based on the prevalidated predictive classifications. Compute the empirical treatment effect in IU, $\widehat{\Delta}(IU)$ and take that as an approximation to the treatment effect in using the full sample classifier C(A,D) with new cases in the future. Simulation studies have shown that this estimator is much better than the resubstitution estimator but somewhat conservative (Freidlin et al. 2010). An alternative approach was described by Zhang et al. (2017).

A confidence interval for treatment effect among future patients classified positive using C(A,D) is approximated by repeating the entire cross-validation procedure with different partitions.

Summary

Developments in cancer genomics and biotechnology are dramatically changing the opportunities for development of more effective cancer therapeutics and molecular diagnostics to guide the use of those treatments. These opportunities can have enormous benefits for patients and for containing health care costs. One of the greatest opportunities is developing predictive biomarkers for the patients who require treatment and are likely to benefit from specific drugs. Co-development of drugs and companion diagnostics add complexity to the development process, however. New paradigms emphasize narrow eligibility enrichment designs when the biology of the target is well understood and which otherwise incorporates prospectively specified analysis plans that enable adaptive identification of the appropriate intended use population in a manner that preserves the study-wise false positive error rates.

These methods have been developed and applied earlier for oncology than for other diseases because of the discovery of strong predictive biomarkers (somatic mutations) in tumors. The effectiveness of many of the methods depends on the existence of strong candidate predictive biomarkers. It is likely, however, that other diseases will be able to use some of the information-rich designs described here.

References

Brannath W, Zuber E, Branson M, Bretz F, Gallo P, Posch M, Racine-Poon A (2009) Confirmatory adaptive designs with Bayesian decision tools for a targeted therapy in oncology. Stat Med 28: 1445–1463

Freidlin B, Simon R (2005) Adaptive signature design: an adaptive clinical trial design for generating and prospectively testing a gene expression signature for sensitive patients. Clin Cancer Res 11:7872–7878

Freidlin B, Jiang W, Simon R (2010) The cross-validated adaptive signature design. Clin Cancer Res 16:691–698

Freidlin B, Korn EL, Gray R (2014) Marker Sequential Test (MaST) design. Clin Trials 11:19–27

Höfling H, Tibshirani R (2008) A study of pre-validation. Ann Appl Stat 2:643–664

Jennison C, Turnbull BW (2007) Adaptive seamless designs: selection and prospective testing of hypotheses. J Biopharm Stat 17:1135–1161

Jiang W, Freidlin B, Simon R (2007) Biomarker-adaptive threshold design: a procedure for evaluating treatment with possible biomarker-defined subset effect. J Natl Cancer Inst 99: 1036–1043

Karuri SW, Simon R (2012) A two-stage Bayesian design for development of new drugs and companion diagnostics. Stat Med 31:901–914

Lievre A, Bachet J-B, Le Corre D, Boige V, Landi B, Emile J-F, Côté J-F, Tomasic G, Penna C, Ducreux M (2006) KRAS mutation status is predictive of response to cetuximab therapy in colorectal cancer. Cancer Res 66:3992–3995

Magnusson BP, Turnbull BW (2013) Group sequential enrichment design incorporating subgroup selection. Stat Med 32:2695–2714

Maitournam A, Simon R (2005) On the efficiency of targeted clinical trials. Stat Med 24:329–339

Mehta CR, Gao P (2011) Population enrichment designs: case study of a large multinational trial. J Biopharm Stat 21:831–845

Mi G (2017) Enhancement of the adaptive signature design for learning and confirming in a single pivotal trial. Pharm Stat 16:312–321

Paik S, Tang G, Shak S, Kim C, Baker J, Kim W, Cronin M, Baehner FL, Watson D, Bryant J (2006) Gene expression and benefit of chemotherapy in women with node-negative, estrogen receptor-positive breast cancer. J Clin Oncol 24:3726–3734

Pusztai L, Anderson K, Hess KR (2007) Pharmacogenomic predictor discovery in phase II clinical trials for breast cancer. Clin Cancer Res 13:6080–6086

Scher HI, Nasso SF, Rubin EH, Simon R (2011) Adaptive clinical trial designs for simultaneous testing of matched diagnostics and therapeutics. Clin Cancer Res 17:6634–6640

Simon R (2012) Clinical trials for predictive medicine. Stat Med 31:3031–3040

Simon RM (2013) Genomic clinical trials and predictive medicine. Cambridge University Press, Cambridge, UK

Simon R (2014) Stratification and partial ascertainment of biomarker value in biomarker-driven clinical trials. J Biopharm Stat 24:1011–1021

Simon R, Maitournam A (2004) Evaluating the efficiency of targeted designs for randomized clinical trials. Clin Cancer Res 10:6759–6763

Simon N, Simon R (2013) Adaptive enrichment designs for clinical trials. Biostatistics 14:613–625

Simon N, Simon R (2018) Using Bayesian modeling in frequentist adaptive enrichment designs. Biostatistics 19:27–41

Simon R, Wang S-J (2006) Use of genomic signatures in therapeutics development in oncology and other diseases. Pharmacogenomics J 6:166–173

Slamon DJ, Leyland-Jones B, Shak S, Fuchs H, Paton V, Bajamonde A, Fleming T, Eiermann W, Wolter J, Pegram M (2001) Use of chemotherapy plus a monoclonal antibody against HER2 for metastatic breast cancer that overexpresses HER2. N Engl J Med 344:783–792

Song Y, Chi GYH (2007) A method for testing a prespecified subgroup in clinical trials. Stat Med 26:3535–3549

Wang S-J, James Hung HJ, O'Neill RT (2009) Adaptive patient enrichment designs in therapeutic trials. Biom J 51:358–374

Zhang Z, Li M, Lin M, Soon G, Greene T, Shen C (2017) Subgroup selection in adaptive signature designs of confirmatory clinical trials. J R Stat Soc C 66:345–361

Zhou C, Wu Y-L, Chen G, Feng J, Liu X-Q, Wang C, Zhang S, Wang J, Zhou S, Ren S (2011) Erlotinib versus chemotherapy as first-line treatment for patients with advanced EGFR mutation-positive non-small-cell lung cancer (OPTIMAL, CTONG-0802): a multicentre, open-label, randomised, phase 3 study. Lancet Oncol 12:735–742

Clinical Trials in Children

121

Gail D. Pearson, Kristin M. Burns, and Victoria L. Pemberton

Contents

Introduction	2380
Why Should We Do Trials in Children?	2380
Historical Perspectives and Protections for Children in Research	2382
Modern Protections and Ethical Considerations	2384
Pediatric Trials: Attitudes and Action	2385
Trial Design	2387
Challenges	2389
Summary and Conclusions	2392
Key Facts	2392
Cross-References	2392
References	2392

Abstract

Clinical trials in children are important and challenging. Many advances in pediatric health have occurred as a result of clinical trials, ranging from the polio vaccine to chemotherapy for childhood leukemia. Nevertheless, the majority of medications prescribed to children have never been evaluated in them. Relatively recent programs to encourage testing of drugs in children have yielded important new information about pharmacokinetics and pharmacodynamics in pediatric populations, often contrary to what might have been expected. Trials are required, therefore, in order to determine not only the effects of drugs but also

---

The content of this chapter is solely the responsibility of the authors and does not necessarily represent the official views of the National Heart, Lung, and Blood Institute or the National Institutes of Health.

G. D. Pearson (✉) · K. M. Burns · V. L. Pemberton
National Heart, Lung, and Blood Institute, National Institutes of Health, Bethesda, MD, USA
e-mail: Gail.pearson@nih.gov; Kristin.burns@nih.gov; Victoria.pemberton@nih.gov

© Springer Nature Switzerland AG 2022
S. Piantadosi, C. L. Meinert (eds.), *Principles and Practice of Clinical Trials*,
https://doi.org/10.1007/978-3-319-52636-2_259

safe doses of medications in light of developmental changes throughout childhood. In addition, clinical trials are necessary in children because they have conditions that adults may not have. Finally, as in the case of early treatment for childhood leukemia, trials in children can help inform treatment in adults with similar conditions. In the current era, there are multiple regulations and strategies to optimize safety of pediatric participants in trials. Trial design in children follows the same principles as any other trial, although particular attention needs to be paid to burden on the child and family and understanding parental perceptions of clinical trials. Pediatric drug formulations and devices may be particularly challenging to develop.

Keywords

Clinical trials · Pediatric · IRB · DSMB · Safety · Intermediate endpoints

Introduction

Clinical trials in children have gone from being completely unregulated to nearly prohibited, to now being carefully overseen and promoted as a public good. There are many reasons why clinical trials should be done in children, including addressing differences from adults in their developing physiology and drug metabolism and the fact that they have diseases that don't occur in adulthood. The volatile past of pediatric clinical research, before the advent of regulations, remains an object lesson for those designing ethical clinical trials today. However, there have been many exciting breakthroughs from research in children, including the polio vaccine and treatment for acute lymphoblastic leukemia. Even with current safeguards, it can be a challenge to persuade caregivers to introduce the topic of trials and to encourage parents to consider allowing their child to participate in a trial. Stimulating pharmaceutical companies to conduct trials in children has required legislation providing significant incentives for drug studies, and yet such incentives are lacking for pediatric device trials. The number of pediatric clinical trials represents a mere fraction of the number of clinical trials in adults (Pasquali et al. 2012). Nevertheless, many dedicated researchers and committed families and children do participate in well-designed trials, resulting in a great deal of valuable information that improves the care of children. This chapter will provide an overview of the history, regulation, and current conduct of clinical trials in children.

Why Should We Do Trials in Children?

The most obvious reason to conduct trials in children is that they are not simply smaller adults. Newborns, infants, and children have physiological responses that change as they grow and are often different from those of adults. As just one example, maturation of the clotting cascade occurs over the first several months to years of life, and at a variable pace, depending on the clotting protein involved. To use antithrombotic agents effectively in children, therefore, clinical trials are needed to assess pharmacokinetics (PK), pharmacodynamics, and effectiveness at several ages.

A corollary of this is that the correct dose of medication for a child cannot be determined by simply adjusting the standard adult dose for body size and weight. Absorption, distribution, metabolism, and elimination differ across the lifespan. In studies of gabapentin, a seizure medication, children less than 5 years of age needed higher doses to achieve a therapeutic state than children over 5, a result that was not intuitive (Haig et al. 2001). Even within a class of drugs, medications can behave differently. For example, tetracyclines demonstrated an increased toxicity in infants and children, while aminoglycosides showed decreased toxicity in newborns. Among antibiotics cleared by the renal system, clearance is decreased in neonates and infants, which could lead to increased exposure and toxicity if dosing is based on adult doses (Le and Bradley 2018). Another example is cyclosporin. Shortly after it was approved for use in adults to suppress the immune response to rejection of an organ transplant, it began to be used in children without performing pediatric clinical trials. When it became clear that it was not as effective in children as in adults, studies found that cyclosporin was metabolized much more quickly in children, and thus different dosing regimens were needed (Hoppu et al. 1991). In fact, the majority of drugs given to children are used off-label, meaning that they have not been tested in children. A median of 9 years passes from approval of adult-use drugs to the inclusion of pediatric data in product labels (Bogue et al. 2016). These examples illustrate the potential dangers of off-label use of drugs.

Another major reason to do trials in children is that children have diseases and conditions that do not occur in adults. With rare exceptions, polio occurs only in children, primarily children ages 5–9 years. The largest medical experiment in history, the Francis Field Trial, began in 1954 and included 750,000 children in a placebo-controlled trial of the polio vaccine and more than one million children in an observational study. Somewhat miraculously for the size of the trial, the results were reported only 14 months later in 1955 (Francis 1955). By 1979, the number of new cases of polio in the United States had dropped to zero (Centers for Disease Control and Prevention 2017), from a 1952 high of 58,000. Sudden infant death syndrome (SIDS) occurs primarily in infants before 4 months of age and has been the subject of research for decades. While the exact causes are still unknown, research has shown that babies who sleep prone have 1.7–12.9 times the risk of SIDS than those who sleep on their backs. Public health campaigns that promote back sleep positions have dramatically reduced the rate of SIDS by >50% in the United States (American Academy of Pediatrics Task Force on Sudden Infant Death 2005). Ongoing research focuses on causes and factors associated with SIDS to further reduce occurrence. Kawasaki disease is another condition that primarily affects children. With the decline in rheumatic heart disease, Kawasaki disease is now the most common acquired pediatric cardiovascular disease in the United States. It is an inflammatory condition of unknown etiology that affects the small- and medium-sized blood vessels, including the coronary arteries. One of its most dangerous sequelae is coronary artery aneurysms, which can thrombose and cause a fatal myocardial infarction in childhood. In the late 1980s, the National Heart, Lung, and Blood Institute funded a clinical trial that demonstrated that the rate of coronary artery aneurysms could be significantly reduced with a regimen of high-dose aspirin and intravenous gamma globulin (Newburger et al. 1986). This trial led to important changes in practice, which are followed to this day.

Clinical trials conducted in children can also benefit adults. One key example is that of acute lymphoblastic leukemia (ALL), which occurs in children as well as in adults. Before the 1960s, survival with childhood ALL was unheard of. However, survival began to improve in the 1960s, when Frei and his colleagues demonstrated the potential for chemotherapy using a combination of two drugs to achieve 2-year survival of about 20% in children (Frei et al. 1961). Subsequent clinical trials are built on this knowledge, and in the present day, pediatric survival is about 90%. These successes with pediatric ALL influenced treatment of adult leukemia by identifying the benefit of combination chemotherapy, as well as the effectiveness of phasing induction, consolidation, and maintenance chemotherapy. In addition, the methodology of relentlessly comparing the standard-of-care chemotherapy regimen with the best long-term survival against the standard plus a particular modification has resulted in the steady rise in cure rate over 50 years (Pui and Evans 2013).

Experience with heart surgery also began in children, and lessons learned from it have benefitted adults. Aside from rare attempts to suture a battlefield laceration, operating on the heart was considered impossible until physicians began thinking about how to palliate congenital heart disease. The first such operation was in 1938, when Robert Gross successfully ligated a patent ductus arteriosus, a remnant of the fetal cardiovascular system that had not closed spontaneously and was causing significant symptoms in a child (Gross and Hubbard 1939). In 1944, Alfred Blalock did the opposite: he created an artificial ductus arteriosus using part of a subclavian artery to provide needed additional pulmonary blood flow in a child with the cyanotic condition known as tetralogy of Fallot (Blalock 1945). This procedure inaugurated not only a new era for congenital heart disease but also effectively launched the entire field of cardiac surgery. Neither of these was a clinical trial, but one could think of them as N-of-1 trials, in which the magnitude of the effect was so large that conventional trials were not needed.

Historical Perspectives and Protections for Children in Research

Many cite the first report of a clinical trial as that of teenage Daniel, as reported in the Bible. Daniel and three other Israelite youths of royal bearing were captured, and a steward was placed in charge of their care by the Babylonian king. To the steward was proposed: "Please test your servants for ten days: Give us nothing but vegetables to eat and water to drink. Then compare our appearance with that of the young men who eat the royal food, and treat your servants in accordance with what you see" (Holy Bible: New International Version 2011). As in a clinical trial, the servants were subjected to a standardized intervention, and data was collected on their outcome.

Early reports of pediatric research included that of Dr. William Watson, the physician who, while caring for abandoned children at the Foundling Hospital in London, tested inoculation strategies to protect against smallpox, the leading cause of death among children (Boylston 2002). In 1767, he conducted a series of experiments in children to determine the best source of the inoculum and whether pretreatment with mercury enhanced survival. He randomized children into small groups, administered three different pretreatments before inoculation, and then compared the number of pocks. His approach to quantitative data was unique for the times in that most previous outcomes were reported qualitatively such as "all the subjects did well" or "half got smallpox."

The nineteenth and early twentieth centuries saw increased experimentation with children in the United States and abroad. While some concerns were expressed about how children were "used" in experiments, particularly orphaned, poor, and institutionalized children, few guidelines on the ethical treatment of children in research existed or were enforced. The first known regulations on the protections of children in research were developed in Prussia in 1900 after healthy children were inoculated with syphilis serum. The directives stated that research should not be conducted in minors or those incompetent for other reasons. A similar incident in the early 1930s, in which healthy German children died or contracted tuberculosis during vaccine studies (1932), spawned the "Guidelines for Human Experimentation" in 1931. The guidelines addressed such issues as voluntary consent, risk commensurate with benefits, and exploitation of disadvantaged persons. They specifically stated that "experimentation involving children or young persons under 18 years of age shall be prohibited if it in any way endangers the child or young person" (Reich 1995). Although these laws remained in effect throughout Germany, they were ignored by the Nazi regime under whose direction, egregious "medical experimentation," was conducted. After World War II, the Nuremberg Code (Shuster 1997) established ten tenets of clinical research ethics that are considered foundational for research conduct today; however, children were not specifically mentioned in the Code. Furthermore, the primary principle stated that "the person involved should have the legal capacity to give consent," which gave rise to controversy about the participation of children in research over the ensuing decades.

The Declaration of Helsinki in 1964 likewise did not mention children or minors but did propose that legal guardians could consent to the participation of "nontherapeutic" research in those who could not legally provide consent (Field and Behrman 2004). It was not until 1973 that the US Department of Health, Education, and Welfare issued a working document on experimentation with children and proposed a number of special protections, but formal regulations were not enacted until 1983. Except for limited revisions, these regulations still govern pediatric research in the United States today. In addition to the regulations, other components essential to the protection of children in research are pediatric-trained investigators and study personnel, institutional review boards (IRBs) with pediatric expertise, well-informed parents and healthcare providers, and research sponsors that support the safety of child participants.

Modern Protections and Ethical Considerations

Based on lessons learned from early research, modern clinical research studies have developed safeguards to protect participants, including IRBs, informed consent/assent, data and safety monitoring boards (DSMBs), and monitoring. Some of these elements warrant additional attention in studies involving children. The Federal Policy for the Protection of Human Subjects, also known as the "Common Rule," describes some of these safeguards, and Title 45, Subpart D of these regulations outlines some additional protections for children as research participants (45 CFR Part 46), including clarifying the circumstances in which it may be permissible to conduct research in children that is more than minimal risk.

IRBs are another critical feature of modern clinical research studies. Independent review of a study by an IRB is a requirement of all studies funded by the NIH and regulated by the FDA, as described in the Code of Federal Regulations, Title 45, Part 46. IRBs are responsible for performing independent review of research protocols, informed consent forms, and patient-facing materials to ensure that the study is ethically appropriate and in compliance with laws and regulations. In addition to the requirement for including a diversity of experience, it is extremely important in pediatric research for IRBs to include expertise in the unique needs of pediatric populations and diseases.

Subpart D of the Code of Federal Regulations also outlines the requirements for obtaining assent, an important feature of pediatric research that respects a child's autonomy despite their status as a minor. In addition to providing one or both parents with information necessary to perform informed consent, children of a certain age (which varies by location) are given the opportunity to indicate their willingness to participate in research by giving assent. When parents and children disagree about participation, a child's dissent overrides parental consent in studies that do not entail direct benefit to the participant. In such situations of disagreement between parents and children about participation of the child in a research study, it is incumbent upon the investigator to carefully broker noncoercive conversations to preserve the process of informed consent and assent.

To ensure the safety of participants and the integrity of the study, DSMBs or data monitoring committees (DMCs) are another standard feature of modern clinical trials. Such boards are comprised of independent experts responsible for periodically evaluating available data and recommending cessation of a study if overwhelming benefit or harm is identified. A DSMB may also recommend stopping a trial if the trial is futile and will not achieve its goals, in order to protect participants from prolonged exposure to an intervention in the setting of a study that will never answer its question. For studies involving children, it is important to include appropriate pediatric expertise on DSMBs to enable identification of safety signals that may be unique to children compared to adults. The NIH-funded Pediatric Heart Network also includes a parent of a child with heart disease on its DSMB, acknowledging the important role that families play in understanding the burden of research participation and identifying potential risks to their children.

Monitoring of studies should be performed to a degree that is commensurate with the degree of risk in the study. For small studies with minimal risk, monitoring by the principal investigator may be adequate, whereas for larger studies that involve vulnerable populations and include more than minimal risk, independent DSMBs are recommended.

Pediatric Trials: Attitudes and Action

Attitudes about children participating in research continue to be diverse. For decades, children were viewed as medication naïve, thus a preferable population for testing new compounds. After a few tragedies resulting in disability and death to children, attitudes shifted, and children were largely excluded from research. Today, most agree that research in children is important to ensure that treatments are safe and effective, acknowledging the differences between children and adults. Current regulations and policies [European Union (European Parliament 2006), United States (Department of Health and Human Services 2018; National Institutes of Health 1998; Food and Drug Administration 2018b), and Japan (Tsukamoto et al. 2016)] address and promote pediatric research, particularly in the arena of drug testing.

Parental perceptions of pediatric research are influenced by many factors, among them risks and benefits, familiarity with research processes, trial uncertainties (e.g., does the doctor know what is best for my child, limited familiarity with the treatment being tested, concern about the "experimental nature" of the study), study burden, and endorsement by their primary care provider (Tait et al. 2004; Miller et al. 2005; Hoberman et al. 2013). While most parents agree that clinical research is necessary to advance treatment of pediatric diseases (Hoffman et al. 2007; Morris et al. 2007), a poll of US adults showed that only one in four would consider allowing their children to participate in clinical research studies (Guary 2004). In addition to the burden of decision-making on behalf of a child, other research indicates that this contradiction may also be related to how parents of sick versus healthy children view the benefits and value of research (Caldwell et al. 2003; Maayan-Metzger et al. 2008). In fact, parents are often confused about the role of healthy children in research, expressing concerns about exposing them to unnecessary procedures or testing (Marceau et al. 2016). Minority parents' decisions about participating in research are influenced by their attitudes about the healthcare system in general, level of trust in medical researchers, cultural beliefs, and incentives to participate (Braunstein et al. 2008; Rajakumar et al. 2009; Cunningham-Erves et al. 2019).

When children are asked about their attitudes related to participating in research, they are largely positive and cite helping themselves and others and financial incentives as key motivators. While parents focus on benefits, risks, and harms, child participants tend to consider things that might cause physical discomfort or disrupt their schedules and lives (Varma et al. 2008; Unguru et al. 2010; Greenberg et al. 2018).

Pediatricians and pediatric nurses agree that research is important but report that, because their primary responsibility is to care for an individual patient, they feel conflicted about encouraging parents to consider research, an activity that provides no guarantee of benefit to any individual child. Pediatricians also cite time burden, lack of resources, fear of losing patients, and lack of incentives among reasons for not referring families to research opportunities (Caldwell et al. 2002; Singhal et al. 2004; Mudd et al. 2008).

Stakeholders agree that pediatric research is essential to improving the health of children. The contradiction between this belief and actual agreement to participate continues to plague researchers. Potential participants see the value in the forms of increased health awareness, potential for extra care and attention, making a valued contribution to help themselves and others, and access to new treatment options (Hoberman et al. 2013; Cunningham-Erves et al. 2019; Pemberton and Pearson 2019a). Although several factors are known to be associated with willingness to participate in research, such as educational level, race, socioeconomic status, risks and study burdens, and benefits and trust, testing strategies to improve recruitment into pediatric clinical trials is still needed.

An important strategy may be educating families, healthcare providers, and pediatric researchers about pediatric research. Development of educational programs could improve trust in medical researchers (Cunningham-Erves et al. 2019). Traditional educational approaches have included study brochures, consent forms, face-to-face discussions, and presentations; but accessibility to information online is quickly replacing or supplementing these more conventional methods. An evaluation of an online education program sponsored by the NIH, Children and Clinical Studies (Pemberton and Pearson 2019a), showed that enabling parents to hear from other parents whose children are involved in research provides a personal connection. In addition, the online education program explained general research concepts such as randomization, blinding, and voluntariness, which they deemed necessary to supplement information received about a specific study (Marceau et al. 2016). Broadcast media may also enjoy a role in educating the public. For instance, participants had significant improvement in knowledge and perceptions of pediatric research across many domains after viewing a broadcast documentary, "If Not for Me" (Marceau et al. 2018). And materials appealing to children, like video games and comics, are important to educating and empowering them to learn about pediatric research (Pemberton and Pearson 2019b).

Pediatric clinical trial networks or consortia can address some of the challenges of pediatric research due to their expertise in conducting studies in children. Networks can focus on specific diseases (e.g., the Children's Oncology Group and the Pediatric Heart Network), or they can conduct research in specific care settings (e.g., Pediatric Research in Office Settings, Pediatric Emergency Care Research Network, Collaborative Pediatric Critical Care Network), on a specific age group (e.g., Neonatal Research Network), or on some aspect of child health like medication testing (e.g., Pediatric Trials Network). These collaborative entities typically incorporate hospitals and practices that specialize in the care of children and have robust research infrastructure with experienced research coordinators, nurses, and doctors.

Conducting safe, transparent research within ethical and regulatory guidelines in pediatric-friendly environments is a hallmark of these networks and can foster trust among participants.

Patient advocacy groups can also play a role in promoting pediatric research. In congenital heart disease research, these groups often partner with investigators to support and disseminate information about pertinent studies and provide a forum for parents to ask questions and discuss their experiences in research. Leveraging the expertise of parents and patient advocates to create proper messaging and make appropriate connections is a helpful strategy that can benefit participants and research teams.

Trial Design

Clinical trial design for children follows the same principles as for adults, described in detail elsewhere in this book. Investigators must have a clinically relevant research question, a suitable hypothesis, accurate information about effect size, an appropriate statistical analysis approach, a valid recruitment plan, and drug or device supply and regulatory approval as needed. However, there are a number of challenges for trial design and execution in children that are unique to this population.

In both pediatric and adult trials, a clinically relevant research question may differ depending on whether you are the researcher or the parent/participant. For example, in a survey of adult patients with congenital heart disease and their physicians, research priorities were different. Patients were interested in research questions that affect them directly, including topics like insurance and exercise. Physicians wanted answers to questions that arise regularly in their clinical practice (Cotts et al. 2014). Many rare pediatric conditions have active patient advocacy groups that can be an excellent source of input when choosing a research question.

The most important consideration in designing a trial involving children is safety. Families and providers need to be absolutely certain that all appropriate safeguards have been brought to bear. Compared to trials in adults, this may mean additional monitoring visits, safety labs, study measures focused on growth and development, and different monitoring strategies in a single trial. If a new drug is being tested, a child may need to be monitored for a longer period of time after their first dose in the study clinic than an adult. DSMBs or DMCs should have expertise in pediatrics and pediatric research and ethics. When medical monitors are appointed, they also should be pediatricians with expertise in clinical research.

Perhaps the most important thing to consider after safety is burden on the child and family. When a child is enrolled in a trial, the burden falls not only on the child but also on the parents, and possibly siblings, and these factors need to be taken into careful consideration. The majority of children attend school, and parents may need to take off work to bring the child for study visits, so the number and length of visits should be considered very carefully and minimized. When possible, strategies for obtaining data remotely should be incorporated into the trial design, either via telehealth strategies, the electronic health record, sensors, or wearables or by a visiting medical research service. When visits to the research center are required, the visit schedule should be adjusted to accommodate school and parental work schedules. Adequate reimbursement should be provided to the family for travel and lodging, and ideally some arrangements may be provided for daycare for siblings. Again, this is an area where parents and patient advocacy groups can be extremely helpful and their advice should be sought.

The gold standard for any trial is an endpoint that can be readily measured and clearly contributes to health outcomes, such as cancer recurrence, clinically significant anemia, or death. Because children are generally healthy, even those with rare diseases, such so-called hard endpoints are not common. Moreover, some other endpoints that are well-accepted for adult studies are not feasible, such as the 6-min walk test to measure cardiorespiratory fitness, which cannot be performed by young children.

Endpoint selection has been addressed in pediatric cardiovascular drug trials, and the principles are broadly applicable to other pediatric research (Torok et al. 2018). When intermediate endpoints, rather than hard endpoints, are required, such endpoints should have been shown to predict a potential benefit of the therapy. In addition, combining several intermediate endpoints may be more informative in identifying a treatment response. Although it is not a hard endpoint, quality of life is an example of a relevant endpoint for the pediatric population and their parents. Pediatric quality-of-life assessment tools have been evaluated and validated in children and are being used more and more in pediatric clinical trials. Finally, the FDA has established a process, "Accelerated Approval of New Drugs for Serious or Life-Threatening Illnesses" (Food and Drug Administration 2018b), that permits drug approval based on a credible intermediate endpoint, but has not been used very much in pediatric studies.

Designing trials for children with rare diseases, particularly those that can be fatal at a young age, can be particularly challenging. In many cases, randomization is neither possible nor palatable to families. In the extreme example of progeria, a very rare condition associated with rapidly accelerated aging and death before adulthood, the number of possible trial participants is less than 100, and no family will accept being enrolled into a placebo arm. On the other hand, families are very motivated to include their children in a trial of any promising therapy. In a situation like this with a small sample size, it is important to collect measurements repeatedly over time, allowing for assessment of within-patient changes.

A number of innovative trial designs have gained currency in recent years, including the use of remote monitoring through devices and wearables, trials within a registry, precision medicine trials, and the use of real-world evidence and real-world data in trials. Most of these approaches have had limited application in children. The STRESS trial (STeroids to REduce Systemic Inflammation After Neonatal Heart Surgery; NCT03229538) is one of the first pediatric trials to use a registry, in this case the Society of Thoracic Surgeons Congenital Heart Surgery Database (STS-CHSD), to provide a significant amount of data for the trial. New technologies are emerging rapidly for monitoring physiological parameters using smartphones and wearable sensors, but there has been little or no application to pediatric research. A good review of pediatric precision medicine trials, which to date have found their greatest applicability in oncology, is provided by Suzanne Forrest and her colleagues (Forrest et al. 2018). These trials require clinical genomic sequencing, actionable targets, and evidence indicating that identified genetic variants are responsive to therapy. A number of precision medicine trials are underway in pediatric oncology. Such trial designs may be useful in other pediatric conditions as well.

Challenges

All clinical trials have challenges, but pediatric trials have to overcome some unique challenges not present in trials of adults.

Consent and assent. A child's participation in a clinical trial requires that the parents provide informed consent. In many cases, this can be done by only one parent, but in cases in which the research presents more than minimal risk and offers no prospect of direct benefit to a child, then both parents may be asked to consent, if they are available.

In addition to parents consenting to a child's participation in a trial, children also must agree, or assent, to be in a trial, which requires an additional, age-appropriate informed assent form. The age at which assent is required varies by state, country, institution, and IRB; in some cases it can be as young as 7 years old. The age at which children reach majority also varies by state. In most cases, the age is 18 years, but there are also exceptions at younger ages for pregnancy and marriage. In studies that include adolescents who will reach the age of majority during the study, there must also be provisions to re-consent participants when they reach the age of majority. This is an additional administrative burden for trials, and participants may withdraw when they are required to consent for themselves.

Recruitment and retention. Recruitment is the Achilles heel of most clinical trials. It is made more difficult by the fact that most physicians and patients do not understand what is involved with participating in a trial. The NIH has developed resources to provide families and children with accessible information, including from families and children themselves, about participating in clinical research (Pemberton and Pearson 2019a).

For pediatric trials in rare diseases or life-threatening conditions, recruitment of families and children to participate may be easier than for trials in other pediatric conditions or in adults. In addition, many childhood diseases have one or more patient advocacy groups with whom recruitment partnerships can be very productive. Social media may be used to direct families to clinical trial sites and potentially to obtain and complete the informed consent process electronically.

Once children are enrolled in a trial, the next challenge is retaining them. Retention, like recruitment, can be affected by the type of condition under study. Parents of children with rare or serious conditions are likely to be more motivated to continue in the trial in order to help advance the science. Retention is also heavily affected by the burden imposed by the trial. A trial with several visits a year will be hard to manage with school and activity schedules. In addition, if the parent needs to bring other children in the family not participating in the trial, provisions may need to be made for supervision for those children during the study visit. Therefore, it behooves the designers of pediatric trials to work hard to minimize visits and other aspects of trial burden while still being able to answer the scientific question. Until pediatric wearables and other sensors become more widespread, one way to address this issue is to use companies that can send professionals to the home and conduct study visits there. Another approach is to make use of data in electronic health records to populate study data where possible. Many older children and adolescents have requirements for community service in their schools, and participation in a clinical trial can fulfill some of these requirements. Finally, parents and members of advocacy groups may be helpful in designing a study that is scientifically rigorous while being child and family friendly.

Formulations and pharmacokinetics. Creating drug formulations that are appropriate for children can add quite a bit of time and expense to a trial and has been one of the barriers to testing adult therapies in children. Creating a liquid formulation often requires extensive work to identify a safe and effective vehicle and then may require lengthy stability testing under various conditions before it can be used in a trial. Among the reasons that the US FDA's oversight powers were increased in 1938 to require that drugs be demonstrated to be safe before public distribution was a disaster arising from a toxic diluent. At the dawn of the antimicrobial era, several companies made preparations of the first effective antibiotic, sulfanilamide. One company recognized the need for a liquid preparation and formulated Elixir Sulfanilamide, which underwent no toxicity testing. Unfortunately, the diluent was 72% diethylene glycol, a sweet-tasting liquid known at the time as an excellent solvent. More than 350 patients received this formulation, and 105 of them, including 34 children, died from renal and liver failure (Wax 1995).

When a liquid preparation is not available, another option may be to use pills that can be dissolved in a small amount of food. This is often a successful strategy, but it requires the child to consume all of the drug-containing food (Food and Drug Administration 2018a). Chewable pills are yet another option. These and other challenges help explain why the majority of drugs that children receive are not labeled for pediatric use.

In addition to challenges with formulation, identifying the correct dose to give to children at different ages and developmental stages requires detailed PK testing, because dosing cannot just be extrapolated from adults. This means that blood must be drawn from children multiple times, and a method must exist for quantitating the drug in a small amount of blood. Multiple factors affect drug absorption and disposition in children, including size and body composition, physiology, and biochemistry. Study of pediatric PK has been accelerated by the passage of the 1997 FDA Modernization Act, the 2002 Best Pharmaceuticals for Children Act, and the 2003 Pediatric Research Equity Act, all of which recognized the unique needs of children. Through studies conducted since passage of these laws, a great deal of information has been learned about differential drug absorption, distribution, metabolism, and elimination in children at different ages (Lu and Rosenbaum 2014). These laws have made it easier to identify the appropriate dose for drugs administered to children clinically and in a trial and also have provided much-needed incentives to industry to develop and study pediatric therapies.

Devices. Just as with drugs, research on pediatric devices is hampered by the absence of devices suitable for children and the challenges in developing such devices. Such devices often will have a small market compared to similar use in adults, and thus companies perceive a low return on investment, coupled with the increased risk of pediatric research. Miniaturizing any device involves multiple unique design considerations, many of which may take considerable time and expense, with no guarantee of success. Recognizing this, Congress passed legislation in 2007 providing for the FDA to fund consortia to stimulate research on pediatric medical devices. The FDA-funded Pediatric Device Consortia Grants Program started in 2009. Since then, about 20 devices have been studied and have made it to market.

Study visits and monitoring. Study visits in pediatric trials are likely to require more time and potentially more staff than for trials in adults. Measuring an infant, for example, may require more than one person, whereas an adult can get on a scale and stadiometer independently. Children may be less compliant with study procedures, which will then require more time to complete. When starting a new study drug, children, particularly young children, may require more extensive on-site monitoring, which also requires more time spent during the study visit. Although there are a number of wearable sensors for adults now that can be employed in trials, there are few, if any, for children, so that more monitoring needs to be done at the study site rather than remotely.

Follow-up. Another aspect of monitoring is longitudinal follow-up. Because children are growing and developing, effects of an intervention, particularly a drug, may not be seen for years. An example is drugs that could affect somatic growth. An effect on final height would not be known until the completion of puberty. It may also be important to follow children longitudinally if they have undergone a procedure or had extensive therapy at an early age to see what the long-term effects might be. The Pediatric Heart Network conducted a trial comparing two surgical strategies in newborns with single ventricle heart disease, which showed that one of the strategies conferred improved 1-year transplant-free survival compared to the other (Ohye et al. 2010). However, longer-term follow-up revealed that this survival advantage disappeared within a few years and that the initially preferred strategy was associated with an excess of additional procedures (Newburger et al. 2018). Another example is the Childhood Cancer Survivor Study, first funded by the National Cancer Institute in 1994 (Robison et al. 2009). This study has enrolled nearly 25,000 individuals who were treated in childhood in two different treatment eras and a small number of their siblings. In addition to identifying late effects of both the underlying condition and the treatments, these two cohorts provide useful information about the transition from childhood to adulthood, a phase of increasing interest to researchers and policy-makers.

Summary and Conclusions

Children deserve to have the best medical care and the best science applied to their health. One way to accomplish this is to conduct well-designed, robust clinical trials on conditions that affect children. We now have the tools to study children safely in trials, including strategies to recruit and retain children in studies and regulations conferring protections for children during trial participation. As an additional benefit, trial results in children may also help adults. Pediatric healthcare providers and pediatric clinical investigators need to continue efforts to educate families about the availability and importance of clinical trials in children.

Key Facts

- Clinical trials are important tools to improve pediatric health.
- Tensions between believing pediatric research is critical to improved health, and actual willingness to participate must be addressed through education and information.
- Children's developmental trajectories mean that adult treatments cannot just be downsized.
- Robust regulations and other tools have been developed to optimize safety in pediatric trials.

Cross-References

▶ Orphan Drugs and Rare Diseases

References

(1932) BERLIN: appeal taken from the decision in the Luebeck case. JAMA 98(15):1316–1317
American Academy of Pediatrics Task Force on Sudden Infant Death (2005) The changing concept of sudden infant death syndrome: diagnostic coding shifts, controversies regarding the sleeping environment, and new variables to consider in reducing risk. Pediatrics 116(5):1245–1255
Blalock ATH (1945) The surgical treatment of malformations of the heart. JAMA 128(3):189–202
Bogue C, DiMeglio LA, Maldonado S, Portman RJ, Smith PB, Sullivan JE, Thompson C, Woo H, Flinn S (2016) Special article: 2014 pediatric clinical trials forum. Pediatr Res 79(4):662–669
Boylston AW (2002) Clinical investigation of smallpox in 1767. N Engl J Med 346(17):1326–1328
Braunstein JB, Sherber NS, Schulman SP, Ding EL, Powe NR (2008) Race, medical researcher distrust, perceived harm, and willingness to participate in cardiovascular prevention trials. Medicine (Baltimore) 87(1):1–9
Caldwell PH, Butow PN, Craig JC (2002) Pediatricians' attitudes toward randomized controlled trials involving children. J Pediatr 141(6):798–803
Caldwell PH, Butow PN, Craig JC (2003) Parents' attitudes to children's participation in randomized controlled trials. J Pediatr 142(5):554–559

Centers for Disease Control and Prevention (2017) Polio elimination in the United States. https://www.cdc.gov/polio/us/index.html. Accessed 14 June 2019

Cotts T, Khairy P, Opotowsky AR, John AS, Valente AM, Zaidi AN, Cook SC, Aboulhosn J, Ting JG, Gurvitz M, Landzberg MJ, Verstappen A, Kay J, Earing M, Franklin W, Kogon B, Broberg CS, Alliance for Adult Research in Congenital Cardiology (2014) Clinical research priorities in adult congenital heart disease. Int J Cardiol 171(3):351–360

Cunningham-Erves J, Deakings J, Mayo-Gamble T, Kelly-Taylor K, Miller ST (2019) Factors influencing parental trust in medical researchers for child and adolescent patients' clinical trial participation. Psychol Health Med 24(6):691–702

Holy Bible: New International Version (2011) Daniel 1:12–16. Biblica

Department of Health and Human Services (2018) Electronic code of Federal Regulations. https://www.ecfr.gov. Accessed 30 May 2019

European Parliament (2006) Regulation (EC) No 1901/2006 of the European Parliament and of the Council on Medicinal Products for Paediatric Use: L 378/371–319. https://ec.europa.eu/health/sites/health/files/files/eudralex/vol-1/reg_2006_1901/reg_2006_1901_en.pdf. Accessed 30 May 2019

Field MJ, Behrman RE (eds) (2004) Ethical conduct of clinical research involving children. National Academies Press, Washington, DC

Food and Drug Administration (2018a) FDA guidance, use of liquids and/or soft foods as vehicles. https://www.fda.gov/downloads/Drugs/GuidanceComplianceRegulatoryInformation/Guidances/UCM614401.pdf. Accessed 30 May 2019

Food and Drug Administration (2018b) Code of federal regulations title 21: subpart H–accelerated approval of new drugs for serious life threatening illnesses. https://www.accessdata.fda.gov/scripts/cdrh/cfdocs/cfcfr/CFRSearch.cfm?CFRPart=314&showFR=1&subpartNode=21:5.0.1.1.4.8. Accessed 29 May 2019

Forrest SJ, Geoerger B, Janeway KA (2018) Precision medicine in pediatric oncology. Curr Opin Pediatr 30(1):17–24

Francis TJ (1955) Evaluation of the 1954 poliomyelitis vaccine field trial: further studies of results determining the effectiveness of poliomyelitis vaccine (Salk) in preventing paralytic poliomyelitis. J Am Med Assoc 158:1266–1270

Frei E, Freireich EJ, Gehan E, Pinkel D, Holland JF, Selawry O, Haurani F, Spurr CL, Hayes DM, James GW, Rothberg H, Sodee DB, Rundles RW, Schroeder LR, Hoogstraten B, Wolman IJ, Traggis DG, Cooper T, Gendel BR, Ebaugh F, Taylor R (1961) Studies of sequential and combination antimetabolite therapy in acute leukemia: 6-mercaptopurine and methotrexate. Blood 18:431–454

Greenberg RG, Gamel B, Bloom D, Bradley J, Jafri HD, Nambiar S, Wheeler C, Tiernan R, Smith PB, Roberts J, Benjamin DK Jr (2018) Parents' perceived obstacles to pediatric clinical trial participation: findings from the clinical trials transformation initiative. Contemp Clin Trials Commun 9:33–39

Gross RE, Hubbard JP (1939) Surgical ligation of a patent ductus arteriosus: report of first successful case. JAMA 112:729–731

Guary J (2004) Only a quarter (25%) of U.S. adults would consider allowing a child of theirs to participate in a clinical research study. Health Care News 4(17):1–8

Haig GM, Bockbrader HN, Wesche DL, Boellner SW, Ouellet D, Brown RR, Randinitis EJ, Posvar EL (2001) Single-dose gabapentin pharmacokinetics and safety in healthy infants and children. J Clin Pharmacol 41(5):507–514

Hoberman A, Shaikh N, Bhatnagar S, Haralam MA, Kearney DH, Colborn DK, Kienholz ML, Wang L, Bunker CH, Keren R, Carpenter MA, Greenfield SP, Pohl HG, Mathews R, Moxey-Mims M, Chesney RW (2013) Factors that influence parental decisions to participate in clinical research: consenters vs nonconsenters. JAMA Pediatr 167(6):561–566

Hoffman TM, Taeed R, Niles JP, McMillin MA, Perkins LA, Feltes TF (2007) Parental factors impacting the enrollment of children in cardiac critical care clinical trials. Pediatr Cardiol 28(3):167–171

Hoppu K, Koskimies O, Holmberg C, Hirvisalo EL (1991) Pharmacokinetically determined cyclosporine dosage in young children. Pediatr Nephrol 5(1):1–4

Le J, Bradley JS (2018) Optimizing antibiotic drug therapy in pediatrics: current state and future needs. J Clin Pharmacol 58(Suppl 10):S108–S122

Lu H, Rosenbaum S (2014) Developmental pharmacokinetics in pediatric populations. J Pediatr Pharmacol Ther 19(4):262–276

Maayan-Metzger A, Kedem-Friedrich P, Kuint J (2008) Motivations of mothers to enroll their newborn infants in general clinical research on well-infant care and development. Pediatrics 121 (3):e590–e596

Marceau LD, Welch LC, Pemberton VL, Pearson GD (2016) Educating parents about pediatric research: children and clinical studies website qualitative evaluation. Qual Health Res 26 (8):1114–1122

Marceau LD, Cho E, Coleman J, Liao W, Dennin S (2018) Evaluating the film if not for me: children and clinical studies. Clin Pediatr (Phila) 328–335. https://doi.org/10.1177/0009922818817799

Miller VA, Drotar D, Burant C, Kodish E (2005) Clinician-parent communication during informed consent for pediatric leukemia trials. J Pediatr Psychol 30(3):219–229

Morris MC, Besner D, Vazquez H, Nelson RM, Fischbach RL (2007) Parental opinions about clinical research. J Pediatr 151(5):532–537, 537 e531–535

Mudd LM, Pham X, Nechuta S, Elliott MR, Lepkowski JM, Paneth N, Michigan Alliance for the National Children's Study (2008) Prenatal care and delivery room staff attitudes toward research and the National Children's Study. Matern Child Health J 12(6):684–691

National Institutes of Health (1998) NIH policy and guidelines on the inclusion of children as participants in research involving human subjects. https://grants.nih.gov/grants/guide/notice-files/not98-024.html. Accessed 30 May 2019

Newburger JW, Takahashi M, Burns JC, Beiser AS, Chung KJ, Duffy CE, Glode MP, Mason WH, Reddy V, Sanders SP et al (1986) The treatment of Kawasaki syndrome with intravenous gamma globulin. N Engl J Med 315(6):341–347

Newburger JW, Sleeper LA, Gaynor JW, Hollenbeck-Pringle D, Frommelt PC, Li JS, Mahle WT, Williams IA, Atz AM, Burns KM, Chen S, Cnota J, Dunbar-Masterson C, Ghanayem NS, Goldberg CS, Jacobs JP, Lewis AB, Mital S, Pizarro C, Eckhauser A, Stark P, Ohye RG, Pediatric Heart Network Investigators (2018) Transplant-free survival and interventions at 6 years in the SVR trial. Circulation 137(21):2246–2253

Ohye RG, Sleeper LA, Mahony L, Newburger JW, Pearson GD, Lu M, Goldberg CS, Tabbutt S, Frommelt PC, Ghanayem NS, Laussen PC, Rhodes JF, Lewis AB, Mital S, Ravishankar C, Williams IA, Dunbar-Masterson C, Atz AM, Colan S, Minich LL, Pizarro C, Kanter KR, Jaggers J, Jacobs JP, Krawczeski CD, Pike N, McCrindle BW, Virzi L, Gaynor JW, for the Pediatric Heart Network Investigators (2010) Comparison of shunt types in the Norwood procedure for single-ventricle lesions. N Engl J Med 362(21):1980–1992

Pasquali SK, Lam WK, Chiswell K, Kemper AR, Li JS (2012) Status of the pediatric clinical trials enterprise: an analysis of the US ClinicalTrials.gov registry. Pediatrics 130(5):e1269–e1277

Pemberton VL, Pearson GD (2019a) Children and clinical studies. http://www.childrenandclinicalstudies.org/. Accessed 29 May 2019

Pemberton VL, Pearson GD (2019b) Children and clinical studies – the kids files. http://www.childrenandclinicalstudies.org/the-kids-files. Accessed 29 May 2019

Pui CH, Evans WE (2013) A 50-year journey to cure childhood acute lymphoblastic leukemia. Semin Hematol 50(3):185–196

Rajakumar K, Thomas SB, Musa D, Almario D, Garza MA (2009) Racial differences in parents' distrust of medicine and research. Arch Pediatr Adolesc Med 163(2):108–114

Reich WT (1995) Encyclopedia of bioethics. Macmillan, New York. Appendix 2762–2763

Robison LL, Armstrong GT, Boice JD, Chow EJ, Davies SM, Donaldson SS, Green DM, Hammond S, Meadows ST, Mertens AC, Mulvihill JJ, Nathan PC, Neglia JP, Packer RJ, Rajaraman P, Sklar CA, Stovall M, Strong LC, Yasui Y, Zeltzer LK (2009) The Childhood Cancer Survivor Study: a National Cancer Institute-supported resource for outcome and intervention research. J Clin Oncol 27(14):2308–2318

Shuster E (1997) Fifty years later: the significance of the Nuremberg Code. N Engl J Med 337(20):1436–1440

Singhal N, Oberle K, Darwish A, Burgess E (2004) Attitudes of health-care providers towards research with newborn babies. J Perinatol 24(12):775–782

Tait AR, Voepel-Lewis T, Malviya S (2004) Factors that influence parents' assessments of the risks and benefits of research involving their children. Pediatrics 113(4):727–732

Torok RD, Li JS, Kannankeril PJ, Atz AM, Bishai R, Bolotin E, Breitenstein S, Chen C, Diacovo T, Feltes T, Furlong P, Hanna M, Graham EM, Hsu D, Ivy DD, Murphy D, Kammerman LA, Kearns G, Lawrence J, Lebeaut B, Li D, Male C, McCrindle B, Mugnier P, Newburger JW, Pearson GD, Peiris V, Percival L, Pina M, Portman R, Shaddy R, Stockbridge NL, Temple R, Hill KD (2018) Recommendations to enhance pediatric cardiovascular drug development: report of a multi-stakeholder think tank. J Am Heart Assoc 7(4):e007283. https://doi.org/10.1161/JAHA.117.007283

Tsukamoto K, Carroll KA, Onishi T, Matsumaru N, Brasseur D, Nakamura H (2016) Improvement of pediatric drug development: regulatory and practical frameworks. Clin Ther 38(3):574–581

Unguru Y, Sill AM, Kamani N (2010) The experiences of children enrolled in pediatric oncology research: implications for assent. Pediatrics 125(4):e876–e883

Varma S, Jenkins T, Wendler D (2008) How do children and parents make decisions about pediatric clinical research? J Pediatr Hematol Oncol 30(11):823–828

Wax PM (1995) Elixirs, diluents, and the passage of the 1938 Federal Food, Drug and Cosmetic Act. Ann Intern Med 122(6):456–461

Trials in Older Adults

122

Sergei Romashkan and Laurie Ryan

Contents

Introduction	2398
Ethics in Geriatric Clinical Trials	2398
Barriers to Participation, Recruitment, and Retention of Older Adults in Clinical Trials	2400
Selection of Outcomes Important to Older Adults	2403
Effects of Multimorbidity and Polypharmacy on Trial Design	2404
Time to Benefit, Time to Harm, and Life Expectancy	2405
Multifactorial Interventions	2406
Selecting Modifiable Risk Factors to Target	2407
Selecting Components of a Multicomponent Intervention	2407
Defining Eligibility Criteria	2407
Treatment Allocation, Outcome Assessment, and Adjudication	2407
Assignment of Components of the Intervention	2408
Sample Size Calculations	2408
Estimating Individual Component Effects	2408
Considerations for Trials for Alzheimer's Disease and Other Age-Related Dementias	2409
Background	2409
Target Population/Stage of Disease	2409
Challenges for Clinical Meaningfulness in Predementia Populations	2410
Participation, Recruitment, Retention in AD and Related Dementia Trials	2410
Conclusion	2412
Key Facts	2413
References	2413

S. Romashkan (✉) · L. Ryan
National Institutes of Health, National Institute on Aging, Bethesda, MD, USA
e-mail: romashks@nia.nih.gov; ryanl@mail.nih.gov

© This is a U.S. Government work and not under copyright protection in the U.S.;
foreign copyright protection may apply 2022
S. Piantadosi, C. L. Meinert (eds.), *Principles and Practice of Clinical Trials*,
https://doi.org/10.1007/978-3-319-52636-2_260

Abstract

This chapter discusses several unique features of clinical trials in older adults such as ethics in geriatric medicine research; recruitment and retention, including barriers to participation by older adults in clinical trials; selection of outcomes that are important to this population; effects of polypharmacy and multimorbidity on trial design; time to benefit, time to harm and life expectancy; and multimodal interventions targeting numerous risk factors and/or pathways for diseases and conditions associated with aging. This chapter also discusses unique features of trials in patients with Alzheimer's Disease (AD) and AD-related dementias (ADRD).

Keywords

Alzheimer's Disease (AD) · AD-related dementias (ADRD) · Barriers to participation · Multifactorial interventions · Multimorbidity · Polypharmacy · Time to benefit · Time to harm · Universal outcomes · Older adults

Introduction

Worldwide, the population of adults 65 years of age and older (the generally accepted definition of an older adult) is expected to almost double to 1.6 billion from 2025 to 2050, while growth of the overall population is not expected to exceed 34% during this period (He et al. 2016). In its 2018 press release, the US Census Bureau notes that "The aging of baby boomers means that within just a couple decades, older people are projected to outnumber children for the first time in U.S. history. By 2035, there will be 78.0 million people 65 years and older compared to 76.7 million under the age of 18." As people age, their utilization of health care resources increases significantly. US Centers for Medicare and Medicaid Services (2018) estimate that, in 2012, per capita health care expenses for adults 65 years of age and older were $18,988 versus $3,552 per child, and $6,632 per working age individual. The elderly, who, in 2012, accounted for just 14% of the US population, utilized about 34% of all health care spending. Therefore, there is an urgent need to develop the effective and safe interventions addressing the needs of older adults. Objectives of such interventions are to increase the health span and to reduce health care costs in this population. Such interventions are not limited to drugs and devices but include behavioral, nutritional, and social interventions.

Ethics in Geriatric Clinical Trials

US Code of Federal Regulations (CFR) establishes additional protections for children (21CFR50 and 45CFR46), pregnant women, human fetuses, neonates, and prisoners involved in research, but not for older adults. The Declaration of Helsinki does not consider older adults a vulnerable group of research subjects either but requires that "All vulnerable groups and individuals should receive specifically considered protection." While all ethical considerations of the Good Clinical Practice guidelines apply to clinical trials in older adults, it is not surprising that the regulations and research guidelines do not consider elderly a vulnerable group because only a small percentage of them will have difficulties understanding information about the study and will be unable to give a truly informed consent (Vellinga et al. 2004).

The European Forum's Ethical Guidance for Good Clinical Practice on "Medical Research for and with Older People in Europe" (Diener et al. 2013) provide that consent should be sought from all older adults who are capable of giving a consent. A consent document should be short, easy to understand, accompanied by information sheet and printed in a font that is suitable for older people. Several important issues should be considered when developing a consent process for elderly participants. This population may confuse the research risks with the inconveniences and discomforts associated with participation in a clinical trial (e.g., risk of visiting a clinical site is usually not greater than that of going to a grocery store, but a site could be 5 or 10 or more miles away, while a grocery store is just around the corner). The inconvenience of driving a longer distance or the need to arrange for transportation could be perceived by an older person as an increased risk of research. While focusing on the need to arrange for transportation, older adults may not recognize risks of developing serious adverse events described in consent documents. Because many older people are taking medications for years, they may consider adverse events a remote possibility or a "normal inconvenience" of taking a medication. Therefore, a consent document and any study information materials should unambiguously identify the risks (e.g., exposure to radiation, known adverse effects, etc.) and inconveniences and discomforts (the need to arrange for transportation, wait time at a clinic, total visit duration, etc.) of research participation and describe measures that the will be taken to mitigate the risks and minimize the inconveniences and discomforts.

The issue of comprehension is closely related to the quantity and quality of information provided in the consent document. It is not unusual for a consent form to be 15, 20, or more pages long while an older person could be fatigued after reading just half of such a lengthy document because an average time needed to read 15- or 20-page long consent is about 60 min. Legal and medical terms further reduce comprehension and affect true "informativeness" of the consent process. Quorum Review IRB (2018) notes that "legalese and other complex wording" is one of the two most common consent form problems. Comprehension of a consent document could be improved by using short sentences with fewer than ten words, organizing long paragraphs into bulleted lists, offering layperson-friendly synonyms for complex terminology and by never copying text directly from a protocol or investigator's brochure.

When seeking informed consent from older participants, investigators should use simple tools such as vignettes to confirm understanding of the consent. If understanding of the study's procedures, risks, discomforts, and other crucial information is not adequate, a consent by proxy should be obtained. In such instances, an older adult still should sign an assent based upon simplified and shortened information about the study. Participant's competence to consent could be assessed using several subjective and objective approaches. Subjective approaches include judgments of physicians, caregivers, and family members; objective – such commonly used screening instruments for dementia as Mini Mental Status Exam and Modified Mini-Mental State test (Vellinga et al. 2004). Given significant inconsistencies in assessing the same individuals by physicians, caregivers, and family members, the subjective approaches are seldom, if ever, used.

There are several other important considerations related to informed consent process in older individuals. One of them is independence of older adults consenting to participate in a clinical trial. While many remain physically and financially independent, a significant proportion of this population is dependent upon relatives, caregivers, federal, state, and local governments for their mobility, living arrangements, and financial support. Investigators should pay close attention to the issue of paternalism and protect decisions by older adults to participate in clinical trials from undue influence by their caregivers. This is a crucial issue to consider when a study involves institutionalized older adults whose decisions could be made on their behalf by the facility administration and staff. It is also important to recognize that because of depression, exhaustion, anxiety, fatigue, or similar reasons, older adults suffering from serious and debilitating diseases may not be weighing the risks and benefits the same way their healthier peers do. Therefore, IRBs and Ethics committees reviewing research in elderly should include members with expertise in geriatric research to ensure that clinical trials in this population adhere to the highest ethical standards.

Barriers to Participation, Recruitment, and Retention of Older Adults in Clinical Trials

Older adults taking many more medications than their younger peers, but few participate in clinical trials of drugs, biologics, and devices. While such studies included some elderly, they were not sufficiently powered for subgroup analysis to provide definitive evidence on the effects of interventions in this population. Analysis of demographic data from 105 applications to FDA for cancer drugs show that of 224,766 patients enrolled in trials supporting the submissions, just 12% were 75 years of age and older, while this population accounted for 29% of all cancer cases (Singh et al. 2017). Of 440 trials on effects of drugs for treating type 2 diabetes, 65.7% excluded significant proportion of older adults by establishing the upper age eligibility limit usually ranging from 65 years of age and older to 85 years of age and older (Cruz-Jentoft et al. 2013).

There are several reasons for underrepresentation of older adults in clinical trials. One of the most important barriers to participation is the study design that excludes older adults to reduce heterogeneity, which reduces treatment response and, thus, decreases power. While eligibility criteria rarely specify the upper age limit, many trials of drugs, biologics, and devices exclude older people because of safety concerns (e.g., hematologic, pulmonary, renal, or cardiovascular abnormalities); comorbidities; polypharmacy (taking several drugs); impaired cognitive function; or being unable to carry out activities of daily living without the caregivers' help.

Health care providers are another reason for underrepresentation of older adults in clinical trials. When asked why they do not enroll or recommend against participation by the elderly in clinical trials, providers often note a lack of resources; inexperience recruiting and working with this population; the need for caregiver; lack of coverage for some procedures related to participation in clinical trials; physicians' believe one treatment arm being more effective than the other, or not considering trial interventions as effective as other treatment options; poor health status of prospective participants; and too short life expectancy in this population.

The most common barriers noted by the elderly include ability to choose their own treatment (dislike of randomization) and lengthy and confusing consent documents. Antonoio Cherubini, professor of geriatrics at Perugia University and a member of the European Medicines Agency's (EMA) geriatric expert group, noted that "We cannot necessarily use the same consent form for a 90-year-old person as for a 40-year-old one. We need simplified explanations (Watts 2012)." Other barriers noted by older trial participants include small support network, lack of transportation, and relationship to their primary care provider. Some feel that their provider could be offended if they join the study or saw another physician. The most important barriers to participation by ethnic minorities are mistrust of research rooted into a general mistrust of society, mistrust of health care system, and mistrust of researchers. In areas with significant immigrant populations, investigators should consider mistrust of authorities, cultural, literacy, and language barriers. Institutionalization of older adults adds administrative complexity to the already complex process of recruiting and retaining elderly in clinical trials. During the trial planning phase, investigators should ensure that the study is accepted by a facility's administration and staff.

It is important to know what motivates older adults to enroll in clinical trials. Members of the focus groups indicate that home-based outcome collection, participation encouraged by their own doctors, convenient appointment times, and reimbursement of transportation costs encourage their participation in clinical trials. They list curiosity, or interest in finding out more about the study, "a desire to support research," and anticipated personal benefits, such as health screening, among the most important motivators for generating initial interest in a trial. Use of mobile technology-based assessments will not affect participation, if investigators take measures to ensure data security and reduce burden (Lenze et al. 2016). Investigators should focus on "simplified protocols, fewer exclusion criteria, more training for research staff, more emphasis to patients on the benefits of participation, easier physical access to research institutions, the possibility of home visits, more frequent follow-up and contact (Watts 2012)" to increase participation by older adults in clinical trials.

There are several other crucial factors to consider. One of them is selection of endpoints important to older adults. Among these are independence, activities of daily living, and quality of life. Philippe Guillet, Sanofi-Aventis's head of healthcare technologies for ageing, noted that "We need to understand the unmet needs of the older population to ensure that whatever we look for in the preclinical animal models is translatable into relevant measures in clinical studies (Watts 2012)." In pragmatic trials, the research team should provide support to prescribers on drug administration and dose adjustment. Receiving personal results from the study after it ends is "very" important to older adults (Lenze et al. 2016).

Retention is as important as recruitment and participants who feel as though they are partners, not subjects in the research enterprise, usually complete the studies. The warning signs for participants dropping out from the trial include missing visits, difficulties contacting a participant, interpersonal or communication difficulties, animosity toward the research team, worsening of the target or concomitant condition or disease, intercurrent illness requiring treatment with a protocol-prohibited medication, and persistent adverse events. The most successful mitigation strategy for the retention challenges is personalized attention by the study staff including more frequent contacts with a participant, increased time with a site investigator, clinic visits with a different study coordinator, and keeping primary care provider informed about participant's journey through the study. Keeping participants informed about the progress of the study is important for maximizing the retention of older adults in long-term trials. Participants in the "Prospective Study of Pravastatin in the Elderly at Risk (PROSPER)" indicated that ongoing health monitoring was the most important recruitment and retention motivator. The role of retention incentives remains unclear and the social aspect of an incentive could be more important to older adults than the incentive itself. PROSPER participants noted that the social aspect of participation in a lunch was more important to them then the food itself. They also valued the newsletter more than other incentives because of information about the study progress (Tolmie et al. 2004). Treatment of an intercurrent illnesses and/or adverse events at the trial facility could decrease time burden and inconvenience of participation and increase retention.

The following tips should help increase recruitment and retention of older adults in clinical trials:

1. Engage all stakeholders (participants, caregivers, healthcare providers, and administrators) in the trial development process.
2. Convene the focus groups to establish what motivates prospective participants to join the study and what barriers are the most important to them.
3. Minimize selection criteria and align them with the research question.
4. Chose outcomes important to the target population. Whenever possible, avoid invasive, uncomfortable, or time-consuming outcome measures.
5. As much as feasible, employ technology-based and/or home-based outcome collection to reduce participant burden.
6. Simplify consent documents and study information materials, and streamline the consent process. Consider two simpler consents: one – for screening, second – for randomization and treatment. Seek input from prospective participants on the consent documents and process.

7. Provide transportation to and from the sites.
8. Pilot test recruitment and retention strategies.
9. Develop a study social-support network by enhancing social interactions with the study staff and among participants. Consider holiday parties, study newsletters, and wellbeing telephone calls.
10. Minimize or eliminate out of pocket costs (e.g., provide reimbursement for transportation and parking, etc.).

Selection of Outcomes Important to Older Adults

Importance of outcomes to target population is a key factor guiding their selection in clinical trials in elderly because it affects recruitment, retention and adherence to the intervention. Other factors informing outcome selection include intervention goal (treatment or prevention trial), importance to healthcare system and to the society, ability to be measured (objectively or subjectively), the outcome event rate, and responsiveness to intervention over time. The outcome measures, especially in older adults with multiple chronic conditions (MCC), should minimize participant burden (ideally be administrable in under 15 min) and should yield meaningful health information which is readily interpretable by both patients and their providers. The outcomes should be responsive to change within a relatively short period of time which is not exceeding the life expectancy of the target population, the investigators should consider the feasibility of proxy-reporting, costs associated with administration of the measurements, and feasibility of incorporating the outcome measures into electronic health records. Older adults have no difficulties completing the technology-based assessments but are worried about data security and test burden.

A survey of participants enrolled into cardiovascular trials showed significant differences in perception of importance of outcomes by younger (median age 23) and older (median age 73) individuals. For older adults, the most important outcome was stroke followed by dementia, death, admission to a nursing home, and myocardial infarction. Younger adults viewed death as the most important outcome, followed by dementia, stroke, myocardial infarction, and institutionalization (Canavan et al. 2016). Adults 60 years of age and older with treatment-resistant depression noted that psychological well-being and symptomatic remission were outcomes that matter most to them: "Life isn't worth much without a certain level of satisfaction" one participant said (Lenze et al. 2016). Measuring risks associated with the intervention is as important as measuring intervention benefits. In the same study, participants noted that falls and fall-related injuries, cognitive function, and mobility limitations were among the most important outcomes for antidepressant trials.

Given that majority of older adults have more than one chronic disease or condition, it is important to assess how treatment for one disease or condition affects comorbid diseases and conditions. Therefore, effects of intervention on the overall health status of an older individual could be a more clinically relevant outcome than the effect of the intervention on a disease-specific outcome. Several universal health outcomes such as self-rated health, basic and instrumental activities of daily living, disability, and death have been used in clinical trials in the elderly (Tinetti et al. 2011). Trial eligibility criteria should consider the floor and ceiling effects of the instruments measuring physical function, cognition, and disability. Because disability states vary in both directions across time in older adults, measures of disability should account for such transitions. Accordingly, persistent disability is more meaningful than the incident disability outcome. In participants with impaired cognitive function reliability of such patient-reported outcomes as self-rated health and basic and instrumental activities of daily living is quite low because cognitively impaired individuals often overestimate their functional abilities comparing to reports by proxies (Neumann et al. 2000).

While the universal health outcomes are appealing, there are challenges designing trials with such outcomes and interpreting their results. Incident diseases, worsening of comorbid conditions requiring adjustment in dose, discontinuation, change in dose or administration of additional concomitant medications, and evolution of treatment guidelines significantly increase heterogeneity of study population and so increase variability in response to intervention. If a composite outcome is used, its components are often of different clinical importance and could differentially respond to the intervention. Designs of trials in elderly should consider the issue of competing risk of death which is progressively increasing as the trial population gets older during the follow-up period.

Effects of Multimorbidity and Polypharmacy on Trial Design

Multimorbidity, defined as coexistence of several chronic diseases or conditions, is highly prevalent in older adults. Among adults 65 to 84 years of age and those 85 and older, 64.9% and 81.5%, respectively, had been diagnosed with several chronic conditions (Barnett et al. 2012). Many of the comorbid diseases are treated with at least one drug and some conditions, quite prevalent in this population including hypertension, congestive heart failure, and type 2 diabetes mellitus, often require administration of several drugs to manage a single condition. As a result, in 2010, 39% of adults 65 years of age and older in the United States were taking five or more medications (Charlesworth et al. 2015). Accordingly, multimorbidity leads to polypharmacy (defined as a simultaneous administration of multiple drugs) and trial designs in this population should account for multiple drug-drug, drug-disease, and disease-disease interactions.

Drug-drug interactions are the most common, can result in hospitalizations and, in some instances, in death. For example, administration of Bactrim (sulfamethoxazole and trimethoprim) to adult 66 years of age and older who are treated with angiotensin-converting enzyme inhibitors or angiotensin receptor blockers results in a sevenfold increase risk of hospitalization due to hyperkalemia, compared with amoxicillin. Drugs metabolized using cytochrome P450 mechanism, including amlodipine, diltiazem, colchicine, verapamil, and clarithromycin, may affect serum concentration of lipophilic statins such as lovastatin, simvastatin, and atorvastatin.

Another commonly prescribed drug spironolactone to older adults should not be administered to patients with porphyria because of the risk of acute attack. Among disease-disease interactions, hospitalizations associated with adverse events often lead to functional decline and loss of independence. Drug-drug, drug-disease, and disease-disease interactions could increase the incidence of geriatric syndromes such as falls and delirium that are not routinely monitored in clinical trials but are important to older adult's safety outcomes.

Therefore, it is often difficult or impossible to attribute adverse event to a specific drug or a condition. As the number of conditions increases, the symptom burden rises, and symptom management becomes an important treatment goal and a major trial outcome. The infinite number of combinations of drugs further increases the risk of adverse events and makes their assessment and management challenging, which prompts investigators to restrict participation by individuals with MCCs in clinical trials. A combination of factors such as high symptom burden, increased risk of adverse events, and the need to take multiple drugs could decrease compliance with the investigational medication regimen.

Time to Benefit, Time to Harm, and Life Expectancy

The Time to Benefit (TTB) in a clinical trial is defined as "...the amount of time required to observe a significant, measurable effect in a group of patients treated with a therapy compared to a control group" (Holmes et al. 2013). Accordingly, the Time to Harm (TTH) is defined as "...the time until a statistically significant adverse effect is seen in a trial for the treatment group compared to the control group." The TTB could be either shorter or longer than TTH and the benefits and harms could be immediate or delayed, becoming apparent months and even years after the intervention was discontinued. For example, a single administration of ceftriaxone and azithromycin would cure an uncomplicated gonococcal infection of the cervix, urethra, or rectum, while antibiotics should be taken for months to treat tuberculosis. Anaphylaxis could develop as early as first administration of an antibiotic, while with pseudomembranous colitis it might be as late as 8 weeks after treatment was completed. Preventive interventions have the longest TTB – benefits of colon cancer screening (colonoscopy) become apparent in 10 years, while effects of statins for secondary prevention could be seen as early as in 6 months.

Older adults have limited life expectancy (LE). Accordingly, TTB, TTH, estimated LE, and the magnitude of expected benefits and harms become important considerations in the design of trials in this population. Conversely, trials should be designed to yield as much information about the TTB and TTH as feasible to inform clinical decision making. Such data would provide for selecting treatments based upon patients' LE with the most favorable TTB and TTH profiles. It will also inform decisions about when to stop preventive interventions to reduce polypharmacy. In trials using composite outcomes or testing effects of intervention on several outcomes, TTB and TTH for different components or outcomes could be different and could exceed the trial duration for some of them. If a composite outcome includes death or one of the outcomes is mortality, determining TTB and TTH for other components or outcomes becomes more difficult because of competing risk. Another limitation is that trials stopped early for efficacy could miss harms because TTH could be longer than TTB for one or more components or outcomes. Not only the trial duration and outcome selection, but the sample size, frequency of interim analyses, the stopping rules, and characteristics of the study population affect the TTB and TTH.

The TTB could be determined by statistical process control (SPC) as was shown using data from the Fracture Intervention Trial testing efficacy of alendronate versus placebo for reducing fracture risk in postmenopausal women (van de Glind et al. 2016). This method identified the time point from which the cumulative difference in the number of clinical fractures remained greater than the upper control limit on the SPC chart. For preventive interventions with short-term harms and long-term benefits such as aspirin, colonoscopy, and prophylactic vascular surgeries, the "payoff time" could be calculated by dividing a patient's probability of being harmed due to the intervention by the reduction in mortality attributable to the intervention and that then determines when the benefits will exceed harms (Braithwaite et al. 2009). Participants' LE could be estimated using mortality indexes accounting for multimorbidity, functional status and age.

Multifactorial Interventions

Geriatric syndromes are prevalent, multifactorial in etiology, clinical conditions that cannot be attributed to any specific disease category. Among such syndromes are falls, frailty, delirium, urinary incontinence, and some other. Accordingly, when more than one risk factor is involved in the development of a syndrome, a multifactorial intervention modifying all contributing factors could be the best treatment strategy to improve health outcomes. It is well-established that the risk of falls is increasing with the increase in number of contributing factors. "Strategies to Reduce Injuries and Develop Confidence in Elders (STRIDE)" clinical trial is a good example of a study testing the efficacy of a multifactorial fall injury prevention strategy on reducing fall-related injuries in older adults. Falls care managers assess each trial participant for seven modifiable risk factors for fall injuries (strength, balance, gait impairment; fall risk increasing drugs; vitamin D deficiency; home safety; orthostatic hypotension; visual impairment; foot problems or unsafe footwear; and osteoporosis), explain the identified risks to the participant and caregiver, and suggest interventions, based on the identified risk factors, and according to study algorithms for each such factor (Bhasin et al. 2018).

While the multifactorial intervention approach offers a great promise of effective, highly targeted individualized medicine, generating evidence of efficacy and safety of such interventions is difficult because of the following complexities involved in the design and analysis of trials of such interventions (Allore et al. 2005).

Selecting Modifiable Risk Factors to Target

The investigators should carefully consider prevalence of risk factors, their relative contribution to the development of a condition (high or low risk factors), potential response to the intervention, and correlation of risk factors. Prevalence, high-low risk, and response to treatment will affect the sample size and generalizability of the study results. The correlation between the risk factors could either positively or negatively influence the effect of another factor on the health outcome. Therefore, the chosen risk factors should be as independent as possible from each other.

Selecting Components of a Multicomponent Intervention

Ideally, each component of the intervention should target a single risk factor, but this is rarely achievable in real life because often one component modulates more than one risk factor. In the STRIDE study, an exercise component of the intervention improves strength, balance, and gait. There are other reasons for selecting components of the intervention that address more than one factor. A large number of components increases intervention delivery costs, affects treatment compliance, and scalability of the multifactorial intervention. Investigators interested in effects of individual components on specific risk factors could elucidate such effects in secondary analysis. Overall, the magnitude of effect of an individual component could be estimated by comparing the degree of change in a risk factor it targets in intervention and control groups.

Defining Eligibility Criteria

Selection of eligibility criteria depends upon objectives of a trial testing the efficacy and safety of a multifactorial intervention. Broad eligibility with few exclusions increases heterogeneity, thus, generalizability of the study findings, but dilutes the treatment effect. If investigators are interested in the effects of individual components, they may need to increase the sample size to ensure that the study is sufficiently powered for the subgroup analysis. Restricting eligibility to a subset of population increases the treatment effect and protects those who could be harmed by one or more components of the intervention, but restricted eligibility decreases generalizability of the study findings and could affect scalability of the intervention.

Treatment Allocation, Outcome Assessment, and Adjudication

Because many multifactorial interventions include components such as behavior modification (exercise or diet), change in home environment or medication, alternative approaches to health care delivery (office-based vs. home-based), and similar, double blinding of participants and investigators is not possible. Therefore, trials of multifactorial interventions are prone to significant bias arising from participant preferences affecting adherence to intervention or its select components, and investigators' expectations. Single blinding of the interventionists, outcome assessors, and adjudicators as well as designs accounting for participant preferences could decrease bias.

Assignment of Components of the Intervention

With a global design, all the participants are assigned all components of the multifactorial intervention. This approach simplifies intervention delivery and reduces costs, but it is rarely clinically justified because not all the participants have all the risk factors, thus some components are not needed, they could harm participants and/or increase participant burden. There are also significant analytical challenges in determining the effects of individual components because of the collinearity and heterogeneity of the study population (i.e., significant variation in a number and type of risk factors across participants). Therefore, the standardly or individually tailored interventions are more commonly used. Such designs assign components based upon a priori determined risk factors and assign only those components that modulate factors present in a participant (e.g., STRIDE trial). Such designs are clinically meaningful, but there remain issues with determining the effects of individual components on specific risk factors because a component could modulate more than one factor (e.g., exercise improving strength, balance, and gait).

Sample Size Calculations

There are significant challenges in calculating the sample size arising from differential assignment of components across study population, variations in effect size of individual components, and multiple comparisons, if effects of individual risk factors are determined. Cluster randomized designs have an added complexity of accounting for the intracluster correlation or similarity among participants within their preexisting clusters. Such a similarity reduces the variability of responses and decreases power to detect differences between the treatment groups. The correlation is presented as the intracluster coefficient of correlation which compares the intragroup variance with the intergroup variance.

Estimating Individual Component Effects

In addition to challenges related to determining the individual component effects discussed above, the investigators face the issues of collinearity and of defining the appropriate control group. Collinearity of two or more components increases variance and decreases precision of effect estimates. In an individually tailored design, the control group for estimating effect of a component should include only participants who have a risk factor that would be targeted by such a component. When a global design is used, all participants in the intervention arm receive all the components regardless of the number of risk factors present. Accordingly, only participants with the risk factor of interest should be identified and included in a subgroup analysis.

Considerations for Trials for Alzheimer's Disease and Other Age-Related Dementias

Background

Dementias of aging including Alzheimer's disease (AD) impact an estimated almost 50 million people worldwide currently and that figure is projected to grow threefold to approximately 132 million by 2050 (Prince et al. 2015). AD (late-onset, sporadic) is the most common cause of dementia in those aged 65 and older, and it is estimated that it currently affects more than five million people in the USA and is the sixth leading cause of death (Alzheimer's Association 2018). Frontotemporal Degeneration, another age-related dementia, is the leading cause of dementia in people under the age of 60. Other AD-related dementias include, Lewy body dementia, corticobasal degeneration, progressive supranuclear palsy, vascular dementia, and Parkinson's dementia. Mixed dementia (multiple pathologies such as AD and vascular disease) is more common than previously thought and its likelihood increases with age.

Despite a substantial R&D investment for AD and related dementias and advances made in our understanding of disease pathogenesis, safe and effective treatments for patients are still lacking. Currently there are only a few interventions that have been approved by the Food and Drug Administration for the treatment of AD, and those approved have demonstrated only modest effects in modifying the clinical symptoms for relatively short periods of time. None has shown a clear effect on disease progression. There are no approved treatments for the other related dementias. Currently most trials for AD are focusing on disease-modifying therapies to delay or slow disease progression. It is now well recognized that researchers should target selected therapeutics to specific stages of AD and consider the disease in terms of primary, secondary, and tertiary prevention (Sperling et al. 2011). A review of the AD drug pipeline in 2018 revealed that trials are increasingly focused on the earliest disease stages, in particular on prevention trials in individuals in the preclinical stage with biomarker evidence of disease but without clinical symptoms.

Target Population/Stage of Disease

Identifying the appropriate target population is critical for trials investigating disease modifying therapies. In AD, there are stages of disease that although not distinct, represent a progression from a high-risk preclinical stage in which amyloid is present in the brain, to a prodromal AD stage with mild cognitive impairment and biomarker evidence of AD, to the AD dementia stage with more significant cognitive impairment as well as functional impairment (Cummings et al. 2018). Appropriate assessments and outcome measures vary by stage of disease and must be carefully selected.

The US Food and Drug Administration (FDA) recently updated its draft guidance for industry to assist sponsors in the clinical development of drugs for the treatment of the stages of AD that occur before the onset of overt dementia (FDA 2018). The guidance outlines the following four categories for the design and evaluation of clinical trials in different stages of AD and include discussion of suitable outcome measures:

> Stage 1: Patients with characteristic pathophysiologic changes of AD but no evidence of clinical impact. These patients are truly asymptomatic with no subjective complaint, functional impairment, or detectable abnormalities on sensitive neuropsychological measures. The characteristic pathophysiologic changes are typically demonstrated by assessment of various biomarker measures.
> Stage 2: Patients with characteristic pathophysiologic changes of AD and subtle detectable abnormalities on sensitive neuropsychological measures, but no functional impairment. The emergence of subtle functional impairment signals a transition to Stage 3.
> Stage 3: Patients with characteristic pathophysiologic changes of AD, subtle or more apparent detectable abnormalities on sensitive neuropsychological measures, and mild but detectable functional impairment. The functional impairment in this stage is not severe enough to warrant a diagnosis of overt dementia.
> Stage 4: Patients with overt dementia. This diagnosis is made as functional impairment worsens from that seen in Stage 3. This stage may be refined into additional categories (e.g., Stages 4, 5, and 6, corresponding with mild, moderate, and severe dementia).

Challenges for Clinical Meaningfulness in Predementia Populations

Historically, the effectiveness of AD treatments in symptomatic patients had to be established for approval not only based on a treatment effect on cognition but also on a global or functional scale. Having a coprimary functional measure was established to ensure that any beneficial cognitive effects would also be clinically meaningful to patients and their families/caregivers (FDA 2018). As trials have moved into earlier predementia stages with little or no identifiable functional impairment, the establishment of clinical meaningfulness has become more challenging. While biomarkers of early AD processes and sensitive neuropsychological measures that can detect subtle cognitive change are now available, it is not yet known if a beneficial treatment effect would ultimately translate into a delay in the onset of cognitive decline/dementia (Aisen et al. 2017).

Participation, Recruitment, Retention in AD and Related Dementia Trials

Recruitment and retention of participants in AD and related dementias clinical trials is a long-standing challenge and is a major factor in increasing clinical trial duration and costs. While recruitment challenges are not unique to dementia trials, studies of Alzheimer's disease research participation have identified a number of barriers that inhibit recruitment (Watson et al. 2014):

Barriers for primary care physicians. Most individuals experiencing changes in cognition will first present to a primary care provider. Research has demonstrated that lack of time, lack of available diagnostic clinical tools, concern over risks to patients in experimental protocols, and lack of proximity to a research center, along with patient comorbidities, are among the barriers physicians report as challenges to referral for AD and related dementia clinical trials. Additionally, to refer a patient for a clinical trial, the provider must recognize that the patient might have or be at risk for cognitive impairment. Yet some studies show that physicians are unaware of cognitive impairment in more than 40% of their cognitively impaired patients (Galvin et al. 2009).

Barriers for under-represented populations. Clinical trials for dementia struggle to include people from diverse racial and ethnic backgrounds that have traditionally been under-represented in research participation. Barriers to their participation may include understandable and long-standing mistrust of the medical establishment overall and of particular local academic research institutions; language; logistical barriers and cost; lack of cultural sensitivity and ethnic and cultural similarity of staff to participants; and invasive study procedures. This is particularly troublesome given that many of these under-represented groups are at higher risk for developing dementia. Additionally, many trials exclude individuals with comorbid conditions that are prevalent in some racial or ethnic groups, such as diabetes and vascular disease, thus impacting participation (Watson et al. 2014).

Study partner requirement. AD and related dementia trials typically require the participation of a study partner, that is, someone (spouse, partner, adults child, friend, or caregiver) who knows the participant well enough to provide accurate information about daily functioning, as well as report on cognitive changes in the participant, assure compliance with study procedures, and be available to assist with managing study risks and even informed consent in later disease stages (Watson et al. 2014; National Institute on Aging 2018). A retrospective analysis of several AD trials by Grill and colleagues (2013) found that a majority of study partners were spouses. This is problematic given that recent data suggest that an increasing number of older people with dementia do not have a spouse or live alone. As the researchers noted, their data did not explain why participants with non-spousal study partners were underrepresented. However, they found that compared with spouses, adult child study partners were more likely to be working and living apart from the patient and that this suggested that patients with AD who have adult child caregivers face increased logistical challenges to research participation.

Invasive procedures. Although clinical trials for other diseases involve invasive procedures, current AD and related dementias studies often involve both brain scans with radioactive materials and lumbar punctures. In many cases, these procedures are part of screening for inclusion in the study before a potential participant is even accepted into a trial. Further, such procedures may occur on multiple occasions throughout a study. Additionally, some of the therapeutic candidates currently being evaluated require infusions to administer, which can take many hours. Finally, because AD and related dementias impact cognition, there are frequently hours of neuropsychological assessments, also repeated throughout the course of the investigation. The extensive time and effort involved in taking part in AD and related dementia studies can give pause and ultimately deter potential volunteers and their study partners (Watson et al. 2014). Willingness to participate in AD trials was lower in predementia populations compared to dementia populations especially for trials requiring frequent visits and using biomarker testing procedures.

In October 2018, the National Institute on Aging, part of the National Institutes of Health, released the national strategy for Alzheimer's and related dementias research recruitment and participation (National Institute on Aging 2018). This national strategy was developed with facilitation by the Alzheimer's Association, and a collaborative of government, private, academic, and industry stakeholders, as well as from individuals, caregivers, and study participants to address the challenges to recruiting participants for trials and other studies to prevent or treat Alzheimer's and its related dementias. The strategy has four major themes:

1. Increase awareness and engagement at a broad, national level: Focus on policies and activities at the national level that help identify and support strategies for successful recruitment and retention.
2. Build and improve capacity and infrastructure at the study site level: Focus on how study sites and multisite networks do business and how they can be most effectively structured and staffed for the number and types of clinical studies currently underway as well as for future studies.
3. Engage local communities and support participants: Focus on connecting at the local level, identifying and implementing best practices to build trusting relationships with communities and individuals toward the shared goal of making a difference for people and families affected by AD and related dementias.
4. Develop an applied science of recruitment: Focus on research on recruitment to establish evidenced-based practices.

The overarching goal of the strategy is to engage broad segments of the public in the Alzheimer's and related dementias research enterprise, with a particular focus on underrepresented communities, so that studies can successfully and more rapidly enroll and retain individuals to better understand and ultimately treat these disorders in all those affected.

Conclusion

There are several unique features that should be considered while designing clinical trials in the elderly. When enrolling older adults into clinical trials, it is important to find the right balance between the quantity and quality of information provided in the consent documents. Comprehension of the study details should be assessed and, if it is questionable, a proxy consent should be sought. Given that the elderly are often dependent upon relatives, caregivers, and/ or federal, state, and local governments, it is important to ensure that the consent process is free from coercion or undue influence. To reach the recruitment goals, the investigators should identify and eliminate or minimize the impact of any barriers to participation and select the outcomes that are important to older adults. As LE becomes limited with increasing age, TTB, TTH, estimated LE, and the magnitude of expected benefits and harms become important considerations in the design of trials in this population. Identifying the appropriate target population is critical for trials investigating AD modifying therapies because stages of disease represent a progression from a high-risk preclinical stage to a prodromal AD stage with mild cognitive impairment and biomarker evidence of AD, to the AD dementia stage with more significant cognitive impairment as well as functional impairment. Recruitment and retention of participants in AD and related dementias clinical trials is a long-standing challenge and is a major factor in increasing clinical trial duration and costs. Participation in AD and related dementia trials typically require a study partner who knows the participant well enough to provide accurate information about daily functioning, report on cognitive changes in the participant, and assure compliance with study procedures.

Key Facts

Worldwide, the population of adults 65 years of age and older is expected to almost double to 1.6 billion from 2025 to 2050; dementias of aging including Alzheimer's disease (AD) impact an estimated almost 50 million people worldwide currently and that figure is projected to grow threefold to approximately 132 million by 2050; physicians are unaware of cognitive impairment in more than 40% of their cognitively impaired patients; in 2012, per capita health care expenses for adults 65 years of age and older were $18,988 versus $3,552 per child and $6,632 per a working age individual; an average time needed to read 15- or 20-page long consent is about 60 min; of 224,766 patients enrolled in trials supporting the FDA submissions, just 12% were 75 years of age and older, while this population accounted for 29% of all cancer cases; the most common barriers noted by the elderly include ability to choose their own treatment (dislike of randomization) and lengthy and confusing consent documents; among adults 65 to 84 years of age and those 85 and older, 64.9% and 81.5%, respectively, had been diagnosed with several chronic conditions.

References

Aisen P, Touchon J, Amariglio R, Andrieu S, Bateman R, Breitner J, Donohue M, Dunn B, Doody R, Fox N, Gauthier S, Grundman M, Hendrix S, Ho C, Isaac M, Raman R, Rosenberg P, Schindler R, Schneider L, Sperling R, Tariot P, Welsh-Bohmer K, Weiner M, Vellas B, Task Force Members (2017) EU/US/CTAD task force: lessons learned from recent and current Alzheimer's prevention trials. J Prev Alzheimers Dis 4(2):116–124

Allore HG, Tinetti ME, Gill TM, Peduzzi PN (2005) Experimental designs for multicomponent interventions among persons with multifactorial geriatric syndromes. Clin Trials 2:13–21

Alzheimer's Association (2018) Alzheimer's disease facts and figures. Alzheimers Dement 14(3):367–429

Barnett K, Mercer SW, Norbury M, Watt G, Wyke S, Guthrie B (2012) Epidemiology of multimorbidity and implications for health care, research, and medical education: a cross-sectional study. Lancet 380:37–43. https://doi.org/10.1016/S0140-6736(12)60240-2

Bhasin S, Gill TM, Reuben DB, Latham NK, Gurwitz JH, Dykes P, McMahon S, Storer TW, Duncan PW, Ganz DA, Basaria S, Miller ME, Travison TG, Greene EJ, Dziura J, Esserman D, Allore H, Carnie MB, Fagan M, Hanson C, Baker D, Greenspan SL, Alexander N, Ko F, Siu AL, Volpi E, Wu AW, Rich J, Waring SC, Wallace R, Casteel C, Magaziner J, Charpentier P, Lu C, Araujo K, Rajeevan H, Margolis S, Eder R, McGloin JM, Skokos E, Wiggins J, Garber L, Clauser SB, Correa-De-Araujo R, Peduzzi P (2018) Strategies to reduce injuries and develop confidence in elders (STRIDE): a cluster-randomized pragmatic trial of a multifactorial fall injury prevention strategy: design and methods. J Gerontol A Biol Sci Med Sci 73:1053–1061. https://doi.org/10.1093/gerona/glx190

Braithwaite RS, Fiellin D, Justice AC (2009) The payoff time: a flexible framework to help clinicians decide when patients with comorbid disease are not likely to benefit from practice guidelines. Med Care 47:610–617. https://doi.org/10.1097/MLR.0b013e31819748d5

Canavan M, Smyth A, Robinson SM, Gibson I, Costello C, O'Keeffe ST, Walsh T, Mulkerrin EC, O'Donnell MJ (2016) Attitudes to outcomes measured in clinical trials of cardiovascular prevention. QJM 109:391–397. https://doi.org/10.1093/qjmed/hcv132

Charlesworth C, Smit E, Lee DSH, Alramadhan F, Odden MC (2015) Polypharmacy among adults aged 65 years and older in the United States: 1988–2010. J Gerontol A Biol Sci Med Sci 70:989–995. https://doi.org/10.1093/gerona/glv013

Cruz-Jentoft AJ, Carpena-Ruiz M, Montero-Errasquín B, Sánchez-Castellano C, Sánchez-García E (2013) Exclusion of older adults from ongoing clinical trials about type 2 diabetes mellitus. J Am Geriatr Soc 61:734–738. https://doi.org/10.1111/jgs.12215

Cummings J, Ritter A, Zhong K (2018) Clinical trials for disease-modifying therapies in Alzheimer's disease: a primer, lessons learned, and a blueprint for the future. J Alzheimers Dis 64:S3–S22

Diener L, Hugonot-Diener L, Alvino S, Baeyens JP, Bone MF, Chirita D, Husson JM, Maman M, Piette F, Tinker A, von Raison F, European Forum for Good Clinical Practice Geriatric Medicine Working Party (2013) Guidance synthesis. Medical research for and with older people in Europe: proposed ethical guidance for good clinical practice: ethical considerations. J Nutr Health Aging 17:625–627. https://doi.org/10.1007/s12603-013-0340-0

Galvin JE, Meuser TM, Boise L, Connell CM (2009) Predictors of physician referral for patient recruitment to Alzheimer disease clinical trials. Alzheimer Dis Assoc Disord 23(4):352–356

He W, Goodkind D, Kowal P (2016) U.S. Census Bureau, international population reports, P95/16-1. An aging world. U.S. Government Publishing Office, Washington, DC, p 2015

Holmes HM, Min LC, Yee M, Varadhan R, Basran J, Dale W, Boyd CM (2013) Rationalizing prescribing for older patients with multimorbidity: considering time to benefit. Drugs Aging 30:655–666. https://doi.org/10.1007/s40266-013-0095-7

Lenze EJ, Ramsey A, Brown PJ, Reynolds CF, Mulsant BH, Lavretsky H, Roose SP (2016) Older adults' perspectives on clinical research: a focus group and survey study. Am J Geriatr Psychiatry 24:893–902. https://doi.org/10.1016/j.jagp.2016.07.022

National Institute on Aging (2018) Together we make the difference: national strategy for recruitment and participation in Alzheimer's and related dementias clinical research. https://www.nia.nih.gov/sites/default/files/2018-10/alzheimers-disease-recruitment-strategy-final.pdf. Accessed 19 Oct 2018

Neumann PJ, Araki SS, Gutterman EM (2000) The use of proxy respondents in studies of older adults: lessons, challenges, and opportunities. J Am Geriatr Soc 48:1646–1654

Prince M, Wimo A, Guerchet, M, Ali G, Wu Y, Prina M (2015) World Alzheimer report 2015: the global impact of dementia. Alzheimer's Disease International. https://www.alz.co.uk/research/WorldAlzheimerReport2015.pdf. Accessed August 2015

Quorum Review IRB. Two common consent form problems (And how to fix them). https://www.quorumreview.com/two-common-consent-form-problems-and-how-to-fix-them/. Accessed 16 Nov 2018

Singh H, Kanapuru B, Smith C, Fashoyin-Aje L, Myers A, Kim G (2017) FDA analysis of enrollment of older adults in clinical trials for cancer drug registration: a 10-year experience by the U.S. Food and Drug Administration. J Clin Oncol 35(15_suppl):10009–10009. https://doi.org/10.1200/JCO.2017.35.15_suppl.10009

Sperling RA, Jack CR Jr, Aisen PS (2011) Testing the right target and right drug at the right stage. Sci Transl Med 3(111):111cm33. https://doi.org/10.1126/scitranslmed.3002609

Tinetti ME, McAvay G, Chang SS, Ning Y, Newman AB, Fitzpatrick A, Fried TR, Harris TB, Nevitt MC, Satterfield S, Yaffe K, Peduzzi P (2011) Effect of chronic disease-related symptoms and impairments on universal health outcomes in older adults. J Am Geriatr Soc 59:1618–1627. https://doi.org/10.1111/j.1532-5415.2011.03576.x

Tolmie EP, Mungall MM, Louden G, Lindsay GM, Gaw A (2004) Understanding why older people participate in clinical trials: the experience of the Scottish PROSPER participants. Age Ageing 33:374–378. https://doi.org/10.1093/ageing/afh109

U.S. Centers for Medicare and Medicaid Services. National Health Expenditure Fact Sheet. Projected 2017–2026. https://www.cms.gov/research-statistics-data-and-systems/statistics-trends-and-reports/nationalhealthexpenddata/nhe-fact-sheet.html. Accessed 2 Nov 2018

U.S. Food and Drug Administration (2018) Early Alzheimer's disease: developing drugs for treatment: draft guidance for industry. 83 Fed Regist 7060–7061

van de Glind EM, Willems HC, Eslami S, Abu-Hanna A, Lems WF, Hooft L, de Rooij SE, Black DM, van Munster BC (2016) Estimating the time to benefit for preventive drugs with the statistical process control method: an example with alendronate. Drugs Aging 33:347–353. https://doi.org/10.1007/s40266-016-0344-7

Vellinga A, Smit JH, van Leeuwen E, van Tilburg W, Jonker C (2004) Competence to consent to treatment of geriatric patients: judgements of physicians, family members and the vignette method. Int J Geriatr Psychiatry 19:645–654. https://doi.org/10.1002/gps.1139

Watson JL, Ryan L, Silverberg N, Cahan V, Bernard MA (2014) Obstacles and opportunities in Alzheimer's clinical trial recruitment. Health Aff 33:574–579

Watts G (2012) Why the exclusion of older people from clinical research must stop. BMJ 344:e3445. https://doi.org/10.1136/bmj.e3445

Trials in Minority Populations

123

Otis W. Brawley

Contents

Introduction	2418
The Applicability of Clinical Findings	2419
Defining and Categorizing Populations	2419
The Importance of Race	2421
Federal Laws Regarding Inclusion	2422
The NIH Interpretation of the Inclusion Law	2423
Potential Harms Caused by the Law	2424
Inclusion Is Important	2424
Summary and Conclusion	2426
Key Facts	2426
References	2427

Abstract

It is a widely held belief that race is a biological categorization. This is not true. Indeed, race encompasses a broad group of people and is a socio-political categorization. There is biologic genetic diversity (genetic differences) within populations, when populations are defined by race, area of geographic origin, or ancestry. Race is complicated by admixture such that racial self-identity often does not correlate with genetic ancestry. While race does not matter biologically, it does matter sociopolitically. Race often correlates with exposures that can cause disease. Certain populations as defined by race are also less likely to receive quality care. The NIH Revitalization Act of 1993 requires NIH-funded research include racial minorities and women such that "valid subset analyses" can be done to distinguish differences. The implementation of the law has stimulated a movement encouraging minority accrual and a focus on assessment of differences in outcomes by race. The Federal rules imply that biologic racial differences

---

O. W. Brawley (✉)
Johns Hopkins School of Medicine, and Johns Hopkins Bloomberg School of Public Health, Baltimore, MD, USA
e-mail: Otis.Brawley@jhu.edu

© Springer Nature Switzerland AG 2022
S. Piantadosi, C. L. Meinert (eds.), *Principles and Practice of Clinical Trials*,
https://doi.org/10.1007/978-3-319-52636-2_171

account for differences in outcomes. What is needed is diversity of enrollment in clinical trials and open mindedness in assessment and interpretation of data. Populations should be defined with attention to distribution of genetic markers. Some scientific study should be targeted to specific populations as defined by those genetic markers. In certain instances, clinical trials with diverse populations can be assessed in meta-analysis, and some differences in metabolism of disease can be found. It is more useful to try to associate these differences with the area of geographic origin or ancestry versus race.

Keywords

Race · Minority health · Disparities · Biological categorization · Clinical trials · Minority inclusion · Subset analysis · Genomic markers

Introduction

Interest in minority health and the differences in healthcare outcomes by race grew out of the US civil rights movement of the 1950s and 1960s. This was a time when sickle cell disease was gaining attention as a genetic disease primarily affecting people of African origin. It was widely believed that there are biological differences among populations as defined by race. In the early 1970s, the US National Cancer Institute began a surveillance program and published cancer incidence, mortality, and survival by race (Howard et al. 1992). The documentation of disparities caused even greater interest in cancer disparities.

It has been a long-held view that the biology of blacks or Negroes is different from that of whites or Caucasians. Even in medicine today, it is common folklore that angiotensin-converting enzyme (ACE) inhibitors are better for treatment of hypertension in whites, and diuretics such as hydrochlorothiazide are the preferred therapy for blacks (Flack et al. 2000). Many clinical laboratories have race-adjusted renal values and lung function norms (Eneanya et al. 2019; Lujan and DiCarlo 2018; Cerdeña et al. 2020).

It is fact that a substantial number of clinical studies and trials in the USA have few or no black or African American participants. This has supported the belief that blacks have not enjoyed much of the progress in American medicine because they have not been included in clinical studies. That belief has resulted in laws and regulations mandating minority inclusion in US government-funded research and in privately funded research presented to the US Food and Drug Administration for drug and treatment approval (Freedman et al. 1995).

While these laws are met to improve health for a large group of Americans who do suffer disparately, some are based on erroneous assumptions and ignoring important facts. The concept of race is often used in a naïve, simplistic way (Baker et al. 2017). While populations do have biologic differences, racial categorization is inappropriate in studying these differences (Rotimi 2004) (Yudell et al. 2016). While race is less important biologically, race does matter sociopolitically. It is important to appreciate that a substantial proportion of especially black, but also poor, Americans receive less than optimal healthcare (Shavers and Brown 2002).

The Applicability of Clinical Findings

The clinical trialist must respect the rules of the research funders and medical regulators while trying to conduct good science and assure/ensure that clinical research addresses the health needs of all Americans (Freedman et al. 1995). Applicability is an issue that must be approached logically and rationally. Diverse inclusion in clinical trials is appropriate and important for it can help define the distribution of specific genomic markers in the population. In some cases, targeted study of populations with a specific marker is appropriate (Ellison et al. 2008).

One can view interventional clinical studies (treatment and prevention) as a spectrum from efficacy to effectiveness. An efficacy study assesses the intervention in close to an ideal environment. It often can be thought of as addressing the question "does an intervention work?" An effectiveness study assesses the intervention in the real world. It asks the question "how well does the intervention work in the population?" There is no such thing as a pure effectiveness study, but larger population-based phase 3 studies are close to pure effectiveness studies (Wells 1999).

The effectiveness question is best assessed on a large population with few entry criteria or barriers to entry. It should not have just broad racial representation, but broad representation by as many factors as possible, socioeconomic status (SES), clinical site of care, and even geography. The expansion of the NCI clinical trials network beyond academic cancer centers to include community centers was in part an effort to improve estimates of effectiveness (Kaluzny et al. 1994).

Again, outcomes from large clinical trials with a diverse representative population of subjects and providers speak to the population and not to the individual. The result tells us how well the intervention works on the entire population. It is limited in how it addresses the issue of how well the intervention works on an individual or group of individuals. This is a constant tension in the politics regarding clinical trials.

Defining and Categorizing Populations

A great problem is the focus on race as a biological categorization and biological differences between the races. American society has struggled with the concept of race ever since slaves were brought to the new world in 1619. Slavery was justified based on the belief that Africans were less than human. Later, the racial terms Negroes or blacks were applied to people of African heritage. Even in the twentieth century, race has been viewed as a defining biological difference. In the 1930s, it was commonly believed that syphilis affected whites, the more human race, more so and differently than blacks. Officially entitled "The Study of Untreated Syphilis in the Negro Male," and better known as "The Tuskegee Syphilis Trial," it compared 401 men with tertiary syphilis to 199 men who did not. This trial lasted more than 40 years. The study is famous for its many ethical affronts such as lying to subjects to make them stay in the study, unnecessary and painful testing such as lumbar punctures, and withholding treatment for syphilis once a cure was available (Brawley 1998). Indeed, this trial and the fact it could go on for more than four decades are major reasons that many minorities are suspicious of American medicine and hesitant to seek basic medical care, not just enter clinical trials (Baker et al. 2005).

Race as used in US databases is defined by the US Office of Management and Budget (OMB) in the Office of the President just before every decennial census (https://obamawhitehouse.archives.gov/omb/fedreg_directive_15). These definitions are to be used in the collection of all US government data, including health data (Friedman et al. 2000). The document defining race for every census since 1960 states that race is a sociopolitical categorization and is not based in biology. The US government racial definitions have changed over time. The categories have changed, as have the definition of the categories.

The racial categories used in the 2000, 2010, and 2020 censuses are:

- White or Caucasian
- Black or African American
- Asian
- American Indian/Alaskan Native
- Native Hawaiian or other Pacific Islander (Friedman et al. 2000)

In some censuses, Hawaiians were considered Native Americans. In others, Pacific Islanders were combined with Asians, and in yet others they were separated from Asians and combined into a category "Native Hawaiian or other Pacific Islander." The 1990 census allowed for an individual to select only one race. A major change in the 2000 and later censuses is people were instructed to select one or more races to indicate what the individual considered themselves to be. This was an acknowledgment of the many multiracial Americans.

The US OMB recognizes only two ethnicities, non-Hispanic and Hispanic. In truth, there are numerous ethnicities among people originating in Europe, Africa, Asia, or even among Hispanics. These multiple ethnicities could be used as scientific categorizations as they relate to cultural factors such as diet and lifestyle. These are health behaviors that influence not just risk of disease, but type of disease (Friedman et al. 2000; Parker and Makuc 2002). The anthropologic community has noted that race has no taxonomic significance (Baker et al. 2017). It is a very broad categorization that is loosely associated with area of geographic origin. Caucasian refers to people from 840 areas of geographic origin. Negro refers to people from 109 defined areas (Dai et al. 2020). As understanding grows, the number of defined areas of geographic origin is likely to grow.

Racial self-identity often does not correlate with genetic ancestry (Foster and Sharp 2002; Ntzani et al. 2012. Interestingly, most Americans who identify as black have some European genetics, and a good proportion of Americans identifying as white have African genetics. Centuries of admixture undermine the use of labels that group individuals into discrete nonoverlapping categories. A noted social scientist once said, "trying to categorize populations by race is like trying to slice soup"(2002).

While race has been medicalized, area of geographic origin, ancestry, and family history are scientifically important and less appreciated. There are certain genetic predispositions associated with specific areas of geographic origin. Examples include:

- Glucose-6-phosphate dehydrogenase (G6PD) deficiency is particularly common in certain parts of Africa, Asia, the Mediterranean, and the Middle East. Specific mutations of the gene coding for G6PD are specific to specific geographic regions (Howes et al. 2013).
- The HLA-B*15:02 allele has a strong association with carbamazepine-induced Stevens-Johnson syndrome. This allele has a very high prevalence among persons living along the Thai-Myanmar border (Jaruthamsophon et al. 2017).
- Aldehyde dehydrogenase deficiency causes flushing with alcohol consumption. Most Aldehyde dehydrogenase deficiency is due to inheritance of variants in gene coding for the ALDH enzyme due to single-nucleotide polymorphisms (SNPs). By some estimates, one in three people with east Asian (Chinese, Japanese, and Korean) ancestry has it (Harada 2001).
- Sickle cell disease is a group of disorders affecting hemoglobin. Each disorder is due to a specific single nucleotide polymorphism. Sickle cell anemia is due to a SNP causing HgS. This SNP is most common among people originating in malaria-prone regions of sub-Saharan Africa but is also found in people originating in the Mediterranean (including Italy and Greece), the Middle East, and India (Mangla et al. 2020).
- Lung cancers with mutations of the epidermal growth factor receptor (EGFR) are often responsive to growth factor inhibitors such as erlotinib. These mutations are more common in lung cancer patients from East Asia (Zhang et al. 2016).

It is important to note that these are genomic markers each with a higher prevalence in people from a specific area, and in people with ancestral history from a specific area. In no case should we assume people from a specific area monopolize the genomic markers above. The clinician caring for a patient might be tempted to engage in a sort of "benevolent profiling" and test for a specific marker because a patient appears from a specific geographic area or of a specific descent. Patients who do not fit the profile would still be harmed. This is an argument in support of whole genome sequencing of all patients with a serious illness. Whole genome sequencing to find novel therapeutic approaches for cancer patients with relapsed or newly diagnosed advanced disease is increasingly common in many academic practices and fast becoming the standard of care in the USA (Marquart et al. 2018).

The Importance of Race

While race is not a biological categorization, it is a political and socioeconomic categorization in the USA with black more often meaning poor. Socioeconomics can influence risk of disease and even epigenetics of disease. Socioeconomic status (SES) often correlates with race and can make race appear to be an appropriate category (Coughlin 2019). Indeed, research has shown that the predominant reason for racial disparities is differences in SES. In the case of drugs for common acute and chronic diseases, more often, it is not that the drug does not work in racial minorities, rather that the drug is not available, not prescribed, and/or not taken. Studies demonstrate disparities in care from preventative, to screening, to diagnostic, to therapeutic, and to end of life care using such SES variables as household income, insurance status, or maximum education (Siegel et al. 2011). SES can also correlate with some environmental exposures that cause epigenetic changes (Lara et al. 2020). Epigenetic influences are environmental effects on genetics that can be passed from one generation to the next.

Federal Laws Regarding Inclusion

The NIH first published regulations mandating minority inclusion in NIH-sponsored clinical trials in 1994 (Freedman et al. 1995). The US Food and Drug Administration and the European Medicines Agency have since published guidance aimed at improving diversity in clinical trials (Baird 1999). The published purpose of these efforts is to ensure that the discoveries, treatments, interventions, and prevention strategies derived from clinical trials are relevant to minority populations.

A brief review of the history leading up to this legislation and subsequent rules is helpful in understanding how to appropriately design and conduct clinical trials. The Physicians' Health Study was designed in the late 1970s and started in 1982 (1989). The initially unnamed trial was to randomize more than 20,000 people to daily beta carotene, aspirin, or placebo to determine if these drugs prevented cardiac disease and cancer. Trial participants would need to be followed for a long time. It was decided to enroll physicians as they are easy to follow long term. In 1981, most physicians were male, and it was decided the trial would be most efficient as a study of male physicians. In 1989, the study found that an aspirin per day reduces relative risk of myocardial infarction in men by 44%. This, of course, led to the question "what about women?"

Revitalization acts are federal laws that give US government institutions guidelines to carry out their work. The NIH Revitalization Act of 1993 was being written at the time of the uproar (Freedman et al. 1995). Language was put into the act saying that women must be included in NIH-sponsored clinical research, to include clinical trials, if women get the disease being studied. Furthermore, the trial must be designed and carried out in a manner sufficient to provide for "valid analysis" of whether the variables being studied in the trial affect women differently.

The early 1990s was a time when healthcare differences among racial groups were becoming even more appreciated. Numerous studies had demonstrated that black Americans had higher rates of death from cancer, diabetes, cardiovascular disease, and stroke (Ruffin 1995). As noted above, many believed and the law says that many disparities are due to the lack of blacks in clinical trials, and newly developed drugs and treatments simply did not work or did not work as well in blacks. The proposed legislation was changed to say, "women or members of minority groups" wherever it said "women." Hence the legislation mandated subgroup analysis to evaluate the differences among minority groups. This version of the legislation was passed by both houses of congress and signed into law by President William Clinton on June 10, 1993.

There were no hearings or attempt at fact-finding before the language was adapted. Some aspects of the law are very nonscientific. There is also ambiguous language in the act. The call for valid subgroup analysis implied that any subgroup analysis could provide statically significant meaningful findings. It is clear "members of minority groups" refer to racial minorities. Many of the well-meaning legislators and many in the US population including scientists were and still are of the belief that race is a biological categorization.

The NIH Interpretation of the Inclusion Law

The NIH Director facing a legislation with some ambiguity and some conflict with the conduct of good science commissioned a group of biostatisticians, epidemiologists, and clinicians representing all the NIH institutes to give perspective for NIH-funded clinical trialists. This was published as the "NIH Guidelines" in the Federal Register on March 28, 1994. These experts interpreted the act "as demanding appropriate representation of subjects of different gender and race/ethnicity in clinical trials so as to provide the opportunity for detecting major qualitative differences," if they exist" among gender and racial/ethnic subgroups and to identify more subtle differences that might, if warranted, be explored further in specifically targeted studies" (Freedman et al. 1995).

The experts defined certain terms in the legislation:

- "Clinical trials" refer to phase 3 clinical investigations.
- "Valid analysis" means an unbiased assessment. Valid analysis is interpreted as not meaning "statistically valid analysis."
- "Significant difference" is understood as the meaning of a difference which is of clinical or public health import. It does not mean a "statistically significant difference."

The NIH has updated its guidance three times over the past 25 years. It has required the clinical trialist to address the issue of minority inclusion and generalization of findings in the protocol and to have a plan for minority accrual. Funding has been cut or even terminated in extreme cases where investigators have not taken the issue seriously. Peer review has generally rewarded those who can put race, culture, socioeconomic status, and area of geographic origin in proper perspective and properly design clinical studies looking for important leads and having a plan to diversify recruitment as much as possible (Teh 2019).

The US Food and Drug Administration (FDA) has issued guidance asking collection of racial and demographic data in registry trials (https://www.fda.gov/media/75453/download). For new drug applications, sponsors must present a summary of safety and effective data by demographic subgroups which include age and race.

Potential Harms Caused by the Law

There are some potentially harmful outcomes to the legislation and resulting policies that mandate racial inclusion. First, subset analysis,, even when done correctly, can be wrong. This can lead to the unexpected harm of a wrong conclusion. Subset analysis by its nature is underpowered and should be used only to support a hypothesis for future research. If a clinical trial were powered to have valid subset analysis, it would require oversampling of the minority populations. As a clinical trial involves some risk, oversampling would mean increased risk for members of especially smaller racial groups who would have to be disproportionately accrued. This poses an ethical challenge.

Rumor of a racial difference or good science misinterpreted can cause harm. In 1991, a subset analysis was performed in one of the first studies to show the efficacy of zidovudine, also known as AZT, in the treatment of advanced HIV disease (Easterbrook et al. 1991; Lagakos et al. 1991; Smith 1991). Non-Hispanic whites had a 40% 2-year survival, Hispanics had a 39% survival, and blacks had a lower 2-year survival of 27%. The authors were concerned about the finding and very specifically noted that there was no racial difference in outcome when there was adjustment for severity of disease at the start of the trial and medication compliance. Blacks were, as a group, sicker than whites and Hispanics at the start of the trial and less adherent to the prescribed drug regimen. This is a case of good science followed by racial stereotyping and public disinformation leading to harm. The news media failed to convey the complete finding. The finding that blacks did not do as well led to a wide-scale rumor in black communities that AZT was a "white people's drug." Nearly 30 years later, it is common to hear in many black communities that AIDs treatments work better in whites than blacks (Bogart et al. 2010). All due to incomplete conveyance of this clinical finding. HIV treatment has improved to the point that Zidovudine is not even used anymore.

The requirement for minority inclusion creates another ethical challenge. The physician and clinical trials data manager should offer every eligible patient the opportunity to participate in an available trial and respect the patient's decision. However, the NIH can withdraw funding for a trial that has inadequate minority accrual. This means the physician and data manager are incentivized to recruit minority candidates to trial more so than majority candidates. While consenting the minority candidate, even the most well-meaning person knows that recruitment of the minority keeps them employed. The law encourages them to give the minority candidate the hard sell and give the white candidate a choice.

Inclusion Is Important

We should prioritize inclusion while respecting an individual's right not to participate. Pharmacogenetics is associated with area of geographic origin. The key to benefiting as many people as possible is to know as much as possible about the pharmacology/metabolism of the drug as well as the drug's mechanism of action and target (Teh

2019). We should then study the variance of these factors across the population at large. This does require study of a broad diverse group of people. In some instances, there should be a targeted study of specific populations. These populations should not be described by race, but by area of geographic origin or better yet by a molecular marker. The existence of people of mixed descent should be accepted. In this author's opinion, this has not happened well enough in American research.

Tamoxifen was developed in the 1970s. It was approved by the US FDA in 1977, after a clinical trial showed that some women with metastatic disease had regression of tumor. The drug was approved before subset analysis by race was mandated and before the introduction of the estrogen receptor assay (Manni et al. 1980). Under today's rules, the drug might have been approved for whites and not for blacks. Appreciation of tamoxifen pharmacology and the development of robust estrogen receptor assays allow us to now know that breast cancer patients of African descent are less likely to have estrogen receptor positive disease compared to women from Europe. However, tamoxifen is a fine drug for the 70% or so who do have estrogen receptor positive disease (Kong et al. 2020).

Many of today's precision cancer medicines are developed in smaller phase 2 trials or umbrella trials enrolling patients based on molecular abnormalities in tumors. Enrollment in precision medicine studies requires assessment of genetic or molecular abnormalities in the patient's cancer. These findings often require next-generation sequencing (Nassar et al. 2020). This is expensive. Poor or underinsured patients often do not get these tests. It is most concerning that individuals of European descent comprise well over 90% of participants in genome-wide association studies. These molecular studies have become standard of care, and large numbers of minorities are unable to participate for SES reasons (Adigbli 2020).

NIH-sponsored trials, especially, are rigorously peer reviewed, meaning the patients receive good care as defined by experts. Kaluzny and colleagues have demonstrated that participation in clinical trials is a way of assuring receipt of state-of-the-art, adequate care (Kaluzny et al. 1993). Meta-analysis of clinical trials that enroll a large proportion of minority patients has been helpful in dismissing some of the race-based theories by demonstrating that equal treatment generally yields equal outcome among equal patients. There is social and scientific value in grouping a number of trials with diverse inclusion together and studying them carefully. For example, in a study of multiple clinical trials of men from the VA, DOD, SEER, and 4 RTOG trials that rigorously adjusted for demographic data, black race was not associated with inferior stage-for-stage prostate cancer-specific mortality (Dess et al. 2019). Other meta-analyses have tried to do this but failed to adequately adjust for socioeconomic status (Dignam 2010).

Ironically, the emphasis on difference in biology by race has taken emphasis away from the fact that there is not equal treatment by race. Patterns of care studies demonstrate that a substantial number of minorities receive substandard care (DeSantis et al. 2019). Indeed, considerable numbers of minority and poor Americans could be saved if all received adequate available care (Ma et al. 2019). Study after study shows that black women with breast cancer are less likely to receive appropriate surgery or radiation compared to whites. Black women are also less likely to receive appropriate hormonal therapy or chemotherapy, and when treated with chemotherapy they are less likely to be dosed appropriately (Short et al. 2010). These disparities are usually more closely correlated with socioeconomic status than race, but race is often correlated with socioeconomic status (DeSantis et al. 2016).

There is also benefit in seeing physicians and clinical practices who offer clinical trials. Doctors who participate in clinical trials take better care of all their patients, not just the 3–5% they put on clinical trials, compared to doctors who do not participate in clinical trials (McFall et al. 1996). This is an especially important issue when there is significant data showing that a large proportion of minorities in the USA get less than optimal standard care.

Summary and Conclusion

Race as used in the USA is a flawed concept that is often used in naïve, simplistic ways. There is also limited understanding of clinical trials and clinical research among physicians and the lay public. There is misunderstanding of how trials are conducted and how trials can be beneficial. These misunderstandings lead to patient distrust of research and a reluctance to participate in clinical trials especially among minority patients. Ironically, the existence of the NIH Revitalization Act of 1993 and the mandating of racial inclusion can increase distrust.

Institutions and individuals who have success recruiting minority patients to clinical trials have a reputation for providing compassionate service to their communities. Many institutions have found it easier to recruit minority patients to interventional treatment trials as compared to recruiting well subjects to nontherapeutic trials, that is, it is easier to recruit patients who have an illness to treatment studies versus well patients to a study trying to develop a prevention or screening tool. The addition of navigators and data managers who can spend time talking and explaining to candidates is helpful (Cook et al. 2010).

Scientists do need to be attentive to the question "How can we best serve the needs of the entire population?" It is a fact that science and society have slighted the health needs of women and minorities. Focusing only on racial inclusion in clinical trials is not enough. Serving all requires a very focused logical effort at defining populations and their biologic differences, as well as defining the reasons for disparities in outcome (Trant et al. 2020). When it comes to health disparities, "race" is not the appropriate categorization in terms of biology although it is an appropriate category in terms of access to quality care. Indeed, there is legitimate reason to stress racial equity using race as a socioeconomic not a biologic categorization. Health equity is a matter of human rights and social justice.

Key Facts

Race is and should be viewed as a sociopolitical categorization of populations. It is not a valid biological categorization of populations. By federal law, racial inclusion must be collected and reported for NIH-funded clinical trials. Racial demographics should also be reported for FDA registration trials. While racial subset analysis is required for NIH-funded phase 3 clinical trials, one should look at the data with a broad open mind. One should look for the distribution genomic markers of drug metabolism or drug targets in a population defined by area of geographic origin or ancestry.

References

(1989) Final report on the aspirin component of the ongoing Physicians' Health Study. N Engl J Med 321(3):129–135
(2002) Slicing soup. Nat Biotechnol 20(7):637
Adigbli G (2020) Race, science and (im)precision medicine. Nat Med 26(11):1675–1676
Baird KL (1999) The new NIH and FDA medical research policies: targeting gender, promoting justice. J Health Polit Policy Law 24(3):531–565
Baker SM, Brawley OW, Marks LS (2005) Effects of untreated syphilis in the negro male, 1932 to 1972: a closure comes to the Tuskegee study, 2004. Urology 65(6):1259–1262
Baker JL, Rotimi CN, Shriner D (2017) Human ancestry correlates with language and reveals that race is not an objective genomic classifier. Sci Rep 7(1):1572
Bogart LM, Wagner G, Galvan FH, Banks D (2010) Conspiracy beliefs about HIV are related to antiretroviral treatment nonadherence among african american men with HIV. J Acquir Immune Defic Syndr 53(5):648–655
Brawley OW (1998) The study of untreated syphilis in the negro male. Int J Radiat Oncol Biol Phys 40(1):5–8
Cerdeña JP, Plaisime MV, Tsai J (2020) From race-based to race-conscious medicine: how antiracist uprisings call us to act. Lancet 396(10257):1125–1128
Cook ED, Arnold KB, Hermos JA, McCaskill-Stevens W, Moody-Thomas S, Probstfield JL, Hamilton SJ, Campbell RD, Anderson KB, Minasian LM (2010) Impact of supplemental site grants to increase African American accrual for the Selenium and Vitamin E Cancer Prevention Trial. Clin Trials 7(1):90–99
Coughlin SS (2019) Social determinants of breast cancer risk, stage, and survival. Breast Cancer Res Treat 177(3):537–548
Dai CL, Vazifeh MM, Yeang CH, Tachet R, Wells RS, Vilar MG, Daly MJ, Ratti C, Martin AR (2020) Population histories of the United States revealed through fine-scale migration and haplotype analysis. Am J Hum Genet 106(3):371–388
DeSantis CE, Siegel RL, Sauer AG, Miller KD, Fedewa SA, Alcaraz KI, Jemal A (2016) Cancer statistics for African Americans, 2016: progress and opportunities in reducing racial disparities. CA Cancer J Clin 66(4):290–308
DeSantis CE, Miller KD, Goding Sauer A, Jemal A, Siegel RL (2019) Cancer statistics for African Americans, 2019. CA Cancer J Clin 69(3):211–233
Dess RT, Hartman HE, Mahal BA, Soni PD, Jackson WC, Cooperberg MR, Amling CL, Aronson WJ, Kane CJ, Terris MK, Zumsteg ZS, Butler S, Osborne JR, Morgan TM, Mehra R, Salami SS, Kishan AU, Wang C, Schaeffer EM, Roach M 3rd, Pisansky TM, Shipley WU, Freedland SJ, Sandler HM, Halabi S, Feng FY, Dignam JJ, Nguyen PL, Schipper MJ, Spratt DE (2019) Association of Black race with prostate cancer-specific and other-cause mortality. JAMA Oncol 5(7):975–983
Dignam JJ (2010) Re: Racial disparities in cancer survival among randomized clinical trials of the Southwest Oncology Group. J Natl Cancer Inst 102(4):279–280; author reply 280–272
Easterbrook PJ, Keruly JC, Creagh-Kirk T, Richman DD, Chaisson RE, Moore RD (1991) Racial and ethnic differences in outcome in zidovudine-treated patients with advanced HIV disease. Zidovudine Epidemiology Study Group. JAMA 266(19):2713–2718
Ellison GT, Kaufman JS, Head RF, Martin PA, Kahn JD (2008) Flaws in the U.S. Food and Drug Administration's rationale for supporting the development and approval of BiDil as a treatment for heart failure only in black patients. J Law Med Ethics 36(3):449–457

Eneanya ND, Yang W, Reese PP (2019) Reconsidering the consequences of using race to estimate kidney function. JAMA 322(2):113–114

Flack JM, Mensah GA, Ferrario CM (2000) Using angiotensin converting enzyme inhibitors in African-American hypertensives: a new approach to treating hypertension and preventing target-organ damage. Curr Med Res Opin 16(2):66–79

Foster MW, Sharp RR (2002) Race, ethnicity, and genomics: social classifications as proxies of heterogeneity. Genome Res 12(6):844–850

Freedman LS, Simon R, Foulkes MA, Friedman L, Geller NL, Gordon DJ, Mowery R (1995) Inclusion of women and minorities in clinical trials and the NIH Revitalization Act of 1993–the perspective of NIH clinical trialists. Control Clin Trials 16(5):277–285; discussion 286–279, 293–309

Friedman DJ, Cohen BB, Averbach AR, Norton JM (2000) Race/ethnicity and OMB Directive 15: implications for state public health practice. Am J Public Health 90(11):1714–1719

Harada S (2001) Classification of alcohol metabolizing enzymes and polymorphisms–specificity in Japanese. Nihon Arukoru Yakubutsu Igakkai Zasshi 36(2):85–106

Howard J, Hankey BF, Greenberg RS, Austin DF, Correa P, Chen VW, Durako S (1992) A collaborative study of differences in the survival rates of black patients and white patients with cancer. Cancer 69(9):2349–2360

Howes RE, Dewi M, Piel FB, Monteiro WM, Battle KE, Messina JP, Sakuntabhai A, Satyagraha AW, Williams TN, Baird JK, Hay SI (2013) Spatial distribution of G6PD deficiency variants across malaria-endemic regions. Malar J 12:418

Jaruthamsophon K, Tipmanee V, Sangiemchoey A, Sukasem C, Limprasert P (2017) HLA-B*15:21 and carbamazepine-induced Stevens-Johnson syndrome: pooled-data and in silico analysis. Sci Rep 7:45553

Kaluzny A, Brawley O, Garson-Angert D, Shaw J, Godley P, Warnecke R, Ford L (1993) Assuring access to state-of-the-art care for U.S. minority populations: the first 2 years of the Minority-Based Community Clinical Oncology Program. J Natl Cancer Inst 85(23):1945–1950

Kaluzny AD, Lacey LM, Warnecke R, Morrissey JP, Sondik E, Ford L (1994) Using a community cancer treatment trials network for cancer prevention and control research: challenges and opportunities. Cancer Epidemiol Biomark Prev 3(3):261–269

Kong X, Liu Z, Cheng R, Sun L, Huang S, Fang Y, Wang J (2020) Variation in breast cancer subtype incidence and distribution by race/ethnicity in the United States from 2010 to 2015. JAMA Netw Open 3(10):e2020303

Lagakos S, Fischl MA, Stein DS, Lim L, Volberding P (1991) Effects of zidovudine therapy in minority and other subpopulations with early HIV infection. JAMA 266(19):2709–2712

Lara OD, Wang Y, Asare A, Xu T, Chiu HS, Liu Y, Hu W, Sumazin P, Uppal S, Zhang L, Rauh-Hain JA, Sood AK (2020) Pan-cancer clinical and molecular analysis of racial disparities. Cancer 126(4):800–807

Lujan HL, DiCarlo SE (2018) Science reflects history as society influences science: brief history of "race," "race correction," and the spirometer. Adv Physiol Educ 42(2):163–165

Ma J, Jemal A, Fedewa SA, Islami F, Lichtenfeld JL, Wender RC, Cullen KJ, Brawley OW (2019) The American Cancer Society 2035 challenge goal on cancer mortality reduction. CA Cancer J Clin 69(5):351–362

Mangla A, Ehsan M, Maruvada S (2020) Sickle Cell Anemia. StatPearls, Treasure Island

Manni A, Arafah B, Pearson OH (1980) Estrogen and progesterone receptors in the prediction of response of breast cancer to endocrine therapy. Cancer 46(12 Suppl):2838–2841

Marquart J, Chen EY, Prasad V (2018) Estimation of the percentage of US patients with cancer who benefit from genome-driven oncology. JAMA Oncol 4(8):1093–1098

McFall SL, Warnecke RB, Kaluzny AD, Ford L (1996) Practice setting and physician influences on judgments of colon cancer treatment by community physicians. Health Serv Res 31(1):5–19

Nassar SF, Raddassi K, Ubhi B, Doktorski J, Abulaban A (2020) Precision medicine: steps along the road to combat human cancer. Cells 9(9):2056

Ntzani EE, Liberopoulos G, Manolio TA, Ioannidis JP (2012) Consistency of genome-wide associations across major ancestral groups. Hum Genet 131(7):1057–1071

Parker JD, Makuc DM (2002) Methodologic implications of allocating multiple-race data to single-race categories. Health Serv Res 37(1):203–215

Rotimi CN (2004) Are medical and nonmedical uses of large-scale genomic markers conflating genetics and 'race'? Nat Genet 36(11 Suppl):S43–S47

Ruffin J (1995) Forging alliances to meet future research and research training needs. J Natl Med Assoc 87(8 Suppl):624–626

Shavers VL, Brown ML (2002) Racial and ethnic disparities in the receipt of cancer treatment. J Natl Cancer Inst 94(5):334–357

Short LJ, Fisher MD, Wahl PM, Kelly MB, Lawless GD, White S, Rodriguez NA, Willey VJ, Brawley OW (2010) Disparities in medical care among commercially insured patients with newly diagnosed breast cancer: opportunities for intervention. Cancer 116(1):193–202

Siegel R, Ward E, Brawley O, Jemal A (2011) Cancer statistics, 2011: the impact of eliminating socioeconomic and racial disparities on premature cancer deaths. CA Cancer J Clin 61(4): 212–236

Smith MD (1991) Zidovudine. Does it work for everyone? JAMA 266(19):2750–2751

Teh BT (2019) The importance of including diverse populations in cancer genomic and epigenomic studies. Nat Rev Cancer 19(7):361–362

Trant AA, Walz L, Allen W, DeJesus J, Hatzis C, Silber A (2020) Increasing accrual of minority patients in breast cancer clinical trials. Breast Cancer Res Treat 184(2):499–505

Wells KB (1999) Treatment research at the crossroads: the scientific interface of clinical trials and effectiveness research. Am J Psychiatry 156(1):5–10

Yudell M, Roberts D, DeSalle R, Tishkoff S (2016) SCIENCE AND SOCIETY. Taking race out of human genetics. Science 351(6273):564–565

Zhang YL, Yuan JQ, Wang KF, Fu XH, Han XR, Threapleton D, Yang ZY, Mao C, Tang JL (2016) The prevalence of EGFR mutation in patients with non-small cell lung cancer: a systematic review and meta-analysis. Oncotarget 7(48):78985–78993

Expanded Access to Drug and Device Products for Clinical Treatment

124

Tracy Ziolek, Jessica L. Yoos, Inna Strakovsky, Praharsh Shah, and Emily Robison

Contents

Introduction	2432
Expanded Access to Investigational Drugs	2433
Single-Patient Treatment Use of an Investigational Drug Product	2434
Single-Patient Emergency Use of an Investigational Drug Product	2435
Intermediate-Size Population and Treatment Use of an Investigational Drug Product	2436
Expanded Access to Investigational Devices	2437
Single-Patient Emergency Use of an Investigational Device	2438
Individual Patient/Small Group Compassionate Use of an Investigational Device	2440
Treatment Use of an Investigational Device	2441
Treatment with a Humanitarian Use Device	2443
International Regulations for Expanded Access to Drug and Device Products for Clinical Treatment	2446
Australia	2447
Brazil	2448
Canada	2449
Summary and Conclusion	2449
Key Facts	2450
Cross-References	2450
References	2450

Abstract

Historically, patient access to investigational products (drugs or devices) has been limited to enrollment in clinical trials. However, enrollment of a patient into a clinical trial is not always possible for various reasons. Demand from patients and

---

T. Ziolek (✉) · J. L. Yoos · I. Strakovsky · P. Shah
University of Pennsylvania, Philadelphia, PA, USA
e-mail: ziolekt@upenn.edu; tracy_ziolek@uhg.com; jessyoos@upenn.edu; innastr@upenn.edu; prahp@upenn.edu

E. Robison
Optum Labs, Las Vegas, NV, USA
e-mail: Emily_robison@uhg.com

© Springer Nature Switzerland AG 2022
S. Piantadosi, C. L. Meinert (eds.), *Principles and Practice of Clinical Trials*,
https://doi.org/10.1007/978-3-319-52636-2_172

physicians for access to investigational products is due to the (sometimes remote) potential benefit to patients who have no other therapeutic alternatives.

There are various options for the use of investigational drugs and devices in patient treatment through the Food and Drug Administration's (FDA) expanded access program. These are outlined, along with criteria for use, submission requirements, approval processes, and associated practical guidance.

There are four expanded access pathways for the use of investigational drugs: single-patient emergency use, single-patient treatment use, intermediate-size population treatment use, and treatment use. There are three expanded access pathways for the use of investigational devices: single-patient emergency use, single-patient or small group compassionate use, and treatment use. Additionally, treatment of a rare disease or condition with a Humanitarian Use Device (HUD) under a Humanitarian Device Exemption (HDE) is also possible.

Keywords

Expanded access · Emergency use · Compassionate use · Treatment use · Humanitarian use · Investigational drug · Investigational device · FDA · Life-threatening

Introduction

The most common avenue of access to investigational products (drugs and devices) occurs by enrolling into an approved clinical trial. The volume of clinical trials being conducted in a variety of targeted medical conditions continues to increase. There is more access now than ever before to innovative and cutting-edge products as they are being formally investigated within the context of a clinical trial. While this does offer a potential for benefit from a clinical care perspective on an individual patient level, the overall intention of most clinical trials is to collect initial or additional information related to safety and effectiveness of a product. Therefore, any benefit to those willing to participate is not guaranteed (at least in the earliest phases of clinical research). However, even with the more expansive options for clinical trial participation in the current medical setting, there remains a need to provide opportunity for the receipt of investigational drugs and devices on either an individual patient basis or for smaller groups of patients.

The regulations governing the use of investigational drugs and devices allow for scenarios in which an investigational product may be utilized for the purposes of clinical care. These pathways may be used when an appropriate argument can be made that it is in the best interest of the patient to do so, and when the investigational product is known to be the only option for the patient (either due to no other therapies being available for that condition, or the therapies are known to be subpar). This treatment option for individual and small groups of patients has been a part of FDA regulation for some time and has been often utilized by those who were aware of the options and the approval process.

However, despite these available pathways, some patients have been unable to gain access to investigational products at all or in a timely manner. Product manufacturers are not required to allow access to their products for these purposes, and some have refused to do so. This led to the initiation of Right to Try laws in various states. The Right to Try movement created political pressure to improve access to investigational products. FDA thus worked towards facilitating the expanded access submission process. Subsequently, the 21st Century Cures Act (United States (US) Government Publishing Office (GPO) 2016) was signed into law in 2016. The purpose of the 21st Century Cures Act is to facilitate the development of new products so that patients may get access to them faster. The Act also allocates funds to the FDA to implement related changes. More recently, the federal Right to Try Act was signed into law.

Previously, FDA regulations limited the use of data from those who receive an investigational drug for treatment use purposes. The motive behind this limitation was twofold. First, it was based on the idea that the use of the drug or device in a single patient was for altruistic purposes only. Moreover, given the data was not collected in the context of a controlled clinical trial, it was thought that the data could not be used in support of the safety or efficacy of the drug or device.

However, recent regulatory updates related to the 21st Century Cures Act now allow for data from single patients and small groups of patients via expanded access to be included in support of drug and device approval to the FDA. Such data may be considered appropriate "real world evidence" that the FDA may be able to consider in support of product approval. This was a critical update, as previously it was necessary, from a human subjects' protections standpoint, to clearly state that data would not be used or shared for this purpose. Now, under the new allowances, it should be the exact opposite scenario that is shared in the consent form provided to the patient(s).

In order to better understand which options are available for use of investigational products for treatment and what the processes are to seek these approvals, each type of access scenario will be broken down. Practical guidance is provided related to seeking these options from the FDA, the manufacturer of the product, and the local ethical review entity (as well as any other ancillary review entities that may be required).

There are four expanded access pathways for the use of investigational drugs: single-patient emergency use, single-patient treatment use, intermediate-size population treatment use, and general treatment use. There are three expanded access pathways for the use of investigational devices: single-patient emergency use, single-patient or small group compassionate use, and treatment use. Additionally, treatment of a rare disease or condition with a Humanitarian Use Device (HUD) under a Humanitarian Device Exemption (HDE) is also possible. Key definitions that apply to both drugs and devices, as well as criteria for emergency use, compassionate use, and exception from informed consent are outlined in Table 1.

Expanded Access to Investigational Drugs

Access to investigational drugs are typically limited to clinical trial use through an Investigational New Drug (IND) application. A physician may treat a patient with an investigational drug outside of the context of an IND clinical trial through the FDA's

Table 1 Key definitions and criteria

	Criteria
Emergency use	1. The patient has a life-threatening or serious disease or condition that needs immediate treatment 2. No generally acceptable alternative treatment for the condition exists 3. Because of the immediate need to use the drug/device, there is no time to use existing procedures to obtain FDA approval for the use
Compassionate/ treatment use	1. The patient has a life-threatening or serious disease or condition 2. No generally acceptable alternative treatment for the condition exists
Exception from informed consent	1. The patient has a life-threatening or critical illness that requires the investigational product 2. Informed consent cannot be obtained due to the patient being unable to communicate or provide legally effective consent 3. There is inadequate time to obtain permission from the patient's legally authorized representation 4. There is no other approved or recognized treatment that would afford the same or greater probability of saving the patient's life
Life-threatening	1. The likelihood of death is high unless the course of the disease is interrupted 2. A disease or condition with a potentially fatal outcome, where the end-point is survival 3. The disease or condition causes major irreversible morbidity

expanded access program. However, the use of an investigational drug in this manner is restricted to patients with serious or life-threatening illnesses for which there is no alternative therapy. There are four expanded access pathways for the use of investigational drugs: single-patient treatment use, single-patient emergency use, intermediate-size population compassionate use, and treatment use.

Single-Patient Treatment Use of an Investigational Drug Product

One of the most common access options, and the one that clinicians are most familiar with, is the single-patient treatment use. Single-patient treatment use allows for use of an investigational drug in one patient. However, it must be confirmed that the investigational product is the best option for the patient's clinical care based on the current standard of care options available. Moreover, the patient must not have any options in terms of a locally available clinical trial, either due to the fact that there is not a local clinical trial or the patient does not qualify for the trial, and an exception to include them into the trial is not appropriate. Once it is determined that an investigational drug is the best option for the patient, the following steps must occur in order to move forward. The timing of these steps carries great importance as well:

- Determine availability of the drug as well as the manufacturer's willingness to provide the drug for the single-patient treatment use.

Please note: The drug may be available on site already if there is a clinical trial being conducted (however, appropriate permissions to use the drug (or any other product) for this purpose must be sought prior to use). Alternatively, the drug may need to be requested from the manufacturer to be sent to the site, if the drug is not available from the on-site pharmacy or clinical trial supply.
- If the drug availability/approval to use the drug has been secured, the application to the FDA may be completed. This requires submission of Form 3926 (or a standard Form 1571 may be used) along with all required corresponding supportive documentation.

    Please note: it is essential to select the appropriate option on the FDA Form to ensure that local ethical review can occur via a facilitated review (expedited review), as it is common in these scenarios to need to begin therapy quickly.
- After submission to the FDA, the local ethical review entity [likely an Institutional Review Board (IRB)] should be contacted to determine the local application needed to grant approval to the use of the investigation drug for this individual patient.

    Please note: This local application will require submission of the consent form that will be utilized for the patient for receipt of the investigational drug. If there is a local clinical trial, the clinical trial consent may be revised to reflect the single-patient treatment use scenario. If there is not a local clinical trial, the manufacturer may have a consent template for the drug that they can provide for local revisions to fit the request for the single-patient use. As a final option, a consent can be drafted by the clinician (or appropriate delegated personnel) to outline the necessary information to provide to the patient related to receipt of the investigational drug for treatment purposes.
- Once all appropriate approvals are in place, the patient may be approached for consenting to receive the investigational drug for their treatment. A standard consenting process should mostly be used. The physician should ensure the consent discussion clarifies that the patient is not joining a clinical trial, but is being offered the investigational drug as part of their clinical care. The consent discussion should also explain that it is felt by those engaged in the patient's care to be his/her best clinical option and why this is the case.

Single-Patient Emergency Use of an Investigational Drug Product

Another potential avenue for individual patient access to an investigational drug for treatment purposes is emergency use. Emergency use is similar to single-patient treatment use, with the following distinct differences.

The first difference is that the treating clinician and an unbiased second clinician must determine, per FDA requirements, that the patient's condition is life-threatening. Life-threatening, for the purposes of section 56.102(d), includes the scope of both life-threatening and severely debilitating, as defined in Table 1. The criteria for life-threatening do not require the condition to be immediately life-threatening or to immediately result in death. Rather, the subjects must be in a life-threatening situation requiring intervention before review at a convened meeting of the IRB is feasible. "Examples of severely debilitating conditions include blindness, loss of arm, leg, hand or foot, loss of hearing, paralysis or stroke." (FDA 2010).

The second substantial difference between single-patient treatment use and emergency use is the review of the treatment by the local ethical review entity (again, likely an IRB) in advance of the administration may not be required with emergency use. This is due to the emergent nature of the request. In addition, consent may or may not be able to obtained, given the medical condition of the patient and whether there is an appropriate surrogate available to provide permission for the patient to receive the investigational drug because it is thought to be the best option in this emergent situation.

Please note: FDA approval for requests of this nature can be sought at any time via phone.

Another point to consider is that emergency use of a drug is generally only possible when the drug is already present at the location where the emergency use is going to occur. However, there is still a requirement to seek approval from the manufacturer to utilize the drug for the emergency use purpose. However, practical judgement related to patient care takes precedent over administrative/logistical requirements.

Once the emergency use has occurred, the local ethical review entity should be provided with a status report of the patient's condition within five business days. This should occur regardless of whether the local ethical review entity was engaged in the original decision for the emergency use or consulted for concurrence with the decision. If consent was obtained either prior to the use of the investigational drug or permission/notification occurred after the drug was used, the 5-day report should indicate this.

Intermediate-Size Population and Treatment Use of an Investigational Drug Product

During the course of an IND trial, data may suggest that the drug product may be effective. A separate treatment protocol may be developed to make the drug available to seriously ill patients. This could be for a smaller group (intermediate size population) or a larger group of patients (treatment use). This may occur after trials have been completed or while trials are still ongoing. The criteria for treatment use as defined in Table 1 applies.

Prospective review of the protocol by the FDA would be required. The IND application would be required to include a full clinical trial protocol with a description of the drug's use, patient selection criteria, rationale for the use of the drug, as well as procedures and other measures that will be used to evaluate and monitor patient outcomes. A data safety monitoring plan would also be required. The sponsor should determine if a data safety monitoring board should be established. Product labelling and related information about safety and effectiveness must also be submitted to the FDA. This may be incorporated by reference through a letter of

Table 2 Review requirements by expanded access pathway for drug products

Type of expanded access	IRB review	Prior FDA approval
Single-patient emergency use	Post hoc notification	Yes
Single-patient treatment use	Convened review, unless box 10b is checked on FDA form 3926	Yes
Intermediate-size population Compassionate use	Convened review	Yes
Treatment use	Convened review	Yes

authorization from the drug manufacturer. Administrative information is also required, such as the sponsor's contact information and commitments to adhere to applicable regulations [21 CFR 312 (IND regulations), 21 CFR 56 (IRB regulations), and 21 CFR 50 (obtaining informed consent)] and the investigator(s') information on the 1572 form. The sponsor is responsible for submitting IND annual reports to the FDA as well as all other reports specified in 21 CFR 312.

Submission to the local ethical review entity and the FDA in tandem can make the submission process more efficient. A treatment IND protocol must be reviewed by an Institutional Review Board (IRB) at a convened meeting. Physicians should contact their local IRB or ethical review entity to determine institution specific submission requirements.

Prospective informed consent or permission from a legally authorized representative would be required unless criteria for an exception from informed consent were met. The consent discussion should be appropriately documented by way of an informed consent form. The consent discussion and associated form should clearly convey the investigational nature of the drug and the goal of treatment, rather than research (Table 2).

Expanded Access to Investigational Devices

Access to investigational devices that may pose significant risk to the health of a patient are typically restricted for clinical trial use through an Investigational Device Exemption (IDE). However, enrollment of a patient into a clinical trial is not always possible. This could be due to patient ineligibility or the lack of an active clinical trial with the device.

A physician may treat a patient with an investigational device outside of the context of an IDE clinical trial through the FDA's expanded access program. However, the use of an investigational device in this manner is restricted to patients with serious or life-threatening illnesses (see Table 1) for which there is no alternative therapy. There are three expanded access pathways for the use of investigational devices: emergency use, compassionate use, and treatment use. Additionally, a physician may treat a patient with a rare disease or condition with a Humanitarian Use Device (HUD) under a Humanitarian Device Exemption (HDE).

Single-Patient Emergency Use of an Investigational Device

The emergency use pathway for the use of an investigational device is restricted to emergency situations. The emergency use must meet specific criteria outlined by the FDA:

- The patient must have a life-threatening or serious illness that requires urgent treatment.
- There must be no other satisfactory therapies to treat the condition.
- Given the need for immediate treatment, there is no time to obtain FDA approval prior to the use of the device.

Requirements to Meet the Use of the Product

There are certain requirements that must be met before the emergency use of an investigational device to treat a single patient may take place. Once it has been confirmed that the above criteria are met, the device manufacturer must give authorization for the use of the device in this manner. If this authorization is received, an investigational device may be used through the emergency use expanded access pathway. This is permitted before an IDE for the device is approved, while the device is being investigated under an IDE, and when a device is not being investigated in a clinical trial.

FDA approval of the emergency use of an investigational device is not required prior to device administration, given the previously outlined criteria are met. However, FDA holds expectations for physicians using investigational devices in an emergency. The FDA expects the treating physician to confirm that the criteria for emergency use are met. Moreover, there should be potential benefit to the patient, and the physician should have appropriate rationale to support this.

The FDA also expects physicians to engage in as many patient protection measures as possible prior to the administration of the device. These include:

- Obtaining an impartial assessment from a physician not involved in the patient's care
- Following local institutional policies, including obtaining any necessary institutional approvals
- Obtaining informed consent from the patient or their legally authorized representative
- Obtaining concurrence from the Institutional Review Board (IRB) chair

Obtaining Informed Consent

Prospective informed consent or permission from a legally authorized representative would be required unless certain criteria are met. If consent can be obtained, a consent form should be used to document the consent discussion. The consent discussion and associated form should clearly convey the investigational nature of the device. Moreover, the use of the device should not be confused with research because the purpose is treatment.

If consent cannot be obtained, an exception from informed consent requirements may be possible [21 CFR 50.23(a)]. An exception may be granted when the following criteria are met:

- The patient has a life-threatening or critical illness that requires the investigational product.
- Informed consent cannot be obtained due to the patient being unable to communicate or provide legally effective consent.
- There is inadequate time to obtain permission from the patient's legally authorized representative.
- There is no other approved or recognized treatment that would afford the same or greater probability of saving the patient's life.

If these criteria are met, the physician should document the rationale for the determination. The rationale should be reviewed by an independent physician not involved in the patient's care. This review by an independent physician should occur before the administration of the device when possible. Otherwise, it should occur within 5 business days of the administration of the product.

Federal Review Requirements

Although FDA approval is not required in advance of the emergency use of an investigational device, the Center for Devices and Radiological Health (CDRH) at FDA requires notification of the device administration within 5 business days [see (21 CFR 812.35(a)(2)]. If an IDE has been approved by the FDA for the device, the IDE sponsor (e.g., the device manufacturer) is responsible for FDA notification. If there is no clinical trial approved under an IDE for the use of the device, the physician who administered the device is required to submit the follow-up report.

The follow-up report is required to include the following information: details about the patient and an outline of the emergency situation, patient protection measures that were implemented, information about the patient outcome, and (if no IDE exists) a description of the device.

Local Review Requirements

The FDA expects physicians to obtain local ethical review entity concurrence as a patient protection measure whenever possible. If obtaining chair concurrence in advance of device administration is not possible due to situational urgency, investigators should follow the reporting requirements outlined by their local or commercial IRB. Best practice would involve providing a follow-up report to the IRB within the required FDA reporting timeline (5 business days).

Investigators should consult their local or commercial IRB regarding specific information required for chair concurrence and IRB reporting. Investigators should include a description of the patient protection measures implemented, along with details about the patient, the emergency situation, and (if providing a follow-up report) the patient outcome.

Individual Patient/Small Group Compassionate Use of an Investigational Device

Sometimes there are nonemergency situations where a patient is faced with a serious or life-threatening disease or condition and use of investigational device is the only option available for patient. The compassionate use provision makes an unapproved/ uncleared (investigational) device available to the patient. This pathway can be used: (1) when patient does not qualify for a clinical trial in which the device is being used and the use of that device can be beneficial, per patient's treating physician and (2) for devices that are not being studied in a clinical investigation (i.e., an IDE for the device does not exist).

Usually compassionate use is approved by FDA for individual patients but may be approved to treat a small group of patients. Prior FDA approval is required before compassionate use may occur.

The compassionate use must meet specific criteria outlined by the FDA:

- The patient has a life-threatening or serious disease or condition.
- No generally acceptable alternative treatment for the condition exists.

Requirements for Compassionate Use
If a licensed physician wants to obtain an investigational device for an individual patient or small group of patients, all compassionate use criteria must be met, and the medical device company must first agree to provide the investigational device for compassionate use. If the device manufacturer agrees to provide the device for compassionate use, there are two different pathways to obtain FDA approval, depending on whether there is an IDE for a clinical trial for the device.

1. If there is an IDE for the device, the sponsor of the IDE should submit an IDE supplement requesting approval for a compassionate use to treat the patient or group of patients (21 CFR 812.35(a)).
    The IDE supplement should include:
    (i) A description of the patient's condition and the circumstances requiring treatment
    (ii) Number of patients to be treated (when requesting use for group of patients)
    (iii) A discussion of why alternative therapies are unsatisfactory and why the probable risk of using the investigational device is no greater than the probable risk from the disease or condition
    (iv) Identification and listing of any deviations from the approved clinical protocol that are required in order to treat the patient(s)
    (v) A description of the appropriate patient protection measures that will be followed, including:
        - A draft of the informed consent document that will be used
        - A description of any local institutional policies that will be followed, including obtaining any necessary institutional approvals
        - Concurrence from the Institutional Review Board (IRB) chair

- An impartial assessment from a physician not involved in the patient's care
- Authorization from the device manufacturer on the use of the device

In some cases, the Institutional Review Board will not approve the request until they have approval from the FDA. In such cases, the original request to the FDA should indicate that IRB approval will be obtained prior to use of the device and proof of the approval by IRB chair will be required to be submitted with the follow-up report after the patient is treated.

2. If there is no IDE for the device, the device manufacturer or the physician should submit the following information to the FDA:
   - All information listed in i, ii, iii, and v above and
   - A description of the device to be provided by the manufacturer

Local Requirements

Physicians should consult their local or commercial IRB regarding specific information required for chair concurrence and IRB reporting. However, IRB reporting requirements should align with FDA reporting requirements. Physicians should include a description of the patient protection measures implemented, along with details about the patient(s), and (if providing a follow-up report) the patient outcome.

FDA Review of Compassionate Use Request

FDA reviews submitted information to determine whether the preliminary evidence of safety and effectiveness justifies the compassionate use and whether compassionate use would interfere with the conduct of a clinical trial to support marketing approval.

After a compassionate use request is received, FDA will approve, approve with conditions, or disapprove the request. When there is an IDE for the device, compassionate use request IDE supplements have the same statutory 30-day review cycle as other IDE submissions. However, the patient need is considered when reviewing these requests and they are often expedited if necessary.

Post-approval Requirements

After the approval of the request, the treating physician should design an appropriate schedule for monitoring the patient depending on the investigational nature of the device and the specific requirements of the patient(s). The patient(s) should be monitored to detect any possible problems arising from the use of the device.

Follow-up information on the use of the device should be submitted to FDA by whoever submitted the original compassionate use request in a report after all compassionate use patients have been treated. The report should contain summary information regarding patient(s') outcomes. If there were any problems as a result of device use, these should be discussed in follow-up report and reported to the reviewing IRB as soon as possible.

Treatment Use of an Investigational Device

During the course of an IDE trial for a serious or life-threatening disease or condition, there may be data suggesting that the device is effective. If so, the trial may be expanded to include additional patients with life-threatening or serious diseases. Alternatively, a separate treatment protocol may be developed. This is done to make promising new devices available to seriously ill patients as early in the device development process as is possible. Generally, a device may be made available for treatment of a serious condition after all trials have been completed; if patients have a life-threatening condition, a device may be made available while trials are still ongoing.

Requirements to Meet the Use of the Product

The criteria for treatment use as defined in Table 1 applies. The additional following criteria must be met for treatment use to be approved:

- The device is under investigation in a clinical trial with an approved IDE for the same use, or all such trials have been completed.
- The sponsor the clinical trial is pursuing marketing approval or clearance of the device.

Obtaining Informed Consent

Prospective informed consent or permission from a legally authorized representative would be required unless criteria for an exception from informed consent (see Table 1) are met. If consent can be obtained, a consent form should be used to document the consent discussion. The consent discussion and associated form should clearly convey the investigational nature of the device. Moreover, the description of the use of the device should clearly convey that it is for treatment purposes and not research.

Federal Review Requirements

An application for a treatment IDE to the FDA must include the following items in the following order:

1. Sponsor's contact information.
2. A written protocol, including a description of the device's use and patient selection criteria.
3. Rationale for the device's use, including an explanation of treatments that should be tried before using the device in question or an explanation of why device use is preferable to any other available treatment.
4. A description of procedures, tests, or other measures that will be used to evaluate the device's effects and minimize risk.
5. A description of how the treatment use will be monitored and by whom.
6. Instructions for device use and labeling, as required under 21 CFR 812.5 (a) and (b).
7. Information about device safety and effectiveness as related to the proposed treatment use (Note that information from another application may be incorporated by reference through a letter of authorization).

8. A statement of the sponsor's commitment to meet all applicable requirements in 21 CFR 812 (IDE regulations), 21 CFR 56 (IRB regulations), and 21 CFR 50 (obtaining informed consent).
9. An example of the agreement to be signed by all investigators participating in the treatment IDE and a certification that no investigator will be added before such an agreement is signed.
10. If the device will be sold, the price that will be charged and a statement confirming that the price is based on manufacturing and handling costs only (i.e., not promotion).

The sponsor is responsible for submitting progress reports twice a year to the FDA. The FDA has a suggested format for an IDE Progress Report (FDA 2018d). The sponsor is also responsible for all other reports specified in 21 CFR 812.150.

Local Review Requirements
A treatment IDE protocol must be reviewed by an Institutional Review Board (IRB) at a convened meeting. Physicians should contact their local IRB or ethical review entity to determine institution specific submission requirements.

Treatment with a Humanitarian Use Device

A Humanitarian Use Device (HUD) is intended to benefit patients with rare diseases or conditions. A rare disease is defined by the Orphan Drug Act (ODA) (97th U.S. Congress 1983) as a "condition that affects fewer than 200,000 people in the United States." There are approximately 7,000 known rare diseases. Only a fraction of these have approved treatments in the United States. Given the small number of patients affected by these rare conditions, obtaining evidence of safety and efficacy through the research IDE pathway can be challenging.

Hence, the Safe Medical Devices Act (101st U.S. Congress 1989) created the Humanitarian Device Exemption (HDE) Program, a regulatory pathway for devices intended to treat rare diseases. An HDE is a marketing application to the FDA for the use of a Humanitarian Use Device (HUD). An HUD is a medical device intended to treat or diagnose rare diseases that afflict no more than 8,000 individuals in the United States on a yearly basis (United States (US) Government Publishing Office (GPO) 2016).

Federal Application Regulations Review

HUD Designation
A device to treat rare diseases must first receive a Humanitarian Use Device designation from the Office of Orphan Products Development (OOPD). The application should include information about the rare disease in which the device is intended to be used, rationale for why the treatment is necessary, a description of the

device, and rationale for the use of the device in the patient population. The application should establish how the device meets the definition of an HUD.

HDE Application

Once an HUD designation has been given, a manufacturer may submit an HDE to the FDA. The HDE submission to the FDA should include the HUD designation made by the FDA's OOPD. Rationale is also required for making the product available under an HDE. This should explain why the device would otherwise be unavailable outside of the HDE marketing pathway. The submitter should also confirm the lack of similar devices to treat the disease. The risks and benefits of any other therapies currently accessible in the United States should be outlined.

Moreover, rationale for the probable benefit to patients and how it outweighs the risks of the device is necessary. This rationale should be in the context of the product's mechanism of action and the underlying disease. An HDE submission to the FDA requires much of the same information and documentation required for a Premarket Approval Application (PMA) to market a significant risk device [21 CFR 814.20(b)]. However, the FDA does not require a summary of clinical trials for HDE marketing. Instead, the device manufacturer should summarize clinical experience or investigations that are related to the potential risks and benefits of the device. HDE applications do not require effectiveness supporting data. The HDE applicant is also required to inform the FDA of the device cost. The cost of the device should not be greater than the cost to develop, research, manufacture, and distribute the device. FDA will review an HDE application within 75 days. Separate HDE applications are not required for pediatric populations (21 years or younger); pediatric populations may be included in the adult population HDE.

Post-approval Reporting

The FDA requires the submission of an HDE supplement when modifications are made to the device that affect the safety and probable benefit of the device (21 CFR 814.108). Moreover, the FDA's Pediatric Advisory Committee (PAC) conducts annual reviews of approved HDEs and adverse events for HDE devices used in pediatric populations, when the manufacturers are permitted to make a profit.

Adverse Device Effect Reporting

Adverse device effects are required to be submitted to the FDA according to the Medical Device Reporting (MDR) Regulation, at 21 CFR Part 803:

- "may have caused or contributed to a death or serious injury, or
- has malfunctioned and would be likely to cause or contribute to a death or serious injury if the malfunction were to recur."

The FDA considers a serious injury an event that: threatens the life of a patient; permanently impairs a body function or inflicts permanent damage to a body structure; or requires medical or surgical care to avoid permanent impairment or damage. Adverse events should also be reported to the IRB of record.

Periodic Reports

FDA requires periodic reports on the HUD device after the approval of an HDE has been issued. The required frequency of these reports is communicated to the HDE holder in the HDE approval. FDA expects these reports to include current, revised documentation establishing that the HUD designation still applies (21 CFR 814.126 (b)). The FDA also requires a report on the number of devices shipped or sold since the initial approval from the FDA.

Local Review Requirements

An HUD can only be used clinically in a facility that has an IRB. Federal regulations require initial review of an HUD to be performed at a convened meeting (21 CFR 56.108). IRB review should consider whether risks to subjects are minimized and reasonable in relation to the proposed treatment benefit. A blanket approval may be issued by the IRB for the use of the device. Alternatively, the IRB may require approval on a case-by-case basis.

Clinicians should clarify submission requirements with their local or commercial IRB. While the FDA does not require the submission of a protocol to use an HUD according to its marketed indications, some IRBs may require a protocol. IRBs may consider the following documentation during an initial review of an HUD per FDA recommendations:

- The HDE approval from the FDA
- A narrative describing the device
- The device labeling
- A description of the proposed use of the device, including screening processes, ancillary procedures to use the device (e.g., surgery), plans for follow-up, and any other related tests and procedures

Likewise, federal regulations do not dictate informed consent must be obtained for the use of an HUD. However, some IRBs may require informed consent. Many HUD manufacturers develop patient information packets that include information about potential risks and benefits of the device, as well as associated procedures. The FDA has determined that such information, when available, should be provided to patients prior to the use of the device. HUD patient information packets are available online on FDA's website by searching with the HDE number.

If no patient information packet is available, the FDA recommends the following information be provided in an informed consent form:

- The purpose of the device (to diagnose or treat), along with the HDE approved indications
- A description about how the device is expected to work for the disease or condition
- A statement that there is a lack of similar devices to treat the disease or condition
- A statement indicating that the device has an HUD designation and that the effectiveness of this device is unknown or not well-established

Table 3 Review requirements by expanded access pathway for device products

Type of expanded access	IRB review	Prior FDA approval
Single-patient emergency use	Chair concurrence when possible or post hoc notification	Post hoc notification
Single patient/small group Compassionate use	Convened review or chair concurrence	Yes
Treatment use	Convened review	Yes
Humanitarian use	Convened review[a]	Yes

[a]Continuing review for Humanitarian Use Devices may be conducted at the expedited level, per FDA guidance

- A description of any procedures required for the use of the HUD such as surgery
- A description of how the device will be used
- Potential risks to the patient

When an HUD is used for treatment or diagnosis purposes under its approved HDE, HIPAA authorization for the use or disclosure of protected health information (PHI) is not required (45 CFR Parts 160 and 164).

Once an HDE is approved by the FDA and the IRB, a treating physician may use the HUD. Ongoing continuing review and approval by the IRB is required for the use of a HUD. IRBs may use the expedited review procedures (21 CFR 56.110) to conduct continuing review because the device is legally marketed and there is no systematic collection of safety and efficacy data. Risk benefit information as well as any adverse device effects should be available for the IRB's consideration.

Using a HUD in a Clinical Investigation

An HUD may be studied in a clinical trial under its approved HDE for its approved indication. This investigational use to collect safety and effectiveness data is subject to IRB review and the Common Rule regulations. Informed consent as outlined in 21 CFR Part 50 is required when an HUD is being investigated in a clinical trial. Likewise, HIPAA authorization are required for the use and disclosure of PHI for the purpose of research, unless otherwise waived by the IRB of record.

If the investigational use is for another indication not approved in the HDE, then an IDE is required. When applicable, an IRB may review the clinical use of an HUD for treatment purposes as well as the investigational use of an HUD in a clinical trial concurrently. If an IDE is required and the sponsor has not yet obtained IDE approval from the FDA, the IRB may need to make a device risk determination (21 CFR 812.66) (Table 3).

International Regulations for Expanded Access to Drug and Device Products for Clinical Treatment

While the details of expanded access to drugs and devices in the United States is made fairly transparent through FDA managed online resources, obtaining the same level of understanding internationally was more of a challenge.

In terms of the European Union, it is made clear that the European Medicines Agency (EMA) provides comprehensive support and guidance to its member states but does not create a legal framework. The EMA works to support Member States by facilitating a centralized procedure for access to compassionate use programs meant for groups of patients in order to standardize the access across the EU. Individual applicants must contact the relevant drug authority in their country as a liaison to EMA opinions and resources for compassionate use. These programs are for therapies expected to help patients with life-threatening, long-lasting, or seriously debilitating illnesses, which cannot be treated satisfactorily with any currently authorized medicine.

The medicine must be undergoing clinical trials or have entered the marketing-authorization application process, and while early studies will generally have been completed, its safety profile and dosage guidelines may not be fully established.

The EMA clarifies that access through a clinical trial should be prioritized, followed by compassionate use program access. They also reference individual requests as "named patient basis" requests; however, the details for how those individual requests should be managed is left to the individual European countries. EMA states they do not need to be informed of those requests for an individual patient which are placed directly with the manufacturer by a treating physician.

Comprehensive information for the EMA oversight of compassionate use programs in the European Union is available here: https://www.ema.europa.eu/en/human-regulatory/research-development/compassionate-use

To better understand how EU member countries engage in expanded access, individual policies were researched on a country-by-country basis. Most countries are clear that their policies for multi-patient compassionate use programs align with the EMA. However, the procedures for seeking expanded access for a single patient was much less consistent and at times completely absent. What we found were vastly differing approaches by many countries and some countries with no transparent processes at all. An objective account of the variable availability of information related to expanded access programs in the EU is available here: https://www.ncbi.nlm.nih.gov/pmc/articles/PMC5116859/

While the European Union was found to be difficult to identify and digest, other countries outside of Europe have developed comprehensive programs and provide increased transparency.

Australia

The Australian Therapeutic Goods Administration (TGA) manages expanded access to drugs and devices via their comprehensive Special Access Scheme (SAS). Complete details are available here; https://www.tga.gov.au/special-access-scheme-guidance-health-practitioners-and-sponsors

In summary, the SAS allows individual patients access to unapproved therapies where:

- Critically ill patients require urgent, early access to therapeutic goods including experimental and investigational therapeutic goods.

- Therapeutic goods have been withdrawn from the Australian market for commercial or other reasons.
- Therapeutic goods are initially provided to patients through a clinical trial while a marketing application is being considered.
- Therapeutic goods are available overseas but not marketed in Australia.

Under the scheme are three categorized pathways encompassing drugs, devices, and biologics under the title of "therapeutic goods":

Category A is a notification only pathway which can be accessed for patients who are seriously ill with a condition from which death is reasonably likely to occur within a matter of months, or from which premature death is reasonably likely to occur in the absence of early treatment.

Category B is for patients who do not fit the description of Category A pathway requirements AND the sought-after therapy does not have an established history of use. Category B requires a comprehensive application and an approval letter from the TGA must be received prior to access.

Category C is also notification only and is reserved for therapies that have an established history of use but are not currently authorized in Australia. The TGA maintains a list of medicines, medical devices, and biologics that qualify for access under Category C.

Brazil

In Brazil, the Brazilian Health Regulatory Agency (Anvisa) has created both compassionate use and expanded access programs. In summary:

Expanded access is specific to groups of patients who are carriers of serious debilitating and/or life-threatening diseases and with no satisfactory therapeutic alternative with products registered in Brazil. The program is for providing new, promising drug, still without Anvisa's registration or not commercially available in Brazil, that is in developing or completed phase III study.

Compassionate use applies provision of new promising drug, for personal use of patients and nonparticipants of expanded access program or clinical trial. Compassionate use is limited to single patients who are carriers of serious debilitating and/or life-threatening diseases and with no satisfactory therapeutic alternative with products registered in Brazil.

Brazil defines a serious debilitating disease as "one that substantially impairs its carriers in the performance of daily life tasks and chronic disease that, if not treated, will progress in most of the cases, leading to cumulative loss of autonomy, to sequels or death."

Comprehensive guidance on both programs is available here: https://abracro.org.br/pdfs/04_RA_RDC38-2013_MANUAL_acesso%20exp_uso%20compas_JUL.pdf

Canada

Health Canada has an organized Special Access Program divided into two directorates, one for drugs and one for devices.

In summary, Health Canada conducts all reviews of special access programs on a case-by-case basis based on the rationale and background information provided by the requesting physician. Drug requests are for access to non-marketed drugs to treat patients with serious or life-threatening conditions. Special access to drugs is only considered when conventional therapies have failed, are unsuitable, or are unavailable. Special access for devices is given for emergencies or when conventional therapies have failed, are unavailable, or are unsuitable to treat a patient.

Special access authorization is required for all medical devices that have not been approved for use in Canada, as well as some custom-made devices.

Comprehensive guidance for special access drugs in Canada is available here: https://www.canada.ca/content/dam/hc-sc/documents/services/drugs-health-products/special-access/drugs/guidance/guidance-eng.pdf

Comprehensive guidance for special access devices in Canada is available here: https://www.canada.ca/content/dam/hc-sc/migration/hc-sc/dhp-mps/alt_formats/hpfb-dgpsa/pdf/acces/sap-md-dg-as-im-ld-eng.pdf

Summary and Conclusion

There are several scenarios that allow the use of investigational drugs and devices for the purposes of clinical care. These pathways may be used when it is in the best interest of the patient to do so, and when the investigational product is known to be the only option for the patient. Recent regulatory updates have allowed data from single patients and small groups of patients in expanded access trials to be included in support of marketing applications.

For investigational drugs, there are four expanded access pathways:

1. Single-patient emergency use
2. Single-patient treatment use
3. Intermediate-size population treatment use
4. General treatment use

For investigational devices, there are three expanded access pathways:

1. Single-patient emergency use
2. Single-patient or small group compassionate use
3. Treatment use

Additionally, for a rare disease or condition, there is the possibility of using a Humanitarian Use Device (HUD) under a Humanitarian Device Exemption (HDE).

Key Facts

- The most common avenue of access to investigational products (drugs and devices) occurs by enrolling into an approved clinical trial.
- There remains a need to provide opportunity for the receipt of investigational drugs and devices on either an individual patient basis or for smaller groups of patients.
- Product manufacturers are not required to allow access to their products for expanded access purposes.
- FDA approval for emergency requests can be sought, and obtained, via phone.

Cross-References

▶ Clinical Trials, Ethics, and Human Protections Policies
▶ Consent Forms and Procedures
▶ Device Trials
▶ Institutional Review Boards and Ethics Committees
▶ Investigator Responsibilities

References

101st U.S. Congress (1989) H.R. 3095: Safe Medical Devices Act of 1990. Accessed 2/9/2019 from https://www.govinfo.gov/content/pkg/STATUTE-104/pdf/STATUTE-104-Pg4511.pdf

97th U.S. Congress (1983) H.R. 5238: Orphan Drug Act. Accessed 2/9/2019 from https://www.govinfo.gov/content/pkg/STATUTE-96/pdf/STATUTE-96-Pg2049.pdf

United States (US) Department of Health and Human Services (DHHS) (2019) Security and privacy, 21 CFR Part 164. Washington, DC.

United States (US) Department of Health and Human Services (DHHS) (2019) General administrative requirements, 21 CFR Part 160. Washington, DC

United States (US) Food and Drug Administration (FDA) (2010) Guidance for HDE Holders, Institutional Review Boards (IRBs), Clinical Investigators, and FDA Staff – Humanitarian Device Exemption (HDE) Regulation: Questions and Answers. Accessed 2/9/2019 from: http://www.fda.gov/MedicalDevices/DeviceRegulationandGuidance/HowtoMarketYourDevice/PremarketSubmissions/HumanitarianDeviceExemption/ucm563322.htm

United States (US) Food and Drug Administration (FDA) (2018a) Humanitarian use devices, 21 CFR Part 814, Subpart H. Washington, DC

United States (US) Food and Drug Administration (FDA) (2018b) Institutional review boards, 21 CFR Part 56. Washington, DC

United States (US) Food and Drug Administration (FDA) (2018c) Investigational device exemptions, 21 CFR Part 812. Washington, DC

United States (US) Food and Drug Administration (FDA) (2018d) IDE Reports. https://www.fda.gov/MedicalDevices/DeviceRegulationandGuidance/HowtoMarketYourDevice/InvestigationalDeviceExemptionIDE/ucm046717.htm. Accessed 3/10/2019

United States (US) Food and Drug Administration (FDA) (2018e) Medical device reporting, 21 CFR Part 803. Washington, DC

United States (US) Food and Drug Administration (FDA) (2018f) Protection of human subjects, 21 CFR Part 50. Washington, DC

United States (US) Food and Drug Administration (FDA) (2018g) Expanded access for medical devices. Washington, DC

United States (US) Food and Drug Administration (FDA) (2018h) Supplemental applications, 21 CFR part 812.35. Washington, DC

United States (US) Government Publishing Office (GPO) (2016) 21st Century Cures Act (Public Law 114–255). Washington, DC. Accessed 2/9/2019 from http://www.congress.gov

Van Norman GA (2018) Expanding patient access to investigational drugs: single patient investigational new drug and the "Right to try." JACC Basic Transl Sci 3(2):280–293. https://doi.org/10.1016/j.jacbts.2017.11.007

A Perspective on the Process of Designing and Conducting Clinical Trials

125

Curtis L. Meinert and Steven Piantadosi

Contents

Introduction	2454
Funding	2458
Design Issues	2460
Who to Study	2460
Design Structure	2460
Design Variable	2461
Primary Outcome	2461
Treatment	2461
Length of Follow-Up	2461
Closeout Design	2462
Single Center Versus Multicenter	2462
Randomization Design	2462
Masking (Blinding)	2463
Governance and Organizational Issues	2464
Apportioning Monies	2464
Who Is in Charge	2464
Authorship Policy	2465
Publication Policy	2465
Results Blackout	2465
Data and Safety Monitoring	2465
Masked Data Monitoring	2466
Problems in Execution	2466
Recruitment Shortfalls	2466
Early Stops	2467

C. L. Meinert (✉)
Department of Epidemiology, School of Public Health, Johns Hopkins University, Baltimore, MD, USA
e-mail: cmeiner1@jhu.edu

S. Piantadosi
Department of Surgery, Division of Surgical Oncology, Brigham and Women's Hospital, Harvard Medical School, Boston, MA, USA
e-mail: spiantadosi@bwh.harvard.edu

© Springer Nature Switzerland AG 2022
S. Piantadosi, C. L. Meinert (eds.), *Principles and Practice of Clinical Trials*,
https://doi.org/10.1007/978-3-319-52636-2_175

Changes to the Study Protocol 2467
Changes to Data Procedures or Data Forms 2467
Adding or Subtracting Treatments 2467
Adding Study Clinics 2468
Withdrawal of Clinics 2468
Drug Supply and Packaging 2468
Plagiarism, Data Fabrication, and Fraud 2468
Issues in Publishing 2469
Data Acquisition 2469
When to Freeze Data Files 2469
Counting 2470
Quality Control 2470
Interim Publications 2470
When the Primary Outcome Is Trumped by a Higher-Order Outcome 2471
Rejections 2471
Data Sharing 2471
Closing Word 2471
References 2472

Abstract

Trials are not for the faint of heart. As noted by Donald Fredrickson (Director of the NIH: 1 July 1975 to 30 June 1981), "they lack glamor, they strain our resources and patience, and they protract the moment of truth to excruciating limits" (Fredrickson 1968). This chapter addresses issues in design and conduct of trials including who to study, choice of treatments to be tested, choice of outcome measures, and issues in monitoring and governance of the trial.

Keywords

Design issues · Organization · Governance

Introduction

Trials are not for the faint of heart. As noted by Donald Fredrickson (Director of the NIH: 1 July 1975 to 30 June 1981), "they lack glamor, they strain our resources and patience, and they protract the moment of truth to excruciating limits" (Fredrickson 1968). Trials are expensive, unwieldy, and cumbersome and cannot be applied to many questions of major importance due to limitations based on ethics, practicality, and cost. The phases of a trial, all of which can be tribulations, from the perspective of a person undertaking one might be as shown in Table 1.

The modern day equivalent of a controlled trial was done by James Lind almost 275 years ago:

> On the 20th of May 1747, I took twelve patients in the scurvy, on board the Salisbury at sea. Their cases were as similar as I could have them. . . . Two of these were ordered each a quart of cyder a-day. Two others took twenty-five gutts of elixir vitriol three times a day, upon an empty stomach;

Table 1 Stages of a clinical trial

Stage	Feature
Euphoria	Fleeting; prompted by news that the trial will be funded
Holy s___!	Marked by realization now you must do what you proposed; stage can last months marked by bouts of despair and depression
Anxiety	Marked by bickering, sniping, and squabbles with colleagues; generally regarded as starting with and lasting throughout screening for enrollment
Max Q	Space age term indicating the point of maximum dynamic pressure; in trials generally arising during the period of enrollment in presence of short falls in enrollment and realization that the event rate used for sample size calculations is unrealistically high
Doldrums	Marked by tedium and boredom arising, in large measure, from realization that the trial still has a long time to run before there is anything to publish
Accolade	Comes on publication of results; transitory at best; may not exist at all if results are not what the world wants to hear or the authors want to tell the world
Bunker	May last years after publication if trial receives "brickbats" of criticism

using a gargle strongly acidulated with it for their mouths. Two others took two spoonfuls of vinegar three times a day, upon an empty stomach; having their gruels and their other food well acidulated with it, as also the gargle for their mouth. Two of the worst patients, with the tendons in the ham rigid, (a symptom none of the rest had), were put under a course of seawater. ... Two others had each two oranges and one lemon given them every day. ... The two remaining patients, took the bigness of a nutmeg three times a-day. ... The consequence was, that the most sudden and visible good effects were perceived from the use of the oranges and lemons; one of those who had taken them, being at the end of six days fit for duty. (Lind 1753)

So the British Navy equipped their ships with fresh fruits as soon as word of Lind's experiment got around? Not quite. It would be 50 years after Lind before that happened. The reason was Lind and others believed scurvy was the result of living in damp quarters and ill-digested food.

For all intents and purposes, Lind woke up one day and decided to do his trial. He did not need approvals. He did not have to register the trial before he started nor was he required to post results after he finished. He did not have to have an independent monitoring committee to advise him as to when to stop.

In current times, it would be months before Lind could take *twelve patients in the scurvy* and do his trials. He would have to be IRB and HIPAA trained and certified before he could do anything. He would not have any standing in front of his IRB without those certifications. After certification he would be eligible to submit his proposed protocol and a draft consent for his sailors to sign before enrollment. He would have to justify, in dialog with his IRB, why he was studying only males. He would have to have an independent data monitoring committee to advise him as to when to stop the trial unless he could convince the IRB that he did not need one.

The time spent doing trials is only a fraction of the total time required to do them. Much of the time required will be spent before the first person is enrolled and after the last data collection visit. Table 2 gives rough estimates of times required for the various activities of a trial. Some of the activities overlap so the total time required from beginning to end of a trial will be less than the sum of times listed.

Table 2 Timeline for clinical trial elements

Activity	Time estimate	Comments
Funding	Months to years; 6 months under best of circumstance; 3–4 years if investigator-initiated dependent on grant funding from governmental agency	Time will depend on amount of funding needed; usually more complicated and time-consuming for multicenter trials and when multiple funding sources involved; time longer if trial is investigator initiated rather than sponsor initiated
Protocol development	6–12 months	Time generally less for investigator-initiated trials than for sponsor-initiated trials because much of the development work has been done in relation to funding requests
IRB submissions and approvals	2–6 months; sometimes longer	Amount of time will depend on the number of submissions required for approval; can expect one or two submissions to address issues concerning consent and consent form
Drug acquisition and packaging	6–12 months	Not all trials involve drugs, but if they do, acquisition may be problematic, especially if the treatments are to be masked. Getting the drug from the manufacturer may be the easiest part of the acquisition. Usually, getting a placebo to match the drug is the most complicated part of acquisition
Form development	6–9 months	Development of data collection forms is tedious and time-consuming. Enrollment cannot start until forms are developed and are IRB approved. The truth is forms are never "final"; always subject to change over the course of the trial. An issue is whether forms are to be "paper" or electronic
Data system development	6–9 months	There is not much that can be done developing a data system until data collection forms are done and approved. Data on study forms must be harvested into some data system. An issue is how the information is harvested; by people at study clinics keying directly as data are generated, from paper forms, or centrally at the data center from forms transmitted from clinics; the usual default is keying at the place of generation

(continued)

Table 2 (continued)

Activity	Time estimate	Comments
Training and certification of study personnel	Collectively months	All study personnel required to be IRB and HIPAA certified either by having active certifications or by taking required didactic courses before being allowed to participate in the trial
Registration	1–3 days	Registration on ClinicalTrials.gov or some other acceptable registration site before the start of enrollment; required by some journals to be eligible for publication of results when trial is finished
Enrollment	Months to years	Enrollment cannot start until the trial is IRB approved and data collection forms and all measurement methods are ready and, if the trials involves drug treatment, until drug has been distributed to clinics. Enrollment never goes as fast as investigators expect. Typically, enrollment continues until the sample size requirement has been met, but there are lots of trials stopped short of that because of funding, results of interim analyses, or inability to get the required sample size
Follow-up	Months to years	Typically, the period of follow-up is for a fixed period following enrollment or ends for all persons regardless of when they were enrolled. The period will be years if follow-up is, say, 5 years after the last person was enrolled meaning that the minimum period of follow-up will be 5 years and the maximum will be the time represented for the first person enrolled
Closeout of data collection	1–3 months; maybe longer if there is an event adjudication process that takes place after the end of follow-up	Period required to empty data pipelines after the last data collection visit
Final dataset	1–4 months; maybe longer if there is an event adjudication process that takes place after the end of follow-up	Time needed to produce a "clean" dataset for paper writing after final editing
Posting "tabular results"	Days to a month	Required under FDA regulations for trials under FDA control; to be done within 1 year of completion of the trial

(continued)

Table 2 (continued)

Activity	Time estimate	Comments
Paper writing	0 for groups choosing to not write up results; otherwise 1–3 years; maybe more for groups producing multiple publications	Minimum time from analyzable dataset to a submission ready manuscript 6–9 months; time to publication will depend on number of revisions or rejections before acceptance
Data de-identification	3–6 months	Data shared must be de-identified per HIPAA requirements
Data sharing	Indeterminate	Unfunded mandate; especially when having to deal with requests after funding for the trial has ended

Many of the tribulations we sketch in this chapter are discussed fully in other sections of this book. However, it is useful to see the challenging list of details that the modern investigator must address, even in condensed form, and be made alert to potential unhealthy diversions that can occur. Every trial, the multicenter trial especially, is a microcosm of the issues we sketch.

Funding

Except in more simple times like Lind's, the hard truth is "no money, no trial." Starting work on a trial on the promise of money or that the "check is in the mail" is a mistake. Obviously, the issue of funding must be addressed and solved before anything can be done to implement a trial. Funding is always a tribulation: for sponsors if the trial is sponsor-initiated and for investigators if investigator-initiated. From the investigator perspective with a sponsor-initiated trial, the battle for funding will be fought and won before would-be investigators know of plans to fund the trial. Even if the sponsor is a drug company, somebody in the corporate structure wanting to do the trial will have to convince people in the board room that the trial is worth doing.

Anyone wanting to do a trial for an important question can wait for one to appear and make application to join it, or they can try to initiate one on their own. The easier road is to try to be part of one being formed by a sponsor by applying for a role when the trial is announced. The NIH has two vehicles for organizing and funding trials: request for proposal (RFP) and request for application (RFA). The major differences are in who runs the trial and how centers are funded. Funding via RFPs is by contract with the funding agency and with that agency playing a major role in design and conduct of the trial. Funding via RFAs is through grants with a partnership role between the funding agency and investigators regarding trial design and conduct.

Both RFPs and RFAs will have hard deadlines for response. The trial may or may not be initiated depending on whether the funding agency received enough viable applications to warrant initiating the trial.

RFAs and RFPs issued by the NIH are the product of consensus conferences or advice from the scientific community. Indeed, RFAs and RFPs may be due, in part to urgings of people who, when issued, respond to them. Hence, one option for investigators wishing to initiate a trial is to urge funding agencies to release an RFP or RFA calling for the trial and then respond to the request when released and hope their application is successful.

The other option for investigators wishing to initiate a trial is to be the initiator, or at least try. The option, in that case, is to seek funding via a wealthy donor, a foundation, a drug company, or a governmental agency. In the case of the United States, governmental agencies mean the NIH or other government entities like the FDA, CDC, or the Department of Defense.

One funding option is traditional grant support as available from the NIH, but that may be difficult. The options for investigators trying to do a multicenter trial are to apply for a planning grant and hope they can parlay that into a full-sized trial or by a letter of request to the funding agency seeking permission to submit a full-blown proposal.

The trouble with planning grants is that they may not lead to the promised land. There is no guarantee of funding when the planning grant is finished. Even if successful in getting the definitive trial funded, there is likely to be a hiatus of a year or more between cessation of funding under the planning grant and full-blown funding.

The other option is a proposal for funding involving a period of planning and implementation as well as the actual trial. The catch here is that, under current policies, investigators need permission to submit an application for any trial involving $500,000 in direct cost for any year of funding:

> Effective with the January 1, 2002 receipt dates, applicants must seek agreement to accept assignment from Institute/Center staff at least 6 weeks prior to the anticipated submission of any application requesting $500,000 or more in direct costs for any year. (NIH notice: 6 Oct 2001)

The limit remains at $500,000, even though now the equivalent of $325,000 in 2019 after adjustment for inflation.

If approval is granted, the investigators may submit a grant application for review and possible funding. Typically funding, if granted, will be under a cooperative agreement between investigators and the funding agency. Cooperative agreements are partnership between the funding agency and investigators giving, in effect, an equal relationship between the two parties.

Negotiations to get the trial funded may lead to compromises in the size or length of the trial or transition from a hard clinical outcome to a surrogate measure to reduce sample size requirements and trial duration.

Investigators are notorious for underestimating the time it will take for recruitment in trials. Invariably, when the trial is being planned, estimates are that recruitment will be a cake walk, and when the trial starts, the patients mysteriously disappear. The result is that the trial period may need to be extended, which can have significant budgetary consequences or the trial simply may be judged infeasible and work may be stopped.

Usually funding is for a specified period. The time may be what is assumed to be enough or only for a specified period with expectation of renewals of funding over the course of the trial.

Design Issues

Who to Study

You must study people with the condition or disease you are trying to prevent or treat. But who among those? Samples of convenience may be skewed – males only, females only, infants and adolescents, adults, and elderly. Active samples that create a study cohort of given composition or specification are guaranteed to be much more expensive than convenience samples. Who should be excluded from the trial for safety or other reasons? The answer to this question has at various times in the past been pregnant women, women of childbearing potential, minors, or the elderly. Quite appropriately, we are protective of our children and so are IRBs. Studies involving children will be subject to greater scrutiny by IRBs than studies involving free-living adults.

Focusing on one gender group if the condition or disease is common to both gender groups is not viable, especially if women are excluded. The argument that the number of certain individuals is too small for meaningful subgroup analyses is not a convincing rationale for exclusion. The more restrictive the enrollment criteria, the harder and longer it will take to recruit. Therefore, unless there are good medical or practical reasons for exclusions, they should not be imposed. The same can be said for exclusions based on age.

Presently trialists and sponsors alike are attempting to eliminate as many eligibility restrictions as possible to broaden the composition of study cohorts. This is a matter of both social justice and generalizability of results and applies especially to comorbidities and age. Eligibility and exclusion criteria are intended to serve two purposes. One is safety – to be sure that medical and other circumstances of participants do not place them at additional risk. Second is reduced variability, which has the benefit of revealing treatment effects with a minimal number of study subjects. We have yet to achieve the ideal balance in these competing needs.

Design Structure

A modern clinical trial will likely not be designed or described as easily as one of the past few decades. The list of possible design types is extensive and bewildering to new investigators. While all RCTs of recent years have data monitoring processes and the explicit flexible options for early stopping for either efficacy, safety, or futility, the concept of "adaptive trials" has new meaning and includes many options such as adaptive randomization, cluster randomization, stepped wedge designs, adding or dropping treatments, and sample size re-estimation to name a few. Flexibilities come with additional complexities and costs. The needs of patients and emphasis on precision medicine therapeutics have also reoriented how we look at trials, particularly whether they are "treatment centric" or "patient centric" (Biankin et al. 2015).

Design Variable

The design variable is the variable used for determining sample size in a trial. The variable may be change from baseline after a specified period of treatment or may be an event like occurrence or recurrence of a cancer or some clinical event like stroke or myocardial infarction or death. The choice of the design variable will have profound implications for the time it takes to do the trial. Generally, event-type outcomes will require larger sample sizes and longer periods of follow-up than designs based on change measures.

Primary Outcome

The primary outcome, in the jargon of trials, is synonymous to "design variable," meaning that the analysis in the primary results publication is focused on the measure specified in the sample size calculation. Exceptions are when the trial produces unexpected results, for example, as in a trial designed to measure change when the variable is trumped by some higher-order outcome, like a clinical event or death.

Treatment

The treatment schedule should mimic real-life as closely as possible. Treatment may be applied in a single application, for example, as in a surgical trial; in discrete time periods, for example, once a week for diet counseling in a weight loss trial; or daily, for example, in a blood pressure trial in which persons are expected to take the assigned medicine daily. If the treatment does not mimic actual practice, various complications are likely to result, including issues of adherence and protocol deviations.

One might argue that trials are and have been "treatment centric" in the sense that the science and design have revolved around the properties, risks, and promises of the treatment under study. Perhaps this is only indirectly a focus on the patient or participant. This could change with precision or personalized therapeutic approaches that offer a more direct patient focus.

Length of Follow-Up

Length of follow-up is the time people are followed to observe the effects of the treatments studied. The time will be driven by the amount of time judged reasonable for observing treatment effects and funding. The judgment will depend on the design variable. For example, if the measure is weight change in a diet trial, the follow-up period can be shorter than if the outcome is an event, like stroke, in a blood pressure trial. The decision taken has major effects on the cost of the trial. The longer the period of follow-up, the greater the cost of the trial. Here also, an ill-fitting follow-up interval can damage the power, credibility, or external validity of the trial.

Closeout Design

Broadly there are two options: anniversary closeout or common date closeout. Anniversary closeout designs are those in which persons are separated from trials after specified periods of time following enrollment, for example, separation of persons 6 weeks after enrollment. The downside is that the closeout process lasts as long as the enrollment process and, hence, that clinics may be closing out follow-up while still enrolling others.

Common closeout designs involve separating everybody from the trial at the same time, regardless of when they enrolled, for example, after the last person enrolled has been followed for 2 years. The upside of the design is that it allows clinics to concentrate closeout in a confined period rather than stringing it out in anniversary closeouts. It also generates more follow-up information than anniversary closeouts as some are followed for longer than their "anniversary."

Single Center Versus Multicenter

A key design question has to do with how you will find people to study. How many clinics do you need to achieve the enrollment goal in the time proposed – one or several? The more clinics, the greater the logistical complexities in organizing and running the trial, so the preferred number is one. That may work for a small trial involving a commonplace condition but will not work for rare conditions or when large numbers are needed. You will need multiple clinics to have any hope of achieving the enrollment goal.

The necessary number of clinics is akin to grandma telling you how much sugar she uses for her "to kill for" apple strudel. "Not too much and not too little." Not too many clinics and not too few. Too few and you will have trouble if the few you have do not recruit as promised (they rarely do). Too many and you will run up the cost of the trial and have clinics fighting for a piece of the recruitment and money pie.

Every clinic adds to the overhead cost of the trial and to the logistic complexities of the trial. The "sweet spot" is to have enough clinics to achieve the enrollment goal in the time proposed knowing that some clinics will "over" recruit and others will "under" recruit.

Randomization Design

The randomization design is the bedrock of a trial. Properly designed and administered, it ensures that study subjects and clinic personnel have no way of predicting or influencing assignments. To achieve bias-free assignments, it is imperative to have a system in which assignments remain unknown to all concerned until issued, that persons for whom assignments are intended have consented to being enrolled and have agreed to accept whatever treatment is assigned, and that when randomized the person is counted as enrolled, even if they walk out of the clinic the instant the assignment is issued.

These requirements are why "envelope" systems of assignment are not recommended. Envelope systems are where clinics are provided with sealed numbered envelopes, to be opened in numbered order as persons are enrolled. The trouble with any self-administered system is that assignments are discoverable before issue and that there is no way to know if assignments were issued in numbered order. In other words, no way to be sure that clinics did not take occasional "peeks" to ensure that persons get the "right" assignments.

An issue to be addressed in constructing the randomization design is whether to "block" assignments so that the desired ratio of assignments is met in intervals over enrollment. For example, in a trial involving two treatment groups issued in blocks of 16, there will be exactly 8 assignments issued to the two treatment groups after the 16th person is enrolled, exactly 16 in the two treatment groups after the 32nd enrollment, and so on. The advantage to blocking is that it protects against wide variations from the desired assignment ratio over the course of enrollment. If a single block size is utilized, small block sizes of 2 or 4 are easily discovered and best avoided. Large block sizes can also be problematic due to the possibility of large imbalances within unfilled blocks at the completion of randomization. An alternative is permuted block designs which use more than one block size and put the blocks in random order.

Another issue is whether to stratify assignments. The usual practice is to stratify assignments by clinic in multicenter trials to ensure balance in the ratio of assignments within clinics. Chance imbalances in assignments by clinic could make treatment comparisons problematic if the ratios of assignments are disparate and if clinic is an important predictor of outcome. When some centers will accrue only a very small number of persons, they may be grouped in the stratification.

Stratification on other variables, like gender or age, on top of clinic is usually not done because of the complications involved and because it has the potential of negating the benefits of blocked randomization. Too many strata essentially place each person into their own stratum, undoing the balancing effect.

For more on randomization, see Piantadosi 2017, Chap. 13, Meinert 2012b, Chap. 17, and Meinert 2013, Section VII.

Masking (Blinding)

Masking in the context of treatments in trials is the act or procedure of keeping information regarding treatments assigned from designated persons in a trial: single-masked if only persons enrolled are blocked from having that information and double-masked if also persons responsible for treatment and care of persons enrolled are blocked from having that information.

A decision that must be made when designing a trial is whether treatments are masked. Masking is not always possible, as in most surgery trials. It is possible in drug trials if the medicine represented in the different treatment groups looks the same or can be made to look the same, for example, by placing the medicines in identically appearing capsules. The importance of masking diminishes in trials with hard outcomes like death because the likelihood of bias in reporting is low.

Governance and Organizational Issues

Apportioning Monies

Typically funding of study clinics is on an FTE (full time equivalent) or per unit basis. If on an FTE basis, a clinic is funded to pay the salaries and fringe benefits for the fractions of personnel deemed necessary for effort associated with screening, enrolling, and following study participants. Funding is for a fixed period, typically a year, and may be increased or reduced in following time periods depending on workload. If funding is on a per unit basis, clinics will be paid a specified amount when a person is enrolled and corresponding amounts for each follow-up visit completed. The budget, whether on an FTE or per unit basis, will also include per unit cost for laboratory tests or other procedures required for data collection.

Other costs that must be covered are those associated with monitoring clinic performance and data quality control, data processing, data monitoring, and data analysis. Most of these activities, at least in multicenter trials, are housed in coordinating centers, separate and distinct from clinics, and are usually covered by separate awards to those centers. The costs for these activities in a well-balanced budget can be expected to be between 10 and 20 percent of the overall study budget, depending on duties performed.

Who Is in Charge

Every trial is collaborative, even if done on board the Salisbury at sea as with Lind's scurvy trial. It no doubt involved people to help Lind carry out his trial. Clearly Lind was in charge, but what about multicenter trials with dozens of centers all headed by co-equal people? Then who is in charge?

Typically, the issue of governance is addressed before the trial is funded or is the first issue addressed when the group comes together at its initial organizational meetings. The usual approach is to establish a steering committee comprised of directors of centers in the trial. To be functional, its size should be 15 or less, meaning that in the case of trials involving dozens of centers, there has to be some way of choosing among heads. This was almost exactly the size of the National Emphysema Treatment Trial (NETT) Steering Committee. Because that study compared a surgical treatment to medical management, there was tendency for additional politics between the surgeons and pulmonologists. One of each was selected from each clinical center, and the high-quality result is a testament to their mutual respect and collaboration (Fishman et al. 2003).

Authorship Policy

Often, investigators do not confront the issue of authorship for papers coming from the trial until there is a paper to be written – a mistake. Paper writing is a process that, to be successful, has to begin early in the course of the trial, before there are any papers to write.

The issue of authorship is reasonably straightforward in single center trials but not when there are multiple centers involved in the trial. Even the approach of listing just center directors can lead to mastheads with dozens of "authors." A policy should be established early and from first principles rather than being left to argument later.

Publication Policy

An issue to be addressed before there are papers to write is whether results are presented at scientific meeting before publication. The preferred policy, as discussed in a chapter in "Publication and Related Issues," is to publish first and present later.

Results Blackout

A results blackout is a state of conduct in which investigators are shielded from seeing interim results by treatment group, imposed to protect against treatment-related bias in observation and collection of study data. Blackouts are not to be confused with masked treatment administration. Masking of treatment assignments precludes investigators from knowing the treatment administered. It does not preclude them from seeing interim results by treatment group.

A downside of blackouts is that they rob investigators of insights into data being collected during the trial and perhaps reduce their acumen when it comes to writing up results for publication after the trial is finished. It also means that there must be procedures for lifting the mask if there is a stop before the normal end of the trial so persons, when exiting the trial, can be informed of results.

Data and Safety Monitoring

The assumption is that results must be monitored as they accumulate over time to stop the trial if results indicate the trial is futile or that a treatment is harmful or superior to others being tested. IRBs will assume the need for monitoring unless investigators can present convincing arguments that it is not necessary. The options for monitoring are study investigators or a specially constituted subgroup of them or appointment of a group specially created to do the monitoring. An issue with both options is whether monitors see results identified to treatment group or are masked.

Masked Data Monitoring

Masked data monitoring is when persons responsible for monitoring are shown data by treatment group, but the treatments are not identified until or unless differences arise in which monitors decide to lift the mask. Investigator may not have any say in the matter of masking if the monitoring body is appointed by the sponsor and reports to the sponsor. The only thing in those cases investigators can do is to object to the practice. The reason to object is that it dumbs down the monitors by denying them access to the most important variable in the trial – treatment assignment.

Masking is often preferred by sponsors because of the perception that it reduces the risk of bias in how results are viewed. But masking complicates the production of monitoring reports and reduces the combined competence of monitors in exploring study data (Meinert 1998).

The issues with specially appointed monitors are:

1. Who makes the appointment: (a) the sponsor, (b) the investigators, or (c) the two together? The last option is preferred because the body serves both the sponsor and investigators.
2. Who the monitor body reports to: (a) the sponsor, (b) the investigators, or (c) the sponsor and investigators simultaneously? Again, the third option is preferred for reason stated in (1).
3. Investigator involvement: Is the body appointed to include selected study investigators, e.g., the study chair and director of the coordinating center? This is preferred again because the activity is a shared activity.

Problems in Execution

Recruitment Shortfalls

If one listens to investigators when a trial is being planned, to a person, they will tell you that recruitment will be a piece of cake. "We see patients like those all the time." Yet they seem to disappear when the trial gets started.

Recruitment is always a troublesome issue. Investigators are notorious for overestimating availability as well as underestimating the time it will take to recruit. Invariably the rule of twos applies: It will take you twice as long to do the project as originally planned; the budget will be half of what is needed; the achieved sample size will be half that planned; it will take twice as long to enroll half the number planned; the control event rate used for sample size calculation will be twice as large as that actually observed.

The tendency to miss the mark is due to investigators failing to take account of the exclusions to enrollment as specified in the study protocol. But some of it is "grantsmanship" by "saving" money to make the trial more appealing to funding agencies by shaving corners on what is really required by way of time to recruit by being overly optimistic.

Early Stops

An early stop is an instance of a trial being stopped prior to its scheduled end because accumulated data suggesting benefit or harm associated with one of the study treatments or because it is considered futile to continue. These judgments are based on statistical analyses conducted during a trial to assess the likelihood of a current null result becoming a non-null informative result if the trial continued to its appointed end.

Early stops can also occur because of lack of unwillingness of the sponsor to continue funding or because funding runs out. Early stops, because of benefit or harm associated with the study treatment, can come out of the blue any time during the trial. The obligation is to publish and to do as quickly as possible consistent with allowing enough time for data pipeline to clear and careful analysis.

Changes to the Study Protocol

There is virtually no study protocol that does not undergo changes during the trial. Any change to treatment schedules or treatment dosages, or changes having the potential of effecting the safety or benefit of being studied, including changes to data collection schedules, constitute amendments to the protocol and require IRB review and approval before implementation.

The concern with any protocol change is the possibility of introducing biasing effects on data if the changes affect the treatment groups differentially – unlikely in trials with balanced randomization over the course of enrollment.

Changes to consent forms or to the wording in consent forms, as well as changes in study procedures adding to the nuisance or risk of being studied, must be reviewed and approved by IRBs before they can be implemented.

Absent a central IRB structure, changes must be reviewed by individual IRBs. It can take months before the change is cleared by all IRBs. Investigators must decide whether to implement the change on a clinic-by-clinic basis as they are approved or wait on implementation until the change has been approved by all IRBs.

Changes to Data Procedures or Data Forms

Minor changes to data collection forms can be implemented without IRB approval. Addition of questions considered "sensitive" must be reviewed before the form can be used.

Adding or Subtracting Treatments

Adding a new treatment or changing dose is major. They will involve changes to consent form and to the randomization schedule. The likelihood is that all patients, including those already enrolled, will have to be informed of the change and reconsented.

Adding Study Clinics

Adding clinics in multicenter trials after they are underway is relatively common. Additions may be planned, for example, as in the Coronary Drug Project starting with five clinics and ultimately expanding to 55 (Coronary Drug Project Research Group 1973) or may come about because of shortfalls in patient enrollment. Generally, randomizations in multicenter trials are stratified by clinic meaning that assignment ratios are robust to additions or subtractions.

Clinics may not be cleared for enrollment without IRB approval.

Withdrawal of Clinics

Cessation of clinic operations occurs naturally when the trial comes to a normal end. Under those circumstances, there is time to plan for orderly separations of study participants from the trial. It is a different story if it is necessary to cease operations because of poor performance of a clinic or because of withdrawal of the clinic. The main issue in those cases is what to do with persons enrolled and under follow-up in the trial. The best option is for someone else in the institution where the clinic is located to assume responsibility for the clinic. The next best option is to transfer responsibilities to some other medical institutions in the area. That option may exist in multicenter trials with another study clinic in the same city.

Drug Supply and Packaging

A major problem in mounting a placebo-controlled masked trial is finding a placebo to match the study drug. The study drug may be supplied or purchased from the manufacturer, but the placebo will have to be obtained elsewhere. If the study drug is in pill form embossed with the makers mark, it is illegal to produce a placebo with the same marking. The best that can be done is to manufacture a pill of the same size but without the marking. Study patients may not notice the difference unless they have opportunity to compare, but study personnel will notice.

The usual course in such cases is to encapsulate, achieved by placing the study drug and placebo pills in similar colored and sized capsules. Generally, this means that both kinds of pills must be shipped to a packaging firm to load the capsules and to bottle and label medications for dispensing in the study. It can take up to a year or longer to complete all the steps necessary before clinics will be supplied with study drug to start enrollment.

Plagiarism, Data Fabrication, and Fraud

These are a trialist's worst nightmares (see Research Integrity Standards and Consequences of Violations; "Special Topics"). Any occurrence must be reported to IRBs and to funding agencies and dealt with accordingly.

Issues in Publishing

Data Acquisition

Getting IRB approval of the data collection schedule and data forms is key. Enrollment cannot start until that is done, but that is only part of the data collection process. A good deal of study data in typical trials come from laboratory tests or other procedures like fundus photography, ECGs, or x-rays, processed after a person's clinic visit. Investigators have to devise ways to connect that information to participants' data records and devise mechanisms for data to flow back to clinics and the study data processing sites.

The logistics and mechanics of creating data flows and connecting the data to study participants is every bit as tedious and vexing as creating the actual data collection forms for enrollment and follow-up. Though the tests and procedures are done during a study participant's clinic visit, results of the tests or procedures may not be available until days or weeks later.

The mechanics of flow can be simplified if it is direct from the processing site to the study data center bypassing clinics, but that leaves clinic personnel and study participant in the dark as to results and hence not advisable if the information is necessary in caring for study participants. The flow can be simultaneous to a participant's study clinic and study data center, but that can lead to medical-legal issues if data flowing to the two sites does not match. The best practice is for flows to study clinics and from there to study data processing sites.

An issue in flow is with "batched" readings, for example, as with x-ray readings by a committee for consensus readings done in face-to-face meetings or via conference telephone. The difficulty with "batching" is that it may be months after the close of a trial before there is a finished dataset for analysis with readings and the reality of early stops that can come out of the blue. The preferred practice is to avoid batching.

When to Freeze Data Files

The answer is when everything needed for a paper is in the data system and the data have been edited and cleaned. Analysis for paper writing must be done using a fixed dataset for counts and analyses to agree in the manuscript. The dataset cannot be frozen until data pipelines in the trial have been emptied. It may take weeks or months before that happens depending on how data are captured and on how long it takes for data flow through study pipelines. The final dataset is the one used to perform the analysis that will be published.

A problem in closing datasets is gathering information on people lost to follow-up. Unless there has been a system in the trial to account for dropouts and people lost to follow-up when the dropout or loss occurs, that tracking will have to be done at the end of data collection before the dataset can be frozen. That can delay closing the dataset by months until the tracking is finished. The tracking should be enough to indicate when a person was lost to follow-up and why. If tracking is not done until the trial closes trails may be cold. Then it may take special efforts to find where people are and whether alive or dead. Death is an important event even if not the design variable for the trial. Counts of deaths by treatment group must be included in publications.

Counting

It can be said that counting is the hardest part of doing trials. To count accurately and to be able to reproduce counts, there must be clear operational definitions. Even such a seemingly simple count of number enrolled requires a crisp definition of what it means to be "enrolled." What is the specific act that defines enrollment? When the patient consents to enrollment? When the treatment assignment is issued to the clinic? When the assignment is revealed to the person being enrolled? When the person takes the first dose of treatment? What if the person consents and the clinic receives the assignment, but the person decides at the last minute against enrollment. Then what? Do you count the person as enrolled? If you do then when counting treatment dropouts, do you count the person as a dropout even though the person never received any study drug?

The best way to ensure reproducible counts is by having written definitions of desired counts and then to ask two people, independent of each other, to make the counts and then to adjudicate differences.

Quality Control

The last thing one wants is to publish a paper only to discover errors after publication. There are lots of ways to make mistakes; some are potentially career ending. One of those is to mislabel the treatment groups. Basically, all it takes to make that mistake is for the person creating the analysis dataset to mix up the treatment codes. After that, unless detected, the paper will be submitted with the coding error. Prudent quality control procedures involve independent checks on coding used to create the analysis dataset.

Also essential is having an independent analyst recreate essential analyses and tables included in the manuscript before submission.

Interim Publications

Assuming the trial is long-term and not operated under a blackout mode of operation (as discussed above), investigators have the option of producing one or more interim publications summarizing results up to points in the trial. They may be motivated to produce such publication simply as a way of keeping the trial in the eye of the public, to counter published results of a sister study, or simply to sharpen their own acumen in analysis and interpretation of the accumulating data.

The downside of such publications is that whatever is said may have to be taken back or revised when the trial is finished and results published. Hence, all in all, probably best to forego such publications even if possible.

When the Primary Outcome Is Trumped by a Higher-Order Outcome

Consider the case of the University Group Diabetes Program (University Group Diabetes Program Research Group 1970). A multicenter long-term trial is designed to determine if commonly accepted treatments for type 2 diabetes were effective in preventing the morbidity typically associated with the condition. Was it appropriate for investigators to stop one of the treatments, tolbutamide, because of excess mortality in the treatment group?

Critics argued it was not because mortality was not the design variable for the trial. Taken on its face, the argument means one would ignore deaths because they were not used in designing the trial. That argument is tantamount to ignoring serious events because they were not mentioned in the protocol, an untenable ethical position.

Rejections

Rejections are part of the publication process. If you have not had a paper rejected, you have not submitted many.

Broadly, there are two kinds of rejections: cold (thank you for the submission but try somewhere else) and warm (we cannot accept your manuscript but are willing to reconsider if appropriately revised). The best authors can hope for with cold rejections are quick rejections.

Data Sharing

Data sharing is (1) an arrangement in which data generated from a research project are made available for others outside the investigator group under specified conditions, e.g., as specified in data use agreements, or (2) an arrangement involving the deposit of supplemental tables, source code, details of methods, or raw data supporting a publication as required by some journals. Data sharing in either form involves de-identification and making data HIPPA compliant.

Increasingly the expectation is that data will be shared in the sense of definition (1) when the trial is finished. That expectation poses burden on investigators in preparing data for deposit and in answering questions that invariably arise when used by others.

Closing Word

We opened this treatise with a quote from Donald Fredrickson in a speech before the New York Academy of Medicine in 1968, reminding us that trials are ordeals and that they lack glamor, but in that same speech, he also recognized trials as being "among the most challenging tests of our skills" and asks "If, in major medical dilemmas, the alternative is to pay the cost of perpetual uncertainty, have we really any choice?"

The world needs trials and people to do them. Our effort here has been to enlighten trialists of the issues and challenges they face in doing trials, not to discourage them from undertaking them. We are not futurists and cannot say with certainty what clinical trials of the future will look like. It seems unlikely to us that they will omit design fundamentals like strong random error control, removal of bias using randomization and masking, and control over extraneous influences. They will also likely require similar governance, organization, and attention to details as trials have in the last 50 years. Science and therapeutics will advance, and new measures and outcomes will appear in trials. Wearable technology (Gresham et al. 2018), for example, holds great promise to meet the needs for accuracy, reliability, patient relevance, and convenience for many emerging therapeutic questions. We expect that many who read this book will see much more of that in the future.

The two of us have been involved in dozens of trials, sometimes as heads of coordinating centers in multicenter trials and sometimes as members of data monitoring committees for trials. Every trial is a new adventure; no two alike. The joy is in the discoveries that come from the data; the joy of being among the first to see new results and discover new insights.

We have yet to meet anyone who regrets their involvement in trials. They all have tales and war stories, but no regrets, and itching for the next trial. Invariably people, when they finish, characterize their involvement as among the most enriching and educational experience of their professional lives.

References

Biankin AV, Piantadosi S, Hollingsworth SJ (2015) Patient-centric trials for therapeutic development in precision oncology. Nature 526:361

Coronary Drug Project Research Group (1973) The Coronary Drug Project: design, methods, and baseline results. Circulation 47(Suppl I):I-1–I-50

Fishman A et al (2003) A randomized trial comparing lung-volume-reduction surgery with medical therapy for severe emphysema. N Engl J Med 348(21):2059–2073

Fredrickson DS (1968) The field trial: some thoughts on the indispensable ordeal. Bull NY Acad Med 44:985–993

Gresham G et al (2018) Wearable activity monitors in oncology trials: current use of an emerging technology. Contemp Clin Trials 64:13–21

Lind J (1753) A treatise of the scurvy (Reprinted in Lind's treatise on scurvy, edited by Stewart CP, Guthrie D, Edinburgh University Press, Edinburgh, 1953). Sands, Murray, Cochrane, Edinburgh, 1753

Meinert CL (1998) Masked monitoring in clinical trials – blind stupidity? N Encl J Med 338:1381–1382

Meinert CL (2012a) Clinical trials dictionary: terminology and usage recommendations. Wiley, Hoboken

Meinert CL (2012b) Clinical trials: design, conduct, and analysis, 2nd edn. Oxford University Press, New York

Meinert CL (2013) Clinical trials handbook: design and conduct. Wiley, New York

Piantadosi S (2017) Clinical trials: a methodological perspective, 3rd edn. Wiley, Hoboken

University Group Diabetes Program Research Group (1970) A study of the effects of hypoglycemic agents on vascular complications in patients with adult-onset diabetes: II. Mortality results. Diabetes 19(Suppl 2):785–830

Appendix 1

Nüremberg Code
Description: The 10 principles of the original Nüremberg Code (1947) are transcribed below (Anonymous 1949). The code and history of the Nüremberg trials are described further in the 1997 *NEJM* article by Evelyne Shuster for the 50th anniversary of the Nüremberg Code (Shuster 1997).

1. *The voluntary consent of the human subject is absolutely essential. This means that the person involved should have legal capacity to give consent; should be so situated as to be able to exercise free power of choice, without the intervention of any element of force, fraud, deceit, duress, over-reaching, or other ulterior form of constraint or coercion; and should have sufficient knowledge and comprehension of the elements of the subject matter involved, as to enable him to make an understanding and enlightened decision. This latter element requires that, before the acceptance of an affirmative decision by the experimental subject, there should be made known to him the nature, duration, and purpose of the experiment; the method and means by which it is to be conducted; all inconveniences and hazards reasonably to be expected; and the effects upon his health or person, which may possibly come from his participation in the experiment. The duty and responsibility for ascertaining the quality of the consent rests upon each individual who initiates, directs or engages in the experiment. It is a personal duty and responsibility which may not be delegated to another with impunity.*
2. *The experiment should be such as to yield fruitful results for the good of society, unprocurable by other methods or means of study, and not random and unnecessary in nature.*
3. *The experiment should be so designed and based on the results of animal experimentation and a knowledge of the natural history of the disease or other problem under study, that the anticipated results will justify the performance of the experiment.*
4. *The experiment should be so conducted as to avoid all unnecessary physical and mental suffering and injury.*

5. No experiment should be conducted, where there is an a priori reason to believe that death or disabling injury will occur; except, perhaps, in those experiments where the experimental physicians also serve as subjects.
6. The degree of risk to be taken should never exceed that determined by the humanitarian importance of the problem to be solved by the experiment.
7. Proper preparations should be made and adequate facilities provided to protect the experimental subject against even remote possibilities of injury, disability, or death.
8. The experiment should be conducted only by scientifically qualified persons. The highest degree of skill and care should be required through all stages of the experiment of those who conduct or engage in the experiment.
9. During the course of the experiment, the human subject should be at liberty to bring the experiment to an end, if he has reached the physical or mental state, where continuation of the experiment seemed to him to be impossible.
10. During the course of the experiment, the scientist in charge must be prepared to terminate the experiment at any stage, if he has probable cause to believe, in the exercise of the good faith, superior skill and careful judgement required of him, that a continuation of the experiment is likely to result in injury, disability, or death to the experimental subject.

References

Anonymous (1949) Trials of war criminals before the Nüremberg military tribunals under Control Council Law No. 10, vol 2. U.S. Government Printing Office, Washington, DC, pp 181–182

Shuster E (1997) Fifty years later: the significance of the Nüremberg Code. NEJM 337:1436–1440

Appendix 2

The Belmont Report (1979)
Description: This Appendix includes the Basic Ethical Principles of the Belmont Report established by the National Commission at the Belmont Conference Center in Maryland in 1976, published in 1978, and reprinted in the Federal Register April 18, 1979 (National Commission for the Protection of Human Subjects of Biomedical and Behavioral Research 1978). Related documents describing the history and impact the Belmont Report has had on medical research are cited at the end of this Appendix for further reading (Rothman 1991; Lederer 1996; Beecher 1996; Department of Health, Education, and Welfare and National Commission for the Protection of Human Subjects of Biomedical and Behavioral Research 2014; Beauchamp et al. 2014).

The following text (italics) is a reproduction of the Belmont report obtained from reference National Commission for the Protection of Human Subjects of Biomedical and Behavioral Research (1978):

Basic Ethical Principles

The expression "basic ethical principles" refers to those general judgments that serve as a basic justification for the many particular ethical prescriptions and evaluations of human actions. Three basic principles, among those generally accepted in our cultural tradition, are particularly relevant to the ethics of research involving human subjects: the principles of respect of persons, beneficence and justice.

1. ***Respect for Persons.*** *— Respect for persons incorporates at least two ethical convictions: first, that individuals should be treated as autonomous agents, and second, that persons with diminished autonomy are entitled to protection. The principle of respect for persons thus divides into two separate moral requirements: the requirement to acknowledge autonomy and the requirement to protect those with diminished autonomy.*

    An autonomous person is an individual capable of deliberation about personal goals and of acting under the direction of such deliberation. To respect autonomy is to give weight to autonomous persons' considered opinions and choices while refraining from obstructing their actions unless they are clearly detrimental to others. To show lack of respect for an autonomous agent is to repudiate that person's considered judgments, to deny an individual the freedom to act on those considered judgments, or to withhold information necessary to make a considered judgment, when there are no compelling reasons to do so.

However, not every human being is capable of self-determination. The capacity for self-determination matures during an individual's life, and some individuals lose this capacity wholly or in part because of illness, mental disability, or circumstances that severely restrict liberty. Respect for the immature and the incapacitated may require protecting them as they mature or while they are incapacitated.

Some persons are in need of extensive protection, even to the point of excluding them from activities which may harm them; other persons require little protection beyond making sure they undertake activities freely and with awareness of possible adverse consequence. The extent of protection afforded should depend upon the risk of harm and the likelihood of benefit. The judgment that any individual lacks autonomy should be periodically reevaluated and will vary in different situations.

In most cases of research involving human subjects, respect for persons demands that subjects enter into the research voluntarily and with adequate information. In some situations, however, application of the principle is not obvious. The involvement of prisoners as subjects of research provides an instructive example. On the one hand, it would seem that the principle of respect for persons requires that prisoners not be deprived of the opportunity to volunteer for research. On the other hand, under prison conditions they may be subtly coerced or unduly influenced to engage in research activities for which they would not otherwise volunteer. Respect for persons would then dictate that prisoners be protected. Whether to allow prisoners to "volunteer" or to "protect" them presents a dilemma. Respecting persons, in most hard cases, is often a matter of balancing competing claims urged by the principle of respect itself.

2. **Beneficence**. — Persons are treated in an ethical manner not only by respecting their decisions and protecting them from harm, but also by making efforts to secure their well-being. Such treatment falls under the principle of beneficence. The term "beneficence" is often understood to cover acts of kindness or charity that go beyond strict obligation. In this document, beneficence is understood in a stronger sense, as an obligation. Two general rules have been formulated as complementary expressions of beneficent actions in this sense: *(1)* do not harm and *(2)* maximize possible benefits and minimize possible harms.

The Hippocratic maxim "do no harm" has long been a fundamental principle of medical ethics. Claude Bernard extended it to the realm of research, saying that one should not injure one person regardless of the benefits that might come to others. However, even avoiding harm requires learning what is harmful; and, in the process of obtaining this information, persons may be exposed to risk of harm. Further, the Hippocratic Oath requires physicians to benefit their patients "according to their best judgment." Learning what will in fact benefit may require exposing persons to risk. The problem posed by these imperatives is to decide when it is justifiable to seek certain benefits despite the risks involved, and when the benefits should be foregone because of the risks.

The obligations of beneficence affect both individual investigators and society at large, because they extend both to particular research projects and to the entire enterprise of research. In the case of particular projects, investigators and members of their institutions are obliged to give forethought to the maximization of benefits and the reduction of risk that might occur from the research investigation. In the case of scientific research in general, members of the larger society are obliged to recognize the longer term benefits and risks that may result from the improvement of knowledge and from the development of novel medical, psychotherapeutic, and social procedures.

The principle of beneficence often occupies a well-defined justifying role in many areas of research involving human subjects. An example is found in research involving children. Effective ways of treating childhood diseases and fostering healthy development are benefits that serve to justify research involving children – even when individual research subjects are not direct beneficiaries. Research also makes it possible to avoid the harm that may result from the application of previously accepted routine practices that on closer investigation turn out to be dangerous. But the role of the principle of beneficence is not always so unambiguous. A difficult ethical problem remains, for example, about research that presents more than minimal risk without immediate prospect of direct benefit to the children involved. Some have argued that such research is inadmissible, while others have pointed out that this limit would rule out much research promising great benefit to children in the future. Here again, as with all hard cases, the different claims covered by the principle of beneficence may come into conflict and force difficult choices.

3. **Justice**. — Who ought to receive the benefits of research and bear its burdens? This is a question of justice, in the sense of "fairness in distribution" or "what is deserved." An injustice occurs when some benefit to which a person is entitled is denied without good reason or when some burden is imposed unduly. Another way of conceiving the principle of justice is that equals ought to be treated equally. However, this statement requires explication. Who is equal and who is unequal? What considerations justify departure from equal distribution? Almost all commentators allow that distinctions based on experience, age, deprivation, competence, merit and position do sometimes constitute criteria justifying differential treatment for certain purposes. It is necessary, then, to explain in what respects people should be treated equally. There are several widely accepted formulations of just ways to distribute burdens and benefits. Each formulation mentions some relevant property on the basis of which burdens and benefits should be distributed. These formulations are **(1)** to each person an equal share, **(2)** to each person according to individual need, **(3)** to each person according to individual effort, **(4)** to each person according to societal contribution, and **(5)** to each person according to merit.

Questions of justice have long been associated with social practices such as punishment, taxation and political representation. Until recently these questions have not generally been associated with scientific research. However, they are foreshadowed even in the earliest reflections on the ethics of research involving human subjects. For example, during the 19th and early 20th centuries the burdens of serving as research subjects fell largely upon poor ward patients, while the benefits of improved medical care flowed primarily to private patients. Subsequently, the exploitation of unwilling prisoners as research subjects in Nazi concentration camps was condemned as a particularly flagrant injustice. In this country, in the 1940's, the Tuskegee syphilis study used disadvantaged, rural black men to study the untreated course of a disease that is by no means confined to that population. These subjects were deprived of demonstrably effective treatment in order not to interrupt the project, long after such treatment became generally available.

Against this historical background, it can be seen how conceptions of justice are relevant to research involving human subjects. For example, the selection of research subjects needs to be scrutinized in order to determine whether some classes (e.g., welfare patients, particular racial and ethnic minorities, or persons confined to institutions) are being systematically selected simply because of their easy availability, their compromised position, or their manipulability, rather than for reasons directly related to the problem being studied. Finally, whenever research supported by public funds leads to the development of therapeutic devices and procedures, justice demands both that these not provide advantages only to those who can afford them and that such research should not unduly involve persons from groups unlikely to be among the beneficiaries of subsequent applications of the research.

References

Beauchamp TL, Walters L, Kahn JP, Mastroianni AC (2014) Contemporary issues in bioethics, 8th edn. Cengage Learning, Boston, pp 22–27

Beecher HK (1996) Ethics and clinical research. NEJM 274:1354e66

Department of Health, Education, and Welfare, National Commission for the Protection of Human Subjects of Biomedical and Behavioral Research (2014) The Belmont report. Ethical principles and guidelines for the protection of human subjects of research. J Am Coll Dent 81(3):4–13

Lederer SE (1996) Subjected to science: human experimentation in America before the Second World War. Johns Hopkins University Press, Baltimore

National Commission for the Protection of Human Subjects of Biomedical and Behavioral Research (1978) The Belmont report: ethical principles and guidelines for the protection of human subjects of research. The Commission, Bethesda

Rothman DJ (1991) Strangers at the bedside: a history of how law and bioethics transformed medical decision making. Basic Books, New York

Appendix 3

Declaration of Helsinki
Description: This Appendix includes the earliest version of the Declaration of Helsinki, first issued at the meeting of the World Medical Association (WMA) in Helsinki in 1964 ("Declaration of Helsinki* (1964)") and the most recent version from the 64th WMA General Assembly in 2013 ("Declaration of Helsinki* (2013)"), having undergone seven revisions during this time (World Medical Association 1964; World Medical Association 2013). A description of the various revisions that have been made to the Declaration of Helsinki and its role in clinical research over time can be found in the additional references listed at the end of this Appendix (Krleza-Jerić and Lemmens 2009; Millum et al. 2013; Ndebele 2013).

Declaration of Helsinki* (1964)

World Medical Association (1964)

Introduction

> It is the mission of the doctor to safeguard the health of the people. His knowledge and conscience are dedicated to the fulfilment of this mission.
>
> The Declaration of Geneva of the World Medical Association binds the doctor with the words, "The health of my patient will be my first consideration"; and the International Code of Medical Ethics which declares that "Any act or advice which could weaken physical or mental resistance of a human being may be used only in his interest."
>
> Because it is essential that the results of laboratory experiments be applied to human beings to further scientific knowledge and to help suffering humanity, the World Medical Association has prepared the following recommendations as a guide to each doctor in clinical research. It must be stressed that the standards as drafted are only a guide to physicians all over the world. Doctors are not relieved from criminal, civil, and ethical responsibilities under the laws of their own countries.

In the field of clinical research a fundamental distinction must be recognized between clinical research in which the aim is essentially therapeutic for a patient, and clinical research the essential object of which is purely scientific and without therapeutic value to the person subjected to the research.

I. Basic Principles

1. Clinical research must conform to the moral and scientific principles that justify medical research, and should be based on laboratory and animal experiments or other scientifically established facts.
2. Clinical research should be conducted only by scientifically qualified persons and under the supervision of a qualified medical man.
3. Clinical research cannot legitimately be carried out unless the importance of the objective is in proportion to the inherent risk to the subject.
4. Every clinical research project should be preceded by careful assessment of inherent risks in comparison to foreseeable benefits to the subject or to others.
5. Special caution should be exercised by the doctor in performing clinical research in which the personality of the subject is liable to be altered by drugs or experimental procedure.

II. Clinical Research Combined with Professional Care

1. In the treatment of the sick person the doctor must be free to use a new therapeutic measure if in his judgment it offers hope of saving life, re-establishing health, or alleviating suffering.

    If at all possible, consistent with patient psychology, the doctor should obtain the patient's freely given consent after the patient has been given a full explanation. In case of legal incapacity consent should also be procured from the legal guardian; in case of physical incapacity the permission of the legal guardian replaces that of the patient.
2. The doctor can combine clinical research with professional care, the objective being the acquisition of new medical knowledge, only to the extent that clinical research is justified by its therapeutic value for the patient.

III. Non-therapeutic Clinical Research

1. In the purely scientific application of clinical research carried out on a human being it is the duty of the doctor to remain the protector of the life and health of that person on whom clinical research is being carried out.
2. The nature, the purpose, and the risk of clinical research must be explained to the subject by the doctor.
3a. Clinical research on a human being cannot be undertaken without his free consent, after he has been fully informed; if he is legally incompetent the consent of the legal guardian should be procured.
3b. The subject of clinical research should be in such a mental, physical, and legal state as to be able to exercise fully his power of choice.
3c. Consent should as a rule be obtained in writing.' However, the responsibility for clinical research always remains with the research worker; it never falls on the subject, even after consent is obtained.
4a. The investigator must respect the right of each individual to safeguard his personal integrity, especially if the subject is in a dependent relationship to the investigator.
4b. At any time during the course of clinical research the subject or his guardian should be free to withdraw permission for research to be continued. The investigator or the investigating team should discontinue the research if in his or their judgment it may, if continued, be harmful to the individual.

Declaration of Helsinki* (2013)

World Medical Association (2013)

Preamble

1. The World Medical Association (WMA) has developed the Declaration of Helsinki as a statement of ethical principles for medical research involving human subjects, including research on identifiable human material and data.

    The Declaration is intended to be read as a whole and each of its constituent paragraphs should not be applied without consideration of all other relevant paragraphs.

2. Consistent with the mandate of the WMA, the Declaration is addressed primarily to physicians, the WMA encourages others who are involved in medical research involving human subjects to adopt these principles.

General Principles

3. The Declaration of Geneva of the WMA binds the physician with the words, "The health of my patient will be my first consideration," and the International Code of Medical Ethics declares that, "A physician shall act only in the patient's interest when providing medical care."
4. It is the duty of the physician to promote and safeguard the health, well-being and rights of patients, including those who are involved in medical research. The physician's knowledge and conscience are dedicated to the fulfilment of this duty.
5. Medical progress is based on research that ultimately must include studies involving human subjects.
6. The primary purpose of medical research involving human subjects is to understand the causes, development and effects of diseases and improve preventive, diagnostic and therapeutic interventions (methods, procedures and treatments). Even the best current interventions must be evaluated continually through research for their safety, effectiveness, efficiency, accessibility and quality.
7. Medical research is subject to ethical standards that promote and ensure respect for all human subjects and protect their health and rights.
8. While the primary purpose of medical research is to generate new knowledge, this goal can never take precedence over the rights and interests of individual research subjects.
9. It is the duty of physicians who are involved in medical research to protect the life, health, dignity, integrity, right to self-determination, privacy, and confidentiality of personal information of research subjects. The responsibility for the protection of research subjects must always rest with the physician or other health care professionals and never with the research subjects, even though they have given consent.
10. Physicians must consider the ethical, legal and regulatory norms and standards for research involving human subjects in their own countries as well as applicable international norms and standards. No national or international ethical, legal or regulatory requirement should reduce or eliminate any of the protections for research subjects set forth in this Declaration.
11. Medical research should be conducted in a manner that minimises possible harm to the environment.
12. Medical research involving human subjects must be conducted only by individuals with the appropriate ethics and scientific education, training and qualifications. Research on patients or healthy volunteers requires the supervision of a competent and appropriately qualified physician or other health care professional.
13. Groups that are underrepresented in medical research should be provided appropriate access to participation in research.

14. Physicians who combine medical research with medical care should involve their patients in research only to the extent that this is justified by its potential preventive, diagnostic or therapeutic value and if the physician has good reason to believe that participation in the research study will not adversely affect the health of the patients who serve as research subjects.
15. Appropriate compensation and treatment for subjects who are harmed as a result of participating in research must be ensured.

Risks, Burdens and Benefits

16. In medical practice and in medical research, most interventions involve risks and burdens.

    Medical research involving human subjects may only be conducted if the importance of the objective outweighs the risks and burdens to the research subjects.
17. All medical research involving human subjects must be preceded by careful assessment of predictable risks and burdens to the individuals and groups involved in the research in comparison with foreseeable benefits to them and to other individuals or groups affected by the condition under investigation.

    Measures to minimise the risks must be implemented. The risks must be continuously monitored, assessed and documented by the researcher.
18. Physicians may not be involved in a research study involving human subjects unless they are confident that the risks have been adequately assessed and can be satisfactorily managed.

    When the risks are found to outweigh the potential benefits or when there is conclusive proof of definitive outcomes, physicians must assess whether to continue, modify or immediately stop the study.

Vulnerable Groups and Individuals

19. Some groups and individuals are particularly vulnerable and may have an increased likelihood of being wronged or of incurring additional harm.

    All vulnerable groups and individuals should receive specifically considered protection.
20. Medical research with a vulnerable group is only justified if the research is responsive to the health needs or priorities of this group and the research cannot be carried out in a non-vulnerable group. In addition, this group should stand to benefit from the knowledge, practices or interventions that result from the research.

Scientific Requirements and Research Protocols

21. Medical research involving human subjects must conform to generally accepted scientific principles, be based on a thorough knowledge of the scientific literature, other relevant sources of information, and adequate laboratory and, as appropriate, animal experimentation. The welfare of animals used for research must be respected.
22. The design and performance of each research study involving human subjects must be clearly described in a research protocol.

    The protocol should contain a statement of the ethical considerations involved and should indicate how the principles in this Declaration have been addressed. The protocol should include information regarding funding, sponsors, institutional affiliations, other potential conflicts of interest, incentives for subjects and information regarding provisions for treating and/or compensating subjects who are harmed as a consequence of participation in the research study. In clinical trials, the protocol must also describe appropriate arrangements for post-trial provisions.

Research Ethics Committees

23. The research protocol must be submitted for consideration, comment, guidance and approval to the concerned research ethics committee before the study begins. This committee must be transparent in its functioning, must be independent of the researcher, the sponsor and any other undue influence and must be duly qualified. It must take into consideration the laws and regulations of the country or countries in which the research is to be performed as well as applicable international norms and standards but these must not be allowed to reduce or eliminate any of the protections for research subjects set forth in this Declaration.

    The committee must have the right to monitor ongoing studies. The researcher must provide monitoring information to the committee, especially information about any serious adverse events. No amendment to the protocol may be made without consideration and approval by the committee. After the end of the study, the researchers must submit a final report to the committee containing a summary of the study's findings and conclusions.

Privacy and Confidentiality

24. Every precaution must be taken to protect the privacy of research subjects and the confidentiality of their personal information.

Informed Consent

25. Participation by individuals capable of giving informed consent as subjects in medical research must be voluntary. Although it may be appropriate to consult family members or community leaders, no individual capable of giving informed consent may be enrolled in a research study unless he or she freely agrees.

26. In medical research involving human subjects capable of giving informed consent, each potential subject must be adequately informed of the aims, methods, sources of funding, any possible conflicts of interest, institutional affiliations of the researcher, the anticipated benefits and potential risks of the study and the discomfort it may entail, post-study provisions and any other relevant aspects of the study. The potential subject must be informed of the right to refuse to participate in the study or to withdraw consent to participate at any time without reprisal. Special attention should be given to the specific information needs of individual potential subjects as well as to the methods used to deliver the information.

    After ensuring that the potential subject has understood the information, the physician or another appropriately qualified individual must then seek the potential subject's freely-given informed consent, preferably in writing. If the consent cannot be expressed in writing, the non-written consent must be formally documented and witnessed.

    All medical research subjects should be given the option of being informed about the general outcome and results of the study.

27. When seeking informed consent for participation in a research study the physician must be particularly cautious if the potential subject is in a dependent relationship with the physician or may consent under duress. In such situations the informed consent must be sought by an appropriately qualified individual who is completely independent of this relationship.

28. For a potential research subject who is incapable of giving informed consent, the physician must seek informed consent from the legally authorised representative. These individuals must not be included in a research study that has no likelihood of benefit for them unless it is intended to promote the health of the group represented by the potential subject, the research cannot instead be performed with persons capable of providing informed consent, and the research entails only minimal risk and minimal burden.

29. When a potential research subject who is deemed incapable of giving informed consent is able to give assent to decisions about participation in research, the physician must seek that assent in addition to the consent of the legally authorised representative. The potential subject's dissent should be respected.
30. Research involving subjects who are physically or mentally incapable of giving consent, for example, unconscious patients, may be done only if the physical or mental condition that prevents giving informed consent is a necessary characteristic of the research group. In such circumstances the physician must seek informed consent from the legally authorised representative. If no such representative is available and if the research cannot be delayed, the study may proceed without informed consent provided that the specific reasons for involving subjects with a condition that renders them unable to give informed consent have been stated in the research protocol and the study has been approved by a research ethics committee. Consent to remain in the research must be obtained as soon as possible from the subject or a legally authorised representative.
31. The physician must fully inform the patient which aspects of their care are related to the research. The refusal of a patient to participate in a study or the patient's decision to withdraw from the study must never adversely affect the patient-physician relationship.
32. For medical research using identifiable human material or data, such as research on material or data contained in biobanks or similar repositories, physicians must seek informed consent for its collection, storage and/or reuse. There may be exceptional situations where consent would be impossible or impracticable to obtain for such research. In such situations the research may be done only after consideration and approval of a research ethics committee.

Use of Placebo

33. The benefits, risks, burdens and effectiveness of a new intervention must be tested against those of the best proven intervention(s), except in the following circumstances:
    – Where no proven intervention exists, the use of placebo, or no intervention, is acceptable; or.
    – Where for compelling and scientifically sound methodological reasons the use of any intervention less effective than the best proven one, the use of placebo, or no intervention is necessary to determine the efficacy or safety of an intervention.
    – and the patients who receive any intervention less effective than the best proven one, placebo, or no intervention will not be subject to additional risks of serious or irreversible harm as a result of not receiving the best proven intervention.
        Extreme care must be taken to avoid abuse of this option.

Post-Trial Provisions

34. In advance of a clinical trial, sponsors, researchers and host country governments should make provisions for post-trial access for all participants who still need an intervention identified as beneficial in the trial. This information must also be disclosed to participants during the informed consent process.

Research Registration and Publication and Dissemination of Results

35. Every research study involving human subjects must be registered in a publicly accessible database before recruitment of the first subject.
36. Researchers, authors, sponsors, editors and publishers all have ethical obligations with regard to the publication and dissemination of the results of research. Researchers have a duty to make publicly available the results of their research on human subjects and are accountable for the completeness and accuracy of their reports. All parties should adhere to accepted guidelines for ethical reporting. Negative and inconclusive as well

as positive results must be published or otherwise made publicly available. Sources of funding, institutional affiliations and conflicts of interest must be declared in the publication. Reports of research not in accordance with the principles of this Declaration should not be accepted for publication.

Unproven Interventions in Clinical Practice

37. In the treatment of an individual patient, where proven interventions do not exist or other known interventions have been ineffective, the physician, after seeking expert advice, with informed consent from the patient or a legally authorised representative, may use an unproven intervention if in the physician's judgement it offers hope of saving life, re-establishing health or alleviating suffering. This intervention should subsequently be made the object of research, designed to evaluate its safety and efficacy. In all cases, new information must be recorded and, where appropriate, made publicly available.

References

Krleza-Jerić K, Lemmens T (2009) 7th revision of the Declaration of Helsinki: good news for the transparency of clinical trials. Croat Med J 50(2):105–110

Millum J, Wendler D, Emanuel EJ (2013) The 50th anniversary of the Declaration of Helsinki: progress but many remaining challenges. JAMA 310(20):2143–2144

Ndebele P (2013) The Declaration of Helsinki, 50 years later. JAMA 310(20):2145–2146

World Medical Association (1964) Human experimentation: code of ethics of W.M.A. Br Med J 2 (5402):177

World Medical Association (2013) Declaration of Helsinki ethical principles for medical research involving human subjects. JAMA 310(20):2191–2194

Appendix 4

Hippocratic Oath and Related Documents
Description: The text from the classical and modern versions of the Hippocratic Oath is included below. The Classical version originally written Ionic Greek, circa 400 BCE, was translated into English in the 1700s (section "Classical Version") (NLM 2002). The Hippocratic Oath was rewritten by Louis Lasagna in 1964 and is considered the Modern version of the Hippocratic Oath (section "Modern Version"). Third, the most recent version of the Declaration of Geneva (2017), intended as a revision of the Hippocratic Oath, is included as section "World Medical Association Declaration of Geneva" (World Medical Association 2018).

Classical Version

National Library of Medicine of the National Institutes of Health (2002):

> *I swear by Apollo Physician and Asclepius and Hygieia and Panaceia and all the gods and goddesses, making them my witnesses, that I will fulfill according to my ability and judgment this oath and this covenant:*
> *To hold him who has taught me this art as equal to my parents and to live my life in partnership with him, and if he is in need of money to give him a share of mine, and to regard his offspring as equal to my brothers in male lineage and to teach them this art—if they desire to learn it—without fee and covenant; to give a share of precepts and oral instruction and all the other learning to my sons and to the sons of him who has instructed me and to pupils who have signed the covenant and have taken an oath according to the medical law, but no one else.*
> *I will apply dietetic measures for the benefit of the sick according to my ability and judgment; I will keep them from harm and injustice.*
> *I will neither give a deadly drug to anybody who asked for it, nor will I make a suggestion to this effect. Similarly I will not give to a woman an abortive remedy. In purity and holiness I will guard my life and my art.*
> *I will not use the knife, not even on sufferers from stone, but will withdraw in favor of such men as are engaged in this work.*
> *Whatever houses I may visit, I will come for the benefit of the sick, remaining free of all intentional injustice, of all mischief and in particular of sexual relations with both female and male persons, be they free or slaves.*

What I may see or hear in the course of the treatment or even outside of the treatment in regard to the life of men, which on no account one must spread abroad, I will keep to myself, holding such things shameful to be spoken about.

If I fulfill this oath and do not violate it, may it be granted to me to enjoy life and art, being honored with fame among all men for all time to come; if I transgress it and swear falsely, may the opposite of all this be my lot.

Modern Version

Louis Lasagna (1964):

I swear to fulfill, to the best of my ability and judgment, this covenant:

I will respect the hard-won scientific gains of those physicians in whose steps I walk, and gladly share such knowledge as is mine with those who are to follow.

I will apply, for the benefit of the sick, all measures [that] are required, avoiding those twin traps of overtreatment and therapeutic nihilism.

I will remember that there is art to medicine as well as science, and that warmth, sympathy, and understanding may outweigh the surgeon's knife or the chemist's drug.

I will not be ashamed to say "I know not," nor will I fail to call in my colleagues when the skills of another are needed for a patient's recovery.

I will respect the privacy of my patients, for their problems are not disclosed to me that the world may know. Most especially must I tread with care in matters of life and death. If it is given me to save a life, all thanks. But it may also be within my power to take a life; this awesome responsibility must be faced with great humbleness and awareness of my own frailty. Above all, I must not play at God.

I will remember that I do not treat a fever chart, a cancerous growth, but a sick human being, whose illness may affect the person's family and economic stability. My responsibility includes these related problems, if I am to care adequately for the sick.

I will prevent disease whenever I can, for prevention is preferable to cure.

I will remember that I remain a member of society, with special obligations to all my fellow human beings, those sound of mind and body as well as the infirm.

If I do not violate this oath, may I enjoy life and art, respected while I live and remembered with affection thereafter. May I always act so as to preserve the finest traditions of my calling and may I long experience the joy of healing those who seek my help.

World Medical Association Declaration of Geneva

World Medical Association (2018):

The Physician's Pledge
AS A MEMBER OF THE MEDICAL PROFESSION:
I SOLEMNLY PLEDGE to dedicate my life to the service of humanity;
THE HEALTH AND WELL-BEING OF MY PATIENT will be my first consideration;
I WILL RESPECT the autonomy and dignity of my patient;
I WILL MAINTAIN the utmost respect for human life;
I WILL NOT PERMIT considerations of age, disease or disability, creed, ethnic origin, gender, nationality, political affiliation, race, sexual orientation, social standing or any other factor to intervene between my duty and my patient;
I WILL RESPECT the secrets that are confided in me, even after the patient has died;

I WILL PRACTISE my profession with conscience and dignity and in accordance with good medical practice;

I WILL FOSTER the honour and noble traditions of the medical profession;

I WILL GIVE to my teachers, colleagues, and students the respect and gratitude that is their due;

I WILL SHARE my medical knowledge for the benefit of the patient and the advancement of healthcare;

I WILL ATTEND TO my own health, well-being, and abilities in order to provide care of the highest standard;

I WILL NOT USE my medical knowledge to violate human rights and civil liberties, even under threat;

I MAKE THESE PROMISES solemnly, freely, and upon my honour.

References

Edelstein L (1967) The Hippocratic Oath: text, translation and interpretation. In: Temkin O, Temkin CL (eds) Ancient medicine: selected papers of Ludwig Edelstein. Johns Hopkins University Press, Baltimore, pp 3–64

Lasagna L (1964) Hippocratic Oath – modern version. WGBH Educational Foundation for PBS and NOVA Online. http://www.pbs.org/wgbh/nova/body/hippocratic-oath-today.html. Accessed 6 Mar 2018

Markel H (2004) "I Swear by Apollo" – on taking the Hippocratic Oath. NEJM 350(20):2026–2029

National Library of Medicine, National Institutes of Health (2002) The Hippocratic Oath (trans: Michael N). http://www.nlm.nih.gov/hmd/greek/greek_oath.html. Retrieved 6 Mar 2018

Orr RD, Pang N, Pellegrino ED, Siegler M (1997) Use of the Hippocratic Oath: a review of twentieth century practice and a content analysis of oaths administered in medical schools in the U.S. and Canada in 1993. J Clin Ethics 8(4):377–388

World Medical Association (2018) WMA Declaration of Geneva. https://www.wma.net/policies-post/wma-declaration-of-geneva/. Accessed 6 Mar 2018

Appendix 5

Consolidated Standards of Reporting Trials (CONSORT) 2010

Description: The CONSORT statement was first published in 1996 with the purpose of improving the quality of Randomized Controlled Trial (RCT) reports (CONSORT 2010). It was revised again in 2001 and the most recent version was published on March 24, 2010. The CONSORT statement (2010) was published simultaneously by eight journals and the Explanation and Elaboration was published in two additional journals (Moher et al. 2010a, b; Schultz et al. 2010). The 2010 CONSORT statement describes the intent of CONSORT 2010, provides a summary of changes in the most recent statement, and includes the CONSORT reporting checklist and the CONSORT flowchart. It is available in multiple languages and can be used as a tool for authors, reviewers, and consumers. The CONSORT 2010 checklist includes 25 items sorted by sections or topics that represent the minimum set of recommendations for reporting randomized trials (Fig. 1). The CONSORT flow diagram (Fig. 2) is used for documenting the flow of participants through a trial especially for two group parallel designs (Schultz et al. 2010). Extensions of the CONSORT Statement are also available for different types of trial designs in Table 1.

Additional information on CONSORT is available at: http://www.consort-statement.org

CONSORT 2010 checklist of information to include when reporting a randomised trial*

Section/Topic	Item No	Checklist item	Reported on page No
Title and abstract			
	1a	Identification as a randomised trial in the title	_____
	1b	Structured summary of trial design, methods, results, and conclusions (for specific guidance see CONSORT for abstracts)	_____
Introduction			
Background and objectives	2a	Scientific background and explanation of rationale	_____
	2b	Specific objectives or hypotheses	_____
Methods			
Trial design	3a	Description of trial design (such as parallel, factorial) including allocation ratio	_____
	3b	Important changes to methods after trial commencement (such as eligibility criteria), with reasons	_____
Participants	4a	Eligibility criteria for participants	_____
	4b	Settings and locations where the data were collected	_____
Interventions	5	The interventions for each group with sufficient details to allow replication, including how and when they were actually administered	_____
Outcomes	6a	Completely defined pre-specified primary and secondary outcome measures, including how and when they were assessed	_____
	6b	Any changes to trial outcomes after the trial commenced, with reasons	_____
Sample size	7a	How sample size was determined	_____
	7b	When applicable, explanation of any interim analyses and stopping guidelines	_____
Randomisation:			
Sequence generation	8a	Method used to generate the random allocation sequence	_____
	8b	Type of randomisation; details of any restriction (such as blocking and block size)	_____
Allocation concealment mechanism	9	Mechanism used to implement the random allocation sequence (such as sequentially numbered containers), describing any steps taken to conceal the sequence until interventions were assigned	_____

Fig. 1 (continued)

Implementation	10	Who generated the random allocation sequence, who enrolled participants, and who assigned participants to interventions
Blinding	11a	If done, who was blinded after assignment to interventions (for example, participants, care providers, those assessing outcomes) and how
	11b	If relevant, description of the similarity of interventions
Statistical methods	12a	Statistical methods used to compare groups for primary and secondary outcomes
	12b	Methods for additional analyses, such as subgroup analyses and adjusted analyses

Results

Participant flow (a diagram is strongly recommended)	13a	For each group, the numbers of participants who were randomly assigned, received intended treatment, and were analysed for the primary outcome
	13b	For each group, losses and exclusions after randomisation, together with reasons
Recruitment	14a	Dates defining the periods of recruitment and follow-up
	14b	Why the trial ended or was stopped
Baseline data	15	A table showing baseline demographic and clinical characteristics for each group
Numbers analysed	16	For each group, number of participants (denominator) included in each analysis and whether the analysis was by original assigned groups
Outcomes and estimation	17a	For each primary and secondary outcome, results for each group, and the estimated effect size and its precision (such as 95% confidence interval)
	17b	For binary outcomes, presentation of both absolute and relative effect sizes is recommended
Ancillary analyses	18	Results of any other analyses performed, including subgroup analyses and adjusted analyses, distinguishing pre-specified from exploratory
Harms	19	All important harms or unintended effects in each group (for specific guidance see CONSORT for harms)

Discussion

Limitations	20	Trial limitations, addressing sources of potential bias, imprecision, and, if relevant, multiplicity of analyses
Generalisability	21	Generalisability (external validity, applicability) of the trial findings
Interpretation	22	Interpretation consistent with results, balancing benefits and harms, and considering other relevant evidence

Other information

Registration	23	Registration number and name of trial registry
Protocol	24	Where the full trial protocol can be accessed, if available
Funding	25	Sources of funding and other support (such as supply of drugs), role of funders

Fig. 1 CONSORT 2010 checklist

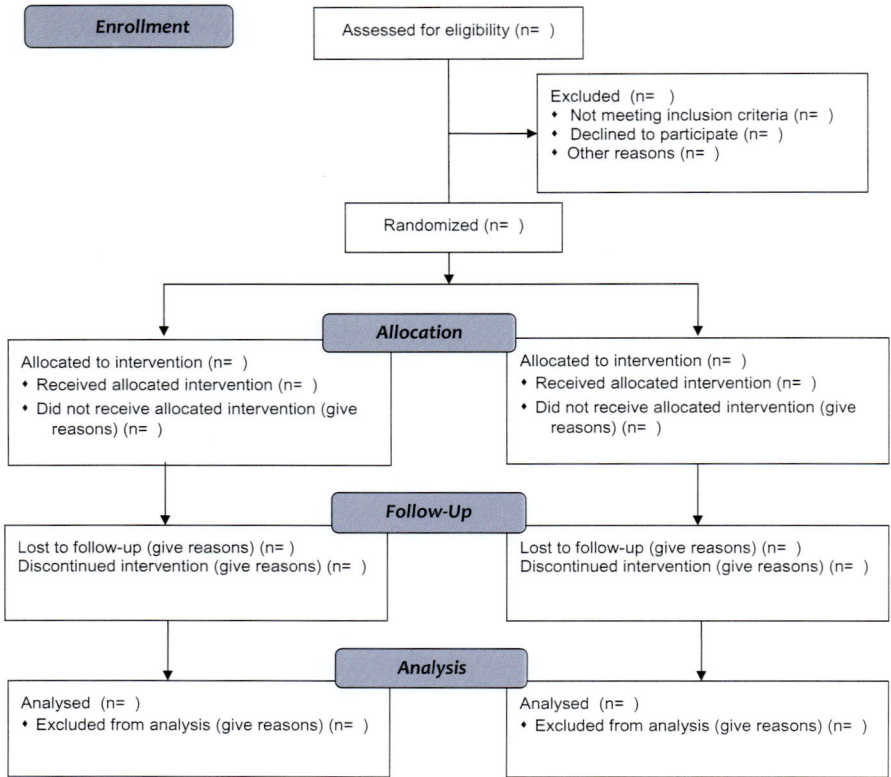

Fig. 2 CONSORT 2010 flow diagram

Table 1 Extensions of CONSORT 2010[a]

Designs	Cluster Trials
	Non-Inferiority and Equivalence Trials
	Pragmatic Trials
	N-of-1 Trials
	Pilot and Feasibility Trials
	Within Person Trials
Interventions	Herbal Medicinal Interventions
	Non-Pharmacologic Treatment Interventions
	Acupuncture Interventions
	Chinese Herbal Medicine Formulas
Data	CONSORT-PRO (Patient-Reported Outcomes)
	Harms
	Abstracts
	Equity

[a]Adapted from Table: http://www.consort-statement.org/extensions

References

CONSORT Transparent Reporting of Trials (2010). http://www.consort-statement.org/. Accessed May 2018

Moher D, Hopewell S, Schulz KF, Montori V, Gøtzsche PC, Devereaux PJ, Elbourne D, Egger M, Altman DG (2010a) CONSORT 2010 explanation and elaboration: updated guidelines for reporting parallel group randomised trials. J Clin Epi 63(8):e1–e37

Moher D, Hopewell S, Schulz KF, Montori V, Gøtzsche PC, Devereaux PJ, Elbourne D, Egger M, Altman DG (2010b) CONSORT 2010 explanation and elaboration: updated guidelines for reporting parallel group randomised trials. BMJ 340:c869

Schulz KF, Altman DG, Moher D, CONSORT Group (2010a) CONSORT 2010 statement: updated guidelines for reporting parallel group randomised trials. Ann Int Med 152

Schulz KF, Altman DG, Moher D, CONSORT Group (2010b) CONSORT 2010 statement: updated guidelines for reporting parallel group randomised trials. BMC Med 8:18

Schulz KF, Altman DG, Moher D, CONSORT Group (2010c) CONSORT 2010 Statement: updated guidelines for reporting parallel group randomised trials. BMJ 340:c332

Schulz KF, Altman DG, Moher D, CONSORT Group (2010d) CONSORT 2010 Statement: updated guidelines for reporting parallel group randomised trials. J Clin Epi 63(8):834–840

Schulz KF, Altman DG, Moher D, CONSORT Group (2010e) CONSORT 2010 statement: updated guidelines for reporting parallel group randomized trials. Obstet Gynecol 115(5):1063–1070

Schulz KF, Altman DG, Moher D, CONSORT Group (2010f) CONSORT 2010 Statement: updated guidelines for reporting parallel group randomized trials. Open Med 4(1):60–68

Schulz KF, Altman DG, Moher D, CONSORT Group (2010g) CONSORT 2010 statement: updated guidelines for reporting parallel group randomised trials. PLoS Med 7(3):e1000251

Schulz KF, Altman DG, Moher D, CONSORT Group (2010h) CONSORT 2010 statement: updated guidelines for reporting parallel group randomised trials. Trials 11:32

Appendix 6

ICMJE Recommendations

Description: This Appendix provides an overview and highlights key characteristics and developments of the ICMJE recommendations. The establishment and purpose of ICMJE recommendations is provided in section "International Committee of Medical Journal Editors (ICMJE) Recommendations" followed by a list of ICMJE journal members in section "ICMJE Journal Members and List of Journals That Follow ICMJE Recommendations". The definition of the author's roles and responsibilities is transcribed in section "ICMJE Roles and Responsibilities of Authors". Additional topics covered in the ICMJE recommendations are listed in Table 1. Lastly, the ICMJE policy for trial registration is covered in section "Clinical Trial Registration".

ICMJE Recommendations

ICMJE recommendations (also known as the "Vancouver Convention") were first published as "Uniform Requirements for Manuscripts Submitted to Biomedical Journals (URMs)" in 1978 (ICMJE 2017). The most recent version of the recommendations was updated December 2017: "Recommendations for the Conduct, Reporting, Editing, and Publication of Scholarly Work in Medical Journals." The ICMJE recommendations were developed to provide guidance on best practice for the conduct and reporting of research with an intended audience of journal editors, authors, and reviewers. The primary use for the recommendations is intended for authors who submit their work for publication to ICMJE member journals.

ICMJE Journal Members and List of Journals That Follow ICMJE Recommendations

ICMJE member journals include:

- *Annals of Internal Medicine*
- *British Medical Journal*
- *Bulletin of the World Health Organization*

- *Deutsches Ärzteblatt*
- *Ethiopian Journal of Health Sciences*
- *Iranian Journal of Medical Sciences*
- *JAMA*
- *Journal of Korean Medical Science*
- *New England Journal of Medicine*
- *New Zealand Medical Journal*
- *PLOS Medicine*
- *The Lancet*
- *Revista Médica de Chile*
- *Ugeskrift for Laeger*

Additional journals that have stated that they follow the ICMJE recommendations are listed at the following link: http://www.icmje.org/journals-following-the-icmje-recommendations/

ICMJE Roles and Responsibilities of Authors

ICMJE recommendations cover the Roles and Responsibilities of authors, Publishing and Editorial issues, and Manuscript Preparation guidelines. Additional topics covered by the ICMJE recommendations are provided in Table 1.

Table 1 ICMJE Recommendations: Table of Contents[a]

Topics	Subtopics
About the Recommendations	Purpose of the Recommendations Who Should Use the Recommendations History of the Recommendations
Roles & Responsibilities	Defining the Role of Authors and Contributors Author Responsibilities – Conflicts of Interest Responsibilities in the Submission and Peer-Review Process Journal Owners and Editorial Freedom Protection of Research Participants
Publishing and Editorial Issues	Corrections, Retractions, Republications, and Version Control Scientific Misconduct, Expressions of Concern, and Retraction Copyright Overlapping Publications Correspondence Fees Supplements, Theme Issues, and Special Series Sponsorship or Partnership Electronic Publishing Advertising Journals and the Media Clinical Trials
Manuscript Preparation	Preparing for Submission Sending the Submission

[a]The complete document including ICMJE requirements is available at: http://www.icmje.org/recommendations/

An important component of the ICMJE requirements includes the definition and description of the role of authors and contributors. An individual should meet all four criteria as stated below to be considered a contributing author:

1. *Substantial contributions to the conception or design of the work; or the acquisition, analysis, or interpretation of data for the work; AND*
2. *Drafting the work or revising it critically for important intellectual content; AND*
3. *Final approval of the version to be published; AND*
4. *Agreement to be accountable for all aspects of the work in ensuring that questions related to the accuracy or integrity of any part of the work are appropriately investigated and resolved.*

Clinical Trial Registration

The ICMJE issued a policy that clinical trial registration, including pre-specification of primary and secondary outcome measures, at or before time of first patient enrolment is required for consideration of publication in ICMJE journals (ICMJE 2005, 2007; Laine et al. 2007; Groves 2008). Implementation of this policy resulted in increased trial registration and acceptance of the need for structured summary results (Zarin et al. 2017).

References

Groves T (2008) Mandatory disclosure of trial results for drugs and devices. BMJ 336(7637):170

ICMJE (2005) Update on trials registration: is this clinical trial fully registered? A Statement from the International Committee of Medical Journal Editors. http://www.icmje.org/news-and-editorials/update_2005.html. Accessed 26 May 2018

ICMJE (2007) Clinical trial registration: looking back and moving forward. http://www.icmje.org/news-and-editorials/clincial_trial_reg_jun2007.html. Accessed 26 May 2018

International Committee of Medical Journal Editors (2017) Recommendations for the conduct, reporting, editing and publication of scholarly work in medical journals. http://www.ICMJE.org. Accessed 26 May 2018

Laine C, Horton R, DeAngelis CD, Drazen JM, Frizelle FA, Godlee F et al (2007) Clinical trial registration. BMJ 334:1177–1178

Zarin DA, Tse T, Williams RJ, Rajakannan T (2017) Update on trial registration 11 years after the ICMJE Policy Was Established. N Engl J Med 376(4):383–391

Appendix 7

Standard Protocol Items: Recommendations for Interventional Trials (SPIRIT)
Description: The SPIRIT guidelines are defined as "recommendations for a minimum set of scientific, ethical, and administrative elements that should be addressed in a clinical trial protocol."[1] The guidelines include a 33-item checklist of recommended items to include in clinical trial protocols and related documents. The most recent version of the checklist (Chan et al. 2013a) is displayed below (Table 1). Related documents including the 2013 SPIRIT statement and example template of the schedule of enrolment, interventions, and assessments are available at the following links:

SPIRIT statement[1]: http://www.spirit-statement.org/spirit-statement/
SPIRIT statement 2013 explanation and elaboration[2]: https://www.bmj.com/content/346/bmj.e7586.full?ijkey=QpAJnYI57zIwVr3&keytype=ref
SPIRIT checklist[3]: http://www.spirit-statement.org/title/
SPIRIT schedule of enrolment figure: http://www.spirit-statement.org/schedule-of-enrolment-interventions-and-assessments/

Table 1 SPIRIT 2013 checklist: Recommended items to address in a clinical trial protocol and related documents[a]

Section/item	Item No	Description
Administrative information		
Title	1	Descriptive title identifying the study design, population, interventions, and, if applicable, trial acronym
Trial registration	2a	Trial identifier and registry name. If not yet registered, name of intended registry
	2b	All items from the World Health Organization Trial Registration Data Set
Protocol version	3	Date and version identifier
Funding	4	Sources and types of financial, material, and other support
Roles and responsibilities	5a	Names, affiliations, and roles of protocol contributors
	5b	Name and contact information for the trial sponsor

(continued)

Table 1 (continued)

Section/item	Item No	Description
	5c	Role of study sponsor and funders, if any, in study design; collection, management, analysis, and interpretation of data; writing of the report; and the decision to submit the report for publication, including whether they will have ultimate authority over any of these activities
	5d	Composition, roles, and responsibilities of the coordinating centre, steering committee, endpoint adjudication committee, data management team, and other individuals or groups overseeing the trial, if applicable (see Item 21a for data monitoring committee)
Introduction		
Background and rationale	6a	Description of research question and justification for undertaking the trial, including summary of relevant studies (published and unpublished) examining benefits and harms for each intervention
	6b	Explanation for choice of comparators
Objectives	7	Specific objectives or hypotheses
Trial design	8	Description of trial design including type of trial (e.g., parallel group, crossover, factorial, single group), allocation ratio, and framework (e.g., superiority, equivalence, noninferiority, exploratory)
Methods: Participants, interventions, and outcomes		
Study setting	9	Description of study settings (e.g., community clinic, academic hospital) and list of countries where data will be collected. Reference to where list of study sites can be obtained
Eligibility criteria	10	Inclusion and exclusion criteria for participants. If applicable, eligibility criteria for study centres and individuals who will perform the interventions (e.g., surgeons, psychotherapists)
Interventions	11a	Interventions for each group with sufficient detail to allow replication, including how and when they will be administered
	11b	Criteria for discontinuing or modifying allocated interventions for a given trial participant (e.g., drug dose change in response to harms, participant request, or improving/worsening disease)
	11c	Strategies to improve adherence to intervention protocols, and any procedures for monitoring adherence (e.g., drug tablet return, laboratory tests)
	11d	Relevant concomitant care and interventions that are permitted or prohibited during the trial
Outcomes	12	Primary, secondary, and other outcomes, including the specific measurement variable (e.g., systolic blood pressure), analysis metric (e.g., change from baseline, final value, time to event), method of aggregation (e.g., median, proportion), and time point for each outcome. Explanation of the clinical relevance of chosen efficacy and harm outcomes is strongly recommended

(continued)

Table 1 (continued)

Section/item	Item No	Description
Participant timeline	13	Time schedule of enrolment, interventions (including any run-ins and washouts), assessments, and visits for participants. A schematic diagram is highly recommended
Sample size	14	Estimated number of participants needed to achieve study objectives and how it was determined, including clinical and statistical assumptions supporting any sample size calculations
Recruitment	15	Strategies for achieving adequate participant enrolment to reach target sample size
Methods: Assignment of interventions (for controlled trials)		
Allocation:		
Sequence generation	16a	Method of generating the allocation sequence (e.g., computer-generated random numbers), and list of any factors for stratification. To reduce predictability of a random sequence, details of any planned restriction (e.g., blocking) should be provided in a separate document that is unavailable to those who enrol participants or assign interventions
Allocation concealment mechanism	16b	Mechanism of implementing the allocation sequence (e.g., central telephone; sequentially numbered, opaque, sealed envelopes), describing any steps to conceal the sequence until interventions are assigned
Implementation	16c	Who will generate the allocation sequence, who will enrol participants, and who will assign participants to interventions
Blinding (masking)	17a	Who will be blinded after assignment to interventions (e.g., trial participants, care providers, outcome assessors, data analysts), and how
	17b	If blinded, circumstances under which unblinding is permissible, and procedure for revealing a participant's allocated intervention during the trial
Methods: Data collection, management, and analysis		
Data collection methods	18a	Plans for assessment and collection of outcome, baseline, and other trial data, including any related processes to promote data quality (e.g., duplicate measurements, training of assessors) and a description of study instruments (e.g., questionnaires, laboratory tests) along with their reliability and validity, if known. Reference to where data collection forms can be found, if not in the protocol
	18b	Plans to promote participant retention and complete follow-up, including list of any outcome data to be collected for participants who discontinue or deviate from intervention protocols
Data management	19	Plans for data entry, coding, security, and storage, including any related processes to promote data quality (e.g., double data entry; range checks for data values). Reference to where details of data management procedures can be found, if not in the protocol

(continued)

Table 1 (continued)

Section/item	Item No	Description
Statistical methods	20a	Statistical methods for analysing primary and secondary outcomes. Reference to where other details of the statistical analysis plan can be found, if not in the protocol
	20b	Methods for any additional analyses (e.g., subgroup and adjusted analyses)
	20c	Definition of analysis population relating to protocol non-adherence (e.g., as randomised analysis), and any statistical methods to handle missing data (e.g., multiple imputation)
Methods: Monitoring		
Data monitoring	21a	Composition of data monitoring committee (DMC); summary of its role and reporting structure; statement of whether it is independent from the sponsor and competing interests; and reference to where further details about its charter can be found, if not in the protocol. Alternatively, an explanation of why a DMC is not needed
	21b	Description of any interim analyses and stopping guidelines, including who will have access to these interim results and make the final decision to terminate the trial
Harms	22	Plans for collecting, assessing, reporting, and managing solicited and spontaneously reported adverse events and other unintended effects of trial interventions or trial conduct
Auditing	23	Frequency and procedures for auditing trial conduct, if any, and whether the process will be independent from investigators and the sponsor
Ethics and dissemination		
Research ethics approval	24	Plans for seeking research ethics committee/institutional review board (REC/IRB) approval
Protocol amendments	25	Plans for communicating important protocol modifications (e.g., changes to eligibility criteria, outcomes, analyses) to relevant parties (e.g., investigators, REC/IRBs, trial participants, trial registries, journals, regulators)
Consent or assent	26a	Who will obtain informed consent or assent from potential trial participants or authorised surrogates, and how (see Item 32)
	26b	Additional consent provisions for collection and use of participant data and biological specimens in ancillary studies, if applicable
Confidentiality	27	How personal information about potential and enrolled participants will be collected, shared, and maintained in order to protect confidentiality before, during, and after the trial
Declaration of interests	28	Financial and other competing interests for principal investigators for the overall trial and each study site
Access to data	29	Statement of who will have access to the final trial dataset, and disclosure of contractual agreements that limit such access for investigators

(continued)

Table 1 (continued)

Section/item	Item No	Description
Ancillary and post-trial care	30	Provisions, if any, for ancillary and post-trial care, and for compensation to those who suffer harm from trial participation
Dissemination policy	31a	Plans for investigators and sponsor to communicate trial results to participants, healthcare professionals, the public, and other relevant groups (e.g., via publication, reporting in results databases, or other data sharing arrangements), including any publication restrictions
	31b	Authorship eligibility guidelines and any intended use of professional writers
	31c	Plans, if any, for granting public access to the full protocol, participant-level dataset, and statistical code
Appendices		
Informed consent materials	32	Model consent form and other related documentation given to participants and authorised surrogates
Biological specimens	33	Plans for collection, laboratory evaluation, and storage of biological specimens for genetic or molecular analysis in the current trial and for future use in ancillary studies, if applicable

[a]It is strongly recommended that this checklist be read in conjunction with the SPIRIT 2013 explanation and elaboration for important clarification on the items (Chan et al. 2013b). Amendments to the protocol should be tracked and dated. The SPIRIT checklist is copyrighted by the SPIRIT Group under the Creative Commons "Attribution-NonCommercial-NoDerivs 3.0 Unported" license

References

Chan A-W, Tetzlaff JM, Altman DG, Laupacis A, Gøtzsche PC, Krleža-Jerić K, Hróbjartsson A, Mann H, Dickersin K, Berlin J, Doré C, Parulekar W, Summerskill W, Groves T, Schulz K, Sox H, Rockhold FW, Rennie D, Moher D (2013a) SPIRIT 2013 statement: Defining standard protocol items for clinical trials. Ann Intern Med 158:200–207

Chan A-W, Tetzlaff JM, Gøtzsche PC, Altman DG, Mann H, Berlin J, Dickersin K, Hróbjartsson A, Schulz KF, Parulekar WR, Krleža-Jerić K, Laupacis A, Moher D (2013b) SPIRIT 2013 explanation and elaboration: guidance for protocols of clinical trials. BMJ 346:e7586

Appendix 8

Protection of Human Subjects (45 CFR 46)
Description: The Table of Contents for the Code of Federal Regulations, Title 45, is transcribed below. The complete document can be accessed and read on the Department of Health and Human Services webpage at the following link:

https://www.hhs.gov/ohrp/regulations-and-policy/regulations/45-cfr-46/index.html

45 CFR 46 Table of Contents (*transcribed*):

Code of Federal Regulations TITLE 45 PUBLIC WELFARE DEPARTMENT OF HEALTH AND HUMAN SERVICES PART 46 PROTECTION OF HUMAN SUBJECTS *** Revised January 15, 2009 Effective July 14, 2009 ***
Subpart A. Basic HHS Policy for Protection of Human Research Subjects
§46.101 To what does this policy apply?
§46.102 Definitions
§46.103 Assuring compliance with this policy – research conducted or supported by any Federal Department or Agency
§46.104 –
§46.106 [Reserved]
§46.107 IRB membership
§46.108 IRB functions and operations
§46.109 IRB review of research
§46.110 Expedited review procedures for certain kinds of research involving no more than minimal risk, and for minor changes in approved research
§46.111 Criteria for IRB approval of research
§46.112 Review by institution
§46.113 Suspension or termination of IRB approval of research

(continued)

§46.114	Cooperative research
§46.115	IRB records
§46.116	General requirements for informed consent
§46.117	Documentation of informed consent
§46.118	Applications and proposals lacking definite plans for involvement of human subjects
§46.119	Research undertaken without the intention of involving human subjects
§46.120	Evaluation and disposition of applications and proposals for research to be conducted or supported by a Federal Department or Agency
§46.121	[Reserved]
§46.122	Use of Federal funds
§46.123	Early termination of research support: Evaluation of applications and proposals
§46.124	Conditions
Subpart B. Additional Protections for Pregnant Women, Human Fetuses and Neonates Involved in Research	
§46.201	To what do these regulations apply?
§46.202	Definitions
§46.203	Duties of IRBs in connection with research involving pregnant women, fetuses, and neonates
§46.204	Research involving pregnant women or fetuses
§46.205	Research involving neonates
§46.206	Research involving, after delivery, the placenta, the dead fetus or fetal material
§46.207	Research not otherwise approvable which presents an opportunity to understand, prevent, or alleviate a serious problem affecting the health or welfare of pregnant women, fetuses, or neonates
Subpart C. Additional Protections Pertaining to Biomedical and Behavioral Research Involving Prisoners as Subjects	
§46.301	Applicability
§46.302	Purpose
§46.303	Definitions
§46.304	Composition of Institutional Review Boards where prisoners are involved
§46.305	Additional duties of the Institutional Review Boards where prisoners are involved
§46.306	Permitted research involving prisoners
Subpart D. Additional Protections for Children Involved as Subjects in Research	
§46.401	To what do these regulations apply?
§46.402	Definitions
§46.403	IRB duties
§46.404	Research not involving greater than minimal risk
§46.405	Research involving greater than minimal risk but presenting the prospect of direct benefit to the individual subjects
§46.406	Research involving greater than minimal risk and no prospect of direct benefit to individual subjects, but likely to yield generalizable knowledge about the subject's disorder or condition
§46.407	Research not otherwise approvable which presents an opportunity to understand, prevent, or alleviate a serious problem affecting the health or welfare of children
§46.408	Requirements for permission by parents or guardians and for assent by children
§46.409	Wards

(continued)

Subpart E. Registration of Institutional Review Boards

§46.501 What IRBs must be registered?

§46.502 What information must be provided when registering an IRB?

§46.503 When must an IRB be registered?

§46.504 How must an IRB be registered?

§46.505 When must IRB registration information be renewed or updated?

Authority: 5 U.S.C. 301; 42 U.S.C. 289(a)

Appendix 9

FDA Institutional Review Boards (21 CFR 56)
Description: The Table of Contents for 21 CFR 56 covering Institutional Review Boards is transcribed in this Appendix. There are five subparts covering: General Provisions; Organization and Personnel; IRB Functions and Operations; Records and Reports; Administrative Actions for Noncompliance. The most up-to-date Subchapter 21 CFR 56 can be accessed online at the following link:

https://www.ecfr.gov/cgi-bin/text-idx?SID=c0f612ad3a3137f7e96da5971a3953a2&mc=true&node=pt21.1.56&rgn=div5

TITLE 21 – FOOD AND DRUGS
CHAPTER I – FOOD AND DRUG ADMINISTRATION
DEPARTMENT OF HEALTH AND HUMAN SERVICES
SUBCHAPTER A – GENERAL
PART 56 INSTITUTIONAL REVIEW BOARDS
Subpart A – General Provisions
§ 56.101 – Scope
§ 56.102 – Definitions
§ 56.103 – Circumstances in which IRB review is required
§ 56.104 – Exemptions from IRB requirement
§ 56.105 – Waiver of IRB requirement
Subpart B – Organization and Personnel
§ 56.106 – Registration
§ 56.107 – IRB membership
Subpart C – IRB Functions and Operations
§ 56.108 – IRB functions and operations
§ 56.109 – IRB review of research
§ 56.110 – Expedited review procedures for certain kinds of research involving no more than minimal risk, and for minor changes in approved research

(continued)

§ 56.111 – Criteria for IRB approval of research	
§ 56.112 – Review by institution	
§ 56.113 – Suspension or termination of IRB approval of research	
§ 56.114 – Cooperative research	
Subpart D – Records and Reports	
§ 56.115 – IRB records	
Subpart E – Administrative Actions for Noncompliance	
§ 56.120 – Lesser administrative actions	
§ 56.121 – Disqualification of an IRB or an institution	
§ 56.122 – Public disclosure of information regarding revocation	
§ 56.123 – Reinstatement of an IRB or an institution	
§ 56.124 – Actions alternative or additional to disqualification	

Appendix 10

Health Insurance Portability and Accountability Act of 1996
Description: The Health Insurance Portability and Accountability Act (HIPAA) was enacted in 1996 with the purpose of protecting the privacy and security of health information. It was modified further in 2003 and referred to as the Privacy Rule (45 CFR Sections 160 and 164). In 2013 the Department of Health and Human Services issued the Final rule to modify the HIPAA Privacy, Security, and Enforcement Rules under the Health Information Technology for Economic Clinical Health Act (HITECH Act).

The 2013 version of the Privacy Rule is available at: https://www.hhs.gov/sites/default/files/hipaa-simplification-201303.pdf

This Appendix is divided into three sections: The definition of protected health information (PHI) and de-identification of PHI ("Protected Health Information (PHI)"); a list of Authorization Core elements and required statements ("Authorization Core Elements and Required Statements"); and sample language for an Authorization form ("Sample Authorization Language").

Additional topics covered by HIPAA can be found on the website (https://www.hhs.gov/hipaa/for-professionals/index.html):

- Privacy
- Security
- Breach Notification
- Compliance and Enforcement
- Special topics (e.g., Mental health and substance use disorders; De-identification methods, Research, Genetic information, etc.)
- Patient Safety
- Covered Entities and Business Associates
- Training and Resources

Protected Health Information (PHI)

Definition: *"Individually identifiable health information transmitted or maintained by a covered entity or its business associates in any form or medium (45 CFR 160.103)."*

PHI includes demographic information as information that relates to:

- The individual's past, present, or future physical or mental health or condition
- The provision of health care to the individual
- The past, present, or future payment for the provision of health care
- Common identifiers (name, address, birth date, Social Security Number)

Methods for the de-identification of PHI are specified on the HHS.gov website: https://www.hhs.gov/hipaa/for-professionals/privacy/special-topics/de-identification/index.html#rationale

There are two methods for de-identifying PHI in accordance with HIPAA: (1) Expert Determination and (2) Safe Harbor (Fig. 1)

The first method is described as determination by a qualified expert who determines that PHI is not individually identifiable if:

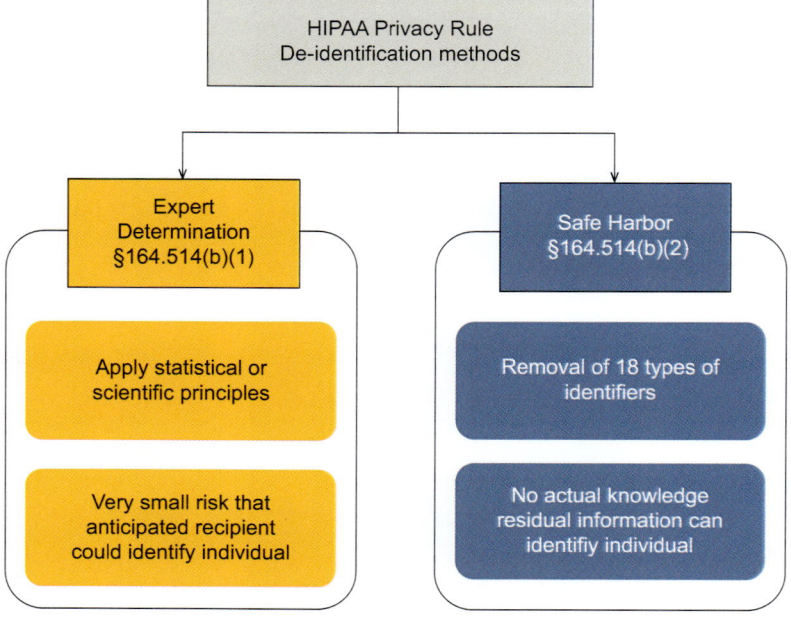

Fig. 1 HIPAA Privacy Rule De-Identification Methods Schema (Source: https://www.hhs.gov/sites/default/files/ocr/images/deidentification_fig_1.jpg)

(1) A person with appropriate knowledge of and experience with generally accepted statistical and scientific principles and methods for rendering information not individually identifiable:

Applying such principles and methods, determines that the risk is very small that the information could be used, alone or in combination with other reasonably available information, by an anticipated recipient to identify an individual who is a subject of the information; and
Documents the methods and results of the analysis that justify such determination.

The second method involves de-identification of 18 identifiers:

(A) Names
(B) All geographic subdivisions smaller than a state, including street address, city, county, precinct, ZIP code, and their equivalent geocodes, except for the initial three digits of the ZIP code if, according to the current publicly available data from the Bureau of the Census:
(C) All elements of dates (except year) for dates that are directly related to an individual, including birth date, admission date, discharge date, death date, and all ages over 89 and all elements of dates (including year) indicative of such age, except that such ages and elements may be aggregated into a single category of age 90 or older
(D) Telephone numbers
(L) Vehicle identifiers and serial numbers, including license plate numbers
(E) Fax numbers
(M) Device identifiers and serial numbers
(F) Email addresses
(N) Web Universal Resource Locators (URLs)
(G) Social security numbers
(O) Internet Protocol (IP) addresses
(H) Medical record numbers
(P) Biometric identifiers, including finger and voice prints
(I) Health plan beneficiary numbers
(Q) Full-face photographs and any comparable images
(J) Account numbers
(R) Any other unique identifying number, characteristic, or code
(K) Certificate/license numbers

Authorization Core Elements and Required Statements

Information on Authorizations for Research is available at: https://www.hhs.gov/hipaa/for-professionals/special-topics/research/index.html

The Authorization Core elements (Privacy Rule, 45CFR164.508 (c)(1)) include:

- *Description of PHI to be used or disclosed (identifying the information in a specific and meaningful manner).*
- *The name(s) or other specific identification of person(s) or class of persons authorized to make the requested use or disclosure.*
- *The name(s) or other specific identification of the person(s) or class of persons who may use the PHI or to whom the covered entity may make the requested disclosure.*
- *Description of each purpose of the requested use or disclosure. Researchers should note that this element must be research study specific, not for future unspecified research.*
- *Authorization expiration date or event that relates to the individual or to the purpose of the use or disclosure (the terms "end of the research study" or "none" may be used for research, including for the creation and maintenance of a research database or repository).*
- *Signature of the individual and date. If the Authorization is signed by an individual's personal representative, a description of the representative's authority to act for the individual.*

The Authorization required statements (Privacy Rule, 45CFR164.508. (c)(2)) are:

- *The individual's right to revoke his/her Authorization in writing and either (1) the exceptions to the right to revoke and a description of how the individual may revoke his/her Authorization or (2) reference to the corresponding section(s) of the covered entity's Notice of Privacy Practices.*
- *Notice of the covered entity's ability or inability to condition treatment, payment, enrollment, or eligibility for benefits on the Authorization, including research-related treatment, and, if applicable, consequences of refusing to sign the Authorization.*
- *The potential for the PHI to be re-disclosed by the recipient and no longer protected by the Privacy Rule. This statement does not require an analysis of risk for re-disclosure but may be a general statement that the Privacy Rule may no longer protect health information.*

Sample Authorization Language

Sample authorization language for research uses for both required and optional elements is transcribed below and available at: https://privacyruleandresearch.nih.gov/authorization.asp.

SAMPLE AUTHORIZATION LANGUAGE FOR RESEARCH USES AND DISCLOSURES OF INDIVIDUALLY IDENTIFIABLE HEALTH INFORMATION BY A COVERED HEALTH CARE PROVIDER

Authorization to Use or Disclose (Release) Health Information that Identifies You for a Research Study

REQUIRED ELEMENTS:

If you sign this document, you give permission to [name or other identification of specific health care provider(s) or description of classes of persons, e.g., all doctors, all health care providers] at [name of covered entity or entities] to use or disclose (release) your health information that identifies you for the research study described below:

[Provide a description of the research study, such as the title and purpose of the research.]

The health information that we may use or disclose (release) for this research includes [complete as appropriate]:

[Provide a description of information to be used or disclosed for the research project. This may include, for example, all information in a medical record, results of physical examinations, medical history, lab tests, or certain health information indicating or relating to a particular condition.]

The health information listed above may be used by and/or disclosed (released) to:

[Name or class of persons involved in the research; i.e., researchers and their staff]

[Name of covered entity] is required by law to protect your health information. By signing this document, you authorize [name of covered entity] to use and/or disclose (release) your health information for this research. Those persons who receive your health information may not be required by Federal privacy laws (such as the Privacy Rule) to protect it and may share your information with others without your permission, if permitted by laws governing them.

Please note that [include the appropriate statement]:

- You do not have to sign this Authorization, but if you do not, you may not receive research-related treatment. **(When the research involves treatment and is conducted by the covered entity or when the covered entity provides health care solely for the purpose of creating protected health information to disclose to a researcher)**

- [Name of covered entity] may not condition (withhold or refuse) treating you on whether you sign this Authorization. **(When the research does not involve research-related treatment by the covered entity or when the covered entity is not providing health care solely for the purpose of creating protected health information to disclose to a researcher)**

Please note that [include the appropriate statement]
- You may change your mind and revoke (take back) this Authorization at any time, except to the extent that [name of covered entity(ies)] has already acted based on this Authorization. To revoke this Authorization, you must write to: [name of the covered entity(ies) and contact information]. **(Where the research study is conducted by an entity other than the covered entity)**
- You may change your mind and revoke (take back) this Authorization at any time. Even if you revoke this Authorization, [name or class of persons at the covered entity involved in the research] may still use or disclose health information they already have obtained about you as necessary to maintain the integrity or reliability of the current research. To revoke this Authorization, you must write to: [name of the covered entity(ies) and contact information]. **(Where the research study is conducted by the covered entity)**

This Authorization does not have an expiration date [or as appropriate, insert expiration date or event, such as "end of the research study."]

_____
Signature of participant or participant's personal representative

_____
Printed name of participant or participant's personal representative

_____
Date

_____
If applicable, a description of the personal representative's authority to sign for the participant

SAMPLE AUTHORIZATION LANGUAGE FOR RESEARCH USES AND DISCLOSURES OF INDIVIDUALLY IDENTIFIABLE HEALTH INFORMATION BY A COVERED HEALTH CARE PROVIDER

Authorization TO Use OR Disclose (RELEASE) Health Information THAT IDENTIFIES YOU FOR A RESEARCH STUDY

OPTIONAL ELEMENTS:

Examples of optional elements that may be relevant to the recipient of the protected health information:

- Your health information will be used or disclosed when required by law.

- Your health information may be shared with a public health authority that is authorized by law to collect or receive such information for the purpose of preventing or controlling disease, injury, or disability, and conducting public health surveillance, investigations or interventions.

- No publication or public presentation about the research described above will reveal your identity without another authorization from you.

- If all information that does or can identify you is removed from your health information, the remaining information will no longer be subject to this authorization and may be used or disclosed for other purposes.

- **When the research for which the use or disclosure is made involves treatment and is conducted by a covered entity:** To maintain the integrity of this research study, you generally will not have access to your personal health information related to this research until the study is complete. At the conclusion of the research and at your request, you generally will have access to your health information that [name of the covered entity] maintains in a designated record set, which means a set of data that includes medical information or billing records used in whole or in part by your doctors or other health care providers at [name of the covered entity] to make decisions about individuals. Access to your health information in a designated record set is described in the Notice of Privacy Practices provided to you by [name of covered entity]. If it is necessary for your care, your health information will be provided to you or your physician.

- If you revoke this Authorization, you may no longer be allowed to participate in the research described in this Authorization.

Appendix 11

NIH Revitalization Act of 1993
Description: The NIH Revitalization Act was signed into law by William Clinton in June 1993 to establish guidelines for the inclusion of women and minorities in clinical research (Chen et al. 2014; Freedman et al. 1995; Institute of Medicine (US) Committee on Ethical and Legal Issues Relating to the Inclusion of Women in Clinical Studies et al. 1994). The 1993 Revitalization Act is available at: https://orwh.od.nih.gov/sites/orwh/files/docs/NIH-Revitalization-Act-1993.pdf.

It specifies that:

> In conducting or supporting clinical research for the purposes of this title, the Director of NIH shall ... ensure that (a) women are included as subjects in each project of such research; and (b) members of minority groups are included in such research. 492B(a)(1)
> The statute further directed the NIH to establish guidelines to specify:
>
> (a) the circumstances under which the inclusion of women and minorities as subjects in projects of clinical research is inappropriate ... ;
> (b) the manner in which clinical trials are required to be designed and carried out; and
> (c) the operation of outreach programs, 492B(d)(1).

and further states that:

> In the case of any clinical trial in which women or members of minority groups will be included as subjects, the Director of NIH shall ensure that the trial is designed and carried out in a manner sufficient to provide for valid analysis of whether the variables being studied in the trial affect women or members of minority groups, as the case may be, differently than other subjects in the trial.

Source: https://grants.nih.gov/grants/funding/women_min/guidelines.htm

References

Chen MS Jr, Lara PN, Dang JH, Paterniti DA, Kelly K (2014) Twenty years post-NIH Revitalization Act: enhancing minority participation in clinical trials (EMPaCT): laying the groundwork for improving minority clinical trial accrual: renewing the case for enhancing minority participation in cancer clinical trials. Cancer 120(Suppl 7):1091–1096

Freedman LS, Simon R, Foulkes MA, Friedman L, Geller NL, Gordon DJ, Mowery R (1995) Inclusion of women and minorities in clinical trials and the NIH Revitalization Act of 1993 – the perspective of NIH clinical trialists. Control Clin Trials 16(5):277–285; discussion 286–9, 293–309

Institute of Medicine (US) Committee on Ethical and Legal Issues Relating to the Inclusion of Women in Clinical Studies, Mastroianni AC, Faden R, Federman D (eds) (1994) Women and health research: ethical and legal issues of including women in clinical studies, vol I. National Academies Press (US), Washington, DC. B, NIH Revitalization Act of 1993 Public Law 103–143. https://www.ncbi.nlm.nih.gov/books/NBK236531/

Appendix 12

Clinical Trials Registries
Description: This Appendix includes a list of clinical trial registries and their web link (Table 1) as well as a list of the 20 data items for a registry to be considered acceptable by ICMJE requirements first identified by the World Health Organization in 2006 (WHO 2018) (Table 2).

Additional information regarding the World Health Organization Primary Registries is available at: http://www.who.int/ictrp/network/primary/en/.

Table 1 Clinical trial registries and their web links (URL)

Registry	URL
Australian New Zealand Clinical Trials Registry[a]	http://www.anzctr.org.au/
Brazilian Clinical Trials Registry[a]	http://www.ensaiosclinicos.gov.br
Health Canada's Clinical Trials Database	https://health-products.canada.ca/ctdb-bdec/index-eng.jsp
Chinese Clinical Trials Registry[a]	http://www.chictr.org.cn/index.aspx
Cuban Public Registry of Clinical Trials[a]	http://registroclinico.sld.cu/en/home
EU Clinical Trials Register[a]	https://www.clinicaltrialsregister.eu/
German Clinical Trials Register[a]	https://www.drks.de/drks_web/
India Clinical Trials Registry[a]	http://ctri.nic.in/Clinicaltrials/login.php
Iranian Registry of Clinical Trials[a]	http://www.irct.ir/
Italian Clinical Trials Database	http://www.agenziafarmaco.gov.it/en/content/clinical-trials
Japan Primary Registries Network[a]	http://www.umin.ac.jp/ctr/index-j.htm http://www.japic.or.jp/ http://www.jmacct.med.or.jp/en/
The Netherlands National Trial Register[a]	http://www.trialregister.nl/trialreg/index.asp
Pan African Clinical Trials Registry[a]	https://pactr.samrc.ac.za/
Peruvian Clinical Trial Registry[a]	https://ensayosclinicos-repec.ins.gob.pe/en/
Republic of Korea – Clinical Research Information Service[a]	http://cris.nih.go.kr/cris/en/use_guide/cris_introduce.jsp

(continued)

Table 1 (continued)

Registry	URL
Sri Lanka Clinical Trials Registry[a]	http://www.slctr.lk/
Thai Clinical Trials Registry[a]	http://www.clinicaltrials.in.th/
Turkey Clinical Trials database	http://vistaar.makrocare.com/reg-updates/59-turkey-develops-clinical-trials-turkey-database
United States Clinical Trials database[a]	www.Clinicaltrials.gov
World Health Organization[a]	http://apps.who.int/trialsearch/
ISRCTN[a]	http://www.isrctn.com/

[a]ICMJE acceptable database

Table 2 WHO and ClinicalTrials.gov registration data elements

WHO trail registration data set (v 1.3)[1]	ClinicalTrials.gov registration data element(s)[2]
1. Primary Registry and Trial identifying Number	ClinicalTrials.gov Identifier (NCT Number) – *assigned by system*
2. Date of Registration in Primary Registry	*Generated by system*
3. Secondary Identifying Numbers	Unique Protocol Identification Number, Secondary IDs
4. Source(s) of Monetary or Material Support	Name of the Sponsor, Collaborators
5. Primary Sponsor	Name of the Sponsor
6. Secondary Sponsor(s)	Collaborators
7. Contact for Public Queries	Facility Contact OR Central Contact Person
8. Contact for Scientific Queries	Overall Study Officials
9. Public Title	Brief Title
10. Scientific Title	Official Title
11. Countries of Recruitment	Facility Information – Country
12. Health Condition(s) or Problem(s) Studied	Primary Disease or Condition Being Studied in the Trial, or the Focus of the Study
13. Intervention(s)	Intervention Type, Intervention Name(s), Intervention Description, Arm or Group/Interventional Cross Reference, Arm Title, Arm Type, Arm Description
14. Key Inclusion and Exclusion Criteria	Eligibility Criteria, Sex/Gender, Age Limits, Accepts Healthy Volunteers
15. Study Type	Study Type, Allocation, Masking, Interventional Study Model, Primary Purpose, Study Phase
16. Date of First Enrollment	Study Start Date
17. Sample Size	Enrollment
18. Recruitment Status	Overall Recruitment Status
19. Primary Outcome(s)	Primary Outcome Measure information – Title, Description, Time Frame

(continued)

Table 2 (continued)

WHO trail registration data set (v 1.3)[1]	ClinicalTrials.gov registration data element(s)[2]
20. Key Secondary Outcomes	Secondary Outcome Measure information – Title, Description, Time Frame
21. Ethics Review	Human Subjects Review
22. Completion Date	Study Completion Date
23. Summary Results	ClinicalTrials.gov Results Data Elements
24. IPD Sharing Statement	IPD Sharing Statement

[1]https://www.who.int/clinical-trials-registry-platform
[2]https://prsinfo.clinicaltrials.gov/definitions.html
Reproduced from: https://prsinfo.clinicaltrials.gov/trainTrainer/WHO-ICMJE-ClinTrialsgov-Cross-Ref.pdf

Reference

World Health Organization (2018) International Clinical Trials Registry Platform (ICTRP). http://www.who.int/ictrp/network/primary/en/. Accessed 1 Oct 2018

Appendix 13

Society for Clinical Trials
Description: The Society for Clinical Trials (SCT) is an international organization that was founded in 1978 with a primary focus on the design, conduct, and analysis of clinical trials and health care research methodologies (https://www.sctweb.org). Dr. Curtis Meinert was founding member of the Society for Clinical Trials, served on the first Board of the Directors and was Editor of the Journal from 1980 until 1993.

This Appendix includes information regarding the SCT Annual Meetings (section "Society of Clinical Trials Annual Meetings"), a table of trials that were selected for the SCT David Sackett Trial of the Year (section "David Sackett Trial of the Year") and information about the Journal of the Society for Clinical Trials (section "Journal of the Society for Clinical Trials"). The Society for Clinical Trials webpage can be accessed at the following link: http://www.sctweb.org/public/home.cfm

Society of Clinical Trials Annual Meetings

The Society of Clinical Trials has had 40 Annual Meetings as of May 2019. The meeting includes contributed sessions (oral and poster presentations), invited sessions (thematically linked talks and panels), and educational sessions (workshops and tutorials). There are several awards presented at the Annual Meetings including the Chalmers Students Scholarships, Sylvan Green Travel Award, Fellow of the Society for Clinical Trials, and the David Sackett Trial of the Year Award which will be described in greater detail in section "David Sackett Trial of the Year". Since 2000, the keynote address of the meeting is recognized as "The Curtis Meinert lecture." Each year, abstracts can be submitted to the following link: http://www.sctweb.org/meeting/#abstract

Abstracts from previous meetings can be located at: http://www.sctweb.org/public/search/results.cfm

David Sackett Trial of the Year

Each year, a trial has been selected to receive the David Sackett Trial of the Year Award. Since 2007, 12 trials have been selected to receive the award and are presented at the Society for Clinical Trials Annual Meeting. The trials are described in Table 1.

Selection criteria for award includes the following:

The awarded trials are recognized as advancing the field significantly and meet the following standards: http://www.sctweb.org/public/about/toty.cfm

- *Improves the lot of humankind*,
- *Provides basis for a substantial, beneficial change in health care*,
- *Reflects expertise in subject matter, excellence in methodology, and concern for study participants*,
- *Overcame obstacles in implementation*
- *Presentation of its design, execution, and results is a model of clarity and intellectual soundness*.

Journal of the Society for Clinical Trials

The journal of the Society for Clinical Trials was founded in 1980 by Dr. Curtis Meinert who served as editor of the journal from its inception until 1993. The name of the journal was changed to *Clinical Trials* in 2004 and published by SAGE publications (previously published by Elsevier). The current editor of *Clinical Trial* is Colin Begg of Memorial Sloan Kettering Center. It has an impact factor of 2.715 as of 2016 and covers topics related to the design, conduct, analysis, synthesis and evaluation of clinical trials. The journal website can be accessed at the following web link: http://journals.sagepub.com/home/ctj

Appendix 13

Table 1 Clinical trials selected for the David Sackett Trial of the Year Award

SCT award year	Sponsor	Trial title	Registration number	Design	Enrollment
2018	NIAID	Scleroderma: Cyclophosphamide or Transplantation (SCOT) (Sullivan et al. 2018)	NCT00114530	Randomized, parallel 2-group, open label, clinical trial	75
2017	Medical Research Council	The Systemic Therapy in Advancing or Metastatic Prostate Cancer: Evaluation of Drug Efficacy (STAMPEDE) (Parker et al. 2018)	NCT00268476	Randomized, parallel, multi-arm multi-state, platform clinical trial	11,200[a]
2017	Spark Therapeutics	Efficacy and Safety of Voretigene Neparvovec (AAV2-hRPE65v2) in Patients with RPE65-mediated Inherited Retinal Dystrophy (Russell et al. 2017)	NCT00999609	Randomized, parallel 2-group, open-label, clinical trial	31
2016	Hoffman-La Roche	A Phase III, Multicentre, Randomized, Parallel-group, Double-blind, Placebo Controlled Study to Evaluate the Efficacy and Safety of Ocrelizumab in Adults With Primary Progressive Multiple Sclerosis (Montalban et al. 2017)	NCT01194570	Randomized, parallel 2-group, double-masked placebo-controlled trial	732
2015	National Institute of Allergy and Infectious Diseases (NIAID)	Induction of Tolerance Through Early Introduction of Peanut in High-Risk Children (LEAP) (Du Toit et al. 2015)	NCT00329784	Randomized, parallel 2-group, open-label trial	640
2014	Health Technology Assessment Programme (UK)	Cluster randomised controlled trial of the LUCAS™ mechanical chest compression device for out of hospital cardiac arrest (PARAMEDIC) (Perkins et al. 2015)	ISRCTN0823394	Cluster-randomized, 2-group open-label pragmatic trial	4471
2013	Johns Hopkins University	Randomized Trial Of Achieving Healthy Lifestyles In Psychiatric Rehabilitation (ACHIEVE) (Daumit et al. 2013)	NCT00902694	Randomized, parallel 2-group, double-masked controlled trial	291

(continued)

Table 1 (continued)

SCT award year	Sponsor	Trial title	Registration number	Design	Enrollment
2012	Robert Silbergleit	A Double-blind Randomized Clinical Trial of the Efficacy of IM Midazolam Versus IV Lorazepam in the Pre-hospital Treatment of Status Epilepticus by Paramedics (RAMPART) (Silbergleit et al. 2011)	NCT00809146	Randomized, parallel 2-group, double-masked noninferiority trial	1024
2011	The George Washington University	Myelomeningocele Repair Randomized Trial (MOMS) (Adzick et al. 2011)	NCT00060606	Randomized, parallel, 2-group, open-label surgical trial	183
2010	The Institute of Child Health (UK)	The Ekjut Trial in Jharkhand and Orissa (Tripathy et al. 2010)	ISRCTN21817853	Cluster-randomized, 2-group, open-label trial	36 clusters
2009	Europe Against Cancer	The European Randomized Study of Screening for Prostate Cancer (Schröder et al. 2009)	ISRCTN49127736	Randomized, parallel, 2-group, open-label trial	182,000
2008	Imperial College London	he Hypertension in the Very Elderly Trial (HYVET) (Beckett et al. 2008)	NCT00122811	Randomized, parallel, 2-group, double-masked placebo-controlled trial	3845
2007	McMaster University	Efficacy and Safety of Methylxanthines in Very Low Birthweight Infants (Schmidt et al. 2007)	NCT00182312	Randomied, parallel, 2-group, triple-masked placebo-controlled trial	2006

[a]Estimated

References

Adzick NS, Thom EA, Spong CY, Brock JW 3rd, Burrows PK, Johnson MP, Howell LJ, Farrell JA, Dabrowiak ME, Sutton LN, Gupta N, Tulipan NB, D'Alton ME, Farmer DL, MOMS Investigators (2011) A randomized trial of prenatal versus postnatal repair of myelomeningocele. N Engl J Med 364(11):993–1004. https://doi.org/10.1056/NEJMoa1014379. Epub 2011 Feb 9. PubMed PMID: 21306277

Beckett NS, Peters R, Fletcher AE, Staessen JA, Liu L, Dumitrascu D, Stoyanovsky V, Antikainen RL, Nikitin Y, Anderson C, Belhani A, Forette F, Rajkumar C, Thijs L, Banya W, Bulpitt CJ, HYVET Study Group (2008) Treatment of hypertension in patients 80 years of age or older. N Engl J Med 358(18):1887–1898. https://doi.org/10.1056/NEJMoa0801369. Epub 2008 Mar 31. PubMed PMID: 18378519

Daumit GL, Dickerson FB, Wang NY, Dalcin A, Jerome GJ, Anderson CA, Young DR, Frick KD, Yu A, Gennusa JV 3rd, Oefinger M, Crum RM, Charleston J, Casagrande SS, Guallar E, Goldberg RW, Campbell LM, Appel LJ (2013) A behavioral weight-loss intervention in persons with serious mental illness. N Engl J Med 368(17):1594–1602. https://doi.org/10.1056/NEJMoa1214530. Epub 2013 Mar 21

Du Toit G, Roberts G, Sayre PH, Bahnson HT, Radulovic S, Santos AF, Brough HA, Phippard D, Basting M, Feeney M, Turcanu V, Sever ML, Gomez Lorenzo M, Plaut M, Lack G, LEAP Study Team (2015) Randomized trial of peanut consumption in infants at risk for peanut allergy. N Engl J Med 372(9):803–813. https://doi.org/10.1056/NEJMoa1414850. Epub 2015 Feb 23. Erratum in: N Engl J Med. 2016 Jul 28;375(4):398. PubMed PMID: 25705822; PubMed Central PMCID: PMC4416404

Montalban X, Hauser SL, Kappos L, Arnold DL, Bar-Or A, Comi G, de Seze J, Giovannoni G, Hartung HP, Hemmer B, Lublin F, Rammohan KW, Selmaj K, Traboulsee A, Sauter A, Masterman D, Fontoura P, Belachew S, Garren H, Mairon N, Chin P, Wolinsky JS, ORATORIO Clinical Investigators (2017) Ocrelizumab versus placebo in primary progressive multiple sclerosis. N Engl J Med 376(3):209–220. https://doi.org/10.1056/NEJMoa1606468. Epub 2016 Dec 21

Parker CC, James ND, Brawley CD, The Systemic Therapy for Advanced or Metastatic Prostate Cancer: Evaluation of Drug Efficacy (STAMPEDE) Investigators (2018) Radiotherapy to the primary tumour for newly diagnosed, metastatic prostate cancer (STAMPEDE): a randomised controlled phase 3 trial. Lancet 392(10162):2353–2366. https://doi.org/10.1016/S0140-6736(18)32486-3. Epub 2018 Oct 21. PubMed PMID: 30355464; PubMed Central PMCID: PMC6269599

Perkins GD, Lall R, Quinn T, Deakin CD, Cooke MW, Horton J, Lamb SE, Slowther AM, Woollard M, Carson A, Smyth M, Whitfield R, Williams A, Pocock H, Black JJ, Wright J, Han K, Gates S, PARAMEDIC Trial Collaborators (2015) Mechanical versus manual chest compression for out-of-hospital cardiac arrest (PARAMEDIC): a pragmatic, cluster randomised controlled trial. Lancet 385(9972):947–955. https://doi.org/10.1016/S0140-6736(14)61886-9. Epub 2014 Nov 16

Russell S, Bennett J, Wellman JA, Chung DC, Yu ZF, Tillman A, Wittes J, Pappas J, Elci O, McCague S, Cross D, Marshall KA, Walshire J, Kehoe TL, Reichert H, Davis M, Raffini L, George LA, Hudson FP, Dingfield L, Zhu X, Haller JA, Sohn EH, Mahajan VB, Pfeifer W, Weckmann M, Johnson C, Gewaily D, Drack A, Stone E, Wachtel K, Simonelli F, Leroy BP, Wright JF, High KA, Maguire AM (2017) Efficacy and safety of voretigene neparvovec (AAV2-hRPE65v2) in patients with RPE65-mediated inherited retinal dystrophy: a randomised, controlled, open-label, phase 3 trial. Lancet 390(10097):849–860. https://doi.org/10.1016/S0140-6736(17)31868-8. Epub 2017 Jul 14. Erratum in: Lancet. 2017 Aug 26;390(10097):848. PubMed PMID:28712537; PubMed Central PMCID: PMC5726391

Schmidt B, Roberts RS, Davis P, Doyle LW, Barrington KJ, Ohlsson A, Solimano A, Tin W, Caffeine for Apnea of Prematurity Trial Group (2007) Long-term effects of caffeine therapy for apnea of prematurity. N Engl J Med 357(19):1893–1902. PubMed PMID: 17989382

Schröder FH, Hugosson J, Roobol MJ, Tammela TL, Ciatto S, Nelen V, Kwiatkowski M, Lujan M, Lilja H, Zappa M, Denis LJ, Recker F, Berenguer A, Määttänen L, Bangma CH, Aus G, Villers A, Rebillard X, van der Kwast T, Blijenberg BG, Moss SM, de Koning HJ, Auvinen A, ERSPC Investigators (2009) Screening and prostate-cancer mortality in a randomized European study. N Engl J Med 360(13):1320–1328. https://doi.org/10.1056/NEJMoa0810084. Epub 2009 Mar 18. PubMed PMID:19297566

Silbergleit R, Lowenstein D, Durkalski V, Conwit R, Neurological Emergency Treatment Trials (NETT) Investigators (2011) RAMPART (Rapid Anticonvulsant Medication Prior to Arrival Trial): a double-blind randomized clinical trial of the efficacy of intramuscular midazolam versus intravenous lorazepam in the prehospital treatment of status epilepticus by paramedics. Epilepsia 52(Suppl 8):45–47. https://doi.org/10.1111/j.1528-1167.2011.03235.x

Sullivan KM, Goldmuntz EA, Keyes-Elstein L, McSweeney PA, Pinckney A, Welch B, Mayes MD, Nash RA, Crofford LJ, Eggleston B, Castina S, Griffith LM, Goldstein JS, Wallace D, Craciunescu O, Khanna D, Folz RJ, Goldin J, St Clair EW, Seibold JR, Phillips K, Mineishi S, Simms RW, Ballen K, Wener MH, Georges GE, Heimfeld S, Hosing C, Forman S, Kafaja S, Silver RM, Griffing L, Storek J, LeClercq S, Brasington R, Csuka ME, Bredeson C, Keever-Taylor C, Domsic RT, Kahaleh MB, Medsger T, Furst DE, SCOT Study Investigators (2018) Myeloablative autologous stem-cell transplantation for severe scleroderma. N Engl J Med 378(1):35–47. PubMed PMID: 29298160

Tripathy P, Nair N, Barnett S, Mahapatra R, Borghi J, Rath S, Rath S, Gope R, Mahto D, Sinha R, Lakshminarayana R, Patel V, Pagel C, Prost A, Costello A (2010) Effect of a participatory intervention with women's groups on birth outcomes and maternal depression in Jharkhand and Orissa, India: a cluster-randomised controlled trial. Lancet 375(9721):1182–1192. https://doi.org/10.1016/S0140-6736(09)62042-0. Epub 2010 Mar 6. PubMed PMID: 20207411

Appendix 14

Sketches of Selected Trials

Introduction

This Appendix includes a selection of landmark trials that helped shape the clinical trial landscape. This Appendix includes a list and brief description of selected landmark trials (section "Selected Trials from Project ImpACT") as well as more recent trials that were not part of Project ImpACT (section "Additional Summaries of Selected Trials Not Included in Project ImpACT").

Selected Trials from Project ImpACT

Description: Trials were selected and extracted from Project ImpACT, which includes over 200 profiles of clinical trials across 23 disciplines up to 2007. All Project ImpACT trials went through a nomination and review process, which involved soliciting nominations from field experts and societies. A nomination team and advisory board was responsible for entering nominated studies into the Project ImpACT database and assigning to a team member for further development and drafting of trial profiles. Profiles include detailed information about the trial designs, composition, methods, and results in addition to their relevance and impact in their respective fields. Trial profiles underwent a review and vetting process, for which 30 have been reviewed and 13 have been vetted. Project ImpACT is an ongoing process for which clinical trials continue to be nominated, reviewed, and vetted.

Authors (Steven Goodman, Karen Robinson) can be contacted for further information regarding Project IMPACT and access to the complete list of the trials included in the trial database.

From the list of reviewed trials, a selection of nine trials from Project ImpACT have been listed and summarized in the tables below in chronological order (Tables 1 and 2).

Table 1 List of trials selected from Project ImpACT

Trial	Appendix number
Project ImpACT trials	
Polio vaccine trials (1954)	A.14.1
UGDP (1961)	A.14.2
Gastric Freeze (1963)	A.14.3
MRFIT (1973)	A.14.4
NSABP B-06 (1976)	A.14.5
PHS (1987)	A.14.6
CAST (1989)	A.14.7
WHI (1993)	A.14.8
Nigral Graft (1994)	A.14.9
Additional trials (not part of Project Impact)	
Linxian nutrition studies (1986)	A.14.10
RE-LY (1994)	A.14.11
ERSPC (1994)	A.14.12
Crizotinib (2009)	A.14.13
BIA 10-2474 (2015)	A.14.14

Table 2 Selected trial summaries from Project ImpACT

14.1: Salk Polio Vaccine Trials	
Design Feature	Description
Trial Name	Salk Vaccine Trials
Design Summary	Incorporated 2 studies: 1. Randomized, double-masked, placebo-controlled trial 2. Single-group observational study
Start year	April 26 1954
Study center(s)	44 US states; 15,000 public schools, 217 areas shown to have previously high poliovirus attack rates.
Investigators	Thomas Francis, Jr.; The Vaccine Evaluation Center, University of Michigan
Sponsor	Funded entirely through public donations to the National Foundation for Infantile Paralysis (NFIP), or the March of Dimes
Trial Registration number	Not Applicable
Primary Research Question	Is the Salk preparation of formalin-inactivated poliovirus vaccine effective for use in preventing paralytic polio?
Study Population	School children aged 6–9 years enrolled in 1st, 2nd, or 3rd grade
Number of treatment groups	The Salk Vaccine Trials incorporated two studies: 1. RCT: 2 2. Observational: 1
Study Treatment	Salk vaccine (Formalin-inactivated poliovirus), series of 3
Control Group	1. RCT: Saline shot, series of 3 (placebo) 2. Observational: No comparison group

(continued)

Table 2 (continued)

Primary Outcomes	Confirmed cases of paralytic and nonparalytic polio. Serum antibody titers
Sample size	1. RCT: 455,474 children 2. Observational study: 567,210 children
Key Findings	RCT: 82 of all polio cases were reported among 200,745 who were vaccinated versus 162 cases among the 201,229 who received the placebo (attack rates were 41 per 100,000 vs 81 per 100,000, respectively; $p < 0.001$) RCT: Significant difference between the two treatment arms with respect to the incidence of paralytic polio as 33 cases were diagnosed among the vaccinated vs 115 among the placebo controls ($p < 0.001$), corresponding to respective attack rates of 16 and 57 per 100,000 Observational study: 38 vaccinated children vs 330 observed controls were diagnosed with paralytic polio (respective attack rates were 17 vs 46 per 100,000, $p < 0.001$) Throughout the course of this trial, polio incidence in the randomized study (428 cases in 749,236; attack rate of 57 per 100,000) was similar to that in the observational study (585 cases in 1,080,680; attack rate of 54 per 100,000) No major differences between the two populations with regard to the distribution of paralytic vs nonparalytic classifications
Issues encountered	Walter Winchell unfavorable broadcast warning against trial participation (NFIP) resulted in 10% of trial pool being dissuaded Difficulty diagnosing nonparalytic cases of polio leading to re-assessment by the advisory committee Evaluation center was under intense pressure to release results causing the timeline to be shortened Virus isolation was difficult
Impact	Considered "the biggest public health experiment ever" Large public demand for the Salk vaccine as a result of the trials' findings Vaccine was approved for license by the US Public Health Service on the same day the field trial results were released and a nationwide vaccination program began 2 weeks later The rush to provide mass quantities of the vaccine resulted in off-protocol production by some manufacturers and subsequent vaccine-related cases of polio The results of this trial confirmed that vaccine effectiveness varies by individual age and previous exposures The study established that effectiveness may vary by poliovirus strain, clinical outcome (paralytic vs. nonparalytic), and vaccine lot. This knowledge of poliovirus epidemiology and serology helped shape future vaccine studies The level of public involvement in this trial was unprecedented and has not been seen since. The trial enlisted over 200,000 volunteers and enrolled over 1 million children
14.2: UGDP	
Design Feature	Description
Trial Name	A Study of the Effects of Hypoglycemic Agents on Vascular Complications in Patients with Adult-onset Diabetes Group Diabetes

(continued)

Table 2 (continued)

Design Summary	Randomized, double-masked (Tolbutamide, phenformin, and placebo groups only), placebo-controlled
Enrollment start year	1961–1975
Study center(s)	12 clinics across the United States
Investigators	University Group Diabetes Program: CL Meinert
Sponsor	National Institute for Arthritis and Metabolic Diseases
Trial Registration number	N/A
Primary Research Question(s)	Do standard strategies for blood glucose control prevent long-term vascular complications in adult-onset, non-insulin dependent diabetics?
Study Population	Individuals with a diagnosis of diabetes within 1 year prior to their entry into the study
Number of study groups	5 groups (4 treatment, 1 control)
Control	Lactose Placebo (equivalent doses in form of tablets or capsules that were indistinguishable from oral hypoglycemic agents

Primary Outcome(s)	Original outcomes of interest:
	  Neurological, retinal, renal, and vascular complications
	  Mortality
	Additional outcome of interest:
	  Cardiovascular mortality

Sample size	Total = 1,027

Key Findings	Tolbutamide results:
	  26 cardiovascular deaths in the tolbutamide group vs. 10 in the placebo group ($p < 0.005$)
	  All-cause mortality in the tolbutamide group was not significantly different than the placebo group (30 vs. 21 deaths, $p > 0.17$)
	Phenformin results:
	  27 cardiovascular deaths in the phenformin group vs. 3 in the placebo group ($p < 0.08$)
	  All-cause mortality in the phenformin group was not significantly different than the placebo group (34 vs. 7 deaths, $p > 0.36$)
	There was no evidence that insulin treatment, either standard or variable, was superior to (or worse than) diet alone in reducing the risk of cardiovascular disease or mortality

Issues encountered	Phenformin was added to the study in 1962 after the FDA approved the drug for clinical use An interim analysis in 1969 revealed an excess of cardiovascular deaths in the tolbutamide group compared to the placebo group and that tolbutamide was no better than a placebo in preventing vascular complications The UGDP investigators voted 21-5 to discontinue treatment with tolbutamide in 1969 because cardiovascular risks associated with the drug no longer justified its continued inclusion in the trial The phenformin arm was discontinued in 1971 due to an excess of cardiovascular deaths among those receiving it compared to those treated with insulin and diet or diet alone

(continued)

Table 2 (continued)

	In 1977, the FDA banned phenformin, deeming it an "imminent hazard" due to the risk of death from lactic acidosis
Impact	Clinicians and statisticians challenged both the merits of the clinical findings and the validity of the study
	The NIH selected the Biometric Society to assess the validity of the study and the UGDP's conclusions
	In 1975, the Biometric Society released the results of their investigation, finding in favor of the UGDP
	Based on the 1970 report of the cardiovascular risks associated with tolbutamide, the FDA made the decision to revise the package labeling of the drug. Prominent diabetologists organized to protest the decisions made by the UGDP and the FDA concerning tolbutamide. Due to the ensuing protracted political and legal battles, the FDA was unable to issue new labeling guidelines until 1984
	A group of clinicians filed Freedom of Information Act (FOIA) requests with the Department of Health, Education, and Welfare (HEW) to obtain the UGDP's original data and records. In 1980, the U.S. Supreme Court ruled 7-2 in the case of *Forsham* vs. *Harris* that federally funded investigators were *not* considered federal agencies and therefore not subject to disclosure requirements under the FOIA
Primary reference(s)	1. (1970) Effects of hypoglycemic agents on vascular complications in patients with adult-onset diabetes. I. Design, methods, and baseline results. Diabetes 19(Suppl 2):747–783
	2. Meinert CL, Knatterud GL, Prout TE, Klimt CR (1970) A study of the effects of hypoglycemic agents on vascular complications in patients with adult-onset diabetes. II. Mortality results. Diabetes 19 (Suppl):789–830
14.3: Gastric Freeze Trial	
Design Feature	Description
Trial Name	A Co-operative Double-Blind Evaluation of Gastric "Freezing" in the Treatment of Duodenal Ulcer
Design Summary	Double-masked, sham-controlled randomized clinical trial
Enrollment start year	1963
Study center(s)	5 USA Institutions: University of Chicago School of Medicine, Duke University Medical Center, Louisiana State University School of Medicine, the Scott and White Clinic and Vanderbilt University School of Medicine
Investigators	Jullian M. Ruffin, M.D., James E. Grizzle, Ph.D., Nicholas C. Hightower, M.D., Gordon McHardy, M.D., Harrison Shull, M.D., and Joseph B. Kirsner, M.D.
Sponsor	NIH
Trial Registration number	Not Applicable
Primary Research Question(s)	1. What are the effects of gastric freezing on the natural history of duodenal ulcer and gastric secretion?
	2. What are the hazards and complications of the procedure of gastric freezing?
Study Population	Adults with active ulcers

(continued)

Table 2 (continued)

Number of study groups	2
Experiment	Gastric freeze treatment
Control	Sham control
Primary Outcomes	Recurrences Morbidity (perforation, hospitalization for ulcer pain, partial or complete obstruction, hemorrhage, surgery for ulcer, repeat hypothermia, x-ray therapy to the stomach Mortality
Sample size	Total: 160 Experimental: 82 Control: 78
Key Findings	No statistical difference between experimental and control groups By second year of follow-up, 35 patients in the "freeze" group and 30 in the "sham" group had experienced one of the predefined complications of the procedure or had died. The difference in effect between treatment groups was not statistically significant
Issues encountered	All 160 followed for 12 months, 151 followed for 18 months, and 141 followed for 24 months. However, there was no statistical evidence that failure to appear at follow-up was related to treatment group.
Impact	This was the largest randomized controlled trial to demonstrate the ineffectiveness of gastric freezing The results from the trial officially put an end to the practice of gastric freezing, although its popularity had largely diminished by the time of its publication This properly designed and well conducted clinical trial gave definitive results and confirmed physicians' growing distrust of gastric freezing.
Primary reference	Ruffin JM, Grizzle JE, Hightower NC, McHardy G, Shull H, Kirsner JB (1969) A co-operative double-blind evaluation of gastric "freezing" in the treatment of duodenal ulcer. N Engl J Med 281(1): 16–19

14.4: MRFIT

Design Feature	Description
Trial Name	Multiple Risk Factor Intervention Trial for Prevention of Coronary Heart Disease (MRFIT)
Design Summary	Randomized, controlled, non-masked trial
Enrollment start year	1973
Study center(s)	22 clinical centers (university clinics, public health clinics and HMOs)
Investigators	Multiple Risk Factor Intervention Trial Research Group
Sponsor	National Heart, Lung and Blood Institute
Trial Registration number	Not Applicable
Primary Research Question	Do behavioral interventions that target multiple modifiable cardiovascular risk factors (cigarette smoking, elevated serum cholesterol, and hypertension) lower mortality due to coronary heart disease (CHD)?

(continued)

Table 2 (continued)

Study Population	Men aged 35–57 with increased risk of death from CHD
Number of study groups	2
Experiment	Special program targeted at smoking cessation, reduction in cholesterol, and reduction in blood pressure
Control	Usual care (referral to community physicians for whatever treatment of their risk factors was deemed individually necessary)
Primary Outcome(s)	Mortality due to Coronary heart disease
Key Findings	No statistical difference in outcomes between men in specialized intervention arm versus men in usual arm
At 7 years post-randomization, occurrence of CHD mortality and cardiovascular disease mortality was lower in specialized intervention group compared to control, but not statistically significant
An observation study conducted 10.5 years post-randomization showed a mortality benefit in the men who were randomized to the specialized intervention, which persisted 16 years post-randomization with 11.4% lower CHD mortality (95% CI: −23% to 1.9%)
Issues encountered	Lower than expected mortality in usual care arm has been cited as primary reason or lack of statistical significance in primary outcomes
Possible explanations for lower mortality include the participants' and their physicians' knowledge of participation in a federally funded study about their risk factors as well as their high-risk status. Thus, their usual care and symptom management may have been more thorough and comprehensive than investigators anticipated
There have been comments about the need for an analogous study to evaluate CHD outcomes and risk factors in women ("MSFIT")
Impact	This was the earliest and largest CHD prevention trial to assess a a multicomponent behavioral intervention for prevalent symptoms
MRFIT contributed to the clinical understanding of the extent to which controlling CHD risk factors decreases CHD outcomes
MRFIT had large impact, including approximately 300,000 subjects in either the prevention trial or observational study for over a decade
Primary reference(s)	1. Multiple Risk Factor Intervention Trial Research Group (1982) Multiple risk factor intervention trial. Risk factor changes and mortality results. JAMA 248(12):1465–1477
2. (1976) The multiple risk factor intervention trial (MRFIT). A national study of primary prevention of coronary heart disease. JAMA 235(8):825–827
14.5: NSABP B06	
Design Feature	Description
Trial Name	Comparison of Total Mastectomy and Lumpectomy With or Without Radiation
Design Summary	Randomized controlled trial
Enrollment start year	1976
Study center(s)	Approximately 80 NSABP member institutions in Canada and the United States
Investigators	The NSABP Investigators (85) from Canada and the United States
Sponsor	National Cancer Institute (NCI-U10-CA-12027 and NCI-U10-CA-35211) and the American Cancer Society (ACS-RC-13)

(continued)

Table 2 (continued)

Trial Registration number	N/A
Primary Research Question(s)	In women with breast cancer, what is the effectiveness of lumpectomy (segmental mastectomy) for breast preservation? Does radiation therapy reduce the incidence of tumor in the ipsilateral breast after lumpectomy? Does breast conservation result in a higher risk of distant disease and death than does mastectomy? What is the clinical importance of tumor multicentricity?
Study Population	Women undergoing treatment for primary operable breast cancer
Number of study groups	2
Experiment	Total Mastectomy and Lumpectomy with radiation
Control	Total Mastectomy and Lumpectomy without radiation
Primary Outcome(s)	Disease-free survival Distant-disease-free survival Overall survival
Sample size	Total enrolled: 2,122 Total analysed: 1,843 Total mastectomy: 586 Segmental mastectomy: 632 Segmental mastectomy+ radiation therapy: 625
Key Findings	There were 2.5 myocardial infarctions per 1000 person-years among those receiving aspirin versus 4.4 myocardial infarctions per 1000 person-years among those taking the aspirin placebo, translating into a 44% reduction in risk (relative risk 0.56; 95% CI, 0.45–0.70) The reduction in the risk of myocardial infarction associated with aspirin use was evident only in those 50 years of age or older The beneficial effects of aspirin were observed at all cholesterol levels but were greatest at low levels
Issues encountered	Of the 2163 entered into the trial, 41 (1.9%) of women refused to participate in the trial. Of the remaining 2,122, 1.5% were deemed ineligible because of noninvasive tumors and 1.9% were found to be ineligible for protocol exclusion reasons 8% of women (174) did not accept randomly assigned treatment but did agree to be followed. Reasons for exclusion included in the data analyses included: non-invasive tumor (32), ineligible (40), follow-up data not available (24) and nodal status unknown (9) When the protocol was initiated, consent was required preceding randomization. Due to low enrollment rates, the protocol was changed to allow randomization before consent (prerandomization). This change was accompanied by a six-fold increase in enrollment rates. This practice provoked considerable ethical debate At St. Luc Hospital, Dr. Poisson admitted fraud after a routine audit revealed that records had been altered. He believed that the treatment provided by the NSABP protocol was beneficial to potential participants
Impact	Findings from this trial along with the findings of the B-04 trial repudiated the Halstedian principles of breast cancer treatment and provided support for the theory that breast cancer is a systemic disease

(continued)

Table 2 (continued)

	Lumpectomy was shown to be an acceptable alternative to mastectomy for women with Stage I and II breast cancer Radiation therapy was shown to be beneficial in reducing local recurrence of tumor in lumpectomy patients. These findings provided women with valuable information so that they could make an informed choice Publicity generated by the report of the committed fraud by Dr. Poisson alarmed women and their physicians resulting in disciplinary actions against the principal investigators (later vindicated) and increased oversight from regulatory authorities and the NCI Delayed publication of the reanalysis of the B-06 data (excluding the improperly enrolled patients) resulted in deeply concern about the validity of results. Reasons for the delay included waiting for the result of the NCI audit and a belief that the results would not change significantly. Reanalysis revealed that the findings did not change This trial raised ethical issues regarding both informed consent, fraud, and the appropriateness of actions against the investigators after the fraud had been detected
Primary reference(s)	1. Fisher B et al (1985) Five-year results of a randomized clinical trial comparing total mastectomy and segmental mastectomy with or without radiation in the treatment of breast cancer. N Engl J Med 312(11):665–673 2. (1994) NCI issues information on falsified data in NSABP trials. J Natl Cancer Inst 86(7):487–489
14.6: Physician's Health Study (PHS)	
Design Feature	Description
Trial Name	A Randomized Trial of Aspirin and β-Carotene among U.S. Physicians
Design Summary	Randomized, double-masked, placebo-controlled, 2 × 2 factorial trial
Enrollment start year	1982
Study center(s)	USA physicians
Investigators	Charles Hennekens and the Physicians' Health Study Research Group
Sponsor	National Cancer Institute; National Heart, Lung, and Blood Institute; Bristol Meyers; and BASF
Trial Registration number	NCT00000500
Primary Research Question(s)	In a population free from prior myocardial infarction and stroke, does alternate-day consumption of 325 mg aspirin over a period of 4 years reduce total cardiovascular mortality by 20% and death from all causes by 10%? Does alternate-day consumption of beta-carotene over a period of 4 years reduce cancer rates by 30%?
Study Population	U.S. male physicians, ages 40–84 years, who responded to an invitational questionnaire and completed a run-in phase of the trial
Number of study groups	4
Experiment	Active aspirin and active beta-carotene Active aspirin and beta-carotene placebo

(continued)

Table 2 (continued)

Control	Aspirin placebo and active β-carotene
	Aspirin placebo and beta-carotene placebo
Primary Outcome(s)	Cardiovascular mortality (The final results reported myocardial infarction and stroke as the primary outcomes)
	Incidence of cancer
Sample size	Total: 22,071
	Active aspirin and active beta-carotene: 5,517
	Active aspirin and beta-carotene placebo: 5,520
	Aspirin placebo and active β-carotene: 5,519
	Aspirin placebo and beta-carotene placebo: 5,515
Key Findings	There were 2.5 myocardial infarctions per 1000 person-years among those receiving aspirin versus 4.4 myocardial infarctions per 1000 person-years among those taking the aspirin placebo, translating into a 44% reduction in risk (relative risk 0.56; 95% CI, 0.45–0.70)
	The reduction in the risk of myocardial infarction associated with aspirin use was evident only in those 50 years of age or older
	The beneficial effects of aspirin were observed at all cholesterol levels but were greatest at low levels
Issues encountered	In December 1987, the Data Monitoring Board recommended that the randomized aspirin component of the trial be terminated, and the Steering Committee accepted this recommendation
Impact	The American Heart Association and the US Preventive Services Task Force recommended a regimen of low-dose aspirin for individuals with an increased risk of a first coronary events
	Physicians and researchers continued to voice concerns over the study's findings. In particular, they questioned (1) whether the trial's duration was long enough to make meaningful conclusions about the effectiveness of aspirin in reducing cardiovascular disease (2) the generalizability of the findings to more general, less healthy populations; and (3) the risk-benefit ratio of aspirin use in certain sub-populations, especially those at increased risk for stroke
	This trial was cited as an example of how NIH-funded studies failed to include sufficient numbers of women, and as a result, how many key questions concerning women's health remained unaddressed
Primary reference(s)	1. Hennekens CH, Eberlein K (1985) A randomized trial of aspirin and beta-carotene among U.S. physicians. Prev Med 14(2):165–168
	2. Physicians' Health Study Research Group (1998) Preliminary report: findings from the aspirin component of the ongoing physicians' health study. N Engl J Med (1988) 318(4):262–264
14.7: Cardiac Arrhythmia Suppression Trial (CAST)	
Design Feature	Description
Trial Name	Effect of Encainide and Flecainide on Mortality in a Randomized Trial of Arrhythmia Suppression After Myocardial Infarction: Cardiac Arrhythmia Suppression Trial
Design Summary	Multicenter, randomized, placebo-controlled trial
Enrollment start year	1986
Study center(s)	Over 100 research centers in the U.S., Canada and Europe
Investigators	CAST study investigators
Sponsor	National Heart, Lung and Blood Institute

(continued)

Table 2 (continued)

Trial Registration number	NCT00000526
Primary Research Question(s)	Will the suppression of mildly symptomatic or asymptomatic ventricular arrhythmias with Class Ic antiarrhythmic drugs reduce mortality in patients with arrhythmias following a myocardial infarction?
Study Population	Patients with mild to moderate arrhythmias were eligible for CAST between 6 days and 2 years after acute myocardial infarction
Number of study groups	3
Experiment	Encainide or flecainide Moricizine
Control	Placebo
Primary Outcome(s)	Arrhythmia related mortality incidence rate Non-fatal cardiac arrest incidence rate Total mortality rate
Sample size	Total: 1,727 Encainide or flecainide: 730 Placebo: 725 Moricizine: 272
Key Findings	There were 2.5 myocardial infarctions per 1000 person-years among those receiving aspirin versus 4.4 myocardial infarctions per 1000 person-years among those taking the aspirin placebo, translating into a 44% reduction in risk (relative risk 0.56; 95% CI, 0.45–0.70) The reduction in the risk of myocardial infarction associated with aspirin use was evident only in those 50 years of age or older The beneficial effects of aspirin were observed at all cholesterol levels but were greatest at low levels
Issues encountered	In December 1987, the Data Monitoring Board recommended that the randomized aspirin component of the trial be terminated, and the Steering Committee accepted this recommendation
Impact	The American Heart Association and the US Preventive Services Task Force recommended a regimen of low-dose aspirin for individuals with an increased risk of a first coronary events Physicians and researchers continued to voice concerns over the study's findings. In particular, they questioned (1) whether the trial's duration was long enough to make meaningful conclusions about the effectiveness of aspirin in reducing cardiovascular disease (2) the generalizability of the findings to more general, less healthy populations; and (3) the risk-benefit ratio of aspirin use in certain sub-populations, especially those at increased risk for stroke This trial was cited as an example of how NIH-funded studies failed to include sufficient numbers of women, and as a result, how many key questions concerning women's health remained unaddressed
Primary reference(s)	1. The Cardiac Arrhythmia Suppression Trial (CAST) Investigators (1989) Preliminary report: effect of encainide and flecainide on mortality in a randomized trial of arrhythmia suppression after myocardial infarction. N Engl J Med 321:406–412 2. Ruskin JN (1989) The cardiac arrhythmia suppression trial. N Engl J Med 321:386–388

(continued)

Table 2 (continued)

14.8: Women's Health Initiative (WHI)	
Design Feature	Description
Trial Name	Women's Health Initiative: Risks and Benefits of Estrogen Plus Progestin in Healthy Postmenopausal Women
Design Summary	Randomized, double-masked, placebo-controlled, clinical trial
Enrollment start year	1993
Study center(s)	40 U.S. clinical centers
Investigators	Ross L. Prentice; Garnet L. Anderson
Sponsor(s)	National Heart, Lung and Blood Institute (NHLBI)
Trial Registration number	NCT00000611
Primary Research Question(s)	What are the major health benefits and risks of combined progestin and estrogen replacement therapy among healthy postmenopausal women in the U.S.?
Study Population	Healthy postmenopausal women with an intact uterus aged between 50–79 years at initial screening.
Number of study groups	2
Experiment	Estrogen+progestin
Control	Placebo
Primary Outcome(s)	Coronary heart disease (CHD): nonfatal myocardial infarction and CHD death Primary adverse outcome: invasive breast cancer
Sample size	Total = 16,608 Estrogen+progestin ($n = 8{,}506$) Placebo ($n = 8{,}102$)
Key Findings	Cancer: HR of invasive breast cancer was 1.26 (nominal 95% CI: 1.00–1.59) with hormone use Cardiovascular disease: Hazard ratio and nominal 95% CI of CHD events was 1.29 (1.02–1.63) and most of the excess was in non-fatal MI There were no statistically significant differences in rates of CHD deaths or revascularization procedures (95% CI: 0.84–1.28) Stroke rates were increased by 41% (7–85%) and venous thromboembolism, PE and DVT were significantly increased by two-fold. In addition, there was a 22% increase in total cardiovascular disease including other events requiring hospitalization Difference in rates of in situ breast cancers but rates of colorectal cancer were reduced by 37% (nominal 95% CI 8–57%) in the combined hormone group. No significant differences in incidence of endometrial, lung or total cancer.
Issues encountered	In December 1987, the Data Monitoring Board recommended that the randomized aspirin component of the trial be terminated, and the Steering Committee accepted this recommendation
Impact	This trial demonstrated that combined estrogen plus progestin was not effective but rather harmful for primary prevention of cardiovascular diseases among healthy, postmenopausal women The findings were shocking and extremely surprising to many

(continued)

Appendix 14

Table 2 (continued)

	clinicians who had believed HRT to be beneficial Publication of trial results led to a significant decrease in the initiation of HRT as well as a marked discontinuation among current users[8] Also, the American College of Obstetricians and Gynecologists (ACOG), the North American Menopause Society (NAMS) and the U.S. Preventive Services Task Force (USPSTF) issued recommendations against the routine use of hormone therapy for the prevention of chronic conditions in postmenopausal women The trial reinforced the importance of conducting large scale RCTs to investigate the effect of health interventions despite having observational data support its use
Primary reference(s)	1. Rossouw JE, Anderson GL, Prentice RL, LaCroix AZ, Kooperberg C, Stefanick ML, Jackson RD, Beresford SA, Howard BV, Johnson KC, Kotchen JM, Ockene J, Writing Group for the Women's Health Initiative Investigators (2002) Risks and benefits of estrogen plus progestin in healthy postmenopausal women: principal results from the women's health initiative randomized controlled trial. JAMA 288(3):321–333 2. Grady D, Rubin SM, Petitti DB, Fox CS, Black D, Ettinger B, Ernster V, Cummings SR (1992) Hormone therapy to prevent disease and prolong life in postmenopausal women. Ann Intern Med 117: 1016–1037 3. Hemminki E, McPherson K (1997) Impact of postmenopausal hormone therapy on cardiovascular events and cancer: pooled data from clinical trials. BMJ 315:149–153
14.9 Nigral Graft Transplantation trial	
Design Feature	Description
Trial Name	Embryonic Dopamine Cell Implants for Parkinson's Disease: A Double-Masked Study
Design Summary	Randomized, sham-controlled clinical trial
Enrollment start year	1995
Study center(s)	University Hospital, the University of Colorado Health Sciences Center Denver, Colorado, United States The Movement Disorder Center, Columbia-Presbyterian Hospital New York, New York, United States North Shore University Hospital, Manhasset, New York, United States
Investigators	Curt R. Freed
Sponsor	National Institute of Neurological Diseases and Stroke National Center for Research Resources Parkinson's Disease Foundation Program to End Parkinson's Disease
Trial Registration number	NCT00038116
Primary Research Question(s)	Does transplantation of human embryonic dopamine neurons into specific areas of the brain (putamen) of patients with Parkinson's disease have an effect on disease severity, and is this effect modified by patient age?

(continued)

Table 2 (continued)

Study Population	Healthy postmenopausal women with an intact uterus aged between 50–79 years at initial screening
Number of study groups	2
Experiment	Embryonic Dopamine cell implant surgery
Control	Sham control: Holes drilled in the skull without penetration of the dura
Primary Outcome(s)	Patient's subjective global rating of the change in the severity of disease at 12 months after intervention
Sample size	Total: 40 Transplantation: 20 Sham control: 20
Key Findings	Overall, the implant of embryonic tissue was not associated with a significant change in patient's assessment of the severity of parkinsonism at 1-year follow-up: The mean (±SD) subjective global rating score was 0.0 ± 2.1 among patients receiving transplantation, and -0.4 ± 1.7 among those in the sham-surgery group ($p = 0.62$) Patients ≤60 years old in the transplantation group had a non-significant improvement in subjective global rating scores compared to the control group: Mean (±SD) 0.5 ± 2.1 and -0.3 ± 1.7, respectively Patients >60 years had negative scores in both intervention groups, not differing significantly (-0.7 ± 2.0 surgery vs. -0.4 ± 1.7 sham)
Impact	This was the first masked randomized trial of transplantation of embryonic neurons in Parkinson's disease using sham surgery as control The design of the study documented the considerable placebo effects surgery produces in Parkinson's disease patients, and reinforced the appropriateness of this type of design when such effects are expected The trial generated much debate and encouraged methodological/ethical discussion regarding the use of sham surgery as a justifiable control intervention[14–16]
Primary reference(s)	Freed CR, Greene PE, Breeze RE, Tsai W-Y, DuMouchel W, Kao R, Dillon S, Winfield H, Culver S, Trojanowski JQ et al (2001) Transplantation of embryonic dopamine neurons for severe Parkinson's disease. N Engl J Med 344(10):710–719

Additional Summaries of Selected Trials Not Included in Project ImpACT

Description: This section includes other landmark trials, especially occurring within the last 20 years, that were not included in PROJECT IMPACT. These trials were selected based on their contribution to the field, design, relevance and impact. Many of these trials involve more contemporary designs (e.g., platform designs, step-wedge, group sequential) A summary of each trial can be found below.

14.10 Linxian Nutrition trial	
Design Feature	Description
Trial Name	Nutrition intervention Linxian trials in the general population
Design Summary	Randomized fractional 2^4 factorial design
Enrollment start year	1986
Study center(s)	Linxian China, 4 Linxian communes
Investigators	Bing Li
Sponsor	NCI Intramural Program (DCEG)
Trial Registration number	N/A
Primary Research Question(s)	What is the effect of multiple vitamin and mineral supplements on esophageal/gastric cardia cancer incidence and mortality in the general population of Linxian?
Study Population	General population of Linxian: All adults between the ages of 40 and 69 years in Yaocun, Rencun, and Donggang communes in Linxian who were not already participating in the Dysplasia Trial
Number of study groups	8 factor combinations
Experiment(s)	Retinol + zinc Riboflavin + niacin Ascorbic acid + molybdenum Selenium + β-carotene + α-tocopherol
Primary Outcome(s)	Esophageal cancer All-cause mortality
Sample size	29,584
Key Findings	Lower total mortality was observed among those receiving supplementation with beta carotene, vitamin E, and selenium (RR) = 0.91; 95% confidence interval [CI] = 0.84–0.99, $p = 0.03$) Reduction in mortality was due to lower cancer rates (RR = 0.87; 95% CI = 0.75–1.00), especially stomach cancer (RR = 0.79; 95% CI = 0.64–0.99), with the reduced risk beginning to arise about 1–2 years after the start of supplementation with these vitamins and minerals 86% of all participants took over 90% of their pills (range: 85–87% across groups by treatment factor) while just 5% were poor compliers (i.e., <50% of pills taken) Reduction in risk was still apparent in 10-year follow-up
Issues encountered	Issues were raised regarding the selection of doses and combination of micronutrients, duration of intervention The assumption about lag time to effect in disease rates observed in the population may have been underestimated Given the unique characteristics of the population of Linxian, authors stated that generalizability of results to other populations are limited
Impact	This is the second trial of two randomized nutrition trials in Linxian, China, where the first was a double-blind randomized trial in patients with esophageal dysplasia and the second was a factorial design in the general population

(continued)

	These trials were conducted in a distinctive setting, where rates of esophageal cancer were among the highest
	These were some of the largest chemoprevention trials to evaluate cancer at any site
	The General Population Trial used a fractional factorial design that had not been previously employed in clinical trials and demonstrated its utility in these types of trials
	During the time of the trial, few nutrition and prevention studies had been conducted
	Excellent compliance was documented throughout the study
	Findings from these trials helped advance the understanding of nutrition and cancer in general, as well as for esophageal carcinogenesis
Primary reference(s)	1. Li B, Taylor PR, Li JY, Dawsey SM, Wang W, Tangrea JA, Liu BQ, Ershow AG, Zheng SF, Fraumeni JF Jr et al (1993) Linxian nutrition intervention trials. Design, methods, participant characteristics, and compliance. Ann Epidemiol 3(6):577–585 2. Blot WJ, Li JY, Taylor PR, Guo W, Dawsey S, Wang GQ, Yang CS, Zheng SF, Gail M, Li GY et al (1993) Nutrition intervention trials in Linxian, China: supplementation with specific vitamin/mineral combinations, cancer incidence, and disease-specific mortality in the general population. J Natl Cancer Inst 85(18):1483–1492

14.11 ERSPC

Design Feature	Description
Trial Name	The European Randomized Study of Screening for Prostate Cancer
Design Summary	Randomized, multicenter, unmasked trial
Enrollment start year	1994
Study center(s)	Seven European Countries (Netherlands, Belgium, Sweden, Finland, Italy, Spain, Switzerland)
Investigators	Fritz Schroder and ERSPC investigators
Sponsor	Supported by grants from Europe Against Cancer and 5th and 6th framework program of the European Union
Trial Registration number	ISRCTN49127736
Primary Research Question(s)	Does screening with PSA reduce the risk of death from prostate cancer in men?
Study Population	Men between the ages of 50 and 74 years
Number of study groups	2
Experiment	PSA screening at an average of once every 4 years
Control	Usual care, did not receive PSA screening
Primary Outcome(s)	Prostate cancer mortality
Sample size	Total: 182,000 Screening group: 82,816 Control: 99,184

(continued)

Key Findings	82% of men in screening group were screened at least once
	Cumulative incidence of prostate cancer was 8.2% in the screening group vs. 4.8% in the control group
	Rate ratio for death from prostate cancer in the screening group was 0.80 (95% CI 0.65, 0.98, $p = 0.04$) compared to control group
	Absolute risk difference was 0.71 deaths per 1000 men (1410 men would be needed to be screened to prevent one death from PC)
	Rate Ratios for death from prostate cancer by age group
	Overall: 0.85; 95% CI 0.73–1.00
	50–54 years: 1.47; 95% CI 0.41–5.19
	55–59 years: 0.73; 95% CI 0.53–1.00
	60–64 years: 0.94; 95% CI 0.69–1.27
	65–69 years: 0.74; 95% CI 0.56–0.99
	70–74 years: 1.26; 95% CI 0.80–1.99
	No deaths reported as complications associated with biopsy procedure
Issues encountered	Some criticisms included the fact that mortality benefit was evident after 7–8 years, thus longer follow-up needed to lead to mortality benefit
	Choice of 4 years screening was based on prostate cancer lead time of 5–10 years
	There were variations in methodology between countries due to local policies and guidelines
	E.g., PSA screening in Sweden every 2 years vs. Screening in Belgium every 4–5 years; Finland biopsy different thresholds than Italy
	High rate of overdiagnosis of likely asymptomatic prostate cancer
Impact	Largest randomized study on screening for Prostate Cancer
	Answered important and controversial public health questions regarding prostate cancer screening
	Despite the increased risk reduction for death from prostate cancer by 20%, there was also a high risk of overdiagnosis
	Combined with results from the PLCO prostate screening trials, these findings lead to the 2012 USPSTF recommendation against PSA screening altogether
Primary reference(s)	Schröder FH, Hugosson J, Roobol MJ, Tammela TL, Ciatto S, Nelen V, Kwiatkowski M, Lujan M, Lilja H, Zappa M, Denis LJ, Recker F, Berenguer A, Määttänen L, Bangma CH, Aus G, Villers A, Rebillard X, van der Kwast T, Blijenberg BG, Moss SM, de Koning HJ, Auvinen A, ERSPC Investigators (2009) Screening and prostate-cancer mortality in a randomized European study. N Engl J Med 360(13):1320–1328

14.12 RE-LY	
Design Feature	Description
Trial Name	Dabigatran versus Warfarin in Patients with Atrial Fibrillation
Design Summary	Randomized non-inferiority trial
Enrollment start year	1994
Study center(s)	951 clinical centers in 44 countries

(continued)

Investigators	S.J. Connolly and members of the Randomized Evaluation of Long-Term Anticoagulation Therapy (RE-LY) Study Group
Sponsor	Boehringer Ingelheim
Trial Registration number	NCT00262600
Primary Research Question(s)	Among individuals with chronic atrial fibrillation, how does dabigatran at two different does compare to warfarin in terms of stroke risk and the risk of major bleeding?
Study Population	Patients with atrial fibrillation and risk of stroke
Number of study groups	3
Experiment	Fixed doses (110 mg or 150 mg twice daily) of dabigatran
Control	Warfarin (open-label)
Primary Outcome(s)	Stroke or systemic embolism
Sample size	18,113 Dabigatran 110 mg: 6,015 Dabigatran 150 mg: 6,076 Warfarin: 6,022
Key Findings	Rates of the primary outcome were 1.69% per year in the warfarin group, as compared with 1.53% per year in the group that received 110 mg of dabigatran (relative risk with dabigatran, 0.91; 95% confidence interval [CI], 0.74–1.11; $p < 0.001$ for noninferiority) and 1.11% per year in the group that received 150 mg of dabigatran (relative risk, 0.66; 95% CI, 0.53–0.82; $p < 0.001$ for superiority) Myocardial infarction and gastrointestinal side effects were significantly more common with dabigatran than with warfarin. Rates of myocardial infarction were 0.72% and 0.74% with 110 mg and 150 mg of dabigatran, respectively, and 0.53% with warfarin The lower dose of dabigatran (110 mg twice daily) caused fewer hemorrhages
Issues encountered	There was risk for reporting and observer biases because patients randomized to the warfarin treatment group were not masked and had regular follow-up visits for INR purposes To minimize this issue, events were adjudicated by two independent investigators who were unaware of the treatment assignments and all hospital records were reviewed
Impact	Prior to RE-LY, warfarin was the primary anticoagulant used in the prevention of thromboembolic stroke among patients with atrial fibrillation While the study was designed to test non-inferiority of the two dabigatran doses compared to warfarin, the final analysis demonstrated superiority of the high-dose (150 mg) dabigatran resulting in FDA approval of the high-dose for nonvulvular atrial fibrillation The lower dose was approved for use in individuals with renal impairment, although this was not studied in a clinical trial
Primary reference(s)	1. Connolly SJ, Ezekowitz MD, Yusuf S, Eikelboom J, Oldgren J, Parekh A, Pogue J, Reilly PA, Themeles E, Varrone J, Wang S, Alings M, Xavier D, Zhu J, Diaz R, Lewis BS, Darius H, Diener HC, Joyner CD, Wallentin L, RE-LY Steering Committee and

(continued)

	Investigators (2009) Dabigatran versus warfarin in patients with atrial fibrillation. N Engl J Med 361(12):1139–1151 2. Gage BF (2009) Can we rely on RE-LY? N Engl J Med 361(12): 1200–2. https://doi.org/10.1056/NEJMe0906886

14.13 Crizotinib vs. chemotherapy in NSCLC

Design Feature	Description
Trial Name	Crizotinib versus Chemotherapy in Advanced *ALK*-Positive Lung Cancer
Design Summary	Randomized open-label trial
Enrollment start year	2009
Study center(s)	264 study locations in the United States
Investigators	Alice Shaw and A8081007 investigators
Sponsor	Pfizer
Trial Registration number	NCT00932893
Primary Research Question(s)	Does Crizotinib reduce progression free survival in patients with ALK-Positive advanced non-small cell lung cancer compared to standard of care?
Study Population	Patients With Advanced Non-small Cell Lung Cancer (Nsclc) Harboring A Translocation Or Inversion Event Involving The Anaplastic Lymphoma Kinase (Alk) Gene Locus
Number of study groups	2
Experiment	Crizotinib (PF-02341066)
Control	Pemetrexed or Docetaxel
Primary Outcome(s)	Progression-Free Survival
Sample size	Total: 347
Key Findings	PFS was significantly longer in the crizotinibarm, with medianPFS of 7.7 and 3.0 months in the crizotinib and chemotherapy arms (hazard ratio for progression or death with crizotinib, 0.49; 95% confidence interval [CI], 0.37–0.64; $p < 0.001$) The response rates were 65% (95% CI, 58–72) with crizotinib, as compared with 20% (95% CI, 14–26) with chemotherapy ($p < 0.001$) Common adverse events associated with crizotinib were visual disorder, gastrointestinal side effects, and elevated liver aminotransferase levels, whereas common adverse events with chemotherapy were fatigue, alopecia, and dyspnea
Issues encountered	A lack of survival benefit was observed, possibly due to confounding effects of crossover High crossover rate was observed among patients in the chemotherapy group, thus complicating the analysis of overall survival in a prespecified interim analysis
Impact	Approval of Crizotinib was granted while both phase 1 and 2 trials were ongoing Accelerated approval of Crizotinib was based on two single-arm trials in 2011

(continued)

	Crizotinib then received FDA approval for the treatment of patients with locally advanced or metastatic non-small cell lung cancer that is ALK-positive based on confirmation of benefit in this trial The approval was accomplished in record time, from drug development in 2007 to its initial accelerated approval in 2011
Primary reference(s)	1. Shaw AT, Kim DW, Nakagawa K et al (2013) Crizotinib versus chemotherapy in advanced ALK-positive lung cancer. N Engl J Med 368:2385–2394 2. Kazandjian D, Blumenthal GM, Chen HY, He K, Patel M, Justice R, Keegan P, Pazdur R (2014) FDA approval summary: crizotinib for the treatment of metastatic non-small cell lung cancer with anaplastic lymphoma kinase rearrangements. Oncologist 19(10): e5–e11

14.14 BIA 10-2474

Design Feature	Description
Trial Name	A double-blind, randomised, placebo-controlled, combined single and multiple ascending dose study including food interaction, to investigate the safety, tolerability, pharmacokinetic and pharmacodynamic profile of BIA 10-2474, in healthy volunteers
Design Summary	A double-blind, randomised, placebo-controlled, combined single and multiple ascending dose study (Phase 1)
Enrollment start year	2015
Study center(s)	Single center- Rennes University Hospital
Investigators	Bial/BioTrial investigators
Sponsor	Biotrial
Trial Registration number	Not available
Primary Research Question(s)	What is the safety and tolerability of BIA 10-2474 after single and multiple oral doses What is the effect of food on the PK and PD of BIA 10-2474
Study Population	Healthy volunteers
Number of study groups	The trial involved four parts: 　1. A single ascending dose (SAD) part comprising 8 cohorts of 8 healthy volunteers receiving a single-oral dose of BIA 10-2474 (6 subjects) or placebo (2 subjects) ($n = 64$) 　2. A cross-over part to evaluate the fed versus fasting state of 12 healthy volunteers, each receiving either a single or multiple dose of BIA 10-2474 in either the fed or fasting state in an open-label, two-way crossover design ($n = 32$) 　3. A multiple ascending dose (MAD) part comprising of 4 cohorts of 8 healthy volunteers receiving an oral dose of BIA 10-2474 (6 subjects) or placebo (2 subjects) once daily for 10 days ($n = 12$) 　4. Pharmodynamics Part comprising of 1 cohort of 20 healthy male volunteers in a double-blind, placebo-controlled, cross-over design to assess PD effects of BIA 10-2474 (did not start)
Experiment	BIA 10-2474
Control	Placebo

(continued)

Primary Outcome(s)	Safety and tolerability of BIA 10-2474
Sample size	Total: 128
Key Findings	In the single dose study neither 50 mg nor 100 mg of BIA 10-274 produced adverse events Prior to study termination, 116 subjects had been recruited and 84 other volunteers had received the drug during the trial without serious adverse events being reported SAEs occurred in 6 subjects from the fifth dose cohort (50 mg/day) ascending from 40 mg/day in the previous cohort
Issues encountered	On the fifth day of the fifth cohort (50 mg/day), the first subject of the fifth cohort experienced neurological side effects and died 1 week following admission on January 17th, 2016 An additional five participants from the same cohort were hospitalized of five others in January 2016, before the trial was stopped Errors were attributed to the dose itself, specificity of the drug, the trial design, and possible human error Details of results of preclinical and Phase 1 part of the trial were not available and trial was not registered resulting in difficulty reaching a conclusion as to what went wrong
Impact	This was a first-in human trial planned to include 128 healthy male and female volunteers that resulted in the death of a healthy volunteer and hospitalization of 5 others This trial received extensive media coverage and outcry as a result of the tragic events as well as a lawsuit As a result of this trial mishap, the European Medicines Agency (EMA) issued stricter guidelines that emphasize the requirement for comprehensive preclinical tests of new compounds including its off-target effects. Additional guidance on dosing and safety monitoring has also been provided to minimize risk at each step Questions about the design used as well as the design of Phase 1 trials in general have also been raised where better designs and methods could be used to accomplish the study objectives There is a need for improvement in the extrapolation of preclinical data and findings from animals to humans as well as making these data publicly available It remains unclear what happened to cause the BIA 10-274 toxicity, however, cannabinoid-related research has been impacted as a result of this trial with a negative perception from public Little information regarding the study findings are available for both preclinical data as well as from BIA 10-274 This trial along with the highlights the importance of trial registration, safety monitoring and reporting in a timely manner to prevent harm
Primary reference(s)	1. Kaur R, Sidhu P, Singh S (2016) What failed BIA 10-2474 Phase I clinical trial? Global speculations and recommendations for future Phase I trials. J Pharmacol Pharmacother 7(3):120–126 2. Moore N (2016) Lessons from the fatal French study BIA-10-2474. BMJ 353:i2727. https://doi.org/10.1136/bmj.i2727. Erratum in: BMJ. 2016 May 24;353:i2956 3. Protocol available at: Clinical Study Protocol N° BIA-102474-101 (Version 1.2, 1 July 2015)" (PDF). (ANSM) 1 July 2015

Appendix 15

Clinical Trials-Related Websites
Description: This section includes a list of web resources related to clinical trials in addition to search terms that can be entered into search engines (e.g., Google). This list is meant to serve as a starting point to help navigate readers to trials-related websites that are currently available.

Trial/Topic	Web link	Search term (s)
History		
James Lind library	http://www.jameslindlibrary.org/	James Lind Library; James Lind
The Classics in Medicine: Summaries of the Landmark Trials Online Edition	https://www.2minutemedicine.com/the-classics-directory/	Landmark trials; The Classics in Medicine
Clinical Trials timeline	http://ictd2015.lillycoi.com/	History of Clinical trials; Clinical Trials timeline
The Doctors Trial: The Medical Case of the Subsequent Nüremberg proceedings	https://www.ushmm.org/information/exhibitions/online-exhibitions/special-focus/doctors-trial	Nuremberg doctor's trial; Holocaust memorial museum Nuremberg code
Ethics		
HHS Ethical Codes and Research Standards	https://www.hhs.gov/ohrp/international/ethical-codes-and-research-standards/index.html	HHS ethics codes; HHS research standards; OHRP ethics codes
The Belmont Report	https://www.hhs.gov/ohrp/regulations-and-policy/belmont-report/read-the-belmont-report/index.html	The Belmont Report; Read the Belmont Report; The Belmont Principles
Nüremberg Code	https://history.nih.gov/about/timelines/nuremberg.html	Nuremberg code document; Nuremberg code PDF; Office of history Nuremberg code

(continued)

Trial/Topic	Web link	Search term (s)
Declaration of Helsinki	https://www.wma.net/policies-post/wma-declaration-of-helsinki-ethical-principles-for-medical-research-involving-human-subjects/	WMA Declaration of Helsinki; WMA Helsinki
Code of Federal Regulations- Title 45	https://www.hhs.gov/ohrp/regulations-and-policy/regulations/45-cfr-46/index.html	45 CFR 46; Common Rule; CFR human research protections
Code of Federal Regulations Title 21, Part 11	https://www.accessdata.fda.gov/scripts/cdrh/cfdocs/cfcfr/CFRSearch.cfm?CFRPart=11	21 CFR Part 11; Code of federal title 21;
Council for International Organizations of Medical Science (CIOMS)	https://cioms.ch/	CIOMS; Council for International Organizations of Medical Science; CIOMS guidelines
Health Insurance Portability and Accountability Act (HIPAA)	https://www.hhs.gov/hipaa/index.html	HHS HIPAA; Health Information Privacy; Privacy Rule
Agencies and Health Organizations		
U.S. Food and Drug Administration	https://www.fda.gov/default.htm	FDA; US Food and Drug; Food and Drug Association
National Institutes of Health	https://www.nih.gov/	NIH; National Institutes of Health; US Department of Health and Human Services=
U.S. Department of Health and Human Services	https://www.hhs.gov/	US Department of Health and Human Services; Health and Human Services; HHS
World Health Organization	www.who.int/	WHO; World Health Organization; World Health
National Health Services	https://www.nhs.uk/	NHS; National Health Service; UK health
World Medical Association	https://www.wma.net/	WMA; World Medical Association
Resources for Trialists		
Clinical Trials Transformation Initiative	https://www.ctti-clinicaltrials.org/	AACT; AACT CTTI; Clinical Trials Transformation Initiative
Cochrane Collaboration	https://www.cochrane.org/	Cochrane; Cochrane Collaboration; Cochrane Systematic Reviews
PubMed	https://www.ncbi.nlm.nih.gov/pubmed/	PubMed; NCBI article search; US NLM database
Clinical Trials Registries	Please see full list in Appendix 12	Clinical trials registry; clinical trials database;

(continued)

Trial/Topic	Web link	Search term (s)
Society for Clinical Trials	http://www.sctweb.org/public/home.cfm	SCT; Society for Clinical Trials; Clinical Trials Society; SCT annual meeting
International Society for Computational Biology (ISCB)	https://www.iscb.org/	International Society for Computational Biology; ISCB
Retraction Watch	https://retractionwatch.com/	Retraction watch; retraction watch journals
Examples of online statistical calculators	http://powerandsamplesize.com/ http://biostat.mc.vanderbilt.edu/wiki/Main/PowerSampleSize http://www.sample-size.net/ https://biostatistics.csmc.edu/ewoc/ewocWeb.php	Online power and sample size calculator; clinical trial sample size calculators; study sample size calculator; online power calculation
International Clinical Trial Center Network	https://www.icn-connect.org/	International Clinical Trials; ICN; International trial network
UK Clinical Trials Gateway	https://www.ukctg.nihr.ac.uk/	UK clinical trials gateway; NHS trials; UK clinical trials
Clinical Trials Registries	Please see full list in Appendix 12	Clinical trials registry; clinical trials database; clinicaltrials.gov
Trials Resources for Patients		
NIH Clinical Research Trials and You	https://www.nih.gov/health-information/nih-clinical-research-trials-you/basics	NIH The Basics; Clinical Trials and you
FDA for patients	https://www.fda.gov/forpatients/approvals/drugs/ucm405622.htm	FDA what patients need to know; FDA for patients
OHRP About Research Participation	https://www.hhs.gov/ohrp/education-and-outreach/about-research-participation	HHS about research participation; OHRP research participation
Medline Plus Clinical Trials	https://medlineplus.gov/clinicaltrials.html	Medline plus trials; Medline clinical trials
ClinicalTrials.gov: Learn about Clinical Trials	https://clinicaltrials.gov/ct2/about-studies/learn	clinicaltrials.gov learn about trials; clinicaltrials.gov about studies
Patient-Centered Outcomes Research Institute	https://www.pcori.org/	PCORI; Patient-Centered Outcomes Research
Patient Advocacy Groups		
Alliance Professional Health Advocates	https://aphadvocates.org/	Patient advocacy groups; Patient advocates; Professional patient health advocates;
National Association of Healthcare Advocacy Consultants	https://www.nahac.com/#!event-list	NAHAC; National Association of Healthcare Advocacy; Healthcare advocacy group

(continued)

Trial/Topic	Web link	Search term (s)
List of Cancer Advocacy Organizations	https://www.aacr.org/Funding/PAGES/STAND%20UP%20TO%20CANCER/ADVOCACY-ORGANIZATIONS-WITH-CLINICAL-TRIAL-INFORMATION.ASPX	AACR advocacy groups; Clinical Trial Patient Advocacy
National patient Advocate Foundation	https://www.npaf.org/	National patient Advocate Foundation; NPAF; Patient Foundation
Other Patient Advocacy Sites	See Google terms	Patient Advocacy Organizations; Patient advocacy groups; Healthcare Advocacy Organizations; Professional advocacy groups
Clinical Trials Reporting and Publication		
CONSORT statement	http://www.consort-statement.org/	CONSORT; Consort statement; CONSORT extensions
International Committee of Medical Journal Editors	http://www.icmje.org/	ICMJE; International committee of journal editors; ICMJE recommendations
International Council for Harmonisation	https://www.ich.org/home.html	ICH; Council for Harmonisation of Technical Requirements;
SPIRIT Statement	http://www.spirit-statement.org/	SPIRIT protocol statement; SPIRIT statement
Clinical Trials Journals		
Clinical Trials: Journal of the Society for Clinical Trials	https://journals.sagepub.com/home/ctj	Clinical Trials journal; Journal of the Society for Clinical Trials
Contemporary Clinical Trials	https://www.journals.elsevier.com/contemporary-clinical-trials	Contemporary Clinical Trials Journal; Contemporary Trials Journal
Trials	https://trialsjournal.biomedcentral.com/	BMC trials journal; Trials; Trials Journal
International Journal of Clinical Trials	http://www.ijclinicaltrials.com/index.php/ijct	International Journal of Clinical Trials
List of journals that are ICMJE members	http://www.icmje.org/about-icmje/faqs/icmje-membership/	ICMJE journals; ICMJE membership; Journals following ICMJE recommendations
Other trial-related websites		
Trials Meinert's Way	https://jhuccs1.us/clm/default.asp	Meinert clinical trials; Trials Meinert's Way
CenterWatch	http://www.centerwatch.com/	CenterWatch; CenterWatch trials;

(continued)

Trial/Topic	Web link	Search term (s)
List of "Famous Trials" by Professor Douglas O. Linder	http://famous-trials.com/	Famous trials; Nuremberg trials;
Catalog of Bias	https://catalogofbias.org/	Bias catalog; Bias types;
Clinical Trials Registration Campaign: AllTrials	http://www.alltrials.net/	All Trials; All Trials registered and reported
List of Clinical Trials Websites	http://mastersinclinicalresearch.com/blog/	Top clinical trials websites; Masters in clinical research blog

Appendix 16

Clinical Trials Related Bibliography
Description: This Appendix includes a list of selected books related to clinical trials for further reading. Books are sorted by author, in alphabetical order, where only the most recent edition is listed.

References

Brody T (2012) Clinical trials: study design, endpoints and biomarkers, drug safety, and FDA and ICH guidelines. Elsevier, London
Buyse ME, Staquet MJ, Sylvester RJ (eds) Cancer clinical trials: methods and practice. Oxford University Press, Oxford
Chow SC, Liu JP (2013) Design and analysis of clinical trials: concepts and methodologies, 3rd edn. Wiley, New Jersey
Cook TD, DeMets DL (2008) Introduction to statistical methods for clinical trials. Taylor & Francis Group, Boca Raton
Crowley J (ed) (2000) Handbook of statistics in clinical oncology. Marcel Dekker, New York
Day S (1999) Dictionary for clinical trials. Wiley, Chichester
DeMets DL, Furberg CD, Friedman LM (2006) Data monitoring in clinical trials: a case studies approach. Springer Science and Business Media, New York
Fairclough DL (2002) Design and analysis of quality of life studies in clinical trials. CRC Press, Andover
Fayers PM, Hays R. (eds) (2006) assessing quality of life in clinical trials: methods and practice, 2nd edn. Oxford University Press, Oxford
Friedman LM, Furberg CD, DeMets DL, Reboussin DM, Granger CB (2015) Fundamentals of clinical trials, 5th edn. Springer, London
Girling DJ, Parmar MKB, Stenning SP, Stephens RJ, Steward LA (2003) Clinical trials in cancer. Oxford University Press, Oxford
Green S, Crowley J, Smith A (2010) Clinical trials in oncology. Chapman and Hall, New York
Hill AB (1948) Principles of medical statistics, 4th edn. The Lancet Ltd., UK
Hollon SD (2014) Randomized clinical trials. The encyclopedia of clinical psychology
Jadad A (1998) Randomised controlled trials. British Medical Journal, London
Jennison C, Turnbull BW (2000) Group Sequential methods with applications to clinical trials. Chapman & Hall, Boca Raton, FL
Julious SA (2010) Sample sizes for clinical trials. Taylor and Francis Group, LLC, Boca Raton
Kelly WK, Halabi S (2018) Oncology clinical trials: successful design, conduct, and analysis. Springer Publishing Company, LLC

Kotz S, Johnson HL, Read CB (1998) Encyclopedia of statistical sciences. 1982
Machin D, Campbell MJ (2005) Design of studies for medical research. Wiley, Chichester
Machin D, Campbell MJ, Fayers PM, Pinol APY (1997) Sample size tables for clinical studies. Blackwell Science, Oxford
Machin D, Day S, Green S (2006) Textbook of clinical trials, 2nd edn. Wiley, Chichester
Matthews JNS (2006) Introduction to randomized controlled clinical trials, 2nd edn. Taylor and Francis Group, LLC, Boca Raton
McFadden ET (1997) Management of data in clinical trials. Wiley, New York
Meinert CL (2011) An insider's guide to clinical trials. Oxford University Press, Oxford
Meinert CL (2012a) Clinical trials dictionary: terminology and usage recommendations, 2nd edn. Wiley, New Jersey
Meinert CL (2012b) Clinical trials: design, conduct, and analysis, 2nd edn. Oxford University Press, New York
Meinert CL (2013) Clinical trials handbook: design and conduct. Wiley, New Jersey
O'Grady J, Joubert PH (1997) Handbook of phase I/II clinical drug trials. CRC Press, London
Piantadosi S (2017) Clinical trials: a methodologic perspective, 3rd edn. Wiley, New York
Pocock SJ (2013) Clinical trials: a practical approach. Wiley
Redmond C, Colton T (eds) (2001) Biostatistics in clinical trials. Wiley, Chichester
Senn SJ (1993) Cross-over trials in clinical research. Wiley, Chichester
Shih WJ, Aisner J (2016) Statistical design and analysis of clinical trials: principles and methods. Taylor & Francis Group, Boca Raton
Tygstrup N (1982) Randomized clinical trial and therapeutic decisions, 1st edn. CRC Press
Wang D, Bakhai A (eds) (2006) Clinical trials: a practical guide to design, analysis and reporting. Remedica, London
Whitehead J (1997) Design and analysis of sequential clinical trials, revised 2nd edn. Wiley, Chichester
Wooding WM (1994) Planning pharmaceutical clinical trials. Wiley, New York
Ziegel ER (2000) Encyclopedia of biostatistics. Technometrics 42(2):222–222

Index

A
Ablation, 1421
Absolute neutrophil count (ANC), 1246
Accelerated approval pathway, 2301
Acceptable distance, 1423
Acceptable subset selection, 1051–1052
  for LRL procedures, 1057–1058
Accept-reject method, 1565
Accountability, 179, 183–185
Actelion-451840, 1948
Active control trials, 2202
Acupuncture, 2264, 2270, 2271, 2280
Acute lymphoblastic leukemia (ALL), 887, 2380, 2382
Acute myeloid leukemia (AML), 578
Acute respiratory distress syndrome (ARDS), 694
ADAGIO trial, 1209
ADAPTABLE trial, 2309
Adaptive combination tests, 1090–1091
Adaptive design, 1084, 1085, 1088, 1474, 1567, 2372–2373
  adaptive parallel Simon two-stage design, 1163–1164
  adaptive patient enrichment design, 1162–1163
  adaptive signature design, 1159–1160
  adaptive threshold enrichment design, 1161–1162
  multi-arm multi-stage design, 1164–1165
  outcome-based adaptive randomization design, 1160–1161
Adaptive Gauss-Hermite quadrature, 1434
Adaptive intervention, *see* Dynamic treatment regimen (DTR)
Adaptive seamless designs, 1088, 1092, 1097
Adaptive signature design, 1159–1160, 2375
Adaptive threshold determination, 2374–2375
Adding/subtracting treatments, 12, 2467

Add-on tests, 1189
Adeno-associated viral (AAV) vectors, 2304
Adherence, 1263, 1265, 1266, 1270, 1271, 1274, 2276–2277
  monitoring, 2276
Adherence adjusted estimates
  RCM (*see* Rubin causal model)
  structural mean models, 1841–1842
Administration of study treatments
  eligibility checking and randomization, 283–284
  end of treatment, 292
  inclusion and exclusion criteria, treatment administration, 283
  monitoring early treatment discontinuation and tracking reasons for discontinuation, 289–290
  monitoring treatment adherence, 287–289
  participants, 285–286
  promoting treatment adherence, 286–287
  study team, treatment adherence, 290–292
  training, 282
  verification of site readiness, 283
Administrative censoring, 1646
AD related dementias (ADRD), 2409
Adult AIDS Clinical Trials Group (AACTG), 2104
Adverse drug events (ADEs), 1971
Adverse drug reaction (ADR), 1967
Adverse events, 114, 470, 605, 928
  safety signals, 1966
Advisory committee, 566
Age-Related Eye Disease Study (AREDS), 1379
Age-related macular degeneration (AMD), 1383, 2202
Aging and cognitive health evaluation in elders (ACHIEVE) trial, 847
Albendazole, 2217

ALCOA, 373
Aldehyde dehydrogenase deficiency, 2421
Aliskiren Trial on Acute Heart Failure Outcomes (ASTRONAUT) trial, 2246
Aliskiren Trial to Minimize Outcomes in Patients with Heart Failure (ATMOSPHERE) trial, 693
Allocation concealment, 742
  See also Double-blinding
Alpha and beta (or power) levels, 773
Alpha level, 1622
Alternative hypothesis, 1621
Alzheimer's disease (AD), 1200, 1271, 2409
  biomarkers, 2410
  invasive procedures, 2411
  primary care physicians, barriers for, 2411
  study partner requirement, 2411
  target population/stage of disease, 2409–2410
  under-represented populations, barriers for, 2411
Alzheimer's Disease Anti-inflammatory Prevention Trial (ADAPT), 2108
American College of Rheumatology (ACR), 1248
American Society of Clinical Oncology (ASCO), 2322
Amery-Dony design (AD design), 1442, 1445–1446
Aminoglycosides, 2381
Analgesic, Anesthetic, and Addiction Clinical Trial Translation, Innovations, Opportunities and Network (ACTTION), 1650
Analysis, 322
  database, 2091–2092
Analysis of covariance (ANCOVA), 838, 1652, 1772
Analysis of variance (ANOVA), 1289, 1710
Analysis principles, in complex trials, 1593–1594
Ancillary studies, 565
Anesthesia, 2323
Anganwadi Centers (AWCs), 2217
Angiotensin-converting–enzyme (ACE) inhibitors, 1719
Anti-kickback statute, 532
Antisense oligonucleotides (ASOs), 2304
Antithrombotic agents, 2381
Anturane reinfarction trial, 1590
Apparent validation, 2017
Applications, 505, 515
Apportioning monies, 2464

Approval, 460–462, 464, 466, 467, 469, 472, 473, 475, 477
Approved Personnel List (APL), 246
Approximations, 1853, 1858, 1860–1862
Archiving, 638, 641
  data collection schedule, 642
  documentation, 638
  electronic, 638
  guidelines, 638
  multicenter trials, 642
  NEJM expressions, 638
  protocol, 641, 642
  randomization procedure, 639
  sponsor and investigator, 646
  tolbutamide, 639
  trials, 322, 646
Area under the response vs. time curve (AUC), 1242
Artificial intelligence (AI), 1271, 1272
Aspirin Dosing: A Patient-centric Trial Assessing Benefits and Long-Term Effectiveness (ADAPTABLE) trial, 2252, 2255
Assay sensitivity, 1306, 1311–1312
Assent, 392, 393
Assignment bias, 742
Association for the Accreditation of Human Research Protection Programs (AAHRPP), 662
Association of Clinical Research Professionals (ACRP), 129–131
As treated (AT) populations, 1606
Asymptomatic subclinical assessments, 846
Attributable/absolute risk reduction (ARR), 1972
Attributable risk (AR), 1972
Attributable toxicity, 1011–1016
Attrition bias, 795–797
Authorship models, 2092, 2094, 2098
  conventional form, 2109
  corporate, 2109
  modified conventional form, 2109
  modified corporate, 2109
  POS research group, 2110
  recognition, 2110
Authorship policy, 2465
Authors per publication, 2111
Autism, 2198
Automated data management, 562
Availability, 353
Average treatment effect, 1683–1685, 1687, 1690
Averted infections ratio, 1319

Index

B

Balanced factorial design, 1356
Barriers to participation, 2400–2403
Baseline covariates, 1780, 1783
Baseline disease risk, 1264
Baseline information, 1326
Baseline measurement, 490
Baseline observation carried forward (BOCF), 1639
Bayes factors, 990–992
Bayesian, 974, 976, 977, 981, 983
    adaptive clinical trial designs, 1939
    adaptive design, 1410
    adaptive randomization, 1478
    analysis, 1290
    approaches, 1316–1317
    designs, 1035
    forecasting, 1955–1956
    hierarchical modeling, 1141
    methods, 1425
    model-free approaches, 1125–1127
    statistics, 576
Bayesian Confidence Propagation Neural Network (BCPNN), 1967
Bayesian design, for device trials
    Bayesian adaptive design, 1410–1411
    operating characteristics, 1411
    prior information, 1410
Bayesian optimal interval design (BOIN), 956
Bcrm package, 1112
BCX-34, 2322
Belief disconfirmation bias, 2218
Belmont Report, 86, 93, 660, 661, 664, 669
Benchmarking, 259, 265, 266
Beneficence, 57
Beneficiary inducements statute, 532
Benefit-less-risk analysis (BLRA), 1972, 1973
Benefit-risk assessment (BRA), 1970
Benefit-risk framework (BRF), 1970
Benefits, 348
Benford's law, 2329
Bernoulli distribution, 1790
Beta-binomial distribution, 1037–1038
Beta-carotene, 2220
Better-than-placebo (BTP) subset, 1059
Between-subject information, 1326, 1340, 1348–1350
Bias, 884–885, 2198, 2199, 2201
    information, 885–886
    selection, 885

Bias control
    chronological bias (*see* Chronological bias)
    patient allocation, 857
    predictability (*see* Predictability)
    random walk, 858, 860
    robust hypothesis tests, 869
    selection bias, 857
Biased coin, 751
    designs, 955
Big data and clinical trials, 2249
    CDMs, research networks with, 2251–2253
    individual health systems, pragmatic trials within, 2253–2254
    machine learning, 2257–2260
    multiple healthcare systems, 2254
    patient recruitment and consent, 2255–2256
    registries, 2254–2255
Big stick design, 864
Billing compliance, 527–531
Binary data, 2181
Binary logistic regression
    bias correction, 1792
    confidence interval, 1794
    estimation, 1791
    interpretation of model, 1794–1796
    skewness coefficient, 1793
    test statistics, 1793
Binary outcome, 1175, 1394, 1876
Binary response, 1791
Bioassay, 1254
Biocreep, 1318
Bioequivalence, 1242
Biological categorization, 2419, 2421, 2423
Biological models, 2236
Biologics, 1238
Biologics license application (BLA), 2297
Biologics licensing application/new drug application (BLA/NDA), 461, 464, 472
Biologics Price and Competition (BPCI) Act, 1239, 1249
Biomarker(s), 893, 896–897, 943, 1138–1139, 1146, 1361–1363, 2368
    adaptive designs, 2372–2373
    adaptively determining predictive classifier, 2375–2376
    adaptive threshold determination, 2374–2375
    clinical utility, 1150
    clinical validity, 1150
    discovery and analytical validity, 1149–1150
    enrichment design, 2370
    life course of, 1149–1150

Biomarker(s) (*cont.*)
  predictive, 1148
  predictive biomarkers, 2368, 2369
  predictive classifiers, 2369
  prognostic, 1147, 2368
  test positive and test negative patients, in clinical trial, 2370–2372
  types of, 1147
Biomarker guided trials
  adaptive designs, 1159–1165
  analysis of, 1166
  designs, 1150–1151
  non-adaptive (*see* Non-adaptive biomarker-guided trial designs)
  operational considerations, 1165–1166
Bio-materials, international trials
  future research, 355
  obtaining materials, 355
  retaining materials, 355
  shipping materials, 355
  translational research, 355
Biometric identifiers, 2128
Biopharma, 579
Biosimilar drug development, *see* Biosimilarity
Biosimilarity
  analytical similarity, 1245, 1246
  clinical efficacy studies, 1251–1253
  clinical studies, 1246, 1247
  definition, 1239
  efficacy assessment, 1256
  equivalence, 1243–1245
  equivalent efficacy, 1247–1249
  global development programs, 1256
  interchangeability, 1249–1251
  non-clinical studies, 1245
  operational challenges, 1254–1255
  originator products, 1238, 1255
  regulatory requirements, 1255
  small molecule drugs, 1238
  statistical issues, 1256
  steps, 1240
  stepwise approach, 1240–1243
Biospecimen sharing, 633, 634
Biostatisticians, 2327
Blackouts, paper writing
  approval authority, 2035
  database freeze, 2035
  event adjudication, 2035
  insider trading, 2036
  reviews, 2035
  sign-offs, 2036
Blind, 816
Blinding, 829

Body mass index, 790
Bonferroni correction, 732, 733, 2280
Bootstrap
  model selection in replication, 1905–1907
  non-parametric, 1904–1905
Bootstraping, 2019
Botanical Drug Development Guidance, 2267
Breakthrough therapy designation (BTD), 577
Breast cancer prevention trials, 1269
Brief Pain Inventory Short Form (BPI-SF), 922
Broad-based screening technology, 576
Budget, 412
  considerations, 417
  contract and, 413
  evaluation, 422
  format, 418
  proposal and, 417

C

Cacchillo v. Insmed Inc., 2363
Calcium polyp prevention trial, 1269
Canadian Critical Care Trials Groups, 2110
Cancer, 1223, 1226
Cancer clinical trials, 616
Cancer Imaging Archive, 2131
Cardiac resynchronization therapy (CRT), 1405
Carry across effect, 1380, 1382
Case-control design, 1173
Case-control studies, 1798, 1808
Case report forms (CRFs), 306, 348, 359, 360
Cataract surgery trial, 1386
Categorial outcomes, 897
Causal effect models, 1609
Causal inference, 1635
Causal models, 1835, 1836
Causation, 2357–2358
Cause-specific hazards, 1758, 1764–1767
Censoring, 1718–1720, 1722, 1723, 1726, 1729
Centers for Medicare and Medicaid Services, 523, 524
Central laboratory, 98, 102, 563
Central reading center, 563
Central statistical monitoring, 2328, 2329, 2332
Certification, 113
Certified Clinical Research Coordinator (CCRC), 130, 131
Change management, 230, 231, 235
Chemical/structural similarity, 2295
Chemoprevention trials, 1273
Chemotherapy, 1247, 2382
Chen's design, 860
Childhood Cancer Survivor Study, 2391

Chiroprastic therapy, 2264, 2270, 2271, 2280
Chi-square (χ^2) test, 1711–1713
Chondroitin, 2265
Choroidal Neovascularization Prevention Trial (CNVPT), 1393
Chronic back pain, 2277
Chronic diseases, 1249
Chronic myelomonocytic leukemia, 1136
Chronological bias
 power, 868
 randomization tests, 870
 suspectibility, 868
 time trend, 866
Cisplatin, 1113
Citation bias, 2048, 2060
Clinical & Translational Science Awards Program (CTSA), 129
Clinical centers, 562
 certification and training, 112, 113
 clinical coordinator, 111, 112
 ethical approval, 112
 failure, 566
 funding, 99, 102, 110
 implementation phase, 110
 non-traditional sites, 109
 organization binders/files, 112
 principal investigator, 109, 111
 responsibilities, 103–106
 site organization, 110, 111
 study team, 111
 team interactions, 112
Clinical coordinating centers (CCC), 99, 594, 595
 clinical trial, 597
 clinical trial operations, 594, 595
 competitive environment, 608
 data collection and data submission, 597
 and DCC, 599
 development, 595
 FDA debarment database, 598
 management, 610
 management and quality improvements, 608
 multi-site clinical trial, 609
 multi-site investigator-initiated, 594
 and participating sites, 609
 protocol document, 597
 quality management, 594
 regulatory compliance, 594
 research administration, 595
 resources, 597
 responsibilities and management, 595, 605

 risk management, 609
 site management, 594, 599
 site selection, 597
 trial development, 595
Clinical Data Acquisition Standards Harmonization project (CDASH), 444, 445
Clinical data management system (CDMS), 211, 213, 234, 430–434
Clinical Data Research Networks (CDRN), 2251
Clinical equipoise, 59–60
Clinically meaningful effect sizes, 772
Clinically recognized outcomes, 846
Clinically superior drugs, 2296
Clinical outcome assessment, 2304
Clinical research, 2340
Clinical Research Associate (CRA), 262
Clinical Research Coordinator (CRC), 125–127, 129–131
Clinical Research Organizations (CROs), 586, 604
Clinical research staff
 credentialing organizations, 129–131
 history of, 124–126
 qualifications, 126–128
 training, 128–129
Clinical scenario evaluation (CSE) approach, 1566
Clinical significance, 1817
Clinical study reports (CSRs), 475, 2059, 2060, 2064
Clinical trial(s), 6, 37, 74, 75, 77–80, 834, 836, 839, 1386, 1418, 1814, 2340
 analysis by assigned treatment vs. per protocol analysis, 52
 baseline vs. baseline period, 51
 bias, 52–53
 blind vs.mask, 49
 blocking vs. stratification, 40
 clinical investigator vs. investigator, 46
 consent, 43
 contractual disputes, 2358–2359
 controlled, 42
 criminal actions, 2362
 database, 484, 493
 data monitoring vs. data monitoring committee, 46
 design variable vs. primary outcome measure, 50
 development, 579
 dropout, 49

Clinical trial(s) (*cont.*)
  early history of, 4–5
  in early twentieth century, 6–7
  employment lawsuits, 2361–2362
  end of followup *vs.* end of trial, 52
  ethics, 9–11
  intellectual property disputes, 2359–2360
  lawsuits demanding medicines or treatment, 2362–2363
  legal duties of participants, 2344–2358
  lost to followup, 49
  methodology, 1590
  minority populations (*see* Minority populations, clinical trials)
  name of, 38
  nominal stop *vs.* early stop, 53
  open, 41
  outcome *vs.* endpoint, 48
  pharmaceutical and medical device mass tort litigation, 2363–2364
  pilot *vs.* feasibility study, 37
  placebo, 42–43
  policy, 524–526
  primary *vs.* secondary outcome, 47
  principal investigator *vs.* study chair, 46
  quotafication, 41
  randomization *vs.* randomized, 44
  random *vs.* haphazard, 46–47
  registration, 483
  registration *vs.* enrollment, 44
  research subject, 39
  role of governments in institutionalization, 8–9
  screened *vs.* enrolled, 51–52
  securities litigation, 2360–2361
  single-center *vs.* multicenter, 45
  steering *vs.* executive committee, 46
  vs. study, 37
  study group, treatment group or arm, 39
  theories of liability (*see* Theories of liability)
  treatment failure *vs.* treatment cessation, 48
  treatment or intervention, 38–39
  trial protocol *vs.* manual of operations, 40
  withdrawing from, 50
Clinical Trial Agreement (CTA), 420
Clinical trial application (CTA), 178
Clinical trial authorization (CTA), 471–475
Clinical trial data
  ethical principles, 2117
  identifiers in, 2119–2120
Clinical trial management system (CTMS), 179, 598

Clinical trial networks, 144
  benefits, 147
  limitations, 147
  structure examples, 144–146
Clinical trials, children
  challenges, 2389–2391
  drug metabolism, 2380
  heart surgery, 2382
  medical experimentation, 2383
  medication, 2381
  nontherapeutic research, 2383
  pediatric research, 2380, 2385–2387
  physiology, 2380
  polio vaccine, 2381
  protections and ethical considerations, 2384–2385
  tested inoculation strategies, 2383
  trail design, 2387–2389
ClinicalTrials.gov
  database, 493–494
  downloading content, 492–493
  history, 480–484
  quality control review, 491–492
  registration process, 484
  results reporting, 489–490
  results submission process, 490–491
  trial registration, 486–489
  website content, 484–486
Clinical Trials Facilitation and coordination Group (CTFG), 471–472
Clinical Trials Regulation (CTReg), 475–476
Clinical Trials Transformation Initiative (CTTI), 575
Clinical utility, 2015–2017
Clinician-reported outcomes, 907
Closed report, 824
Close out, 282, 292, 334, 336
Closeout design, 2462
Clustering, 1419, 1420, 1424, 1426, 1427, 1429, 1432–1433, 1435
Cluster-level methods, 1500–1501
Cluster randomized controlled trial (CRCT), 1429–1430
Cluster-randomized-crossover-trials, 1432
Cluster randomized trial, 1435, 1436
  analysis population, 1491–1492
  characteristics of, 1489–1490
  cluster specification, 1493–1494
  definition, 1488
  effects, 1492–1493
  ethics and data monitoring, 1502
  highly constrained randomization, 1496
  matching and stratification, 1494

randomization, 1494–1496
sample size and power, 1497–1500
statistical analysis, 1500–1501
stepped wedge design, 1497
variability across clusters, 1490–1491
CMS reimbursement
  Category A, 525, 529
  Category B, 525, 529
  clinical trial policy, 524–526
  coverage with evidence development, 526
  device categorization, 523, 525
  Medicare Advantage plans, 531
  Medicare area contractor, 528
  Medicare Secondary Payer (MSP) rule, 534
  national coverage determination, 526
  reasonable and necessary, 523, 525, 527, 529
CobWEB, 2083
Cochran-Mantel-Hanzel (CMH) test, 1779
Cockcroft-Graf formula, 1941
Code of Federal Regulations (CFR), 460, 463–467, 470, 586, 599
Coefficient of variation (CV), 835
Coenzyme Q, 2265
Cognitive behavioral therapy (CBT), 2275
Coherence, 961, 962
Cohort studies, 1798
Co-investigators (CO-I), 126
Coledronic acid, 1953
Collaborative clinical trial system, 575
Collaborative Ocular Melanoma Study (COMS), 102, 107
Collective investigation, 5
Commercial funding, 501
Commissioned calls, 508
Commission on Accreditation of Allied Health Education Programs (CAAHEP), 129
Committee accountability, 565
Committee chair, 564
Committee charge, 564
Committee failure, 567
Committee members, 564
Committee staff, 564
Common Data Model (CDM), 2251–2253
Common effect meta-analysis, 2182–2183
Common Rule, 86, 661–669, 673, 674, 676
Common Technical Document (CTD), 467
Communications, 114
  adverse events, 643
  and correspondences, 643
  Directives, 643
  formats, 268
  IRBs, 643
  queries, 643
Community-based participatory research (CBPR), 573
Companion diagnostics, 943
Comparability
  analytical similarity with residual uncertainty, 1241
  analytical studies, 1240
  binding and functionality, 1241
  equivalence margins, 1248
  fingerprint-like analytical similarity, 1241
  insufficient analytical similarity, 1241
  PK/PD level, 1242
  tentative analytical similarity, 1241
Comparative designs, 1090
Comparative observational study, 1412
Comparative selection design, 1059
Compassion, 203
Compassionate use, 2433, 2440
  FDA review of, 2441
  program access, 2447
  requirements for, 2440–2441
COMPASS trial, *see* Comprehensive post-acute stroke services (COMPASS) trial
Competency, 246
Competent Authority (CA), 170, 350, 351
Competent regulatory authority, 178
Competing risks, 1756
  estimable quantities, 1758
  estimators, 1759–1761
  nonidentifiability problem, 1757–1758
  nonparametric tests, 1761–1765
  observations, 1757
  regression models for, 1765–1767
Complementary health approach, 2265
  See also Integrative health approach
Complete randomization (CR), 858
Complete two-period design, 1207
Complex interventions, 1435, 1436
  characteristics, 1420
  components, 1419, 1421
  definition, 1419
  delivery of, 1420
  evaluation/statistical methods, 1425–1433
  factors, 1421
  feasibility/early phase studies, 1424
  implementation, 1435
  issues, 1419
  model fitting and analysis, 1433, 1434
  package development, 1422
  pragmatic trials, 1420

Complex interventions (*cont.*)
  provider, 1419
  public health, 1419, 1420
  quantitative and qualitative research, 1420
  reporting, 1434
  scientific quality, 1420
  surgical trial design, 1420
  timing evaluation, 1423–1424
Compliance, 178, 184, 185, 196, 1606, 1608, 1639, 1640, 2269, 2384
Complier average causal effect (CACE), 1840
  Bayesian models, 1845–1846
  dichotomous outcomes, 1842–1843
  longitudinal outcome, 1844
  maximum likelihood method, 1843–1844
Composite outcomes, 908–909
Composite strategy, 1642
Comprehensive portfolio database, 617, 623–624
Comprehensive post-acute stroke services (COMPASS) trial, 847
Comprehensive Statistical Reporting, 624
Computable phenotype, 2313
Computerization, 28
Concurrent controls, 1464–1467
Concurrently-controlled futility design, 1074–1075
Concurrent treatment *vs.* Sequential treatment, 1385
Confidence interval, 979, 980, 987
  anti-conservative, 1620
  approach, 1244
  arbitrary confidence level, 1618
  calculation, 1616
  and declaring noninferiority, 1626
  definition, 1617
  estimation, 1619
  and hypothesis testing, 1616, 1620
  null value, 1622
  population proportion, 1618
Conflicts of interest (COIs), 682
  characteristics, 542
  Committee, 544, 548–551
  definition, 542
Confounding, 1986, 1988, 1991, 1995
Congenital heart disease, 2382, 2387
Consent, 653
Consent form, *see* Informed consent
Consenting, 259
Consolidated Standards of Reporting Trials (CONSORT), 1290, 1307, 1434, 2280–2283
  for abstracts, 2080, 2081
  checklist and guidance, 2093
  checklist with manuscript, 2093

CONSORT 2010 statement, 2075, 2076
  extensions of, 2079
  flow diagram, 2075, 2078
  future plans, 2084
  guidelines, 1384
  history and development, 2074
  impact of, 2081–2083
  initiatives, 2083–2084
  objectives, 2074
  recommendations, 2096, 2097
  statement, 808
Contamination, 2269, 2277
Context, 2210, 2218–2221
Continual reassessment method (CRM), 957, 1107
  criteria, 1005, 1013, 1015
  extensions to, 1122–1123
  time-to-event, 1112
Continuation-ratio approach, 1120
Continuing education unit (CEU), 590
Continuous data, 2181
Continuous outcome, 1876
Continuous screen design, 1227
Continuous variables
  functional form, 1902–1903
  interaction of treatment with, 1913
  linear effect of, 1912–1913
Contract, 412, 2344
  content, 420
  research organizations, 2354–2356
Contractual disputes, 2358–2359
Control groups, 4, 2202, 2203, 2206
Controlled Clinical Trials, 79
Controlled direct effect (CDE), 1997
Controlled substances, 174, 180
Controversy, 2217, 2221
Conventional frequentist approach, 1938
Conventional meta-analysis, 1290
Conventional randomized clinical trial, 1444–1445
Conventional treatment, 1391
Convergence strategy (CS), 861, 863
Cooperative group clinical trials, 144
Coordinating Center Models Project (CCMP), 76–78, 101
Coordinating centers, 75–77, 79, 80, 98, 563, 567
  clinical, 99
  data, 99–101
Core outcome sets (COS), 443
Coronary artery aneurysms, 2382
Coronary artery bypass grafting, 2324
Coronary Artery Surgery Study (CASS), 2031
Coronary Drug Project (CDP), 74, 2031, 2106
Corporate authorship formats, 2110

Correlated data, 1500
Cost-effectiveness analysis, 1192
Costs, of clinical trials
   financial cost, 2247–2248
   opportunity cost, 2248–2249
Council for International Organizations of Medical Sciences (CIOMS), 675
Counting, 2470
Courts, 2340, 2342, 2345, 2351, 2352, 2355
Covariance matrices, 1369
Covariate-adaptive randomization, 754
Covariate adjustment, 1775
Covariate balance, 1495
Coverage analysis, 527, 536
Coverage with evidence development (CED), 524, 526, 530
COVID-19, 436
COVID-19 vaccine trials, 2229, 2239
Cox model, 1766, 1779, 1780
Cox proportional hazard regression model, 2005, 2016, 2020
Cox proportional hazards regression, 1230
CReDECI guidelines, 1434
Credible interval, 985
Credible intervals, 986, 987
Credit roster, 2092, 2098
Credits, 2111
Cross-classified designs, 1428–1429
Crossover, 287
   design, 837
Cross-over trials, 1285, 1289, 1290
   carry-over effect, 1328
   to compare 3 treatments, 1341
   to compare 4 treatments, 1341
   designing, 1329
   parallel groups design, 1333
   sequence of treatments, 1326
   2×2, 1327
   trial procedures, 1327
   with five treatments, 1342–1345
Cross-validated Adaptive Signature Design, 2376
CTI Clinical Trial Services v. Gilead Sciences, 2359
Cubic spline function, 1018, 1019
Cumulative cohort design (CCD), 955
Cumulative distribution functions (CDF), 947, 948
Cumulative hazard, 1925
   function, 1727–1728
Cumulative incidence function, 1761, 1763, 1765
Current Good Manufacturing Practices (CGMPs), 171, 175, 178
Curriculum vitaes (CV), 645

Cutaneous T-cell lymphoma (CTCL), 2322
Cyclosporin, 2381
Cytochrome P450 mechanism, 2404

D
Darke v. Estate of Isner, 2349
Data/safety monitoring board, 566
Data/statistical coordinating centers
   allocation (randomization) process, 100
   operations/procedures, 101
   personnel, 101
   principal investigator, 100
   requirements, 101
   responsibilities, 100, 101, 103–106
   telephone interviews, 101
   trial phase, 101
Data and safety monitoring, 2465
Data and safety monitoring boards (DSMB), 680, 681, 695, 824, 825, 829, 1234, 2354, 2384
   ad-hoc meetings, 686
   charter, 684–690
   closed session, 692–693
   confidentiality, 688–689
   executive session, 693
   final results/end-of-trial meeting, 687
   first patient first visit, 686
   formation, 682–684
   government-sponsored trials, 683
   guideline documents, 681
   independence, 688
   industry-sponsored trials, 683
   initial/organizational/kick-off meeting, 684–686
   interim analysis review meetings, 686
   meeting settings, 687
   meeting types, 684–687
   open session, 691–692
   organization, 681–684
   quorum, 687–688
   recommendations and follow-up, 693
   safety review meetings, 686
   structure of meetings, 690–691
Data and safety monitoring plan (DSMP), 680
Database lock, 324, 334, 336, 337, 344
Data capture
   case report form, 306
   data management lifecycle, 304
   methods, 305–306
Data collection, 115, 305
   forms, 566
   strategies, 359–360
Data collisions, 2329
Data Coordinating Center (DCC), 280, 281

Data extraction, 230, 232, 233
Data files freezing, 2469
Data inconsistency score (DIS), 2329, 2331, 2332
Data management, 308, 357–360, 616–617, 2275
　centers, 98, 115
　CRF completion guidelines, 314
　data management plan, 314
　data review, 312–314
　future considerations, 318
　quality control tools, 311–312
　risk-based monitoring (RBM), 308–309
　in single *vs.* multi-center trials, 317
　site and sponsor communication, 316–317
　system user, 315
　training of staff and system users, 315–316
Data management plan (DMP), 435
Data mining algorithms, 1967
Data Monitoring Committees (DMCs), 46, 824, 827, 829, 1095, 1315, 2384
　See also Data and safety monitoring boards (DSMB)
Data propagation, 2329
Data protection officer (DPO), 363
Data quality assessment, 838–839
Data quality control/assurance, 2330
Data reduction, 2235
Data repositories, 443, 446–448, 2142–2143
Data retention, regulatory obligations for, 428–435
Data reuse, 2140, 2142, 2145
Data safety monitoring boards (DSMBs), 66, 291, 552
Data Safety Monitoring Committee (DSMC), 625
　interim analysis strategies, 632
　standard report formatting, 630
　structure, 629
Dataset, 644
Data sharing, 339, 344, 436–439, 441, 442, 446, 448–451, 633, 2471
　accessibility, 2147–2148
　costs and sustainability, 2153
　culture of, 2151–2153
　FAIR data sharing principles, 2140–2151
　findability, 2144–2145
　funder platforms, 2144
　future issues, 2153–2154
　institutional platforms, 2143
　interoperability, 2148–2150
　reusability, 2150–2151
　study-specific platforms, 2143

Data source availability, 2119
Data standards, 225, 235, 443–446, 448–451
Data Transfer Agreement, 423
Data Usage Agreement (DUA), 633
Data use agreements, 442–443
Data validation plan (DVP), 314
Decision making, 500, 507, 518
Decision models, 1193
Decision points, 1545
Decision rules, 1546
Declaration of Helsinki, 153, 165, 659
Defense-in-depth approach, 624
Degarelix, 1947–1948
Deidentified data, 644
De-identifying clinical trial data
　commercial software and automated tools, 2124
　definition, 2118–2119
　ethical context, 2117–2118
　expert determination, 2127–2129
　governance, 2131–2133
　implementing, 2123–2125
　protected health information, 2120–2123
　"Safe Harbor" de-identification, 2125–2127
　structured data, 2124
Delayed screen design, 1228
Delayed start design, 1204, 1205
Delegation of Authority Log, 587–588
Delegation of tasks, 88, 89
Demarcated research procedures, 59, 60
Density function, 1720
Deployment options, 215
Design effect (DE), 1432
Design issues, 2460–2464
Design structure, 2460
Design synopsis, 2036
Design variable, 2461
Desirability of outcome ranking (DOOR), 1317
Destruction and return, 354–355
Detection bias, 794–795
Development safety update report (DSUR), 475
DEVTA study, 2217–2219
Diabetes Control and Complications Trial (DCCT), 436
Diabetic neuropathy, 1384
Diagnostic device, 1407
　companion diagnostic device, 1408–1409
　complementary diagnostic device, 1409
　imaging devices, 1408
　NGS, 1409
Diagnostic prediction models, 2005

Diagnostic trials, 1172
    accuracy, 1180
    add-on tests, 1189
    area under the ROC curve, 1178–1179
    discordant test results trial design, 1186
    economic analysis, 1192–1193
    explanatory vs. pragmatic approaches for, 1191
    multiple tests, 1186–1191
    paired trial, 1175
    positive and negative predictive values., 1177
    random disclosure trial, 1184–1186, 1189
    randomized controlled trial, 1174
    randomized controlled trial of testing, 1183
    sample size calculation, 1179–1180
    sensitivity and specificity, 1176
    statistical analysis and sample size calculation, 1192
    test-treatment trial design, 1182
    triage/parallel strategies, 1189
    type I, 1173–1181
    type II, 1182–1193
DicomCleaner™, 2131
Dietary supplements, 2264–2266, 2269
Differential dropout, 2278
Direct endpoints, 894
Directors, 78, 80
Disclosures, 2112
    of income and payments, 549
    of payment, 546
    of potential, 548
    up-to-date, 549
Discount prior method, 1577
Disease committee structure
    PRC, 619
    protocol development process, 619
    RaPID review meeting, 619
    Statistical Center, 617–619
Disease control rates (DCR), 1140
Disease-drug-trial models, 1940
    components of, 1940
    mechanistic models, 1940
    semi-mechanistic and empirical models, 1940
    study design, 1943–1945
Disease modification, 1200
Disease-modifying effect, 1201–1204, 1209
Disparities, 2418, 2422, 2426
Distinguishability, 2119
Distribution, 354
    function, 1720
Divergence strategy (DS), 862

Documentation, 370, 585, 586, 588–590
    definition, 372
    ICH guidelines, 373
    participating site, 375
    sponsor, 373–375
Dose-escalation
    cancer trial, 1110–1111
    of cisplatin in pancreatic cancer, 1113
    dual-agent, 1122, 1123
Dose-finding
    algorithm, 1108, 1121
    combination of agents, 964–965
    ease of implementation and adaptability, 961
    goals, 952
    heterogeneity of participants, 965–967
    interval-based method, 955–957
    model-based method, 957–959
    operating characteristics, 960–961
    principle of coherence, 961
    semiparametric and order restricted methods, 959
    time-to-event CRM, 963
    two drugs with, 1025
Dose limiting toxicity (DLT)
    minimum available dose combination, 1008
    probability, 1004
    target probability, 1006
    taxotere, 1012
Dose-ranging
    3+3 algorithm, 954–955
    See also Dose-finding
Dose toxicity surface models, 1123
Double-blinding, 856
Double mask, 807, 816
Double-masked vs. single-masked trials, 2274
Doubly robust, 1689–1690
Drop out, 297, 298
Drug accountability, 89
Drug combinations
    model based designs for, 1025
    treatment protocols, 1027
    trials use, 1004
Drug development, 1939
    life cycle, 1964
    process, 570, 571
Drug Enforcement Administration (DEA), 174
Drug formulations, 2390
Drug management, 179
Drug safety
    benefit and risk assessments, 1969–1977
    guidelines, 1962
    passive and proactive models, 1964–1965

Drug safety (*cont.*)
　pharmacovigilance, 1963
　vs. post-marketing surveillance, 1963–1965
　signal detections and regulatory interventions, 1965–1969
Drug supply and packaging, 2468
Duchenne muscular dystrophy, 572
Duke Clinical Research Institute (DCRI), 2252
Dunnett's test, 1473
Duplicate publication bias, 2048
Duplicate reporting, 2055
Dynamic treatment regimen (DTR), 1544, 1547
　scientific questions, 1547

E

Early-phase testing, 2267
Early physical therapy vs. usual care, 2276
Early stopping, 1085, 1093, 1094, 2467
Early Treatment of Retinopathy of Prematurity (ETROP), 1391
Eastern Cooperative Oncology Group (ECOG), 2104
Ebola, 436
Ebola *ça suffit!* trial, 1494
Ebola outbreak of 2014, 1049
EchoCRT study, 1405
Education, 124, 128, 131, 132
　control, 2270
Effectiveness, 2308
Effect preservation, 1303, 1312–1313, 1319
Effect size, 772, 781, 782
Efficacy, 1084, 1085, 1087–1090, 1092, 1095–1098, 1600–1601, 1982–1986, 2308
EffTox design, 1116
Efron's biased coin design (EBCD), 859
Electrical stimulation, 1421
Electronic case report form (CRF), 618
Electronic data capture (EDC), 181, 305, 622
Electronic data collection (EDC), 359, 642
Electronic health record (EHR), 2254, 2259, 2390
　challenges, 2310
　data concordance, 2314–2315
　data latency, 2314
　definition, 2249
　emergence of, 2250
　gaps in patient data, 2313
　patient identification, 2311
Electronic medical record (EMR), 318, 881–884
Electronic remote data capture (eRDC), 214, 235

Electronic Trial Master File (eTMF), 179
Electronic version of the CTD (eCTD), 467, 468, 473
El Emam and Malin methodology, 2130
Eligibility and exclusion, 735–736
Emergency use, 2433
　single patient, 2435, 2438
Empathy, 111, 203
Empirical model, 1940
Employment lawsuits, 2361–2362
End of Trial, 324, 332, 334
Endpoints, 565
Enforcement strategies, 198
Enrichment designs, 1092, 1152, 2370
Enrichment strategies, 735, 736
Enrichment trials, 1449–1451
Enrollment, 44
　batches *vs.* ongoing, 271
　competitive *vs.* allocated, 271
　definition, 260
　monitoring, 271
　procedures, 271
Entry criteria, 2200
Environmental Protection Agency (EPA), 185
EP06-301, 1246
EP06-302, 1246
EPAD PoC study, 1476–1477
Epidermal growth factor receptor (EGFR), 1362, 2369, 2421
EQUATOR network, 1181, 1308
Equipoise, 199
Equivalence
　confidence interval approach, 1244
　hypotheses, 1244
　logarithmic transformation, 1243
　mean values, 1245
　measurements, 1243
　testing approach, 1243
　test statistics, 1244
　TOST approach, 1244
Equivalence margins, 1244
　ACR20 responder rates, 1248
　comparability, 1248
　efficacy endpoint, 1247
　historical data, 1248
　PK bioequivalence, 1247
　regulatory authorities, 1249
Escalation with overdose control (EWOC), 1005, 1108–1109
　conditional, 1025
　dose-escalation cancer trial, 1110–1111
　feasibility bound, 1111
　method, 958

Index

principle, 1007
software packages, 1112
toxicity-dependent feasibility bounds, 1111–1112
Essential documents, 372
Estimands, 1592, 1637, 1982, 1985
  benefit risk, 1648
  causal inference, 1635
  clinical trial planning team, 1633
  complex designs, 1646
  covariates, 1644
  estimators, 1647, 1648
  framework, 1635, 1636
  intercurrent events, 1637–1643
  ITT, 1636
  meta-analysis, 1646
  missingness types, 1644, 1645
  network meta-analysis, 1646
  NI, 1647
  planning stage, 1643
  randomization and randomized clinical trials, 1634
  regulators, 1633
  safety, 1645
  time-to-event endpoints, 1645
Estimators, 1635, 1647, 1648
Ethics, 9–11, 27
Ethics Committees (ECs), 350, 666, 675
Ethics of clinical trials
  clinical equipoise, 59–60
  conception of trials, 57–58
  conduct, 66
  demarcated research procedures, 60
  fair subject selection, 62–63
  ICD, 65
  inclusion, 63–64
  maximizing efficiencies, 62
  research without informed consent, 65
  respect for persons, 64
  risk/benefit, 59
  riskless research, high risk research comparative effectiveness trials, 61–62
  valid informed consent, elements of, 64–65
Ethnicity, 13
Ethnic representation, 2238
EU clinical trials, regulatory affairs
  amendments, 474–475
  CTA submission, 473
  CTFG, 471–472
  CTReg, 475–476
  EMA, 472
  EudraLex, 471
  evolution, 470–471
  safety reporting and annual reporting, 475
  VHP, 473–474

EudraLex, 471
EU European Medicines Agency (EMA), 1963
European Heart Journal, 2323
European Medicines Agency (EMA), 173, 461, 467, 472, 1248, 2064, 2422
European Organization for Research and Treatment of Cancer (EORTC) QLQ-30 questionnaire, 925
European public assessment reports (EPARs), 1248
European Union Clinical Trial Register (EUCTR), 2064
European Union General Data Protection Regulation, 348, 361–363
Evaluation of randomization procedures for design optimization (ERDO), 869
Evidence-based decision-making, 2047
Evidence-based therapies, 2242
Ewoc package, 1112
Execution, problems in, 2466–2468
Executive Committee, 561, 565
Expanded access
  international regulations for, 2446–2447
  investigational devices, 2437–2442
  to investigational drugs, 2433
  pathways, 2433
  review requirements by, 2437
  submission process, 2433
Expanded disability status scale (EDSS), 901, 908
Expectation-maximization (EM) algorithm, 1844
Expert cross-disease teams (cores)
  clinical trials, 621, 622
  FDA application core, 621
  PROs, 621
  Rave study-build, 622
  recruitment and retention, 621
  standardized publication policy, 623
  training opportunities, 623
  translational medicine methods, 622
Expert determination, 2127–2129
  aggregation, 2129
  encoding, 2129
  guidance, 2128
  implementation of, 2127
  masking, 2128
  perturbation, 2129
  removal, 2128
  risk of re-identification, 2129
Exploratory analyses, 1426, 1431
ExTENd SMART study, 1548–1551
External validity, 2232, 2233

Extracorporeal membrane oxygenation (ECMO), 694
Extrapolation, 1239, 2228

F
Fabrication, 2320, 2322, 2327, 2328
Facility resources, 194–195
Factorial designs, 1370–1372
    characteristics, 1355–1358
    consequential features, 1364
    efficiencies, 1357–1358
    ethical and toxicity constraints, 1374
    hazard rates, 1359
    incomplete, 1373
    interactions/efficiency, 1355
    partial, 1372–1373
    structure, 1355–1357
    treatment effects, 1357
Factorial trials, 1358
    analysis of, 1363–1364
    biomarkers, design with, 1361–1363
    interaction, design with, 1360–1361
    interaction, design without, 1358–1360
    principle of, 1364
Failure-free survival (FFS), 1511
Fair allocation, 6
False Claims Act (FCA), 535–536, 2362
False discovery rate (FDR), 1409, 2280, 2332
Falsification, 2320–2322, 2327, 2328
Family-wise error rate (FWER), 909, 1473, 1661
Family-wise type I error rate (FWER), 1523–1524
Fast Healthcare Interoperability Resources (FHIR), 2254
FDA adverse event reporting system, 1965
FDA Adverse Event Reporting Systems (FAERS), 1964
FDA Amendments Act (FDAAA), 2064
FDA regulation
    adverse device effect reporting, 2444
    approval process, 2432
    compassionate use request, 2441
    device cost, 2444
    emergency use of investigational device, 2438
    expanded access program, 2437
    federal Right to Try Act, 2433
    HDE submission, 2444
    IND annual reports to, 2437
    local ethical review entity, 2435
    OOPD, 2444
    patient's condition, life-threatening, 2435
    periodic reports, 2445
    post approval reporting, 2444
    post approval requirements, 2441
    protocol by, 2436
    recommendations, 2445
    reporting timeline, 2439
Feasibility study, 38
Federal Controlled Substances Act (CSA), 180
Federal Policy for the Protection of Human Subjects, 2384
Federal wide Assurance (FWA), 664
Fidelity, 1421
File, 585–590
Financial compliance
    billing compliance, 527–531
    CMS reimbursement, 523–527
    non-compliance, 531–536
Financial conflicts of interest (FCOIs)
    in clinical trials, 543
    disclosures of potential, 548
    in human subject research, 548
    influence of, 555
    management, 546
    in medical research, 542
    recruitment and consent, 552
    risks, 543, 551
Financial cost, 2247–2248
Findable, accessible, interoperable and reusable (FAIR), 437
First in human studies, 1945–1946
Fischer and White approach, *see* Structural mean model approach
Fisher combination test, 2331
Fisher information matrix (FIM), 1121
Fisher's exact test, 1713, 1714, 1857
Fisher's information, 1514, 1515
Fish oil, 2265
Fixed effects, 1426
    model, 1349
    model parameters, 1942
    random effects, 1328
Fixed subset size procedure, 1050
Fixed versus random subset sizes, 1052–1053
Fleming approach, 1135
Flexibility, 2301
Flexible designs, 1085, 1088
Flexible machine learning models, 2011, 2019
Flexible randomization programs, 791
Flying squad, 2218
FOCUS4 study in metastatic colorectal cancer, 1479–1480
Follow-on biologics, *see* Biosimilarity

Follow-up, 2391
Food and Drug Administration (FDA), 44, 460, 462, 464–470, 472, 600, 660, 1239, 1241, 1408, 1410–1412, 2290, 2410
Food and Drug Administration Amendments Act (FDAAA), 483
Food and Drug Administration Modernization Act (FDAMA), 480, 2063, 2301
Food and Drug Administration Safety and Innovation Act (FDASIA), 2302
Forced titration studies, 1951
Forcing index (FI), 866
Forecasting, 353
Forest plots, 2184
Fourth International Study of Infarct Survival (ISIS-4), 1370
Fraud
  case studies, 2321–2325
  center scoring, 2331
  detection, 2328–2329
  misconduct, 2320
  on-site audit, 2332
  predisposing factors, 2325, 2326
  prevalence, 2326–2328
  statistical monitoring, 2329–2331
Fraud Recovery Plan, 2334
Fraudulent medical research, 2199
Fredrickson, Donald S., 74
Frequentist, 974–982, 985
Frequentist statistical approaches, 1939
Frequentist two-stage design
  vs. Bayesian predictive probability approach, 1043
  description, 1033–1035
  disadvantages, 1035
Friter v. Iolab Corp., 2352
Full time equivalent (FTE), 2464
Functional specification, 219, 222, 226, 227
Funder bias, 2048
Funder policies
  remits, 505–506
  on research culture, 506–507
Funding, 2458–2460
  decisions, 498, 504, 516
  models, 500, 507–508
  organizations, 514
  sources, 562
Futility, 1085, 1088, 1089, 1099
  monitoring, 1134, 1135
Futility design
  calibration control, 1073
  concurrently-controlled, 1074–1075

creatine and minocycline in early Parkinson disease, 1073–1075
intracerebral hemorrhage deferoxamine (i-DEF), 1075–1080
methodology, 1069
null hypothesis, 1071
sample size, 1077
sequential futility design, 1080
single-arm, 1071–1073
treatment-trial confounding, 1072

G
Gabapentin, 2381
GBM AGILE study in glioblastoma, 1478–1479
GCP contract service providers, 586–587
General Data Protection Regulation (GDPR), 361–363, 439, 2122, 2123
Generalized linear models, 1425, 1434
Generalized pairwise comparison (GPC)
  inference, 1874–1875
  measures of treatment effect, 1873–1874
  outcomes (*see* Prioritized outcome)
  stratification, 1875–1876
  Wilcoxon-Mann-Whitney test, 1872
Generalizing clinical trial results
  accounting for new findings and old data, 2233–2234
  COVID-19 vaccine trials, 2229
  harmful effects double standard, 2237–2238
  mechanistic models, 2230
  reduced variation, 2230
  sampling, 2231–2233
  shared biology, 2230, 2235–2237
General linear mixed model, 1818–1820
Generally Recognized as Safe (GRAS), 177
Generic manufacturing, 174
Generics, 1238, 1247, 1255
Genomic markers, 2419, 2421
Globalization, 12
Glucosamine, 2265
Glucose-6-phosphate dehydrogenase (G6PD) deficiency, 2421
Good clinical practice (GCP), 95, 124, 129, 131, 244, 356, 363, 429–431, 462
  critical aspect, 653
  definition, 650
  development, 651
  documents, 654, 655
  goals, 650
  guideline, 651
  historical timeline, 651, 652

Good clinical practice (GCP) (*cont.*)
 ICH, 651
 IRB/EC, 653
 principles, 655
 privacy, 654
Good distribution practice (GDP), 650
Good documentation practice (GDoP), 650
Good manufacturing practice
  (GMP), 462, 650
Governance and organizational issues,
  2464–2466
Governance models, 27
Government-sponsored trials, 683
Gray's tests, 1763–1765
Greenberg Report, 74, 75
Group/cluster randomized trials (GRT),
  2272, 2273
Group sequential methods, 1085, 1090
Group Statistician, 617
Guidance for Clinical Trials, 1591
Guidelines for Human Experimentation, 2383
Gumbel copula model, 1117

H

Hamiltonian Monte Carlo algorithm, 1933
Hard endpoints, 2388
Hawthorn effect, 2214
Hazard function, 1720
Hazard rate, 1720
Hazard ratio (HR), 887, 1269, 1512, 1513
Health Authorities (HA), 350, 351
Health Care Finance Administration, 523, 524
Healthcare providers, 1419, 1422, 1436
Healthcare systems, 579
Health Insurance Portability and Accountability
  Act (HIPAA), 439
Health-related quality of life (HRQOL),
  924–925
Health-related research, 504
Health status, 923–925
Health technology assessment (HTA), 923
Heart muscle regeneration, 2325
Hematopoetic stem cells, 2304
Hepatotoxicity, 2280
Herbal/botanical products, 2264, 2267, 2268
Hereditary transthyretin-mediated amyloidosis
  (hATTR), 2304
Heterogeneity, 2183–2187
Hierarchical/nested design, 1426
High costs, clinical trials
  financial cost, 2247–2248
  opportunity cost, 2248–2249

High-dose chemotherapy, 2322
HIPAA Privacy Rule, 2120, 2122, 2124–2126,
  2130, 2132, 2134
HIP breast cancer study, 1601–1602
Historical controls/comparators, clinical trials,
  879, 1463–1464
 analytic methods, 886–887
 data sources, 881–882
 information bias, 885–886
 quality, 880
 selection bias, 885
 test efficacy, 887–888
Historical information, 1251, 1252
Hochberg procedure, 733, 2280
Holm procedure, 733, 2280
Hommel procedure, 733
Hormone therapy, 2204
Hosmer-Lemeshow test, 1799, 2013
Human health, 2207
Humanitarian Device Exemption (HDE), 2433,
  2437, 2443
Humanitarian Use Device (HUD), 2433,
  2437, 2443
Human protections policies, 61, 62
Human trial, 944
Hybrid Bayes-frequentist methodology, 1253
Hydroxyethyl starch (HES), 2324
Hypotheses, 2201
Hypothesis testing, 979, 991, 993, 998, 1448,
  1593, 1704–1706
 controversies in, 1627
 definition, 1620
 framework, 1621
 of null hypothesis, 1622
 power, 1622
Hypothetical Factorial Trial, 1366
Hypothetical platform trial, experimental
  treatment arms and control, 1464, 1465
Hypothetical strategy, 1639

I

Idea, Development, Exploration,
  Assessment and Long-term study
  (IDEAL), 1422
Imaging committee, 565
Immunogenicity, 1242
Imputation
 Markov Chain Monte Carlo, 1694–1696
 multiple, 1692–1694
 multiple imputation using chained
  equations, 1696–1697
 regression, 1690–1692

Incentives
    orphan drug exclusivity, 2295–2296
    orphan drug grants, 2298
    PRV, 2296–2297
    tax credits, 2298
    user fee exemption, 2299
    written protocol assistance, 2299
Incomplete block
    analysis of, 1347
    cross-over design, 1346
    design, 1345
    type, 1326
Incomplete factorial designs, 1373
Incremental net health benefit (INHB), 1975
Incremental risk-benefit ratio (IRBR), 1976
Independent data monitoring committee (IDMC), 249, 378, 1533
Independent Ethics Committees (IECs), 196
Independent Statistical Center, 378
Independent Statistical Reporting Group (ISRG), 682
Independent trial steering committee (TSC), 249
Indexed medical journals, 2031
Indifference-zone approach, 1050
Individual-level regression methods, 1500
Individually randomized designs, 1425–1428
Individually randomized group-treatment (IRGT), 2272, 2273
Individual organizational units, 562, 563
Individual paper approach, 2032
Individual participant data (IPD), 435–437, 448–449, 2192
    general preparation, 449
    study-specific activity, 450–451
Individual participant-level data (IPD), 2140, 2147, 2150
Industry-sponsored clinical trials, 2059
Industry-sponsored trials, 683
Infectious disease trials, 1637
Informal trials of therapy, 1282
Information bias, 885–886
Information component (IC), 1966
Informed assent, 2384, 2389
Informed consent, 64, 113, 283, 652, 658, 659, 661, 663, 666, 667, 669, 670, 676, 1221, 2117, 2384, 2389, 2438
    assessment of comprehension, 403
    in Canada, 404–405
    community approval, 393
    context, 402
    definition, 390
    discussion, 401
    documentation, 394–401, 669–673
    ICD, 65
    lack capacity, 391
    materials, 401
    non-native speaker, 392
    parental permission, 392
    process, 91–92
    re-consent, 403
    research without, 65
    termination of, 404
    understandable Language, 402
    in United Kingdom, 406–409
    valid informed consent, elements of, 64–65
    waivers of, 673–674
Informed consent document (ICD), 65
Informed presence, 2313
In-house tools
    automatic monthly study reports, 627
    comprehensive statistical reporting tool, 625, 626
    site performance metrics reports, 628
    specimen tracking application, 626, 627
    statistical design calculators, 627
Initiative on Methods, Measurements, and Pain Assessments in Clinical Trials (IMMPACT), 1650
Institutional conflicts of interest (Institutional COIs), 549
Institutional Performance Report (IPR), 628
Institutional Review Boards and Ethics Committees (IRBs/ECs), 651
Institutional review boards (IRBs), 66, 90, 91, 175, 196, 350, 391, 531, 659, 2049, 2351–2354, 2383, 2384
    criteria for IRB approval, 668–669
    ethics violations, 661–662
    functions and operations, 663–669
    informed consent, 669–674
    National Commission and Belmont Report, 659–661
    records, 667–668
    review levels, 666–667
    review of research and definitions, 664–666
    revision of Common Rule, 662–663
    single IRB review and IRB reliance, 674–675
Instrumental variables methods, 1986, 1999
Integrated hazard function, 1721
Integrative health approach
    conventional medical care, 2264
    efficacy outcomes assessment, 2279–2280
    mind and body, 2270–2278
    natural products, 2266–2270

Integrative health approach (*cont.*)
  participant recruitment and retention, 2278, 2279
  reporting research results, 2280
  safety outcomes assessment, 2280
Intellectual property disputes, 2359–2360
Intention to treat (ITT), 1590–1593, 1636
  analysis, 1310, 2277
  approach, 796
  design considerations, 1610–1611
  missing data, 1607–1608
  noninferiority or equivalence trials, 1609
  plan, 1271
  principle, 1604–1605
Interaction, 1148
Interactive voice/web response system (IxRS), 270, 271
Interchangeability, 1247
  BPCI Act, 1249
  EMA, 1251
  FDA's study design, 1250
  immune system complications, 1250
  parallel groups design, 1249
  statistical methodologies, 1251
  switching and non-switching sequences, 1250
  therapeutic equivalence, 1250
  treatment-naive patients, 1249
Intercurrent events
  composite strategy, 1642
  dropouts, 1643
  hypothetical strategy, 1639
  principal stratification, 1639–1642
  treatment policy strategy, 1638, 1639
  treatment strategy, 1643
Inter-eye correlation, 1381, 1387, 1389
Interim analysis, 630, 632, 824, 827, 1458, 1471
  applications, 1087–1089
  data types in, 1086–1087
  methods of, 1089–1092
Interim monitoring, 1084, 1134–1135, 1138
  See also Interim analysis
Interim publications, 2470
Intermediate endpoints, 2388
Intermediate outcome, 1511, 1514, 1515, 1517, 1521, 1528, 1533, 1538
Internal review, 2093, 2096, 2098
Internal validation, 2017–2019
International Agency for Research on Cancer (IARC), 2237
International Air Transport Association (IATA), 185

International Association of Clinical Research Nurses (IACRN), 125
International Classification of Diseases (ICD) code, 530
  ICD10 code Z00.6, 530
International Clinical Trials Registry Platform (ICTRP), 2064
International Committee of Medical Journal Editors (ICMJE), 530, 2063, 2110
International Conference on Harmonization (ICH), 152
International Council for Harmonization (ICH), 197, 463, 1633
International Ethics Committee (IEC), 179
International regulatory authorities, 173
Interoperability, 2148–2150
Interpretation, 2210, 2221
Interrater reliability, 902
Inter-subject reliability, 903
Interventional study, 484
Intervention group allocation, 2275
Intervention specific appendix (ISA), 1460
Intracerebral hemorrhage deferoxamine (i-DEF), 1075
Intra-class Correlation Coefficient (ICC), 1424
Intracluster correlation coefficient, 1491
Intraocular pressure (IOP), 1381
Inventory management, 181, 182
Inverse probability weighting, 1686–1689
Inverse variance meta-analysis, 2182
Investigational device
  expanded access to, 2437–2442
  individual patient/small group compassionate, 2440
  single patient emergency use, 2438
  treatment use, 2441
  use of, 2433
Investigational device exemption (IDE), 523, 2437
Investigational drug
  expanded access pathways, 2433
  expanded access to, 2433
  FDA regulations, 2433
  intermediate-size population and treatment use, 2436–2437
  single patient emergency use, 2435–2436
  single patient treatment use of, 2434–2435
Investigational medicinal product (IMP)
  distribution, 354
  forecasting, 353
Investigational new drug (IND), 171, 197, 462, 468–469, 2267
  amendments, 469–470

annual reporting, 470
application, 524, 526, 662, 2292
safety reporting, 470
Investigational product (IP), 198
  blinded, 171
  distribution, 170, 178–187
  guidelines, 170
  manipulation, 171
  pharmacy, 171
  placebo, 170
  procurement, 172–178
  safety and efficacy, 170
Investigational Product Procurement Planning, 177
Investigative team
  motivation, 199
  research experience and past performance, 200, 201
  site team dynamics, 199
Investigator, 88
  commitments, 198
  definition, 87
  IRB, 91
  protocol noncompliance and misconduct, 92–93
  qualification, 198
  research study design and conduct, 87–90
  responsibilities, 87, 197–198
  safeguards to protect research participants, 90–92
  selection plan, 193, 194, 196
Investigator Brochure (IB), 601
Investigator-initiated, 605, 606, 610
Investigator-Initiated Clinical Trials, 609
Investigator's Brochure, 642
Investigatorship, 584
  external teams, 589
  GCP CSPs, 586–587
  Investigator site team, 587–589
  training documentation and files, 589–590
  training meetings, 589
  trial sponsor team, 584–586
Investigator site team, 587, 650
  PI Delegation of Authority, 587–588
  site monitoring visits, 588–589
IP distribution
  accountability, 183–185
  controlled substances, 180
  inventory management, 181, 182
  qualified sites, 179
  quality assurance, 187
  shipping and receipt, 185, 187
iPLEDGE® program, 1969

IP procurement
  blinded trials manipulation, 173, 174
  blinded trials manufacturing and packaging, 176, 177
  controlled substances, 174
  generic drug, 173
  international clinical trials, 177, 178
  packaging considerations, 176
  planning, 172
  qualified vendors, 175
I-SPY COVID-19 trial, 1477
Issues in publishing, 2469
16-item Stroke impact scale (SIS-16), 847

J

James Lind Library Initiative, 2046
Japanese Society of Anesthesiologists (JSA), 2323
Joint modeling approach, 1694–1696
Joint probability distribution, 1921
Joint Task Force (JTF) for Clinical Trial Competency, 129, 130
Journal club, 2228
Journal supplement *vs.* regular issue, 2032
Justice, 57, 62–64

K

Kaplan-Meier estimator, 1760
  of survival function, 1722–1726
Kawasaki disease, 2381
Kernke v. The Menninger Clinic, 2347
Kershaw v. Reichert, 2353
Key opinion leaders (KOLs), 584, 589
Key risk indicators, 2330
KRAS-wild-type tumors, 1138
Kruskal-Wallis test, 1711
Kullback-Leibler divergence, 945, 948
Kus v. Sherman Hospital, 2351

L

Laboratory committee, 565
Laboratory (preclinical) experiments, 2229
Language bias, 2048, 2053, 2054
Last observation carried forward (LOCF) analysis, 1609, 1633
Latent ignorability, 1641
Lead time, 1223, 1225
Learning assessments, 1422

Length bias, 1224, 1225
Length of follow-up, 2461
Levin-Robbins-Leu (LRL) family, 1053
　of sequential subset selection procedures, 1055
Levin-Robbins-Leu procedure, 1050
Levin-Robbins-Leu selection procedures, 1060
Life expectancy (LE), 2405
Life-table estimator, of survival function, 1726–1727
Life-threatening illnesses
　and clinician, FDA requirement, 2435
　expanded access, 2448
　intervention before review, 2436
　investigational drug, 2434
Lifetime prevalence, 2327
Likelihood-based methods, 1684–1686
Likelihood ratio (LR), 1062, 2331
Limited data set, 2126
Linear models, 1368–1370
Lipid-altering drugs, 2204
Lipitor multidistrict litigation, 2363
Litigation, 2340, 2341, 2355
　pharmaceutical and medical device mass tort, 2363–2364
　securities, 2360–2361
Liu v. Janssen Research & Development, 2348
Location bias, 2048
Log hazard ratio, 1512, 2373
Logistic regression, 1790
　binary (*see* Binary logistic regression)
　case study, 1804–1808
　fitted model, 1798–1804
　model, 1920, 1923, 1931
　multivariable, 1796–1798
　sampling design, 1798
Logrank tests, 1734–1737, 1739–1740, 1761
　multiple groups, 1737–1738
　stratified logrank test, 1738–1739
Longitudinal data
　individual dynamic prediction, 1932
　joint modelling, 1923–1933
　model specification and estimation, 1921–1923
　population prediction supporting clinical trial design, 1923–1932
Longitudinal growth modeling, 1819–1820
Longitudinal studies
　benefits, 911
　description, 910
　drawbacks and complications, 911–912
Looney v. Moore, 2357
Lotronex (alosetron), 1969

Low enrollment rate, clinical trials, 2244
　consequences of, 2246
　patient perspective, 2244
　site investigator/site perspective, 2245
Lower-bound formula, 1057
Lung cancers, 2421

M

Machine learning, clinical trials
　patient recruitment and engagement, 2259–2260
　phenotyping complex diseases, 2257–2259
　risk prediction, 2259
Macromolecules, 2295
Macular photocoagulation study (MPS), 2104
Major adverse cardiovascular events (MACE), 690
Management plan, 548, 552, 554, 555
Mann-Whitney test, 1709
Mann-Whitney Wilcoxon test, 1594
Manual of operations, 40
Marginal Quasi-Likelihood (MQL), 1434
Marginal structural model, 2277
Margin of non-inferiority, 1298, 1302–1305
Marketing authorization, 173, 460, 465–467, 476, 477
Marketing authorization application (MAA), 461, 464, 467, 471, 472
Markov Chain Monte Carlo, 1694–1696
Masked data monitoring, 2466
Masking, 816–820, 825, 826, 828–830
　in clinical trials, 816
　of drugs, 818
　effect of, 817
　goals of, 817
　participants, 817, 818
　purpose of, 816
Masking (blinding), 806, 2463
　randomized trials, 806–810
Mask investigators, randomized trials, 810–813
Massage, 2264, 2270, 2271
Mass spectrometry, 1241
Master protocols, 576, 1135, 1456
MAST method, 2372, 2373
Matched/paired design, 837
Matchpoint trial, 1118–1119
Material Usage Agreement (MUA), 633
Maternal mortality, 2219–2220
Maximum acceptable risk (MAR), 1977
Maximum likelihood (ML), 1641
Maximum likelihood estimate (MLE), 1444–1447, 1536

Maximum likelihood method, 1843–1844
Maximum tolerated dose (MTD)
  curve, 1005
  definition, 1004
  dose combination, 1006
  estimation, 1010
  recommendation, 1016
  reparametrization, 1006
  tolerable dose combination, 1023
McNemar test, 1392–1395
Mean body temperatures, 2333
Measurement errors, 835, 836
Mechanistic models, 2230
Mechanistic pharmacodynamic models, 1943
Mediation analysis, 1983, 1993
Medical device
  Bayesian design, for device trials, 1409–1411
  blinding/masking, 1403
  definition, 1400
  diagnostics, special considerations for, 1407–1409
  drugs vs. devices, 1400–1403
  implants, 1402–1403
  mechanism of action, 1401
  observational (non-randomized) clinical studies, 1411–1414
  placebo effect and sham control, 1403
  safety and efficacy/effectiveness assessment, 1401–1402
  skill of the user, 1402
  therapeutic device trials, design considerations for, 1403–1407
Medical dictionary for regulatory activities (MedDRA) coding system, 900
Medical product, 1251
Medical Research Council (MRC), 1420
Medical therapy, 2250
Medicare coverage, see CMS reimbursement
Meditation, 2264, 2265, 2270, 2272, 2274, 2276
Meeting conduct, 565
Melatonin, 2265
Mendelian genetics, 2207
Meta-analysis, 1646, 2161, 2163, 2167, 2172, 2180
  binary data, 2181
  common effect, 2182–2183
  continuous data, 2181
  heterogeneity, 2183–2187
  IPD, 2192
  meta-regression, 2188–2190
  NMA, 2192–2193

  random effects, 2183
  small-study effects and publication bias, 2190–2191
  subgroup analysis, 2187–2188
  summary effect, 2182
  time-to-event data, 2181
  within-trial bias, 2190
Metadata, 431, 433, 443, 444, 446–448, 450, 451, 2234
  file, 230
Meta-regression, 2188–2190
95/95 method, 1302–1303
Microarray, 2324
Mind and body, 2264
  adherence, 2276–2277
  contamination, 2277
  design and randomization strategies, 2272
  fidelity, intervention delivery, 2275
  intervention and appropriate controls, 2270–2271
  masking, 2274–2275
  missing data, 2277–2278
  randomization and trial design, 2271–2274
Minimax design, 1033, 1034
Minimization, 754–757
Minimum clinical efficacy (MCE), 1974
Minority health, 2418
Minority inclusion, 2418, 2422–2424
Minority populations, clinical trials
  applicability of clinical findings, 2419
  defining and categorizing populations, 2419–2421
  minority inclusion, 2422, 2424
  NIH, 2423
  race, 2421
  subset analysis, 2424
Misconduct, 2320, 2322, 2327, 2334
Missing at random (MAR), 1213, 1644, 1683, 1685
Missing completely at random (MCAR), 1591, 1644
Missing data, 1605, 1607–1608, 1815, 2204
Missing not at random (MNAR), 1645
Missing observations, 2204
Missing outcome data, 1591–1592
Mitigation of issues, 360–361
Mixed effect model, 1392, 1942
Mixed model repeated measures (MMRM), 1212
Mixed model with repeated measures (MMRM), 1644
Model Agreements & Guidelines International (MAGI), 534

Model-based analysis, 1393
Model calibration, 2012–2013
Model discrimination, 2013–2015
Modifications to the ITT (mITT), 1606
Modified intention-to-treat approach, 797
Modified-ITT (mITT) population, 1310
Modified probability toxicity interval (mTPI) method, 956
Monitoring, 240, 246–248, 252, 586, 588–590, 2391
    and auditing, 356–357
Monographs, 2031
Monotone missingness, 1645
Monte Carlo randomization test, 1855
Monte Carlo simulation (MCS), 1976
Monte Carlo simulations and trial design, 1565–1567
    SPYRAL HTN OFF-MED trial, 1575–1582
    VALOR trial, 1567–1574
Motivation, 199, 275
MOXonidine CONgestive Heart Failure (MOXCON) trial, 694
MRC Complex Intervention guidance, 1422
Multi-arm multi-stage design (MAMS), 1164–1165
Multi-arm multi-stage (MAMS) randomized clinical trial, 1508, 1510, 1537
    advantages, 1510–1511
    analysis at interim and final stages, 1519
    analysis considerations, 1535–1537
    binding/non-binding stopping boundaries, 1523
    conduct considerations, 1535
    correlation structure, 1521–1522
    design considerations, 1532–1535
    design specification, 1513–1517
    family-wise type I error rate, all-pair/any-pair power, 1523–1525
    intermediate and definitive outcomes, 1520–1521
    new research, 1527–1528
    operating characteristics, 1521–1525
    pairwise design significance level and power, 1519–1520
    pairwise type I error rate (PWER) and power, 1522–1523
    selection designs, 1525–1527
    software, 1528–1532
    steps to design, 1518–1519
Multicenter clinical trials (MCCTs), 560, 561
    design considerations, 141–142
    formation, 138–139
    sites in, 142–144
    trial leadership, 140–141

Multicenter collaborations, 28
Multi-center trial, 643
    organizational units, 98
    participant close-out phase, 116
    participant enrollment phase, 113–116
    phases, 102
    post-funding phase, 116
    resource centers, 98–113
Multi-component, 1419, 1422, 1429, 1435
Multi-criteria decision analysis (MCDA), 1976
Multidimensional data, 1272
Multifactorial interventions, 2406
    assignment of components, 2408
    eligibility criteria, 2407
    individual component effects, 2408–2409
    risk factors, 2407
    sample size calculations, 2408
    selecting components, 2407
    treatment allocation, outcome assessment and adjudication, 2407–2408
Multi-item Gamma Passion Shrinker (MGPS), 1966, 1967
Multimorbidity, 2404, 2406
Multiphase optimization strategy (MOST), 1422
Multiple chronic conditions (MCC), 2403, 2405
Multiple comparisons, 1661, 1664
Multiple endpoints, 1594
Multiple imputation, 1592, 1692–1694
Multiple interim analyses, 1576
Multiple measures, outcomes, 907–910
Multiple Membership Multiple Classification (MMMC), 1429
Multiple outcomes
    analysis methods, 1871
    composite pairwise score, 1878
    overall pairwise score, 1878
    prioritized outcome, 1879–1880
Multiple regression analysis, 838
Multiple sclerosis, 572
Multiple sclerosis functional composite (MSFC), 901
Multiplicity, 730–731, 2279
    multiple sources, 734
    single sources, 732–734
    software, 734
Multi-site clinical trial, 601, 608
Multi-site coordinating center, 610
Multi-site investigator-initiated, 605
Multi-sponsor platform trials, 1461–1462
Multi-stage randomized trial, *see* Sequential, multiple assignment, randomized trial (SMART)

Multivariable fractional polynomial interaction
   (MFPI) procedure, 1903, 1910, 1913
Multivariate analysis methods, 1871, 2058
Multivariate normal model, 1696
Myelodysplastic syndrome, 1136
MyHeart Counts Cardiovascular Health
   Study, 2255
Myocardial infarction (MI), 1718, 2203

N
Nasolacrimal mucosa, 1381
National Academy of Medicine
   (NAM), 1271
National Academy of Sciences (NAS), 1633
National Advisory Heart Council, 74
National Breast Cancer Coalition, 575
National Cancer Institute (NCI), 572, 629
National Cancer Trial Network (NCTN),
   616–617, 629
National Center for Advancing Translational
   Sciences (NCATS), 940
National Clinical Trial (NCT) number, 530
National Commission for the Protection of
   Human Subjects of Biomedical and
   Behavioral Research, 659
National Competent Authorities (NCAs),
   471–476
National Conference on Clinical Trials
   Methodology, 78–79
National Cooperative Gallstone Study
   (NCGS), 2106
National Emphysema Treatment Trial (NETT),
   2032, 2109
National Health Interview Survey
   (NHIS), 2264
National Heart, Lung, and Blood Institute
   (NHLBI), 74–79, 2130
National Institute for Health Research
   (NIHR), 500
National Institute of Standards and
   Technology, 2130, 2131
National Institute on Aging, 2412
National Institutes of Health (NIH), 74,
   76–78, 80
National Library of Medicine (NLM), 2110
National lung screening trial (NLST), 1223
National Patient-Centered Clinical Research
   Network (PCORnet), 2251
National Research Council (NRC), 1633
National Surgical Adjuvant Breast and Bowel
   Project (NSABP), 638, 2321
Natural history, 1264, 1267, 1273, 1274
   studies, 2303, 2304

Natural products, 2264
   alternative trial designs, 2269, 2270
   assessing intervention quality, 2268–2269
   biomarkers, 2266
   compliance and contamination, 2269
   intervention and appropriate controls,
      2266–2267
   knowledge base, 2266
   randomization and masking, 2267, 2268
NCI Community Oncology Research Program
   (NCORP), 617
Neaton, James, 79
Negative predictive value, 1177
Negligence, 2341–2343
Nelson-Aalen estimator, of cumulative hazard
   function, 1727–1728
Neovascular age-related macular degeneration
   (AMD), 1880
Net Benefit, 1873–1874
Network meta-analysis (NMA), 1646,
   2192–2193
Network security, 624
Neupogen, 1245
Neutropenia, 1247
New drug application (NDA), 1651, 2297
Next generation sequencing (NGS), 576, 1409
Neyman concept, 1836
NIH 2014 Consensus Response Criteria
   Working Group, 881
NIH-funded Pediatric Heart Network, 2384
NIH Genomic Data Sharing Policy, 2131
NIH PROMIS, 926–927
NIH Revitalization Act, 2422
Nitrate's Effect on Activity Tolerance in
   Heart Failure With Preserved
   Ejection Fraction (NEAT-HFpEF)
   trial, 2257
NLM-Scrubber, 2131
Nocebo effect, 1282
N-of-1 randomized control trial (RCT), 1281,
   1285, 1293
   advanced techniques, 1287
   age restrictions, comorbidity/concurrent
      therapy, 1282
   aggregation, 1289–1290
   anticipated benefits, 1283
   benefits, 1284
   collaboration with pharmacy, 1287
   definition, 1280
   determining appropriateness, 1284–1285
   drug development, 1283
   ethics, 1290–1291
   evidence-based management options, 1283
   history, 1281

N-of-1 randomized control trial (RCT) (*cont.*)
  informal trials of therapy, limitations of, 1282
  mean daily Likert score, 1292
  mean period score, 1292
  medication, 1283
  non-parametric statistical tests, 1288
  outcomes, 1285–1286
  parametric statistical tests, 1289
  randomization, 1287
  reporting, 1290
  treatment and placebo difference scores, 1293
  treatment response, 1282
  trial length, 1286
  t-test results, 1294
  visual inspection, 1288
Non-adaptive biomarker-guided trial designs
  biomarker strategy design, 1154–1157
  enrichment designs, 1152
  hybrid design, 1153–1154
  marker stratified design, 1153
  phase II clinical trial design, 1158–1159
  reverse biomarker-based strategy, 1157–1158
  single-arm designs, 1151
Non-adherence, 1984, 1987, 1988, 1999
Non-comparative designs, 1089
Non-comparative observational study, 1412
Non-compliance, 92, 177, 1641, 1649, 1834, 1838, 1848
  civil money penalties, 532
  subject injury, 533, 534
  waiving of co-pays, 532, 533
Non-identifiability problem, 1757–1758
Non-inferiority (NI) trial, 1211, 1215, 1298, 1308, 1647
  assay sensitivity, 1311–1312
  averted infections ratio, 1319
  Bayesian approaches, 1316–1317
  choice of analysis populations and estimands, 1310–1311
  combination therapies, 1303–1304
  confidence interval and, 1626
  CONSORT, 1307
  definition, 1626
  DISCOVER, 1301
  drawbacks of, 1626
  effect preservation, 1312–1313
  hypotheses and notation, 1299
  and inferiority, 1309
  interim analyses and data and safety monitoring, 1315–1316
  justification of margin in practice, 1315
  95/95 method, 1302–1303
  motivation, 1300
  noninferiority margin, 1626
  pragmatic superiority strategy trial, 1318–1319
  public health clinical criteria, 1304–1305
  regulatory guidelines, 1306–1307
  sample size, 1305–1306
  sensitivity of trial results, 1314–1315
  setting, 1626
  STREAM, 1301–1302
  and superiority, 1313–1314
  three-arm NI design, 1318
  trial designs, 1317
Non-inferiority-type test, 1243
Non-informative prior distributions, 1036–1037
Non-linear mixed effects modeling, 1942
Non-linear Parkinson disease progression model, 1931
NONMEM, 1930
Nonparametric estimation, survival analysis
  hazard function, estimators of, 1728–1730
  Kaplan-Meier estimator, of survival function, 1722–1725
  left-truncated data, estimation for, 1730–1731
  life-table estimator, of survival function, 1726–1727
  Nelson-Aalen estimator, of cumulative hazard function, 1727–1728
  right-truncated data, estimation for, 1731–1733
Non-parametric statistical tests, 1288
Non-parametric test
  for categorical variables, 1713–1715
  for multiple groups, 1711
  t-tests, 1708
Non-pharmacologic treatment strategies, 2284
Non-significant risk (NSR) device, 529
Normal distribution model, 2235
Normality, 1853, 1861, 1862
No test strategy, 1184
Novartis-sponsored phase II open-entry platform trial, 1461
Nuisance parameter, 1086, 1091
Null hypothesis, 863, 866, 870, 1621, 1673
Numbering publications, 2107
Numbering related trials, 2107
Number needed to harm (NNH), 1973, 1974
Number needed to treat (NNT), 1973, 1974
Numerical rating scale (NRS), 1650
Nutrition researchers, 2219
N-year survival rate, 1224

O

Objective performance criterion (OPC), 1412
O'Brien-Fleming efficacy, 1568
Observational (non-randomized) clinical studies, 1411
  bias, 1412–1413
  comparative observational study, 1411–1412
  non-comparative observational study, 1412
  outcome-free design, 1413–1414
Observational study, 2219
Observer-reported outcomes, 907
Ocular Surface Disease Index (OSDI), 1385
Odds ratio, 887, 1794, 1797, 1804
  confidence intervals for, 1795
  fitted multivariable logistic regression model, 1807
  fitted univariable logistic regression model, 1805
Office for Human Research Protections (OHRP), 360, 662
Office for Protection from Research Risks (OPRR), 662
Office of Orphan Products Development (OOPD), 2291, 2443
Office of the Inspector General, 523
Older adults, in clinical trials
  Alzheimer's disease and age-related dementias, 2409–2412
  barriers to participation, recruitment and retention, 2400–2403
  ethics, 2398–2400
  multifactorial interventions, 2406–2409
  multimorbidity and polypharmacy, 2404–2405
  selection of outcomes, 2403–2404
  time to benefit, time to harm and life expectancy, 2405–2406
Oligonucleotide therapy, 2304
Omics models, 2324
Oncology, 2389
Oncology Center of Excellence (OCE), 572
Online education program, 2386
Online Wound Electronic Medical Record (OWEMR), 1610
On-site monitoring, 2328
Open calls, 508
Open platform master protocol, 1458, 1459
Open report, 824
Operating characteristics, 960–961
Operational data model (ODM), 446
Operational efficiency, 608
Ophthalmic trials, 1380

Ophthalmology, 1378, 1383
Opportunity cost, 2248–2249
Optical character recognition system, 623
Optimal design, 1033
Optimal design theory, 1121
OPTIM-ARTS design, 1471
Oral autopsies, 2212
Ordinal outcomes, 898
Organizational units, 562
Organization and management (OM)
  committee roles and structure, 564–566
  committees, 561, 564–566
  funding source and trial operations, 562
  individual organizational units, 562, 563
  threats and failures, 566–567
  trial participants, 560
  trial planning, 560
Organization structure, 563
Orphan diseases, see Rare diseases
Orphan drug(s)
  amendment, 2294
  approved indications, 2290, 2291
  clinical development, 2290
  clinical superiority, 2299
  clinical trials, 2291
  cost recovery, 2299
  designation, 2292
  evidence, 2300–2302
  exclusivity, 2295–2296
  FDA, 2300
  grants, 2298
  incentives, 2294–2299
  natural history studies, 2303, 2304
  ODDRs, 2292–2294
  patient voice, 2302–2303
  sponsor, 2300
Orphan Drug Act (ODA), 2291, 2292, 2299, 2305, 2443
Orphan drug designation requests (ODDRs)
  elements, 2292
  identification of disease/condition, 2292, 2293
  population estimation, rarity of disease/condition, 2294
  scientific rationale for drug usage, 2293
  submission, 2292
Orphan Drug Tax Credit (ODTC), 2298
Orphan subsets, 2293
Osteopathic manipulation, 2264
Osteopenia/osteoporosis, 2204
Outcome-adaptive randomization, 1140–1141
Outcome measurement, 1392
Outcome measures, 1664–1671

Outcome reporting bias, 2050, 2056, 2060, 2062
Outcomes in clinical trials, 892
　biomarkers, 896–897
　categorial, 897
　clinician-reported outcomes, 907
　common measures, 898–899
　definition, 892
　direct endpoints, 894
　longitudinal studies, 910–912
　multiple measures, 907–910
　nominal *vs.* ordinal, 898
　non-statistical and practical considerations, 901
　observer-reported outcomes, 907
　patient-reported outcomes, 906–907
　primary and secondary, 893
　quantitative, 897
　reliability, 902–903
　response shift, 903
　safety, 899–900
　surrogate endpoints, 894–896
　validity, 901–902 (*see also* Trial outcomes)
Overall survival (OS), 1358, 1359, 1362, 1510
Overdiagnosis bias, 1224
Oversight, 240, 241, 246, 248–251

P

Paced auditory serial addition test (PASAT), 903
Package labeling, 353–354
Packaging and shipping, 354
Pain management, 2271, 2280
Pain medications
　acute pain, 1650
　adequate pain, 1650
　chronic pain, 1650
　discontinuations, 1650
　FDA, 1651, 1652
Paired design, 1378
Paired-eye design, 1380
Pairwise type I error rate (PWER) and power, 1522–1523
Paper writing
　blackouts, 2034–2036
　design synopsis and study curriculum vitae, 2036
　presentation *vs.* publication, 2033–2034
　publication imperative, 2028, 2029
　publication issues, 2030–2033
　rules, 2037–2042
　study publications types, 2029
　trialist's oath, 2042

Parallel group trials, 1379
Parameter, 1616
　estimation, 1593
Parametric analyses, 1860–1862
Parametric models, for survival data, 1721–1722
Parametric statistical tests, 1289
Parametric test, 1712
Parkinson's disease, 1200
Partial factorial designs, 1372–1373
Partially nested trials, 1427
Partially ordered CRM (POCRM), 1123
Participant(s), 1263, 1264, 1266–1271, 1273
　close-out phase, 116
　recruitment, 566
Participant enrollment phase
　adverse events, 114
　data collection, 115
　data management, 115
　recruitment, 113
　scheduling and communications, 114
　screening and randomization, 113, 114
　site visits, 115
　study meetings, 116
　treatment and follow-up phase, 114
Participant follow-up, 292–293
　follow-up schedule, trial design, 293–294
　predicting retention, 297–298
　retention monitoring, 296–297
　site staff training, 294–295
　study team, in promoting retention, 298
　trial data collection, 294
Patient advocacy
　capturing and measuring, 577–578
　data generation, 578
　groups, 2387
　trial designs and endpoint selection, 575–577
Patient-centered approach, 570, 573
Patient-centered care, 1814
Patient-Centered Outcomes Research Institute (PCORI), 571, 2251
Patient community, 570
Patient engagement
　barriers, 574–575
　enrollment rates, 571
　research and drug development, 571–573
Patient-focused approach, 573
Patient-focused drug development (PFDD), 572, 2302, 2303
Patient-Powered Research Networks (PPRN), 2251

Index

Patient reported outcome (PRO), 578, 621, 847, 906–907, 1814, 1870, 2267
  area under the curve, 1820, 1821
  clinical trial protocol development, 932–933
  data visualization, 1826
  definitions related to, 917
  endpoint model, 919–920
  Europe, label claims in, 922
  FDA guidance, 931–932
  frequency and duration of assessments, 930–931
  general linear mixed model, 1818–1820
  healthcare utility and cost-effectiveness, 925–926
  health-related quality of life, 924–925
  intent-to-treat and treatment nonadherence, 1815–1816
  label claims in United States, 921–922
  measurement, 1815
  missing data, 1823–1826
  mode of administration and data collection method, 929–930
  multiplicity, 1823
  number of clinical trials with, 920
  PRO-CTCAE, 927–928
  PROMIS, 926–927
  quality-adjusted life years, 1822
  responder analysis, 1817–1818
  role in clinical trials, 919–921
  selection of, 928–929
  time-to-event analysis, 1821
Patient safety, 2327
Pediatric devices, 2391
Pediatric Heart Network, 2391
Pediatricians, 2386
Pediatric research
  drug testing, 2385
  educational programs, 2386
  financial incentives, 2385
  healthy children, 2385
  networks, 2386
  parental perceptions, 2385
  stakeholders, 2386
Peer review, 2094
Penalized Quasi-Likelihood (PQL), 1434
Peptide mapping, 1241
Percent correct selection (PCS), 960
Percutaneous coronary intervention (PCI), 1404
Perez v. Progenics Pharmaceuticals, Inc., 2361
Performance bias, 793–794
Period prevalence, 2327

Permutation test, 762, 1671–1677
  definition, 1854
  generalized, 1856–1858
  Monte Carlo, 1855
  vs. parametric test, 1855
  path dependence, 1858–1859
Permuted block design, 746–750
Permuted block randomization (PBR), 859
Per protocol analysis (PPA), 52
Per-protocol approach, 797
Per-protocol (PP) population, 1310, 1606
Personal injury lawsuits, 2340
  causation, 2357–2358
  damages, 2358
  negligence, 2341–2343
  product liability, 2343–2344
  theories of liability, 2341–2344
Personalized medicine, 1146, 1281, 1660
Pharmaceutical and medical device mass tort litigation, 2363–2364
Pharmaceuticals and Medical Devices Agency (PMDA), 476
Pharmacodynamic model, 1202
Pharmacoepidemiologic studies, 707
Pharmacogenetics, 2424
Pharmacokinetic and pharmacodynamic (PKPD) modeling
  advantages, 1942
  dose-ranging studies, 1948–1954
  first in human studies, 1945–1946
  precision medicine, 1954–1956
  proof of concept, 1946–1948
Pharmacokinetics (PK), 2390
  model, 1926
  pharmacodynamics (PK/PD), 1241, 1242
Pharmacovigilance, 703, 704, 1963
Phase II/III trial designs
  accrual suspension, 1137
  advantage, 1136
  azacitidine, 1136
  experimental *vs.* control comparisons, 1137
  parameters, 1136
  randomized patients, 1136
  time-to-event endpoint, 1137
Phase II clinical trials, 1032
  single-arm *vs.* two-arm, 1032
Phase II design, 1068
Phase II trials
  adaptive pooling, 1141–1142
  biomarkers, 1138–1139
  error-rate requirements, 1134
  interim monitoring, 1134–1135
  oncology, 1134

Phase II trials (*cont.*)
  outcome-adaptive randomization, 1140–1141
  phase III design, 1136–1137
  sample-size reassessment, 1139
Phase I trials, 1106
  cisplatin, 1113
  CRM and most designs for, 1107
  definition, 1107
  dose-escalation cancer trial, 1110–1111
  dual-agent, 1127
  dual-agent and dose-schedule-finding, 1121–1127
  feasibility bound, 1111–1112
  5-fluorouracil, 1109
  goals, 1106
  software, 1112
  toxicity grading, 1114–1116
Physicians' Health Study, 2422
Physiologically based pharmacokinetic (PBPK) model, 1956
Pill count, 284, 287–289
Pilot study, 37
Placebo, 818, 819
Placebo-controlled trial, 2202
Plagiarism, data fabrication, and fraud, 2468
Plagiarism, 2320
Platelet Glycoprotein IIb/IIIa in Unstable Angina: Receptor Suppression Using Integrilin Therapy (PURSUIT) Trial, 1718
Platform trials, 1456
  concurrent controls, 1464–1467
  control arm choice, 1463–1467
  data analysis issues, 1474–1476
  data monitoring and interim decisions rules, 1470–1472
  definition, 1457–1460
  EPAD-PoC study, 1476–1477
  FOCUS4 study, 1479–1480
  GBM AGILE study, 1478–1479
  historical controls, 1463–1464
  I-SPY COVID-19 trial, 1477
  multi-sponsor, 1461–1462
  randomization, 1467–1470
  sample size and power, 1472–1474
  single-sponsor, 1460–1461
  statistical considerations, 1462–1476
Point prevalence, 2327
Poisson-gamma model, 1565
Policy interventions, 4
Policy makers, 12
Polypharmacy, 2401, 2404, 2405

Population enrichment, 1441, 1450
Positive predictive value, 1177
Post approval setting, 701, 703, 704, 706, 709, 712, 715, 719, 721, 722
Post authorization, 701
  efficacy studies, 704, 705
  EMA legislation as, 703
  safety study, 704
Post-funding phase, 116
Post marketing, 701
  requirement, 721
  requirement authorities, 703
  surveillance, 1963, 1964, 1968, 1969
  US regulations as, 702
Postoperative nausea and vomiting (PONV), 2323
Power, 835, 1622–1624
  alternatives to, 782–783
  calculation, 768
  for common trial designs, 773–779
  for fixed sample size studies, 781
  on hypothesis testing, 768
  illustrations of, 769–772
  for non-inferiority studies, 779–780
  practical considerations, 783–784
  precision, 782
  prior approach, 1576
  prior method, 1578
  and sample size, 780–781
  sample size calculations in Bayesian settings, 782
  trade-offs in, 772–773
Pragmatic clinical trial, 2309–2310
  ascertainment and classification of end points, 2312–2313
  clinical trial site investigators vs. practicing physicians, 2315–2316
  electronic health record (*see* Electronic health record (EHR))
  vs. explanatory clinical trial, 2310–2311
  missingness, 2313–2314
Prebiotics, 2265
Precancer Atlas (PCA), 1272
Precision medicine, 1146, 2005
  initiative, 1954–1956
PRECIS wheel, 2310
Predatory journals, 2199
Predictability
  conditional allocation probability, 862–863
  correct guess, 861–862
  multi-arm trials, 865
  type I error probability, 863–866
Prediction intervals, 2186

Prediction models, *see* Risk prediction models
Predictive biomarkers, 1148, 2368, 2369
Predictive classifiers, 2369
Predictive probability (PP) approach, 1039–1042
  oncology example, 1042–1043
Preference zone, least favorable configuration in, 1061
Pregabalin, 1951
Pre-identification, 260
Preliminary exploratory analysis, 1955
Preliminary selection design, 1058
Prerandomization consent, 1221
Prerequisites, documents, 640
Pre-screening, 260
Prescription Drug User Fee Act (PDUFA V), 572
Presentation, 566, 2094, 2098, 2099
Presentation *vs.* publication, 2033, 2034
Press, 253
Prevention trials
  analysis ITT and adherence, 1270–1271
  biomarkers and emerging areas, 1271–1273
  disease process, 1264–1265
  dose, 1267–1268
  duration of exposure/intervention, risk reduction, 1268
  interpreting prevention trials, 1273
  outcomes for, 1269–1270
  sustainability of behavior change, 1265–1266
  time course of intervention, 1266–1267
  trial population, 1263–1264
Primary outcome, 893, 908, 2090–2092, 2094–2096, 2098, 2461
Primary prospective data collection, 881
Principal investigator (PI), 45, 124, 126–128, 130, 197
  definition, 587
  Delegation of Authority Log, 587–588
Principal stratification strategy
  cautions, 1641
  compliance, 1639, 1640
  fixed time, 1642
  noncompliance, 1641
  per protocol analyses, 1642
Prior-data conflict, 1252, 1253
Prior distribution, 983–987, 990
Prior hypothesis, 2232
Prioritized outcome
  benefit/risk assessments, 1886–1888
  binary, 1876
  continuous, 1876–1877
  multiple, 1878–1880
  repeated observations, 1883–1884
  thresholds of clinical relevance, 1880–1881
  time-to-event, 1877
  time-to-event outcome, 1884
Priority review vouchers (PRV), 2296–2297
Prior probability distribution, 1036
Privacy, 2118
Proactive safety surveillance, 1964
Probabilistic simulation methods (PSM), 1976
Probability of correct selection (PCS), 1050
Probiotics, 2264, 2265, 2284
Problems in execution, 2466
Procedural differences, 349–350
Process flow, 195
Process variable, 1989–1991, 1993, 1999
Product liability, 2343–2344
Product masking, 2268
Product of independent beta probabilities dose escalation design (PIPE), 1126
Prognostic biomarkers, 1147, 2368
Prognostic effect, 1662, 1666, 1668, 1670
Prognostic factor(s), 1594, 2368
Prognostic factor analysis, 1772
  improvement in statistical efficiency, 1773–1775
  prognostic factor selection, 1781–1785
  statistical models for, 1777–1780
  treatment effect heterogeneity, 1775–1776
Prognostic modeling, 1756
Prognostic models, 2005
Progression-free survival (PFS), 576, 1510, 1884, 1885, 1923
Proof of concept studies, 1946–1948
Proof-of-concept (PoC) trials, 1460
Propensity score (PS), 880, 887, 888, 1413
Proportional hazards, 1746, 1750–1752
Proportional odds (PO) model, 1115
Proportional reporting ratio (PRR), 1966, 1967
Proposal assessment processes, 508–516
Prospective data collection, 881, 883
Prospective Multicenter Imaging Study for Evaluation of Chest Pain (PROMISE) trial, 1186
Prospective Randomized Open Blinded Endpoint (PROBE) design, 812
Prospective Study of Pravastatin in the Elderly at Risk (PROSPER), 2402
Prostate, lung, colorectal and ovarian (PLCO) cancer screening trial, 1222, 1226, 1227, 1229
Prostate cancer, 1509–1511
Protected health information (PHI), 2120–2123

Protocol, clinical trial, 40
  data collection, 243
  IDMC, 249
  investigator meetings, 253
  planned monitoring visits, 247
  press, 253
  project team, 249
  protocol development, 240–241
  registration/randomisation system, 243
  risk and monitoring, 246–247
  site activation, timing of, 242
  site characteristics, 241–242
  site selection, feasibility and set up, 241
  social media, 252
  TMG, 249
  training, 243–246
  trial monitoring plan, 247
  trial oversight, 248–249
  trial promotion, 251
  trial risk assessment, 247
  trial website, 251–252
  triggered monitoring visits, 248
Protocol development, 616, 619
Protocol Review Committee (PRC), 619
Prototypical SMART design, 1551, 1552
Provider Assessment of Lipid Management (PALM) registry, 2256
Pseudorandom, 47
Psoriasis, 2322
Psychotherapy, 1421
Publication bias, 797–799, 2048–2050, 2055, 2057–2060, 2063, 2065
Publication policy, 2465
Publications, 566
Public health, 2266
  problems, 2219–2220
  professional, 2199, 2201
Public inspection databases, 177
Publicity, 251
Public Registry, 325, 338, 340, 345
Publishing, 324, 325
  issues in, 2469–2471
p-value, 979, 982, 1621, 1622

Q

Q-test, 2185, 2186
Qualifications, clinical research staff, 126–128
Qualified person (QP), 178
Qualifying clinical trials, 526
Qualitative analysis, 2058
Qualitative interaction, 1367

Quality-adjusted life year (QALY), 925–926, 1192, 1973, 1975
Quality-adjusted time without symptoms and toxicity (Q-TWiST), 1973
Quality adjusted time without symptoms of disease and toxicity of treatment (Q-TWIST), 926
Quality assurance, 187, 604
Quality by design, 2328
Quality control, 565, 603, 2470
  centers, 98
  review, 492
Quality management, 602–604, 609, 610, 613
Quality of life (QOL), 1642, 1814
Quality system, 585–587, 590
Quantitative decision making approach, 1243
Quantitative framework for benefit-risk assessment (QFBRA), 1971–1972
Quantitative interaction, 1366, 1367
Quantitative outcomes, 897
Quantitative system pharmacology (QSP) modeling, 1956
Questionnaires, 1815

R

Race, 2418–2421, 2423, 2425, 2426
  and ethnicity, 358
Random allocation rule (RAR), 859
Random assignment, 745–746
Random effects
  fixed, 1347
  independent, 1328
  meta-analysis, 2183
  model, 1339, 1349
  model parameters, 1942
Random errors, 835
Random intercept mixed model, 1819, 1820
Randomization, 114, 741, 759, 837, 856, 858, 1287, 1405–1406, 1467, 1634, 1837
  criteria, 1495
  design, 2462
  equal and fixed unequal, 1467–1469
  errors, 762–763
  invoked population model, 761
  mechanism rules, 1175
  model, 761–762
  population model, 760
  properties and methods, 763
  response-adaptive, 1469–1470
  restricted, 744–754
  simple, 744
Randomization tests, 1855, 1856
  Monte Carlo, 1855

Randomized clinical trial (RCT), 1444–1445,
    1600, 1634, 1682, 1687, 1691, 1834,
    1835, 1838, 2242, 2251, 2260, 2267
  breast cancer, 1601–1602
  childhood mortality, 2212, 2215, 2219
  for chronic disease, 1602–1604
  deficient design and execution, 2213, 2214
  global program, 2217
  health policies, 2210
  health statistics, 2220
  immune response, 2216
  infectious morbidity and mortality, 2216
  insufficient resources, 2214
  measles mortality, Tanzania, 2213
  nutrition, 2210
  protein-energy nutritional status, 2215
  vaccine efficacy, 1600–1604
  vitamin A status, 2214
Randomized community clinical trial,
    2211, 2212
Randomized controlled trial (RCT), 4, 878,
    879, 1220, 1228, 1229, 1419, 1422,
    2050, 2054, 2056, 2062, 2180–2192,
    2232, 2233
  adherence and follow-up, 2203, 2204
  editorial and opinions, 2205
  and evidence-based medicine, 11–12
  frequent citation, 2198
  globalization, 12–13
  hypothesis, 2201
  observations, 2203
  operations, 2203
  outcomes and multiplicity, 2204
  readers, 2199–2200
  research papers, 2198
  social and scientific challenges in, 13–15
  study design, 2202–2203
  study population, 2200
  subgroups, 2205
  variance, 2206
Randomized discontinuation trials (RDTs),
    1440–1442, 1450, 1451
  design, 1441
  enrichment trial designs, 1450–1451
  ethical aspects, 1449
  generalization of results, source population,
    1448–1449
  vs. RCT, 1442
Randomized selection design
  applications of, 1060–1063
  considerations for designing, 1050–1053
  goal of, 1048
  taxonomy of, 1049

Randomized trials, 1422, 1429–1432, 1435, 1436
Randomness, 2329
Random slope mixed model, 1819, 1820
Random subset size selection, with LRL
    procedures, 1058
Ranibizumab, 2202
Rapid enrollment design, 1113
Rare diseases
  challenges, 2300
  definition, 2290
  market products, 2291 (*see also* Orphan
    drugs)
  targeted therapies, 2304–2305
Rare pediatric disease, 2297
Rationalist history and empiric thinking, 27
Readers
  principles, 2199
  types, clinical journals, 2199
Reading center, 98
Real-world (RW) data, 878
Reboxetine, 2047
Receiver operating characteristics (ROC) curve,
    1178, 1407
Re-consent, 403
  See also Informed consent
Recruitment, 113, 195, 258, 565, 621, 2389
  candidates, 267–269
  definition, 259
  funnel, 263, 264
  issues, 260, 275, 276
  low quality, 274
  material, 267, 269
  over-recruitment, 274
  overview, 261
  personalized healthcare, 267
  rate, 264, 265
  risk mitigation, 274, 275
  shortfalls, 2466
  slow/under-recruitment, 274
Recruitment planning
  advisory boards, 263
  assumptions, 260
  benchmarking, 265, 266
  budgeting, 262
  challenges, 263
  geographical distribution, 262
  numbers, 260
  patient involvement, 263
  protocol feasibility, 263
  risk mitigation, 260
  service agencies, 266
  simulation, 266
  timelines, 262

Reduced variation, 2230
Re-engineering protocol implementation and development (RaPID), 619
Registered nurse (RN), 126
Registration, 644
Registry based randomized trials, 2255
Regression imputation, 1690–1692
Regression models, 1641, 1765–1767, 1772, 1776, 1777
Regulations, 8
 and documentation, 354
Regulatory approval, 350–352
Regulatory authorities, 643
Regulatory authority documents, 654
Regulatory compliance, 612, 613
 clinical trials, 599
 FDA regulations, 600
 requirements, 599
Regulatory interventions, 1966, 1968–1969
Regulatory requirements, in clinical trials, 476–477
 CTD Triangle, 468
 in European Union, 470–476
 global regulatory affairs, 462–463
 strategy, 463–465
 in US, 468–470
Rejections, 2471
Relative risk (RR), 1967, 1971
Relative risk reduction (RRR), 1972
Relative value (RV), 1975
Relative-value-adjusted number needed to harm (RV-NNH), 1975
Relative-value-adjusted number needed to treat (RV-NNT), 1975
Relative value units (RVUs), 2245
Repeated measurements design, 837
Replicability, 2119
Replication, 2229
Reporting, 322, 324, 325, 327, 332, 334
Reporting biases, 797–799
 citation bias, 2060
 consequences, 2061–2063
 duplicate reporting, 2055
 fraud, 2063
 language bias, 2053, 2054
 outcome, 2050, 2051
 publication bias, 2048, 2049, 2055, 2057, 2058, 2060
 research syntheses, 2065
 selective reporting, 2050
 spin, 2055, 2056
 time lag bias, 2053, 2054
 trial registration and access to protocols, 2063–2064
 types of, 2047–2048
Reporting odds ratio (ROR), 1966
Reporting of clinical trials
 methods and outcome reporting, 67
 publication and results deposition, 66–67
Reproducible research, 2334
Request for application (RFA), 2458
Request for proposal (RFP), 2458
Re-sampling, 2374
Re-screening, 260
Rescue medication, 1638, 1643, 1651
Research, 87
 fund allocation, 511–512
 groups, 351, 356
Research Administration, 605–607, 613
Research Advocate Training and Support (RATS), 575
Research ethics, 68
 benefits, 59
 origins of, 56–57
 risks, 59
Research ethics board (REB), 66, 1290
Research ethics committees (RECs), 675
Research funding agencies (RFAs), 498, 499
 application route and decision-making processes, 510–515
 assessment criteria, 515–516
 commercial, 501
 democratized model, 502
 funder policies, 505–507
 funding models, 507–508
 impact, 505
 medical research charities, 501
 own account research, 502
 philanthropic, 501
 philosophies and theories of change, 502–504
 politics, 499–500
 priorities, 504
 public, 500
 trans-national, 502
Research Waste and Rewarding Diligence Alliance (REWARD), 506
Residual uncertainties, 1242
Resignation of clinics, 2468
Resource centers, 98
 adjudication centers/committees, 108
 central laboratories, 102
 central pharmacies/procurement and distribution centers, 108

central units/support centers, 98
clinical centers, 109–113
coordinating centers, 99–101
image analysis and interpretation centers, 108
registration system, 108
responsibilities, 102, 109
Respect for persons, 57
Responder analysis, 1817–1818
Response-adaptive randomization (RAR), 1469–1470
Response adjusted for duration of antibiotic risk (RADAR), 1317
Response shift, 903
Restoring Invisible and Abandoned Trials (RIAT), 428
Restricted Maximum Likelihood (REML), 1434
Restricted randomization, 858
Results blackout, 2465
Resveratrol, 2268
Retention, 195, 565, 621, 2389
　partial withdrawal, 272
　participants, 257, 259, 272
　supporting, 273
Retraction/republication, 2330
Retrospective data collection, 882
Reverse biomarker-based strategy design, 1157–1158
Risk/benefit, 824
　assessments, 1871, 1886–1888
Risk Assessment and Categorization Tool (RACT), 609
Risk-based approach, 1241
Risk-based monitoring (RBM), 308–309, 2328
Risk-based monitoring plan, 143
Risk-benefit acceptability threshold (RBAT), 1976
Risk-benefit contour (RBC), 1976
Risk–benefit plane (RBP), 1975
Risk difference (RD), 1972
Risk evaluation and mitigation strategy (REMS), 1963
Risk management, 1964, 1970
Risk management plan (RMP), 1963
Risk of bias
　extracting data and assessing, 2165
　judgment, 2166
Risk prediction models
　apparent validation, 2017
　calibration, 2011
　clinical impact, 2020

continuous predictors, 2009
data collection, 2007–2008
developing of, 2006–2011
discrimination, 2011
external validation, 2019
flexible machine learning methods, 2011
high-dimensional data, 2010–2011
interaction effect, 2009
internal validation, 2017–2019
metrics of model performance, 2011–2017
missing data, 2008
model reporting, 2020
objective and study design, 2006–2007
sample size, 2007
types, 2005–2006
utility, 2011
validation, 2011–2020
variable selection, 2008–2009
Risk ratio, 1971
Rosiglitazone Evaluated for Cardiac Outcomes and Regulation of Glycaemia in Diabetes (RECORD), 2031
Routine on-site monitoring, 604
R software, 734
Rubin causal model, 1837–1838
　application of, 1840
　assumptions, 1838–1840
　Bayesian models, 1846
　CACE (see Complier average causal effect (CACE))
　MLE, 1843–1844
　principle application, 1842
　validity of assumptions, 1846–1847
Rule-based algorithm, 954–955
Rumack-Matthew nomogram, 1956
Run-in, 284

S
"Safe Harbor" de-identification, 2125–2127
Safety, 2383
　monitoring, 1086, 1087, 1089
Safety and Data Monitoring Boards (SDMBs), 824
Salford Lung Study, 2253, 2254
Salk Polio Vaccine Trial, 1600–1601
SALT-ED trial, 2254
Sample size, 835
　calculation of power and, 780–781
　characteristics, 777
　in clinical trials, 768
　determination, 1214

Sample size (*cont.*)
  feasible, 772
  large, 780
  optimal, 769
  reassessment, 1139, 1140
  re-estimation, 1086, 1091, 1098
Scale of measurement, 1366
Scheduling, 114
  meetings, 564
Scientific method, 23, 2200
Scientific misconduct, 93
Score statistics, 1793
Screening, 259, 1442
  activities, 269
  assessments, 269
  definition, 259
  planning, 270
  tools, 270
Screening trial
  continuous screen design, 1227
  delayed screen design, 1228
  design issues, 1220–1223
  endpoints, 1223–1226
  evaluation analysis, 1231–1232
  follow-up analysis, 1229–1230
  monitoring, 1232–1234
  sample size calculation, 1226–1227
  split screen design, 1228
  stop screen design, 1227
  traditional or standard two arm design, 1227
Secondary data use, 435–437
  anonymized *vs.* pseudonymized data, 441
  barriers and issues, 437–438
  consent, role of, 441–442
  data repositories, 446–448
  data standards, scientific value with, 443–446
  data use agreements, role of, 442–443
  de-identification, 439–440
  individual participant data, 448–451
Secondary outcome, 893, 896, 908, 2090, 2095, 2096, 2098
Second International Study of Infarct Survival (ISIS-2), 2231
Securities litigation, 2360–2361
Selection bias, 742, 749, 789–792, 885, 1059
  covariate imbalance, 861
  forcing index, 866
  non-randomized trial, 861
  predictability, 861
  susceptibility, 870
  treatment effect, 869

Selective estrogen receptor modulators (SERMs), 1264
Selective reporting, 2046, 2050, 2051
Self-destructive predilection, 2326
Semi-mechanistic model, 1940
Semi-mechanistic PK, 1927
Semi-parametric and order restricted methods, 959
Semi-parametric model, 1746–1750
Sensitivity analyses, 880, 1633, 1697–1698
  ad hoc, 1649
  anticipated protocol violations, 1648
  composite strategy, 1652, 1653
  data analysis aspects, 1648
  intercurrent events, 1649
  pain medications, 1650–1652
  randomized trials, 1648
  tipping point analysis, 1649, 1653, 1654
Sequential design, 986
Sequential, multiple assignment, randomized trial (SMART), 1547–1551, 1611, 2254
  defining feature of, 1551
  design considerations, 1555–1557
  ExTENd SMART study, 1548, 1550
  implementation, 1555–1557
  power considerations and analytic methods, 1553–1555
  Unrestricted SMART, 1553, 1554
Serious adverse event (SAE), 293, 628
Sham, 818, 819
Shared biology, 2230, 2235–2237
Shortened names (acronyms), 2107
Sickle cell disease, 2421
Šidák procedure, 733
Signal detection algorithms, 1966–1967
Significance, 1621, 1622
Significance level, 1622
Simes procedure, 732
Simon, Wittes, Ellenberg (1985) fixed sample size procedure (SWE), 1053–1054
Simple random variation, 2232
Simulation, 259, 266
Single-arm biomarker exploration design, 1151
Single-arm futility design, 1071–1073
Single center versus multicenter, 2462
Single imputation methods, 1592
Single mask, 807, 816
Single nucleotide polymorphisms (SNPs), 1409, 2421
Single patient trials, 1280
Single site *vs.* multisite trials, 2271
Single-sponsor platform trials, 1460–1461
Site-based end-users, 231

Site initiation visit (SIV), 598
Site management, 607, 613
Site Monitoring and Auditing, 356
    remote audit visit, 356, 357
    remote monitoring, 356, 357
Site qualification visit, 205
Site recruitment, 202
Site selection
    administrative considerations, 195
    facility resources, 194–195
    investigative team, 199–201
    investigator qualification, 198
    investigator responsibilities, 197–198
    recruitment potential, 195
    regulatory and ethics requirements, 196–197
Site teams
    dynamics, 199
    objective items, 203
    qualification visit, 205
    resources, 193, 201
    sponsors, 192
    subjective items, 203
    surveys and questionnaires, 202–204
Small interfering RNAs (siRNAs), 2304
Smallpox, 2383
Social media, 252, 2389
Society for Clinical Trials (SCT), 74, 76
    Controlled Clinical Trials, 79
    Coordinating Center Models Project, 77–78
    coordinating center personnel, meetings of, 76–77
    international participation, 80
    National Conference on Clinical Trials Methodology, 78–79
Society of Clinical Research Associates (SOCRA), 129, 131
Society of Thoracic Surgeons Congenital Heart Surgery Database (STS-CHSD), 2388
Socioeconomic status (SES), 573, 2421
Software, 618, 634
Solid state storage devices, 434
Source data verification, 2328
Sources of funding
    commercial RFAs, 501
    democratized model, 502
    medical research charities, 501
    own account research, 502
    philanthropic RFAs, 501
    public RFAs, 500
    trans-national RFA, 502
Specimen tracking system, 626

Spill-over effect, 1380
Spin, 2055–2057, 2059
Spinal cord injuries (SCI), 1650
Spinal muscular atrophy (SMA), 2304
Split-mouth design, 1378, 1379, 1382
Split screen design, 1228
Sponsor, 192, 193, 197, 200–204, 412, 461–465, 467, 469, 470, 472–477
    of biomedical research, 413
    of clinical trials, 2345–2349
    and Coordinating Centre, 422
    and funder, 416
    oversight, 613
    position, 417
Sponsor's Standard Operating Procedures (SOPs), 177
Spontaneous reporting system (SRS), 1964
SPYRAL HTN OFF-MED trial, 1575
    Bayesian discount prior method, 1575
    discount function, 1578
    discount prior method, 1577
    estimation, 1579
    role of simulation, 1579–1582
    statistical design, 1576–1577
    validation of simulation tools, 1580–1582
Stability investigations, 1905, 1911
Stable unit-treatment value assumption (SUTVA), 1838
Stages, clinical trial, 2455
STAMPEDE trial, 1511, 1531
Standard deviation (SD), 1388
Standard error, 1617, 1618, 1621, 1622
Standardized data collection, 623–624
Standardized mean difference (SMD), 2061
Standard of care (SOC), 878–881
Standard operating procedures (SOPs), 101, 350, 356, 357, 380–382, 435, 449, 452, 567, 602, 633
Standard Protocol Items Recommendations for Interventional Trials (SPIRIT)
    statement, 1308
    administrative information, 153
    assignment of interventions, 159–160
    data collection, 160
    data management, 161–162
    dissemination, 166
    ethics, 165–166
    intervention, 156
    monitoring activities, 162–164
    objectives, 154–155
    outcome measures, 158
    participants, 155

Standard Protocol Items Recommendations for
  Interventional Trials (SPIRIT) statement
  (*cont.*)
 participant timeline, sample size
  recruitment, 158–159
 statistical analysis, 162
 trial design, 155
Standards for Reporting of Diagnostic
  Accuracy Studies (STARD)
  statement, 1181
Standards of operations (SOPs), 195
Stated preference method (SPM), 1977
Statistical advances, 29–30
Statistical analysis, 1392, 1594
 approach, 2387
Statistical analysis plan (SAP), 799, 1595, 1636
Statistical Center
 biospecimen sharing, 633, 634
 communications, 618–619
 data sharing, 633
 disease committee structure, 617, 618
Statistical design, 617
Statistical inference, 974, 981, 983
Statistical method, 1392, 2200
Statistical monitoring
 data error detection, 2328
 implementations, 2330–2331
 principles, 2329–2330
Statistical process control (SPC), 2406
Statistical Research Associates (SRAs), 617
Statistical theory, 2329
Statisticians' Report Worksheet (SRW), 624,
  625, 630
Steering Committee, 561, 564, 565
Steinberg and Venzon (2002) design (SV),
  1054–1055
Stepped wedge design (SWD), 1430–1432,
  1436, 2273
Steroids to Reduce Systemic Inflammation
  After Neonatal Heart Surgery
  (STRESS), 2388
Stochastic approximation expectation-
  maximization (SAEM) estimation
  algorithm, 1930
Stop screen design, 1227
Strategies to Reduce Injuries and Develop
  Confidence in Elders (STRIDE), 2406,
  2407
Stratification, 743
Stratified analysis, 1772, 1779
Stratified Biomarker Trial, 1363
Stratified logrank test, 1738–1739
Stratified medicine, 1146
Stratified randomization, 752–754, 1784

STRengthening Analytical Thinking for
  Observational Studies (STRATOS)
  initiative, 1914
Structural mean model approach, 1841–1842
Structured abstract, 2200
Student's t-test, 1289
Study curriculum vitae, 2036
Study Data Tabulation Model (SDTM), 445
Study definition, 211, 212, 218, 222, 231, 233
Study design, 2200, 2202–2203
Study names
 characteristics, 2107
 reminders, 2106
 trial, 2105
Study population, 2200, 2205
Study protocol, 40
Study publications, 2029, 2030
Study visits, 2391
Subdistribution hazards, 1763, 1764, 1766
Subgroup analysis, 1779, 1785, 2187–2188
Subgroup mixable estimation (SME)
  principle, 1671
Subgroups, 1147, 1150, 1152, 1153, 1156
 biomarker, 1661, 1667
 complementary, 1664
 definition, 1664
 identification, 1663
 null hypothesis, 1662
 survival function, 1670
Subinvestigator, 587
Subject injury, 533–535
Subjective endpoints, 894
Subject remuneration, 531–532
Sub-population selection, 1442
Subset, 2368, 2370, 2371, 2375, 2376
 analysis, 2424, 2425
 selection approach, 1051
Subsetting, 2292
Substantial evidence, 1939, 2301
Sudden Infant Death Syndrome
  (SIDS), 2381
Sulfinpyrazone, 1590
Surgical treatment vs. nonsurgical
  treatment, 1380
Surrogate endpoints, 894–896
Survival analysis, 1719
 hypothesis testing, 1734–1740
 nonparametric estimation, 1722–1734
 parametric models, 1721–1722
Survival function, 1669
Survival modeling, 1746
 exponential, 1745
 parametric, 1748
 roles, 1755

Sustainability, 1263, 1265–1266
Switchability, 1250
SWOG Cancer Research Network, 572
SWOG statistics, 616–617
Sykes v. United States, 2346
Symmetric AD-design, 1446–1447
Symptomatic effect, 1202–1204
Syntactic interoperability, 2149–2150
Systematic error, 835, 836
Systematic review
    clinical trial data, 2171–2172
    definition, 2160
    evidence-based, 2162
    health and healthcare decisions, 2161
    high-quality, 2169
    methodological rigor of, 2169
    methods, 2160
    out of date quickly, 2173
    searchable databases identification, 2170
    steps in, 2161, 2163–2168
System components, 210
System documentation and training, 231
System for Thalidomide Education and Prescribing Safety (STEPS), 1969
Systolic blood pressure, 897

T
Tai chi, 2264, 2270, 2272
Tailoring variable, 1546, 1549
Tamoxifen, 1267, 2425
Targeted therapies, 575, 2304–2305
Target-mediated drug disposition (TMDD) model, 1946
Tax credits, 2298
Technical error (TE), 836
Technical problems, 2333
Technology licensing, 549
Telehealth strategies, 2387
Telithromycin, 2324
Template for Intervention Description and Replication (TIDieR), 1420
Test statistic, 1621–1623, 1674
Test-treatment trial design, 1182
Tetracyclines, 2381
Tetralogy of Fallot, 2382
Thalidomide therapy, 1969
The Lancet, 2218, 2323
Theories of liability
    negligence, 2341–2343
    product liability, 2343–2344
Theory of adaptive designs, 1474
Theory of U-statistics, 1874
Therapeutic area (TA), 444, 445

Therapeutic device trials
    blinding, 1404–1405
    clinical endpoints, 1406
    control group, 1403–1404
    error rate control, 1407
    randomization, 1405–1406
    sample size, 1406–1407
Therapeutic procedures, 59
Thrombus Aspiration in ST-Elevation Myocardial Infarction in Scandinavia (TASTE) trial, 2255
Time and date, 357
Time lag bias, 2048, 2053, 2054
Timeline, for clinical trial elements, 2456
Time to benefit (TTB), 2405–2406
Time-to-event, 1718, 1720
    analysis, 1821
    CRM, 963, 1112
    outcome, 1877, 1884
Time-to-event data
    individual dynamic prediction, 1932
    joint modelling, 1923–1933
    model specification and estimation, 1921–1923
    population prediction supporting clinical trial design, 1923–1932
Time-to-event endpoints, 1112–1113, 1645
    dose-escalation of cisplatin in pancreatic cancer, 1113
Time to harm (TTH), 2405, 2406, 2413
Titling publications
    descriptive type, 2108
    headline type, 2108
Tokenism, 574
TOPCAT trial, 2205
Totality of the evidence, 1239, 1240, 1243, 1252, 1255
Toxicity score approach, 1115
Toxicology, 1241, 1242
Traditional educational approaches, 2386
Traditional/standard two arm design, 1227
Traditional statistical analysis strategy, 2371
Training programme, 243–245
Transcatheter aortic-valve replacement (TAVR), 1406
Translational clinical trial (TCT), 940, 944, 945
    biomarkers, 943
    characteristics of, 942
    companion diagnostics, 943
    definition, 941
    feasibility, 943
    hypothetical prior and outcome probabilities, 945, 946
    safety *vs.* efficacy, 948–949

Translational clinical trial (TCT) (cont.)
    sample size, 946–948
    signaling, 942
    targeting, 942
Translational medicine, 617, 619, 622, 634
Transparency, 325
Treatment, 2461
    crossover, 287–289
    discontinuation, 287, 289–291
    interactions, 1364–1370, 1896
    masking, 792
    options, 1546
    policy strategy, 1638, 1639
    satisfaction, 1814
Treatment-effect-function, 1904
Treatment effect models, 2005
Treatment effect modification, 1989, 1991, 1999
Treatment plus other therapies *vs.* placebo plus other therapies, 1651
Trial Closure Plan, 323, 326, 327, 331, 344
Trial committees, 2328
Trial consortiums, 144
Trial coordination, 349–357
Trial data system, 644
Trial design considerations, 1381
    anti-VEGF, 1382
    bias, 1382
    carry across effect, 1382
    gaining efficiency, 1383
    generalizability, 1383
    within person trials, 1382
    prethreshold ROP, 1384
    randomized trials, 1382
    recruitment, 1382
    requirement, 1383
    subject controls, 1382
Trial Designs and Populations, 359
Trial Management Group (TMG), 249, 450
Trial master file (TMF), 357, 374, 375, 379, 383–386, 429, 639
    clinical, 639
    electronic, 639
    ICH GCP guideline, 639
    intention, 639
    legislation, 639
    planning, 640
Trial monitoring plan, 247, 2328
Trial outcomes
    administrator, 853
    asymptomatic subclinical assessments, 846
    centralized model, 848
    clinical event classification, 851–852
    competing risks, 845
    data capture instrument development, 850–851
    decentralized outcome assessments, 848
    diagnostic data elements, 850
    event ascertainment, 848
    identification of events, 849–850
    informed consent, 852
    major clinically recognized events, 845
    patient reported outcomes, 847
    time-to-event methods, 847
    training in data capture, 851
    treatment assignment, 845
Trial planning, 2270
Trial representativeness, 2247
Trial risk assessment, 247
Trial–specific training, 112
Trial sponsorship
    IND, 601
    Inspection readiness, 602
    intervention, 601
    investigator responsibilities, 601
    quality management, 601
    sponsor oversight, 601, 602
    sponsors, 601
Trial sponsor team, 584
    external training and study specific training, 586
    sponsor quality manual and quality system, 585
Trials types and measurements, 1636
Triple masking, 807
True placebo effect, 1941
T-tests, 1706, 1708
Tumor size model, 1926–1930
Two-one-sided-test (TOST) approach, 1244
Two-period design, 1207, 1214
    ADAGIO trial, 1209, 1210, 1213
    assumptions, 1206, 1207
    delayed start design, 1204
    disease-modifying effects, 1203
    ELLDOPA trial, 1204
    hypothesis, 1212
    missing data, 1212
    missingness mechanism, 1214
    noninferiority, 1211, 1212
    primary analyses, 1210
    rasagiline, 1204
    symptomatic effect, 1204
    withdrawal design, 1203–1207
Two-stage designs, 1033–1035

Type I error, 730, 769, 773, 778, 783, 1252, 1253, 1622
Type II error, 769, 1622

U

UK Breast Cancer Screening Age Trial, 1228
UK Clinical Research Collaboration (UKCRC), 421
Unblinding, 282, 286
Unconditional imputation, 1692
Unified Parkinson's Disease Rating Scale (UPDRS) score, 1943–1945
United Nations Convention on Psychotropic Substances, 180
United Nations Single Convention on Narcotic Drugs, 180
United States Department of Health and Human Services, 2119, 2130
United States Health Insurance Portability and Accountability Act, 2117
Universal health outcomes, 2404
University Group Diabetes Program (UGDP), 74, 2030, 2031, 2106
Unmask, 816, 820
Uppsala Monitoring Center (UMC), 1967
Usage note
    controlled trial, 42
    data monitoring committee., 46
    enrollment, 44
    executive committee, 46
    manual of operations, 40
    open trail, 41
    placebo, 43
    protocol, 40
    randomization, 44
    registration, 44
    steering committee, 46
    study protocol, 40
    treatment failure, 48
U.S. Census Bureau, 2398
U.S. Centers for Medicare and Medicaid Services, 2398
U.S. Code of Federal Regulations (CFR), 2398
U.S. Environmental Protection Agency, 2237
User fee exemption, 2299
US Food and Drug Administration (FDA), 523, 524, 572, 2266, 2322, 2422
US heathcare system, 2250
US National Institutes of Health (NIH) Common Fund, 2253
US Office of Research Integrity (ORI), 2321
US Public Health Service, 2320
U-statistic, 1872
Usual care, 2271

V

Validation, 219, 224, 226–228, 1147
Valid informed consent
    capacity, 64
    understanding, 64
    voluntariness, 64
VALOR trial
    adaptive sample size re-estimation, 1567
    design-stage simulations, 1570–1572
    monitoring-stage simulations, 1572–1573
    practical considerations, operational bias, 1574
    statistical methodology, 1568–1570
Valsartan, 2323
Variable selection, 1899
    candidate variables, 1901–1902
    traditional procedures, 1901
Variance, 834
    in clinical trial, 835
    coefficient of variation, 835
    control, 836–838
    as data quality assessment tool, 838–839
    description, 834
    sources in clinical trial, 835
    technical error, 836
Variance-covariance components, 1424
Variance-covariance matrix, 1444
Vascular endothelial growth factor (VEGF), 1362
Vendors, 172, 175
Verification bias, 1174
Virtual machine (VM), 433
Visit schedule, 281, 292–294
Visit window, 295–297
Visual inspection, 1288, 1291
Visual inspection with acetic acid (VIA), 1175
Visualization techniques, 2145, 2146
Vitamin A supplementation, 2212, 2214, 2215, 2218
Vivli data sharing platform, 2146
Voluntary Harmonization Procedure (VHP), 472–474

W

Waitlist control strategy, 2271
Waiving of co-pays, 532–533
Wald statistics, 1793

Wasting malnutrition, 2213
Wawrzynek v. Statprobe, Inc., 2355
WebCONSORT, 2080, 2083
Website content, 484–486
Weibull discount function, 1578
Whole genome sequencing, 2421
Wholey v. Amgen, Inc., 2345
Wilcoxon-Mann-Whitney test, 1872–1873
Wilcoxon signed rank test, 1288, 1709
WinBUGS, 1037
Win ratio, 1874, 1877
Withdrawal of consent, 290
Within person correlation, 1383, 1388
   advantage, 1381
   heterogeneity, 1381
Within person design, 1378, 1380
   binary outcome, 1389
   carry across effect, 1380
   IOP reduction, 1381
   treatment outcome, 1380
Within person trials, 1378–1380, 1382, 1388, 1389
Within subject controls design, 1378
   alternative designs, 1386

Complications of Age-related Macular Degeneration Treatment Trials (CATT), 1386
   multi-center randomized clinical trial, 1387
Wittes, Janet, 79
Women's Health Initiative (WHI), 1271, 1372
World Health Organization (WHO), 180, 463, 2064
World Medical Association (WMA), 651
Writing team, 2092–2094, 2096, 2098, 2099
Written protocol assistance, 2299

X

Xerophthalmia, 2211, 2213

Y

Y-model, 1689, 1691
Yoga, 2264, 2265, 2270, 2272, 2274, 2276

Z

Zeman v. Williams, 2347, 2350
Z-test statistics, 1516